D0202620

WITHDRAWN-UNL

PATHWAYS OF THE PULP

PATHWAYS OF THE PULP

Edited by

Stephen Cohen, M.A., D.D.S., F.I.C.D., F.A.C.D.
Clinical Professor (Adjunct), Department of Endodontics
University of the Pacific School of Dentistry,
San Francisco, California;
Diplomate, American Board of Endodontics

Richard C. Burns, D.D.S., F.I.C.D., F.A.C.D.
Clinical Professor (Adjunct), Department of Endodontics
University of the Pacific School of Dentistry,
San Francisco, California;
Diplomate, American Board of Endodontics

Sixth Edition

With 45 Contributors, 1773 Illustrations, and 3 Color Plates
Principal Illustrator, Richard C. Burns
Cover Image Created by Gary B. Carr

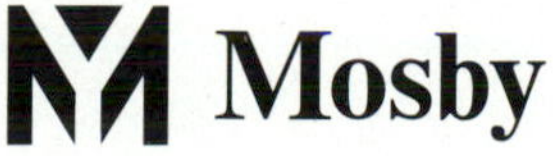

St. Louis Baltimore Boston Chicago London Madrid Philadelphia Sydney Toronto

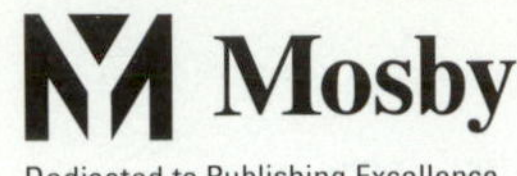

Publisher: George Stamathis
Editor-in-Chief: Don Ladig
Executive Editor: Linda L. Duncan
Developmental Editor: Melba Steube
Project Manager: Linda Clarke
Production Editor: Allan S. Kleinberg
Manufacturing Supervisor: John Babrick
Cover Design: David Zielinski
Cover Art: Gary B. Carr

SIXTH EDITION

Copyright © 1994 by Mosby–Year Book, Inc.

Previous editions copyrighted 1976, 1980, 1984, 1987, 1991

All rights reserved. No part of this publication may be reproduced, stored in a retrieval system, or transmitted, in any form or by any means, electronic, mechanical, photocopying, recording, or otherwise, without prior written permission from the publisher.

Permission to photocopy or reproduce solely for internal or personal use is permitted for libraries or other users registered with the Copyright Clearance Center, provided that the base fee of $4.00 per chapter plus $.10 per page is paid directly to the Copyright Clearance Center, 27 Congress Street, Salem, MA 01970. This consent does not extend to other kinds of copying, such as copying for general distribution, for advertising or promotional purposes, for creating new collected works, or for resale.

Printed in the United States of America
Composition by Clarinda
Printing/binding by Maple Vail

Mosby–Year Book, Inc.
11830 Westline Industrial Drive
St. Louis, Missouri 63146

Library of Congress Cataloging-in-Publication Data

Pathways of the pulp/edited by Stephen Cohen, Richard C. Burns; with 50 contributors; principal illustrator, Richard C. Burns. — 6th ed.
p. cm.
Includes bibliographical references and index.
ISBN 0-8016-7979-6
1. Endodontics. I. Cohen, Stephen, 1938- . II. Burns, Richard C., 1932- .
[DNLM: 1. Dental pulp. 2. Endodontics. WU 230 P297 1994]
RK351.P37 1994
617.6'342—dc20
DNLM/DLC
for Library of Congress 93-42923
CIP

94 95 96 97 98 / 9 8 7 6 5 4 3 2 1

Contributors

Robert E. Averbach, D.D.S., F.I.C.D., F.A.C.D.
President's Teaching Scholar
Dean and Professor of Endodontics
University of Colorado School of Dentistry
Denver, Colorado;
Diplomate, American Board of Endodontics

Richard C. Burns, D.D.S., F.I.C.D., F.A.C.D.
Clinical Professor (Adjunct)
Department of Endodontics
University of the Pacific School of Dentistry
San Francisco, California;
Diplomate, American Board of Endodontics

Joe H. Camp, D.D.S., M.S.D., F.I.C.D., F.A.C.D.
Clinical Associate Professor
Department of Endodontics
University of North Carolina School of Dentistry
Chapel Hill, North Carolina

Gary B. Carr, D.D.S.
Founder and Director
Pacific Endodontic Research Foundation
San Diego, California;
Guest Lecturer in Endodontics
University of California at Los Angeles;
Consultant in Endodontics
VA Hospital
Long Beach, California;
Diplomate, American Board of Endodontics

Noah Chivian, D.D.S., F.I.C.D., F.A.C.D.
Director of Dentistry
Newark Beth Israel Medical Center
Newark, New Jersey;
Diplomate, American Board of Endodontics

Stephen Cohen, M.A., D.D.S., F.I.C.D., F.A.C.D.
Clinical Professor (Adjunct), Department of Endodontics
University of the Pacific School of Dentistry
San Francisco, California;
Diplomate, American Board of Endodontics

Samuel O. Dorn, D.D.S., F.A.C.D.
Clinical Associate Professor
Department of Endodontics
University of Florida College of Dentistry
Gainesville, Florida

Lewis R. Eversole, M.A., D.D.S., M.S.D.
Professor and Chairman
Department of Diagnostic Sciences
UCLA School of Dentistry
Los Angeles, California

Stuart B. Fountain, D.D.S., M.Sc. (Dent.), F.I.C.D., F.A.C.D.
Clinical Associate Professor, Department of Endodontics
University of North Carolina School of Dentistry
Chapel Hill, North Carolina;
Diplomate, American Board of Endodontics

Shimon Friedman, D.M.D.
Associate Professor and Head
Department of Endodontics
Faculty of Dentistry
University of Toronto
Toronto, Ontario
Canada

Arnold H. Gartner, D.D.S.
Clinical Assistant Professor
Department of Endodontics
University of Detroit Mercy
School of Dentistry
Detroit, Michigan

Gerald Neal Glickman, M.S., D.D.S., M.B.A.
Associate Professor and Director of Endodontics
Department of Cariology, Restorative Sciences, and Endodontics
University of Michigan School of Dentistry
Ann Arbor, Michigan;
Diplomate, American Board of Endodontics

Alan H. Gluskin, D.D.S., F.I.C.D., F.A.C.D.
Associate Professor and Chairman
Department of Endodontics
University of the Pacific School of Dentistry
San Francisco, California

Albert C. Goerig, M.S., D.D.S., F.I.C.D., F.A.C.D.
Private Practice in Endodontics
Olympia, Washington;
Diplomate, American Board of Endodontics

Ronald E. Goldstein, D.D.S.
Clinical Professor of Restorative Dentistry
Medical College of Georgia
Augusta, Georgia;
Adjunct Clinical Professor of Prosthodontics
Boston University
Boston, Massachusetts

William W. Y. Goon, D.D.S., F.I.C.D., F.A.C.D.
Associate Professor
Department of Endodontics
University of the Pacific School of Dentistry
San Francisco, California

Daniel B. Green, D.D.S.
Director, Post Graduate Endodontics
University of Louisville School of Dentistry
Louisville, Kentucky;
Attending Faculty
University Pain Control Center
Cincinnati, Ohio

Van B. Haywood, D.M.D.
Associate Professor
Department of Operative Dentistry
University of North Carolina School of Dentistry
Chapel Hill, North Carolina

Harald O. Heymann, D.D.S., M.Ed.
Associate Professor and Chairman
Department of Operative Dentistry
University of North Carolina School of Dentistry
Chapel Hill, North Carolina

James D. Kettering, M.S., Ph.D.
Professor
Department of Microbiology
Schools of Medicine and Dentistry
Loma Linda University
Loma Linda, California

Syngcuk Kim, D.D.S., Ph.D.
L.I. Grossman Professor and Chairman
Department of Endodontics
School of Dental Medicine
University of Pennsylvania
Philadelphia, Pennsylvania

Donald J. Kleier, D.M.D., F.I.C.D., F.A.C.D.
Professor and Chairman, Endodontics and Surgical Dentistry
Department of Surgical Dentistry
University of Colorado School of Dentistry
Denver, Colorado;
Diplomate, American Board of Endodontics

Stanley F. Malamed, D.D.S.
Professor and Chair, Section of Anesthesia and Medicine
University of Southern California School of Dentistry
Los Angeles, California

Leo J. Miserendino, M.S., D.D.S.
Assistant Professor
Department of Oral Biology
University of Illinois at Chicago
College of Dentistry
Chicago, Illinois;
Diplomate, American Board of Endodontics

Kathy I. Mueller, D.M.D.
Assistant Professor
Department of Fixed Prosthodontics
University of the Pacific School of Dentistry
San Francisco, California;
Diplomate, American Board of Prosthodontics

Carl W. Newton, D.D.S., M.S.D.
Professor
Department of Endodontics
Indiana University School of Dentistry
Indianapolis, Indiana;
Diplomate, American Board of Endodontics

Nguyen Thanh Nguyen, D.D.S., F.I.C.D., F.A.C.D., F.A.A.E.
Clinical Professor and Former Chairman
Division of Endodontics
Emeritus Professor of Restorative Dentistry
University of California School of Dentistry
San Francisco, California;
Diplomate, American Board of Endodontics

James B. Roane, B.S., M.S., D.D.S., F.A.C.P.
Professor
Department of Endodontics
University of Oklahoma
College of Dentistry
Oklahoma City, Oklahoma;
Diplomate, American Board of Endodontics

Clifford J. Ruddle, D.D.S., F.I.C.D., F.A.C.D.
Assistant Professor
Department of Graduate Endodontics
University of California-Los Angeles
Los Angeles, California;
Assistant Professor
Department of Graduate Endodontics
Loma Linda University School of Dentistry
Loma Linda, California

James T. Rule, M.S., D.D.S.
Professor and Chairman
Department of Pediatric Dentistry
University of Maryland at Baltimore Dental School
Baltimore, Maryland

Herbert Schilder, D.D.S.
Professor and Chairman
Department of Endodontics
Boston University
Goldman School of Graduate Dentistry
Boston, Massachusetts

James H. S. Simon, A.B., D.D.S., F.I.C.D., F.A.C.D.
Chief, Endodontic Section
Veterans Administrative Medical Center
Long Beach, California;
Professor of Endodontics
Loma Linda University School of Dentistry
Loma Linda, California;
Clinical Associate Professor of Endodontics
University of Southern California School of Dentistry
Los Angeles, California;
Diplomate, American Board of Endodontics

Adam Stabholz, D.M.D.
Professor and Chairman
Department of Endodontics
The Hebrew University
Hadassah Faculty of Dental Medicine
Jerusalem, Israel

H. Robert Steiman, M.S., Ph.D., D.D.S., M.S.D., F.I.C.D.
Professor and Chairman
Department of Endodontics
Director, Postgraduate Endodontics
University of Detroit Mercy
School of Dentistry
Detroit, Michigan;
Diplomate, American Board of Endodontics

David R. Steiner, D.D.S., M.S.D.
Clinical Associate Professor
Graduate Endodontics Program
Department of Endodontics
University of Washington School of Dentistry
Seattle, Washington

Aviad Tamse, D.M.D.
Associate Professor
Department of Endodontology
Maurice and Gabriela Golschlager School of Dental Medicine
Tel Aviv University
Tel Aviv, Israel

Mahmoud Torabinejad, D.M.D., M.S.D.
Professor of Endodontics
Director of Graduate Endodontics
Department of Endodontics
Loma Linda University School of Dentistry
Loma Linda, California

Martin Trope, D.M.D.
Professor and Chairman
Department of Endodontics
University of North Carolina School of Dentistry
Chapel Hill, North Carolina

Henry O. Trowbridge, D.D.S., Ph.D.
Professor of Pathology
University of Pennsylvania School of Dental Medicine
Philadelphia, Pennsylvania;
Attending Staff, Division of Endodontics
Albert Einstein Medical Center
Philadelphia, Pennsylvania

Robert M. Veatch, Ph.D.
Director
Kennedy Institute of Ethics
Georgetown University
Washington, D.C.

Galen W. Wagnild, D.D.S.
Associate Clinical Professor
Department of Restorative Dentistry
University of California
San Francisco, California;
Diplomate, American Board of Prosthodontics

Richard E. Walton, M.S., D.M.D.
Professor and Chairman
Department of Endodontics
College of Dentistry
University of Iowa
Iowa City, Iowa

Leslie A. Werksman, B.S., D.D.S.
Private Practice
Laguna Hills, California

John D. West, D.D.S., M.S.D.
Clinical Associate Professor
Graduate Endodontics Program
Department of Endodontics
University of Washington School of Dentistry
Seattle, Washington;
Clinical Instructor
Boston University
Goldman School of Graduate Dentistry
Department of Endodontics
Boston, Massachusetts;
Guest Faculty
Pacific Endodontic Research Foundation
San Diego, California

Edwin J. Zinman, D.D.S., J.D.
Lecturer, Department of Stomatology
University of California
San Francisco, California

Preface

This sixth edition of *Pathways of the Pulp* has two aims:

- To provide comprehensive and practical discussions and descriptions of what is currently known and practiced by accomplished endodontic clinicians; and
- To introduce those new technologies and theoretical developments in science, medicine and dentistry which will define the future of excellence in the practice of endodontics.

This dual purpose is expressed in the detailed content of each chapter as well as in the editors' selection of chapters and those who author them. Each chapter in this sixth edition has been re-written by a new author, co-author, or team, or substantially revised and updated by its fifth-edition author. Self-assessment quizzes are provided at the end of each chapter to aid the reader in using *Pathways* as a practical, dynamic daily tool in the classroom or in the treatment room. Dr. Daniel B. Green, Dr. H. Robert Steiman, and Dr. Richard E. Walton have carefully prepared each question and reviewed its relevance, clarity, and accuracy.

We gratefully acknowledge the selfless contributions of all of our authors, whose passion for excellence and the highest standards of patient care are evident in their chapters and in their very agreement to take time from their demanding professional lives to share their knowledge and understanding. We are especially grateful as well to Ms. Linda L. Duncan, Ms. Melba Steube, and Ms. Myrna Oppenheim of Mosby for their invaluable assistance with every phase of *Pathways of the Pulp*. The high-quality administrative support provided by Ms. Barbara Leal and Mr. Robert Beirne was also integral to the production of this edition.

The summary statement of this sixth edition is our view that the role of the endodontist is undergoing expansion and redefinition. Endodontic clinicians are necessarily becoming more involved in the diagnosis and treatment of mouth and jaw pain as well as toothache. Technological advancements as well as new information are driving the development of a more integrated approach to patient care and pain resolution. Endodontists now, more than ever, must see themselves as part of a team with the general dentist, other dental specialists, and physicians. To meet this challenge, clinicians and clinicians-in-training need current, reliable, and tested information; the curious mind of the scientist; and the ready heart of the true healer. The sixth edition of *Pathways of the Pulp* is offered as our contribution to this exciting future.

Stephen Cohen
Richard C. Burns

Contents

PART THREE: RELATED CLINICAL TOPICS

PART FOUR: ISSUES IN ENDODONTICS

PART ONE

THE ART OF ENDODONTICS

Chapter 1

Diagnostic Procedures

Stephen Cohen

THE ART AND SCIENCE OF DIAGNOSIS

The dictionary* defines diagnosis as "the art of identifying a disease from its signs and symptoms." Although scientific devices can be used to gather some information, diagnosis is still primarily an art because it is the thoughtful interpretation of the data that leads to a diagnosis. An accurate diagnosis is a result of the synthesis of scientific knowledge, clinical experience, intuition, and common sense.

To be a good diagnostician a clinician must learn the fundamentals of gathering and interpreting clinical information. An inflamed or diseased pulp is a common, straightforward, and nonurgent condition. Systematic recording of a patient's presenting signs and symptoms and careful analysis of the findings from clinical tests inevitably lead to a correct diagnosis. There are instances, however, when a patient presents with an acute situation, conflicting signs and symptoms, or inconsistent responses to clinical testing. Chapter 2 explores the methods for diagnosing and testing these endodontic riddles. Chapter 3 discusses the ostensible toothache of nonodontogenic origin.

Medical History

Even though there are virtually no systemic contraindications to endodontic therapy (except uncontrolled diabetes or a very recent myocardial infarction), a recent and succinct, comprehensive preprinted medical history is mandatory (see box on p. 3). It is only with such a history that the clinician can determine whether medical consultation or premedication is required before diagnostic examination or clinical treatment is undertaken. Some patients require antibiotic prophylaxis before clinical examination because of systemic conditions like heart valve replacement, a history of rheumatic fever, or advanced AIDS. Patients who daily take anticoagulant medications may need to have the dose reduced or dosing suspended if the clinician is to conduct the thorough periodontal examination, which is integral to a complete endodontic workup. When patients report being infected with communicable diseases such as AIDS, hepatitis B, or tuberculosis, dentist and staff need to be especially attentive to the use of protective barriers. In case endodontic therapy is required, the clinician must know what drugs the patient is taking so that adverse drug interactions can be avoided. In such cases, consultation with the patient's physician is recommended. Patients who present with mental or emotional disorders are not uncommon. Some patients are aware of their disorder and inform the dentist. Others may have undiagnosed psychological or emotional problems; abnormal or highly inappropriate behavior may suggest the presence of illness. In these cases, too, medical consultation before the diagnostic examination would be in the best interests of patient, doctor, and staff. A brief summary of these consultations with treating physicians and an outline of their suggestions should be recorded and dated in the patient record.

Dental History

After completing the medical history the clinician should develop the dental history. The purpose of a dental history is to create a record of the chief complaint, the signs and symptoms the patient reports, when the problem began, and what the patient can discern that improves or worsens the condition. The most efficacious way for the clinician to gather this important information is to ask the patient pertinent questions re-

---

Unless otherwise indicated, the illustrations in this chapter were prepared by Dr. Albert Goerig.

**Webster's Third International Dictionary*, Springfield, Mass, 1976, Merriam-Webster Inc.

MEDICAL HISTORY

LAST NAME: ______________ FIRST NAME: ______________

Are you in good health? ______________

Are you presently under the care of a physician? ______

If so, please give reason(s) for treatment ______________

____

Physician's name and address: ______________ Telephone: ______________

Date of last physical exam: ______________

Are you taking any kind of medication (prescribed or non-prescribed), or drug(s) at this time? ______

If so, please give name(s) of the medicine(s) and reason(s) for taking them:

____

____

PLEASE CIRCLE ANY ILLNESS YOU HAVE EVER HAD:

Alcoholism	*Blood Pressure*	*Epilepsy*	*Herpes*	*Mental*	*Sinusitis*
Allergies	*Cancer*	*Glaucoma*	*Immunodeficiency*	*Migraine*	*Ulcers*
Anemia	*Diabetes*	*Head/Neck Injuries*	*Infectious Hepatitis*	*Respiratory*	*Venereal Disease*
Asthma	*Drug/Narcotic Dependency*	*Heart Trouble*	*Kidney or Liver*	*Rheumatic Fever*	*Other*

Allergic to: ______________

Explanation of "Other": ______________

Do you wear a heart pacemaker or any other kind of prosthetic appliance? ______

Have you ever had any trouble with prolonged bleeding after surgery? ______

Have you ever had an unusual reaction to an anesthetic or drug (like penicillin)? ______

Is there any other information that should be known about your health? ______

Signature ______________ Date ______________

garding the chief complaint, and to listen carefully and sensitively to the patient's responses. For example, the doctor might begin by simply asking the patient, "Could you tell me about your problem?" To determine the chief complaint, this question should be followed by a series of other questions, such as "When did you first notice this?" *(inception)*. Affecting factors that improve or worsen the condition should also be determined. "Does heat, cold, biting, or chewing cause pain?" *(provoking factors)*. "Does anything hot or cold relieve the pain?" *(attenuating factors)*. "How often does this pain occur?" *(frequency)*. "When you have pain, is it mild, moderate, or severe?" *(intensity)*. The answers to these questions provide the information the dentist needs to develop a brief narrative description of the problem.

The majority of patients present with evident problems of pain or swelling, so most questions should focus on these areas. For example, "Could you point to the tooth that hurts or the area that you think is swelling?" *(location)*. "When cold (or heat) causes pain, does it last for a moment or for several seconds or longer?" *(duration)*. "Do you have any pain when you lie down or bend over?" *(postural)*. "Does the pain ever occur without provocation?" *(stimulated or spontaneous)*. "What kind of pain do you get? Sharp? Dull? Stabbing? Throbbing?" *(quality)*. Questions like these help the clinician establish the location, nature, quality, and urgency of the problem and encourage the patient to volunteer additional information that completes the verbal picture of the problem. The clinician may be able to formulate a tentative diagnosis while taking a dental history. The examination and testing that follow often corroborate the tentative diagnosis. It is then merely a matter of identifying the problem tooth.[6,7]

In the gathering of a dental history, common sense must prevail. The questions outlined here, along with other questions described in Chapter 2, should be asked if the diagnosis is elusive. If the clinician can see a grossly decayed tooth while sitting and talking with the patient and if the patient points to that tooth, the dental history should be brief because of the obvious nature of the problem. Furthermore, if the patient is suffering from severe distress, with acute symptoms (Chapter 2), the dental history should be brief so the clinician can relieve the pain as soon as possible.

Pain

Because dental pain frequently is the result of a diseased pulp, it is one of the most common symptoms a dentist is required to diagnose.[14a] The source of the pain is usually made evident by dental history, inspection, examination, and testing. However, because pain has psychobiologic components—

physical, emotional, and tolerance—identifying the source is at times quite difficult. Furthermore, because of psychological conditioning, including fear, the intensity of pain perception may not be proportional to the stimulus. When patients present with a complaint of pain that is subsequently determined to be of odontogenic origin, the vast majority of these cases reflect conditions of irreversible pulpitis, with or without partial necrosis.[19,23]

Patients may report the pain as sharp, dull, continuous, intermittent, mild, severe, etc. Because the neural portion of the pulp contains only pain fibers, if the inflammatory state is limited to the pulp tissue it may be difficult for the patient to localize the pain. However, once the inflammatory process extends beyond the apical foramen and begins to involve the periodontal ligament, which contains proprioceptive fibers, the patient should be able to localize the source of the pain. A percussion test at this time to corroborate the patient's perception of the source will be quite helpful.

At times pain is referred to other areas within, and even beyond, the mouth. Most commonly it is manifested in other teeth in the same or the opposing quadrant. It almost never crosses the midline of the head. However, referred pain is not necessarily limited to other teeth. It may, for example, be ipsilaterally referred to the preauricular area, or down the neck, or up to the temporal area. In these instances the source of extraorally referred pain almost invariably is a posterior tooth. Ostensible toothache of nonodontogenic origin (i.e., resulting from neurologic, cardiac, vascular, malignant, or sinus diseases) is described in Chapter 3.

Patients may report that their dental pain is exacerbated by lying down or bending over. This occurs because of the increase in blood pressure to the head, which increases the pressure on the confined pulp.

The dentist should be alert for patients who manifest emotional disorders as dental pain. If no organic cause can be discovered for what appears as dental pain, the patient should be referred for medical consultation. Patients with atypical facial pain of functional rather than organic cause may begin their long journey through the many specialties of the health sciences in the dentist's office.

If the dentist can determine the onset, duration, frequency, and quality of the pain and the factors that alter its perception, and if the dentist can reproduce or relieve the pain by clinical testing, then surely the pain is of odontogenic origin. The patient will usually gain immeasurable psychological benefit if the clinician provides caring and sincere reassurance that, once the source is discovered, appropriate treatment will be provided immediately to stop the pain.

EXAMINATION AND TESTING

The inspection phase of the extraoral and intraoral clinical examination should be performed in a systematic manner. A consistent step-by-step approach, always following the same procedure, helps the clinician develop good working habits and minimizes the possibility of inadvertently overlooking any part of the examination or testing. The extraoral visual examination should begin while the clinician is taking the patient's dental history.

Talking with the patient provides an opportunity to observe the patient's facial features. The clinician should look for facial asymmetry (Fig. 1-1, *A*) or distensions that might indicate swelling of odontogenic origin or a systemic ailment. The patient's eyes should be observed for the pupillary dilation or constriction that may indicate systemic disease, premedication, or fear. Additionally, the patient's skin should be observed for any lesion(s) and, if there is more than one, whether the lesions appear at random or follow a neural pathway.

After a careful external visual examination the clinician should, with the aid of a mouth mirror and the blunt-ended handle of another instrument, begin an oral examination to look for abnormalities of both hard and soft tissues. With a head lamp and good magnification the lips, cheek pouch, tongue, palate, and throat should be briefly examined (Fig. 1-1, *B*). Because it is easier to observe abnormalities when tissues are dry, the liberal use of 2×2 inch gauze, cotton rolls, and a saliva ejector is strongly recommended (Fig. 1-1, *C*). During the visual phase of the examination the clinician should also be checking both the patient's oral hygiene and the integrity of the dentition. Poor oral hygiene and/or numerous missing teeth may indicate that the patient has minimal interest in maintaining a healthy dentition.

Visual inspection of the teeth begins with drying the quadrant under examination and looking for caries, toothbrush abrasion (Fig. 1-1, *D*) (cervical lesions occasionally are overlooked), darkened teeth (Fig. 1-1, *E*), observable swelling (Fig. 1-1, *F*), fractured or cracked crowns (Fig. 1-1, *G*), and defective restorations.

The clinician should observe the color and translucency of the teeth. Are the teeth intact or is there evidence of abrasion, attrition, cervical erosion, or developmental defects in the crowns?

A high index of suspicion must prevail during examination for numerous types of soft-tissue lesions.[8,20] This also means looking for unusual changes in the color or contour of the soft tissues. For example, the clinician should look carefully for lesions of odontogenic origin such as sinus tracts (fistulas) (Fig. 1-2, *A*) or localized redness or swelling involving the attachment apparatus. The presence of a sinus tract may indicate that periapical suppuration has resulted from a pulp that has undergone complete necrosis in at least one root. The suppurative lesion has burrowed its way from the cancellous bone through the cortical plate and finally to the mucosal surface. *All* sinus tracts should be traced with a gutta-percha cone (Fig. 1-2, *B* to *E*) to locate their source, because occasionally the source can be remote.[13]

All observable data indicating an abnormality should be recorded on the treatment chart while the information is still fresh in the clinician's mind. If a tooth is suspected of requiring endodontic treatment, it should be assessed in terms of its restorability after endodontic treatment, its strategic importance, and its periodontal prognosis.

Palpation

When periapical inflammation has developed as an extension of pulpal necrosis, the inflammatory process may burrow its way through the facial cortical bone and begin to affect the overlying mucoperiosteum. Before incipient swelling becomes clinically evident, it may be discerned by both the clinician and the patient using gentle palpation with the index finger (Fig. 1-3, *A*). The index finger is rolled while it presses the mucosa against the underlying bone. If the mucoperiosteum is inflamed, this rolling motion will reveal the existence and degree of sensitivity caused by the periapical inflammation.

To improve tactile skill and learn the full extent of normal

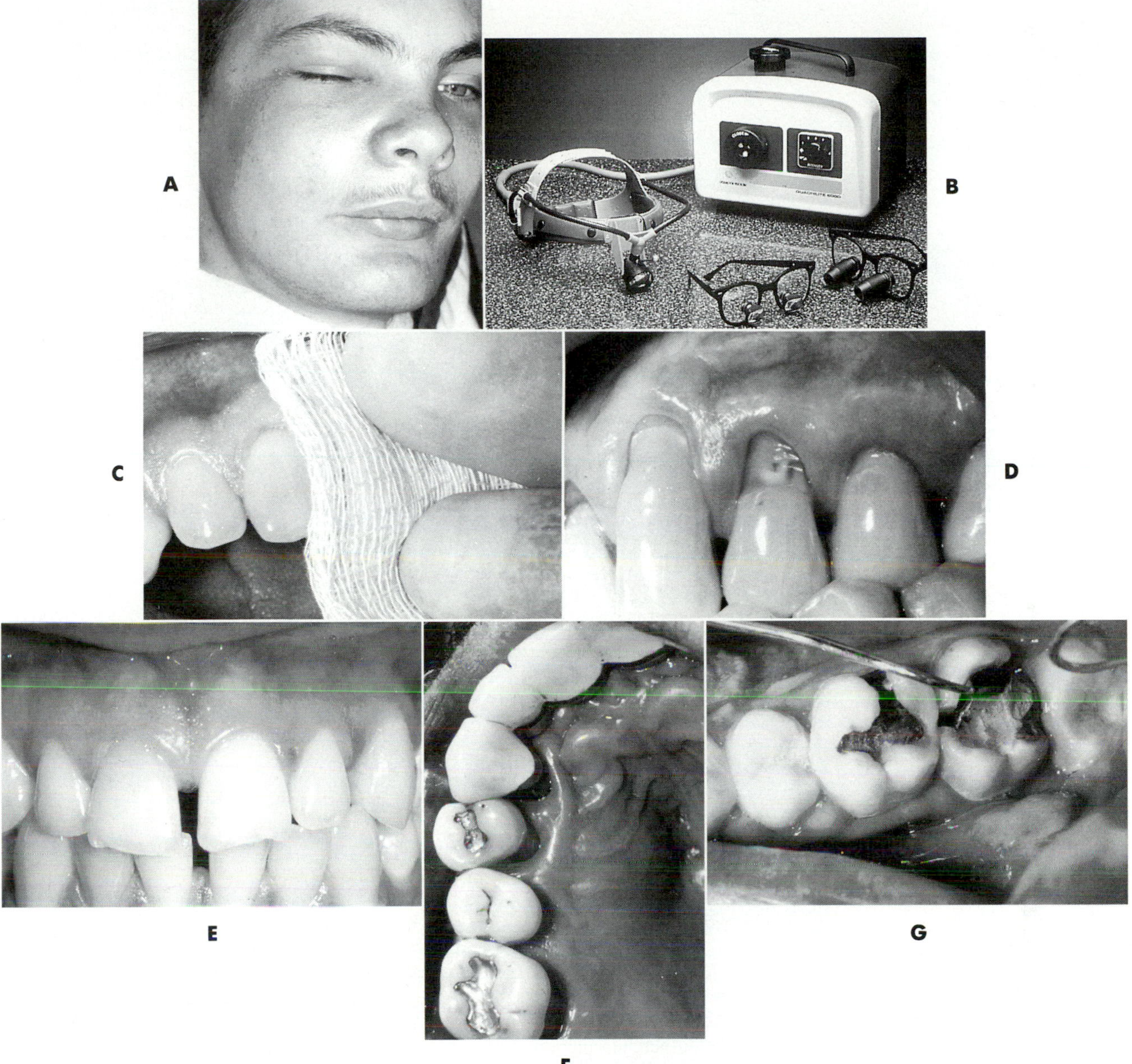

FIG. 1-1 A, Swelling around the right mandible can be readily observed by the clinician while preparing the dental history. **B,** The Designs for Vision fiberoptic headlamp along with 2½ to 3½ × magnification allows the clinician to examine the soft tissues and teeth without any shadows. **C,** A thorough tissue examination is facilitated by drying with cotton rolls, 2 × 2 inch gauze, and a saliva ejector. The initial examination of the teeth and surrounding tissues is conducted with the patient's mouth partly open. With good illumination and magnification, as shown in Fig. 1-1 *B,* changes in color, contour, or texture can be determined by a careful visual examination. **D,** Class V caries lesion, or abrasion, not always detectable radiographically, can be observed. **E,** Tooth discolored following a traumatic incident. Although the tooth appears necrotic, vitality tests should still be conducted because the pulp could remain vital. **F,** Intraoral swelling from periapical disease usually appears around the mucobuccal fold; however, the entire mouth must be thoroughly examined because swelling from periapical disease may occur in unusual locations (e.g., the palate). **G,** With careful visual examination the clinician may observe crown fractures that may not appear in radiographs.

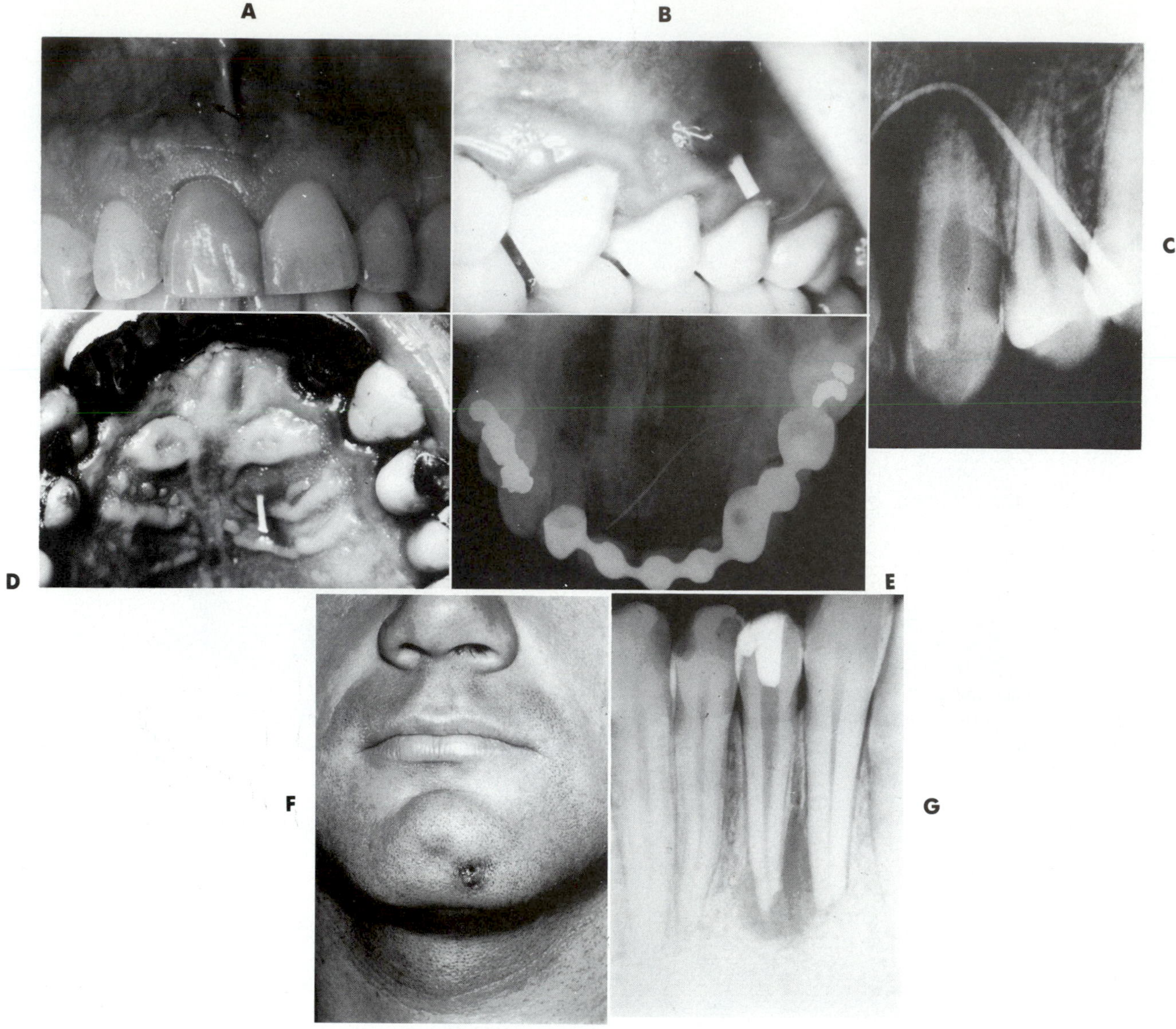

FIG. 1-2 A, Sinus tract (fistula). **B,** When a sinus tract is detected, it should always be traced with a gutta-percha cone to its source. In this case, the sinus tract appeared between the first and second premolars. **C,** The source of the sinus tract was the lateral incisor, as the gutta-percha probe indicates. **D,** Gutta-percha cone used to trace a sinus tract discovered on the palate. **E,** An occlusal jaw radiograph revealed that the sinus tract crossed the midline. The source was a cuspid. **F,** After numerous unsuccessful dermatologic treatments, this patient consulted a dentist. **G,** The dentist discovered the source.

range to be expected, the clinician is urged to perform palpation testing routinely.

Other techniques involving extraoral bidigital or bimanual palpation (e.g., palpating lymph nodes or the floor of the mouth) are described in complete detail by Rose and Kaye.[18]

Occasionally a patient is able to point to a particular facial area that felt tender when shaving or applying makeup. The clinician can follow up by palpating in the mucofacial fold, which may help pinpoint the source of the tenderness. If a site that feels tender to palpation is discovered, its location and extent should be recorded as well as whether or not the area is soft or firm. This provides important information on the possible need for an incision and drainage.

If a mandibular tooth is abscessed, it is prudent also to palpate the submandibular area bimanually to determine whether any submandibular lymph nodes have been affected by extension of the disease process (Fig. 1-3, *B*).

Finally, the cervical lymph nodes should be palpated bidigitally to discern any swollen or firm lymph nodes.

The use of extraoral and intraoral palpation helps the clinician determine the furthest extent of the disease processes.

Percussion

The percussion test may reveal whether there is any inflammation around the periodontal ligament. The clinician should remember that the percussion test does *not* give any indication

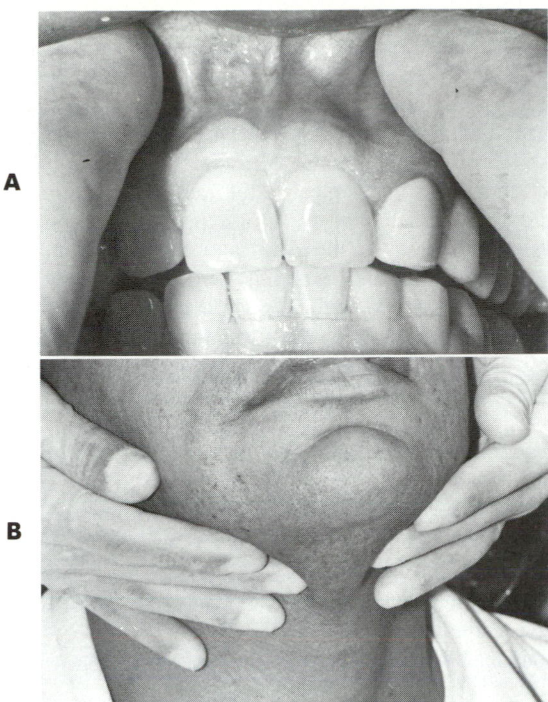

FIG. 1-3 Palpation. **A,** Bilateral intraoral digital palpation aids the clinician in detecting comparative changes in contour or consistency of the soft tissue and underlying bone. A "mushy" feeling detected during palpation around the mucolabial fold may be the first clinical evidence of incipient swelling. **B,** Bimanual extraoral palpation to tactilely search for the extent of lymph node involvement when there is a mandibular dental infection. The clinician should palpate the submandibular nodes (as shown here), the angle of the mandible, and the cervical chain of nodes.

of the health or integrity of the pulp tissues; it indicates only whether there is inflammation around the periodontal ligament. Before the test, the patient should be instructed that making a small audible sound or raising a hand is the best way to let the clinician know when a tooth feels tender, different, or painful with percussion.

Before tapping on the teeth with the handle of a mouth mirror, the clinician is advised to use the index finger to percuss teeth in the quadrant being examined (Fig. 1-4, *A*). Digital percussion is much less painful than percussion with a mouth mirror handle. The teeth should be tapped in a random fashion (i.e., out of sequence) so the patient cannot anticipate when "the tooth" will be percussed. If the patient cannot discern a difference in sensation with digital percussion, the handle of a mouth mirror should be used to tap on the occlusal, facial, and lingual surfaces of the teeth (Fig. 1-4, *B*). Using the most appropriate force for percussing is one of the skills that the clinician will develop as part of the art of endodontic diagnosis. Percussing the teeth too strongly may cause unnecessary pain and anxiety for the patient. The clinician should use the chief complaint and dental history as a guide in deciding how strongly to percuss the teeth. The force of percussion need be only great enough for the patient to discern a difference between a sound tooth and a tooth with an inflamed periodontal ligament. The proprioceptive fibers in an inflamed periodontal ligament, when percussed, help the patient and the clinician locate the source of the pain. Tapping on each cusp can, on occasion, reveal the presence of a crown fracture.

A positive response to percussion, indicating an inflamed periodontal ligament, can be caused by a variety of factors (e.g., teeth undergoing rapid orthodontic movement, a recent high restoration, a lateral periodontal abscess, and, of course, partial or total necrosis of the pulp). However, the absence of a response to percussion is quite possible when there is chronic periapical inflammation.

Mobility

Using the index fingers, or preferably the blunt handles of two metal instruments, the clinician applies alternating lateral forces in a facial-lingual direction to observe the degree of mo-

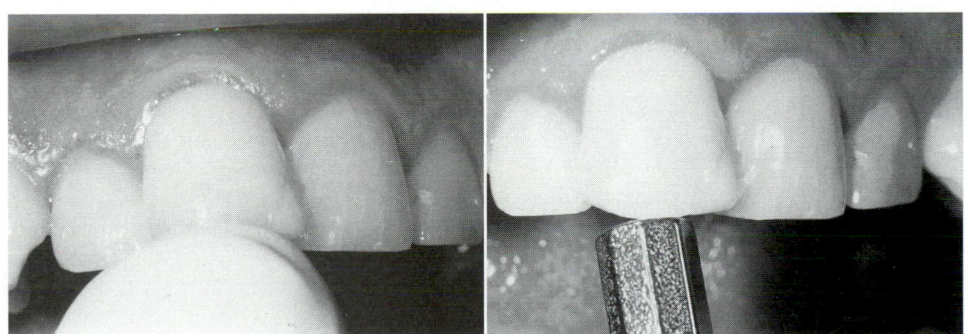

FIG. 1-4 Percussion test to determine whether there is any apical periodontitis. If the patient has reported pain during mastication, the percussion test should be conducted *very gently*. **A,** First only the index finger should be used. The teeth should be percussed from a facial as well as an incisal direction. **B,** If the patient reports no tenderness when the teeth are percussed with the finger, a more definitive, sharper percussion can be conducted with the handle of the mouth mirror.

bility of the tooth within the alveolus (Fig. 1-5). In addition, tests for the degree of depressibility are performed by pressing the tooth into its socket and observing if there is vertical movement. First-degree mobility is barely discernible movement; second-degree is horizontal movement of 1 mm or less; third-degree is horizontal movement of greater than 1 mm, often accompanied by vertical mobility. Tooth movement usually reflects the extent of inflammation of the periodontal ligament.

The pressure exerted by the purulent exudate of an acute apical abscess may cause some mobility of a tooth. In this situation the tooth may quickly stabilize after drainage is established and the occlusion adjusted. There are additional causes for tooth mobility—including advanced periodontal disease, horizontal root fracture in the middle or coronal third, and chronic bruxism or clenching.

Radiographs

Radiographs are essential aids in endodontic diagnosis. Unfortunately, some clinicians rely exclusively on radiographs in their attempt to arrive at a diagnosis. This obviously can lead to major errors in diagnosis and treatment.[2] Because the radiograph is a two-dimensional image of a three-dimensional object, misinterpretation is a constant risk, but with proper angulation of the cone, accurate film placement, correct processing of the exposed film (Fig. 1-6), and good illumination with a magnifying glass, the hazards of misinterpretation can be substantially minimized. The full benefit of periapical radiographs for diagnostic purposes can be achieved if the technique described here is employed.

After correct film placement, either bisected-angle or long-cone methods are effective for film exposure. It is important to expose *two* diagnostic films. By maintaining the same vertical cone angulation and changing the horizontal cone angulation 10 to 15 degrees for the second diagnostic film, the clinician can obtain a three-dimensional impression of the teeth that will aid in discerning superimposed roots and anatomic landmarks. (Refer to Chapter 5 for further discussion of this phase of dental radiology.)

The state of pulpal health or pulpal necrosis cannot be determined radiographically; but any of the following findings should arouse suspicion of degenerative pulp changes: deep carious lesions, deep and extensive restorations, pulp caps, pulpotomies, pulp stones, extensive canal calcification, root resorption, radiolucencies at or near the apex, root fractures, thickened periodontal ligament, and periodontal disease that is radiographically evident.

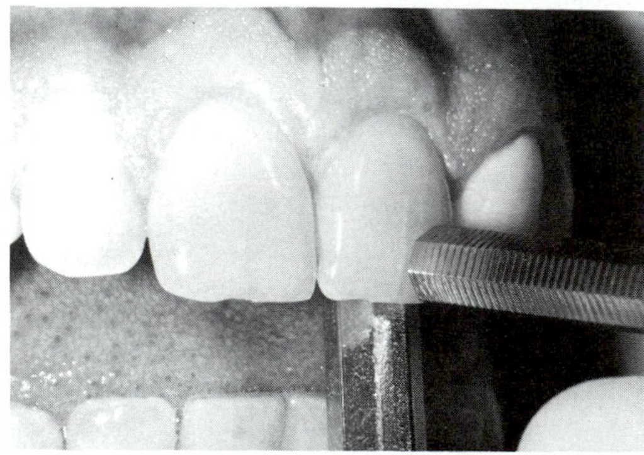

FIG. 1-5 The degree of mobility can be most effectively determined by applying lateral forces with a blunt-handled instrument in a facial-lingual direction.

Radiographic interpretation

Interpretation of good-quality diagnostic radiographs must be done in an orderly and consistent manner. With good illumination and magnification the clinician can detect nuances of change that may reveal early pathologic changes in or around the tooth. First, the crown of each tooth and then the root(s) are carefully observed, then the root canal system, followed by the lamina dura, bony architecture, and finally the anatomic landmarks that may appear on the film. When posterior teeth are being investigated, a bite-wing film provides an excellent supplement for finding the extent of carious destruction, the depths of restorations, the presence of pulp caps or pulpotomies, and dens invaginatus or evaginatus. Generally it is true that the deeper the caries and the more extensive the restoration the greater is the probability of pulpal involvement. Following the lamina dura usually reveals the number and curvature of the roots. A root canal should be readily discernible; if the canal appears to change quickly from dark to light, this indicates that it has bifurcated or trifurcated (Fig. 1-7, *A*). The presence of "extra" roots or canals in all teeth (Fig. 1-7, *B*) is

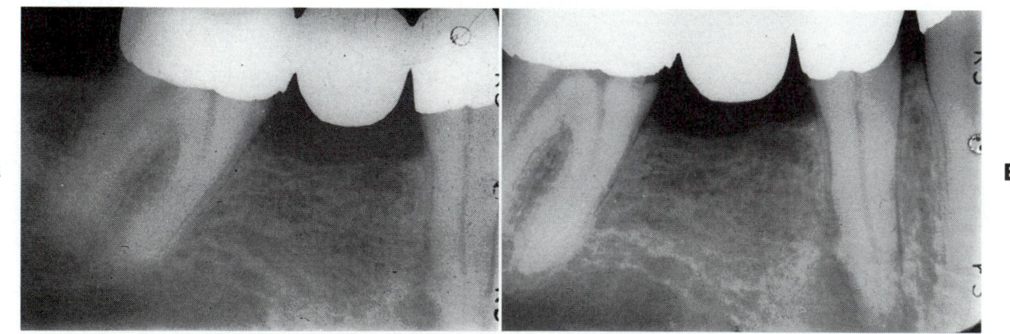

FIG. 1-6 A, An improperly exposed or poorly processed radiograph like this one is difficult or impossible to interpret. **B,** The condition of the crown, roots, and surrounding tissue can be seen only with a properly prepared radiograph.

much more common than was previously believed. If the outline of the root seems unclear or deviates from where it ought to be, an extra root should be suspected.[24] Accordingly, *at least one canal (or root) more than the radiograph shows must always be suspected until clinically proved otherwise*. Three-rooted mandibular molars (Fig. 1-7, *B*) and maxillary premolars as well as two-rooted canines will be found with greater frequency as the examiner's dental anatomic acumen, index of suspicion, and diagnostic sophistication improve.

A necrotic tooth does not cause radiographic changes at the apex until the periapical pathosis has destroyed bony trabeculae at their junction with the cortical plate.[21] Thus a great deal of bone destruction may occur before any radiographic signs are evident. A radiolucent lesion need not be at the apex of the root to indicate pulpal inflammation or degeneration. Toxins of pulp tissue degeneration exiting from a lateral canal can cause bone destruction anywhere along the root. Conversely, a lateral canal can be a portal of entry for potentially harmful toxins in teeth with advanced periodontal disease (Fig. 1-8). If periodontal bone loss extends far enough apically to expose the foramen of a lateral canal, the toxins from the periodontal disease can gain entry into a vital healthy pulp via the lateral canal and cause irritation, inflammation, and even pulpal necrosis in a sound tooth. Periodontal disease extending to the apical foramen definitely causes pathologic pulpal changes (see Chapter 18).

Pulp stones (Fig. 1-9, *A*) and canal calcifications are not necessarily pathologic; they can be mere manifestations of degenerative aging in the pulpal tissue. However, their presence may cause other insults to the pulp and may increase the difficulty of negotiating the root canals. The incidence of calcifications in the chamber or in the canal may increase with periodontal disease, extensive restorations, or aging. As the percentage of the population categorized as elderly increases, clinicians

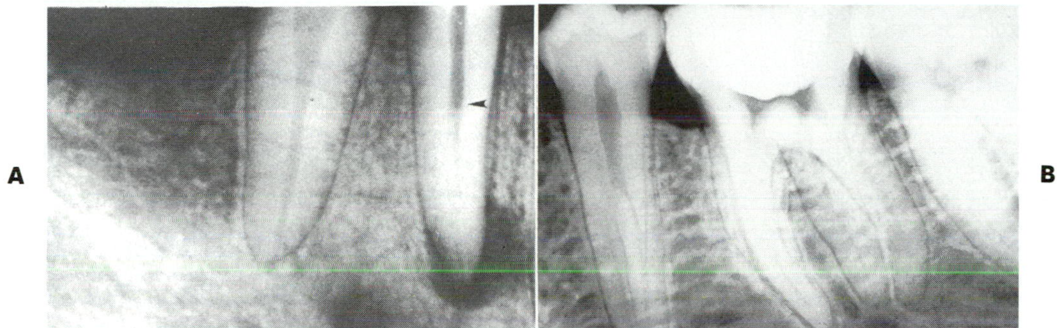

FIG. 1-7 A, A sudden change from dark to light indicates bifurcation or trifurcation of the root canal system *(arrow),* as shown by **B,** premolar with a bifurcated root canal system and a mandibular first molar with three roots.

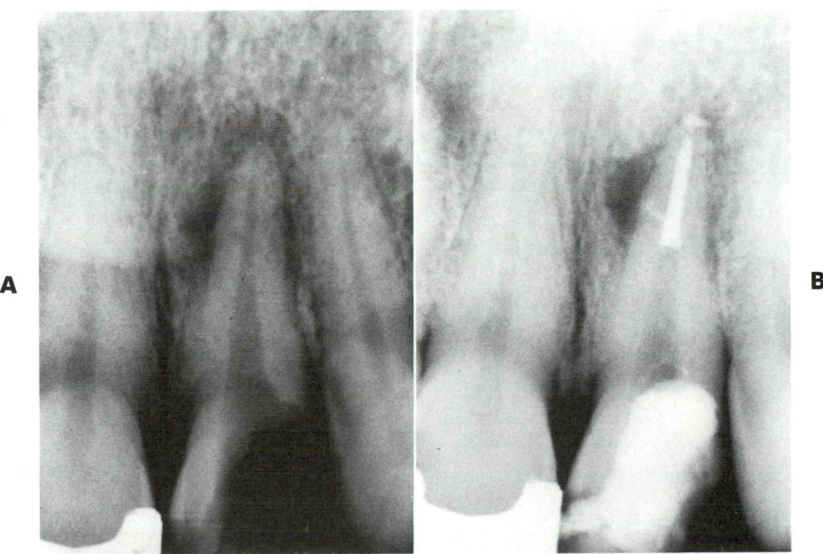

FIG. 1-8 A and **B,** Radiolucent lesions indicates pulp degeneration. These radiographs illustrate how toxins of pulp tissue degeneration may exit from a lateral canal, causing bone destruction along the side. Conversely, this lateral canal could be a portal of entry for toxins that might destroy the pulp and create a periapical lesion.

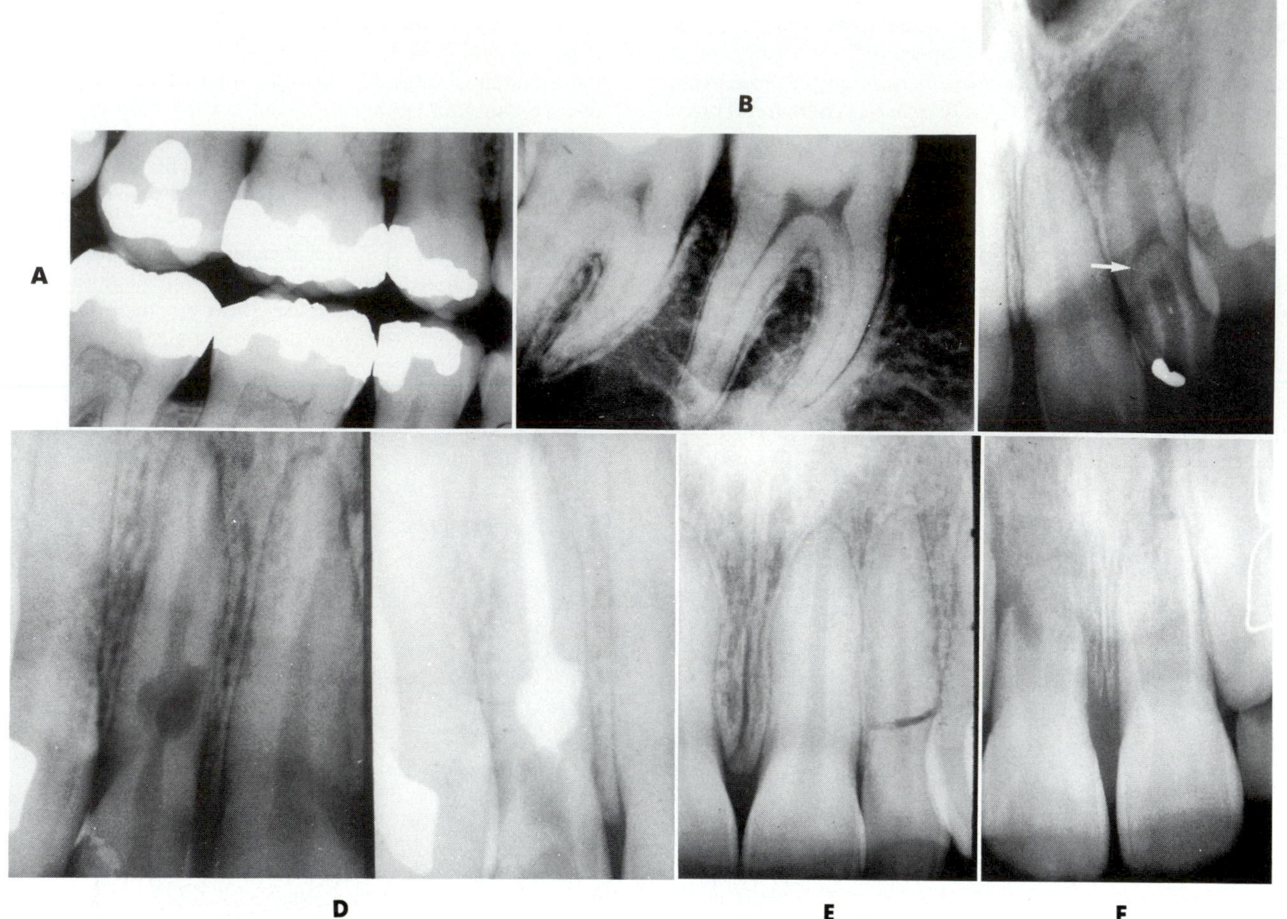

FIG. 1-9 A, Pulp stones and the extent and depth of restorations can be detected more clearly with a bite-wing film. **B,** Periapical osteosclerosis, possibly caused by a mild pulp irritant. **C,** Dens in dente. **D,** Internal resorption, once detected, must be treated promptly before it perforates the root. **E,** Horizontal root fractures can usually be detected with a good-quality radiograph. **F,** Vitality tests on a tooth with an immature apex may yield erroneous results.

should be more attuned to detecting pulp stones and calcification of the canal space[30] (see Chapter 24).

Internal resorption (Fig. 1-9, *D*) (occasionally seen after a traumatic injury) is an indication for endodontic therapy. The inflamed pulp, expanding at the expense of the dentin, must be removed as soon as possible lest a lateral perforation occur. Untreated internal resorption leading to root perforation increases the probability of eventual tooth loss (see Chapter 16).

Radiographs are important for identifying teeth with immature apices (Fig. 1-9, *F*) and teeth with lingual development grooves (Fig. 1-10). The clinician must have this information *before* conducting thermal and electric pulp tests because teeth with immature apices often cause erroneous readings with vitality testing (Chapter 23).

Root fractures may cause pulpal degeneration. Fractures of the root can be difficult to detect on a radiograph. Vertical root fractures (Fig. 1-11, *A* and *B*) are seldom identified with the radiograph except in advanced stages of root separation. Most horizontal root fractures can be readily identified with properly exposed and processed radiographs; however, horizontal fractures may be confused with linear patterns of bone trabeculae. The two phenomena can be differentiated by noting that the lines of bone trabeculae extend beyond the border of the root, whereas a root fracture often causes a thickening of the periodontal ligament.

Finally, the clinician must realize that there are occasions when periapical, bite-wing, and panoramic films may not suffice. Other types of extraoral films, described in greater detail in Chapter 5, may be necessary (especially when there has been a traumatic incident) before a diagnosis can be made.

Radiographic misinterpretation

A dental humorist once claimed that if a clinician looked at a radiograph long enough he would find whatever he was looking for. This overstatement suggests a sound rule for radiographic interpretation: be wary—but not necessarily disbelieving—of what appears to be obvious radiographically. Radiographic interpretation is often quite subjective, as illustrated by a study of more than 250 cases in which the *same* endodontists interpreted

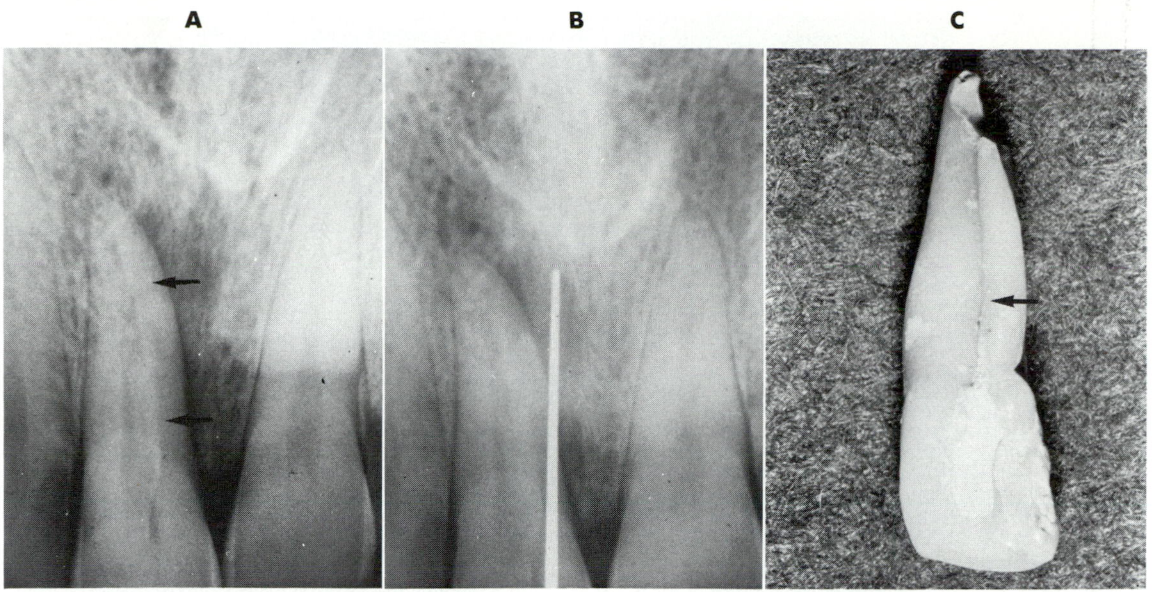

FIG. 1-10 A, Lingual development groove. The radiograph shows the canals of both central incisors to be distinctly different. Arrows point to the groove traced along the root. **B,** Silver cone in the sulcular defect tracing the groove toward the apex. **C,** Although the tooth was vital, only extraction could resolve this problem. In the near future, lasing these grooves may allow these types of teeth to be retained.

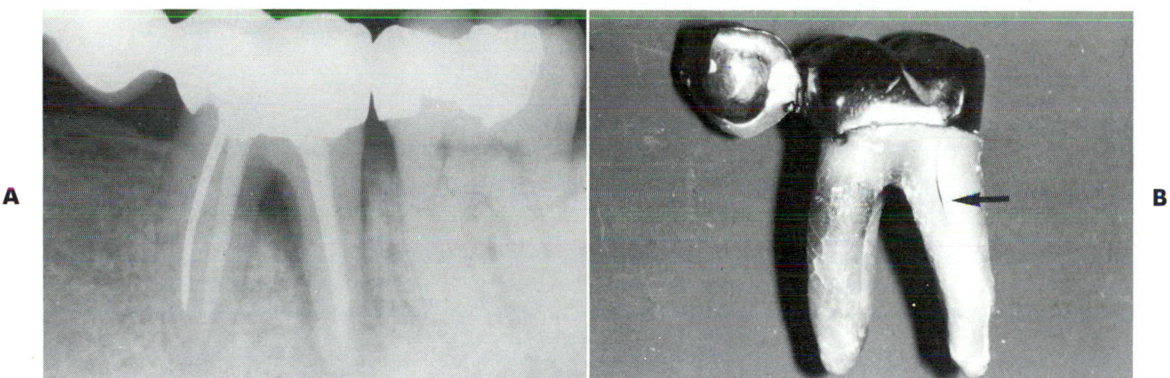

FIG. 1-11 Vertical fractures are rarely evident radiographically until there is advanced root separation. **A,** Distal root with vertical fracture. **B,** Following extraction, the fracture can be seen *(arrow)*.

the *same* radiographs at intervals of 6 to 8 months. The three endodontists in this study agreed with themselves only 72% to 88% of the time.[10] In an earlier study six endodontists all agreed with each other *less than half the time*.[9] The radiographic phenomena that caused misinterpretations were these:

1. Radiolucency at the apex (Fig. 1-12). At first glance this might appear to be a periapical lesion. However, a positive response to vitality tests, an intact lamina dura, the absence of symptoms and probable cause, and the anatomic location clearly show it to be the mental foramen. Only the confirmed absence of pulp vitality will reveal which tooth is the source of the periapical lesion (Fig. 1-13).
2. Well-circumscribed radiolucency at or near the apex (Fig. 1-14, *A-C*). At first glance (Fig. 1-14, *B*) it might appear to be a periapical lesion. However, changing the horizontal angulation and exposing a second radiograph show the lesion to have moved (Fig. 1-14, *C*). Because the tooth was asymptomatic with lack of probable cause and because of a positive response to vitality tests and anatomic location, this was positively identified as the nasopalatine canal.
3. The periapical radiolucency over the lateral incisor suggests the incisor is the source of the lesion, but vitality testing showed it was the canine that was nonvital. Endodontic treatment remineralized the radiolucency over the lateral incisor (Fig. 1-15).

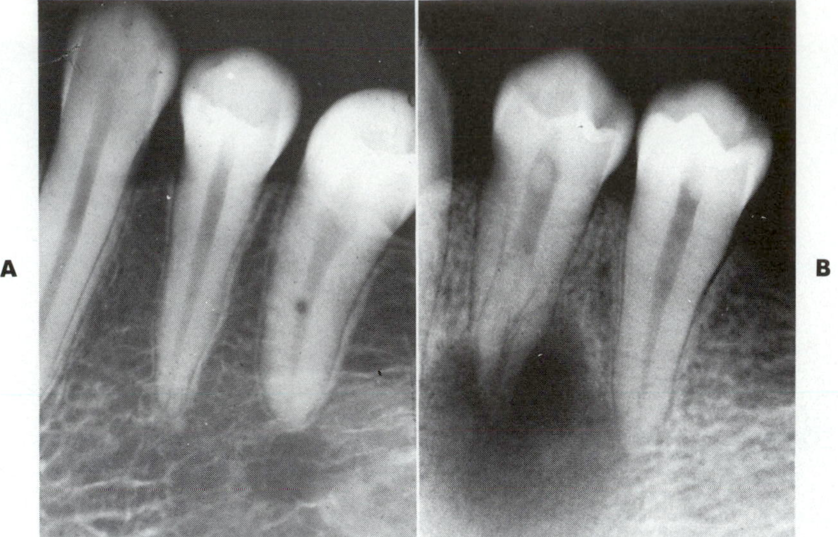

FIG. 1-12 Radiograph misinterpretation. **A,** Mental foramen that might be mistaken for a periapical lesion. Thermal and electric pulp tests and an intact lamina dura revealed that the tooth was vital. **B,** Nonodontogenic lesion surrounding the apex of a vital premolar is too large to be mistaken for a mental foramen.

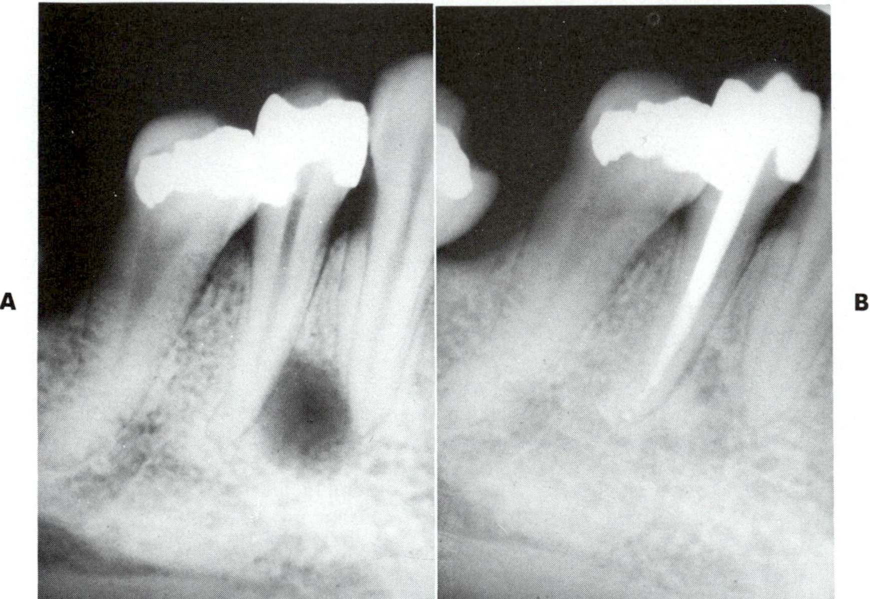

FIG. 1-13 A, Vitality tests indicated that the first premolar and not the cuspid was necrotic. Adjacent teeth tested vital. **B,** One year after completion of endodontic treatment, the bone remineralized.

Accordingly, the clinician should *never* make a clinical diagnosis based merely on the radiograph showing a periapical radiolucency, but should *always* use thermal tests and electric pulp tests for clinical verification.

Thermal Tests

One of the most common symptoms associated with a symptomatic inflamed pulp is pain induced by hot or cold stimulation. Hot and cold tests are valuable diagnostic aids because in certain types of inflamed pulps pain may be induced or relieved by a thermal application. The patient's response to thermal tests frequently provides the clinician with information about whether the pulp is healthy or inflamed; when several teeth in a quadrant are being tested, thermal tests often help pinpoint the thermally symptomatic tooth.

Before testing, the patient should be told what tests are go-

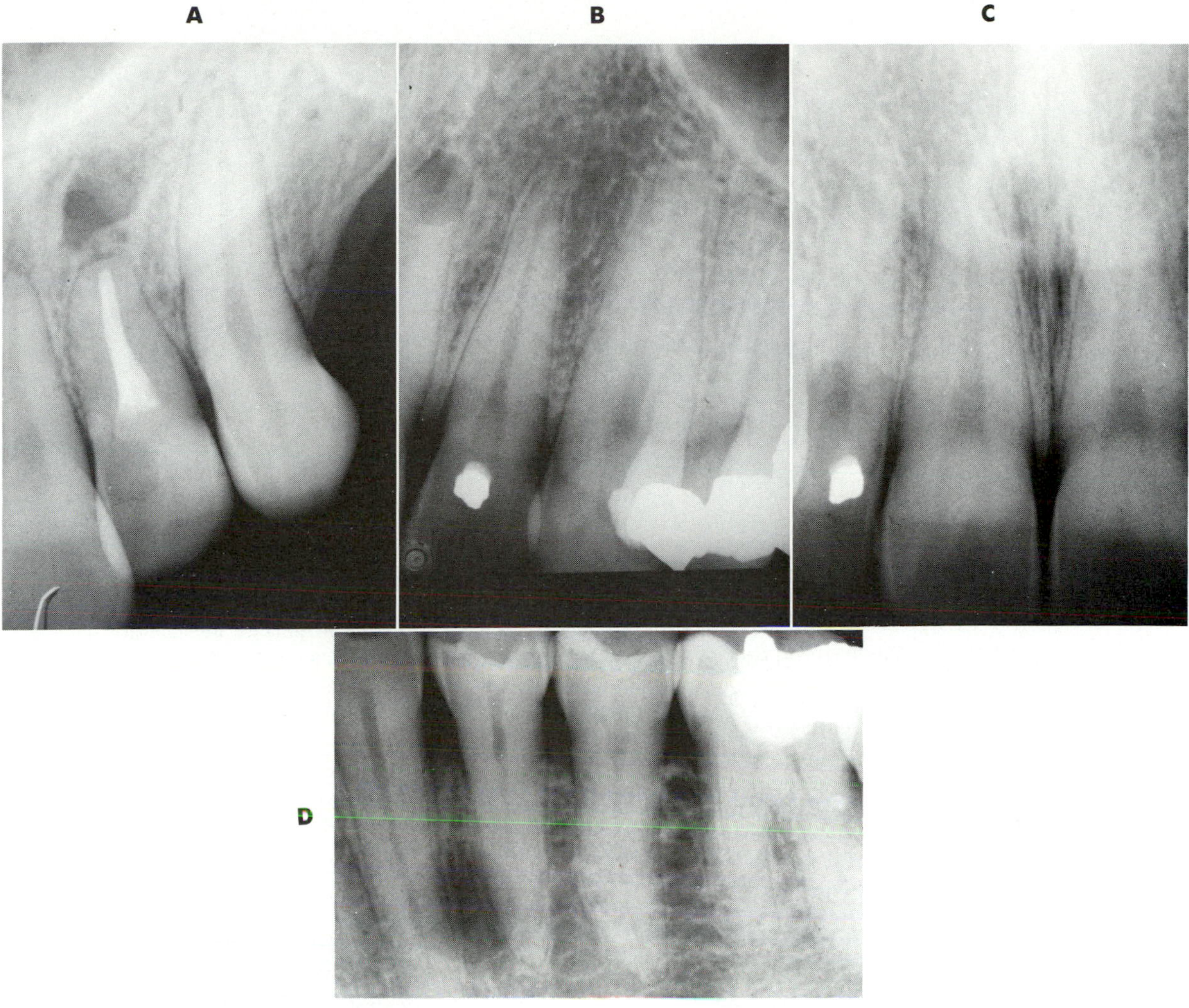

FIG. 1-14 A, Apical scar over lateral incisor. This asymptomatic radiolucency was identified as a scar because the lamina dura is intact and the patient had a history of apical surgery. **B,** Periapical radiolucency that might be mistaken for a periapical lesion *(arrows)*. **C,** Changing the horizontal cone angulation moved the radiolucency toward the midline *(arrows)*. The "lesion" was the nasopalatine foramen superimposed over the apex of the central incisor. **D,** Lateral periodontal cyst. The cuspid and premolar were both vital.

ing to be performed and why. Additionally, the patient should be given some idea of what to expect. One or two teeth on the opposite side of the mouth should be tested first so the patient has an idea of how the tests will feel. If the clinician takes the time to do this, patient anxiety and fear will be substantially reduced.

It is important to inform the patient how to respond when a sensation is experienced, so there will be no thrashing about or other unexpected behavior. For example, the patient should be instructed to raise a hand as soon as any sensation is felt and should be assured that the clinician will remove the stimulus immediately if the patient raises a hand.

The teeth in the quadrant must first be isolated and then dried with 2 × 2 inch gauze, and a saliva ejector placed. The teeth should *not* be dried with a blast of air because the room-temperature air might cause thermal shock and saliva might be sprayed on the clinician or the assistant (Fig. 1-16, *B*).

Heat test

For the heat test, temporary stopping on the blade of a Woodson instrument can be heated over a glass bead sterilizer until the surface becomes glassy (Fig. 1-17, *A*). The heated mass should be applied immediately to the middle third of the tooth surface. The tooth should be lightly lubricated with cocoa butter (or the equivalent) to prevent the stopping from sticking to the tooth.

A second technique for heat testing includes heating a stick of temporary stopping for a few seconds over an alcohol flame until it becomes shiny and sags, but *before* it begins to smoke. The stopping is then immediately placed on the middle third of the facial surface of the crown (Fig. 1-17, *B*). If it is too hot (i.e., the gutta-percha appears to be smoking), it may cause a burn lesion in an otherwise normal pulp. This type of abuse could destroy a debilitated pulp. If the patient has a normal pulp, the response to this test is transient and consists of a mild

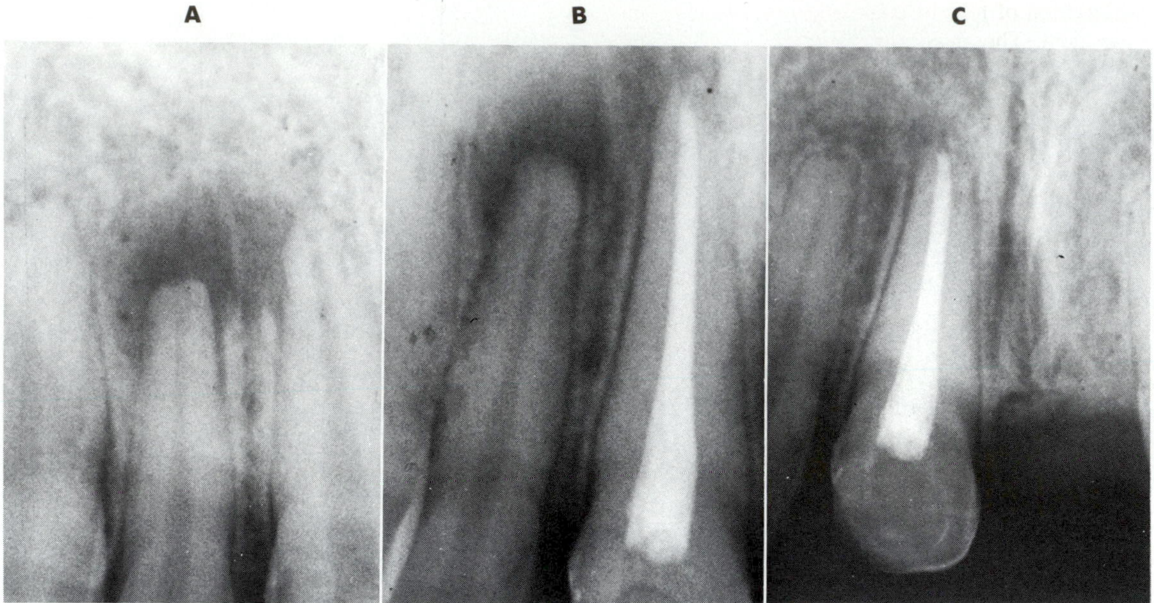

FIG. 1-15 A, The periapical radiolucency over the lateral incisor might indicate the lateral incisors as the source of the lesion. Thermal and electric pulp tests indicated that the lateral incisor was vital and the canine was necrotic. **B,** Endodontic treatment completed for the canine. **C,** Six months after endodontic treatment the canine has completely remineralized over the apex of the lateral incisor. (Courtesy Dr. John Sapone.)

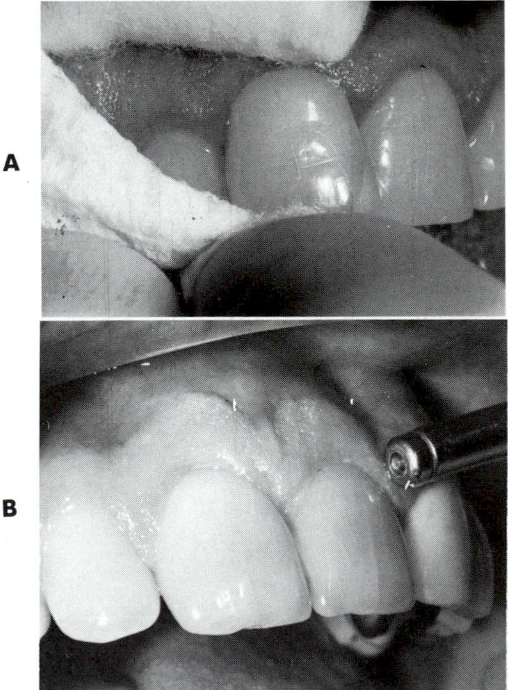

FIG. 1-16 Preparing teeth for thermal and electric pulp testing. **A,** Before testing, the teeth should be isolated with a cotton roll and dried with gauze. **B,** Air should *not* be used to dry the teeth because room temperature air may cause thermal shock. Air drying could also spray saliva on the clinician.

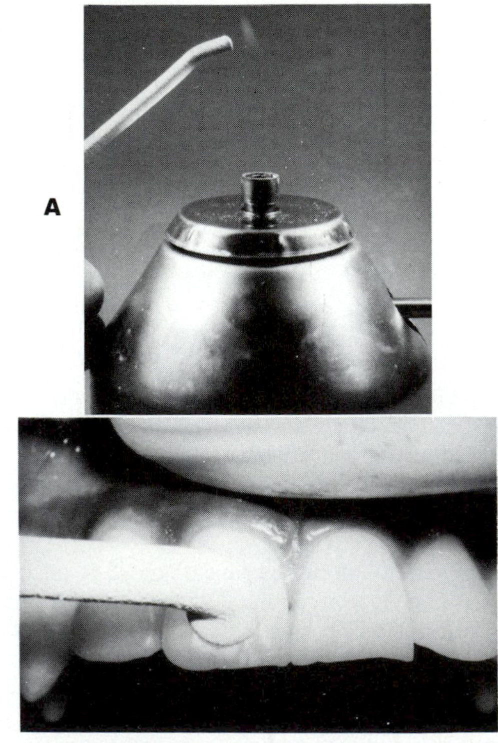

FIG. 1-17 Thermal test with heat. **A,** Temporary stopping is heated over a flame until it becomes soft and begins to bend. **B,** Temporary stopping applied to the dried tooth (lightly coated with cocoa butter to prevent sticking).

to moderate sensation of heat or pain. The patient should not experience any pain. The *most effective* thermal test for any tooth, including a tooth with porcelain or metal full coverage, involves isolating the tooth and bathing in very warm or cold water (Fig. 1-18, *E*). This type of thermal test is clearly the most reliable for reproducing any thermal pain the patient has reported.

Care must be used in applying these and all heat tests, or otherwise the pulp may be damaged by overheating. The preferred temperature for a heat test is approximately 65.5° C (150° F).

Cold test

For cold testing, the teeth must remain isolated and dry. The most common techniques for cold testing utilize ethyl chloride, sticks of ice or carbon dioxide crystals, or Freon 12.[27] Although all methods are generally effective, ethyl chloride is the easiest technique. Sticks of ice require preparation time and, when applied to a tooth surface, may drip onto the gingiva, causing a false-positive response. Carbon dioxide crystals or dry ice is very cold (−77.7° C or −108° F) and can cause infraction lines in enamel because of thermal shock[1] or damage an otherwise healthy pulp.[3]

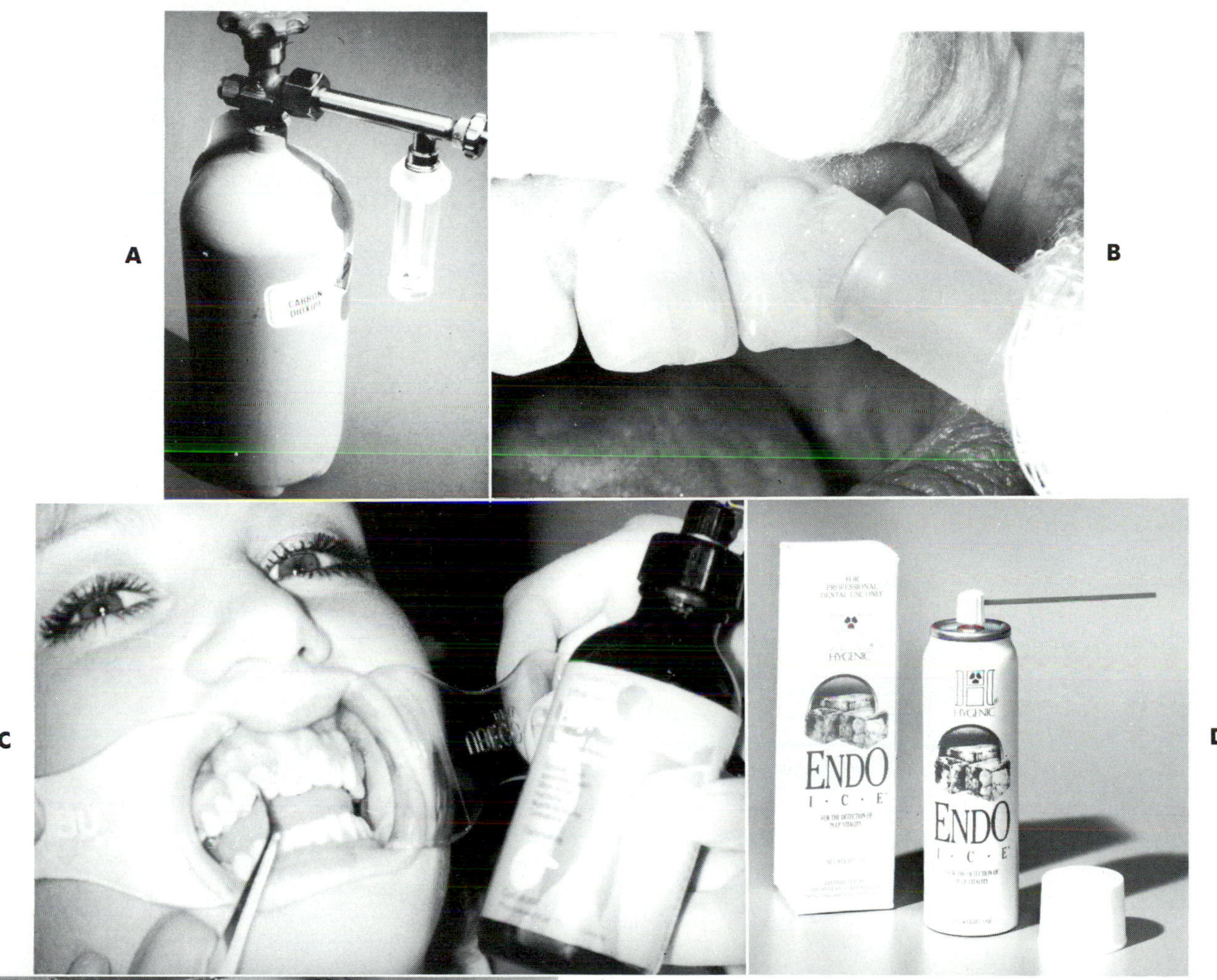

FIG. 1-18 Thermal test with cold. **A,** Carbon dioxide can be used to prepare dry ice sticks for cold testing. **B,** One dry ice stick removed from the cylinder and held with 2 × 2 inch gauze is sufficient to test all teeth. **C,** Endo Ice and ethyl chloride are easy-to-use liquid sprays for cold testing. **D,** Ethyl chloride (or Endo Ice) is sprayed onto a cotton pellet or cotton-wood stick and then applied to the tooth. Excess liquid has been shaken out of the cotton pellet. As soon as crystals form, the pellet is placed on the tooth. **E,** Isolating a tooth with a rubber dam and bathing the tooth with (first) very warm and (then) ice cold water is clearly the most effective and accurate thermal test.

Ethyl chloride is sprayed liberally on a cotton pellet, and the cotton pliers holding the pellet are tapped once or twice to shake out the excess liquid. Without delay the cotton pellet is then placed on the middle third of the facial surface (Fig. 1-18). The pellet should be held in close contact with the tooth surface for several seconds or until the patient has a response of cold with pain. The ethyl chloride technique is effective even on teeth covered with cast metal crowns. Spraying ethyl chloride directly onto a tooth is *not* recommended, because the liquid is a general anesthetic, highly flammable, and potentially dangerous for the patient when used in this manner.

Responses

The patient's responses to heat and cold testing are identical because the neural fibers in the pulp transmit only the sensation of pain. There are four possible reactions the patient may have: (1) no response; (2) a mild to moderate transient thermal pain response; (3) a strong painful response that subsides quickly after the stimulus is removed from the tooth; and (4) a strong painful response that lingers after the thermal stimulus is removed.

If there is no response, the pulp is either nonvital or possibly vital but giving a false-negative response because of excessive calcification, an immature apex, recent trauma, or patient premedication. A moderate transient response is usually considered normal. A painful response that subsides quickly after the stimulus is removed is characteristic of reversible pulpitis. Finally, a painful response that lingers after the thermal stimulus is removed indicates a symptomatic irreversible pulpitis.

Electric Pulp Tests

The electric pulp tester is designed to stimulate a response by electric excitation of the neural elements within the pulp. The patient's response to the electric pulp test does *not* provide sufficient information for a diagnosis. The electric pulp test merely suggests whether the pulp is vital or nonvital and does not provide information regarding the health or integrity of a vital pulp. The electric pulp test does not provide any information about the vascular supply to the tooth, which is the real determinant of vitality. Additionally, a number of situations may cause a false-positive or false-negative response, *so*

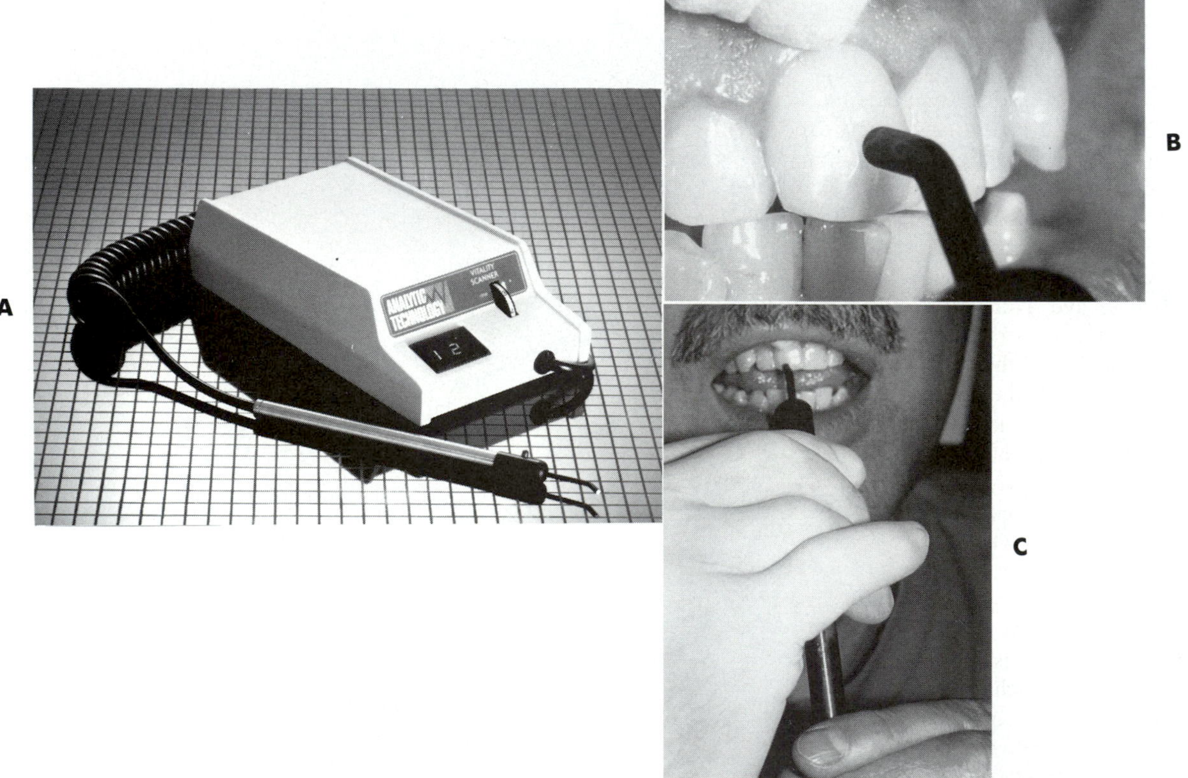

FIG. 1-19 Electric pulp testing. **A,** Analytic Technology pulp tester, a battery-operated instrument of −15 to −300 volts peak and a current from 1050 μamp. Each time the display increases one digit, one burst of 10 pulses of negative polarity is applied to the tooth. When removed and reapplied to the tooth, the tester automatically resets to 0. The newer models include a lip-clip attachment, permitting the clinician to conduct the test with gloves on. **B,** Electrode applied to the dried tooth surface. To ensure good electrical conduction, a generous amount of toothpaste is placed between the electrode and the tooth. **C,** An alternative to using a lip clip is to have the patient gently pinch the metal surface to complete the electrical circuit. As soon as tingling is felt in the tooth, the patient releases the fingers, thereby stopping the electric current.

using other diagnostic tests is essential before arriving at a final diagnosis.

The electric pulp tester (Fig. 1-19) is a valuable tool for diagnosis. Not only does it help the clinician in determining pulp vitality, but with thermal and periodontal tests it can also aid in differentiating among radiographic signs of pulpal, periodontal, or nonodontogenic causes.

The electric pulp test is one of the *last* tests to be performed. The clinician should have a fairly good idea about which tooth is suspect before beginning the electric pulp test. This test merely corroborates what other diagnostic tests have indicated.

Technique

Just as for thermal tests, the teeth must be isolated and dried with 2 × 2 inch gauze and a saliva ejector placed. Furthermore, the patient must be told about the reason for the test and how the test will be performed. One or two teeth on the opposite side of the mouth (preferably the contralateral teeth) should be tested first so that the patient becomes acquainted with the sensation. Testing the opposite side of the mouth also lets the clinician know the patient's normal level of response. The electrode of the pulp tester should be generously coated with a good viscous conductor (e.g., toothpaste). The electrode/conductor is then placed on sound-dried enamel on the middle third of the facial surface.

All restorations should be avoided because they may cause a false reading. Each reading should be recorded in the patient's record. The electrode/conductor can be applied to dried dentin; however, in this situation the clinician should be most careful, and the patient should be cautioned in advance that the sensation may be painful rather than merely warm or tingling, because dentin is an excellent conductor of electricity. The Analytic Technology pulp tester (Fig. 1-19, *A*) and the Neo Sono Pulp Tester are recommended because they *always* start at zero current, do not require manual advancement of any rheostats, and avoid the two problems associated with some other battery-operated pulp testers: an occasional painful electric shock and the inadvertent positioning of the rheostat at a high current when the test is initiated.[5] Patients should be instructed to raise a hand as soon as they begin to feel slight tingling or a sensation of heat. The current flow should be adjusted to increase slowly, because if it increases too quickly the patient may experience pain before he has an opportunity to raise his hand. As with other pulp testers, a complete circuit between the patient and the clinician and tester must be maintained during testing or a false reading may occur. This can be accomplished by either having the patient gently touch the metal stem of the tester and release as soon as sensation is experienced or by attaching a lip clip from the stem to the patient's lip.

Each tooth should be tested two or three times and the readings averaged. The patient's response may vary slightly (which is quite common) or significantly (which suggests a false-positive or false-negative response).

Generally, the thicker the enamel is, the more delayed the response. Accordingly, thin anterior teeth yield a quicker response and broad posterior teeth a slower response because of the greater thickness of enamel and dentin. An additional function of the electric pulp tester is testing vital teeth that have been anesthetized for pulp extirpation. If the vital pulp has been profoundly anesthetized, the electric pulp tester should not be able to stimulate the pulp when maximum current is applied.

Precautions

If the patient's medical history indicates that a cardiac pacemaker has been implanted, the use of an electric pulp tester (as well as electrosurgical units) is contraindicated because of potential interference with the pacemaker.[29]

False reading

The electric pulp tester is usually reliable for indicating pulp vitality; however, there are situations in which a false reading may occur. A *false-positive* reading means the pulp is necrotic but the patient nevertheless signals that he feels sensation. A *false-negative* reading means the pulp is vital but the patient appears unresponsive to electric pulp tests.

Main reasons for a false-positive response

1. Conductor/electrode contact with a larger metal restoration (bridge, Class II restoration) or the gingiva allowing the current to reach the attachment apparatus.
2. Patient anxiety. (Without proper instruction in what to expect, a hyperactive, neurotic, or frightened patient may raise his hand as soon as he thinks the electric pulp tester is turned on or may do so when asked if he "feels anything.")
3. Liquefaction necrosis may conduct current to the attachment apparatus, and therefore the patient may slowly raise his hand near the highest range.
4. Failure to isolate and dry the teeth properly.

Main reasons for a false-negative response

1. Patient heavily premedicated with analgesics, narcotics, alcohol, or tranquilizers.
2. Inadequate contact with the enamel (e.g., insufficient conductor or contact only with a composite restoration).
3. Recently traumatized tooth.
4. Excessive calcification in the canal.
5. Dead batteries or forgetting to turn on the pulp tester.
6. Recently erupted tooth with an immature apex.
7. Partial necrosis. (Although the pulp is still partially vital, electric pulp testing may indicate that it is totally necrotic.)

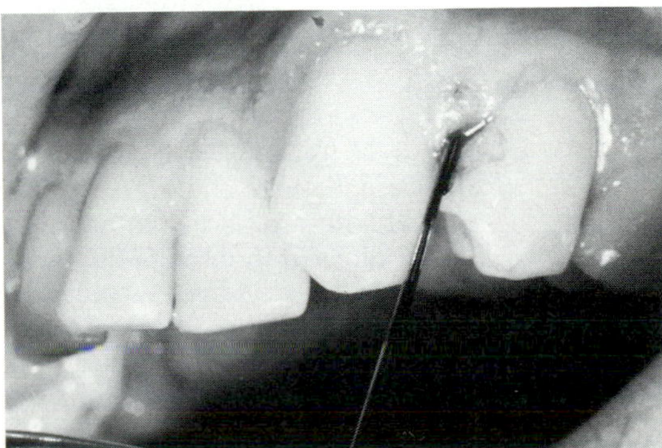

FIG. 1-20 Periodontal examination. A thin calibrated periodontal probe should be used to determine the integrity of the sulcus.

Periodontal Examination

The periodontal probe should be an integral part of all endodontic tray setups. Using a thin, blunt, calibrated periodontal probe, the clinician examines the gingival sulcus and records the depths of all pockets (Fig. 1-20). Multirooted teeth are carefully probed to determine whether there is any furcation involvement. A lateral canal exposed to the oral cavity by periodontal disease may become the portal of entry for toxins that cause pulpal degeneration.

To distinguish lesions of periodontal origin from those of pulpal origin, thermal and electric pulp tests, along with periodontal examination, are essential. For further information regarding the endodontic-periodontal lesion refer to Chapter 17.

Occasionally, for diagnostic or dental-legal reasons, the presence and depth of a periodontal pocket should be confirmed by placing a gutta-percha or silver cone or periodontal probe in the sulcular defect and exposing a radiograph. This type of radiograph can be most effective in assessing periodon-

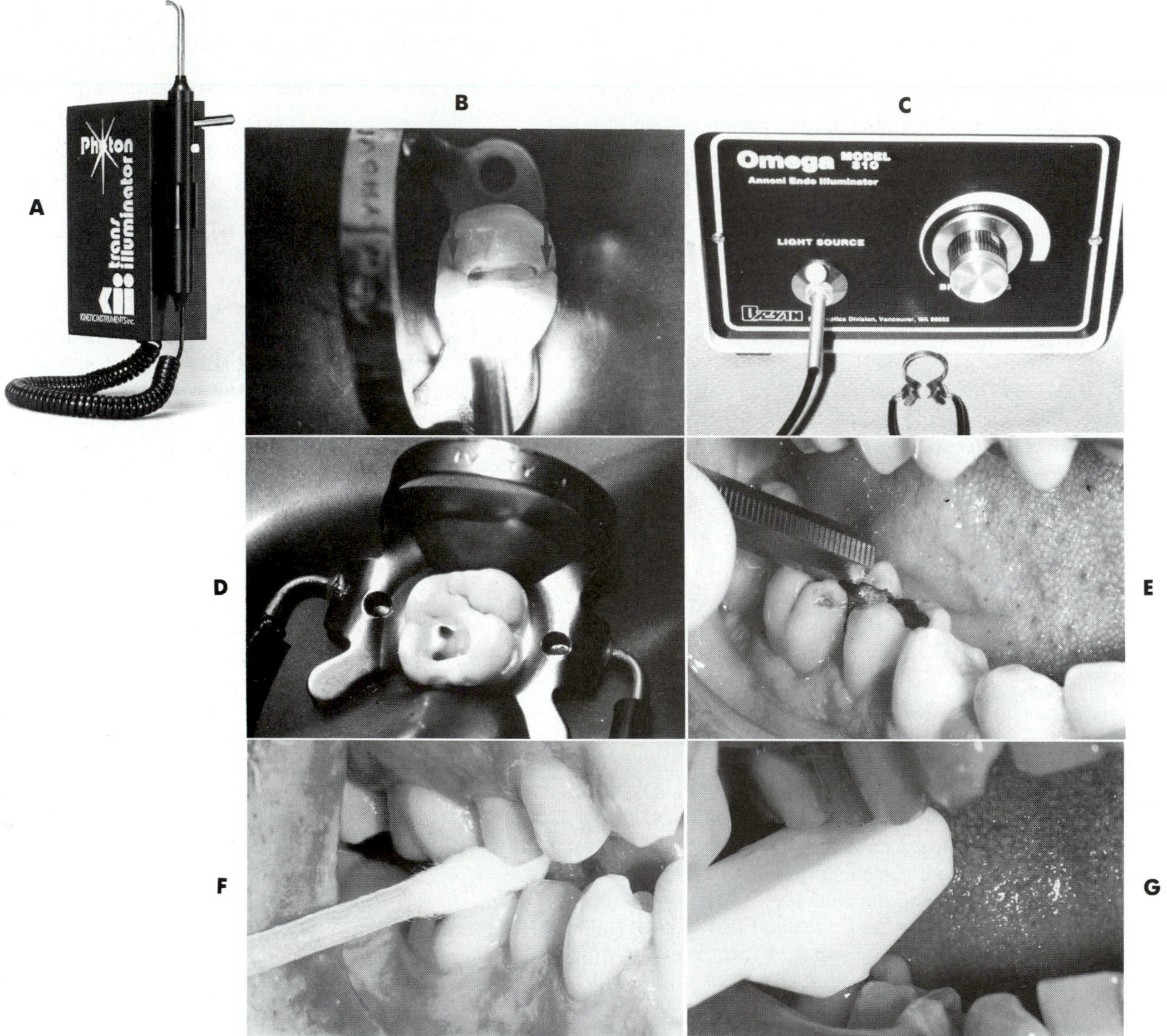

FIG. 1-21 Techniques for detecting vertical crown/root fractures. *Fiberoptic examination.* **A,** Fiberoptic light source. *Transillumination.* **B,** All restorations are removed. The tooth is isolated with a rubber dam and the dentin is dried with cotton pellets. A strong fiberoptic light is directed in through the buccal or lingual wall. A vertical fracture in the dentin may appear as a dark line. **C,** Fiberoptic light sources are available with rubber dam clamp attachments. **D,** When the fiberoptic rubber dam clamp is applied, visualization of vertical fractures (and calcified canal orifices) is enhanced. *Percussion.* **E,** Lateral percussion on individual cusps may provoke a painful response when there is a vertical fracture, whereas vertical percussion may cause no response. **F,** Placing a cotton-wood stock on individual cusps and having the patient masticate may help identify a vertically fractured crown. **G,** The Tooth Slooth, an autoclavable plastic device, can be applied to individual cusps. When biting pressure is applied, a painful response may occur if there is a vertical fracture.

tal repair at a later date or confirming the presence of a vertical root fracture (Fig. 1-21).

Test Cavity

The test cavity involves the slow removal of enamel and dentin to determine pulp vitality. *Without anesthesia* and using a small round bur, the dentist removes dentin as the revolving high-speed bur aims directly at the pulp. If the pulp is vital, the patient will experience a quick sharp pain at or shortly beyond the dentin-enamel junction. This test quickly and accurately determines pulp vitality. However, because it frequently involves drilling a hole through a restoration, the test cavity is employed only when all other means of testing have yielded equivocal results. For example, with patients who have numerous porcelain-fused-to-metal crowns, thermal and electric pulp testing may be inconclusive or ineffective. If percussion, palpation, or radiographic examination suggest one tooth as a suspect, a test cavity to corroborate or negate the results of other tests would certainly be warranted. This test is rarely warranted.

Anesthesia Test

In the uncommon circumstance of diffuse strong pain of vague origin, when all other tests are inconclusive, conduction, selective infiltration, or intraligamentary anesthesia can be employed to help identify the source of the pain. The basis

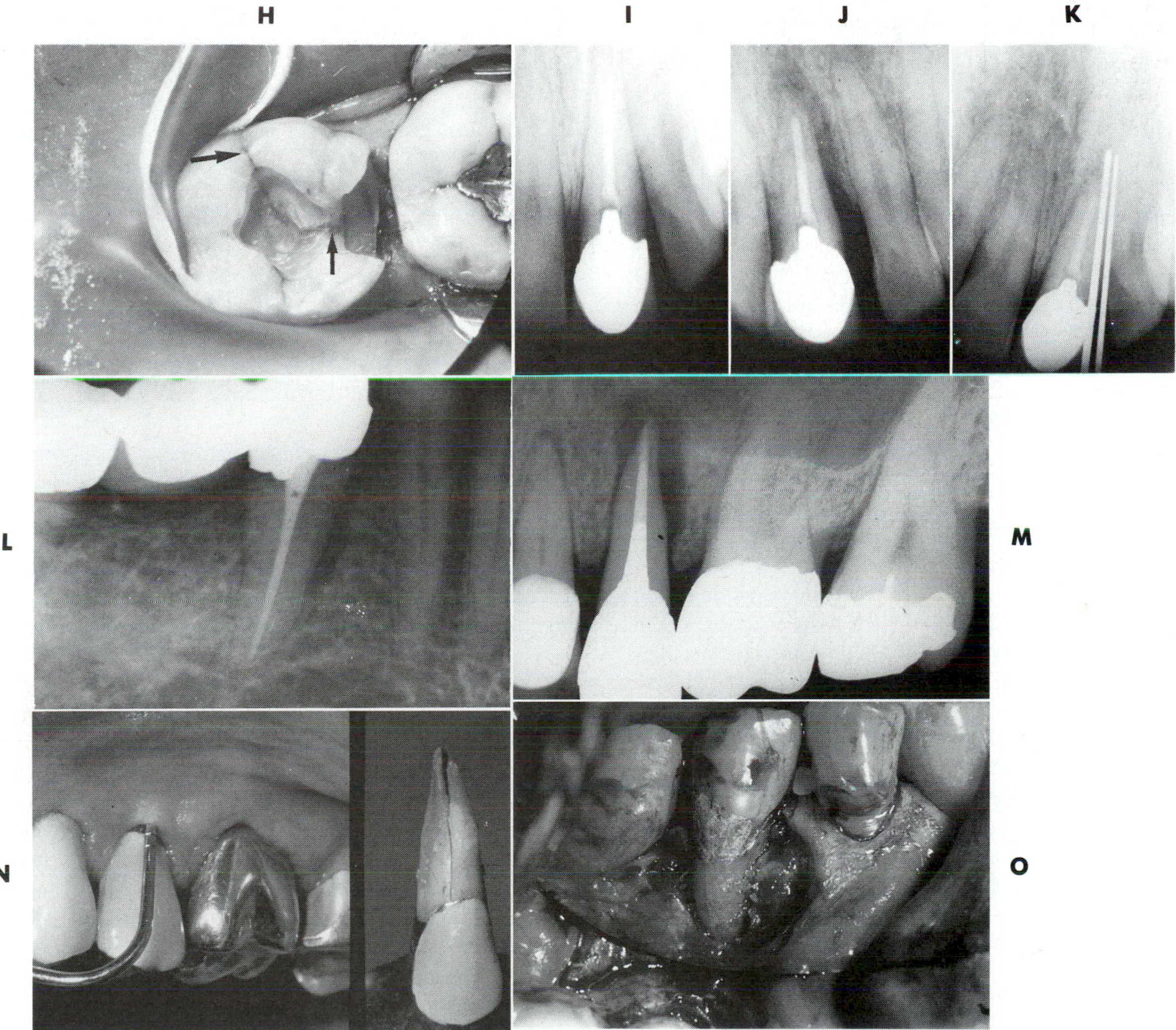

FIG. 1-21, cont'd *Visual inspection.* **H,** After removing restorations, underlying mesial-distal fracture can be seen. **I,** Vertical fracture not evident in an endodontically treated tooth. *Radiography.* **J,** Changing the horizontal angulation reveals a characteristic diffuse demineralized halo around the root. **K,** Diagnostic silver cones trace the periodontal defect to the apex. **L,** A narrow—sometimes teardrop-shaped—radiolucency, as seen on the mesial side of this premolar abutment, is commonly associated with incomplete vertical root fractures. **M,** This patient complained of tenderness to palpation, lateral percussion (horizontal percussion) and pain when chewing. **N,** A deep facial pocket confirmed the suspicion of vertical root fracture. When the tooth was removed, the fracture was evident. **O,** A sinus tract draining through the gingival sulcus and a deep pocket on the facial surface caused suspicion of a vertical root fracture. A full-thickness flap confirmed the diagnosis.

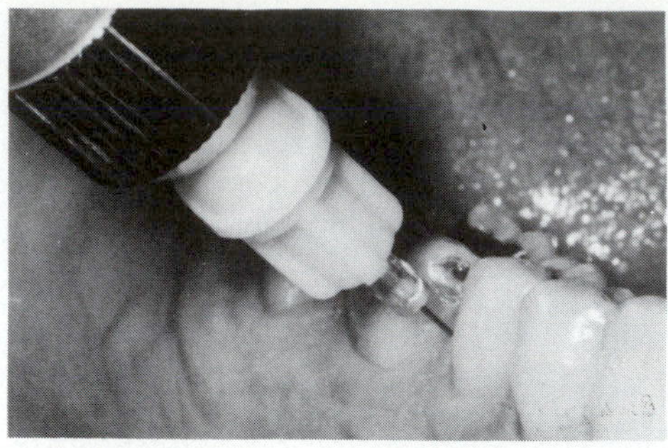

FIG. 1-22 Intraligamentary anesthesia for differential diagnosis. Administering 0.2 ml of local anesthetic (Ligmaject or Peripress) in the distal sulcus stops all pain immediately if the anesthetized tooth is the source of the pain. An ultrashort 30-gauge needle is placed into the sulcus at a 30-degree angle from perpendicular, with the bevel facing away from the tooth.

for this test lies in the fact that pulpal pain, even when referred, is almost invariably unilateral and stems from only one of the two branches of the trigeminal nerve supplying sensory innervation to the jaws.

For example, a patient complains of pain over the entire side of the face and no pathologic changes are evident on the radiographs. If inferior alveolar block anesthesia is employed and the pain completely subsides within 2 to 3 minutes, it can be surmised that a mandibular tooth is the source of the pain. Otherwise, subperiosteal infiltration of the maxillary teeth, starting with the most distal, should be used. After each subperiosteal infiltration (0.25 ml) the clinician should wait 3 minutes. The pain will cease completely with the onset of anesthesia around the source of the pain.

The most effective technique is intraligamentary injection administered in the distal sulcus of each suspect tooth. When the offending tooth is anesthetized by the intraligamentary injection technique, the pain stops immediately (Fig. 1-22),[14,16] for a few minutes.

On the rare occasion when pain still does not subside and the anesthetic has been correctly administered, the clinician must consider other possibilities. For example, pain from mandibular molars is often referred to the preauricular area. If this is truly the case, mandibular block anesthesia quickly stops the pain. If the pain remains, the differential diagnosis should include organic disease of nonodontogenic origin,[4] as described in Chapter 3.

Techniques for Detecting Vertical Crown/Root Fractures

In vital teeth the most common reason for a vertical crown/root fracture is trauma. In nonvital teeth, trauma may also be a contributory factor (if the tooth does not have metal crown protection), but endodontic treatment followed by overzealous post reinforcement[16,28] or a restoration tapped too firmly into place is a common cause.[22,26] There are several ways to determine the presence of a vertical crown or root fracture.

Thorough dental history. If the patient continuously complains of pain with chewing (after frequent occlusal adjustments) or pain with horizontal tapping of the crown, the clinician should suspect a vertical fracture. These symptoms can develop any time—before, during, or after endodontic treatment. A periapical lesion that fails to resolve after a good root canal filling and repeated unsuccessful attempts at apical surgery suggests, as part of the differential diagnosis, a split root. A patient may have a hypersensitive response to thermal change in an otherwise perfectly sound tooth, may recall sudden pain after biting into an unexpected pit or bone, or may present with advanced symptoms of bruxism or clenching. Patients also may report that a restoration continues to fall out after several attempts at replacement or several recementations; before further restorative attempts are made, the remaining tooth should be carefully examined for fracture.

Persistent periodontal defect. Vertical crown/root fracture is suggested when conventional periodontal treatment does not resolve a sulcus defect.[11,17] When an isolated sulcus defect continues to expand, regardless of all treatment attempts, and subsequent bacterial invasion hastens the periodontal breakdown around only one tooth while the other teeth appear periodontally sound, a possible vertical crown/root fracture is implied. Reflecting a full-thickness mucoperiosteal flap with the aid of a strong fiberoptic light may reveal the fine vertical fracture line (Fig. 1-21, *N*).

Fiberoptic examination. As shown in Fig. 1-21, *A* to *D*, pointing a fiberoptic light horizontally at the level of the gingival sulcus in a dimly lit room may reveal a dark, continuous line (in posterior teeth, usually oriented mesiodistally[17]) in an otherwise well-illuminated pulpal floor. This should certainly be considered as a possible vertical fracture. The most reliable results are obtained if preexisting restorations are removed from the tooth before the fiberoptic examination, as shown in Fig. 1-21, *B*.

Wedging and staining. Cracks in teeth can also be discovered by a wedging and staining procedure (Fig. 1-21, *F* and *G*). Wedging force can be used to separate the two halves of the fracture. Whether the fractured tooth is vital or nonvital, there may be pain during mastication. This pain cannot always be detected with vertical percussion; however, having the patient bite on a cotton-wood stick may reveal the split tooth.

If gently and slowly chewing on a cotton roll or a cotton-wood stick still yields inconclusive results, the Tooth Slooth can be applied to the occlusal surfaces of various cusps and the biting/chewing test can be gently repeated. At times this test more readily identifies the split tooth (Fig. 1-21, *G*).

The vertical fracture line can sometimes be more easily identified with food coloring placed on the dried occlusal surface moments before the wedge test. The dye solution stains the fracture line. Immediately after the wedge test, the occlusal surface is cleaned with a cotton pellet lightly moistened with 70% isopropyl alcohol. The alcohol washes away the food coloring on the surface, but the food coloring within the fracture line remains and becomes apparent (Fig. 1-21, *H*).

Radiography. Figure 1-21, *I*, shows a tooth with a vertical fracture that is not apparent. Fig. 1-21, *J*, shows the same tooth at a different horizontal angle. The radiolucent halo is visible from the sulcus to the apex. Fig. 1-21, *K*, shows the periodontal examination, with diagnostic silver cones extending on the labial and palatal aspects from the sulcus to the apex. When the clinician sees a diffuse radiolucent halo around the root, with diagnostic probes extending from the sulcus to the apex, there is a strong probability of a vertical fracture.

For purposes of diagnosing vertical crown/root fractures, no one of the foregoing signs or symptoms may be conclusive; but taking them *in combination* may provide the clinician with the confirmed diagnosis of a vertical crown/root fracture.

Even today the treatment of choice for a vertical fracture in a single-rooted tooth, or a mesial-distal fracture in a multi-rooted mandibular tooth, is still extraction. For some multi-rooted teeth, crown/root amputation may successfully resolve the fracture problem by removing the most mobile segment. The needs of the patient are best served when a crown/root fracture is diagnosed at the outset. Both the clinician and the patient are disappointed when crown/root fracture is seen only after the tooth has been extracted.

Probable Causes

Until the probable cause(s) for pulpal or periapical disease can be ascertained, the signs or symptoms that appear to indicate a dental problem should not be treated. Every dental pathologic entity should have an identifiable cause (e.g., bacterial, chemical, physical, iatrogenic, or systemic). The prudent practitioner should be extremely wary and cautious about treating any ostensible odontogenic problem until the probable cause can be determined. An error in diagnosis may lead to an error in treatment. If cause and effect are unclear, the clinician serves the patient best by referring the case for further consultation with a specialist.

CLINICAL CLASSIFICATION

A clinical classification of pulpal and periapical disease cannot list every possible variation of inflammation, ulceration, proliferation, calcification, or degeneration of the pulp and the attachment apparatus and still remain practical. Besides, this is probably unnecessary, because a clinical classification is meant to provide only a general descriptive phrase that implies the furthest extent of pulpal or periapical disease. The terms used in a clinical classification suggest the signs and symptoms of the disease process. The primary purpose of a clinical classification is to provide terms and phrases that can be used as a means of communication within the dental profession.

In the final analysis, the pulp is either healthy or not and must either be removed or not. The extent of the disease process may affect the method of treatment, from merely a palliative sedative to final pulpectomy. What follows is a series of terms that encompass the clinical signs and symptoms of the various degrees of inflammation and degeneration of the pulp or the nature, duration, and type of exudation associated with periapical inflammation. No attempt is made to associate these terms with histopathologic findings; current knowledge does not allow this to be done accurately.[23,25]

Normal

A normal tooth is asymptomatic and exhibits a mild to moderate transient response to thermal and electric pulpal stimuli; the response subsides almost immediately when such stimuli are removed. The tooth and its attachment apparatus do not cause a painful response when percussed or palpated. Radiographs usually reveal a clearly delineated canal that tapers toward the apex; there is no evidence of canal calcification or root resorption, and the lamina dura is intact.

Reversible Pulpitis

The pulp is inflamed to the extent that thermal stimuli cause a quick, sharp, hypersensitive response that subsides as soon as the stimulus is removed; otherwise the tooth is asymptomatic. Any irritant that can affect the pulp may cause reversible pulpitis (e.g., caries, deep periodontal scaling and root planing, an unbased restoration).

Reversible pulpitis is *not* a disease but merely a symptom. If the cause can be removed, the pulp should revert to an uninflamed state and the symptoms should subside. Conversely, if the cause remains, the symptoms may persist indefinitely or the inflammation may become more widespread, eventually leading to an irreversible pulpitis. A reversible pulpitis can be clinically distinguished from a symptomatic irreversible pulpitis by two methods:

1. With a reversible pulpitis there is a sharp, painful response to thermal stimulation that subsides almost immediately after the stimulus is removed. With an irreversible pulpitis there is a sharp painful response to thermal stimuli, but the pain lingers after the stimulus is removed.
2. With a reversible pulpitis there is no spontaneous pain as there often is with a symptomatic irreversible pulpitis. Most commonly, the clinician can readily diagnose a reversible pulpitis while gathering the patient's dental history (e.g., the patient may report pain when cold liquids come in contact with the tooth or when breathing through the mouth after a recent restoration or prophylaxis and scaling). Nevertheless, the diagnosis should be confirmed by thermal tests to identify the tooth or teeth involved.

Treatment consists of placing a sedative dressing or packing containing zinc oxide and eugenol in or around the tooth. If the pulp can be protected from further thermal shock, it may revert to an uninflamed state. For example, removing all caries or a recent deep amalgam and placing a temporary restoration (e.g., Intermediate Restorative Material) in the cavity for several weeks should provide almost immediate relief. After several weeks the sedative dressing can be replaced with a well-based permanent restoration.

Irreversible Pulpitis

An irreversible pulpitis may be acute, subacute, or chronic; it may be partial or total. The pulp may be infected or sterile. Clinically the acutely inflamed pulp is thought to be symptomatic, the chronically inflamed pulp asymptomatic. These thoughts are often inconsistent with histologic observations (Chapter 12). Clinically the extent of pulp inflammation, partial or total, cannot be determined. Based on present knowledge, irreversible pulpitis in any of its many forms requires endodontic therapy.

Dynamic changes in the pulp are always occurring; the change from quiescent chronicity to symptomatic acuteness may develop over a period of years or in a matter of hours. With pulp inflammation there is an exudate. If the exudate can be vented to relieve the pain that accompanies edema, the tooth may remain quiescent. Conversely, if the exudate that is being continuously formed remains within the hard confines of the root canal, pain will probably occur.

Symptomatic irreversible pulpitis

One type of irreversible pulpitis is characterized by spontaneous intermittent or continuous paroxysms of pain.

"Spontaneous" in this context means that no stimulus is evident. Sudden temperature changes induce prolonged episodes of pain. There may be a prolonged (i.e., remaining after the stimulus is removed) painful response to cold that can be relieved by heat. There may also be a prolonged painful response to heat that can be relieved by cold. There may even be a prolonged painful response to both heat and cold stimulation.

Continuous spontaneous pain may be excited merely by a change in posture (e.g., when the patient lies down or bends over). Commonly, patients recognize this empirically and may spend the night sleeping fitfully in an upright position.

Pain from symptomatic irreversible pulpitis tends to be moderate to severe, depending on the severity of inflammation. It may be sharp or dull, localized or referred (e.g., referred from mandibular molars toward the ear or up to the temporal area), intermittent or constant.

Radiographs alone are of little assistance in diagnosing a symptomatic irreversible pulpitis. They are helpful in detecting suspect teeth (i.e., those with deep caries or extensive restorations). In the advanced stages of an irreversible pulpitis the inflammatory process may lead to development of a slight thickening in the periodontal ligament.

A symptomatic irreversible pulpitis can be diagnosed by a thorough dental history, visual examination, radiographs, and thermal tests. The electric pulp test is of questionable value in accurately diagnosing the disease. An untreated symptomatic irreversible pulpitis may persist or abate if a vent is established for the inflammatory exudate (e.g., the removal of food packed into a deep carious pulp exposure to provide a vent for the inflammatory exudate). The inflammation of an irreversible pulpitis may become so severe as to cause ultimate necrosis. In the transition from pulpitis to necrosis the typical symptoms of irreversible pulpitis are altered according to the extent of the necrosis.

Asymptomatic irreversible pulpitis

Another type of irreversible pulpitis is asymptomatic because the inflammatory exudates are quickly vented. An asymptomatic irreversible pulpitis may develop by the conversion of a symptomatic irreversible pulpitis into a quiescent state, or it may develop initially from a low-grade pulp irritant. It is easily identified by a thorough dental history along with radiographic and visual examination.

An asymptomatic irreversible pulpitis may develop from any type of injury, but it is usually caused by a large carious exposure or by previous traumatic injury that resulted in a painless pulp exposure of long duration.

Hyperplastic pulpitis. One type of asymptomatic irreversible pulpitis is a reddish cauliflower-like overgrowth of pulp tissue through and around a carious exposure. The proliferative nature of this type of pulp is attributed to a low-grade chronic irritation and to the generous vascularity of the pulp that is characteristically found in young people. Occasionally there is some mild, transient pain during mastication. If the apices are mature, complete endodontic therapy should be provided.

Internal resorption. Another type of asymptomatic irreversible pulpitis is internal resorption. This is characterized by the presence of chronic inflammatory cells in granulation tissue and is asymptomatic (before it perforates the root). See Chapter 16 for a complete description of the various types of resorption: their causes, diagnoses, and treatments.

Internal resorption is most commonly diagnosed by radiographs showing internal expansion of the pulp with evident dentinal destruction. In advanced cases of internal resorption in the crown, a pink spot may be seen through the enamel.

The treatment of internal resorption is immediate endodontic therapy; to postpone treatment may lead to an untreatable perforation of the root, resulting in possible loss of the tooth.

Canal calcification. The physical adversity of restorative procedures, periodontal therapy, attrition, abrasion, trauma, and probably some additional idiopathic factors can cause an otherwise normal pulp to metamorphose into an irreversible pulpitis, manifested by deposition of abnormally large amounts of reparative dentin throughout the canal system.[21] The condition is usually first recognized radiographically. Discrete areas of localized pulp necrosis resulting from small infarctions (e.g., caused by deep scaling that interrupts the blood supply into a lateral canal) often initiate localized calcification as a defense reaction. This abnormal calcification occurs in and around pulp vascular channels. The teeth are asymptomatic but may show a slight change in crown color. Several distinct types of calcification (denticles, pulp stones), initiated by a multitude of factors, can occur within the pulp (Chapter 10).

• • •

Irreversible pulpitis may persist for an extended time, but it is common for the inflamed pulp to succumb eventually to the pressures of inflammation and ultimately undergo necrosis.

Necrosis

Necrosis, death of the pulp, may result from an untreated irreversible pulpitis or may occur immediately after a traumatic injury that disrupts the blood supply to the pulp. Whether the necrotic remnants of the pulp are liquefied or coagulated, the pulp is still quite dead. Regardless of the type of necrosis, the endodontic treatment is the same. Within hours an inflamed pulp may degenerate to a necrotic state.

Pulp necrosis can be partial or total. The partial type may exhibit some of the symptoms of an irreversible pulpitis. Total necrosis, before it clinically affects the periodontal ligament, is usually asymptomatic. There is no response to thermal or electric tests. Occasionally with anterior teeth the crown will darken.

Untreated necrosis may spread beyond the apical foramen, causing inflammation of the periodontal ligament; this results in thickening of the periodontal ligament, which may be quite sensitive to percussion.

When there is more than one canal, the diagnostic skill of the clinician is tested. For example, in a molar with three canals the pulp tissue in one canal may be intact and uninflamed, that in the next canal acutely inflamed, and that in the third canal completely necrotic. This accounts for the occasional tooth that causes the patient to respond with confusing inconsistencies to vitality testing.

A natural dichotomy between health and disease does not exist—at least not as far as the pulp is concerned. Pulp tissues may show all degrees of the spectrum from health to inflammation to necrosis. Clinically we can distinguish reversible and irreversible pulpitis from necrosis. A clinically necrotic tooth may still have vascularity in the apical third of the canal, but this can be confirmed only during chemomechanical debridement. When the pulp dies, if the tooth remains untreated, the bacteria, toxins, and protein breakdown products of the pulp may extend beyond the apical foramen and involve the periapical region, thus causing periapical disease.

Periapical Disease

Acute apical periodontitis

Acute apical periodonitis describes inflammation around the apex. The cause may be an extension of pulpal disease into the periapical tissue. It may also be an endodontic procedure that has inadvertently extended beyond the apical foramen. A more chronic variant of this can even be associated with a normal vital pulp in a tooth that has suffered occlusal trauma from a high restoration or from chronic bruxism.

The clinician must therefore recognize that an acute apical periodontitis may be found around vital as well as nonvital teeth. For this reason *thermal and electric testing must be done before treatment is initiated.* Radiographically the apical periodontal ligament may appear normal or perhaps slightly widened, but the tooth is exquisitely tender to percussion. There may even be slight tenderness to palpation. Untreated, the localized acute apical periodontitis may continue to spread, additional symptoms may appear, and an acute apical abscess may develop.

If the pulp is necrotic, endodontic therapy should be started immediately. However, if the pulp is vital, removing the cause (e.g., adjusting the occlusion) should permit quick, uneventful repair.

Acute apical abscess

Acute apical abscess implies a painful, purulent exudate around the apex. Though acute apical abscess is one of the most serious dental diseases, radiographically the tooth may appear perfectly normal or perhaps show only a slightly widened periodontal ligament. Radiographically the periapical tissue may appear normal because fulminating infections may not have had time to erode enough cortical bone to cause a radiolucency. The cause is an advanced stage of acute apical periodontitis from a necrotic tooth, resulting in extensive acute suppurative inflammation.

The acute apical abscess is easily diagnosed by its clinical signs and symptoms: rapid onset of slight to severe swelling, slight to severe pain, pain to percussion and palpation, and possible tooth mobility. In more severe cases the patient is febrile.

The extent and distribution of the swelling are determined by the location of the apex, the location of the adjacent muscle attachments, and the thickness of the cortical plate.

The acute apical abscess is readily distinguishable from the lateral periodontal abscess and from the phoenix abscess.

1. With the lateral periodontal abscess there may be swelling and pain, and radiographically the tooth may appear relatively normal; however, thermal and electric pulp testing indicate that the pulp is vital. Furthermore, there is almost always a periodontal pocket, which upon probing may begin to exude a purulent exudate.
2. With the phoenix abscess there is an apical radiolucency around the apex of the tooth. All other signs and symptoms are identical to those of the acute apical abscess.

Chronic apical periodontitis

Chronic apical periodontitis implies long-standing asymptomatic inflammation around the apex. Although chronic apical periodontitis tends to be asymptomatic, there may be occasional slight tenderness to palpation and percussion. Only biopsy and microscopic examination can reveal whether these apical lesions are dental granulomas, abscesses, or cysts. The dynamic equilibrium standoff between the host's defense mechanisms and the infection oozing out of the canal is manifested by a periapical radiolucency. Of course, this is a matter of radiographic interpretation; what may appear as a widened periodontal ligament to one clinician may appear as a small radiolucency to another.

Because a totally necrotic pulp provides a safe harbor for microorganisms and their noxious allies (no vascularity means no defense cells), only complete endodontic treatment will permit these lesions to be repaired.

Diagnosis is confirmed by the general absence of symptoms, the presence of a radiolucency, and the absence of pulp vitality. Radiographically the lesions may appear large or small, and they may be either diffuse or well-circumscribed.

The additional presence of a sinus tract indicates the production of frank pus. Symptoms are generally absent because the pus drains through the sinus tract as quickly as it is produced. Occasionally patients become aware of a "gum boil."

Periapical dynamic changes are constant. Spontaneously, pus production may cease for a while and the sinus tract may close. After the necrotic contents of a canal are removed during endodontic treatment, the sinus tract closes permanently.

Phoenix abscess

A phoenix abscess is a chronic apical periodontitis that suddenly becomes symptomatic. The symptoms are identical to those of an acute apical abscess, the main difference being that the phoenix abscess is preceded by a chronic condition. Consequently, there is a definite radiolucency accompanied by symptoms of an acute apical abscess.

A phoenix abscess may develop spontaneously, almost immediately after endodontic treatment has been initiated on a tooth diagnosed as having chronic apical periodontitis without a sinus tract. Initiating endodontic treatment may alter the dynamic equilibrium of a chronic apical periodontitis by the inadvertent forcing of microorganisms or other irritants into the periapical tissue and cause a flare-up of pain and swelling.

Periapical osteosclerosis

Periapical osteosclerosis is excessive bone mineralization around the apex. Low-grade, relatively asymptomatic, chronic pulpal inflammation occasionally causes a host response of excessive bone mineralization around the apex. This is most commonly found in young people. Endodontic treatment may convert the periapical radiopacity to a normal trabecular pattern.[12] Conversely, unusual excessive periapical remineralization after endodontic therapy may result in osteosclerosis (Fig. 1-9, *B*). Because this condition is asymptomatic and appears to be self-limiting, the appropriateness of endodontic treatment is arguable.

REFERENCES

1. Andreasen JO: Traumatic injuries of the teeth, ed 2, Philadelphia, 1981, WB Saunders Co.
2. Bavitz JB, Patterson DW, and Sorenson S: Non-Hodgkin's lymphoma disguised as odontogenic pain, J Am Dent Assoc 123:99, 1992.
3. Chambers IG: The role and methods of pulp testing: a review, Int Endod J 15:10, 1982.
4. Cohen S et al: Oral prodromal signs of a central nervous system malignant neoplasm—glioblastoma multiforme: report of a case, J Am Dent Assoc 112:643, 1986.
5. Cooley RL and Lubow RM: Evaluation of a digital pulp tester, J Oral Maxillofac Surg 58:437, 1984.
6. Del Rio C: Endodontic clinical diagnosis, Part 1, Compend Contin Educ 8:56, 1992.
7. Del Rio C: Endodontic clinical diagnosis, Part 2, Compend Contin Educ 8:138, 1992.
8. Eversole LR: Clinical outline of oral pathology: diagnosis and treatment, Philadelphia, 1978, Lea & Febiger.
9. Goldman M, Pearson A, and Darzenta N: Endodontic success—who's reading the radiograph? Oral Surg 33:432, 1972.

10. Goldman M, Pearson A, and Darzenta N: Reliability of radiographic interpretations, Oral Surg 32:287, 1974.
11. Goldstein AR: Periodontal defects associated with root fracture, J Am Dent Assoc 102:863, 1981.
12. Grossman LI, Oliet S, and Del Rio C: Endodontic practice, ed 11, Philadelphia, 1988, Lea & Febiger.
13. Kaufman AY: An enigmatic sinus tract origin, Endodont Dent Trauma 5:159, 1989.
14. Littner MM, Tamse A, and Kaffe I: A new technique of selective anesthesia for diagnosing acute pulpitis in the mandible, J Endod 9:116, 1983.
14a. Lipton, JA, Ship JA, and Larach-Robinson: Estimated prevalence and distribution of reported orofacial pain in the United States, J Am Dent Assoc, 124:115, 1993.
15. Lommel JJ et al: Alveolar bone loss associated with vertical root fractures: reports of 6 cases, Oral Surg 45:909, 1978.
16. Meister F Jr, Lommel JJ, and Gerstein H: Diagnosis and possible causes of vertical root fractures, Oral Surg 49:243, 1980.
17. Polson AM: Periodontal destruction associated with vertical root fracture, J Periodontol 48:27, 1977.
18. Rose LF and Kaye D: Internal medicine for dentistry, ed 2, St Louis, 1990, Mosby–Year Book.
19. Schultz J and Gluskin AH: Rethinking clinical endodontic diagnosis, J Calif Dent Assoc 19:15, 1991.
20. Schwartz S and Cohen S: The difficult differential diagnosis, Dent Clin North Am 36:279, 1992.
21. Schwartz S and Foster J: Roentgenographic interpretation of experimentally produced bony lesions, Oral Surg 32:606, 1971.
22. Schweitzer JL, Gutmann JL, and Bliss RQ: Odontiatrogenic tooth fracture, Inter Endod J 22:64, 1989.
23. Seltzer S and Bender IB: The dental pulp: biologic considerations in dental procedures, ed 3, Philadelphia, 1984, JB Lippincott Co.
24. Slowey RI: Radiographic aids in the detection of extra root canals, Oral Surg 37:762, 1974.
25. Smulson MH: Classification and diagnosis of pulp pathosis, Dent Clin North Am 28:699, 1984.
26. Stewart GG: The detection and treatment of vertical root fractures, J Endod 14:47, 1988.
27. Trowbridge HO: Changing concepts in endodontic therapy, J Am Dent Assoc 110:479, 1985.
28. Wechsler SM et al: Iatrogenic root fractures: a case report, J Endod 4:251, 1978.
29. Woodley L, Woodworth J, and Dobbs JL: A preliminary evaluation of the effects of electric pulp testers on dogs with artificial pacemakers, J Am Dent Assoc 89:1099, 1974.
30. Zakariasen KL and Walton RE: Complications in endodontic therapy for the geriatric patient, Gerodontics 1:34, 1985.

Self-assessment questions

1. A cold test best localizes
   a. pain of pulpal origin.
   b. periodontal pain.
   c. pulp necrosis.
   d. referred pain.
2. Anesthetic testing is most effective in localizing pain
   a. to a specific tooth.
   b. to the mandible or maxilla.
   c. across the midline of the face.
   d. to a posterior tooth.
3. Dental history taking
   a. is less important than x-ray examination.
   b. has as its principal goal to identify the offending tooth.
   c. principally assesses intensity of pain.
   d. focuses heavily on the quality of pain.
4. Percussion testing
   a. differentiates pain of periodontal origin.
   b. stimulates proprioceptive fibers in the periodontal ligament.
   c. indicates tooth fracture.
   d. must be performed with a blunt instrument.
5. Areas of rarefaction are evident on x-ray examination when
   a. the tooth is responsive to cold.
   b. the tooth is responsive to heat.
   c. a tooth fracture has been identified.
   d. the cortical layer of bone has been eroded.
6. An area of rarefaction in the lower premolar area indicates
   a. definite pathology.
   b. torus mandibularis.
   c. possible mental foramen.
   d. root fracture.
7. Percussion, palpation, and thermal testing
   a. are not to be performed on patients with pacemakers.
   b. should involve testing of contralateral teeth for comparison.
   c. are best compared when using ipsilateral teeth.
   d. obviate radiographs.
8. Irreversible pulpitis is often defined by
   a. a moderate response to percussion.
   b. a strong painful response to cold that lingers.
   c. a strong painful response to cold.
   d. a response to heat.
9. Medical history of heart disease is significant
   a. and contraindicates endodontic treatment.
   b. for referred pain to the left mandible indicating possible myocardial infarction.
   c. and indicates the need for premedication with antibiotics.
   d. and contraindicates local anesthetic with epinephrine.
10. The best approach for diagnosis of odontogenic pain is
    a. x-ray examination.
    b. percussion.
    c. visual examination.
    d. a step-by-step sequenced examination and testing approach following the same procedure.
11. Calcification of the pulp
    a. is a response to aging.
    b. does not relate to the periodontal condition.
    c. precedes internal resorption.
    d. indicates the presence of additional canals.
12. Electric pulp tests should not be performed on patients who have a
    a. hearing aid.
    b. hip implant.
    c. dental implant.
    d. pacemaker.
13. A false-negative response to the pulp tester may occur
    a. primarily in anterior teeth.
    b. in a patient heavily premedicated with analgesics, narcotics, alcohol, or tranquilizers.
    c. most often in teenagers.
    d. in the presence of periodontal disease.
14. A test cavity
    a. is the first test in diagnostic sequence.
    b. often results in a dull pain response.
    c. is employed only when all other test findings are equivocal.
    d. should be performed with local anesthetic.

Chapter 2

Orofacial Dental Pain Emergencies: Endodontic Diagnosis and Management

Alan H. Gluskin
William W. Y. Goon

This Is Going to Hurt Just a Bit

One thing I like less than most things is sitting in a dentist chair with my mouth wide open,

And that I will never have to do it again is a hope that I am against hope hopin'.

Because some tortures are physical and some are mental, but the one that is both is dental.[64]

More than a half century after the American poet Ogden Nash felt compelled to aim his satire at the dental profession, today's clinician is still challenged, in the last decade of the twentieth century, to prove how far the practice of dentistry has come in its desire to provide painless and efficient care. No area of dental practice is more susceptible to the charge of inadequacy than the emergency visit for acute orofacial pain.

PATIENT-DOCTOR DYNAMICS

The complex interplay between the patient and doctor has an important effect upon the acute pain emergency. Three basic components of this psychodynamic interaction are meaningful here:

1. The *patient's perspective* of pain based on a multicomponent model
2. The *professional's perception* of the patient in pain
3. The *doctor's decision to treat or refer* the patient in pain.

The patient presents complaints as a series of descriptions and behavioral patterns. The doctor must then understand and interpret this information. This dialogue is often inadequate to manage the patient, even if the source of the problem is identified. To aid in patient management, pain behavior should be viewed from the following perspectives.

Patient Perspectives of Pain

At the most simple and basic level, the patient who seeks care for a "toothache" may be suffering pain from pulpal and periapical tissue inflammation. Other causes, however—referred pain, more complex facial pain, temporomandibular joint (TMJ) pain, nonodontogenic pain in the head and neck—demonstrate that the complaint of toothache is insufficient to diagnose and treat these entities.

When describing their pain, patients offer a descriptive history of their problem and an interpretive narration, both subjective. The dentist must recognize these personal interpretations and distill from them clinically objective terms such as *acute* ("It came outta nowhere") or *chronic* ("I knew it would lead to this"). The patient's actual reaction to the pain can be expressed as body language (e.g., not chewing on one side) and provides valuable behavioral insights, along with the doctor's visual assessment for facial asymmetry, altered constitutional signs (swelling, flushing, pallor), and dysfunctional reflexes or posturing (avoiding trigger zones, massaging the face).

When the clinician needs to determine a cause for the pain, there are a multitude of patient presentations that can occur in the interaction with the dentist. That individuals respond to pain in many different ways is a common and dramatic clinical observation. Patients may show very little evidence of clinical disease but seemingly suffer intolerable and incapacitating pain. Others with serious disease may continue to function at a very high level and think themselves not ill or at risk.[73]

Current models view pain as a complex experience. Pain, by its very nature, is no longer viewed as a single entity; rather, it comprises many overlapping components. "An unpleasant sensory and emotional experience associated with actual or potential tissue damage" defines the physiologic and the psychological components.[55]

The Multicomponent Model of Pain

The pain process involves pain reception (nociception) and its recognition, an emotional-affective component, a cognitive component, and a behavioral component.[73] In recent years, the literature and research have emphasized the importance of the psychological components of orofacial pain.[26,28,36] Today, accommodating the multidimensional components of pain is crucial in diagnosis and treatment of pain entities. To perform triage for urgent care, this distinction is pivotal.

The receptor system recognizes painful stimuli above a threshold by providing afferent information to the perceptual sensory system. The patient's reaction to the experience, in terms of suffering and anxiety, involves the emotional-affective component. Emotional factors such as anxiety can lower the pain threshold and heighten the patient's reaction to pain.

What individuals think about their pain involves the cognitive process. Cognition is implicated in virtually every aspect of the pain experience.[73] What patients understand about their pain is important in modulating how they react to it and this understanding facilitates pain management. Patients, when told that their palatal swelling is from a pulpal disorder and is not life threatening, will react differently to their condition than uninformed patients.

Orofacial pain can generate unreasonable anxiety in a fearful patient. Speaking to the patient in a calm, knowledgeable manner, in words the patient can readily understand, significantly enhances patient management. Providing information about typical procedures and sensations—sights, sounds, smells, vibrations, and other physical stimuli—is an invaluable management tool[41] that removes much of patients' uncertainty about the planned treatment.

How patients perceive their control over pain is another important cognition. Increased tolerance for potentially painful procedures is often seen when the dentist affords the patient a way to stop the operation. Patients who have more control over what happens to them feel more comfortable and show higher tolerance for procedures.[21]

Patients' experience with successful or unsuccessful treatments invariably influences their behavior. Reassurance that the dentist can treat and eliminate acute dental pain efficiently helps to modulate anxiety and fear-related behavior. Personality and cultural factors are additional learned behaviors that can modify a patient's responses to pain and they should be considered in pain management.

The Professional's Perception of the Patient in Pain

In an acute pain emergency the physical problem, as well as the emotional state of the patient, should be considered. The doctor's reactions to the patient is important for both pain and patient management. The patients' needs, their fears about the immediate problem, and their defenses for coping with the situation must be understood. Proper handling of the patient needs to address the psychodynamic interaction between the dentist and patient. This psychodynamic exchange involves five key aspects, elucidated by a number of authors[41,72,73]:

1. The patient is to be treated responsibly. All symptoms and complaints are perceived as real. The patient must see that the dentist is giving the complaint and symptoms serious consideration. Empathy must be shown for the individual. Avoid making negative value judgments. Build patient rapport by saying, "You look as though you have been experiencing a great deal of pain. Let me begin helping you by asking you some questions." This is far more effective than making an impersonal statement that could have easily come out of a tape recording, such as, "You'll be fine, just relax."
2. A show of support for the complaint is reflected through listening and expressing empathy, being nonjudgmental, and establishing and maintaining eye contact with the patient.[41] Such support does not imply absolute agreement. Be thorough in evaluation of the patient's symptoms and complaints. Patients must never feel that the attention is cursory or that less than everything possible is being done to make the diagnosis and provide a solution to the problem.
3. Display a calm and confident professionalism. This demeanor can be expressed verbally and nonverbally. Eye contact, supportive touching of the patient's shoulder, or body contact while moving the patient into the treatment chair is reassuring. Providing care without positive statements or gestures is an obstacle to effective patient management.
4. A positive attitude to the patient's problem can make the individual aware that an efficient and effective treatment or referral will be made to help them. They must never feel that they will be abandoned.
5. Discuss and inform the patient about what to expect, once a diagnosis is made and treatment determined. Discussing the procedures and the physical sensations the patient will feel are very useful. The patient's anxiety should be accepted as common and normal. Do not add guilt to the patient's emotional presentation by telling the patient, "There is nothing to be afraid of." Giving permission to be anxious can help to modulate the emotional responses of an anxious patient in an emergency situation.[41]

Management of the orofacial pain emergency requires a comprehensive understanding of the patient's experience and feelings. The dentist who understands and can actively participate in the dynamic interplay avoids many potential hardships and failures in dental practice.

The Doctor's Decision to Treat or Refer the Patient in Pain

Accommodating an unexpected patient into a busy schedule can be stressfully difficult for both dentist and staff. To ensure that the emergency patient receives appropriate care, the dentist must decide which provider is best able to administer the specific treatment and meet the unique needs of a given patient. The dentist must determine what expertise is required to make a difficult diagnosis or render a complicated treatment. The patient's ability to withstand the procedure, emotionally, physically, or medically, and the availability of time for a complex case may be considerations in referring the emergency.[22]

INTERPRETING THE LANGUAGE OF OROFACIAL PAIN

The Pain Phenomenon[81]

The emergency presentation of orofacial pain may include a series of symptoms in a dental emergency that can be assessed only by evaluating each symptom individually. It may be difficult, however, for the patient to objectively describe the painful experience, because of modulation and crossover in the central neural pathways. Modulation can intensify or suppress pain, giving it a multidimensional character.

At the neurophysiologic level, pain results from noxious stimulation of free nerve endings in orofacial tissues. The peripheral nerve endings, acting as nociceptors or pain receptors, detect and convey the noxious information to the brain, where pain is perceived.

Physiology of Pulpal Pain[47,92]

Odontogenic pain

The sensibility of the dental pulp is controlled by myelinated (A-delta) and unmyelinated (C) afferent nerve fibers. Operating under different pathophysiologic capabilities, both sensory nerve fibers conduct nociceptive input to the brain. Differences between the two sensory fibers enable the patient to discriminate and characterize the quality, intensity, location, and duration of the pain response.

Dentinal pain. The A-delta fibers are large myelinated nerves that enter the root canal and divide into smaller branches, coursing coronally through the pulp. Once beneath the odontoblastic layer, the A-delta fibers lose their myelin sheath and form anastomoses into a network of nerves referred to as the *plexus of Raschkow*. This circumpulpal layer of nerves sends free nerve endings onto and through the odontoblastic cell layer, as well as into dentinal tubules and in contact with the odontoblastic processes. The intimate association of A-delta fibers with the odontoblastic cell layer and dentin is referred to as the *pulpodentinal complex*.

Disturbances of the pulpodentinal complex in a vital tooth initially affect the low-threshold A-delta fibers. Not all stimuli reach the excitation threshold and generate a pain response. Irritants such as incipient dental caries and mild periodontal disease are seldom painful but can be sufficient to stimulate the defensive formation of sclerotic or reparative dentin. When the contents of the dentinal tubules (fluid or cellular processes) are disturbed sufficiently to involve the odontoblastic cell layer, A-delta fibers are excited. The vital tooth responds immediately with symptoms of dentinal sensitivity or dentinal pain.

A-delta fiber pain must be provoked. Nociceptive signals, transmitted through fast conducting myelinated pathways, are immediately perceived as a quick, sharp (bright), momentary pain. The sensation dissipates quickly upon removal of the inciting stimulus, like drinking cold liquids, or biting unexpectedly on an unyielding object.

The clinical symptoms of A-delta fiber pain serve to signify that the pulpodentinal complex is intact and capable of responding to an external disturbance. Many dentists have mistakenly interpreted this symptom to indicate reversible pulpitis; however, they are not mutually exclusive and, thus, dentinal sensitivity or pain should be distinguished from degenerative pulpal inflammation.

Clinical symptoms correlate poorly with the health or histologic status of the pulp. The dentist should be aware that, for the moment, he is dealing with a tooth that is vital. The most appropriate treatment for a vital tooth experiencing apparent A-delta fiber pain can be determined only by the clinical presentation of the involved tooth. While pulp preservation procedures can maintain the vitality of the tooth, the clinical circumstances leading to this decision must be reasonable. Nevertheless, A-delta fiber pain (dentinal sensitivity or pain) warrants consideration of pulp preservation measures as a primary treatment option.

Pulpitis pain. An external irritant of significant magnitude or duration injures the pulp. The injury is localized and initiates tissue inflammation. The dynamics of the inflammatory response determine whether the process can be confined and the tissues repaired, restoring pulp homeostasis. In a low-compliance environment, an intense inflammatory vascular response can lead to adverse increases in tissue pressure, outpacing the pulp's compensatory mechanisms to reduce it. The damaged tissue succumbs by degenerating. The inflammatory process spreads circumferentially and incrementally from this site to involve adjacent structures, perpetuating the destructive cycle.[93]

An injured vital tooth with established local inflammation can also emit symptoms of A-delta fiber pain with provocation. In the presence of inflammation, the response is exaggerated and out of character to the challenging stimulus, quite often thermal (mostly to cold). The *hyperalgesia* is induced by inflammatory mediators. As the exaggerated A-delta fiber pain subsides, however, pain seemingly remains and is now perceived as being a dull, throbbing ache. This second pain symptom signifies the inflammatory involvement of nociceptive C nerve fibers.

C fibers are small, unmyelinated nerves that innervate the pulp much like the A-delta fibers. They are high threshold fibers, course centrally in the pulp stroma, and run subjacent to the A-delta fibers. Unlike A-delta fibers, C fibers are not directly involved with the pulpodentinal complex and are not easily provoked. C fiber pain surfaces with tissue injury and is modulated by inflammatory mediators, vascular changes in blood volume and blood flow, and increases in tissue pressure. When C fiber pain dominates over A-delta fiber pain, pain is more diffuse and the dentist's ability to identify the offending tooth through provocation is reduced. Just as significant, C fiber pain is an ominous symptom that signifies that irreversible local tissue damage had occurred.

With increasing inflammation of pulp tissues, C fiber pain becomes the only pain feature. Pain that may initially start as a short, lingering discomfort can escalate to an intensely prolonged episode or a constant, throbbing pain. The pain is diffuse and can be referred to a distant site or to other teeth. Occasionally, the inflamed vasculature is responsive to cold, which vasoconstricts the dilated vessels and reduces tissue pressure. Momentary relief from the intense pain is provided, and this explains why some patients bring a container of ice water to the emergency appointment. Relief provided by a cold stimulus is diagnostic and indicates significant pulp necrosis.[2] In the absence of endodontic intervention the rapidly deteriorating condition will most likely progress to a periapical abscess.[47]

Stressed pulp syndrome. Not all C fiber pain symptoms are associated with a recent injury or active inflammation of the pulp. In aging persons diffuse pulpal pain is increasingly seen in retained teeth that have been repeatedly or extensively restored. The pathophysiologic process in aging teeth is one of slow deterioration. The pulp of a restored tooth is stressed and is likely undergoing circulatory embarrassment, leading ultimately to ischemic necrosis.[20]

C fiber pain from a stressed pulp is identical to that of degenerative pulpal inflammation. The pain occurs when hot liquids or foods raise intrapulpal pressure to levels that excite C fibers. The process is slow, and the delayed response makes the association with heat provocation difficult. At times, coincidental dental treatment or changes in ambient pressure can initiate symptoms in teeth with degenerative pulpal disease.[20,71] The patient can be confused by the apparently spontaneous appearance of diffuse pain symptoms.

Mediators in pulpal pain[19,88]

Inflammation of pulp tissue can manifest itself as acute pain or no pain at all. Biochemical pathways and immune mechanisms participate directly or indirectly in initiating and sustaining pulpal inflammation.[46] To set the stage for repair of inflamed tissues, activated defenses by the pulp must be able to hemodynamically remove the irritants and moderate the inflammatory process.

Ideally, the inflammatory cycles of vascular stasis, capillary permeability, and chemotactic migration of leukocytes to injured tissues are synchronized with the removal of irritants and drainage of exudate from the area. With moderate to severe injury an aberrant increase in capillary pressure can lead to excessive permeability and fluid accumulation. A progressive pressure front builds and begins to passively compress and collapse all local venules and lymphatic channels,[93] outpacing the pulp tissue's capacity to drain or shunt the exudate.[46,47] Blood flow to the area ceases and the injured tissue undergoes necrosis. Leukocytes in the area degenerate and release intracellular lysosomal enzymes, forming a microabscess of purulent material.

Mediators of vascular inflammation. Metabolites released from specific and nonspecific inflammatory pathways affect directly and indirectly the initiation and control of vascular events, increasing tissue pressure. Pain from pressure heralds the onset of inflammation. Nonspecific biochemical mediators such as histamine, bradykinin, prostaglandins, leukotrienes, and elements of the complement system, dilate blood vessels, increase permeability and thus increase local interstitial pressures. Some mediators are short lived but are constantly replaced through the newly extravasating plasma.[35] The renewed presence of mediators sustains the inflammatory process beyond the initial traumatic event. Fluid leakage diminishes blood flow and results in vascular stasis and hemoconcentration in the vessel. Platelets aggregated in the vessels release the neurochemical serotonin, which is leaked along with plasma into the interstitial tissues.[35] More detailed information on this phenomenon can be found in Chapters 11 and 15.

Mediators of neurogenic inflammation. The neurochemicals, serotonin and prostaglandin, induce a state of *hyperalgesia* in local nerve fiber.[35,92] In the sensitized state, nerve tissues seemingly "overreact" to all low-grade stimulations with acute pain symptoms, which can also occur spontaneously. In addition, neuropeptides such as substance P and calcitonin gene-related peptide (CGRP) are also released by the sensitized nerves.[35] At the local level, the neuropeptides stimulate the release of histamine, which refuels the vascular inflammatory cycle. The sustained inflammatory cycle is detrimental to pulpal recovery, terminating in necrosis of the tissues.

Nonodontogenic pain

It is quite common for orofacial pain from odontogenic and nonodontogenic structures to mimic pulpal-periradicular pain. Pain symptoms are often acute and confusing to the patient, who interprets the pain as a toothache. It is up to the dentist, then, to understand the language of pain and its symptoms, in order to separate out the many subtle clues in the search for a cause. The information that is gleaned from the patient is integrated with the dentist's own knowledge of orofacial disorders that can mimic toothache.

The dentist, with a thorough knowledge of these painful entities, is able to undertake the task of deliberate and selective elimination of nonessential pain characteristics. Through this process, the predominant pathognomonic pain patterns are identified, and a definitive diagnosis is achieved.

Of the many entities that mimic endodontic symptoms, six nonodontogenic conditions that may be seen for urgent care will be briefly reviewed. The emphasis here is on diagnosis. The discussion contrasts pain features that overlap endodontic symptoms with distinctive clinical features that characterize the entity as nonodontogenic. (A thorough review of the causes and management of orofacial pain entities is found in Chapter 3.)

It is best now to put into perspective the overlapping pain features that mimic pulpal or periradicular inflammatory pain. Facial pain typically follows the distribution of blood vessels and/or neural pathways and can arise from the supplied somatic structures. The area of neural involvement may be vastly greater than, or limited to, the trigeminal nerve distribution. The wide region on the face can be confusing to the patient. Pain symptoms are often felt as "diffuse" and, with unilateral confinement, similar to symptoms of irreversible pulpitis. Ultimately, a broadly focused search reveals somatic sensitivity, discloses an area and pattern of cutaneous hypersensitivity, or exposes a psychologically troubled patient or one whose "textbook" description of pain symptoms cannot be substantiated with certainty.

Entities associated with acute jaw pain

Trigeminal neuralgia.[24,54] The onset of trigeminal neuralgia occurs late in life and is most distressing for the patient. Attacks of pain are confined to one side and involve one division of the nerve (though bilateral successive involvements have occurred).[70] The attack produces severe "dental" pain but is described as lancinating, electrical, shocking, shooting, sharp, cutting, or stabbing. When asked, however, the patient traces a line along the distribution of the nerve on the face. Nevertheless, the possibility that these symptoms that resemble trigeminal neuralgia are being triggered by pulpal disease must be ruled out.[70]

A bout of paroxysmal pain in this degenerative neural condition is characteristically short, lasting several seconds but not longer than a minute. There can be secondary pain with a vague burning or aching quality. The patient, usually a female, tells of rigorously massaging the cutaneous site to deaden the pain.

The attacks come in series and can end abruptly. The period of remission is also free from the thermal and periapical sequelae associated with genuine endodontic disease. The patient quickly learns with each episode of painful attacks to avoid the cutaneous or intraoral site that sets off the attack. Some patients are able to identify and describe a vague prodrome of tingling just before an attack. Characteristically, and understandably, the patient is quite reluctant to have the area examined.

Myocardial pain.[24,96] Onset of myocardial pain can involve the jaws. In an imminent myocardial infarct, the pain is both sudden and severe and is not induced by oral stimulation. In coronary (ischemic) artery disease, pain may be less intense and be associated with emotional or physical activity. With cessation of the inducing activity (e.g., resting in the dental chair), pain from ischemia of heart muscle usually dissipates.

Myocardial pain referred to the jaws has often surfaced on the left side, but bilateral involvement has been documented. It is not unusual to find collateral pain in the shoulder(s), back, neck, and especially down the arms. This important feature is generated as sensory impulses cross through several thoracic and cervical dermatomes to reach the sensory pathways of the jaws. Collateral pain may not be readily apparent or present in every case. Here, interpretation of body language (signs and symptoms of shock, nausea, sweats, clammy skin, pallor, etc.) can give a better sense of the gravity of the patient's situation.

With imminent myocardial infarct, pain symptoms are constant and spread to involve vast areas of the maxilla and mandible or travel down into the neck or up into the temporal and zygomatic regions. During this time, the patient becomes anxious and complains of pain that is increasingly unbearable. The cutaneous area over the jaws may be massaged in a desperate attempt to obtund the pain.

Entities associated with acute tooth pain

Maxillary sinusitis. Maxillary sinusitis can produce a constant, dull to moderate aching pain in multiple teeth on the involved side.[24,75] To the exclusion of pulpally involved teeth, the teeth adjacent to the sinus are generally healthy but behave identically to each other, being uniformly hypersensitive to thermal stimulation and sensitive on palpation and percussion. Pain can increase with eating, involve the entire quadrant up to the facial midline, or be referred to the ipsilateral mandibular teeth.

Pain from an inflamed sinus membrane and associated nasal mucosa is characteristically felt in the face. Cutaneous pain features share in the clinical description of this condition and include comments such as fullness in the face, tenderness of the skin overlying the sinus, pain that increases on lying down or bending over, and pain that spreads to the scalp and toward the nose, often in association with postnasal drip.

In the differential diagnosis of maxillary sinusitis the endoantral syndrome and barodontalgia-barosinusitis from chronic pulpal and/or periapical pathosis must be considered, to rule out a coexisting endodontically induced infection of the sinus lining.[71,77]

Atypical orofacial pain. Atypical orofacial pain is a neurologic affliction that can be manifested as toothache pain.[24,33] The "toothache" is characteristically confined in the maxillary region, between the maxillary canine and premolar teeth, but it can involve other sites in either jaw. Pain is felt in the teeth and periodontium and is described as steady and pulsating. In a differential diagnosis, however, the involved tooth or teeth are found to have healthy pulp.

The pain is vague and difficult for the patient to localize, suggestive of a chronic onset. It is a constant, aching, burning, and nagging sensation deep in the tissues. The condition is not associated with any identifiable trigger points and crosses over rather than follows known neurologic boundaries. As pain travels it appears along vascular arborizations into the head region and behind the orbit. Further, the patient often reports that analgesics have no effect.

The intensity of the pain increases with physical exhaustion and general debilitation of the patient, suggestive of an underlying psychogenic foundation to this condition. Early recognition of atypical facial pain spares the patient unwarranted dental treatment and leads to appropriate referral.

Herpes zoster (shingles). A recurrence of herpes zoster infection involving the second and third division of the trigeminal nerve can manifest in a rare prodrome of symptomatic pulpitis.[32] The latent virus resides in the gasserian ganglion following a primary chickenpox (varicella virus) infection. Like any trigeminal nerve involvement, pulp pain is unilaterally confined. Toothache pain can be localized in one or more teeth and is described as sharp, throbbing, and intermittent. *The symptoms are believed to be genuine pulpal pain and not mimicked.*

During the prodrome, which can last for weeks, recognition of a recurrence of zoster is nearly impossible. The symptoms are undeniably those of irreversible pulpitis and the pulpitic teeth are easily identified by the patient. On examination, the dentist can be baffled to find the teeth intact, noncarious, and free of recent trauma.

The dilemma the dentist faces is whether to believe that the symptoms are genuine and benign to the health of the pulpitic teeth. A recent report suggests that intense symptoms are not benign and can lead to adverse pulpal responses, even necrosis.[32] An early decision to intervene endodontically, during the prodrome of a suspected shingles infection, can relieve the intense pulpitis pain. Understandably, the shingles infection may be followed to its clinical conclusion without intervention. Post–shingles infection monitoring for development of pulpal or periapical pathosis is indicated. The clinical merits of each case should dictate the best course of action.

Neoplastic diseases. Neoplastic diseases are extremely rare but can mimic symptoms of a toothache.[75] The nature of the pain can be severe, escalating with time and involving a developing paresthesia.[87] The pain features are out of character to that typically seen with inflammatory pulpal disease and should prompt the prudent dentist to seek consultation with and a referral to an oral surgeon or physician.

Fabricated Pain

Munchausen's syndrome[24]

Munchausen's syndrome is characterized by elaborate description or creation of pain that either is not real or is self-inflicted. The profile of these patients runs the gamut from the psychotic to the neurotic, the pathologic liar, to the chemically dependent addict.

The psychotic or neurotic patient gives a history that is convincingly accurate for orofacial pain but that cannot be substantiated by examination and testing. The preoccupied patient may spend countless hours in a health science library to "research" the condition and boasts of this when questioned. The dentist may be informed that he is the most recent of many professionals the patient has seen. The pain is *real* to the patient, who insists on treatment.

The chemically abusive patient occupies the other extreme and gives detailed textbook descriptions of pain. On examination, the dentist may actually find probable cause for the pain. The situation is self-induced or, at the insistence of the patient, "dentistogenic."

The addicted patient purposely shows up unannounced at inconvenient times in the workday, just before a holiday weekend, or even during the holiday with an "emergency" call to the office. This patient conveys convincing stories, such as: being from out of town and "forgot or lost my pain killers," alleges dissatisfaction with his (or her) dentist, and is seeking someone "new" to take over, or just needs something to "tide me over" until the next workday. The addict may even allow the compassionate dentist to perform treatment. It becomes difficult to deny a prescription to someone who has been rendered urgent care. The patient specifies what type of medication is being sought and abruptly changes demeanor to insist on a strong painkiller.

DIAGNOSIS

As described in Chapter 10, the "standard of care" in dentistry requires that the practitioner provide the quality of care that is expected to be performed by a reasonable and prudent dentist in the community. In order to render care for any orofacial emergency, the dentist must make a prudent and thoughtful diagnosis regarding the etiology and present state of the patient's disease. The dentist's worth as a healer will never be more appreciated than by the patient who has suffered the pain of a throbbing and rapidly degenerating pulpitis that has interfered with his or her eating and sleeping.

The endodontic emergency is a pulpal or periapical pathologic condition that manifests itself through pain, swelling, or both. An urgent endodontic emergency usually interrupts the normal office routine and patient flow. In addition, after-hours accommodations may have to be made to care for the patient.

Triage of the Pain Patient

Emergencies due to orofacial pain demand immediate professional attention. The urgency of the situation, however, should not preclude a thorough clinical evaluation of the patient. Orofacial pain can be the clinical manifestation of a variety of diseases involving the head and neck region. The etiology must be reliably differentiated, odontogenic from nonodontogenic. The task is made needlessly difficult without a comprehensive knowledge of the pathophysiology of inflammatory pain of the pulp and periradicular tissues.

Triage can expedite the differentiation process by systematically sorting through the signs and symptoms of the presenting pain. Each entity is characterized as having a dental or nondental pain feature. Features that are shared and are not exclusive to either source are also noted. With the signs and symptoms collected in this manner, triage is concluded by noting the preponderance of pain features in either the dental or nondental category. A working differential diagnosis is thus methodically begun and directs the dentist to investigate further.

Triage of odontogenic symptoms should discriminate for sensory and proprioceptive sensations that are produced exclusively by inflammatory pulpal and periradicular diseases. Genuine endodontic pain involves nociceptive transmissions in the maxillary and mandibular branches of the trigeminal nerve.

Identifying orofacial pain definitively to be endodontic pain becomes increasingly difficult as the focus shifts away from a more localized and tooth-specific pain to an ever wider area on the face. Numerous orofacial diseases can mimic endodontic pain and produce sensory misperception as a result of overlapping between sensory fibers of the trigeminal nerve and of adjacent cranial and cervical sensory dermatomes. Convergence of signals in the medulla can cause sensory overload to occur and a perceptual error by the cerebral cortex.

Triage of nonodontogenic symptoms should discriminate for pain patterns that are inconsistent with inflammatory pulpal and periradicular diseases. Organic orofacial pain follows many different peripheral neurologic pathways but can also overlay onto the sensory distribution of the trigeminal nerve. Pain can also follow the vascular arborization of head and neck vessels. The interrelationship between the neural and vascular pathways and the orofacial structures they supply produces symptoms that can be readily distinguished as nondental. Pain features that are episodic with painfree remissions, that have trigger points, that travel and cross the midline of the face, that surface with increasing mental stress, that are seasonal or cyclical, or that produce paresthesia are characteristics of nondental involvement.[24]

The process of diagnosis of the endodontic emergency, as set forth in this chapter, will concentrate on the acute emergency, or potentially complex orofacial pain emergency. The practitioner must collect the appropriate data—the set of signs, symptoms and test results—that will lead to a diagnosis.

Careful adherence to the basic principles and a systematic approach to procuring an accurate diagnosis can never be overstressed. A hasty diagnosis, or inappropriate treatment of a suffering patient, are pitfalls with the potential for a litigious aftermath. In procuring diagnostic data, the dentist must generate:

1. A "subjective" interrogatory examination.
2. An "objective" clinical examination.
3. A radiographic examination and evaluation.

The clinician who reviews and prioritizes patient data in all emergencies in a deliberate and thorough manner can avoid the pitfalls of inaccurate diagnosis and inappropriate treatment.

Developing Data: The Medical History

The subjective, interrogatory examination of the patient must include a comprehensive evaluation of the patient's medical history. Although numerous authorities agree that there are almost no medical contraindications to endodontic therapy, it is important to understand how an individual's physical condition, medical history, and current medications might affect the treatment course or prognosis.[86]

A medical history informs the evaluator of any "high-risk patient" whose therapy may have to be modified, for example, a cardiac patient who might tolerate only short appointments. The medical history would also identify patients who require antibiotic prophylaxis for congenital or rheumatic heart disease. Some patients receiving chemotherapy may require antibiotic coverage because of a compromised immune system.[67] The medical history can identify patients for whom healing and repair of endodontic pathosis could be complicated or delayed, such as those who have uncontrolled diabetes or active AIDS.

In situations when owing to systemic illness the prognosis

A

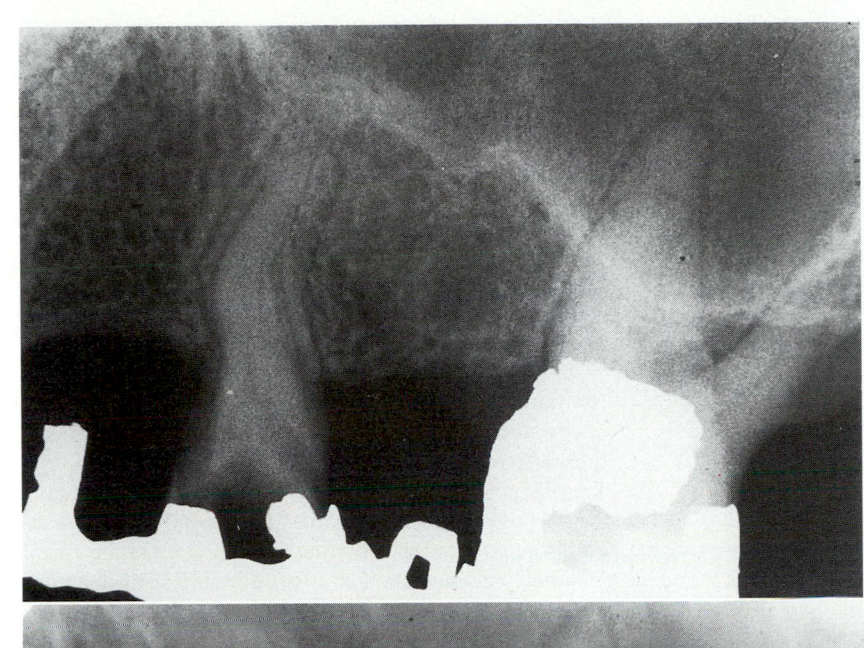

B

C

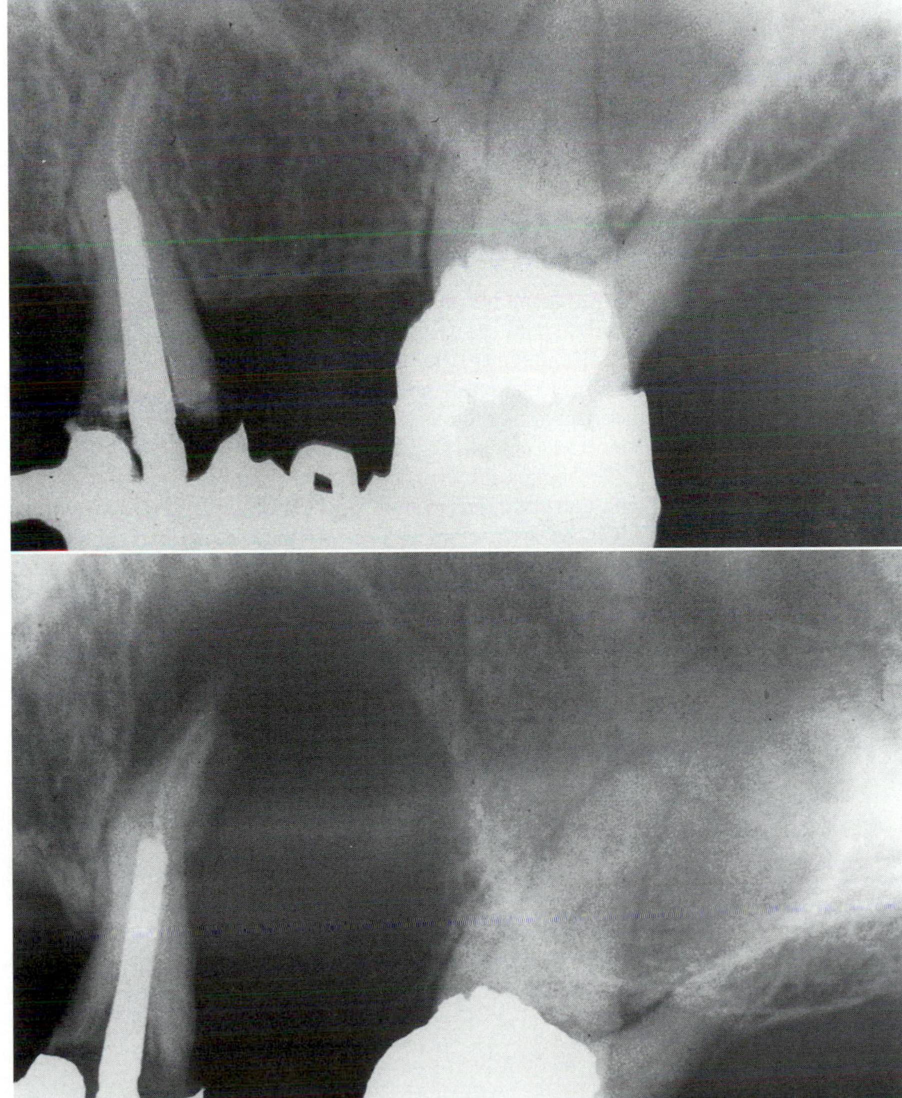

Fig. 2-1 A, Preoperative endodontic involvement of left maxillary first premolar. **B,** Completion of endodontic treatment. **C,** Reexamination at 6 months, radiographic evidence of significant bone loss and apical resorption is seen, which is atypical of endodontic failure. Biopsy revealed multiple myeloma, a malignancy of the lymphoreticular system. The discovery of the systemic disease on the dental films was confirmed by head and chest films that demonstrated widespread involvement. The patient succumbed 7 months later.

is guarded, a second medical consultation with the patient's treating physician is imperative. The use of antibiotic prophylaxis to prevent infective endocarditis is justified in high-risk patients. It is reasonable to mitigate bacteremia in other selected patients at risk because of implanted prosthetic devices, congenital heart disease, hemodialysis, or impaired host defenses.[50,67]

There are also aspects of a patient's medical background that might impact on the chief complaint, the repair potential, or the radiographic appearance of disease. Sickle cell anemia, vitamin D resistant rickets, and herpes zoster have all been implicated in spontaneous pulpal degeneration.[1,10,32] Nutritional disease, stress, and corticosteroid therapy can also decrease the potential for repair.[78]

Forms are available to the dentist that afford quick and efficient evaluation of patient systems in order to provide a simple means of taking a medical history (see suggested forms in Chapters 1 and 9). The dentist should follow up by reviewing what the patient has written and seeking more detailed information that may not impress the patient as important. Some women are reluctant to discuss their use of birth control pills for contraception, yet a number of common antibiotics used to treat endodontic infections significantly decrease the efficacy of oral contraceptives.[3,18] Possible drug interactions between currently prescribed medications and those prescribed for the emergency must be understood by the doctor and noted on the patient's record.

Against the possibility of nondisclosure of important data by the patient, or omission on the medical history form, the diagnostician should ask supplemental questions in the following areas of concern:

1. Current medical condition.
2. History of significant illness or serious injury.
3. Emotional and psychological history.
4. Prior hospitalizations.
5. Current medications, including over-the-counter remedies.
6. Habits (alcohol, tobacco, drugs).
7. Any other noticeable sign or symptom that may indicate an undiagnosed health problem (Fig. 2-1).

All significant medical data should be recorded on the patient's record (Fig. 2-2). In the emergency setting, if possible, the dentist should measure and record the patient's vital signs (pulse rate, blood pressure, respiratory rate, temperature). A hyperventilating patient, one who is febrile, or one who exhibits high blood pressure will require a thoughtful consideration of systemic and/or emotional complications to treatment. If any question exists regarding the patient's current medical status, the appropriate physician should be consulted.

Dental History

The subjective, interrogatory examination continues with the dental history. This is unquestionably the most important aspect of the diagnostic work up and, if carefully done, will build trust in the doctor-patient relationship. This subjective questioning should attempt to provide a narrative from the patient that addresses the following points:

1. *Chief complaint*—as expressed in patient's own words.
2. *Location*—the site(s) where symptoms are perceived.
3. *Chronology*—inception, clinical course, and temporal pattern of the symptoms.
4. *Quality*—how the patient describes the complaint.
5. *Intensity/severity* of symptoms.
6. *Affecting factors*—stimuli that aggravate, relieve, or alter the symptoms.
7. *Supplemental history*—past facts and current symptoms characterizing the difficult diagnosis.

The diagnostician should listen very carefully to the patient's choice of words, remembering that the patient's descriptions are being filtered through a myriad of complex psycho-social and emotional components that affect not only the account of the pain but how it is perceived.

The Chief Complaint

The questions listed below ensure comprehensive and logical evaluation of the chief complaint. When questioning the patient, the dentist may have to rephrase or completely restate a question, to ensure that the patient understands. The dentist should also be prepared to paraphrase the patient's responses, to verify what was heard.

Location

The patient is asked to indicate the location of the chief complaint by pointing to it directly with one finger. Pointing avoids verbal ambiguity, and the dentist can note if the pain is intraoral or extraoral, precise or vague, localized or diffuse. If the symptoms radiate, or if the pain is referred, the direction and extent can also be demonstrated.

The diagnostician should be well aware of referred pain pathways, as referred pain is common with advanced pulpitis when the disease has not yet produced signs or symptoms in the attachment apparatus. In posterior molars, pain can often be referred to the opposing quadrant or to other teeth in the same quadrant. Upper molars often refer pain to the zygomatic, parietal, and occipital regions of the head, whereas lower molars frequently refer pain to the ear, angle of the jaw, or posterior regions of the neck. Corroborating tests and data are necessary to make a definitive diagnosis, or to justify invasive therapy, whenever referred pain is suspected.

MEDICAL HISTORY

Heart Condition angina coronary surgery pacemaker Rheumatic Fever / Murmur Hypertension / Circulatory	Anemia / Bleeding Diabetes / Kidney Hepatitis / Liver Herpes Thyroid / Hormonal Asthma / Respiratory Ulcers / Digestive Migraine / Headaches	Epilepsy / Fainting Sinusitis / ENT Glaucoma / Visual Mental / Neural Tumor / Neoplasms Alcoholism / Addictions Infectious Diseases Venereal Disease	Allergies: penicillin / antibiotics aspirin / Tylenol codeine / narcotics local anesthetic N_2O/O_2 other:	Major Medical Prob: Females: Pregnant _______ mo Recent Hosp. Operation: Current Medical TX: Medications: Initial:

FIG. 2-2 Chart of a medical systems review common to a comprehensive dental record.

Chronology

The dentist must explore the exact nature of the patient's symptoms, because of the extreme variability of patients' descriptions of a complaint.

Inception

The patient should relate when the symptoms of the chief complaint were initially perceived. They may be aware of a history of dental procedures, trauma, or other events such as sinus surgery or tumors in the areas of concern.

Clinical manifestations of disease

Beyond the inception of symptoms, it is extremely important for the dentist to record details of symptoms, emphasizing these features:

1. *Mode*—Is the onset or abatement of symptoms spontaneous or provoked? Is it sudden or gradual? If symptoms can be stimulated, are they immediate or delayed?
2. *Periodicity*—Do the symptoms have a temporal pattern or are they sporadic or occasional? Often, early pulpitis is reported by the patient as recurring symptoms that occur in the evening or after a meal, giving the inflammation a predictable or reproducible quality.
3. *Frequency*—Have the symptoms persisted since they began or have they been intermittent?
4. *Duration*—How long do symptoms last when they occur? Are they "momentary" or "lingering"? If they are persistent, the duration should be estimated in seconds, minutes, hours, or longer intervals. If the symptoms can be induced, are they momentary or do they linger? *By this time, the patient may have provided the dentist with enough data to make an endodontic diagnosis*. However, some cases have far more diffuse symptoms and require a more persistent and astute analysis of key descriptions.

Quality of Pain Descriptions

The patient is asked to render a detailed description of each symptom associated with the presenting emergency. This description is important to differential diagnosis of the pain and for selection of objective clinical tests to corroborate symptoms.

Certain adjectives describe pain of bony origin, such as *dull, drawing,* or *aching*. Other adjectives— *throbbing, pounding,* or *pulsing*—describe the vascular response to tissue inflammation. *Sharp, electric, recurrent,* or *stabbing* pain is usually caused by pathosis of nerve root complexes, sensory ganglia, or peripheral innervation, which is associated with irreversible pulpitis or trigeminal neuralgia. A single episode of sharp, persistent pain can result from acute injury to muscle or ligament, as in temporomandibular joint dislocation or iatrogenic perforation into the periodontal attachment apparatus.

Pulpal and periapical pathosis produce sensations that are described as *aching, pulsing, throbbing, dull, gnawing, radiating, flashing, stabbing,* or *jolting* pain, and many more. Though such descriptions support suspicion of an odontogenic cause, the diagnostician cannot ignore the fact that many of these adjectives can also describe nonodontogenic pathosis.

Intensity

The patient's perception of and reaction to an acute pain emergency, especially one that is odontogenic in origin, is widely variable. For an unremitting toothache the treating clinician usually makes a diagnosis and renders emergency treatment based on its intensity. The dentist, therefore, should try to quantify the intensity of the pain symptoms reported by the patient. There are methods to accomplish this:

1. Try to quantify the pain. Assigning to the pain a degree of 0 (none) to 10 (most severe or intolerable pain) helps monitor the patient's perception of the pain throughout the course of treatment.
2. Have the patient classify the pain as mild, moderate, or severe. This classification has implications for the question, How does the pain affect the patient's lifestyle? The pain can be classified as severe if it interrupts or significantly alters the patient's daily routine. Generally, pain that interferes with sleeping, work, or leisure activities is significant. If bed rest or potent analgesics are required the pain is likewise considered extreme.

Whenever symptoms are clinically reproducible, the intensity of the pain should alert the dentist to which clinical and diagnostic tests are most appropriate. If the clinician can reproduce them, more painful symptoms help locate the chief complaint and provide corroborative information. Reproducing less intense symptoms, though it "creates data," may not help differentiate the involved tooth from those whose responses are within normal limits.

Affecting Factors

The objective of the next part of the interrogatory examination is to identify which factors provoke, intensify, alleviate, or otherwise affect the patient's symptoms. Before any corroborative testing is attempted (such as thermal or percussion tests), it is imperative to know the level of intensity of each affecting stimulus and the interval between stimulus and response. The patient who describes a toothache that manifests itself about halfway through drinking a cup of coffee should alert the diagnostician that the tooth is exhibiting delayed onset of response to heat. This has a significant bearing on how clinical testing should proceed. Unless adequate time between stimulus and response is allowed, coincidence may have the dentist stimulating a second tooth at the same time a previously stimulated tooth is manifesting a delayed response.

The prudent clinician will be cautious and conservative in the use of the percussion test. If by questioning the patient it is learned that percussion may elicit an extreme response, it would be unwise to immediately start percussing teeth and provoke so much discomfort for the patient that the diagnosis is greatly clouded. Symptoms can be more meaningful if the investigator takes the time to hear and understand the circumstances in which they occur:

Local affecting stimulus

The following stimuli are generally associated with odontogenic symptoms:

Heat
Cold
Sweets
Percussion
Biting
Chewing
Manipulation
Palpation

The significance of these provoking factors for the diagnosis of endodontic disease is discussed in Chapter 1. In addition, the patient may experience spontaneous pain of variable quality, intensity, location, and duration.

Predisposing factors

Just as there are factors that can provoke odontogenic pain, there are factors that can precipitate the onset of symptoms that may indicate a nonodontogenic cause:

Postural changes— Head or jaw pain accentuated by bending over, blowing the nose, or jarring one's skeleton (e.g., by jogging) may imply involvement of the maxillary sinuses.

Time of day— Stiffness and pain in the jaws upon waking may indicate occlusal disharmony or temporomandibular joint dysfunction.

Pain with strenuous or vigorous activity may indicate pulpal or periapical inflammation. Pulpal or sinus involvement may also be revealed by changes in barometric pressure, which can occur during skin diving or flying at high altitudes. Another significant implication would be jaw pain associated with exertion, which may be a warning sign of coronary artery disease.

Hormonal change—"Menstrual toothache" or recurring hypersensitivity may occur when there is an increase in body fluid retention.[8]

Supplemental History in the Difficult Diagnosis

For many endodontic emergencies, there is a cause-and-effect relationship. The dentist restores a fractured filling in a patient's lower left first molar, and the patient experiences extreme sensitivity to cold, which lingers several minutes. The diagnosis is uncomplicated: it is irreversible pulpitis, the treatment for which is root canal therapy. However, as biologic variability goes, there will always be cases that perplex and confound even the most astute diagnostician. Every dentist assuredly will be asked to diagnose and treat emergencies whose symptoms are vague and whose cause is far less obvious.

The patient who presents complaining of diffuse, disabling pain is a difficult challenge. There may be a great deal of pain for the patient but very little evidence that constitutes real information for the doctor. If in addition the patient is demanding that something be done, this can compound the stress of the emergency visit. Faced with a dissatisfied, insistent patient, there is a strong temptation to do "something," even before a definitive diagnosis can be made. This situation is to be avoided at all costs. Patients who are made aware of the dentist's concern for their problem and empathy for their suffering will be far more inclined to accept a cautious approach during the diagnostic process. The clinician must emphasize the scientific nature of the diagnosis and the real possibility that it may take more than one visit to identify the problem.

The dentist does well to tell patients that it might be necessary to wait a while for vague symptoms to localize. This is most common in pulpal pathosis confined to the root canal space, which often refers pain to other teeth or extradental sites. It may be necessary to wait for the inflammation to involve the attachment apparatus before it can be localized. Patients generally can be supported with analgesics until a definitive diagnosis can be made.

The Patient Diary

A daily diary can provide valuable information to aid in the difficult diagnosis. Patient's verbal reports are often vague, and can be contradictory. Frequency and severity of symptoms can vary with time, and a patient who is stressed may not report critical information accurately. In these types of cases, especially when the task is to distinguish between odontogenic and nonodontogenic pain, a patient diary provides an hour by hour or day by day narrative. The more chronic or diffuse the complaint, the longer the diary should be kept. Two to three weeks is sometimes common. Information such as the severity of pain (on a 1 to 10 scale), its duration, the time of day, and the type of provocation or activity associated with the discomfort should be recorded. Patients are often surprised to find out when it hurts or what provokes the pain. The patterns of discomfort may provide concise information for the doctor, and also place the problem in perspective for the patient, to help modify their behavior towards their pain.

In the final analysis, after providing descriptive information about the chief complaint, the patient should recount any significant incidents in the affected area—trauma, previous symptoms or treatments, complications. These can be significant elements in an evolving diagnosis. Certain descriptions of pain, such as trigger zones or headaches, as well as medical conditions such as coronary artery disease or a history of neoplasm, are details that should be considered in a differential diagnosis when seeking the cause of pain.

After organizing, analyzing, and assimilating all the pertinent descriptions, facts, and data, the doctor should be ready to proceed with the clinical examination phase of the diagnostic process.

Clinical Examination

Records

If the dentist is to provide a precise and structured appraisal of a patient's chief complaint, an efficient record that quantifies diagnostic data is a mainstay of the clinical examination. Suggested forms appear in Figures 2-3 and 2-4. Details of the comprehensive clinical examination and data acquired from diagnostic tests should be recorded. The clinical examination has three components: (1) physical inspection, (2) diagnostic tests, and (3) radiographic interpretation. In light of this accumulation of clinical data, a graphic is presented in Figure 2-5 to illustrate the now developing systematic approach to the emergency diagnosis.

The clinician is to be reminded that, even in an area with numerous dental problems, in the true endodontic emergency it is most likely that only one tooth is responsible for the acute situation. Clinically it is quite rare that, on a biologic level, the set of circumstances which could produce the odontogenic emergency would occur in two teeth with the same intensity at the same time.

The physical inspection should include observations of periodontal health; tissue color and texture; tooth discoloration; and presence, condition, and extent of restorations, erosion, fractures, caries, sinus tracts, and swelling (Fig. 2-6). A thorough periodontal assessment, with careful probing of the sulcus and attachment apparatus and notation of mobilities, is a standard and essential element of the physical inspection.

Diagnostic tests (described in Chapter 1) enable the practitioner to:

1. Define the pain by evoking reproducible symptoms that characterize the chief complaint.
2. Provide an assessment of normal responses for comparison with abnormal responses which may be indicative of pathosis.

DENTAL HISTORY:	CHIEF COMPLAINT	SYMPTOMATIC	ASYMPTOMATIC			
SYMPTOMS	Location	Chronology	Quality	Affected By	Prior Tx	Initial:
localized diffuse	referred radiating	Inception Clinical Course: constant momentary intermittent lingering	sharp intensity dull + ++ +++ spontaneous pulsating provoked steady reproducible enlarging occasional	hot palpation cold manipulation biting head position chewing activity percussion time of day	Tx: restorative Yes No emergency Yes No RCT Yes No Sx Pre-Tx: Yes No Sx Post-Tx: Yes No	TOOTH R L

FIG. 2-3 A systematic format for charting the dental history.

CLINICAL FINDINGS

EXAMINATION	RADIOGRAPHIC		CLINICAL	
	Tooth	Attachment Apparatus	Tooth	Soft Tissues
	WNL caries restoration calcification resorption fracture perforation / deviation prior RCTx/RCF separated instrument canal obstruction post / build-up open apex	PDL normal PDL thickened alveolar bone, WNL diffuse lucency circumscribed lucency resorption apical lateral hypercementosis osteosclerosis perio:	WNL discoloration caries pulp exposure prior access attrition / abrasion fracture restoration amalgam composite inlay / onlay temporary crown abutment	WNL extra-oral swelling intra-oral swelling sinus tract lymphadenopathy TMJ perio: B M D L

DIAGNOSTIC TESTS						
Tooth #						
perio						
mobility						
percussion						
palpation						
cold						
hot						
EPT						
transillum						
cavity						
bite / chewing						
date:						

FIG. 2-4 Chart for clinical findings and diagnostic data.

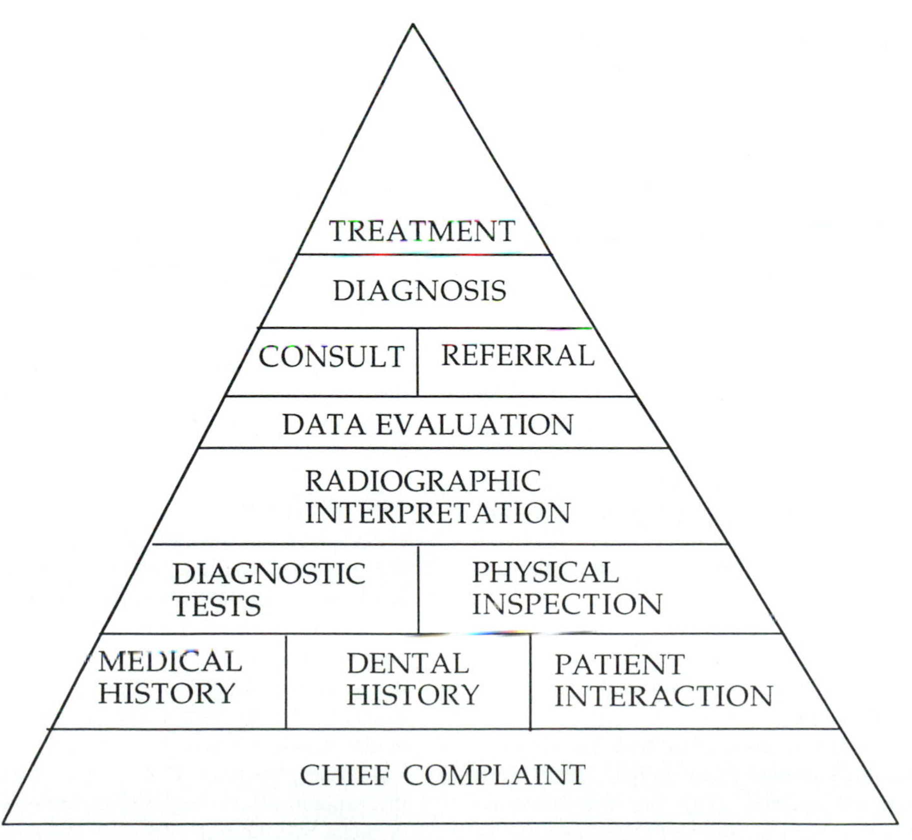

FIG. 2-5 Assembling patient data provides the foundation for determining appropriate treatment of the acute orofacial emergency.

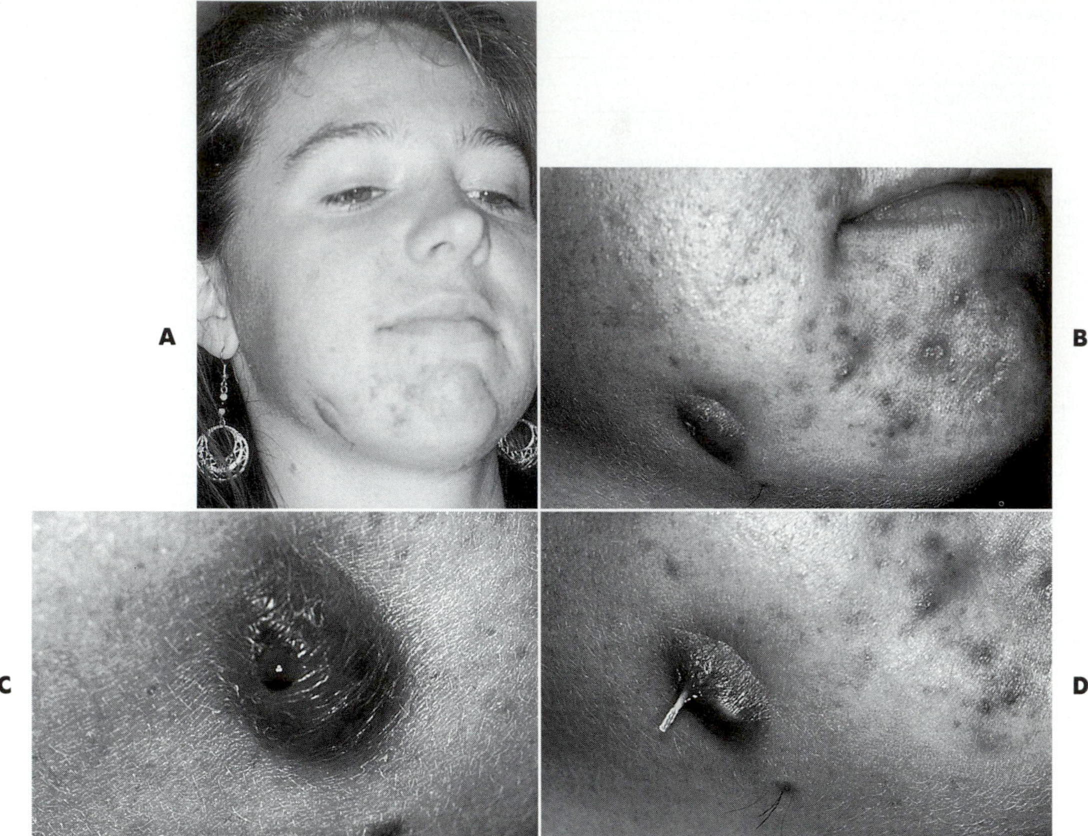

FIG. 2-6 A and **B,** Physical inspection of the skin of a young woman with facial acne. The lesions on the right cheek were found to be resistant to dermatologic therapy. **C,** Closer inspection of a suspicious lesion revealed active drainage. **D,** Presence of an extraoral sinus tract was confirmed by inserting a gutta-percha cone leading to the mandibular first molar. This was confirmed by dental radiographs and pulp vitality testing.

Obviously, the usefulness of diagnostic testing is a function of the clinician's correct and systematic application of those tests and their proper interpretation. Diagnostic tests may include hot and cold thermal testing, tooth percussion, electric pulp testing, tissue palpation, transillumination and magnification, test cavity preparation, and anesthetic tests to localize pain. All of these entities, and the fundamentals of diagnosis, have been discussed in Chapter 1. This discussion focuses on those clinical considerations relative to testing that are requisite to identifying and treating the endodontic emergency.

When diagnostic testing is required to evaluate a patient's chief complaint, the success of the analysis depends on the clinician's

1. Awareness of the limitations of the various tests and how to administer them.
2. Biologic knowledge of the inflammatory process and the pain phenomenon.
3. Knowledge of nonodontogenic entities that mimic pulpal and periapical pathosis.

Investigators have explained why teeth with radiographically discernible periapical lesions retain pulpal innervation, even when necrosis is anticipated.[49] This fact can confound the interpretation of pulp vitality testing and may engender inaction on the part of the dentist when true pathosis is present. This should reinforce our requirement to provide a thorough evaluation and corroborative data before making a definitive diagnosis.

The dentist should include adequate controls for any set of applied test procedures. Several adjacent, opposing and contralateral teeth should be tested prior to the tooth in question, to establish the patient's normal range of response. The dentist should use care not to bias a patient's response by indicating to the patient a suspected culprit tooth before it is evaluated.

Thermal Tests

Endodontists[75] remind us that a misdiagnosis can result from (1) misperception of symptoms, (2) misinterpretation of data, or (3) an incomplete diagnostic examination. They concluded that, in the difficult diagnosis of thermal sensitivity, it is imperative to accurately recreate with thermal tests the conditions that stimulate the pain. They recommend that each tooth be isolated properly with a rubber dam and bathed in hot water, or ice water, to most closely reproduce the environment in which the pain is evoked. This method is also very effective in evaluating teeth with full coverage restorations, porcelain, or metal restorations.

For patients who experience onset of prolonged moderate

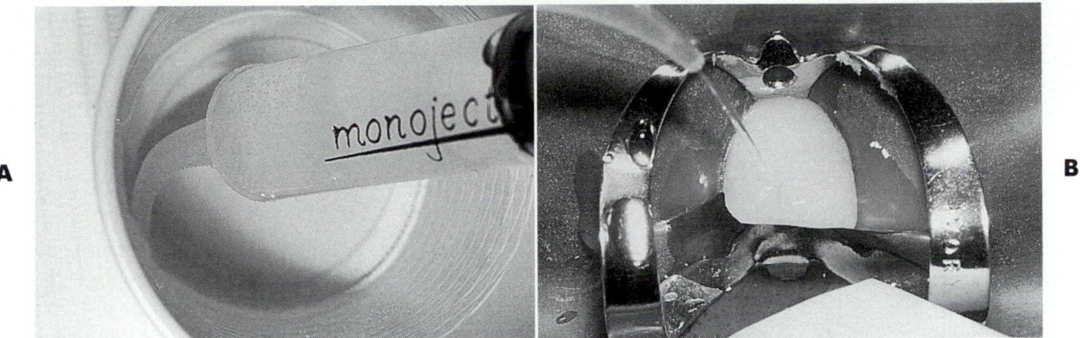

FIG. 2-7 A, Syringe for loading hot water to bathe the suspected tooth. **B,** Rubber dam isolation of a central incisor that is sensitive to heat. The patient should feel the water with a finger to identify the affecting temperature.

or severe pain when taking hot or cold substances into the mouth, rubber dam isolation for thermal testing will reproduce the symptoms more reliably than any other method. Once the complaint is reproduced, the hot or cold fluid should be quickly aspirated away from the patient's tooth to provide humane relief. The dentist must use methodical diagnostic technique to avoid producing conflicting and unreliable responses. The sensory response of teeth is refractory to repeated thermal stimulation. To avoid a misinterpretation of a response, the doctor should wait an appropriate time for tested teeth to respond and recover (Fig. 2-7).

Percussion

If the patient's chief complaint involves pain on biting or chewing, an attempt to identify the initiation of the symptoms can be initially assessed with a soft but resistant object. Having the patient chew on a cotton roll, a cotton swab, or the flexible, reverse end of a low-speed suction straw will identify a single tooth more quickly than simple percussion when the pain is elusive (see Chapter 1). Use of the Tooth Slooth for cuspal and dentinal fractures will readily identify cracks hidden under restorations or those newly developed in the crown or root. Finally, selective percussion from various angles will help identify and isolate teeth with early inflammation in the periodontium of endodontic origin.

Electric Pulp Testing

The clinician should be aware of the limitations of electric pulp testing. The potential for erroneous results—either false-positive or false-negative—is described in Chapter 1. The electric pulp test should be regarded as an aid in detecting pulpal neural response and not as a measure of pulpal health or pathosis. Corroborating tests are also mandatory. Basing a diagnosis of necrosis solely on a nonresponsive electric pulp test ignores errors of technique or a malfunctioning device. In addition, secondary dentin, trauma, restorations, and dystrophic calcification may all contribute to negative responses on a normal tooth.

Transillumination and Magnification

Fiberoptic lighting and chairside magnification have become indispensable in the search for cracks, fractures, and unfound canals and obstructions in root canal therapy.[16] The fact that magnification (e.g., Designs for Vision or a microscope) and transillumination might allow the dentist the only means of diagnosing an offending cracked tooth is becoming an increasing reality.

Radiography

After collecting the details of the chief complaint from the patient's history, physical examination, and clinical or laboratory testing, the doctor should obtain the required radiographic views, those that will contribute to the localization and identification of the patient's stated problem. Occasionally, the contralateral side may need to be viewed, in the event that unusual tooth or alveolar anatomy requires that bilateral symmetry be considered. Though unnecessary use of radiation is definitely discouraged, the attending dentist is cautioned to use discretion in accepting prior diagnostic radiographs from the patient or another dentist, no matter how recently they were made. Such radiographs may not accurately reflect the present condition of the teeth and surrounding bone. Investigations have shown that for a radiograph to exhibit a periapical radiolucency, the lesion must have expanded to the corticomedullary junction and a portion of the bone mineral must have been lost.[9,11] This situation can occur in a short period of time in the presence of an aggressive infection. New radiographs taken when treatment is actually initiated may corroborate a diagnosis or point to a different, unsuspected tooth. Furthermore, prior iatrogenic mishaps such as ledge formation, perforation, or instrument separation are vital for a newly treating dentist to uncover. The dentist who omits taking a new radiograph assumes legal responsibility for the procedural error because there is no documentation that it occurred before the current treatment of the patient. Good radiographic technique includes proper film placement, exposure, processing, and handling. These principles are the foundation for the attainment of a high-quality diagnostic radiograph and may provide the only legal defense in support of treatment outcomes. The interpretation of radiographs can be a source of enlightenment as well as a source of misinformation. A thorough understanding of regional anatomic structures and their variations is critical to proper interpretation. A careful assessment of continuity in the periodontal ligament space, lamina dura, and root canal anatomy will distinguish healthy structures from diseased ones. Changes in the pulp chamber often constitute a record of past

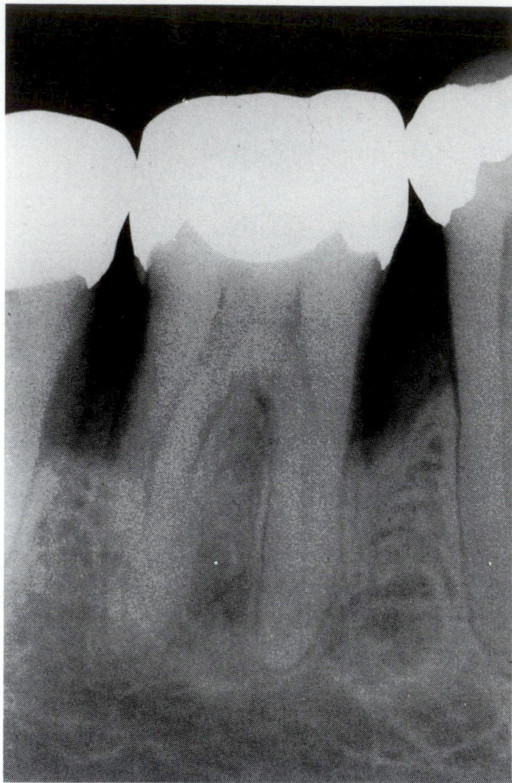

FIG. 2-8 The stressed pulp. A right angle periapical projection reveals complete cusp coverage, dystrophic calcification of the pulp chamber, and chronic periodontal disease with moderate bone loss. This tooth should be a prime suspect when evaluating for vague pain in the area and is a candidate for endodontics if additional restorative treatment is planned.

pulpal inflammation. Caries, secondary dentin under restorations, very large or narrow pulp chambers compared to adjacent teeth, deep bases, calcifications, and condensing osteitis can all indicate pulpal tissue undergoing chronic inflammation (Fig. 2-8). Use of an optical magnifier, as well as proper illumination, will help the examiner discern these subtle and intricate details in the radiographic image. The patient record should provide space for radiographic changes (Fig. 2-4). Subtle radiographic changes can often account for the only changes that might potentially identify an offending tooth. Proper selection of the appropriate type of radiographs (as discussed in Chapter 5) is paramount to complete differential diagnosis.

DETERMINING THE DIAGNOSIS

The final phase of the diagnostic sequence requires a systematic analysis of all pertinent data accumulated from the patient's history, narrative, and clinical and radiographic evaluation. The doctor must be methodical in his or her approach, in order to determine the cause as well as the diagnosis.

Considerations in Treatment Planning

The dentist should begin by determining whether the chief complaint is consistent with an endodontic etiology, and should go through the mental exercise of narrowing down the possibilities to a specific tooth. Tests should be able to confirm whether pulpal pathosis is confined to the root canal space or has progressed and exhibits periapical extension. Specific etiologic factors such as caries, fracture, trauma, restorations, and other, more subtle, initiators of pulpal inflammation (developmental anomalies, orthodontic tooth movement, viral agents[32]) must also be identified.

Diagnostic Determinants

There are specific diagnostic determinants that guide the practitioner into making judgments about diagnosis and treatment. These considerations address whether a given set of symptoms might indicate that treatment should be periodontal, transdentinal, or endodontic.

Periodontal considerations

The acute and painful periodontal abscess can mislead the careful diagnostician into believing that a pulp lesion is the actual cause. Prognosis for long-term tooth retention is usually most dependent on the periodontal status, so before the pulpal status is determined, the results of the periodontal examination should be evaluated. If a significant periodontal condition exists, the extent of involvement and the nature of the problem should be elucidated. If extensive bone loss around a tooth has created acute pulpal symptoms, the practitioner must carefully weigh whether endodontic therapy is in the patient's best interest, even though it may palliate the acute pain. Extraction of the hopeless tooth may be a better treatment. When endodontic pathosis is diagnosed, the clinician should determine whether periodontal factors are also contributing to the chief complaint. Those causal factors that specifically affect periodontal prognosis, such as inadequate epithelial attachment, lingual developmental grooves, and enamel projections, should be explicitly identified in order to separate palliative treatment from definitive therapy.

Dentinal considerations

Probably the most common kind of nonurgent odontogenic pain is pain related to exposure of dentinal tubules to outside stimuli. As the physiology of this type of pain has been discussed previously, it is sufficient to describe the pain as very brief and sharp. Causes range from dentin exposure via caries to trauma of the dentin by enamel fracture. The overriding question for the clinician is whether the brief sharp pain is a "normal" response of a healthy pulp or a sign of pulpal inflammation. Protection and insulation (transdentinal therapy) of exposed dentin in a healthy pulp normally result in complete resolution of the dentinal symptoms. At this point, endodontic therapy is not required unless there is a restorative requirement for such a treatment consideration. The quality of pain described as "dentinal" is usually considered to be normal. Pulp preservation techniques are most commonly indicated in these situations.

Endodontic involvement

Once an endodontic lesion is diagnosed, the dentist must confirm the location and delineate the specific nature of that problem. It is most often seen that irreversible pulpitis without inflammation in the periodontal ligament will exhibit referred pain because of the lack of proprioceptors in the pulp proper. A tooth with a history of deep caries, pulp caps, large and multiple restorations, trauma, or previous painful episodes should be the prime suspect. Once the tooth is identified, endodontic therapy should be instituted as soon as possible. Localization can be achieved by watchful waiting until the inflammation progresses, or it may be delineated by anesthetics or pulpal testing.

Restorative Considerations

In considering the future restorability of the offending tooth, the dentist must assess whether he or she has the requisite skills and knowledge to carry out the treatment without harming the patient. Extraction is sometimes an acceptable and desirable alternative. Extraction has been suggested as a viable choice when no esthetic, masticatory, or space-maintaining function can be attributed to the tooth in question. In addition, it is indicated if the tooth lacks adequate periodontal support, exhibits severe resorption, or is unrestorable, or if the patient refuses endodontic treatment.[58]

Endodontic Treatment Planning

An increasingly enlightened majority of people choose endodontic therapy to alleviate their acute pain and restore their dentition. In order to provide the most biologic strategies for the management of acute odontogenic pain, we must begin considering which areas of treatment afford the practitioner the greatest potential for a successful endodontic outcome. Pulpal and periapical pathoses that result in endodontic emergencies manifest themselves in a variety of ways. Local pain, referred pain, spontaneous pain, provoked pain, thermal sensitivity, and swelling are all common features of pulpal and periapical pathosis. During therapy, operator judgments and iatrogenic treatment factors, pulpal and periapical irritants, and patient factors (such as age, sex, tooth type, allergic history, preoperative pain, periapical lesion size, sinus tracts, and use of analgesics) all have significant bearing on treatment-related emergencies.[91] Many of these complications also affect the incidence of post-obturation pain and swelling and can alter the treatment plan. In the remainder of this chapter we attempt to describe treatment for the odontogenic emergency relative to its clinical presentation. The text focuses on recently investigated areas of emergency management that concentrate on several important themes that are central to efficacious treatment:

1. Pharmacologic control and management of pain and swelling.
2. Complete débridement of the pulpal space.
3. Treatment and prevention of midtreatment and postobturation flare-ups.

MANAGEMENT OF ACUTE DENTAL PAIN

The treatment approaches described next pertain to permanent teeth with mature apices; for a discussion of diagnosis and treatment of primary teeth, immature permanent teeth, and traumatic injuries the reader is referred to Chapters 15 and 22.

Urgent Care for Acute Dentinal Pain

A number of insults can provoke a quick, sharp, momentary tooth pain that initially causes the patient to seek urgent care and consultation. These symptoms of A-delta fiber pain cue the dentist to look for a vital tooth. Ideally, pulp preservation measures should take priority in the management of pain symptoms.

There are overriding factors that become apparent as the individual circumstances present. These factors can alter subsequent treatment decisions. Overriding factors may include significant or obvious stained fracture lines, large or deep areas of decay, recurrent decay, or the chronopathologic status (age and current health) of the tooth in question. The defensive capabilities of the pulp diminish with successive treatment of the aging tooth, which adversely affects pulp vitality.[85] Chronopathologic factors include history of pulp capping (direct/indirect); history of trauma, orthodontic treatment, periodontal disease; history of extensive restorations (pins, buildups, crown); and the restorative treatment planned for the tooth (Fig. 2-8).

As the overriding factors are discovered, each must be carefully assessed because of the adverse impact they can have or may have had on current pulpal health. The dentist must then decide on the most appropriate treatment that will conserve the integrity of the pulpal tissue. At times, this may not be practical. The patient must be informed of the situation in an empathetic and compassionate manner. Treatment may shift radically from pulp preservation measures to deliberate removal of the pulp and sealing of the root canal system in anticipation of long-term restoration. What is important here is for both dentist and patient to realize that urgent care results in the retention of the tooth as a functioning member of the dentition, whether or not the pulp is retained.

Hypersensitive dentin

Exposed cervical dentin from gingival recession, periodontal surgery, toothbrush abrasion, or erosion may result in root hypersensitivity.[12] Any chemical (osmotic gradient), thermal (contraction/expansion), or mechanical (biting or digital scratching) irritant can disturb the fluid content in the dentinal tubules and excite nociceptive receptors in the pulp.[35]

Treatment of hypersensitive dentin has had limited success.[12,82] A number of viable treatment modalities focus on the chemical or physical blockage of the patent dentinal tubules to prevent fluid movement from within. Chemical desensitization attempts to sedate the cellular processes within the tubules with corticosteroids or to occlude the tubules with a protein precipitate, a remineralized barrier, or a crystallized oxalate deposit. Physical techniques attempt to block dentinal tubules with composite resins, varnishes, sealants, soft tissue grafts, and glass ionomer cements. The iontophoresis technique electrically drives fluoride ions deep into dentinal tubules to occlude them. The efficacy of these treatment approaches is temporary, at best, and they must be repeated.

With increasing hypersensitivity, treatment can quickly escalate to the use of physical agents and preparation of the tooth surface.[82] Laser technology may provide the definitive solution for sealing the dentinal tubules permanently. At this time long-term studies of efficacy and safety of these laser applications are yet to come and the equipment is expensive.[82]

Recurrent decay

Teeth with large multisurface restorations can feel sharp pain on eating. Often, an undetected gap has formed in the interface between dentin and restoration, leading to microleakage and recurrent decay. With sufficient occlusal pressure on the defective restoration, pain is produced as saliva in the gap is compressed against the exposed dentin interface.

Treatment of provoked pain, due to recurrent decay, depends on the chronopathologic history of the tooth in question. The tooth may be amenable to pulp conservation measures, provided A-delta fiber pain is the only symptom present and is produced on provocation. Thorough but atraumatic caries removal, placement of indirect pulp capping with calcium hydroxide where indicated, and the temporization of the tooth with a sedative filling like zinc oxide–eugenol material may be beneficial in stabilizing the chronically inflamed pulp. To assess the relative effectiveness of this treatment, the tooth must first be allowed to recover. A more permanent interim restoration is then placed, but with the understanding that pulpal degeneration (stressed pulp syndrome) can occur in the future.

Inadvertent exposure of the pulp or emerging pulpal symptoms following careful caries removal are adverse developments for which endodontic treatment takes precedence over pulp preservation.

Recent restoration

Following a restorative procedure a tooth can sense inflammatory pain in both A-δ and C fibers. The common complaint is of pain that is provoked by a thermal stimulus that would normally not evoke a response. This state of *hyperalgesia* can be produced only by inflammatory mediators and warns that significant local injury to the pulp has occurred.

Historically, postrestorative sensitivity, diagnosed as reversible pulpitis, was routinely managed by immediate removal of the restoration and placement of a sedative filling like zinc oxide eugenol; little thought was given to the consequences. Before submitting the tooth to another insult, the dentist must reassess the situation for answers that only he knows. This may prevent needless removal of the restoration, which increases the likelihood that the pulp will succumb to the inflammatory process. On the other hand, if the sustained injury is significant there is probably little that can be done to reverse the cascading events that lead eventually to pulpal degeneration.

The rendering of urgent care in this situation requires the differentiation between acts of commission and acts of omission. Acts of commission should seek to rectify poor treatment or faulty techniques. This might entail correction of hyperocclusion in a recent restoration, telltale shiny spot(s) in both centric and excursive occlusion.[12] Inadequate or excessive interproximal contacts, which promote food impaction or excessive stresses along the root, must also be corrected.[12] The tight contact must be reduced. The dentist should allow the tooth several weeks to recover from the restorative episode. The inadequate filling can then be removed and the tooth temporized with a sedative filling like zinc oxide–eugenol.[92] This allows the pulp to recover fully before the final restoration is placed. Ligamental injections to induce operative anesthesia are discouraged in vital teeth that are sensitive on preparation. Anesthetics containing high concentrations of a vasoconstrictor can disrupt the flow of blood to the pulp[48] and depress efficient hemodynamic clearing of accumulated inflammatory toxins. A vital tooth whose pulp is compromised may never recover.[94] To complete preparation of a tooth that exhibits a chronopathologically stressed pulp the tooth should be anesthetized through regional and block techniques only.

Acts of omission can be acknowledged only by the provider of the restoration. The detailed technical maneuvers executed in producing the restoration must be honestly assessed for an atraumatic delivery. Use of sharp burs, appropriate preparation depth, ample air and water coolants, application of liners and bases, and avoiding desiccating the dentin are just a few details that, if omitted, can lead to irreversible pulpal injury. If the clinician determines that atraumatic procedures were followed, the tooth should be allowed several weeks to adequately recover before the need for endodontic intervention is assessed.

Cracked tooth syndrome[12]

A cracked tooth feels a sharp momentary pain on mastication, catching the patient by surprise. A tooth that is susceptible to cracking is one that is extensively restored but lacks cuspal protection (cuspal crack) or an intact tooth that has an opposing plunger cusp occluding centrically against a marginal ridge (vertical crack).

Pain, generated only on disclusion, drives oral fluids within the crack in the pulpal direction. This phenomenon is unique to a crack, and it inspired the diagnostic technique of selective closure on the suspected tooth to elicit the pain on release. (See Chapter 1 for tools and techniques used to diagnose the cracked tooth.)

Urgent care of the cracked tooth involves the immediate reduction of its occlusal contacts by selective grinding at the site of the crack or against the cusp(s) of the occluding antagonist.[12]

Definitive treatment of a vertically cracked tooth attempts to preserve pulp vitality by requiring no less than full occlusal coverage for cusp protection.[75] Cusp coverage may seem drastic, but a vertical crack that is left unprotected will migrate "pulpally" and apically. When the aging defect encroaches on the pulp, emerging endodontic symptoms are indicative of the unavoidable need for root canal treatment. A long-standing defect can be betrayed by heavy staining in a tooth that is asymptomatic. It is possible that slow pulp degeneration explains the absence of symptoms.

Endodontic treatment can alleviate pulpal symptoms in a vertically cracked tooth. Tooth retention, however, remains questionable. The apical extension of and future migration of the defect down onto the root will decide the outcome.[75] Full cuspal coverage from this vantage is the most practical approach to treating a tooth with recent symptoms of disclusion pain.

Treatment of cuspal cracking in an extensively restored tooth depends on the chronopathologic history. Consideration should be given to the planned restorative needs and the possible need to perform elective endodontic treatment first. Tooth retention in cuspal cracking is favorable, since the cusp generally separates obliquely in the horizontal plane. The defect usually has no adverse residual effect on the root or on periodontal supporting structures.

Urgent Care for Acute Degenerative Pulpitis and Associated Periapical Pain and Swelling

Pulpal inflammation is responsible for a variety of signs and symptoms seen in an endodontic emergency. The symptom constellation of endodontic C fiber pain has already been described. Identifying the offending tooth is most difficult when the disease is still confined entirely within the pulpal space.[58] Nevertheless, the dentist should proceed in a disciplined and orderly manner to gather subjective, objective, and radiographic data.[58,75]

Selective anesthesia can be the final resort for distinguishing which of adjacent teeth that remain equivocal is the source for the pain but *only if the pain is determined unequivocally to be odontogenic*.[20,58] Delaying treatment would be the prudent course in case of any lingering doubt.[2,58]

An inescapable sequela of pulp inflammation is its eventual spread from the confines of the tooth into the periapical tissue.[58] An inflamed periodontal membrane can be equally painful because of activated A-delta and C nerve fibers in the area. Also activated are proprioceptive mechanoreceptors that enhance the patient's ability to localize the offending tooth. Proprioception is the hallmark of periapical inflammation that signals advanced stages of pulpal disease. As fluid accumulates and pressure increases, the tooth may feel elevated or loose in the socket, and it is increasingly painful on biting or on digital pressure.

Emergency management for the pain of acute degenerative pulpitis involves *initiating root canal treatment* to alleviate pain symptoms and *definitive management* of associated signs and symptoms of soft tissue involvement.

Profound anesthesia[20,95]

Attaining profound anesthesia is paramount to rendering emergency treatment, but this can be elusive even for a seasoned practitioner. Suppression of the nociceptive action potential is hampered by the numerous inflammatory pathways that are operating in the area. As the inflammatory process progresses, local tissue pH falls precipitously. The acidic environment prevents the anesthetic molecule from dissociating into ion form and exerting its pharmacologic activity on the neuron. Further, the inflamed nerve fibers are morphologically and biochemically altered throughout their length by neuropeptides and other neurochemicals. Thus, in a state of hyperalgesia nerve block injections at sites distant from the inflamed tooth are rendered less effective.[14,53]

To be effective, the clinician must gain the advantage by judiciously selecting alternate and supplementary sites for injecting anesthetic solution. Consideration must be given to the type and amount of anesthetic solution required for the conditions. These can be anatomic limitations such as dense bony plates or thick nerve sheaths, aberrant distribution of neural bundles, or accessory innervations, especially in the mandibular regions. The clinician should be skilled in all the various techniques of needle insertion that may be required (see Chapter 19).

Urgent care of an endodontic emergency requires more than routine regional anesthesia of dental structures. Endodontists[20] emphasize that profound anesthesia is mandatory. Only with a complete lack of sensation can definitive treatment be rendered to the patient by the dentist at a stress level that is acceptable to both parties. An anesthetic regimen specific for endodontic emergencies must be planned in advance.

The nerve block injection of a nerve trunk central to an area or tooth is the standard intraoral approach for achieving initial regional anesthesia.[20] A block injection anesthetizes a wider area while avoiding soft tissue areas involved by inflammation and infection. For additional techniques to ensure profound anesthesia the reader is referred to Chapter 19.

Rendering urgent care

It has been said that hindsight often shows what a little foresight might have expedited or even prevented. Nowhere is this truer than in the initial management of the endodontically involved tooth. In a discussion on managing midtreatment pain and swelling, it was pointed out that the symptoms of the interappointment flare-up were in many cases identical to symptoms that first brought the patient in for urgent care.[37] *Thus, the techniques used to manage a midtreatment flare-up, in hindsight, are used more appropriately and advantageously for the initial management of the endodontic emergency.* Although this may not prevent a tooth that is acutely involved from having persistent pain and developing a soft tissue swelling, it is more likely that pain symptoms would be effectively and predictably eliminated with this treatment approach. The healing process can be initiated earlier, and resolution of the inflamed tissues can begin sooner following the urgent care appointment.[4]

Managing acute endodontic pain

The recommendation that emergency treatment is the minimal treatment for alleviating symptoms until definitive therapy can be performed is not entirely sound advice. The clinician is faced with the dilemma of determining the extent of the disease process (irreversible pulpitis, partial necrosis, total necrosis) and deciding on the minimal treatment (pulpotomy, partial pulpectomy, complete pulpectomy) needed to resolve the pain symptoms.

Quite often the treatment decision is determined, not by the urgency, but for expediency and so as to least disrupt a busy schedule. This may be a disservice to the patient. *No one should need reminding that an endodontic emergency has never been an elective visit for the patient in pain.* Pain symptoms can persist or worsen as the inflammatory process extends into the periradicular area. For the dentist, another appointment will be necessary to treat a deteriorating condition that might be complicated by infection and could possibly be fatal.[5,43] "Urgent care" provided in this manner only reinforces the patient's already distorted perception that root canal treatment is the most painful and least desirable of all the dental procedures. A more sobering fact is the increasing number of malpractice suits arising out of endodontic complications and involving generalists and specialists alike.[61,76]

An endodontic emergency is best managed by thorough cleaning and shaping of all the canals. This is the approach that a majority of board-certified endodontists, responding to a survey, routinely used to treat *all* emergencies, regardless of the diagnosis or the particular conditions of the care.[29] The rationale is to impede, if not terminate,[23] the inflammatory reactions by completely removing the irritant (inflamed pulp tissue, infected pulp tissue, necrotic pulpal and bacterial substrate) that is fueling the process and causing pain.[20] Taking time to establish the lengths of the tooth and to completely débride the root canal(s) can obviate a subsequent flare-up or render it more manageable.[37] To make time for this a decision to reschedule an elective procedure may be in order.[58] In most cases, the scheduled patient understands the urgency and needs of the emergency patient. Moreover, the implicit message that the dentist *will not abandon* a patient in pain can be reassuring to the scheduled patient, who one day may also need urgent care.

In most cases instrumentation is confined within the root canal, but it may be passed just beyond the apex to maintain patency and encourage drainage from periapical tissues. Deliberate perforation of the apical foramen or apical trephination should be done only after all canals have been thoroughly cleaned. Specifically, apical trephination is reserved for the pulpless tooth that is manifesting symptoms of periapical tenderness, pressure sensitivity, or a developing swelling.[37] Occlusal reduction or selective adjustment is always indicated for teeth that manifest periapical symptoms, as a palliative measure.[2,20,29,37]

It is the consensus among endodontists that every effort should be made to close the tooth following urgent care.[2,5,29,37] A tooth left open is exposed to new and unwanted oral pathogens and irritants and is frequently involved in midtreatment flare-ups.[79,80] Spontaneous drainage at the beginning of urgent

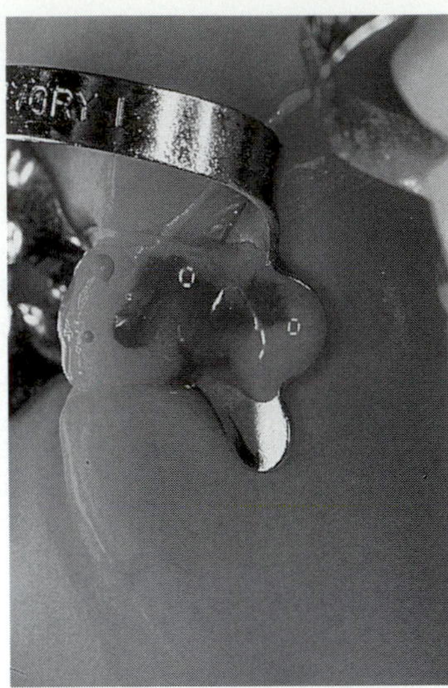

FIG. 2-9 An acute apical abscess relieved by drainage through the access opening. (Courtesy of Dr. Eric Herbranson.)

care should be well under control following thorough cleaning and shaping. Additional chair time may be required to allow the tooth to drain adequately.[2] Observation of serosanguineous fluid, rather than suppurative drainage, is a sufficiently safe indicator for closing the tooth with Cavit or a reinforced zinc oxide–eugenol filling (Fig. 2-9). A notable exception for leaving the tooth open involves the management of a diffuse swelling (with or without drainage) and a hypochlorite accident, which are discussed below.

Managing endodontic swellings

Extension of pulpal disease into the periapical tissues can result in swelling and infection. Tissue swelling can be seen at the initial emergency visit, at an interappointment flare-up, or as a postendodontic complication. Swellings are either localized or diffuse. The cardinal rule for managing these infectious swellings is to attempt to establish drainage[37] and, as indicated, to institute antibiotic therapy.[29] *If no concurrent attempt is made to establish drainage, the use of antibiotics alone is considered inadequate management* (Fig. 2-10).[37,43]

A prerequisite for managing endodontic swellings is the cleaning and shaping of the root canal system, especially at the time of urgent care.[20,29,52] For various reasons this step is often postponed in favor of just establishing soft tissue drainage. This approach may be counterproductive to expeditious resolution of the conditions that are causing pain and swelling. Since toxins remain harbored and continue to seep from the untreated tooth, periapical tissues remain subacutely inflamed. With subsequent instrumentation of the root canal(s), bacteria and toxins can be reinoculated inadvertently into still sensitized periradicular tissues. Thus, the potential exists for initiating a second exacerbation. Another episode of pain can wear heavily on the patient's psyche. With conditions deteriorating, even simple manipulation of the tooth can become a more onerous procedure for the patient to endure.

Localized swelling. Management of a localized soft tissue swelling can be facilitated through incision and drainage of the area. As for any surgical procedure, profound anesthesia is required, but this may not be possible in the presence of swelling. Soft tissue infiltrations around the periphery of the distended tissues can achieve a reasonable degree of anesthesia that permits tissue manipulation with a minimum of discomfort.[2] A long-acting anesthetic solution can provide a margin of comfort until the incised tissues have resolved to a sufficient degree.

An incision is made with a scalpel into the center of the swollen area, down to bone. A purulent discharge usually follows incision of a fluctuant swelling. Running the gloved finger from the periphery of the lesion to the point of incision expresses purulent exudate that has accumulated under the soft tissues. Also, with a thoroughly instrumented tooth, firm but gentle pressure against the alveolar bone can drain periapical exudate back into the patent canal(s).[37] Drainage will continue and resolve on its own. Hot intraoral saline rinses (1 tsp salt in 1 glass of water) can be repeated as necessary to draw out the last vestiges of pus, soothe the tissues, and facilitate healing (Fig. 2-11).[37,43]

A point of contention is whether to incise an indurated swelling or to wait until the tissue becomes fluctuant.[37] Early incision of an indurated swelling can reduce pain from increasing tissue distension, even if only hemorrhagic fluid is obtained.[29] Though we recommend suturing an indwelling drain into place to maintain active drainage until the swelling has resolved significantly, other endodontists do not place any drains into the incision site.

Diffuse swelling (cellulitis). A diffuse swelling can turn into a medical emergency of potentially life-threatening complications. For this reason, most endodontists[37] advise a more aggressive treatment approach, regardless of when the condition is first seen. The diagnostic process should first rule out facial cellulitis caused by nonodontogenic erysipelas or periodontal abscess.[34]

In the absence of drainage through the tooth, soft tissue drainage must be established through incision of the diffusely swollen alveolar tissues.[37] An indwelling drain is sutured into the incision wound to ensure tissue drainage. The tooth is then reduced occlusally and (re)opened, the canal(s) thoroughly (re)instrumented and irrigated. The apical foramen is intentionally instrumented through (under anatomic restrictions) to encourage drainage from the periapical tissues (instruments no larger than a No. 25 file[2] introduced no farther than 1 mm beyond the root end). Until the swelling begins to organize or resolve, the tooth is left open in *all* cases,[37] isolating the chamber from gross contamination with a large cotton pellet.[51]

The patient must be given a course of systemic antibiotics to control the infection and to allow the tissues to fully mobilize an effective defense. While penicillin continues to be the traditional antibiotic of choice for established dental infections,[2,37,43,60] the trend in current clinical therapy finds that erythromycin (500 mg stat, 250 mg qid) may have a greater impact against mixed anaerobic-aerobic cellulitis.[51,52,89] *Hot, intraoral* saline rinses may keep the infection localized until tissue conditions are ready for productive drainage.[37,43] Before dismissing the patient, the endodontist may be consulted by phone for additional instructions or an alternate course of action. Also, an analgesic should be prescribed for the patient; the patient should be monitored closely over the next several days until there is improvement.[37]

The benefit of running an antibiotic sensitivity test may not seem to be an option in rendering urgent care, owing to inad-

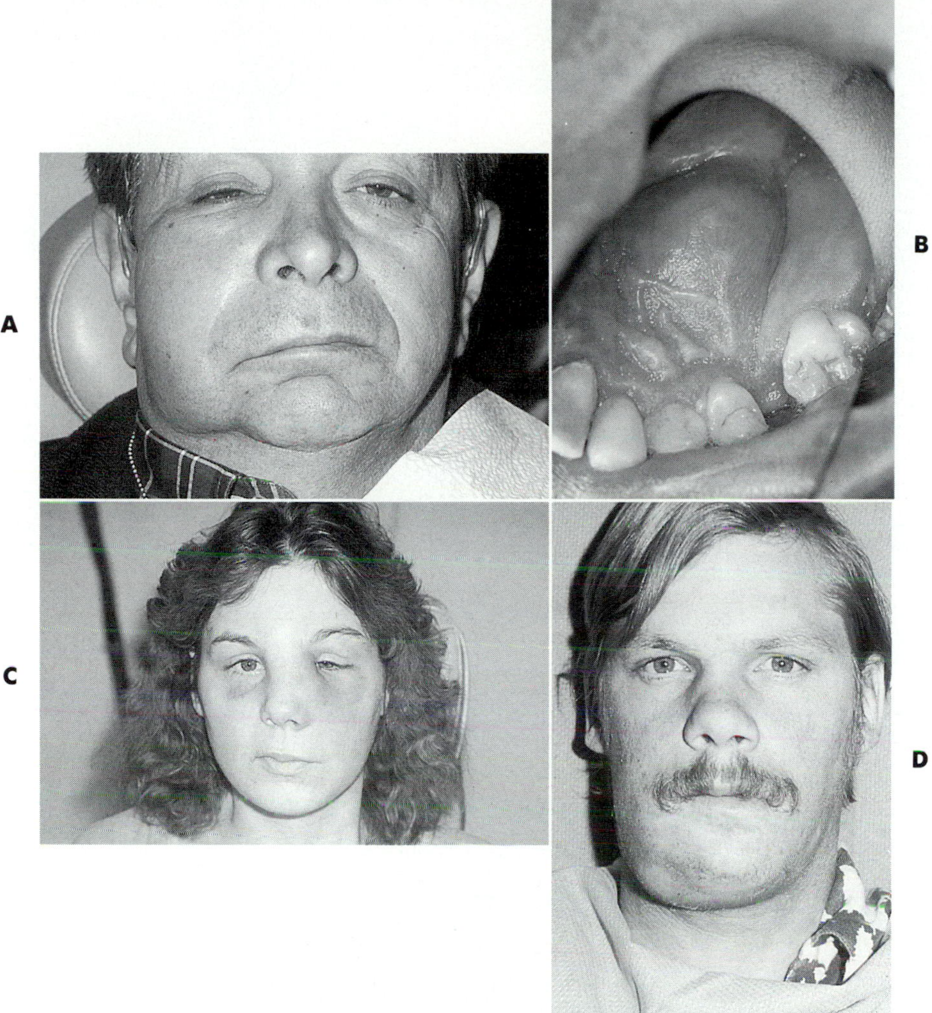

FIG. 2-10 A, Maxillary space infection secondary to an endodontic abscess. **B,** Palatal swelling secondary to a necrotic lateral incisor. (Courtesy of Dr. Joseph Schulz.) **C,** Canine space abscess spreading into the periorbital spaces. **D,** Submandibular space infection from an endodontically involved mandibular molar. (**C** and **D** courtesy of Dr. Mitchell Day.) Cellulitis and space infections require aggressive therapy for resolution. This would include thorough débridement of the root canal space, intraoral drainage whenever possible, and administration of appropriate antibiotics. Culture and antibiotic sensitivity testing, and possibly referral, is strongly recommended for cases that are refractory to initial conventional therapy.

equate sample material or unavailability of appropriate transport media. Nevertheless, prepackaged commercial collection and transport kits are available for in-office storage and use. In addition, during the emergency a commercial laboratory or local hospital can be contacted to supply a collection kit that can isolate anaerobic bacteria (enriched thioglycolate broth[52]) and run an antibiotic sensitivity test. When the infection is extensive or appears difficult to manage or if the patient is at medical risk, purulent samples should be collected and sent immediately to the laboratory for culturing and isolation (Fig. 2-12).[5,37,60]

Progressive deterioration of the patient's condition, as evidenced by increased swelling, a sustained high fever, mental confusion, and difficulty swallowing or breathing, is sufficient reason to hospitalize the patient for more specialized care and around-the-clock monitoring.[60] The laboratory findings can guide the clinician in the subsequent choice of an antibiotic regimen.[5,37,43]

Fortunately, most endodontic infections are controlled through the establishment of drainage.[37] The antibiotics typically administered in dental infections (penicillin or erythromycin) have also been effective against many microorganisms that commonly inhabit pulpless teeth.[37] An uneventful resolution of the crisis can be expected. During this time, swelling usually peaks and the patient begins to show improvement. If, after 48 hours, improvement is slower than expected a switch to a broader-spectrum antibiotic (metronidazole or clindamycin) may be indicated.[5,43,60] Metronidazole is effective against obligate anaerobes; clindamycin, against gram-positive facultative anaerobes.[40,42] Drug toxicity or patient allergy or intol-

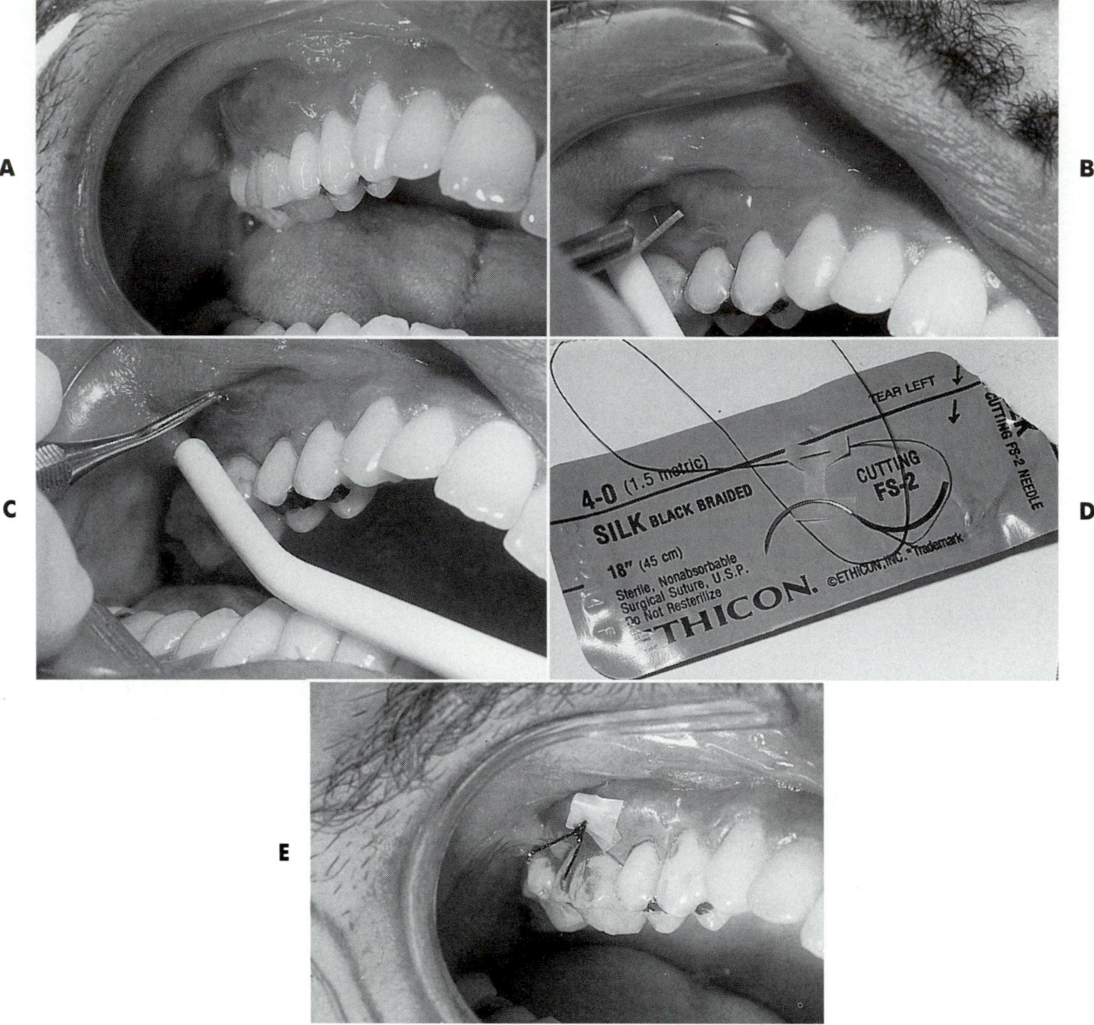

FIG. 2-11 A, Fluctuant intraoral vestibular swelling from a maxillary molar requires incision and drainage. **B,** Horizontal incision made through the swelling to the base of the alveolar bone. **C,** A surgical curette is used to dissect tissue and facilitate drainage. **D,** Suture placement through a rubber dam drain. **E,** The indwelling drain is sutured into place to maintain drainage. Monitor for resolution of swelling. The drain should be removed after 24 to 48 hours. (Courtesy of Dr. Eric Herbranson.)

erance may limit their use.[52] Antibiotic coverage must be maintained until the root canal(s) and pulp chamber can be disinfected and (re)closed.[37] For more details about antibiotic use, the reader is referred to Chapter 12.

Managing midtreatment flare-ups

Flare-up is the term used to describe the onset, persistence, or exacerbation of pain, swelling, or both during the course of root canal treatment. According to one report,[37] the incidence of midtreatment flare-ups is quite low, ranging between 2.5% and 16% for pain and 1.5% and 5.5% for swelling. As infrequent as flare-ups are, the development of interappointment pain and swelling has been universally accepted by dentists as an expected part of endodontic treatment. The clinician who undertakes endodontic treatment must be prepared to deal with these infrequent but painful complications.[37] The best approach to managing the majority of midtreatment flare-ups is prevention.

In vital teeth, the differential diagnosis for persistent or acute onset of pain during midtreatment therapy includes these conditions:

1. *Irreversible pulpitis* from inadequate débridement or overlooked canal(s).
2. *Acute apical periodontitis* from overinstrumentation or overmedication of the canal(s), or a hyperoccluding temporary filling. The condition can progress to an abscess through bacterial contamination of the root canal or coronal leakage through the temporary restoration.

In nonvital teeth, the differential diagnosis for persistent or acute onset of pain during midtreatment therapy includes the following conditions:

1. *Acute apical periodontitis* from a sustained periapical in-

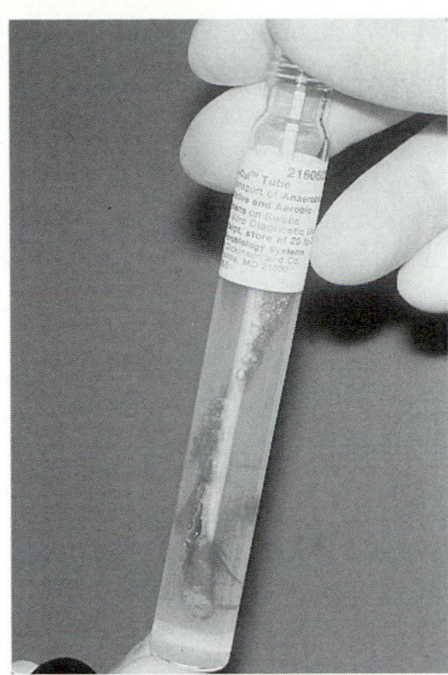

FIG. 2-12 Culture and antibiotic sensitivity testing of pathogenic microorganisms can be conducted with both aerobic and anaerobic techniques. Commercially available sample swabs and transport media are to be used as directed.

flammatory reaction with no infection present can progress into an abscess as a result of less than aseptic treatment, inoculation of apical tissue with infectious debris, or a leaky temporary restoration.

2. *Acute apical abscess* in pulpless teeth with intact periapical tissues can progress to soft tissue swelling.
3. *Phoenix abscess* in pulpless teeth associated with a periapical lesion and absence of a sinus tract can progress into soft tissue swelling.

Sequelae in vital teeth.[37] Normal vital teeth subjected to pulp extirpation and teeth with symptomatic pulpitis should have no pain or slight pain following complete instrumentation of the root canal space. Persistent pain or onset of acute pain often signals the presence of residual pulp tissue in inadequately instrumented or still undetected canal(s). Likewise, overmedicating the tooth can lead to acute onset of pain from medicaments that permeate into the periapical tissues. Thorough débridement of the entire root canal system (especially in multirooted teeth) and copious sodium hypochlorite irrigation are indicated to reduce or eliminate the pain. Also, there is little need for an intracanal medicament in vital teeth that have been thoroughly débrided. The uncommon need for an intracanal medicament is described in Chapter 8.

Advanced stages of pulpal inflammation or inadvertent instrumentation beyond the confines of the canal space can result in persistent pain due to periapical tissue inflammation. Acute pain may also be seen in the hyperoccluding tooth that has been poorly temporized. Inflammatory pain in the bone and attachment apparatus is exacerbated by biting against the tooth. To provide relief, occlusal reduction or selective adjustment in conjunction with complete canal débridement will alleviate many of the periapical symptoms. Instituting nonsteroidal antiinflammatory drug (NSAID) therapy helps counteract a number of inflammatory pathways that are generating the mild to moderate pain.[19,60]

Intense periapical pain is occasionally seen in vital teeth that have been instrumented to the radiographic apex. Treatment-induced acute apical periodontitis is primarily inflammatory pain. Infection usually is not a factor if treatment is rendered using aseptic techniques. In cases of gross overinstrumentation, a serosanguineous exudate and not pus is seen when a sterile paper point is placed into the apical extent of the canal(s). Medicating through the root canal system with a one-time application of topical corticosteroid in suspension (e.g., Decadron, Meticortelone) can suppress the periradicular inflammation and relieve pain.[17,63] In some of these symptomatic canals, a profuse serosanguineous exudate will continue to be discharged despite repeated and thorough reinstrumentation of the root canal(s). The problematic exudation can be controlled by placing a calcium hydroxide preparation (e.g., $Ca(OH)_2$ USP plus anesthetic solution, Calasept, Pulpdent, Hypo-Cal, Calxyl) against or slightly through the perforated foramen. The remainder of the canal is then filled with the calcium hydroxide paste and temporarily sealed. Once the tooth is comfortable, treatment can be continued by removing the paste and reestablishing and maintaining instrumentation within the length of the canal space.

Sequelae in pulpless teeth. Pain may persist following the initial emergency treatment in symptomatic teeth with partial pulp necrosis. Clinical experience has shown that symptomatic teeth can remain problematic throughout the entire endodontic treatment.[38,65,91] While initially mystifying, the explanation lies in the bacterial contamination of the pulpless teeth.[6,37] Teeth with necrotic pulps, with or without associated periradicular lesions, are more predisposed than vital teeth to develop midtreatment flare-ups.[37,62] The prevalence of infectious swelling is reportedly 1.5% after initial treatment and 5.5% for endodontically treated teeth undergoing retreatment.[76]

Thorough débridement of the entire root canal system is a reasonable goal of initial or midtreatment management of all pulpless teeth.[37] Symptoms notwithstanding, canal patency should be achieved to provide possible drainage. In addition, midtreatment management of persistent or acute onset pain requires that the tooth be assessed for early signs of periapical infection, tenderness on biting or palpation, and increasing tissue pressures.[37]

Early stages of an apical abscess can be suspected when pain is severe and little or no exudate is detected in the canal(s).[37] Pain symptoms are likely to continue for another 48 to 72 hours, until the abscess drains spontaneously or can be drained from the bone or soft tissues. It is important to support the patient throughout this *ongoing emergency* with appropriate antibiotics and analgesics. Morse[60] states that antibiotics administered at the first sign of swelling reduce the severity of the infection and shorten the course of therapy from at least a week to 4 days. Judicious occlusal reduction further reduces pain symptoms. Also, leaving the tooth open, with only a cotton pellet inside the pulp chamber, may allow tissue pressures to vent more quickly. With subsequent development of tissue swelling, treatment is the same as that described for urgent care. On rare occasions, surgical trephination into the cortical bone by raising a flap may be the only recourse for relieving intense pain from buildup of intraosseous pressure (see Chapter 19 on Surgical Endodontics).[2,5]

Remember, *midtreatment flare-ups are infrequent,* even for less experienced clinicians.[59] A majority of the patients (some 75% to 96%) experience little or no pain following institution of endodontic treatment.[37] When flare-ups do occur, pulpless teeth are by far the most problematic.[62,91] With prevention in mind, many investigative studies have attempted to identify and understand the factors that contribute to flare-ups. Unfortunately, the findings have generated controversy.[62] Objectivity is sometimes overshadowed by different perspectives in support of a study's conclusion(s). The advice from Gatewood and coworkers[29] is best remembered here: "Individual patient problems are very difficult to place into specific categories, making it impossible to compose a 'cookbook' approach to the treatment of endodontic emergencies [including flare-ups]".

Perhaps the most important factor identified by investigators is that pulpless teeth with associated periradicular lesions are likely to be infected.[6,27,84,97] It is speculated that inadvertent inoculation of the infectious contents from the root canal(s) predisposes the pulpless tooth to periapical exacerbation.[27,37] In an in vitro study, investigators[25] found that instrumenting the canal, whether manually or mechanically, resulted in extrusion of debris through the foramen. One endodontist[60] suggests that a large-dose, short-term antibiotic regimen (identical to the current American Heart Association prophylactic oral dosing schedule) be given one-half hour before treatment is begun, in pulpless teeth with periradicular lesions. The purpose of such antibiotic therapy is not prophylaxis but treatment of an existing quiescent infection.

Others[37] cautioned, however, that it is unreasonable to routinely subject all patients with pulpless teeth and periradicular lesions to a pretreatment antibiotic regimen. In one large case study of 2000 pulpless cases from a patient pool of more than 10,000 cases, ten times more pulpless teeth *did not* flare up following thorough instrumentation of the root canal(s).[91] This study demonstrates a low incidence of flare-ups (9.1%) and, more importantly, that nine of ten patients did just fine without the benefit of pretreatment antibiotics. Therefore, the need for antibiotics should be determined on the basis of the presenting signs and symptoms[37] or overriding host factors that are discussed below.

Operator factors in flare-ups. It is important, then, to consider additional indicators for susceptibility to flare-ups. Operator factors were discussed in the sections on rendering urgent care and managing midtreatment flare-ups. They are most frequently cited when dentists blame themselves for midtreatment emergencies.[62] If treatment is rendered in a conscientious and competent manner, the practitioner will be relieved to know that there is no significant relationship between the incidence of midtreatment emergencies and the treatment he or she has rendered.[91] Investigators[59] similarly found the incidence to be low following treatment by less experienced clinicians.

The concepts of crown-down cleaning and shaping and confirming apical patency (see Chapter 7) are two preeminent factors that can be important in the strategic management of teeth most likely to exhibit midtreatment flare-ups. Symptomatic pulpless teeth and retreatment cases have been determined by numerous investigators to be predisposed to interappointment exacerbations.[62,76,91] When time restrictions at the initial visit truly prevent achieving the ideal goal of measuring and completing canal instrumentation, a crown-down approach can be more expeditious for removing the bulk of infected organic debris from the tooth, thus reducing the potential for a flare-up.[31] If the tooth length can also be established, apical patency should be established and maintained throughout crown-down instrumentation.[13,31] In the event of an exacerbation, the need to trephinate through the apical foramen may be avoided in the canal(s) with confirmed apical patency.

Also, calcium hydroxide paste has become an important adjunct as an interappointment intracanal medicament, along with sodium hypochlorite for dissolving necrotic tissue,[39,56] and for its antimicrobial properties.[15,74] Calcium hydroxide is efficacious against many anaerobic microbes that are harbored in pulpless teeth. In addition, the antimicrobial potency dissipates much more slowly. In case of prolonged or delayed treatment, an intracanal dressing that eliminates the surviving bacterial contaminants is deemed beneficial.[83]

Host factors in flare-ups. Although most patients with systemic disease undergo uneventful endodontic treatment,[62,91] those with allergies were found to have a higher incidence of midtreatment flare-ups.[91] Heightened immunoreactivity to allergens may explain the intense reaction experienced by some of these patients to antigens that may be extruded from the root canal system. Females of all ages were also found to be slightly more susceptible than their male counterparts to flare-ups, for a variety of reasons.[62,91] Plausible explanations may be differences in hormonal makeup and gender roles. Finally, phobic patients are difficult to treat because of their low psychophysiological tolerance. Dental phobias affect patients of both sexes and all ages. Patients with a history of bad dental treatment and those who seem excessively anxious about pain should alert the dentist to potential management problems and, perhaps, the need for chairside pharmacologic interdiction and sedation (see Chapter 19).

Pain control is paramount for this *select group* of patients. The first step of management is informing them of their particular endodontic situation.[20,37,80,91] Patients should be told generally what can be expected during the treatment that is planned and subsequently rendered. These patients must be reassured of the anticipated outcome at the conclusion of treatment, despite unforeseen pain complications that may arise between treatments. Most importantly, the patients must be assured of access to the dentist if the need arises.[37]

For many of these patients, and especially those with pretreatment pain, oral medications administered just before[60,62] and immediately following[91] the urgent care visit were found to reduce the incidence of midtreatment emergencies. Medications should be chosen specifically to counteract pain from either inflammation or a frank infection. Since endodontic pain results from activation of numerous inflammatory and immune pathways,[88,89] most endodontists prefer NSAIDs over narcotics to interfere with this process and reduce pain symptoms.[29] For infectious swelling, antibiotic therapy must be prescribed as well. A large-dose, short-term therapeutic antibiotic regimen, begun at the conclusion of the initial endodontic visit and used at least 4 days, was found to expedite resolution[52] and significantly reduce the incidence of midtreatment flare-ups.[60,61]

The preceding discussion should not be construed as a general endorsement for routine prophylactic predosing of every patient. Clinically it has been reported that infectious flare-ups occurred about 15% of the time and postoperative pain about 25% of the time.[60] The clinician should use discrimination in identifying the pretreatment condition(s) or the one patient in four who is likely to experience pain and possible swelling. Fortunately, some of these patients identify themselves by requesting medication for "pain." Though drugs should never be prescribed to satisfy the patient's desire or addiction,[60] a request that is reasonable must be considered, not only for its pharmacologic effect but for its psychological value.[19] While the pharmacologic benefits may be questionable, based on the clinical assessment, the clinician must look beyond this to consider why the patient is requesting a "pharmacologic crutch." An outright refusal may deprive the patient of the only available control over his or her situation. Seasoned practitioners have learned to routinely encourage direct participation by the patient in selecting an analgesic or antibiotic that is "most effective."[2,29,60,80] By empirically honoring the request that is reasonable, the practitioner recognizes the psychological impact this can have on the patient and may avert an emergency phone call. In most cases, the patient reports back that the prescription was never filled or that the medication was taken for 1 or 2 days only. If the request is for a mood-altering analgesic (a schedule II or III narcotic), one authority[19] advises that a 2-day regimen is *more than sufficient* to manage acute pain in *most clinical situations*. The patient should then take a locally active analgesic such as one of the NSAIDs or (less effective) acetaminophen.

The Hypochlorite Accident

The hypochlorite accident is a comparatively rare occurrence and is associated with severe pain and swelling *as the clinician is irrigating the root canal.*[7,30] The reaction is quite intense, occurring instantly before the clinican's eyes. The reaction is to hypochlorite or hypochlorite–hydrogen peroxide irrigant being forced through the root canal into the periapical tissues. This can happen only by locking the needle of the irrigating syringe in the canal and forcefully injecting the irrigant (Fig. 2-13).

Management

1. Recognize that a hypochlorite accident has occurred.
2. Attend to the immediate problem of pain and swelling. Administer a regional block with a long-acting anesthetic solution. With the irrigant spreading rapidly over a wide region, pain management is difficult because symptoms from distant anatomic structures will continue to cause discomfort. This also explains the extreme pain felt during the incident, despite establishment of adequate local anesthesia before treatment was begun.
3. Assure and calm the patient. The reaction, while alarmingly fast, is still a localized phenomenon and will resolve with time. If available, nitrous oxide sedation can help the patient cope through the remainder of this emergency.
4. Monitor the tooth over the next half hour. There may be discharge back into the canal of a bloody exudate. This bleeding is the body's reaction to the irrigant.[68] Remove the toxic fluid with high-volume evacuation to encourage further drainage from the periapical tissues. If drainage is persistent, consider leaving the tooth open over the next 24 hours until it stops.
5. Consider antibiotic coverage. If the treated tooth is pulp-

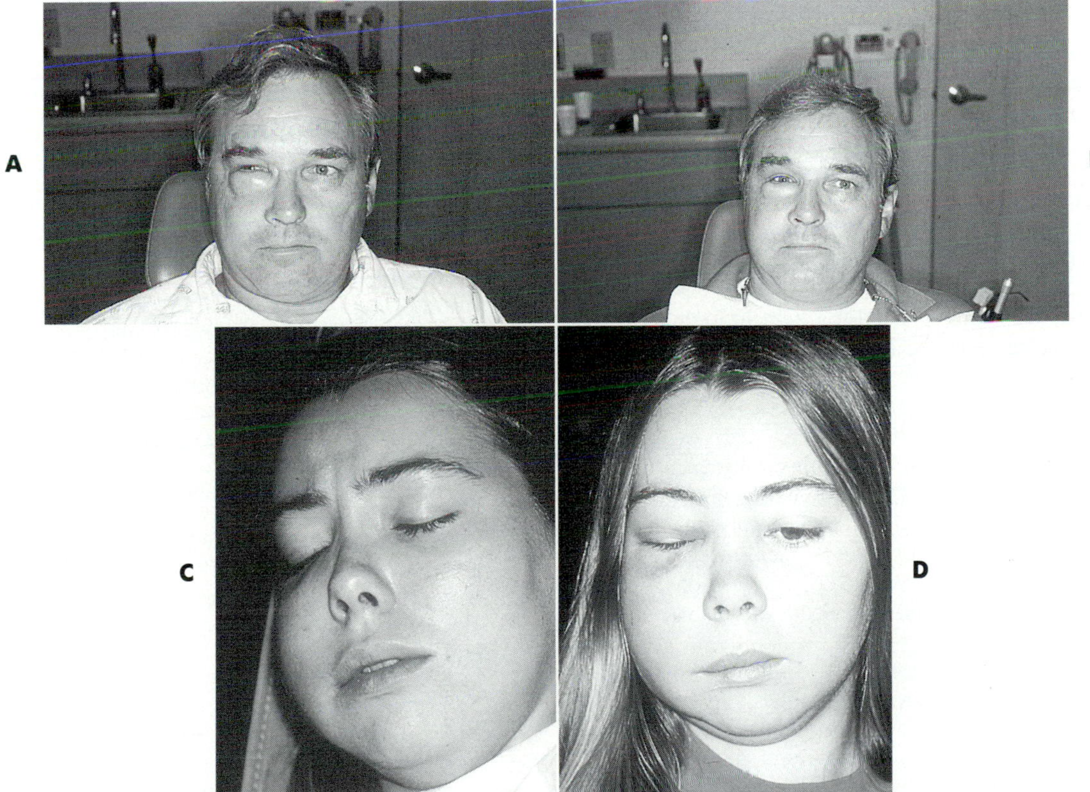

FIG. 2-13 Hypochlorite accident. **A,** Immediate response to a 1.0% solution expressed through the roots of a maxillary premolar. **B,** Presentation 24 hours after the accident. Swelling is evident. (**A** and **B** courtesy of Dr. Peter Chalmers.) **C,** Immediately following mishap through a maxillary canine with a 5.25% solution. The swelling had spread to involve the canine and infraorbital spaces. **D,** Twenty-four hours later, swelling and ecchymosis are evident. (**C** and **D** courtesy of Dr. Ronald Borer.)

less and cleaning and shaping procedures have not been completed, consider prescribing penicillin, 500 mg four times a day, over the next 5 days.

6. Consider an analgesic. Because of possible bleeding complications with aspirin and aspirin derivatives (NSAIDs)[19] an acetaminophen–narcotic analgesic combination may be more appropriate here. If swelling is extensive, it is best to caution the patient to expect bruising or pooling of blood as it subsides.[7,30]
7. Consider referring the patient. If the patient continues to be apprehensive, needs additional reassurance, or develops complications, referral to the oral surgeon or endodontist is appropriate. Informing the specialist about the patient and the nature of the problem will ensure a smooth transition between offices for the patient.

Prevention

A hypochlorite accident is completely avoidable. As an endodontic irrigant, hypochlorite solution is meant only to lavage the pulp chamber clear of noxious debris brought out with instrumentation of the root canal(s). By leaving fresh solution inside the pulp chamber, many endodontists rely on small instruments to effectively and safely bring the fresh irrigant deep into the canal. As canal cleaning and shaping proceeds, coronal flaring of the canal develops. Fresh irrigants passively reach the deeper levels of the canal with little need to deliberately irrigate too deeply.

The following measures are recommended to safeguard against an accident:

1. Bend the irrigating needle at the center to confine the tip of the needle to higher levels in the root canal space and to facilitate access to posterior teeth.
2. Avoid entering deep into a canal where the needle is likely to bind and lock in place.
3. Oscillate the needle in and out of the canal orifice to ensure that the tip is free to express the irrigant.
4. Stop irrigating if the needle jams or if there is any detectable resistance on pressing against the plunger of the syringe.
5. Check the hub of the needle for a tight fit to prevent inadvertent separation and accidental exposure of the irrigant to the patient's eyes.[44]

Postendodontic Complications

The incidence of acute pain or swelling subsequent to the completion of endodontic treatment is extremely low.[80] In cases of midtreatment flare-up conditions resolve in the majority of these teeth (including pulpless ones) to permit sealing of the root canal(s) with no further complications.[4] Postendodontic pain is usually mild, transient, and managed with an appropriate analgesic.

A notable exception may be some teeth that are endodontically completed in a single visit. The popularity of single-visit treatment can be credited to favorable reports that found no difference in the prevalence of treatment complications or success rates when compared with teeth treated in multiple visits.[66,69] The allure of the single-visit approach, however, must be tempered with the understanding that careful case selection and the clinician's expertise figured significantly in achieving the reported outcome. Despite extraordinary treatment precautions and the exceptional skills of the clinician, approximately 10% of the teeth treated in a single visit succumb to complications.[66] It is likely that the prevalence rate is much higher for inexperienced clinicians who are under pressure to properly treat and complete the case within the self-imposed time constraints of the single-visit appointment. For more information on one-visit treatment, the reader is referred to Chapter 3.

With postendodontic flare-ups, serious attention must be given to the patient's description of the pain, in order to identify the cause of the complication. With endodontic therapy, pretreatment pain symptoms will in most cases have decreased or been eliminated if the tooth was accurately identified. A complaint of persistent pain, unremitting pain, or continuing thermal pain should alert the clinician to consider the possibility of misdiagnosis or an overlooked canal.[45,75] A complaint of biting or chewing pain, pressure, or paresthesia in the area should precipitate careful reassessment of the periapical tissues for overinstrumentation, overfilling or underfilling, onset of an apical abscess, or fracture of the crown or root.[57,80]

Emergency management of a postendodontic flare-up is hampered by the presence of the root canal filling. Treatment options are restricted to surgical trephination, root end surgery, and retreatment.[80] The symptomatic tooth that has experienced a procedural mishap, is grossly overfilled, or has developed an apical abscess is best managed by surgical correction supported with appropriate systemic medications. The definitive management of the emergency must follow the same process that was outlined throughout this chapter for diagnosing pain symptoms in any orofacial pain emergency. In the absence of an accurate identification of the problem, the use of analgesics or antibiotics to treat postendodontic complications is considered an inadequate approach.

The art, science, and technology of endodontic diagnosis and treatment have undergone tremendous evolution during the last half of the twentieth century. As a result, the dental profession is strategically positioned to enter into the next century free of the myths, empirical management, and anecdotal remedies that were the resorts of the past.

REFERENCES

1. Andrews CH, England MC, and Kemp WB: Sickle cell anemia: an etiologic factor in pulp necrosis, J Endod 9:249, 1983.
2. Antrim DD, Bakland LK, and Parker MW: Treatment of endodontic urgent care cases, Dent Clin North Am 30:549, 1986.
3. Back DJ, and Orme ML: Pharmacokinetic drug interactions with oral contraceptives, Clin Pharmacokinet 6:472, 1990.
4. Balaban FS, Skidmore AE, and Griffin JA: Acute exacerbations following initial treatment of necrotic pulps, J Endod 10:78, 1984.
5. Baumgartner JC: Treatment of infections and associated lesions of endodontic origin, J Endod 17:418, 1991.
6. Baumgartner JC, and Falkler WA: Bacteria in the apical 5 mm of infected root canals, J Endod 17:380, 1991.
7. Becker GL, Cohen S, and Borer RF: The sequela of accidentally injecting sodium hypochlorite beyond the root apex, Oral Surg Oral Med Oral Pathol 38:633, 1974.
8. Bell WE: Orofacial pains, ed 4, Chicago, 1989, Year Book Medical Publishers.
9. Bender IB: Factors influencing radiographic appearance of bony lesions, J Endod 8:161, 1982.
10. Bender IB, and Naidorf IJ: Dental observations in vitamin D–resistant rickets with special reference to periapical lesions, J Endod 11:514, 1985.
11. Bender IB, and Seltzer S: Roentgenographic and direct observation of experimental lesions in bone, J Am Dent Assoc 62:152, 1961.
12. Blank LW, and Charbeneneau GT: Urgent treatment in operative dentistry, Dent Clin North Am 30:489, 1986.
13. Buchanan LS: Paradigm shifts in cleaning and shaping, Calif Dent Assoc J 19:23, 1991.

14. Byers MR, et al: Effects of injury and inflammation on pulpal and periapical nerves, J Endod 16:78, 1990.
15. Bystrom A, Claesson R, and Sundqvist G: The antibacterial effect of camphorated paramonochlorophenol, camphorated phenol and calcium hydroxide in the treatment of infected root canal, Endod Dent Traumatol 1:170, 1985.
16. Carr GB: Microscopes in endodontics, Calif Dent Assoc J 20:55, 1992.
17. Chance K, et al: Clinical trial of intracanal corticosteroid in root canal therapy, J Endod 13:466, 1987.
18. Ciancio S: Oral contraceptives, antibiotics and pregnancy, Dent Manag 5:54, 1989.
19. Cooper SA: Treating acute pain: do's and don'ts, pros and cons, J Endod 16:85, 1990.
20. Cunningham CJ, and Mullaney TP: Pain control in endodontics, Dent Clin North Am 36:393, 1992.
21. Corah NL: Effect of perceived control on stress reduction in pedodontic patients, J Dent Res 52:1261, 1973.
22. Dietz GC Sr, and Dietz GC Jr: The endodontist and the general dentist, Dent Clin North Am 36:459, 1992.
23. Donnelly JC: Resolution of a periapical radiolucency without root canal filling, J Endod 16:394, 1990.
24. Drinnan AL: Differential diagnosis of orofacial pain, Dent Clin North Am 31:627, 1987.
25. Fairbourn DR, McWalter GM, and Montgomery S: The effect of four preparation techniques on amount of apically extruded debris, J Endod 13:102, 1987.
26. Fricton JR: Recent advances in temporomandibular disorders and orofacial pain, J Am Dent Assoc 122:25, 1991.
27. Fukushima H, et al: Localization and identification of root canal bacteria in clinically asymptomatic periapical pathosis, J Endod 16:534, 1990.
28. Gatchel RJ: Managing anxiety and pain during dental treatment, J Am Dent Assoc 123:37, 1992.
29. Gatewood RS, Himel VT, and Dorn SO: Treatment of the endodontic emergency: a decade later, J Endod 16:284, 1990.
30. Gatot A, et al: Effects of sodium hypochlorite on soft tissues after its inadvertent injection beyond the root apex, J Endod 17:573, 1991.
31. Goerig AC, Michelich RJ, and Schultz HH: Instrumentation of root canals in molars using the step-down technique, J Endod 8:550, 1982.
32. Goon WWY, and Jacobsen PL: Prodromal odontalgia and multiple devitalized teeth caused by a herpes zoster infection of the trigeminal nerve: report of case, J Am Dent Assoc 116:500, 1988.
33. Graff-Radford SB, and Solberg WK: Atypical odontalgia, Calif Dent Assoc J 14:27, 1986.
34. Guinta JL: Comparison of erysipelas and odontogenic cellulitis, J Endod 13:291, 1987.
35. Hargreaves KM, Troullos ES, and Dionne RA: Pharmacologic rationale for the treatment of acute pain, Dent Clin North Am 31:675, 1987.
36. Harness DM, and Rome HP: Psychological and behavioral aspects of chronic facial pain, Otolaryngol Clin North Am 22:1073, 1989.
37. Harrington GW, and Natkin E: Midtreatment flare-ups, Dent Clin North Am 36:409, 1992.
38. Harrison JW, Baumgartner JC, and Svec TA: Incidence of pain associated with clinical factors during and after root canal therapy, Part II, postobturation pain, J Endod 9:434, 1983.
39. Hasselgren G, Olsson B, and Cvek: Effects of calcium hydroxide and sodium hypochlorite on the dissolution of necrotic porcine muscle tissue, J Endod 14:125, 1988.
40. Head TW, et al: A comparative study of the effectiveness of metronidazole and penicillin V in eliminating anaerobes from post extraction bacteremias, Oral Surg Oral Med Oral Pathol 58:152, 1984.
41. Holmes-Johnson E, Geboy M, and Getka EJ: Behavior considerations, Dent Clin North Am 30:391, 1986.
42. Holroyd SV, Wynn RL, and Requa-Clark B: Clinical pharmacology in dental practice, ed 4, St Louis, 1988, CV Mosby Co.
43. Hutter JW: Facial space infections of odontogenic origin, J Endod 17:422, 1991.
44. Ingram TA: Response of the human eye to accidental exposure to sodium hypochlorite, J Endod 16:235, 1990.
45. Keir DM, et al: Thermally induced pulpalgia in endodontically treated teeth, J Endod 17:38, 1991.
46. Kim S: Microcirculation of the dental pulp in health and disease, J Endod 11:465, 1985.
47. Kim S: Neurovascular interactions in the dental pulp in health and inflammation, J Endod 16:48, 1990.
48. Kim S, et al: Effects of local anesthetics on pulp blood flow in dogs, J Dent Res 63:650, 1984.
49. Lin LM, and Skribner J: Why teeth associated with periapical lesions can have a vital response, Clin Prevent Dent 12:3, 1990.
50. Little JW: Prosthetic implants: risk of infection from transient dental bacteremias, Compend Contin Educ Dent 12:160, 1991.
51. Matusow RJ: The acute endodontic cellulitis syndrome: biologic and clinical aspects, J Endod 16:401, 1990.
52. Matusow RJ, and Goodall LB: Anaerobic isolates in primary pulpal-alveolar cellulitis cases: endodontic resolutions and drug therapy considerations, J Endod 9:535, 1983.
53. McMahon RE, Adams W, and Spolnik KJ: Diagnostic anesthesia for referred trigeminal pain: Part 2, Compend Contin Educ Dent 13:980, 1992.
54. Merrill RL, and Graff-Radford SB: Trigeminal neuralgia: how to rule out the wrong treatment, J Am Dent Assoc 123:63, 1992.
55. Merskey H, et al: Pain terms: a list with definitions and notes on usage, recommended by the IASP sub-committee on taxonomy, Pain 6:249, 1979.
56. Metzler RS, and Montgomery S: The effectiveness of ultrasonics and calcium hydroxide for the debridement of human mandibular molars, J Endod 15:373, 1989.
57. Montgomery S: Paresthesia following endodontic treatment, J Endod 2:345, 1976.
58. Montgomery S, and Ferguson CD: Diagnostic, treatment planning, and prognostic considerations, Dent Clin North Am 30:533, 1986.
59. Mor C, Rotstein I, and Friedman S: Incidence of interappointment emergency associated with endodontic therapy, J Endod 18:509, 1992.
60. Morse DR: The use of analgesics and antibiotics in endodontics: current concepts, Alpha Omegan 83:26, 1990.
61. Morse DR, et al: Infectious flare-ups and serious sequelae following endodontic treatment: a prospective randomized trial on efficacy of antibiotic prophylaxis in cases of asymptomatic pulpal-periapical lesions, Oral Surg Oral Med Oral Pathol 64:96, 1987.
62. Morse DR, et al: Endodontic flare-ups: the tape, J Endod 14:106, 1988.
63. Moskow A, et al: Intracanal use of a corticosteroid solution as an endodontic anodyne, Oral Surg Oral Med Oral Pathol 58:600, 1984.
64. Nash O: Face is familiar, Boston, 1938, Little, Brown and Co.
65. O'Keefe EM: Pain in endodontic therapy: preliminary study, J Endod 2:315, 1976.
66. Oliet S: Single-visit endodontics: a clinical study, J Endod 9:147, 1983.
67. Pallasch TJ: Antibiotic prophylaxis: theory and reality, Calif Dent Assoc J 6:27, 1989.
68. Pashley EL, et al: Cytotoxic effects of $NaOCl^-$ on vital tissue, J Endod 11:525, 1985.
69. Pekruhn RB: The incidence of failure following single-visit endodontic therapy, J Endod 12:68, 1986.
70. Pinsawasdi P, and Seltzer S: The induction of trigeminal neuralgia-like symptoms by pulp-periapical pathosis, J Endod 12:73, 1986.
71. Rauch JW. Barodontalgia—dental pain related to ambient pressure change, Gen Dent 33:313, 1985.
72. Rubin JG, Slovin M, and Krochak M: The psychodynamics of dental anxiety and dental phobia, Dent Clin North Am 32:647, 1988.
73. Rugh JD: Psychological components of pain, Dent Clin North Am 31:579, 1987.
74. Safavi KE, et al: A comparison of antimicrobial effects of calcium hydroxide and iodine–potassium iodide, J Endod 11:454, 1985.
75. Schwartz S, and Cohen S: The difficult differential diagnosis, Dent Clin North Am 36:279, 1992.

76. Selbst AG: Understanding informed consent and its relationship to the incidence of adverse treatment events in conventional endodontic therapy, J Endod 16:387, 1990.
77. Selden HS: The endo-antral syndrome, J Endod 3:462, 1977.
78. Seltzer S; Endodontology: biologic considerations in endodontic procedures, ed 2, Philadelphia, 1988, Lea & Febiger.
79. Seltzer S, and Naidorf IJ: Flare-ups in endodontics: I. etiologic factors, J Endod 11:472, 1985.
80. Seltzer S, and Naidorf IJ: Flare-ups in endodontics: II. Therapeutic measures, J Endod 11:559, 1985.
81. Sessle BJ: Neurophysiology of orofacial pain, Dent Clin North Am 31:595, 1987.
82. Sherman A, and Jacobsen PL: Managing dental hypersensitivity: what treatment to recommend to patients, J Am Dent Assoc 123:57, 1992.
83. Sundqvist G: Ecology of the root canal flora, J Endod 18:427, 1992.
84. Sundqvist G, Johansson E, and Sjogren U: Prevalence of black-pigmented *Bacteroides* species in root canal infections, J Endod 15:13, 1989.
85. Takahashi K: Changes in the pulp vasculature during inflammation, J Endod 16:92, 1990.
86. Terezhalmy GT, and McDavid PT: The physical examination, Dent Clin North Am 30:369, 1986.
87. Todd HW, and Langeland K: Pulpal destruction of neoplastic etiology, J Endod 13:299, 1987.
88. Torabinejad M: Mediators of pulpal and periapical pathosis, Calif Dent Assoc J 14:21, 1986.
89. Torabinejad M: Management of endodontic emergencies: facts and fallacies, J Endod 18:417, 1992.
90. Torabinejad M, Eby WC, and Naidorf IJ: Inflammatory and immunological aspects of the pathogenesis of human periapical lesions, J Endod 11:479, 1985.
91. Torabinejad M, et al: Factors associated with endodontic interappointment emergencies of teeth with necrotic pulps, J Endod 14:261, 1988.
92. Trowbridge HO: Intradental sensory units: physiological and clinical aspects, J Endod 11:489, 1985.
93. Van Hassel HJ: Physiology of the human dental pulp, Oral Surg Oral Med Oral Pathol 32:126, 1971.
94. Walton RE: The periodontal ligament injection as a primary technique, J Endod 16:62, 1990.
95. Wong MKS, and Jacobsen PL: Reasons for local anesthesia failures, J Am Dent Assoc 123:69, 1992.
96. Young ER, Saso MA, and Pulver E: Acute chest pain during dental treatment: a case report, J Can Dent Assoc 56:437, 1990.
97. Yoshida M, et al: Correlation between clinical symptoms and microorganisms isolated from root canals of teeth with periapical pathosis, J Endod 13:24, 1987.

Self-assessment questions

1. Pulpal pain response is
   a. dull and throbbing when carried by A-delta myelinated nerve fibers.
   b. dull and throbbing when carried by A-delta unmyelinated nerve fibers.
   c. quick and sharp when carried by A-delta myelinated nerve fibers.
   d. quick and sharp when carried by A-delta unmyelinated nerve fibers.
2. Pulpal pain response is
   a. dull and throbbing when carried by myelinated C fibers.
   b. dull and throbbing when carried by unmyelinated C fibers.
   c. quick and sharp when carried by myelinated C fibers.
   d. quick and sharp when carried by unmyelinated C fibers.
3. Nonspecific biochemical mediators are
   a. pyruvic acid, prostaglandins, and aspartic acid.
   b. arachidonic acid and the complement system.
   c. histamine, bradykinin, prostaglandins, and leukotrienes.
   d. arachidonic acid and serotonin.
4. Neuropeptides such as substance P and calcitonin gene–related peptide (CGRP)
   a. are released from capillaries.
   b. are released from sensitized nerves.
   c. are not part of the inflammatory cycle.
   d. are found in the absence of pain and inflammation.
5. Trigeminal neuralgia differs from odontogenic pain by being
   a. continuous and dull.
   b. sharp and shooting.
   c. sharp, shooting, repetitive, and triggered.
   d. dull and throbbing.
6. Maxillary sinusitis associated with acute tooth pain
   a. is a seasonal phenomenon.
   b. can involve the entire quadrant up to the midline.
   c. can involve the mandible.
   d. is initiated by psychogenic factors.
7. Pain is most commonly referred from
   a. lower anterior teeth to ipsilateral upper molars.
   b. lower molars to upper anteriors.
   c. posterior molars to the opposing quadrant or to other teeth in same quadrant.
   d. upper molars to the contralateral lower quadrant.
8. Odontogenic symptoms are elicited primarily by the following provoking stimuli:
   a. thermal (heat, cold), percussion, palpation.
   b. postural changes.
   c. pain following exertion.
   d. barometric changes.
9. In the presence of an intense inflammatory process, nerve block injections are rendered less effective owing to
   a. distance to source of irritation.
   b. pH changes of inflammation.
   c. length of needle.
   d. prior use of analgesics.
10. For effective urgent care management of the routine endodontic emergency
    a. leave the pulp chamber open for drainage.
    b. pulpotomy will suffice.
    c. after pulpectomy, close the pulp chamber with a temporary dressing.
    d. incise with a scalpel.
11. Localized swelling as an extension of pulpal disease
    a. requires antibiotic therapy alone.
    b. requires analgesics.
    c. is managed using incision, drainage, and an indwelling drain.
    d. resolves without treatment.
12. Flare-ups occur more often
    a. in the afternoon and evening.
    b. in endodontic treatment of vital teeth.
    c. in endodontic treatment of pulpless teeth.
    d. in teenagers.
13. To assess pain intensity, the most useful measure is
    a. how much analgesia the patient requires.
    b. how well the patient eats and sleeps.
    c. zero to ten verbal analogue scale.
    d. the patient's own words.
14. Pain can most frequently be expected as a result of
    a. pulpitis.
    b. a nonvital tooth.
    c. an overinstrumented root canal system.
    d. after routine endodontic therapy.

Chapter 3

Nonodontogenic Facial Pain and Endodontics: Pain Syndromes of the Jaws That Simulate Odontalgia

Lewis R. Eversole

Pain can be the vilest of human experiences. Sometimes it is merely annoying; at other times it is excruciating to the point where the system can no longer handle the experience and the sufferer loses consciousness. Of all the symptoms that the dentist must confront, pain is the most poignant. Ridding the patient of pain is perhaps the most rewarding aspect of practice. The ultimate purpose of the pain response is to inform the patient of a severe or even life-threatening pathologic process. It is, of course, the intent of our pain pathways to inform us of pathologic processes, and in the practice of endodontics, the elimination of pulpal infection is the ultimate goal for odontogenic pain.

To the dismay of the patient, and often the practitioner, this signaling system is occasionally triggered in the absence of noxious stimuli, or it may be exaggerated beyond the severity of the underlying pathologic process. In this regard, the pain experience can be likened to the immune response. Certainly, the intricacies of the immune system were developed to protect the host from foreign agents that have the potential to destroy tissue (i.e., pathogens). In some hosts, however, the immune response is triggered by harmless foreign particles. In the context of a hypersensitivity or allergic reaction, the host immune system is stimulated and the various cellular and biochemical components of this response often result in unpleasant symptoms, including pain. Pain may be analogous to immune hypersensitivity in that symptoms may appear in the absence of a readily identifiable pathologic or detrimental process. Whereas some pain syndromes are associated with a low-grade inflammatory lesion, others seem not to be associated with an underlying disease process. Though many of these pain syndromes are touted as psychogenic problems, the precise cause and pathogenesis have yet to be deciphered. As more research findings unfold and more is learned about various neurotransmitter peptides, eventually we will solve the puzzles of chronic pain for which we now have no explanations.

THE NATURE OF PAIN

Normally, the pain experience is initiated on a physiologic basis by way of the peripheral nervous system. Recall that nerve fibers have a nucleus, the cell body, that is located either within the central nervous system or in ganglia located in the peripheral tissues. Emanating from the cell body are long processes referred to as *axis cylinders*. A single nerve comprises hundreds of individual axis cylinders that are encased in a fibrous capsule known as the perineurium. Each individual axis cylinder is ensheathed by specialized cells, the Schwann cells. Thus, the peripheral nerve can be envisioned as a bundle of electrical cables, all with their own enveloping insulation. Some axis cylinders with their associated Schwann cells have an additional insulating layer known as *myelin,* a specialized lipid synthesized by the Schwann cells. Those fibers capable of transmitting noxious stimuli (i.e., nociceptors) lack a myelin sheath. These nonmyelinated fibers are also referred to as *C fibers* as opposed to certain A or B fibers that transmit nonpainful sensory stimuli. The nerve endings of nociceptor C fibers are found in the skin and mucosa, and of course are prevalent throughout the jaws, teeth, and periodontal tissues. In the region of the jaws, the nociceptor fibers are components of the trigeminal nerve. All of these nociceptors in the trigeminal system have their cell bodies located in the gasserian ganglion, and the afferent axis cylinders that feed into these cell bodies exit the ganglion and extend toward the central nervous system through the trigeminal trunk that enters the pons. These fibers then progress from the pons inferiorly into the upper aspects of the cervical region of the spinal cord. It is in this location where the axis cylinders terminate in a region referred to as the *caudate nucleus of V*. Nerves that are transmitting proprioceptive signals and light touch terminate higher in the spinal cord (mesencephalic nucleus). Fibers that terminate in the caudate nucleus are nociceptors that interdigitate with secondary neurons which then pass superiorly into the brain itself. At this synapse in the caudate nucleus neuropeptides are secreted that are capable of transmitting a noxious impulse from the C fiber across the synapse to the secondary nerve fiber. In addition, other fibers have been identified that modulate this neurotransmitter pathway. Interneurons also have fiber endings that contact the incoming nociceptor fiber and are capable of secreting yet other neurotransmitters that are capable of inhibiting propagation of noxious stimuli. Many of these inhibitory neurosecretory molecules fall into a special class of peptides known as *endorphins*.

Some time ago, a theory was proposed to explain how noxious stimuli became consciously identifiable in the higher centers of the brain. This *gate theory of pain* was based on observation of a variety of interconnections in the region of the synapse. As noxious stimuli became more accentuated, the so-called gate would open and allow the impulses to be transmitted across the synapse. Indeed, neuroscience researchers have provided evidence that the gatekeeper is, in fact, represented by neurotransmitter molecules. Once noxious stimuli, such as chemical moieties in an acutely inflamed dental pulp, stimulate nociceptor fibers and the impulse is transmitted across the synapse in the caudate nucleus, the signal is further propagated through the secondary neuron to the midbrain. In this region, the secondary fibers terminate in the vicinity of the thalamus. This region of the midbrain, the periaqueductal gray matter, is an area under significant neurosecretory molecular influences and is involved in a variety of emotions. It is thus interesting to speculate how some pain syndromes may be modified by the patient's psychological and emotional status. From this area of the brain, tertiary and quaternary neurons synapse and transmit the nerve impulse to the cerebral cortex. It is at this level that the patient actually becomes conscious of the pain symptom.

Nociceptor fibers are stimulated by a variety of physical and chemical stimuli. During an infection or in the face of trauma the tissues release noxious chemicals, including both peptides and lipids. In acute inflammation, the pH often drops below 5, and it is well-documented that both acidic and alkaline solutions stimulate firing of nociceptor fibers. Excessive heat, like that from an electrical burn or thermal injury, stimulates nociceptor fibers as well. In the context of the inflammatory reaction, kinins and prostaglandins, small vasoactive molecules, also have strong nociceptor-stimulating effects. Acute compressive forces on nerve endings may also produce pain, and this compression may be the result of cellular infiltrates into tissues and edema formation. As a rule, the patient is able to localize the specific region of pain where the tissue harbors the pathologic process that has engendered the pain sensation. As clinicians are well aware, severe and acute pain may not always be readily localized. The neuroanatomic basis for the inability to specifically localize severe pain is ill-understood. Eventually, sometimes within 2 or 3 hours, sometimes after 2 or 3 days, the pain becomes more precisely localized.

Sharp pains are precipitated by acute pathologic processes. Alternatively, low-grade or chronic inflammatory conditions frequently manifest as dull aches. Acute infectious or traumatic stimuli tend to cause sudden onset of pain of short duration. *Pain syndromes that fail to show any organic basis commonly present as aching, chronic pains of long duration*. Therefore, pain as a symptom must be precisely characterized in order to arrive at a definitive diagnosis. The clinician is usually confronted with a specific complaint for which more than one entity must be considered. In this chapter we will consider the facial pain syndromes according to the type of pain symptoms that the patient describes, thus constructing a differential diagnoses for specific types of complaints.

Pain may be classified as either acute or chronic. Acute pains are of short duration; chronic pains may last weeks, months, or even years. Another characteristic that must be elicited from the patient is the fluctuating nature of the pain. Some pains that are acute appear for a few days and completely disappear, whereas other acute pains are episodic or paroxysmal, appearing once or twice a day and lasting anywhere from seconds to many minutes. With chronic pain, the pain experience frequently fluctuates from hour to hour or day to day. Some patients may complain of chronic pain that begins as a mere nuisance in the morning and builds to a more severe ache in the late afternoon. Identification of precipitating factors is diagnostically important. Sometimes gravity influences the severity of the pain; simply by placing the head below the knees the patient may experience an exacerbation. Exposure of tooth surfaces to hot and cold certainly is a well-recognized precipitating factor for pulpal pain. Patients may relate exacerbation of pain to emotional stress, jaw clenching, turning the head from left to right, or noting an increase in severity during mealtimes. It is therefore important to explore with the patient any factors that could precipitate an exacerbation of symptoms and to evaluate these in the context of the differential diagnosis.

Anatomic considerations are, of course, extremely important in the differential diagnosis of facial pains, though most pain localized to teeth or the jaw bones is odontogenic in origin. From time to time the clinician may encounter nonodontogenic sources for tooth- and jaw-related pain symptoms. The anatomic sites that must be evaluated in the patient who presents with pain of unknown origin include the teeth, the periodontium, the masticatory musculature, the salivary glands, the sinus linings, the middle ear, and effects within the nerve itself.

In the overall process of patient assessment, particularly when compiling physical findings, it is important to assess the function of cranial nerves. Clinicians are often concerned about the possibility that facial pain is a harbinger of malignancy. In reality, malignant tumors that cause facial pain symptoms are extremely rare.[6a] When they do occur, they often invade areas of the skull and cranial base, with resultant neural compression. Therefore, motor deficits are a common concomitant. A brief evaluation of cranial nerve function takes only 1 minute and is easy to accomplish. Initially, the patient is questioned

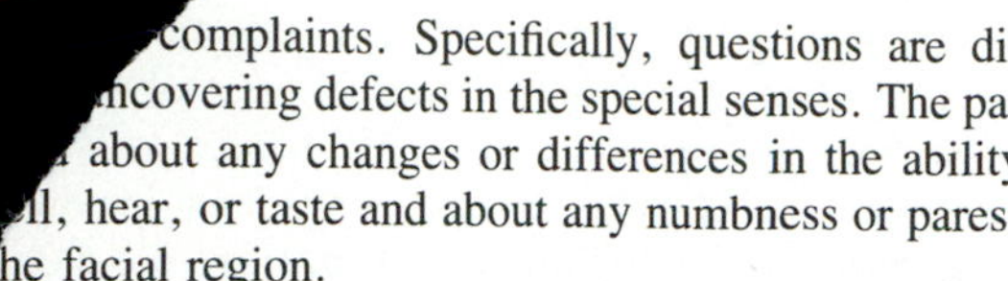

complaints. Specifically, questions are di- ncovering defects in the special senses. The pa- about any changes or differences in the ability ll, hear, or taste and about any numbness or pares- the facial region.

ctive screening of cranial nerves is relatively simple. st, the trigeminal sensory pathways are evaluated by using a cotton tip to test for light touch sensation of the forehead, the cheek, and the chin for all three divisions. This can also be done intraorally along the lateral border of the tongue and the palate as well as on the buccal mucosa. The sensory tract of nerve VII can be evaluated by stimulating the skin around the external auditory meatus. This is quickly followed by an assessment of pain sensation, which can be accomplished using a dental explorer. First, the patient is allowed to experience a brief pinprick on their hand from the explorer, to show what sensation they should expect. Then the same areas of the face are stimulated with a light touch of the sharp explorer point to the skin. The patient should feel all stimuli, and if all sensory pathways are intact the sensation should be the same in one site as in the next.

Once sensory pathways have been evaluated, the objective examination turns to motor function. The cranial nerves that innervate the facial musculature are often grouped together. In this regard, those cranial nerves that innervate the extraocular muscles are evaluated together. Nerves III, IV, and VI can be evaluated by having the patient track a moving object with the eyes. The tracking involves vertical upward and downward movements of the object and side-to-side movements. The object is returned to the center of the patient's gaze and moved down and out in both right and left directions. If the patient's eyes are able to follow the up, down, side-to-side, and down-and-out movements, then nerves III, IV, and VI are intact.

The motor function of nerve VII is assessed by asking the patient to wrinkle the forehead, raise the eyebrows, close the eyes, pucker the lips, and smile. Hypoglossal function is evaluated by having the patient protrude the tongue and move it left and right. Finally, spinal accessory innervation is assessed by having the patient shrug the shoulders against the resistance of a hand placed on the top of the shoulder. Among patients who present with facial pain, should a motor or a sensory deficit be encountered (either paraesthesia or hypoesthesia) a serious organic disease should be suspected.

ACUTE PAIN SYNDROMES OF THE JAWS

Acute pain is defined as pain of sudden onset that either lasts only a few days or exhibits short-lived episodic exacerbations. Patients describe these pains as sharp, stabbing, or lancinating. Such comments as "It feels like a hot poker is jammed into my jaw" or "It feels like a sharp electrical jolt" are commonly related. Once the usual and customary diagnostic approaches have been undertaken to rule out pain of pulpal or periodontal origin, then other disease processes that cause acute pain must be considered. Acute pain syndromes that are episodic or paroxysmal usually represent neuralgias or vasodilatory pain syndromes. Sharp, acute pains that persist for many hours or days are more likely to represent a nociceptor response to organic disease, usually an acute infectious processes. Table 3-1 lists the major pain syndromes subsumed under the rubric of acute pain. For each of these disorders one should consider the clinical features, nature and duration of the pain, and precipitating factors. Some pain syndromes are diagnosed on the basis of exclusion, though most have unique signs and symptoms that allow a definitive diagnosis.

Trigeminal Neuralgia*

Trigeminal neuralgia, or tic douloureux, is a facial pain disorder that has very specific clinical features. The pain involves one or more of the trigeminal nerve divisions, and although the precise cause is unknown, empirical evidence suggests that the symptoms evolve as a consequence of vascular compression of the Gasserian ganglion. The precise neurophysiologic mechanism has not been uncovered, and other theories for this particular disorder include viral infection of either neurons or the Schwann cell sheath.

Two highly characteristic features of tic douloureux allow it to be differentiated from other facial pain syndromes. The character and duration of the symptoms are unique, and a specific anatomic trigger point generally can be identified. The pain tends to involve primarily either the maxillary or the mandibular division, although the ophthalmic division is sometimes involved. The pain is severe and lancinating, shooting into the bone and teeth. Frequently, both patient and dentist are convinced that the source of the pain is pulpal. The electrical quality of the pain is unique and is rarely encountered in

*References 7, 20, 25, 26, 32, 33.

TABLE 3-1. Differentiating acute pains

Condition	Nature	Triggers	Duration
Odontalgia	Stabbing, throbbing, nonepisodic	Hot, cold, tooth percussion	Hours-days
Trigeminal neuralgia	Lancinating, electrical, episodic	1-2 mm locus on skin/mucosa, light touch triggers pain	Seconds
Cluster headache	Severe ache, retroorbital component, episodic	REM sleep, alcohol	30-45 min
Acute otitis media	Severe ache, throbbing, deep to ear, nonepisodic	Lowering head, barometric pressure	Hours-days
Bacterial sinusitis	Severe ache, throbbing in multiple posterior maxillary teeth, nonepisodic	Lowering head, tooth percussion	Hours-days
Cardiogenic	Short-lived ache in left posterior mandible, episodic	Exertion	Minutes
Sialolithiasis	Sharp, drawing, salivary swelling, episodic	Eating, induced salivation	Constant low-level ache, sharp brief episodes when triggered

odontogenic infections. Furthermore, the pain episode lasts only seconds at a time, although paroxysms may occur in rapid succession. Somewhere on the facial skin, or occasionally in the oral cavity, a trigger zone exists. This trigger area may be only 2 mm wide. When it is merely touched with the finger or an instrument the pain paroxysms are triggered. The patient is usually keenly aware of this small anatomic site and will do anything to avoid stimulating the spot.

Treatment modalities are quite varied and include medical intervention with specific drugs that alleviate the neuralgic pain and various surgical interventions. For the dentist, the most salient advice is to establish a diagnosis and avoid any invasive dental procedures. Invariably, patients with trigeminal neuralgia have undergone numerous endodontic procedures and extractions but continue to experience pain since pulpal and periodontal infectious processes have no role in this syndrome. Therefore, despite the insistence by the patient that the symptoms are tooth related, the diagnosis should be established and the patient should be referred to a neurologist for definitive therapy.

Carbamazepine (Tegretol), the standard medical therapy for trigeminal neuralgia, is quite effective. Unfortunately, this particular drug is a bone marrow suppressant and will eventually produce agranulocytosis. This side effect is dose dependent. Therefore, many patients may be maintained on Tegretol without untoward effects if the dose can be restricted to a level where agranulocytosis does not occur yet pain symptoms are alleviated. For patients who do not respond to medical treatment a variety of surgical modalities have been advocated, including peripheral neurectomy, rhizotomy (severance of the nerve trunk at its exit from the ganglion), alcohol injections, and glycerol injections. All of these therapies have met with some degree of success. Two surgical procedures are widely accepted among the neurosurgical community for the relief of trigeminal neuralgia. The hypothesis that vascular compression on the ganglion is a causative factor has met with some acceptance, since surgical decompression of the ganglion often results in prolonged reduction of pain symptoms. Another successful approach is transcutaneous ganglionic neurolysis in which a probe is placed into the ganglion and the neurons are ablated by thermal means. Both of these procedures have resulted in 90% success over a 5-year period. Again, it is stressed that dental extraction or endodontic therapy is contraindicated in trigeminal neuralgia.

Cluster Headache[9,19,23,24]

Cluster headache, also known as *Sluder's neuralgia* or *sphenopalatine ganglion neuralgia,* is an acute paroxysmal pain syndrome of no known cause. The pathogenesis is hypothesized to be a consequence of vasodilatory phenomena that occur on an episodic basis. Presumably, nociceptor fibers that encircle vessels are stimulated during acute vasodilatation. If this is the case, cluster headache is a form of migraine.

Cluster headache is generally encountered among males in their 30s through 50s. Although precipitating factors are not always identifiable, many of these patients report onset of pain after consuming alcohol. There is a tendency for the patients who suffer from cluster headaches to have a unique facial appearance: they are often freckled and have a ruddy complexion. Onset and duration of the pain episodes are quite unique and easily diagnosed. In classic cluster headache, the pain is located unilaterally in the maxilla, sinus, and retroorbital area. It is often mistaken for acute pulpitis or apical abscess of a posterior maxillary tooth. The pain frequen[illegible] ter the patient retires and is entering the early [illegible] sleep. The onset is rather acute and severe with [illegible] cating that it feels like a hot poker has been jamme[illegible] upper jaw and behind the eye. Typically, the pain [illegible] to increase in severity and persists for 30 to 45 minute[illegible] ing this period the patient finds it difficult to remain se[illegible] and tends to pace the floor. The symptoms occur at approximately the same time, once each evening, though some people suffer two such episodes a day. Interestingly, in the classic form of cluster headache, the episodic symptoms persist only 6 to 8 weeks and then spontaneously disappear. Hence the term *cluster headache*. The headache episodes cluster at a certain time of day, and during a certain season. They seem to be more prevalent in spring.

Another form of cluster headache is referred to as *chronic cluster*. These headaches are similar to the classic form in that they occur on an episodic basis and typically last 30 to 45 minutes, but they affect the patient year round rather than seasonally.

In the past, because vasodilatation is involved in their pathogenesis, cluster headaches were managed by prescribing ergotamine tartrate. This medication causes significant side effects, including nausea and vomiting, so it is prescribed as a suppository. Because ergot alkaloids induce vasoconstriction they are contraindicated for patients with hypertension, and many patients with cluster headache are also hypertensive. It was subsequently discovered that oxygen would lessen the headache attacks if administered at the onset of pain. Administration of oxygen is often used as a diagnostic intervention.

The current therapy for cluster headache employs vasoactive drugs, particularly the calcium channel blockers. Nifedipine or one of its related compounds, when prescribed on a regular basis, prevents the pain paroxysms. This medication is of benefit for both classic and chronic cluster headache. In addition, prednisone in combination with lithium has been shown to be effective in alleviating or preventing pain of cluster headache, and more recently serotonin agonists have been demonstrated to be efficacious in clinical trials.

Acute Otitis Media[11]

Infection of the middle ear is common, particularly in children, and is caused by pyogenic micro-organisms, usually streptococci. It is well known that odontogenic infections of posterior teeth may refer pain back to the ear/TMJ area; similarly, middle ear infections may be confused with odontogenic pain, since the symptoms radiate from the ear over the posterior aspects of the maxilla and mandible. It would be unlikely for middle ear infection to be manifested by jaw pain exclusively. The nature of the pain is acute. Patients complain of a severe ache, and throbbing is a frequent accompaniment. Gravitational factors may also come into play. The pain is often exacerbated as the patient lowers the head.

The pathogenesis is straightforward and is, in many ways, similar to that of acute pulp pain. In the dental pulp the noxious components of the inflammatory process and factors secreted by the pathogenic micro-organisms accumulate in a confined space. In otitis media, the infection occurs within the middle ear, which is confined laterally by the tympanic membrane and posteriorly by the oval window; laterally the eustachian tube serves as an outlet. In the process of acute inflammation, with accumulation of neutrophils, exudate, and associated mucosal edema, the eustachian tube lining mucosa swells and …

… Rarely, sy- … nce the diagnosis is established, re- … to an otolaryngologist is recommended.

Acute Maxillary Sinusitis[3,17]

Since the roots of the maxillary teeth extend to the sinus floor, it is axiomatic that acute infectious processes involving the sinus mucous membrane will simulate dental pain. Most forms of sinusitis are allergic and are characterized by chronic pain symptoms as manifested by a dull ache in the malar region and maxillary alveolus.

When maxillary sinusitis is the consequence of an acute pyogenic bacterial infection the symptoms are usually acute. The pain may be stabbing, with severe aching pressure and throbbing. Pain is frequently referred upward under the orbit and downward over the maxillary posterior teeth. Importantly, pain is not referred to a single tooth but is perceived in all teeth in the quadrant. Percussion sensitivity of the molar teeth is a common finding. Typically, when the head is placed below the knees, the pain is exacerbated.

The aforementioned signs and symptoms are rather characteristic; however, other diagnostic approaches can be employed to secure a definitive diagnosis. Transillumination is a diagnostic aid and is easy to perform. A fibro-optic light beam is placed against the palate, and in a darkened room a clear sinus will transilluminate. Antra that are filled with exudate are clouded and will not transilluminate. Radiographic imaging is also of considerable diagnostic utility. Although more advanced imaging such as MRI and CT may be employed, a Water's sinus is usually sufficient.

Since maxillary root apices are separated from the antral floor by a few millimeters of bone, it is understandable that acute periapical infection could spread into the sinus. Therefore, bacterial sinusitis can be a consequence of pulpal infection. It is essential to assess each individual maxillary tooth when a patient presents with acute maxillary sinusitis, since treatment of the sinusitis without management of the dental source will only result in recurrence of symptoms.

Whereas acute bacterial sinusitis is generally readily responsive to antibiotic therapy, induced sinus drainage and lavage may occasionally be necessary when the ostia are closed due to edema. At the time of examination, culture and sensitivity tests should be obtained to select the appropriate antibiotic should preliminary therapy fail to resolve the infection. Referral to an otolaryngologist is recommended.

Cardiogenic Jaw Pain[1,27]

Vascular occlusive disease is one of the most common afflictions of modern society. The accumulation of atherosclerotic plaque in coronary vessels in association with vasospasm will lead to angina pectoris. The most common manifestation of coronary vascular occlusion, particularly in its acute manifestation, is substernal pain with referred pain rotating over the left shoulder and down the arm. This pain is usually precipitated by exertion. Presumably, the pain sensation is transmitted by nociceptor fibers that envelop the coronary vasculature and are stimulated by vasospasm. Of course, angina pectoris … ascertain … symptoms represent a …, angina pectoris is mani- … left shoulder and arm pain without a substernal component. Even less frequent is referral of pain up the neck into the left angle of the mandible. In these instances, the referred pain may mimic odontalgia.

When a patient presents with left posterior mandibular pain and there is no obvious odontogenic source of infection, referred cardiogenic pain should be considered. Importantly, the patient should be questioned about the onset of the symptoms. If they occur after exercise or other exertion, then coronary vascular disease should be an important consideration.

Once suspected, specific diagnostic tests can be performed to assess the potential for coronary vascular occlusive disease. Specifically, electrocardiography or stress tests may be in order. If these findings support a diagnosis of coronary ischemia, cardiac catheterization and angiography are indicated. Treatment consists of a variety of interventions including restricted intake of lipids, administration of aspirin to prevent thrombosis, and surgical intervention by coronary angioplasty or bypass surgery should angiography show significant occlusive disease.

Sialolithiasis[21,28]

Unlike kidney and gallbladder stones, sialoliths are unrelated to increased levels of serum calcium or to dietary factors. The cause is unknown, though the pathogenesis is relatively well understood. Desquamated epithelial cells from the major salivary ducts may accumulate and form complexes with salivary mucin to form a nidus for calcification. The salivary stone evolves by sequential concretion of calcium phosphate salts, much like the growth rings of a tree. Once the stone reaches a critical size, the salivary duct becomes occluded and symptoms develop. Sialolithiasis is significantly more frequent in the submandibular duct, and therefore pain associated with submandibular stones is more prone to mimic endodontic pain in the posterior aspect of the mandible. The occluded duct often leads to swelling of the submandibular area and therefore may mimic lymphadenitis associated with an endodontic infection of a posterior mandibular tooth.

With close examination and questioning, the diagnosis is usually made quite easily, since the pain has characteristic features. Although a chronic ache may extend into the mandible, the primary location is within the submandibular soft tissues. Typically, the pain is exacerbated by salivation (induced by a lemon drop or at mealtimes). The floor of the mouth can be palpated with a milking motion; when the major duct is occluded, no saliva flows from the duct orifice. The nature of the pain is also revealing in that the patient feels a stringent drawing in the area. When pain of this nature is encountered, salivary occlusion should be investigated before each individual tooth in the vicinity is evaluated. Typically, an occlusal radiograph will disclose the presence of a soft tissue calcification along the course of the duct in the floor of the mouth. It should be noted that panoramic radiographs may reveal an opacity in the mandible. In such instances, the soft tissue calcification is simply superimposed though it may mimic focal sclerosing osteomyelitis.

Though sialolithiasis of the parotid duct is quite rare, its pain can be mistaken for toothache. Again, the symptoms are quite similar to those of submandibular sialolithiasis in that the pain is exacerbated during meals and with stimulation of salivation. The sialolith is generally demonstrable with a panoramic radiograph.

Treatment consists of physical attempts to remove the stone by manipulating it out the orifice. Larger stones cannot be removed in this fashion and will require a surgical cutdown to the duct. Indeed, stones of large size and long duration usually culminate in ablation of the secretory component of the gland, and the nonfunctional gland then becomes subject to retrograde bacterial infections. In these instances sialoadenectomy along with removal of the stone is indicated.

CHRONIC PAIN SYNDROMES OF THE JAWS

Internal Derangement of the Temporomandibular Joint and Facial Myalgia[14,15]

Internal derangements of the temporomandibular joint (TMJ) include meniscus displacement, formation of intraarticular adhesions, and various forms of arthritis. A variety of etiologic factors have been implicated, but no single hypothesis has been universally accepted. It has been proposed that stress-related jaw clenching and bruxism may place stress on the meniscus and cause anterior displacement. Alternatively, traumatic events such as yawning and prolonged jaw opening have been suggested to cause overextension of the ligaments with secondary displacement of the meniscus. Once the meniscus has been anteriorly displaced, adhesions may form, the retrodiscal tissues that are not designed for loading become perforated, and bone-to-bone contact progresses to degenerative joint disease. It is highly unlikely that occlusal discrepancies predispose or even cause these events when one evaluates the literature in a nonbiased fashion. See Table 3-2.

Other organic joint diseases may also involve the TMJ and cause pain symptoms in this region. Included here are rheumatoid, gouty, or psoriatic arthritis and arthritis attending collagen diseases. All of these arthritides are quite rare in the TMJ region.

The more common disorders of the TMJ primarily affect young white women[20a] and include meniscus displacement with adhesions and progression to degenerative arthritic changes. It is noteworthy that organic lesions of this nature may develop in the absence of any pain symptoms whatsoever. The chief findings are limitation of jaw opening, deviation upon opening, clicking or crepitus, and pain directly localized to the joint region in front of the tragus of the ear.

The pain associated with internal derangement is generally a dull, boring ache, but it may be more acute when exacerbated by wide opening of the mandible or chewing. In some patients the chronic symptoms become progressively worse and the degree of pain increases. In such instances the pain symptoms may become more generalized. Odontalgia originating from a pulpally or periodontally infected posterior tooth, either maxillary or mandibular, may refer pain back to the TMJ area. In such instances a joint problem may be perceived by the patient as a dental problem or conversely a pulp involvement may be mistaken for a TMJ disorder.

Myalgic pains are the consequence of sustained muscle contraction usually associated with tooth clenching. In this context, facial myalgia is generally considered to be equivalent to tension headache, being a stress disorder. The pain is always dull, aching, and diffuse. In general, most patients complain of symptoms over the mandible and temple. Palpitation of the masticatory muscles will often reveal the presence of so-called "trigger points." These trigger zones are painful foci in the masticatory muscles and should not be confused with the trigger zone of trigeminal neuralgia. Myalgia may exist as an isolated entity, or it may be associated with other pain disorders, including TMJ internal derangement or odontalgia. A pre-existing pain may predispose to muscle posturing and a tendency for jaw clenching. Thus, the pain symptoms become quite variable and confusing to the examiner. In such instances, evaluations of jaw function, auscultation of the TMJ, masticatory muscle palpitation, and endodontic testing must be performed. If an endodontic infection is uncovered, root canal therapy will relieve the primary pain source and secondary myalgia should resolve shortly thereafter.

When odontogenic sources have been ruled out and a diagnosis of internal derangement, myalgia, or internal derangement with myalgia is confirmed, appropriate therapy should be instituted. Muscle relaxants, nonsteroidal analgesics, physical therapy, stress management therapy, and occlusal splints are all noninvasive procedures. Acupuncture has shown some utility in certain populations but is not universally effective. Extensive tooth grinding and fixed prosthetic reconstruction aimed at curing the disorder should be avoided. When intractable pain persists after conservative therapy, arthroscopic examination may be indicated and either arthroscopic surgery or surgical meniscus replacement may be indicated. Even with surgical intervention, severe pain disorders often recur within months after the procedure. Therefore, conservative management is to be encouraged.

TABLE 3-2. Differentiating chronic aching and burning pains

Condition	Nature	Triggers	Duration
Odontalgia	Dull ache	Hot, cold, tooth percussion	Days-weeks
TMJ internal derangements	Dull ache, sharp episodes	Opening, chewing	Weeks-years
Myalgia	Dull ache, degree varies	Stress, clenching	Weeks-years
Atypical facial pain	Dull ache with severe episodes	Spontaneous	Weeks-years
Phantom tooth pain	Dull ache with severe episodes	Spontaneous	Weeks-years
Neuralgia-inducing cavitational osteonecrosis	Dull ache with severe episodes	Spontaneous	Weeks-years
Allergic sinusitis	Dull ache, Malar area, multiple posterior maxillary teeth	Lowering head	Weeks-months Seasonal
Causalgia	Burning	Posttrauma, postsurgical	Weeks-years
Post-herpetic neuralgia	Deep boring ache with burning	Spontaneous after facial shingles	Weeks-years
Cancer-associated facial pain	Variable, motor deficit, paresthesia	Spontaneous	Days-months

Atypical Facial Pain

... conform ... does not represent another ... form of neuralgia. Importantly, there is no identifiable cause. When the pain is localized to the mandible or maxilla without reference to any specific teeth, it is generally termed atypical facial pain. Alternatively, when pain is localized to a given tooth or a group of contiguous teeth in the absence of any pulpal insults or periodontal infection, the condition is termed atypical odontalgia. When pain persists in teeth whose pulp has been extirpated the condition is referred to as *phantom tooth pain,* a phenomenon akin to phantom limb following amputation. These types of atypical pains are chronic and aching. Patients with atypical facial pain feel it deep within the bones and it is hard to localize. Indeed, many patients with atypical facial pain will report that the symptoms seem to wander from site to site. In addition, may of these patients have pain complaints elsewhere in their body. The intensity of these atypical pains varies considerably from one patient to the next. Some complain of a constant nagging ache; others claim that the pain is excruciating at times. The cause of atypical pain has long been a mystery, and many clinicians have emphasized the probability that psychogenic factors play a major role. Some studies have indicated that patients with atypical facial pain also suffer from vascular type headaches such as migraine and cluster headaches; other studies challenge this relationship.

Phantom tooth pain is estimated to occur in less than 1% of patients undergoing root canal therapy. It has been suggested that surgical extirpation of the pulp results in damage to nerve fibers at the apex of the teeth and should be considered a traumatic neuralgia. Another possible mechanism is formation of a small traumatic neuroma in the apical periodontium. Neither of these theories has received any scientific support. Frequently, though these postendodontic pain foci are subjected to surgical procedures, the pain persists. The organic basis for phantom tooth pain remains an enigma.

Atypical pain localized to edentulous foci can sometimes be alleviated with a subperiosteal injection of local anesthetic. In such instances, it has been proposed that small residual inflammatory foci exist within the endosteum and that focal necrosis occurs with neural damage. These so-called pathologic bone cavities are now referred to as *neuralgia-inducing cavitational osteonecrosis.* Large series have been reported in which surgical curettage has alleviated pain. Tissue curetted from these cavities often shows minor pathologic changes such as fibrosis and mild inflammation. The validity of this theory of atypical facial pain arising in edentulous regions is not universally accepted and is somewhat controversial.

Whether atypical facial pains lie in edentulous areas or are poorly localized or centered in teeth, treatment should be approached cautiously. Many patients have submitted to numerous endodontic procedures and extractions for these pains, and subsequent to the invasive procedures the pain has persisted. Many dentists have undertaken such procedures at the insistence of the patient, who firmly believes there is an odontogenic source. When the symptoms are mild, the pain should be managed with analgesics and reassurance. Many patients with atypical facial pain respond favorably to tricyclic antidepres... in more severe ... for trigeminal neuralgia may be indi... In particular, microvascular decompression and transcutaneous thermal neurolysis have been found to be effective in treating the more severe atypical facial pain problems in some, but not all, patients.

Allergic Sinusitis[3,17]

As discussed in the differential diagnosis of acute facial pains, inflammatory disease of the antrum is more often chronic and allergic in nature. Allergies tend to be seasonal since most people with upper airway allergic reactions respond to various seeds and pollens. In more northerly climates the prevalence of sinusitis increases in spring and fall. In warmer climates, such as California and Florida, allergies may be encountered year round, and some are actually more common during the winter months.

The contact of an allergen with the sinonasal mucous membranes results in an immediate-type hypersensitivity reaction that is mediated by an antigen that penetrates the respiratory epithelium, enters the submucosa, and is bound to an IgE antibody. This antibody is complexed with mast cells and, upon binding to the allergen, histamine is released. Vasoactive consequences evolve, with edema formation and transudation of fluids. Involvement of the sinus includes mucosal thickening as well as the presence of a fluid level within the maxillary sinus cavity. As the ostium becomes occluded, pain symptoms evolve. The pain is preceded by a feeling of pressure within the maxilla for a few hours or days, which then evolves into a dull, chronic ache. Frequently the posterior maxillary teeth seem to "itch," and the patient feels compelled to clench. Percussion sensitivity is evident on all of the molar teeth, and frequently the premolars are percussion sensitive as well. This sensitivity is not acute; rather, it is experienced as a dull discomfort. As with acute sinusitis, the symptoms may be accentuated by having the patient place the head between the knees. The gravitational changes shift the fluid in the sinus and the result is increased pain. Maxillary sinus pain is typically accentuated by changes in barometric pressure, so that traveling to high altitudes or flying may exacerbate the pain. Without treatment these symptoms persist throughout the period when allergens circulate in the air.

The diagnosis is supplemented by antral transillumination in which light will not illuminate an affected maxilla in a darkened room. Water's sinus radiographs will disclose either soft tissue membrane thickening of the antral walls or an air-fluid level will be discernable. Mucosal changes are also evident on MRI and CT scans.

Since chronic sinusitis is generally allergic in nature, the treatment differs from that of acute bacterial sinusitis. Decongestants and nasal sprays, along with antihistamines, are the treatment of choice. Identification of the allergen and desensitization may offer relief for some of these patients, and referral to either an otolaryngologist or an allergist should be considered.

CHRONIC BURNING PAIN

Causalgia[16]

Causalgia is a pain syndrome that is rarely encountered in the head and neck. When present, it is unlikely to be confused with odontalgia. Causalgic pain occurs as a consequence of trauma, jaw fracture, or laceration or may evolve after surgery.

It has been hypothesized that nociceptor fibers become retracked in association with sympathetic fibers in causalgia. The skin overlying the painful area often becomes erythematous during pain episodes. Patients have a tendency to rub and scratch the involved area, producing what are known as *trophic foci*. The skin becomes encrusted and keratotic with scaling. The pain is characteristically paroxysmal and burning and may be both superficial and deep. When a deep component is the predominant complaint, it may be confused with toothache.

Thus, in order to arrive at a definitive diagnosis of causalgia, the aforementioned events and clinical features must be identified and administration of an ipsilateral stellate ganglion block will alleviate pain. In these cases, sympathectomy has been advocated.

Postherpetic Neuralgia[4,8,18,29]

Primary infection with varicella zoster virus causes chickenpox, a disease that affects over 95% of the population during early childhood. In its secondary or recurrent form, the disease is referred to as *herpes zoster* or *shingles*. This disease represents a recrudescence of a latent virus that is located in sensory ganglia. In the head and neck area it is the trigeminal ganglion that harbors latent virus. The factors that activate the virus and allow it to exit from the ganglion and enter the axis cylinder are unknown. Importantly, once the virus is liberated from the nerve endings, it enters epithelial cells and induces a rather characteristic vesicular eruption. Unlike herpes simplex, recrudescence of varicella zoster results in a vesicular eruption that outlines the entire distribution of the sensory pathways. Therefore, the vesicles terminate at the midline and involve only one division of the trigeminal nerve, although sometimes more than one division may be involved. Bilateral involvement is extremely rare. The painful lesions of shingles cause a deep boring ache that involves not only the superficial mucosal and cutaneous tissues but also the maxillary or mandibular bones. Before the onset of the vesicular eruption it is common for the patient to experience prodromal pain, and when that happens the diagnosis may be obscured. These prodromal symptoms frequently simulate trigeminal neuralgia in that they last only seconds and have an electrical quality. Once vesicles appear, the diagnosis is straightforward. If any doubts persist, samples of the vesicular fluid collected within the first 3 days can be cultured for virus or subjected to cytologic smear examination with immunoperoxidase staining to identify the specific viral capsid antigen.

In fewer than 5% of varicella zoster infections patients show clearing of vesicles though pain persists. Post-herpetic neuralgia may persist weeks, months, or years. Whereas the prodromal pain is acute and electrical and pain associated with vesicular eruption is a deep boring ache, the pain symptoms of post-herpetic neuralgia differ yet again. Once the vesicles clear, the residual pain has a burning quality and is chronic. Deeper aching pains occasionally may be associated with this burning element and may suggest pain of odontogenic origin. Nevertheless, the classic sequence of events with an antecedent vesicular eruption is sufficient to make the diagnosis.

The management of postherpetic neuralgia is problematic, and there is no way of knowing when the symptoms may resolve of their own accord. A variety of techniques have been used to manage the pain, including transcutaneous electrical nerve stimulation (TENS), antiseizure drugs, analgesics, and topical preparations. Referral to a neurologist is recommended.

FACIAL PAIN SECONDARY TO MALIGNANT NEOPLASIA[12]

Although cancer involving the maxilla and mandible rarely manifests itself with pain, there is a published case report regarding prodromal facial pain from a glioblastoma.[6a] Typically, paresthesia or hypoesthesia is the complaint. Carcinoma arising in the maxillary sinus may proliferate and begin to erode the bony margins of the sinus walls. Encroachment on the infraorbital nerve as the tumor extends into the floor of the orbit induces paresthesia over the malar region and in the maxillary teeth. Similarly, a malignant tumor in the mandible such as metastatic carcinoma from a distant site such as lung, breast, or colon can invade the nerve. Therefore, numbness is the ominous symptom of cancer in the jaws, though occasionally such tumors produce pain symptoms. In particular, multiple myeloma (malignant neoplasia of B-lymphocytes) is notorious for causing intense bone pain. Therefore, in the jaws such lesions could easily mimic toothache. Rarely does myeloma manifest itself only in the jaws, since it is a disseminated disease and pain would be experienced in other bones. The tumor induces "punched-out" radiolucencies that are poorly marginated. Such lesions should be investigated by obtaining a biopsy.

A variety of cancer-associated pain syndromes of the face have been reported in the literature. These are rare conditions and are designated by a host of eponyms. In general, they represent metastatic tumors that have metastasized to the base of the skull, where they encroach on exiting cranial nerves. Most such tumors will invade not only sensory nerves but motor nerves as well. Therefore, muscular weakness or paralysis in conjunction with pain are the usual accompaniments. When tumors affect the upper aspects of the nasopharynx and skull base, upper facial pain is experienced and the third, fourth, and sixth nerve become involved, leading to ophthalmoplegia. Tumors that arise around the exit of the trigeminal nerve generally affect the motor fibers of nerve V and masticatory muscle weakness is identifiable. A combination of atypical facial pain with ocular, facial, or masticatory muscle paresis should alert the clinician that a malignant disease may be present. At this point, more sophisticated imaging studies should be undertaken, such as MRI and CT scans. The tumor will then be localized on such images and referral to an oncologist is recommended.

A variety of pain syndromes involving the head and neck have the potential to refer pain to the jaw areas. In evaluating pulpal and periapical pain, these specific syndromes must be considered in the differential diagnosis, particularly when the usual physical findings fail to implicate a particular tooth. It must always be remembered that individual patients may suffer from more than one disorder. In this context it is certainly possible for a patient who suffers one of these pain disorders also to harbor a dental pulp infection. For this reason one cannot overemphasize the importance of conducting a thorough history with comprehensive physical examination procedures to evaluate the dentition as well as other anatomic sites.

REFERENCES

1. Batchelder BJ, Krutchkoff DJ, and Amara J: Mandibular pain as the initial and sole clinical manifestation of coronary insufficiency: report of case, J Am Dent Assoc 115:710, 1987.
2. Bates RE Jr, and Stewart CM: Atypical odontalgia: phantom tooth pain, Oral Surg Oral Med Oral Pathol 72:479, 1991.
3. Berg O, and Lejdeborn L: Experience of a permanent ventilation and drainage system in the management of purulent maxillary sinusitis, Ann Otol Rhinol Laryngol 99:192, 1990.

4. Bernstein JE, et al. Topical capsaicin treatment of chronic [illegible] postherpetic neuralgia, J Am Acad Dermatol [illegible]
5. Bouquot JE [illegible]
[illegible]
6a. Cohen S, et al: Oral prodromal signs of a central nervous system malignant neoplasm-glioblastoma multiforme, J Am Dent Assoc 121:643, 1986.
7. Dalessio DJ: Management of the cranial neuralgias and atypical facial pain. A review. Clin J Pain 5:55, 1989.
8. De Benedittia G, Besana F, and Lorenzetti A: A new topical treatment for acute herpetic neuralgia and post-herpetic neuralgia: the aspirin/diethyl atner mixture. An open-label study plus a double blind controlled clinical trial.
9. Dechant KL, and Clissold SP: Sumatriptan. A review of its pharmacodynamic and pharmacokinetic properties, and therapeutic efficacy in the acute treatment of migraine and cluster headache.
10. Donlon WC: Neuralgia-inducing cavitational osteonecrosis. Oral Surg Oral Med Oral Pathol 73:319, 1992.
11. Froom J, et al: Diagnosis and antibiotic treatment of acute otitis media: report from International Primary Care network, Br Med J 300:582, 1990.
12. Greenberg HS: Metastasis to the base of the skull: clinical findings in 43 patients, Neurology 31:530, 1981.
13. Harness DM, and Rome HP: Psychological and behavioral aspects of chronic facial pain, Otolaryngol Clin North Am 22:1073, 1989.
14. Harness DM, Donlon WC, and Eversole LR: Comparison of clinical characteristics in myogenic TMJ internal derangement and atypical facial pain patients, Clin J Pain 8:4, 1990.
15. Helms CA, et al: Staging of internal derangements of the TMJ with magnetic resonance imaging: preliminary observations, J Craniomandib Dis 3:93, 1989.
16. Hoffman KD, and Matthews MA: Comparison of sympathetic neurons in orofacial and upper extremity nerves: implications for causalgia, J Oral Maxillofac Surg 48:720, 1990.
17. Kennedy DW, and Loury MC: Nasal and sinus pain: current diagnosis and treatment, Semin Neurol 8:303, 1988.

[illegible] ganglion, J Neurosurg 72:49, 1990.
20a. Lipton JA, Ship JA, and Larach-Robinson D: Estimated prevalence and distribution of reported orofacial pain in the United States, J Am Dent Assoc 124:115, 1993.
21. Lustmann J, Regev E, and Melamed Y: Sialolithiasis. A survey on 245 patients and a review of the literature, Int J Oral Maxillofac Surg 19:135, 1990.
22. Marbach JJ, et al: Incidence of phantom tooth pain: an atypical facial neuralgia, Oral Surg Oral Med Oral Pathol 53:190, 1982.
23. Mathew NT: Advances in cluster headache, Neurol Clin North Am 8:867, 1990.
24. Medina JL, Diamond S, and Fareed J: The nature of cluster headache, Headache 19:309, 1979.
25. Moller AR: The cranial nerve vascular compression syndrome: 1. a review of treatment, Acta Neurochirurgica 113:18, 1991.
26. Moraci M, et al: Trigeminal neuralgia treated by percutaneous thermocoagulation: Comparative analysis of percutaneous thermocoagulation and other surgical procedures, Neurochirurgia 35:48, 1992.
27. Natkin E, Harrington GW, and Mandel MA: Anginal pain referred to the teeth, Oral Surg Oral Med Oral Pathol 40:678, 1975.
28. Pollack CV Jr, and Severance HW Jr: Sialolithiasis: case studies and review, J Emerg Med 8:561, 1990.
29. Robertson DR, George DP: Treatment of post-herpetic neuralgia in the elderly, Br Med Bull 48:113, 1990.
30. Schnurr RR, and Brooke RI: Atypical odontalgia: Update and comment on long-term follow-up, Oral Surg Oral Med Oral Pathol 73:445, 1992.
31. Sicuteri R, et al: Idiopathic headache as a possible risk factor for phantom tooth pain, Headache 31:577, 1991.
32. Taarhj P: Decompression of the posterior trigeminal root in trigeminal neuralgia: A 30-year follow-up review, J Neurosurg 57;14, 1982.
33. Zakrewska JM: Medical management of trigeminal neuralgia, Br Dent J 168:399, 1990.

Self-assessment questions

1. Pain in the absence of identifiable disease is recognized as
   a. acute pain.
   b. inflammation mediated.
   c. hypersensitivity.
   d. chronic pain.
2. Given time, diffuse pain of odontogenic origin
   a. will be referred.
   b. will readily abate.
   c. will localize to specific site.
   d. can be controlled with analgesics.
3. Trigeminal neuralgia can be treated
   a. with analgesics.
   b. by anesthetizing the trigger area.
   c. with lysis of the terminal nerve endings.
   d. with anticonvulsant drugs.
4. Cluster headache differs from migraine in being
   a. unilateral and involving the teeth.
   b. principally a female complaint.
   c. unilateral and involving the eye.
   d. bilateral.
5. Acute maxillary sinusitis
   a. results in referred pain to a single tooth.
   b. results in referred pain to the orbit and maxillary posterior teeth.
   c. is exacerbated by cold testing.
   d. is usually a noninfectious process.
6. Degenerative joint disease most often
   a. results in posterior displacement of the meniscus.
   b. results in irreversible pulpitis.
   c. allows for wide mouth opening.
   d. can lead to adhesions and arthritic changes.
7. TMJ pain can be
   a. sharp, lancinating and electrical.
   b. exacerbated by jaw closing.
   c. the result of ipsilateral maxillary odontalgia.
   d. found in males.
8. Atypical facial pain can be treated most effectively by
   a. microvascular decompression.
   b. radiofrequency gangliolysis.
   c. NSAIDs.
   d. tricyclic antidepressant drugs.
9. Phantom tooth pain or deafferentation pain
   a. can occur briefly after tooth extraction.
   b. is simply a peripheral phenomenon.
   c. can occur for an extended period after pulp extirpation.
   d. is managed by analgesics.
10. A definite diagnosis of facial causalgia can be made
   a. by lidocaine infiltration.
   b. by use of analgesics.
   c. by use of ipsilateral stellate ganglion block.
   d. by observation of symptoms.

Chapter 4

Case Selection and Treatment Planning

Samuel O. Dorn
Arnold H. Gartner

Once a thorough examination has determined that an endodontic problem exists, the process of case selection begins. The dentist must determine whether treatment is indicated for this patient, what treatment will best serve the patient, and whether the patient would be best served by being referred to a specialist or another practitioner. Rating systems have been devised to help dentists decide which cases to treat and which to refer.[34]

EVALUATION OF PATIENT

The patient must be evaluated both physically and mentally. When the patient's physical or mental health is seriously compromised, even the simplest endodontic case can turn into an extremely difficult one. The clinician must use all available knowledge and experience in assessing the patient and the dental problem.

Physical Evaluation

Most medical conditions do not contraindicate endodontic therapy, but the patient's medical condition should be thoroughly evaluated in order to properly manage the case. If the treating dentist does not feel comfortable treating medically compromised patients, such patients should be referred to an endodontist, who may be able to provide more expeditious treatment. The following considerations are offered not as a thorough treatise on the subject, but as ideas that the dentist should consider when planning treatment. For a thorough review of the management of the medically compromised patient the reader is referred to textbooks on the subject.[22,23]

Cardiovascular disease

A history of myocardial infarction within the past 6 months is a contraindication for elective dental treatment.[22] Emergency relief, however, should be provided in consultation with the patient's cardiologist. These patients should be treated with a stress reduction protocol that includes short appointments, psychosedation, and pain and anxiety control. Patients with a history of rheumatic heart disease should be premedicated with amoxicillin, erythromycin, or clindamycin, according to current American Heart Association guidelines.[8]

Bleeding disorders

Laboratory screening tests and physician consultation are necessary for any patient with a bleeding disorder. The dentist should be aware that dialysis patients, alcohol abusers, and patients taking aspirin may have severe bleeding problems. Although endodontic therapy is preferable to extraction in these patients, the dentist should be prepared to handle any bleeding due to impingement of the rubber dam clamp, vital pulp extirpation, or surgical procedures.

Diabetes

An acute endodontic infection can compromise even a well-controlled diabetic; so all diabetes patients must be carefully monitored. Prophylactic antibiotics may be necessary even when there are not yet any signs of periradicular infection. Patients with uncontrolled or brittle diabetes should be monitored carefully for signs of insulin shock or diabetic coma. Appointments should be scheduled so as not to interfere with the patient's normal insulin and meal schedule. A stress reduction protocol should be followed.

Cancer

A thorough history will reveal what type of cancer the patient has and what type of treatment is being rendered. Because some cancers can appear as endodontic lesions, the dentist should biopsy any suspicious ones. Because chemotherapy and radiation to the head and neck region can severely compromise the healing process, endodontic treatment should be done in close consultation with the patient's oncologist.

AIDS

HIV infection, including AIDS, is not a contraindication to endodontic therapy. Indeed, in most instances, the patient is at less risk with endodontic therapy than with extraction.

Pregnancy

Pregnancy is not a contraindication to endodontic therapy. Pain and infection can and should be controlled in consultation with the patient's obstetrician.

Allergies

If the patient is allergic to latex rubber, a dam should be made of vinyl (such as a vinyl glove, which also should be worn over the rubber gloves). A highly allergic patient may be more prone to interappointment flare-ups, which may be preventable by antihistamine premedication.[19a, 41a]

Steroid therapy

Adrenal suppression should be suspected when a patient is receiving steroid therapy. Any patient taking steroids is more susceptible to infection than otherwise and in consultation with his physician, should be appropriately protected with antibiotics.

Infectious diseases

Strict adherence to universal infection control precautions prevents the spread of infectious diseases between patients and dental personnel.

Physical disabilities

Because patients with physical disabilities such as Parkinson's disease, spinal cord injury, or stroke may not be able to hold a radiographic film, the electronic apex locator is recommended.

Psychological Evaluation

Motivation

A patient who shows no incentive to maintain good oral hygiene or one who constantly misses appointments may not be a good candidate for endodontic therapy.

Difficult patients

Fear of ionizing radiation, pain, or needles can impair a patient's ability to behave well in the dental office. Many of these psychological problems can be overcome by a gentle, caring, honest chairside manner.

Economic Evaluation

Endodontic therapy provides good value for treatment rendered.[9] Although 46% of the respondents in a 1987 survey incorrectly perceived endodontic therapy to be more expensive than extraction and replacement with a fixed prosthesis,[3] another survey placed the market value of a tooth at over $300,000.[4]

EVALUATION OF TOOTH

A number of factors should be evaluated to determine (1) whether a tooth should be endodontically treated and (2), if so, by a general dentist or an endodontist.

Morphology

Unusual length

Teeth that are unusually long (greater than 25 mm) or unusually short (less than 15 mm) are more difficult to treat. The general dentist can prudently choose whether an endodontist would better serve the patient.

Unusual canal shapes

Unusual canal shapes (Fig. 4-1) require special techniques. An open apex ("blunderbuss") canal will need either apexification or apexogenesis. C-shaped canals, dens-in-dente, taurodontism, and roots with bulbous ends are more difficult to treat and often require more specialized techniques that are more likely to be acquired by the advanced general dentist or an endodontist.

Dilacerations

Extreme curvature of the root canal (Fig. 4-2) can be difficult for the most experienced clinician to manage. The use of anticurvature filing and nickel titanium files can help avoid strip perforations and ledging.

Unusual number of canals

The treating dentist must always look for and expect extra canals (Fig. 4-3). All molars should be expected to have at least four canals unless proven otherwise. When a large canal stops abruptly on the radiograph, branching into two or more smaller canals should be sought.

Resorptions

Internal resorption can be differentiated from external resorption by its radiographic appearance (Fig. 4-4).[17] External resorption appears to be superimposed on the canal, whereas internal resorption appears to be continuous with the canal. For further information the reader is referred to Chapter 16.

Calcifications

Calcification in the root canal, whether isolated or continuous, can make treatment very difficult for the most skilled clinician. The use of chelating agents, magnification, fiberoptic transillumination, and pathfinding files can help the dentist find and treat calcified canals.

Previous Treatment

Canal blockage

Previously treated teeth may need to be retreated because of persistent disease due to incomplete root canal débridement or obturation (Fig. 4-5). Any material blocking access to the apical extent of the canal must be removed. Ultrasonic instruments have made it much easier to remove posts, silver points, broken instruments, and paste fillings. Care must be taken to avoid ledging or blocking these canals. A dentist inexperienced

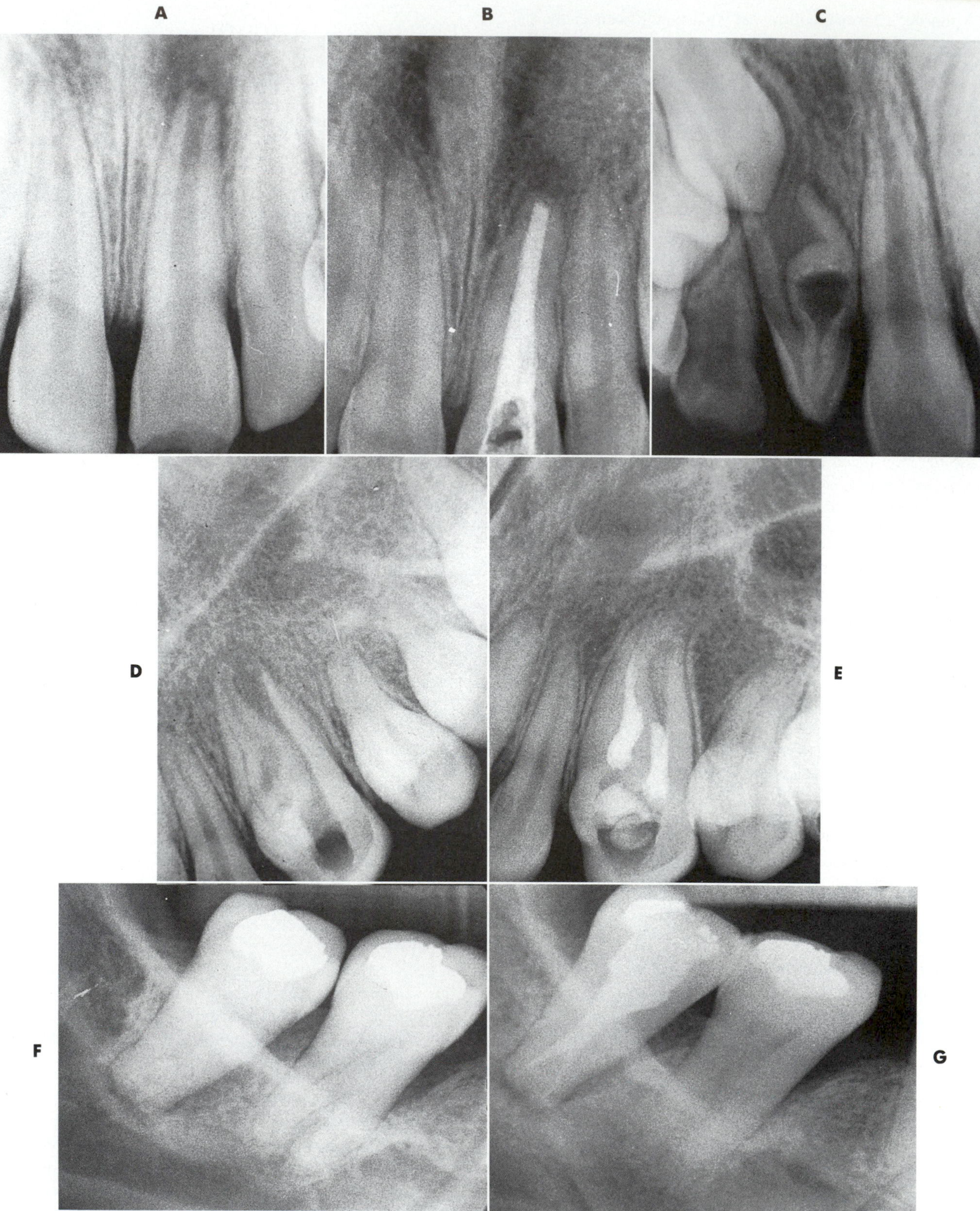

FIG. 4-1 Canal shape. **A** and **B,** Open apex requires apical closure techniques before obturation. **C,** Dens-in-dente. **D** and **E,** Fusion. **F** and **G,** Taurodont teeth have large pulp chambers and short roots, which are often difficult to locate and treat.

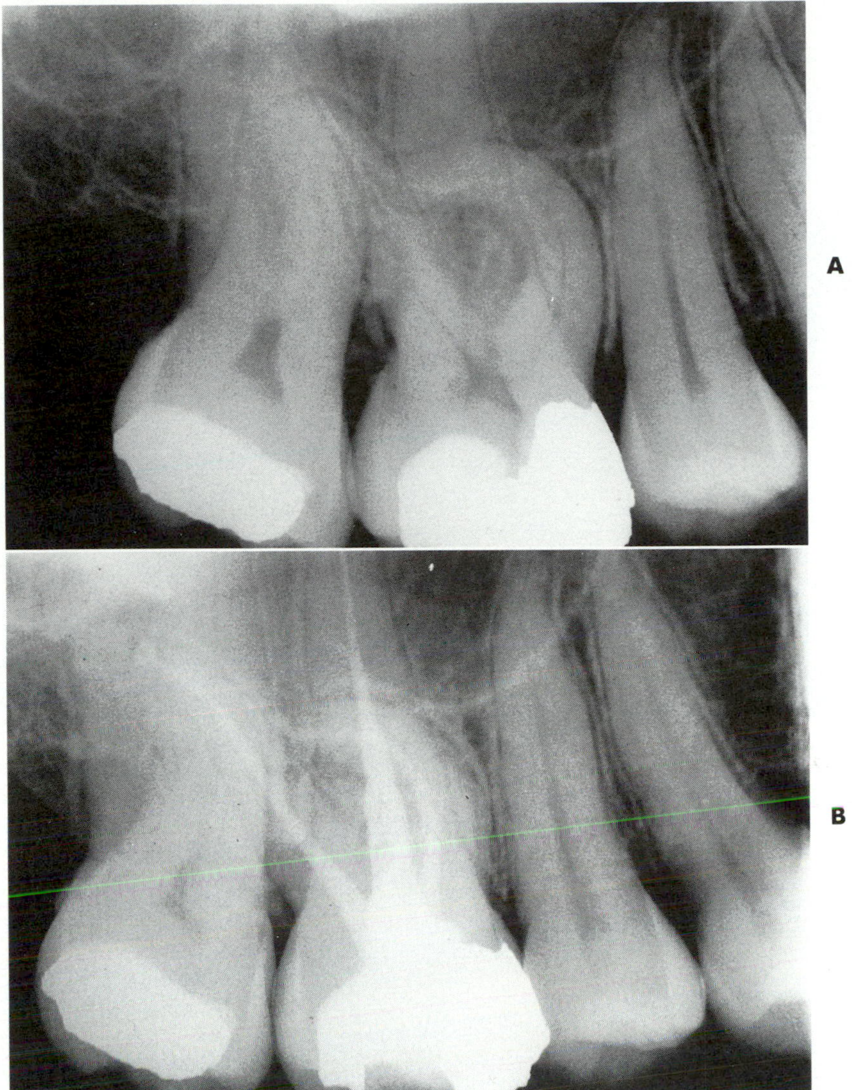

FIG. 4-2 Dilaceration of the mesiobuccal canal. ***A***, Preoperative radiograph. ***B***, Postoperative radiograph.

with retreatment techniques should refer these cases to an endodontist. For further information, the reader is referred to Chapter 24.

Ledging

A previously treated tooth that has a ledge in the canal can be very difficult to treat. Using a file whose apical 2 mm has been bent at a 30-degree angle can help bypass and eliminate the ledge.

Perforations

If a previously treated tooth has a perforation that is improperly sealed, the prognosis may be very poor. When the perforation is in the apical two thirds of the root it may be surgically treatable. If it is in the furcation area it may be possible to pack a matrix of hydroxyapatite and seal the perforation with a glass ionomer cement (Fig. 4-6). If bone loss has already occurred, hemisection, root amputation, or extraction may be indicated.

Location of Tooth

Accessibility

The relative location of a tooth in the arch is directly related to accessibility. The further posterior the tooth, the less accessible are all the canals for visualization and treatment. Limited opening due to trismus, scarring from burns or surgical procedures, or systemic problems such as scleroderma may severely limit access. Angulation of the tooth can also hamper accessibility. Molars that are tipped to the mesial or teeth that are in linguoversion or labioversion can also present problems for less experienced dentists.

Proximity to other structures

Anatomic structures close to the apex of the tooth should give the thoughtful clinician pause. Paresthesia can be caused by overinstrumentation, overfilling, or endodontic disease close to the mental foramen or mandibular canal (Fig. 4-7, *A*). Periradicular infections can cause concomitant infections of the

Text continued on p. 68.

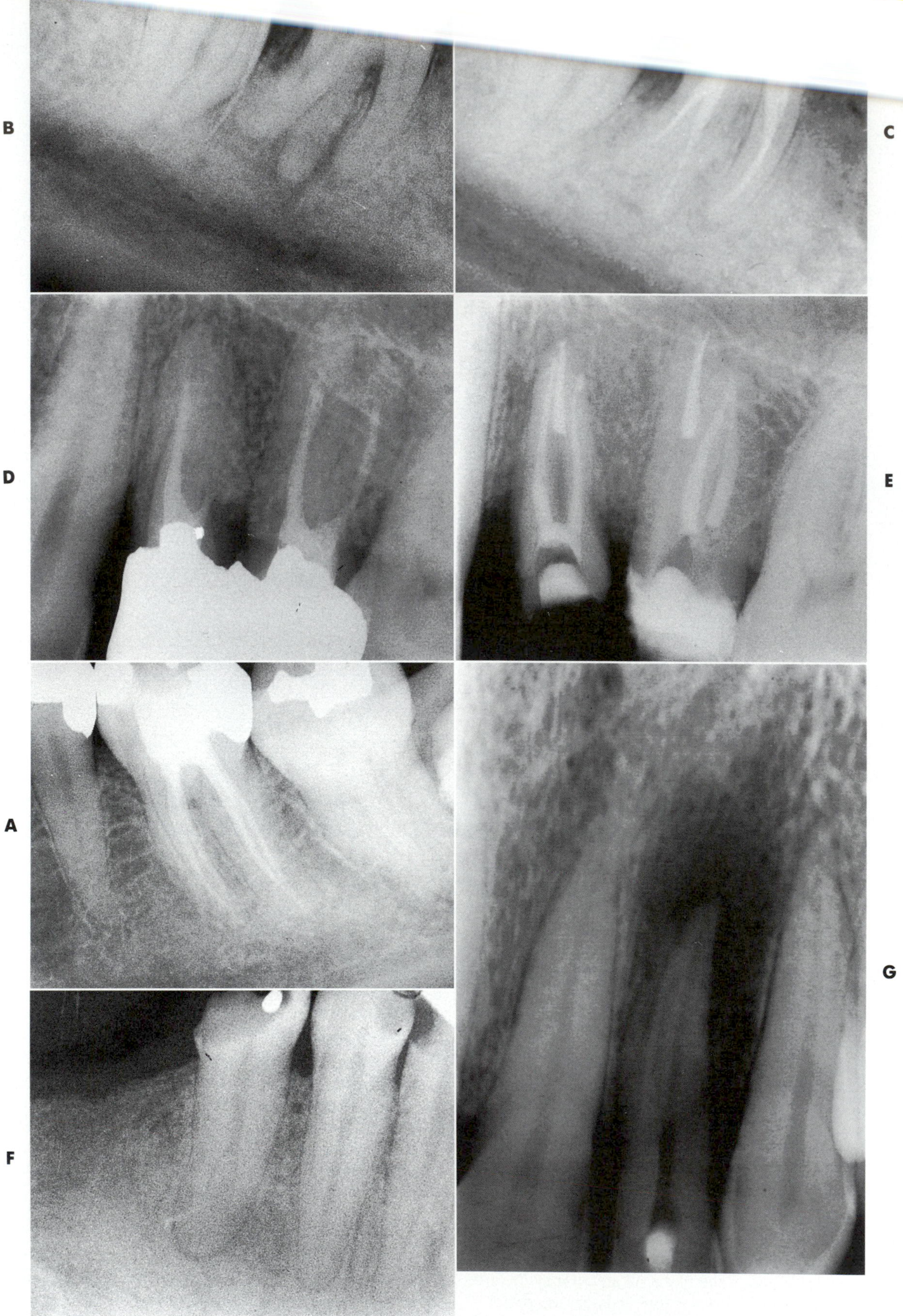

FIG. 4-3 Number of canals. **A,** Mandibular molar with four canals. **B** and **C,** Mandibular molar with extra distal root. **D** and **E,** Maxillary premolars with three roots. Referring dentist thought the canals were calcified. **F,** Mandibular premolar branches in apical third of the tooth. **G,** Maxillary lateral incisor with two roots. The dentist should suspect extra canals until this is ruled out.

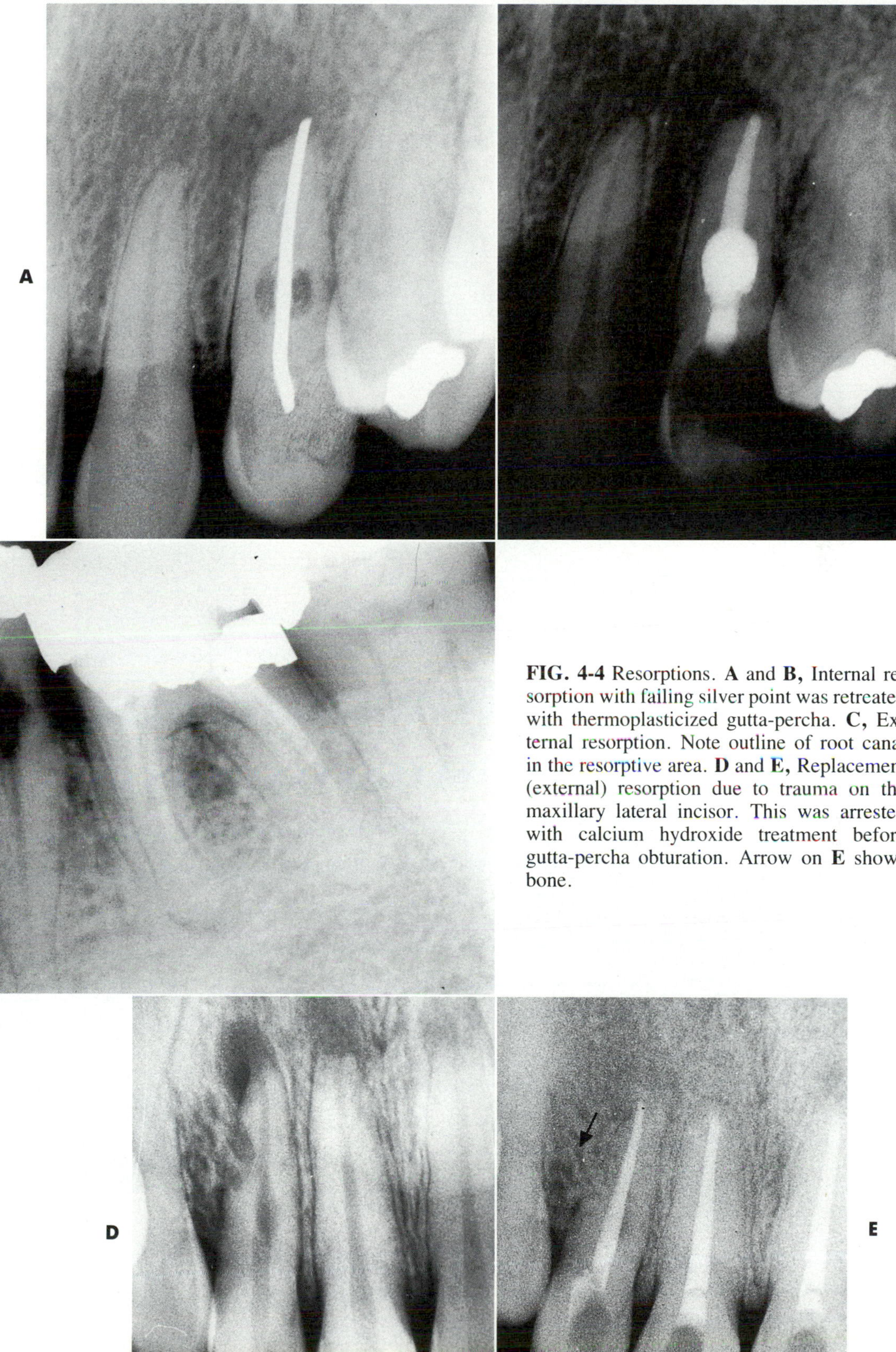

FIG. 4-4 Resorptions. **A** and **B,** Internal resorption with failing silver point was retreated with thermoplasticized gutta-percha. **C,** External resorption. Note outline of root canal in the resorptive area. **D** and **E,** Replacement (external) resorption due to trauma on the maxillary lateral incisor. This was arrested with calcium hydroxide treatment before gutta-percha obturation. Arrow on **E** shows bone.

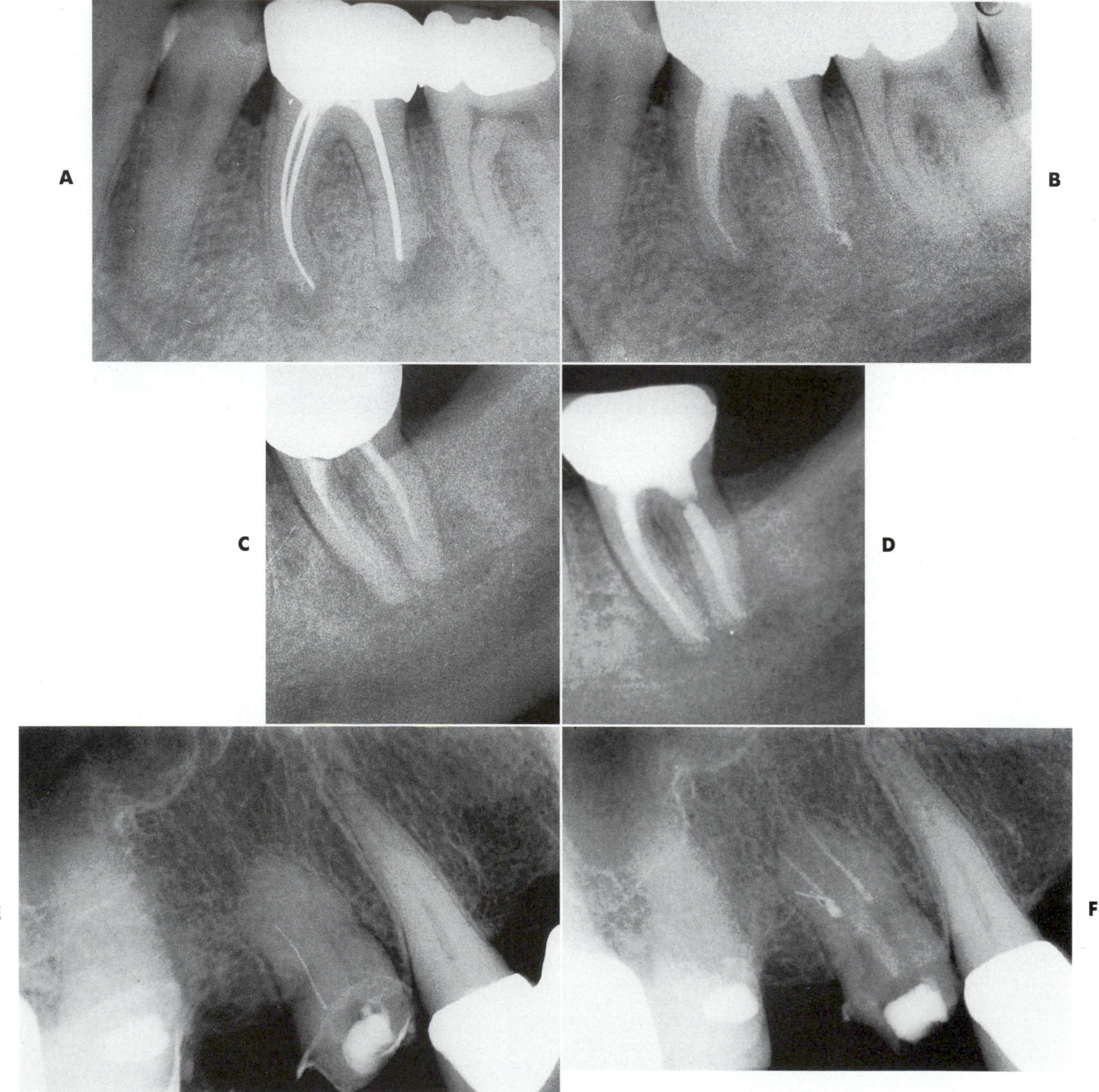

FIG. 4-5 Retreatment. **A** and **B,** Retreatment of a silver point case. **C** and **D,** Retreatment of a poorly obturated gutta-percha case through a crown. **E** and **F,** Retreatment of a maxillary bicuspid with a broken file in the palatal canal. A piece of the file entered the periradicular tissues while being removed with ultrasonics.

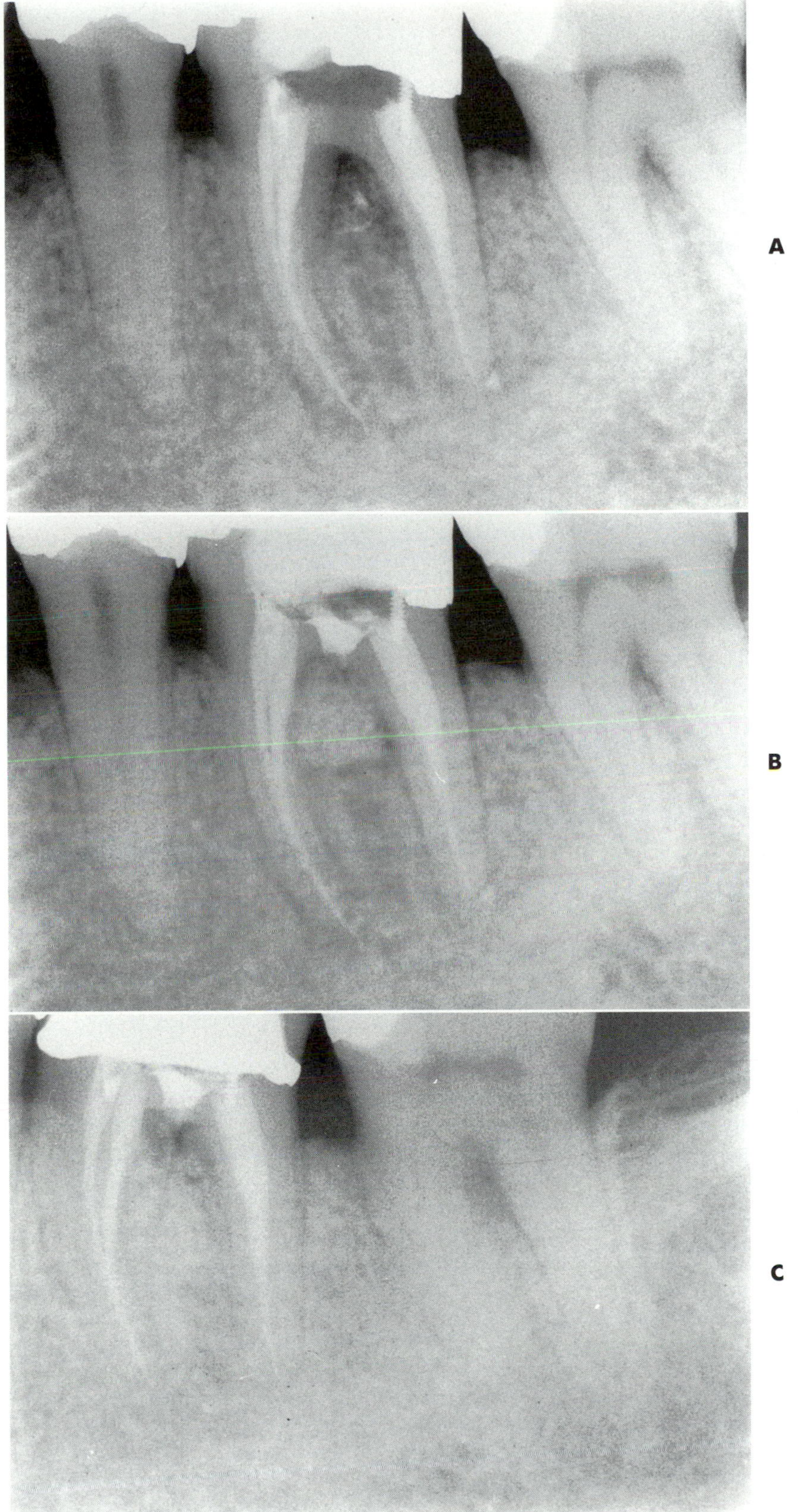

FIG. 4-6 Perforation repair. **A,** Perforation into the furcation area occurred during endodontic treatment 2 years earlier and was repaired with IRM. The patient presents with a sinus tract to the furcation but with no periodontal communication. **B,** The defect is packed tightly with hydroxyapatite through the perforation and covered with Ketac-Silver. **C,** Two years postoperatively, the patient is asymptomatic with no reappearance of the sinus tract.

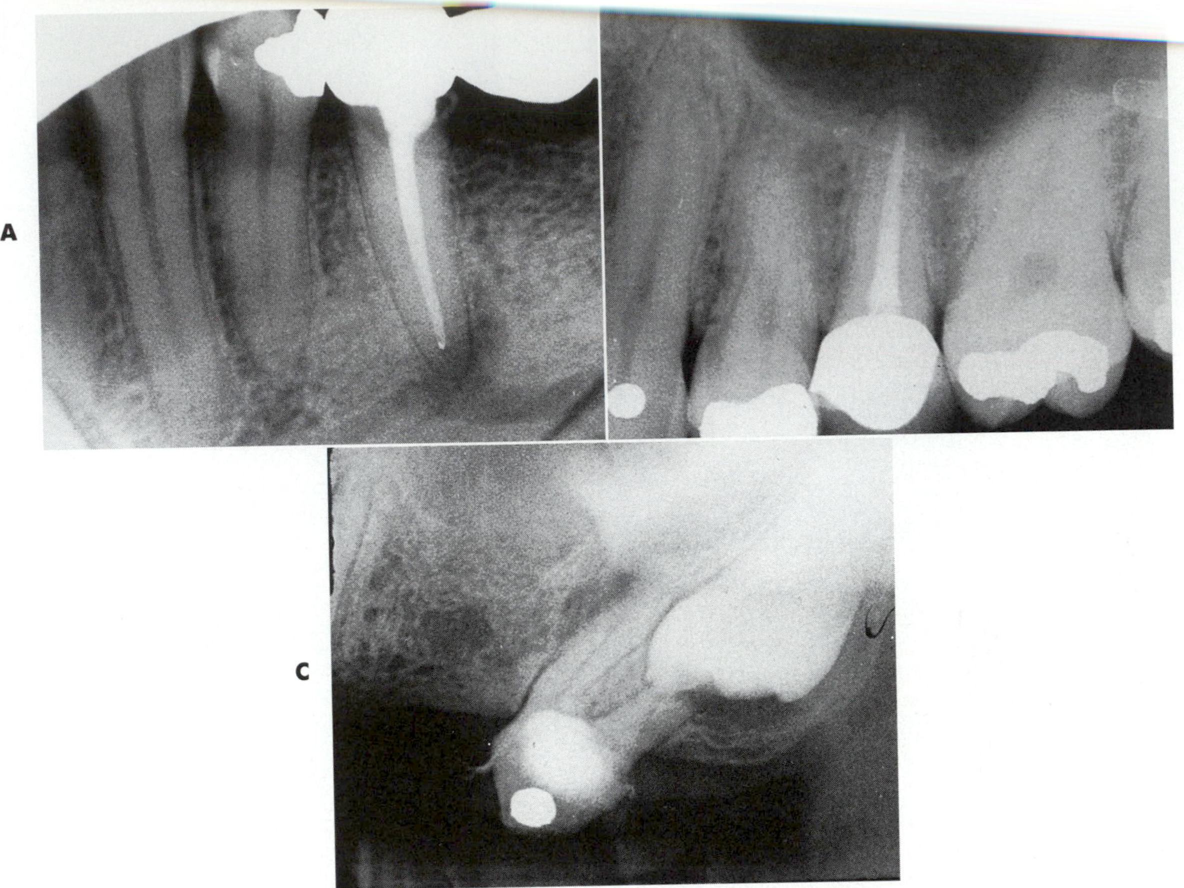

FIG. 4-7 Proximity to other structures. **A,** Mental foramen. **B,** Maxillary sinus. **C,** Malar process and impacted tooth.

maxillary sinus (Fig. 4-7, *B*), nasal cavities, or endosseous implants.

The malar process, impacted teeth (Fig. 4-7, *C*), tori, or overlapping roots (Fig. 4-2) can make radiographic visualization of the apex and periradicular region difficult for both diagnosis and treatment. In these situations the use of electronic apex locators is recommended.

Restorability

The restorability of the tooth must be thoughtfully considered first (Fig. 4-8). All decay should be removed so that the extent of healthy tooth structure can be gauged.

Periodontal status

The prognosis for the endodontically involved tooth should also be evaluated in relation to its periodontal status. A tooth with very little bone support and class III mobility also has a poor endodontic prognosis. An endodontic lesion that is also periodontally involved may never heal.

EVALUATION OF CLINICIAN

Self-evaluation by the clinician should include the following questions:

1. *Do I have the experience to treat this problem?* Complicated treatment procedures should not be attempted until the clinician has had experience with less complex cases of the same type.

2. *Do I have the ability to treat this endodontic case?* Not every clinician has the ability or patience to carefully clean and shape curved, narrow canals or to do surgical procedures. The clinician should honestly evaluate his or her personal ability to treat complicated cases. Clinicians have different interests and preferences.

Patients with medical problems or disabilities might need special or emergency response that is beyond the capability of some clinicians.

3. *Do I have the availability of, and experience with, any special technology that I will need?* Are unusually long or flexible files needed? Does this case call for use of a microscope (Fig. 4-9), ultrasonic device, or electronic apex locator? Will special obturation techniques be necessary because of the canal anatomy?

It is easier to refer a patient to an endodontist before a problem occurs than after the problem creates stress for both the dentist and the patient.

TREATMENT PLANNING

It is essential that a proper diagnosis be made before endodontic therapy is instituted. The most important aspect of endodontics is to properly identify and diagnose the cause of the

A

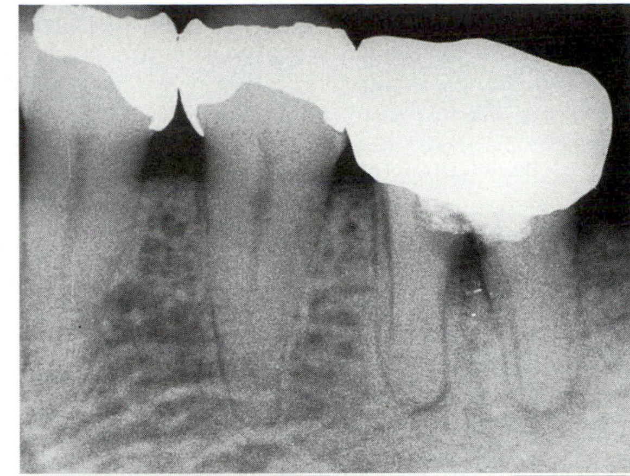

B

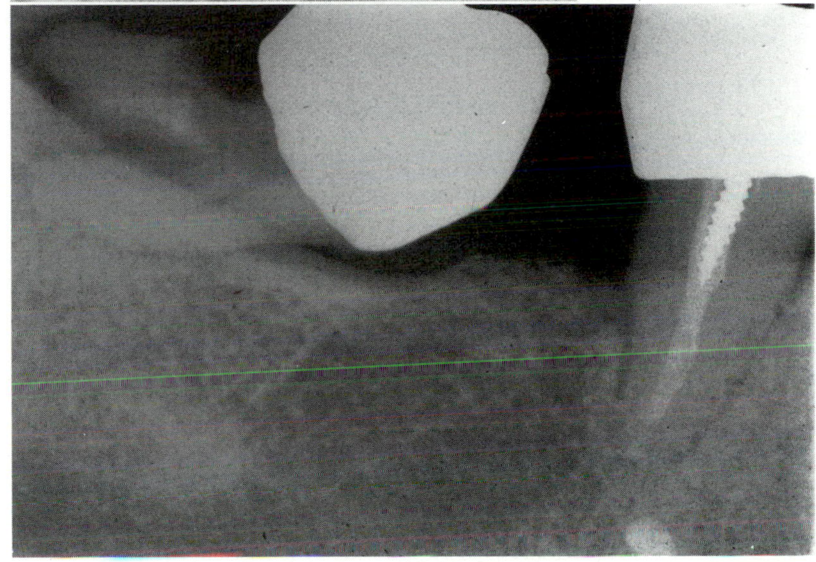

FIG. 4-8 Restorability. **A,** Decay into the furcation may render a tooth untreatable or unrestorable. **B,** Angulation, decay, and lack of bone support render this tooth hopeless.

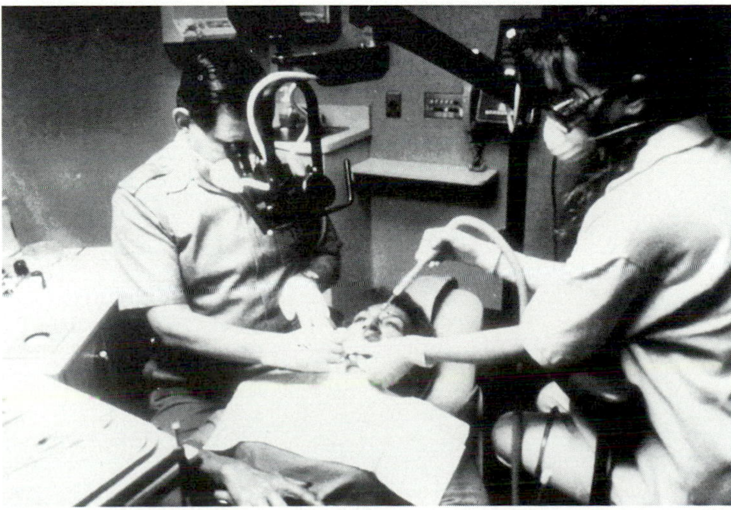

FIG. 4-9 The operating microscope may be necessary to find calcified or additional canals.

patient's pain or discomfort. Incorrect or inadequate diagnostic procedures can lead to improper treatment, and likely legal consequences. Only after the diagnostic procedures discussed in Chapter 1 have been systematically followed and a correct diagnosis has been made should treatment planning begin.

Emergency Treatment

The first goal of endodontic therapy is to relieve acute pain and provide drainage of infection, as described in Chapter 2.

Once the patient's acute symptoms have been alleviated, the completion of the root canal can be set aside while the clinician conducts a comprehensive examination of the patient and develops a customized course of treatment. Following this written treatment plan provides the patient optimal care and helps prevent inappropriate treatment, embarrassment, and patient dissatisfaction. The following sequence is recommended[47]:

1. Management of acute pulp or periodontal pain.
2. Oral surgery for extraction of unsalvageable teeth.
3. Caries control of deep lesions that may threaten the pulp.
4. Periodontal procedures to manage soft tissue.
5. Endodontic procedures for asymptomatic teeth with necrotic pulps and surgical treatment or retreatment of failing root canals.
6. Restorative and prosthetic procedures.

This sequence may be altered if a dental emergency arises or if the patient's systemic health, dental attitude, or financial situation changes.

One-Appointment Root Canal Therapy

History

In recent years, single-appointment endodontics has gained increased acceptance as the best treatment for many cases. Recent studies have shown little or no difference in quality of treatment, incidence of posttreatment complications, or success rates between single-visit and multiple treatment. Not all studies, however, agree about the efficacy of this technique for every case.

Completing endodontic treatment in a single visit is an old concept that can be traced through the literature for at least 100 years. Dodge[10] described various techniques, which included root canal sterilization by hydrogen dioxide and sodium dioxide, hot platinum wire sterilization, potassium permanganate sterilization, or sulfuric acid irrigation. The canals were filled with chloropercha, formopercha, sectional gutta-percha, or zinc oxide and eugenol paste.

Single-visit endodontics enjoyed a resurgence following World War II. However, it was generally performed in conjunction with resection of the root apex immediately after filling the canals. Trephination, or artificial fistulation, was also used in conjunction with single-visit endodontics, to prevent or alleviate postoperative pain and swelling.[30] In many of the early reports opinions were based on limited clinical observations and inadequate scientific studies. In 1959, Feranti[15] reported that there was little difference in postoperative sequelae between single-visit and two-visit root canals. However, relatively few comprehensive studies of one-visit endodontics were published until the 1970s.

In more recent years studies have been published that attempt to answer two basic questions: (1) Is endodontic therapy more painful when performed in a single visit than in multiple visits? (2) Is single-visit endodontic therapy as successful as therapy performed in multiple visits?

Postoperative pain and flare-ups

The reported incidence of postoperative pain following single- and multiple-visit endodontic treatment varies considerably; however, most studies show that one-visit root canal procedures produce no more pain than multiple-visit ones (Table 4-1).

TABLE 4-1. One-visit endodontics: comparative studies on incidence of postoperative pain and flare-ups

				One-visit post-op pain (%)		Multiple-visit post-op pain (%)	
Investigator	**Year**	**No. of cases**	**Pulp status***	**None or slight**	**Moderate to severe**	**None or slight**	**Moderate to severe**
Ferranti[9]	1959	340	N	91.0	9.0	96.2	3.8
Fox et al[10]	1970	270	V-N	90.0	10.0	Not studied	
O'Keefe[20]	1976	55	V-N	98.0	2.0	91.0	7.0
Soltanoff[27]	1978	282	V-N	81.0	19.0	86.0	14.0
Ashkenaz[4]	1979	359	V	96.0	4.0	Not studied	
Rudner, Oliet[24]	1981	98	V-N	88.5	11.5	88.5	11.5
Mulhern et al[18]	1982	30	N	76.5	23.5	73.3	26.7
Oliet[19]	1983	382	V-N	89.0	11.0	93.5	6.5
Roane et al[23]	1983	359	V-N	85.0	15.0	68.8	31.2
Alacam[2]	1985	212	V	86.0	14.0	Not studied	
Mata et al[14] **	1985	150	N	Not studied		98.0	2.0
Morse et al[17] **	1986	200	N	98.5	1.5	Not studied	
Morse et al[16] **	1987	106	N	93.4	6.6	Not studied	
Abbott et al[1] **	1988	195	N	97.4	2.6	Not studied	
Fava[8]	1989	60	V	97.0	3.0	100.0	0.0
Trope[31,33] **	1990	474	V-N	—	—	97.4	2.6
	1991	226		98.2	1.8	—	—
Fava[7]	1991	120	N	95.0	5.0	Not studied	
Walton et al[33] **	1992	935	V-N	97.4	2.6	96.3	3.3

*V, Vital; N, Nonvital.

**Used strict definition for flare-ups.

In 1970, Fox and coworkers[16] treated 291 teeth in single visits and reported severe pain within 24 hours in only 7% of those cases. They found that 90% of the teeth were free of spontaneous pain after 24 hours, whereas 82% had little or no pain on percussion. Wolch[46] also reported in 1970 on more than 5000 nonvital cases treated in one visit. He found severe pain in only 5% of these cases. In 1978, Soltanoff[39] reported that 64% of the single-visit and 38% of the multiple-visit patients experienced postoperative pain, though his figures seem high when compared to those of many studies that followed (Table 4-1). These all confirmed the findings of earlier studies, which suggest that one-visit procedures produce no more pain, and in some cases less pain, than multiple-visit root canals. Most studies showed that when pain occurred it was invariably most intense during the first 24 to 48 hours and declined after the first week.

Recently, the term *flare-up* has become popular for describing posttreatment symptoms, though there is little agreement about at which point pain and swelling become a bona fide flare-up. Morse[26] defines a flare-up as swelling and pain combined or swelling alone that necessitates unscheduled emergency appointments. Pain by itself is not considered a flare-up. Walton's definition of a flare-up is this: "Within a few hours to a few days after a root canal treatment procedure, a patient has either pain or swelling or a combination of both. The problem must be of sufficient severity that there is a disruption of the patient's life style such that the patient initiates contact with the dentist. Required then are both *(a)* an unscheduled visit and *(b)* active treatment (incision and drainage, canal débridement, opening for drainage, etc.)."[45]

Morse and co-workers, in an exhaustive series of clinical studies covering a period of 24 years,[1,24-27] investigated factors that could reduce the incidence of flare-ups and of pain and swelling not associated with flare-up. They concluded that one-appointment endodontics combined with prophylactic administration of antibiotics (penicillin V or erythromycin) and intentional overinstrumentation of the root canal into the approximate center of the bony lesion reduced the prevalence of flare-ups from about 20% to 1.5%. Their strict definition of a flare-up, excluding many cases of "non-flare-up associated pain and swelling," may account for the unusually low incidence of pain in these cases.

These findings are somewhat controversial, since avoiding overinstrumentation has long been a standard of endodontic treatment and prophylactic use of antibiotics, except for cardiovascular or prosthetic replacement premedication, has long been frowned on owing to its questionable value and the possibility of allergic reactions.[36] If Morse's work is correct, however, these techniques should be considered for all one-appointment nonvital cases without sinus tracts. Moderate overinstrumentation past the apex of nonvital cases has long been taught, to increase the likelihood for drainage and relief of pressure. However, from the literature it is quite clear that overinstrumentation of vital cases is to be avoided because it crushes tissue and produces pain and inflammation.[36]

Trope[43] reported that the flare-up rate for one-appointment retreatment cases with apical periodontitis was unacceptably high and this approach to such cases should be avoided. Walton[45] indicated that the overriding factor as to predicting a flare-up was the presence of pain or other symptoms before treatment. If these symptoms exist, it would be reasonable to administer antibiotics in an attempt to control a possible flare-up. One study suggests that single-visit endodontic treatment of posterior teeth seems to produce more postoperative discomfort.[33]

Success rates

Prognostic studies of one-appointment root canal treatment are less numerous than pain studies, but most also indicate that there is no substantial difference in the success rate of one- and two-visit cases (Table 4-2). Despite Soltanoff's[39] report of considerably more pain in association with multiple-visit endodontic treatment, he found that both techniques provided success rates exceeding 85%. Ashkenaz[5] claimed that one-appointment root canals succeeded 97% of the time, but he did not evaluate multiple visits. Rudner and Oliet[35] compared one-visit to multiple-visit treatments and found that both healed with a frequency of about 88% to 90%. Southard and Rooney[40] described total healing of all recalled cases when one-appointment endodontics was combined with incision and drainage and antibiotic therapy. Pekruhn,[31] in a study of 1140 single-visit cases, found a failure rate of only 5.2%. He noted that teeth not previously opened showed three times the number of failures as those that had been previously opened. This was especially true of teeth involved with periapical extension of pulpal disease. There was also a higher incidence of failure in teeth being retreated. Stamos and colleagues[41] described two cases in which total healing occurred following one-visit treatments in which combined hand instrumentation and ultrasonic technique were utilized.

TABLE 4-2. One-visit endodontics: comparative success and failure studies

Investigator	Year	Pulp status*	Total cases	Recall period	One-visit (%)		Multiple-visit (%)	
					Success	Failure	Success	Failure
Soltanoff[26]	1978	V-N	266	6 mo-2 yr	85	15	88	12
Ashkenaz[3]	1979	V	101	1 yr	97	3	Not studied	
			44	2 yr	97.7	1.3		
Rudner and Oliet[24]	1981	V-N	41	6-12 mo	90.2	9.8	85.7	14.3
			27	12-14 mo	88.8	11.2	90.0	10.0
			30	Over 24 mo	90	10.0	91.8	8.2
Oliet[19]	1983	V-N	153	Min 18 mo	88.8	11.2	88.6	11.4
Pekruhn[21]	1986	V-N	925	1 yr	94.8	5.2	Not studied	

*V, vital; N, nonvital.

Survey results

The exact extent of the practice of one-appointment endodontics is not known. In 1980, Landers and Calhoun[20] questioned the directors of postgraduate endodontic programs about one-appointment therapy. Most of the directors saw little difference between single- and multiple-appointment therapy with respect to flare-ups, successful healing, and patient acceptance. One-visit endodontics was taught in 85.7% of the programs, and 91.4% of the directors, faculty, and residents treated some types of cases in one visit. Calhoun and Landers[7] polled 429 endodontists randomly in 1982 and found that 67% would treat vital cases in one visit whereas only 12.8% would so treat necrotic cases. The majority of endodontists thought that there would be more pain if treatment was completed on one appointment.

In a 1985 survey of 35 directors of endodontic programs by Trope and Grossman,[44] 54% indicated that they completed vital cases in one appointment. Only 9% said they would fill teeth with necrotic pulps in one visit. When a periapical lesion was present 70% of the respondents preferred multiple treatments with an intracanal medicament.

Gatewood and co-workers,[18] in a 1990 survey of 568 diplomates, reported that 35% would complete cases in one visit for teeth with a normal periapex whereas only 16% would do so when apical periodontitis was present. Fewer than 10% of the diplomates would complete a nonvital case in one visit, despite the previously cited evidence that there is little difference in pain or healing of multiple- and single-visit root canals. Despite strong evidence to the contrary, the endodontic community seems surprisingly resistant to one-appointment root canal treatment for too many cases.

Advantages and disadvantages

There are many *advantages* to one-visit endodontics[25,26,34]:

1. It reduces the number of patient appointments while achieving predictably high levels of success and patient comfort.
2. It eliminates the chance for interappointment microbial contamination and flare-ups caused by leakage or loss of the temporary seal.
3. For anterior cases it allows immediate use of the canal space for retention of a post and construction of an esthetic temporary crown.
4. It is the most efficient way of performing endodontic treatment, because it allows the practitioner to prepare and fill the canals at the same appointment without the need for the clinician's refamiliarization with the canal anatomy at the next visit.
5. It minimizes fear and anxiety in the apprehensive patient. Few patients ever request to have root canal treatment completed in several appointments!
6. It eliminates the problem of the patient who does not return to have his case completed.

There are a few *disadvantages* to one-appointment endodontics[6,25]:

1. The longer single appointment may be tiring and uncomfortable for the patient. Some patients, especially those with temporomandibular dysfunction or other impairments, may not be able to keep their mouth opened long enough for a one-appointment procedure.
2. Flare-ups cannot easily be treated by opening the tooth for drainage.
3. If hemorrhaging [illegible] to control that and to complete the case at the same visit.
4. Difficult cases with extremely fine, calcified, multiple canals may not be treatable in one appointment without causing undue stress for both the patient and the clinician.
5. The clinician may lack the expertise to properly treat a case in one visit. This could result in failures, flare-ups, and legal repercussions.

Guidelines for one-appointment endodontics

One-appointment endodontics should not be undertaken by inexperienced clinicians. The dentist must possess a full understanding of endodontic principles and the ability to exercise these principles fully and efficiently. There can be no shortcuts to success. The endodontic competence of the practicing dentist should be the overriding factor in undertaking one-visit treatment. *As a guideline, the case should be one that can be completed within 60 minutes.* Treatments that take considerably longer should be done in multiple visits.

Oliet's[30] criteria for case selection include (1) positive patient acceptance, (2) sufficient available time to complete the procedure properly, (3) absence of acute symptoms requiring drainage via the canal and of persistent continuous flow of exudate or blood, and (4) absence of anatomical obstacles (calcified canals, fine tortuous canals, bifurcated or accessory canals) and procedural difficulties (ledge formation, blockage, perforations, inadequate fills).

Within the confines of the clinician's ability, one-appointment root canal therapy should be considered in the following circumstances:

1. Uncomplicated vital teeth.
2. Fractured anterior or bicuspid teeth where esthetics is a concern and a temporary post and crown are required.
3. Patients who are physically unable to return for the completion.
4. Patients with heart valve damage or prosthetic implants who require repeated regimens of prophylactic antibiotics.
5. Necrotic, uncomplicated teeth with draining sinus tracts.
6. Patients who require sedation or operating room treatment.

One-appointment root canal therapy should be avoided in these circumstances:

1. Painful, necrotic tooth with no sinus tract for drainage.
2. Teeth with severe anatomic anomalies or cases fraught with procedural difficulties.
3. Asymptomatic nonvital molars with periapical radiolucencies and no sinus tract.
4. Patients who have acute apical periodontitis with severe pain on percussion.
5. Most retreatments.

Careful case selection and proper and thorough adherence to standard endodontic principles, with no shortcuts, should result in successful one-appointment endodontics. Practitioners should attempt one-visit root canal treatment only after making an honest assessment of their endodontic skills, training, and ability.

Retreatment versus Periradicular Surgery

Retreatment is required when previous endodontic therapy is failing. Retreatment should not be attempted until the cause

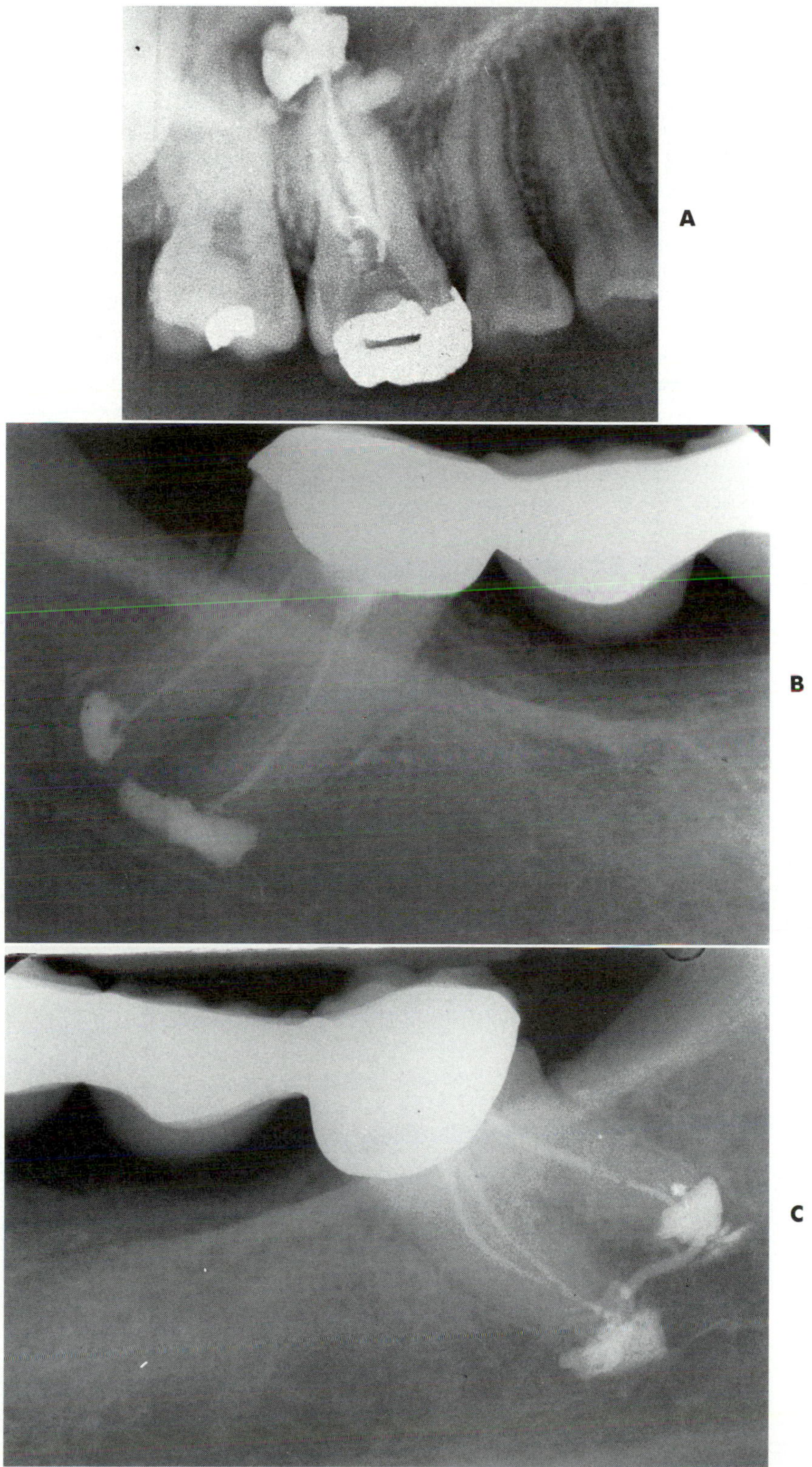

FIG. 4-10 A, Immediate surgery is required to remove extruded N2 from the sinus. **B** and **C,** Extruded N2 from both distal abutments in proximity to the mandibular canal caused bilateral paresthesia. (Courtesy of Dr. Ed Ruiz-Hubard.)

of the patient's symptoms has been ascertained. Often a patient is certain that the symptoms are originating in a previously treated tooth when, instead, an adjacent or nearby tooth is involved. Complaints of hot or cold sensitivity in an existing root canal should be followed up with the appropriate tests. Occasionally a tooth remains sensitive because initially all the canals were not located and treated.

If the failure is obviously caused by poor or incomplete débridement or obturation of all the canals, conventional retreatment should be instituted (Fig. 4-5). Though the success rate for retreatments is high, it may be lower than that for initial endodontic therapy. Removal of failing silver points can be quite easy if the points are small and can be easily grasped. However, large, well-fitted silver points may be very difficult to remove, and the treatment plan may require additional appointments in these cases. Old gutta-percha can be easily removed using Hedstrom files and rectified turpentine as a solvent.

When retreating molars, it is essential to look for additional canals. Despite poor obturation of the major canals, the cause of such failures is often a [illegible] located, débrided, and obturated to achieve success.

Nonsurgical retreatment is generally preferable and should be attempted before resorting to surgery. The presence of a crown is not in itself an indication for choosing surgery over nonsurgical treatment. In certain cases, treatment may be impossible owing to obstructions, calcifications, and prosthetic considerations. The presence of a post is not always an impediment to retreatment. Often the post can be removed utilizing ultrasonics, to allow retreatment of all canals. If only one canal was not previously treated, the access opening can be made alongside the post to locate and treat only the failing canal.

When material that can be harmful to the periradicular tissues, such as N2, is extruded past the apex, it is necessary quickly to enter the area surgically to remove the material (Fig. 4-10). If an innocuous material, such as gutta-percha or the tip of a file, is expelled past the apex, it is not usually necessary to remove it surgically, provided the canal system is adequately débrided and sealed (Fig. 4-5, *D*).

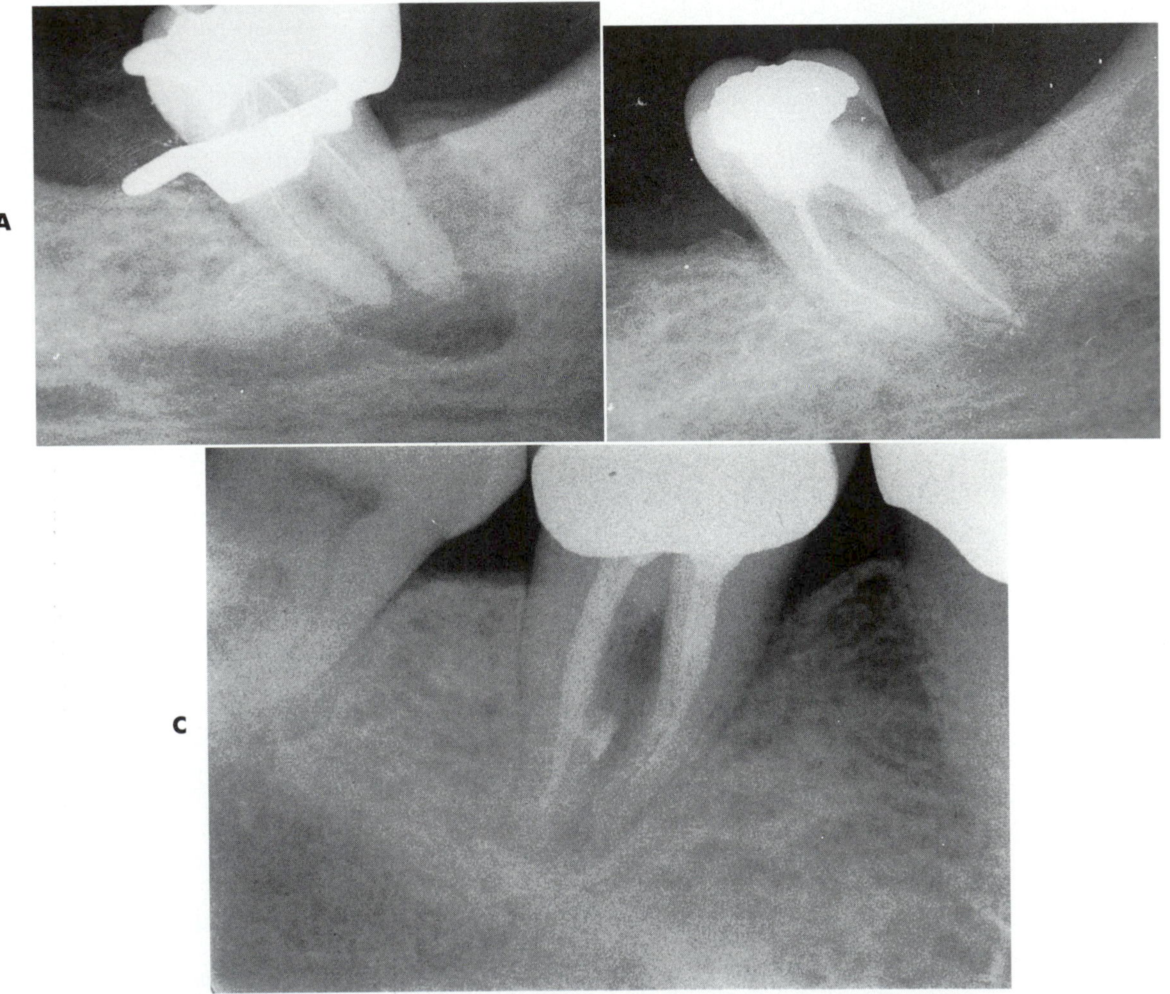

FIG. 4-11 Often lesions that appear to be of periodontal origin are primarily endodontic. **A,** **B,** Successful resolution of an apparent periodontal lesion in a 79-year-old female with a significant history of cardiovascular disease and diabetes. **C,** Furcation involvement often heals following proper endodontic treatment.

Surgery should be planned only when the practitioner is certain that the failing case was treated properly initially and cannot be improved upon, when retreatment is impossible for prosthetic or other reasons, or when the lesion is large and biopsy is prudent. In planning surgeries, the first visit is generally for examination, consultation, and informed consent. Most surgeries are not done as emergencies; they must be scheduled to allow enough time. Often, the profound anesthesia required for periradicular surgery cannot be induced in the presence of severe pain and swelling. Acute symptoms should be alleviated by incision and drainage or trephination before performing periradicular surgery. The surgery can be performed once the patient is comfortable. Many surgical cases are asymptomatic or present with a draining sinus tract and can be scheduled at a time convenient to both dentist and patient.

Coordination with Other Dental Specialists

In some instances cases must be evaluated by other dentists or specialists before endodontic treatment is instituted. The first concern is the restorability of the tooth. Root canal therapy should not be initiated until one is certain that the tooth is restorable. Severe furcation decay or decay below the bony crest may contraindicate endodontics (Fig. 4-8, *A*), or may necessitate root extrusion. Inadequate root structure may not allow for placement of a post following endodontic therapy. It is imperative that coordination with the referring dentist and/or a prosthodontist be done before definitive endodontics is initiated.

Second, periodontal status must be ascertained before endodontic therapy is undertaken (Fig. 4-11), and a periodontist and/or endodontist should be consulted when that status is in question. A periodontal explorer should always be included on the examination tray and should be used in all cases. While endodontic therapy is usually done before periodontal therapy, it is nonetheless essential to be sure that the tooth is periodontally sound. Therapy should not be completed on a tooth whose periodontal status is questionable unless a consultation has taken place. Often, a combination of root canal therapy and resection of periodontally diseased roots is necessary. This should be determined as part of the original treatment plan following necessary consultations.

When careful examination does not reveal the cause of the symptoms, referral is in order. *Endodontic treatment must never be instituted unless the cause of the distress is known with certainty*. It is always wise to refer patients to other specialists rather than to guess and risk making an improper diagnosis. In cases of difficult diagnosis, referral to an endodontist should be considered. When pain of extradental origin is suspected, referral to a neurologist, otolaryngologist, or an orofacial pain clinic is in order.

REFERENCES

1. Abbott AA, et al: A prospective randomized trial on efficacy of antibiotic prophylaxis in asymptomatic teeth with pulpal necrosis and associated periapical pathosis, Oral Surg 66:722, 1988.
2. Alacam T: Incidence of postoperative pain following the use of different sealers in immediate root canal filling, J Endod 11:135, 1985.
3. American Association of Endodontists: Public knowledge and opinion about endodontics, Princeton NJ, 1987, Opinion Research Corp.
4. American Association of Endodontists: Market value of tooth, Princeton, NJ, 1989, Opinion Research Corp.
5. Ashkenaz PJ: One-visit endodontics: a preliminary report, Dent Surv 55:62, 1979.
6. Ashkenaz PJ: One-visit endodontics, Dent Clin North Am 28:853, 1984.
7. Calhoun RL, and Landers RR: One-appointment endodontic therapy: a nationwide survey of endodontists, J Endod 8:35, 1982.
8. Council on Dental Therapeutics and American Heart Association: Preventing bacterial endocarditis: a statement for the dental professional, J Am Dent Assoc 122:87, 1991.
9. Dietz GC, and Dietz GC: The endodontist and the general dentist, Dent Clin North Am 36:459, 1992.
10. Dodge JS: Immediate root-filling in the late 1800's, J Endod 4:165, 1978.
11. Dorn SO, et al: Treatment of the endodontic emergency: a report based on a questionnaire, part I, J Endod 3:94, 1977.
12. Dorn SO, et al: Treatment of the endodontic emergency: a report based on a questionnaire, part II, J Endod 3:153, 1977.
13. Fava LRG: A comparison of one- versus two-appointment endodontic therapy in teeth with non-vital pulps, Int Endo J 22:179, 1989.
14. Fava LRG: One-appointment root canal treatment: incidence of postoperative pain using a modified double flared technique, Int Endo J 24:258, 1991.
15. Ferranti P: Treatment of the root canal of an infected tooth in one appointment: a report of 340 cases, Dent Dig 65:490, 1959.
16. Fox J, et al: Incidence of pain following one visit endodontic treatment, Oral Surg 30:123, 1970.
17. Gartner AH, et al: Differential diagnosis of internal and external root resorption, J Endodon 2:329, 1976.
18. Gatewood RS, Himel VT, and Dorn SO: Treatment of the endodontic emergency: a decade later, J Endod 16:284, 1990.
19. Goerig AC, and Neaverth EJ: Case selection and treatment planning. In Cohen S, and Burns RC, eds: Pathways of the pulp, ed 5, St Louis, 1991, Mosby–Year Book Inc.

19a. Goldman M, et al: Immunological implications and clinical management of the endodontic flare-up, Compend Contin Educ Dent 10:126, 1987.

20. Landers RR, and Calhoun RL: One-appointment endodontic therapy: an opinion survey, J Endod 6:799, 1980.
21. Little JW: Antibiotic prophylaxis for prevention of bacterial endocarditis and infectious major joint prostheses, Current Opin Dentistry 2:93, 1992.
22. Little JW, and Falace DA: Dental management of the medically compromised patient, ed 3. St. Louis, 1988, C.V. Mosby Co.
23. Malamed SF: Handbook of medical emergencies in the dental office, ed 3, St. Louis, 1986, Times Mirror/Mosby College Publishing.
24. Mata et al: Prophylactic use of penicillin V in teeth with necrotic pulps and asymptomatic periapical radiolucencies, Oral Surg 60:201, 1985.
25. Morse DR: One-visit endodontics, Hawaii Dent J 18:12, 1987.
26. Morse DR, et al: Clinical study, infectious flare-ups: induction and prevention, parts 1–5, Int J Psychosomat 33:5, 1986.
27. Morse DR, et al: A prospective randomized trial comparing periapical instrumentation to intracanal instrumentation in cases of asymptomatic pulpal-periapical lesions, Oral Surg 64:734, 1987.
28. Mulhern JM, et al: Incidence of postoperative pain after one-appointment endodontic treatment of asymptomatic pulpal necrosis in single rooted teeth, J Endod 8:370, 1982.
29. O'Keefe EM: Pain in endodontic therapy: preliminary study, J Endod 2:315, 1975.
30. Oliet S: Single-visit endodontics: a clinical study, J Endod 9:147, 1983.
31. Pekruhn RB: Single-visit endodontic therapy: a preliminary clinical study, J Am Dent Assoc 103:875, 1981.
32. Pekruhn RB: The incidence of failure following single visit endodontic therapy, J Endod 12:68, 1986.
33. Roane JB, Dryden JA, and Grimes EW: Incidence of post-operative pain after single- and multiple-visit endodontic procedures, Oral Surg 55:68, 1983.
34. Rosenberg RJ, and Goodis HE: Endodontic case selection: to treat or to refer, J Am Dent Assoc 123:57, 1992.

35. Rudner W, and Oliet S: Single-visit endodontics: a concept and clinical study, Compend Contin Educ 2:63, 1981.
36. Seltzer S: Endodontology: biologic consideration in endodontic procedures, ed 2, Philadelphia, 1988, Lea & Febiger.
37. Seltzer S, and Naidorf IJ: Flare-ups in endodontics: II therapeutic measures, J Endod 11:559, 1985.
38. Simmons NA, et al: Case against antibiotic prophylaxis for dental treatment of patients with joint prostheses, Lancet 339:301, 1992.
39. Soltanoff W: A comparative study of single-visit and multiple-visit endodontic procedures, J Endod 9:278, 1978.
40. Southard DW: Effective one-visit therapy for the acute periapical abscess, J Endod 10:580, 1984.
41. Stamos DE, et al: The use of ultrasonics in single-visit endodontic therapy, J Endod 13:246, 1987.
41a. Torabinejad M, et al: Factors associated with endodontic interappointment emergencies of teeth with necrotic pulps, J Endod 14:261, 1988.
42. Trope M: Relationship of intracanal medicaments to endodontic flare-ups, Endod Dent Traumatol 6:226, 1990.
43. Trope M: Flare up rate of single visit endodontics, Int Endod J 24:24, 1991.
44. Trope M, and Grossman LI: Root canal culturing survey: single-visit endodontics, J Endod 11:511, 1985.
45. Walton R, Fouad A: Endodontic interappointment flare-ups: a prospective study of incidence and related factors, J Endod 18:172, 1992.
46. Wolch I: One-appointment endodontic treatment, J Can Dent Assoc 41:24, 1970.
47. Wood NK: Treatment planning: a pragmatic approach, St Louis, 1978, Times Mirror/Mosby College Publishing.

Self-assessment questions

1. Patients with rheumatic heart disease should
   a. be premedicated with antibiotics per American Heart Association guidelines.
   b. be premedicated with psychosedation.
   c. be premedicated with nonsteroidal antiinflammatory drugs.
   d. postpone elective endodontic therapy.
2. Diabetes patients in need of endodontic therapy
   a. should not receive elective therapy.
   b. should maintain normal insulin and meal schedules.
   c. do well with intracanal steroid therapy.
   d. heal as well as nondiabetics.
3. Patients with HIV infection, including AIDS,
   a. should be premedicated with analgesics.
   b. are at less risk from root canal therapy than from extraction.
   c. are at less risk from extraction than from root canal therapy.
   d. have fewer complications during and after treatment.
4. Pregnant patients in the first trimester
   a. should receive the normal x-ray dose for endodontic therapy.
   b. are not candidates for electronic apex locators.
   c. should delay use of x-ray until the second trimester.
   d. are not at risk from pharmacologic intervention.
5. Patients taking daily steroid therapy (e.g., for systemic lupus erythematosus)
   a. may demonstrate adrenocorticoid depression.
   b. respond well to stress.
   c. are candidates for intracanal corticosteroid therapy.
   d. do not require antibiotic premedication.
6. Extra canals
   a. are rarely found in molar teeth.
   b. are often found in molar teeth.
   c. if not found, have little effect on the success of endodontic therapy.
   d. are often found in upper canines.
7. Treatment consideration(s) for referral are
   a. poor oral hygiene.
   b. a patient who breaks appointments.
   c. calcified and curved root canals.
   d. a patient who does not have dental insurance.
8. Differentiate between external and internal root resorption
   a. internal resorption is contiguous with the canal, and external resorption is superimposed on x-ray examination.
   b. internal resorption appears superimposed, and external resorption appears contiguous with the canal on x-ray examination.
   c. the apex locator is very useful.
   d. internal resorption is larger in size.
9. Crown and root perforations
   a. are not treatable by surgical intervention.
   b. heal after routine root canal therapy.
   c. can respond to a matrix of hydroxyapatite and seal with glass ionomer.
   d. respond whether or not crown/root is sealed.
10. The prognosis is compromised
    a. when patient presents with pain.
    b. when patient experiences interappointment pain.
    c. with class III mobility and loss of bone support.
    d. for molar teeth.
11. The sequence of therapy recommended for emergency treatment is
    a. caries control, pulp/periodontal, oral surgery.
    b. oral surgery, caries, pulp/periodontal.
    c. pulp/periodontal, caries control, extraction.
    d. pulp/periodontal, oral surgery, caries control.
12. Single-visit root canal therapy
    a. is an unacceptable procedure.
    b. should be performed with apicoectomy.
    c. is an acceptable and successful procedure.
    d. requires antibiotic premedication.
13. One-appointment endodontic therapy is not indicated for
    a. fractured anterior teeth where aesthetics is a concern.
    b. patients requiring sedation or operating room procedures.
    c. cases with severe anatomical and procedural difficulties.
    d. when the patient is physically unable to return for completion.
14. Patients scheduled for retreatment
    a. may expect to have less interappointment pain.
    b. should expect successful resolution.
    c. should expect surgical intervention.
    d. may complain of thermal response on an adjacent tooth.
15. Surgical retreatment is indicated
    a. for a persistent area of rarefaction at the apex of a retreated tooth.
    b. for the development of severe periodontal pocket formation.
    c. for juvenile diabetes patients.
    d. before routine endodontic retreatment.

Chapter 5

Preparation for Treatment

Gerald Neal Glickman

Before initiation of nonsurgical root canal treatment, a number of treatment, clinician, and patient needs must be addressed. These include proper infection control and occupational safety procedures for the entire health care team and treatment environment; appropriate communication with the patient, including case presentation and informed consent; premedication, if necessary, followed by effective administration of local anesthesia; a quality radiographic survey; and thorough isolation of the treatment site.

PREPARATION OF OPERATORY

Infection Control

Because all dental personnel risk exposure to a host of infectious organisms that may cause a number of infections, including influenza, upper respiratory tract disease, tuberculosis, herpes, hepatitis B, and AIDS, it is essential that effective infection control procedures be used to minimize the risk of cross-contamination in the work environment.[16,51] These infection control programs must not only protect patients and the dental team from contracting infections during dental procedures but also must reduce the numbers of microorganisms in the immediate dental environment to the lowest level possible.

As the AIDS epidemic continues to expand, it has been established that the potential for occupational transmission of HIV and other fluid-borne pathogens can be minimized by enforcing infection control policies specifically designed to reduce exposure to blood and other infected body fluids.[8-10,51] Since the human immunodeficiency virus (HIV) has been shown to be fragile and easily destroyed by heat or chemical disinfectants, the highly resistant nature of the hepatitis B virus, along with its high blood titers, makes it a good model for infection control practices to prevent transmission of a large number of other pathogens via blood or saliva. Because all infected patients are not readily identifiable through the routine medical history, the American Dental Association (ADA) recommends that each patient be considered potentially infectious; this means that the same strict infection control policies or "universal precautions" apply to all patients.[16,51] In addition, the Occupational Safety and Health Administration (OSHA) of the U.S. Department of Labor, in conjunction with both the ADA and Centers for Disease Control (CDC), has issued detailed guidelines on hazard and safety control in the dental treatment setting.[2,8-10,32,51] In 1992 laws specifically regulating exposure to blood-borne disease became effective through OSHA's Occupational Exposure to Bloodborne Pathogens Standard.[18] Primarily designed to protect any employee who could be "reasonably anticipated" to have contact with blood or any other potentially infectious materials, the standard encompasses a combination of engineering and work practice controls, personal protective clothing and equipment, training, signs and labels, as well as hepatitis B vaccination and authorizes OSHA to conduct inspections and impose financial penalties for failure to comply with specific regulations.[18]

As of early 1993, the ADA, CDC, and OSHA recommended or mandated that infection control guidelines include the following measures:*

1. The ADA and CDC recommend that all dentists and staff who have patient contact be vaccinated against hepatitis B. The OSHA standard requires that employers make the hepatitis B vaccine available to occupationally exposed employees, at the employer's expense, within 10 working days of assignment to tasks that may result in exposure. A declination form, using specific language requested by OSHA,

*References 2, 3, 8-10, 16, 18, 32, 51.

must be signed by an employee who refuses the vaccine. In addition, postexposure follow-up and evaluation must be made available to all employees who have had an exposure incident.

2. A thorough patient medical history, which includes specific questions about hepatitis, AIDS, current illnesses, unintentional weight loss, lymphadenopathy, oral soft tissue lesions, and so on, must be taken and updated at subsequent appointments.
3. Dental personnel must wear protective attire and use proper barrier techniques. The standard requires the employer to ensure that employees use personal protective equipment and that such protection is provided at no cost to the employee.
   a. Disposable latex or vinyl gloves must be worn when contact with body fluids or mucous membranes is anticipated or when touching potentially contaminated surfaces; they may not be washed for reuse. OSHA requires that gloves be replaced after each patient contact and when torn or punctured. Utility gloves for cleaning instruments and surfaces may be decontaminated for reuse if their integrity is not compromised. Polyethylene gloves may be worn over treatment gloves to prevent contamination of objects such as drawers, light handles, or charts.
   b. Hands must be washed with soap before and after gloving and after removal of any personal protective equipment or clothing; for surgical procedures an antimicrobial soap should be used. The standard requires that any body area that has contact with any potentially infectious materials, including saliva, must be washed immediately after contact. Employers must provide washing facilities, including an eyewash, that are readily accessible to employees.
   c. Masks and protective eyewear with solid side shields or chin-length face shields are required when splashes or sprays of potentially infectious materials are anticipated and during all instrument and environmental cleanup activities; it is further suggested that protective eyewear be worn by the patient.
   d. Protective clothing, either reusable or disposable, must be worn when clothing or skin is likely to be exposed to body fluids and should be changed when visibly soiled or penetrated by fluids. OSHA's requirements for protective clothing (i.e., gowns, aprons, lab coats, clinic jackets) are difficult to interpret, since the "type and characteristics [thereof] will depend upon the task and degree of exposure anticipated." The ADA and CDC recommend long-sleeved uniforms, but according to OSHA long sleeves are required only if significant splashing of blood or body fluids to the arms or forearms is expected; thus, endodontic surgery would likely warrant long-sleeved garments. OSHA requires that the protective garments not be worn outside the work area. The standard prohibits employees from taking home contaminated laundry to be washed; it must be washed at the office or by an outside laundry service. Contaminated laundry must be placed in an impervious laundry bag that is colored red or labeled BIOHAZARD. Although OSHA does not regulate nonprotective clothing such as scrubs, such clothing should be handled like protective clothing once fluids have penetrated it.
   e. Patients' clothing should be protected from splashes of caustic materials, such as sodium hypochlorite, with waist-length plastic coverings overlaid with disposable patient bibs.
   f. Use of the rubber dam as a protective barrier is mandatory for nonsurgical root canal treatment, and failure to use such is considered to be below standard care.[11,12,21]
4. OSHA regulates only contaminated sharps. Contaminated *disposable* sharps, such as syringes, needles, and scalpel blades, and contaminated *reusable* sharps, such as endodontic files, must be placed into separate, leakproof, closable, puncture-resistant containers that must be colored red or labeled BIOHAZARD and marked with the biohazard symbol. The standard states that prior to decontamination (i.e., sterilization) contaminated reusable sharps must not be stored or processed in such a manner that employees are required to reach by hand into the containers to retrieve the instruments. The OSHA ruling allows picking up sharp instruments by hand only after they are decontaminated.[32]
   a. A suggested format for handling contaminated endodontic files is this: With tweezers, place used files in glass beaker containing a nonphenolic disinfectant-detergent holding solution; at end of day, discard solution and rinse with tap water; add ultrasonic cleaning solution; place beaker in ultrasonic bath for 5 to 15 minutes (use time adequate for thorough cleaning); discard ultrasonic solution and rinse with tap water; pour contents of beaker onto clean towel; use tweezers to place clean files into metal box for sterilization. Files with any visible debris should be separately sterilized; once sterilized, these files can be picked up by hand and débrided using 2×2 inch sponges; once cleaned, files are returned to metal box for sterilization.
   b. The standard generally prohibits bending or recapping anesthesia needles; however, during endodontic treatment, reinjection of the same patient is often necessary, so recapping is essential. Recapping with a one-handed method or using a mechanical device is the only permissible technique.
5. Countertops and operatory surfaces such as light handles, x-ray unit heads, chair switches, and any other surface likely to become contaminated with potentially infectious materials can be either covered or disinfected. Protective coverings such as clear plastic wrap, special plastic sleeves, or aluminum foil can be used and should be changed between patients and when contaminated. OSHA mandates, however, that work surfaces must be decontaminated and/or recovered at the end of each workshift and immediately after overt contamination. The coverings should be removed by gloved personnel, discarded, and then replaced after gloves are removed with clean coverings. Alternatively, countertops and operatory surfaces can be wiped with absorbent toweling to remove extraneous organic material and then sprayed with an Environmental Protection Agency (EPA)-registered and ADA-accepted tuberculocidal disinfectant such as a 1:10 dilution of sodium hypochlorite, an iodophore, or a synthetic phenol.
6. Contaminated radiographic film packets must be handled in a manner to prevent cross-contamination. Contamination of the film when it is removed from the packet and subsequent contamination of the processing equipment can be prevented either by properly handling the film as it is removed

from the contaminated packet or by preventing the contamination of the packet during use.[24] After exposure "overgloves" should be placed over contaminated gloves to prevent cross-contamination of processing equipment or darkroom surfaces.[31] For darkroom procedures films should be carefully manipulated out of their holders and dropped onto a disinfected surface or into a clean cup without touching them. Once the film has been removed, the gloves are removed and discarded and the film can be processed. All contaminated film envelopes must be accumulated, after film removal, in a strategically positioned impervious bag and disposed of properly. For daylight loaders, exposed film packets are placed into a paper cup; gloves are discarded and hands are washed; a new pair of gloves is donned; paper cup with films and an empty cup are placed into chamber; chamber is entered with gloved hands; packets are carefully opened, allowing the film to drop onto clean surface in chamber; empty film packets are placed into empty cup; gloves are removed and also discarded in cup; films can then be processed.[32] Plastic envelopes such as the ClinAsept Barriers (Eastman Kodak, Rochester, N.Y.) have simplified the handling of contaminated, exposed films by protecting films from contact with saliva and blood during exposure. Once a film is exposed, the barrier envelope is easily opened and the film can be dropped into a paper cup or onto a clean area before processing. The barrier-protected film, however, should be wiped with an EPA-approved disinfectant as an added precaution against contamination during opening.[24]

7. In conjunction with these guidelines for infection control, it has been advocated that prior to treatment patients rinse with a 0.12% chlorhexidine gluconate mouthrinse such as Peridex (Procter & Gamble, Cincinnati, Ohio) to minimize the number of microbes in the mouth and consequently in any splatter or aerosols generated during treatment.[51]
8. Following treatment, all instruments and burs must be cleaned and sterilized by sterilizers monitored with biological indicators. Air/water syringes must be flushed, cleaned, and sterilized. Heavy-duty rubber gloves must be worn during clean-up. The ADA and CDC recommend that all dental handpieces and "prophy" angles be heat-sterilized between patients.[3,32] Water lines must be flushed for 10 to 30 seconds, and all regulated infectious waste must be immediately disposed of in containers that meet specific criteria. Disposal must be in accordance with applicable federal, state, and local regulations.

In 1987, the infection control decision-making process was transferred to the U.S. Government through OSHA.[51] The ongoing goal of OSHA is to establish a routine and practical program of enforcing infection control standards based on published CDC guidelines to ensure the health and safety of all members of the dental health team. According to OSHA,[32,51] dentists must classify personnel and tasks in the dental practice according to levels of risk of exposure and must establish "standard operating procedures" to protect patient and staff from infection transmission. OSHA requires the dentist to provide infection control training for all employees and maintain records of such training; properly label all hazardous substances that employees are exposed to on the job; and have a written hazard communications program with manufacturers' Material Safety Data Sheets (MSDS) for all hazardous substances. With the enactment of OSHA's Bloodborne Pathogens Standard in 1991, employers must make exposure determinations and develop an exposure control plan. As mentioned above, the rule encompasses a number of critical areas: universal precautions, engineering and work practice controls, employee training, specific record keeping, and many others, all ultimately designed to protect employees from exposure to blood-borne pathogens, particularly HIV and the hepatitis B virus. Although the OSHA standard was written principally to protect employees, it does not encompass all of the infection control practices recommended by the ADA and CDC to protect dentists and patients. Therefore, compliance with the OSHA regulations and with the infection control policies of the ADA and CDC will help provide a safer workplace for the entire dental treatment team.[32,51]

PATIENT PREPARATION

Treatment Planning

Aside from emergency situations that require immediate attention, endodontic treatment usually occurs early in the total treatment plan for the patient, so that any asymptomatic but irreversible pulpal and periradicular problems are managed before they become symptomatic and more difficult to handle. The most important rationale for the high priority of endodontics, however, is to ensure that a sound, healthy foundation exists before further treatment is undertaken. A stable root system within sound periradicular and periodontal tissues is paramount for the placement of definitive restorations.

Regardless of the specifics of the case, it is the responsibility of the clinician to explain effectively the nature of the treatment as well as inform the patient of any risks, the prognosis, and other pertinent facts. As a result of bad publicity and hearsay, root canal treatment is reputed to be a horrifying experience. Consequently, some patients may be reluctant, anxious, or even fearful of undergoing root canal treatment. Thus it is imperative that the dentist educate the patient before treatment (i.e., informing before performing)[12] to allay concerns and minimize misconceptions about it.

Good dentist-patient relations are built on effective communication. There is sufficient evidence to suggest that dentists who establish warm, caring relationships with their patients through effective case presentation are perceived more favorably and have a more positive impact on the patient's anxiety, knowledge, and compliance than those who maintain impersonal, noncommunicative relationships.[15] Most patients also experience an increase in anxiety while in the dental chair; a simple but informative case presentation that leaves no question unanswered not only reduces patient anxiety but also solidifies the patient's trust in the dentist.

Case Presentation

The American Association of Endodontists (AAE) and the ADA publish brochures such as "Your Teeth Can Be Saved by Endodontic (Root Canal) Treatment"[1] to help patients understand root canal treatment. Valuable educational aids of this nature should be available to the patient, either before or immediately after the case presentation. This supportive information addresses the most frequently asked questions concerning endodontic treatment. These questions are now reviewed. Accompanying each question is an example of an explanation that patients should be able to understand. In addition, the dentist will find it useful to have a set of illustrations or drawings at hand to help explain the procedure.

What is endodontic (root canal) treatment?

Endodontics is the specialty in dentistry that is concerned with the prevention, diagnosis, and treatment of diseases or injuries to the dental pulp. The pulp, which some people call "the nerve," is the soft tissue inside the tooth that contains the nerves and blood vessels and is responsible for tooth development. Root canal treatment is a safe and effective means of saving teeth that otherwise would be lost.

What causes the pulp to die or become diseased?

When a pulp is injured, diseased, and unable to repair itself it becomes inflamed and eventually dies. The most frequent causes of pulp death are extensive decay, deep fillings, trauma such as a severe blow to a tooth, cracks in teeth, and periodontal or gum disease. When a pulp is exposed to bacteria from decay or saliva that has leaked into the pulp system, infection can occur inside the tooth and, if left untreated, can cause infection to build up at the tip of the root, forming an abscess. Eventually, the bone supporting the tooth will be destroyed, and pain and swelling often accompany the infection. Without endodontic treatment, the tooth would eventually have to be removed.

What are the symptoms of a diseased pulp?

Symptoms may range from momentary to prolonged, mild to severe pain on exposure to hot or cold or on chewing or biting; or, the condition may produce no symptoms at all.

The patient should be informed that the radiographic examination may or may not demonstrate abnormal conditions of the tooth and that sometimes there is radiographic evidence of pulpal and/or periradicular disease in the absence of pain.

What is the success rate for root canal therapy?

Endodontic therapy is one of the few procedures in dentistry that has a predictable prognosis if treatment is performed properly. Studies indicate that root canal treatment is usually 90% to 95% successful. Those in the failure group may still be amenable to retreatment or surgical treatment to save the tooth, though no treatment's success can be guaranteed. In addition, patients must understand that the prognosis may vary depending on the specifics of each case and that, without good oral hygiene and a sound restoration following endodontics, there may be an increased chance for failure. The need for periodic follow-up must be addressed in order to assess the long-term status of the tooth and periradicular tissues.

Will the endodontically treated tooth discolor following treatment?

If the treatment is done correctly, discoloration seldom occurs. Bleaching with heat or chemicals can be used to treat discolored teeth. Some endodontically treated teeth appear discolored because they have been restored with tooth-colored fillings that have become stained or with amalgam restorations that leach silver ions. In these instances the fillings may be replaced, but often the placement of crowns or veneers is indicated.

What are the alternatives to root canal treatment?

The only alternative is to extract the tooth, which often leads to shifting and crowding of surrounding teeth and subsequent loss of chewing efficiency. The patient should understand that often extraction is the easy way out and, depending on the case, may prove to be more costly for the patient in the long run. The patient always reserves the right to do nothing about the problem, provided the associated risks of this decision are explained by the dentist.

Will the tooth need a crown or cap following the treatment?

If there is no previously existing crown, it really depends on the amount of remaining sound tooth structure following endodontic treatment, the type of tooth, and the amount of chewing force to which the tooth will be subjected. Loss of tooth structure significantly weakens the tooth and renders it more susceptible to fracture; as a result, it may be necessary to protect what is left with a restoration such as a crown. Significant loss of tooth structure with a concomitant loss of retentive areas for coronal buildups may necessitate the placement of a metallic post in a canal in order to retain the buildup material (Fig. 5-1, *I* and *J*). For further information on these issues, the reader is referred to Chapter 22.

What does root canal treatment involve?

Treatment may require one to three appointments, depending on the diagnosis, the number of roots, and the complexity of the case. During these appointments the clinician removes the injured or diseased pulp tissue. The root canals are cleaned, enlarged, and sealed to prevent recontamination of the root canal system. The following steps (Fig. 5-1) describe the technical aspects of the treatment (illustrations, diagrams, and radiographs should be used as aids to the presentation):

1. Local anesthesia is usually administered.
2. The tooth is isolated with a rubber dam to prevent contamination from saliva and to protect the patient. This procedure is followed at each subsequent visit.
3. An opening is made through the top of the tooth in order to gain entrance to the root canal system.
4. The pulp tissue is painlessly removed with special instruments called *files*.
5. Periodic radiographs must be taken to ensure that these instruments correspond to the exact length of the root so that the entire tissue can be removed.
6. The root canal is cleaned, enlarged, and shaped, so that it can be filled or sealed properly at the final appointment.
7. Sometimes medications are placed in the opening in order to prevent infection between appointments.
8. A temporary filling is placed in the crown opening between appointments.
9. At the final appointment, the canal is sealed to safeguard it from further contamination.
10. Permanent restoration of the tooth is accomplished after completion of the root canal treatment.

Some additional points should be conveyed to the patient after treatment. The patient should not be given the impression that there will be no pain following the treatment.[49] In most cases, whatever mild discomfort the patient experiences is transitory and can usually be treated with an over-the-counter antiinflammatory or analgesic agent such as aspirin or compound-containing ibuprofen. In fact, prophylactic administration of these drugs before the patient leaves the office will help reduce postoperative discomfort by achieving therapeutic blood levels of analgesic before the local anesthetic wears off (see Chapter 13). In certain cases, simply handing the patient

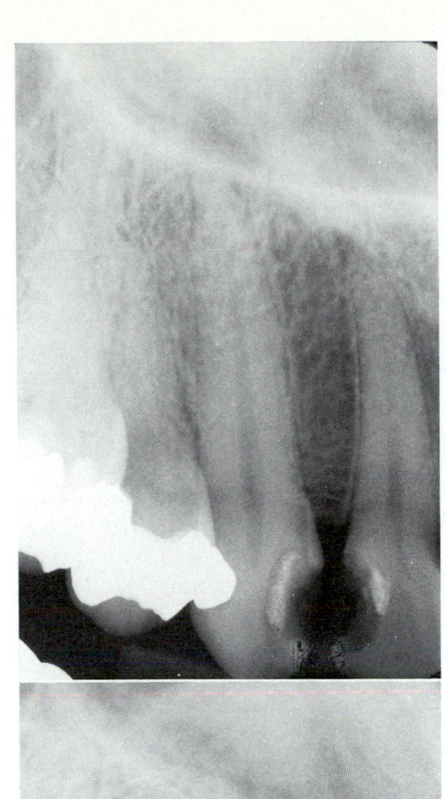

A, B

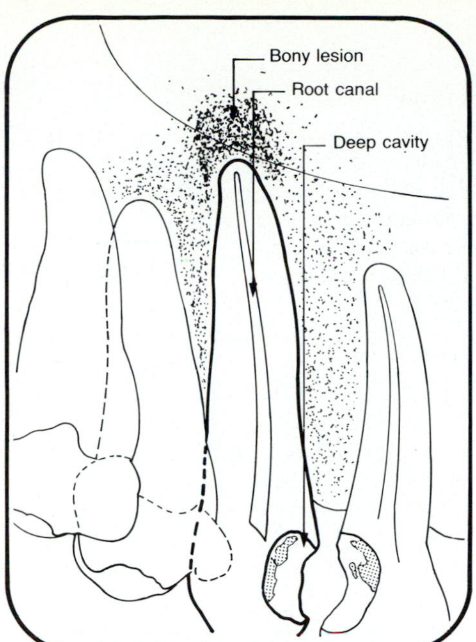

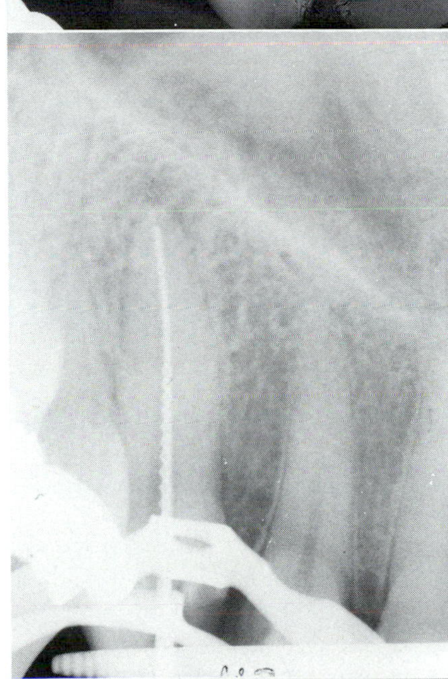

C, D

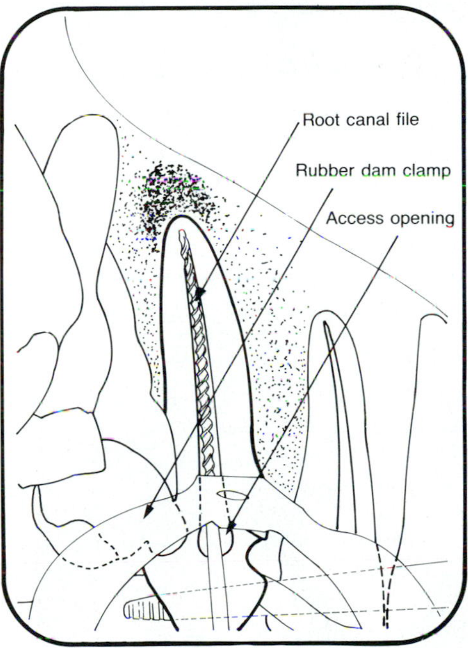

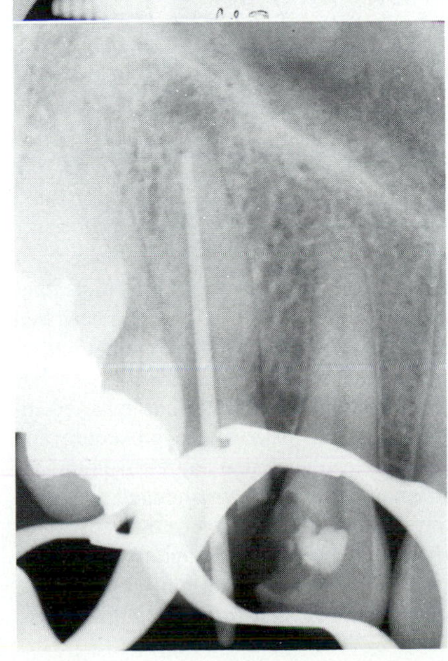

E, F

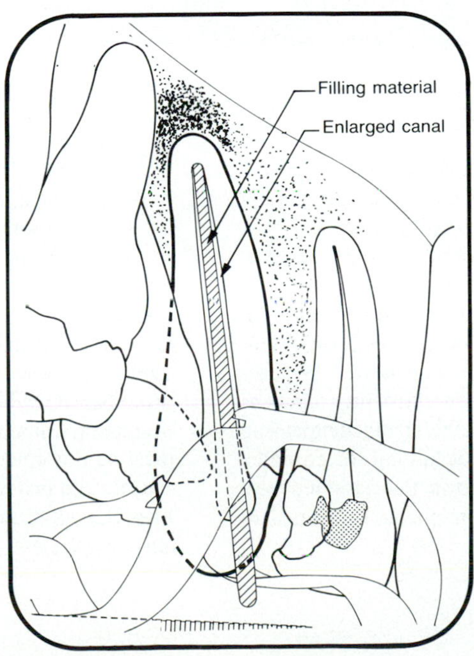

FIG. 5-1 Series of radiographs and illustrations demonstrating root canal treatment and restoration of a maxillary canine. **A** and **B,** Maxillary canine with periradicular lesion of endodontic origin. **C** and **D,** Endodontic file corresponding to length of canal; isolation with rubber dam throughout procedure. **E** and **F,** Endodontic filling material placed after cleaning and shaping of canal.

Continued.

FIG. 5-1, cont'd G and H, Canal system filled and post space made. **I** and **J,** One-year follow-up shows completed restoration and healed periradicular bone.

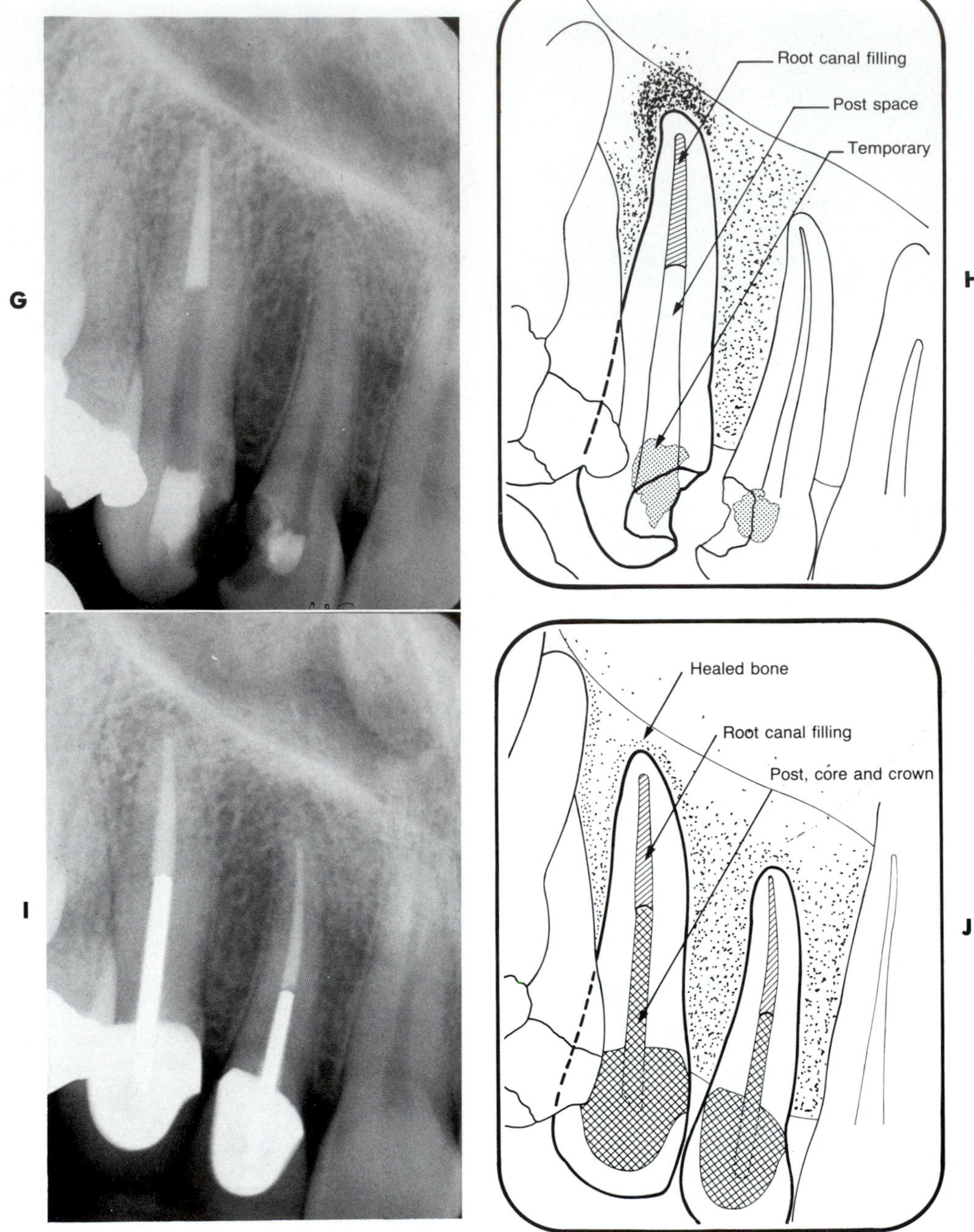

a written prescription for a stronger analgesic, "just in case," conveys a feeling of empathy and caring towards the patient and strengthens the doctor-patient relationship.

If the dentist wishes to refer the patient to an endodontist for treatment, skillful words of encouragement and explanation will convey the caring and concern behind this recommendation. Many patients already feel comfortable with their dentist and thus are fearful of "seeing someone new." In addition, they may not understand why a general dentist chooses not to do the root canal treatment. The referring dentist can only help his or her cause by carefully explaining the complex nature of the case and why it would be in the patient's best interests to visit the endodontist, who is specially trained to handle complex cases.[49]

Informed Consent

A great deal of controversy surrounds the legal aspects of informed consent. The current thinking of the courts holds that, in order for consent to be valid, it must be freely given; that all terms must be presented in language that the patient understands; and that the consent must be "informed."[12,13,41] For consent to be informed, the following conditions must be included in the presentation to the patient: the procedure and prognosis must be described (this includes prognosis in the absence of treatment); alternatives to the recommended treatment must be presented along with their respective prognoses; foreseeable and material risks must be described; and patients must have the opportunity to have questions answered.[41] It is probably in the best interests of the dentist-patient relationship to have the patient sign a valid informed consent form. With today's continuous rise in dental practice litigation, a good rule to follow is to realize that "no amount of documentation is too much and no amount of detail is too little."[41] For further information on this subject, the reader is referred to Chapter 10.

Radiation Safety

A critical portion of the endodontic case presentation and informed consent is educating the patient about the requirement for radiographs as part of the treatment. The dentist must communicate to the patient that the benefits of radiographs in endodontics far outweigh the risks of receiving the small doses of ionizing radiation, as long as techniques and necessary precautions are properly executed.[23] Although levels of radiation in endodontic radiography range from only 1/100 to 1/1000 of the levels needed to sustain injury,[38,47] it is still best to keep ionizing radiation to a minimum, for the protection of both the patient and dental delivery team. A simple analogy can be used to help the patient conceptualize the minimal risk levels with dental radiographs. A patient would have to receive 25 complete full-mouth series (450 exposures) within a very short time frame to significantly increase the risk of skin cancer.[38] Nevertheless, the principles of ALARA (**a**s **l**ow **a**s **r**easonably **a**chievable), which are essentially ways to reduce radiation exposure, should be followed as closely as possible to minimize the amount of radiation that both patient and treatment team receive. ALARA also implies the possibility that no matter how small the radiation dose, there still may be some deleterious effects.[24,38]

Principles of ALARA

In endodontic radiography, one should select fast (sensitive) speed film, either D (Ultraspeed) or E (Ektaspeed).[37] Although E speed film allows for a reduction of approximately 50% of the radiation exposure required for D speed,[19] findings in observer preference studies have been mixed with regards to the quality, clarity, and diagnostic capability of E film compared to D. Processing of the E speed film is also more sensitive.[19,20,30] Specialized radiographic systems such as RadioVisioGraphy[40,42] involve the digitization of ionizing radiation and use considerably smaller amounts of radiation to produce an image that is available immediately after exposure (see section on Digitization of Ionizing Radiation).

Meticulous radiographic technique helps reduce the number of retakes and obviates further exposure. Film-holding devices, discussed later in the chapter, along with correct film and tubehead positioning, are essential for maintaining film stability and producing radiographs of diagnostic quality.[24,38] A quality-assurance program for film processing should also be set up to ensure that films are processed properly.[24,38]

Dental units should be operated using at least 70 kVp. The lower the kilovoltage, the higher the patient's skin dose. Optimally, 90 kVp should be used. Units operating at 70 kVp or higher must have a filtration equivalent of 2.5 mm of aluminum to remove the extraneous low-energy x-rays before they are absorbed by the patient.[24,38]

Collimation also reduces exposure level. Collimation, essentially, is the restriction of the x-ray beam size by means of a lead diaphragm so that the beam does not exceed 2.75 inches (7 cm) at the patient's skin surface. Open-ended circular or rectangular lead-lined cylinders, known as position-indicating devices (PIDs), help direct the beam to the target (Fig. 5-2); however, the rectangular cylinder additionally collimates the x-ray beam by decreasing beam size even more, subsequently reducing the area of skin surface exposed to x-radiation (Fig. 5-3). These PIDs or cones should be at least 12 to 16 inches long because the shorter (8-inch) cones, which provide shorter source-to-film distances, cause more divergence of the beam and more exposure to the patient.[24,38] Pointed cones, illegal in some states, should not be used because of the increased amount of scatter radiation they produce.

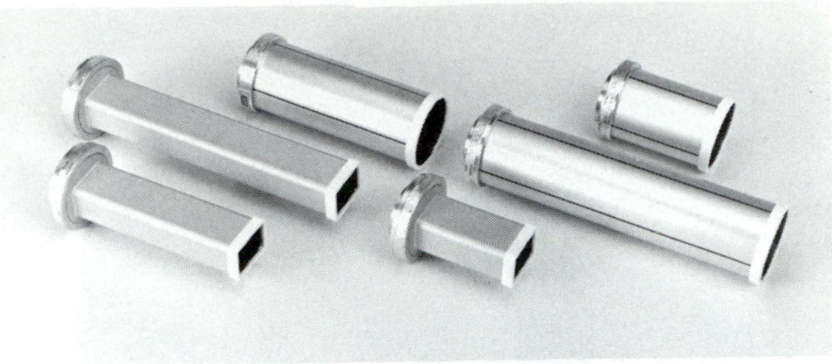

FIG. 5-2 Rectangular and round, collimating, lead-lined position-indicating devices (PIDs). The rectangular PID reduces as much as half the tissue area exposed to radiation. (Courtesy Rinn Corporation, Elgin, Ill.)

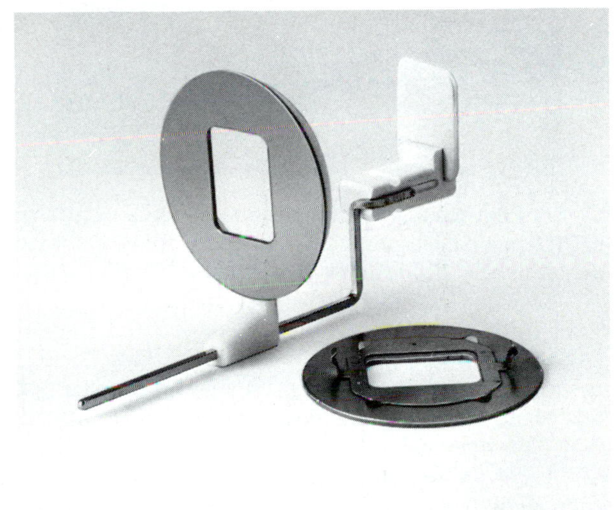

FIG. 5-3 Ring collimator snaps on aiming ring to extend the extra protection of a rectangular collimator to round, open-ended cones. (Courtesy Rinn Corporation, Elgin, Ill.)

The patient should be protected with a lead apron and a thyroid collar at each exposure (Fig. 5-4). When exposing films, the clinician should stand behind a barrier. Plaster, cinderblock, and at least 2.5 inches of drywall provide the necessary protection from the radiation produced by dental units. If there is no barrier, the clinician should stand in an area of minimal scatter radiation: at least 6 feet away from the patient and in area that lies at an angle between 90 and 135 degrees to the beam.[24,38] Film badges for recording occupational exposure should be worn by all dental personnel who might be exposed to occupational x-radiation. If the

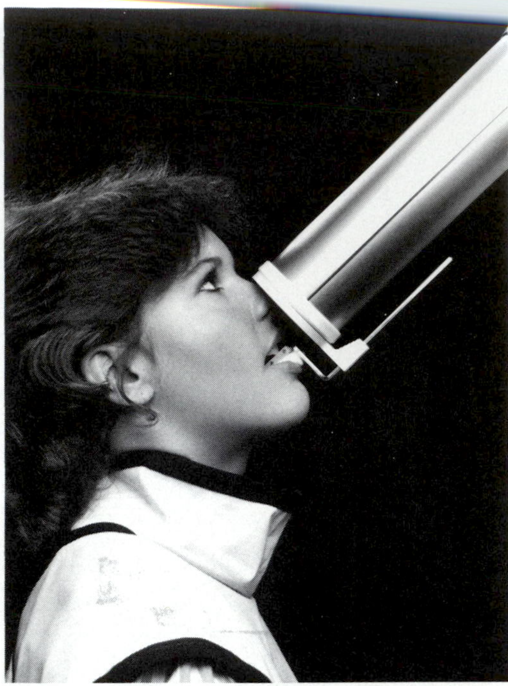

FIG. 5-4 Film holding and aiming device (XCP) instrument with PID on a patient protected with a lead apron and thyroid collar. (Courtesy Rinn Corporation, Elgin, Ill.)

concept of ALARA is strictly adhered to, no member of the dental team should receive doses close to their MPD, or maximum permissible dose (i.e., MPD, 0.02 Sv or 2 rem per year).[24] Every effort should be made to keep the radiation dose to all individuals as low as practicable and to avoid any unnecessary radiation exposure.

Premedication with Antibiotics

Prophylactic coverage with antibiotics or antiinfectives is indicated for patients who are susceptible to systemic disease following bacteremia. Although it has been documented that the incidence of bacteremia associated with nonsurgical root canal treatment is essentially negligible as long as endodontic instruments are confined to the root system,[5,6] the American Heart Association (AHA) recommends prophylactic antibiotic coverage for patients who have prostheses, shunts, or certain diseases to prevent any blood-borne microorganisms from lodging on shunts and prostheses or from multiplying within a depressed system and potentially causing infection and a life-threatening situation.[17,33,39,43]

Patients with certain cardiac conditions are candidates for antibiotic coverage in order to prevent subacute bacterial endocarditis (SBE).[43] These conditions include the presence of prosthetic heart valves, congenital malformations, systemic pulmonary shunts, rheumatic heart disease, idiopathic hypertrophic subaortic stenosis, any history of bacterial endocarditis, and mitral valve prolapse with valvular regurgitation.[17,33]

Patients with Addison's disease, AIDS, chronic alcoholism, blood dyscrasias, and uncontrolled diabetes mellitus should be premedicated as well.[33] Patients with organ transplants, orthopedic prostheses, ventricular-atrial shunts, and indwelling transvenous pacemakers, as well as individuals undergoing ir- [illegible] sives, or antineoplastic drugs, [illegible] propriate antiinfective regimen. The preceding list is not exhaustive but does highlight the cases encountered most often in dental practice.

The AHA has developed a standard prophylactic antibiotic regimen for patients at risk and a set of alternative regimens for those who cannot take oral medications, for those who are allergic to the standard antibiotics, and for those who are not candidates for the standard regimen.[17] The recommended standard prophylactic regimen for all dental, oral, and upper respiratory tract procedures is currently amoxicillin because it is better absorbed by the gastrointestinal tract and provides higher and more sustained serum levels than does penicillin. However, according to the AHA, the choice of penicillin V rather than amoxicillin as prophylaxis against α-hemolytic streptococcal bacteremia following dental procedures is still rational and acceptable.[17] Previous AHA recommendations emphasized the use of special parenteral regimens for persons at high risk for developing endocarditis (i.e., those with prosthetic heart valves, surgically constructed systemic-pulmonary shunts, or a history of endocarditis). The AHA presently recommends the use of the standard regimen for antibiotic coverage for this group of individuals, although it still recognizes that some clinicians may still prefer to use parenteral prophylaxis for these patients at high risk.[17] The official AHA recommendations for prophylactic antibiotic regimens do not specify all clinical situations for which patients may be at risk; thus, it is the responsibility of the clinician to exercise his or her own judgment or consult with the patient's physician before giving treatment.

The AHA guidelines for prophylactic antibiotic coverage are as follows:[17]

Standard regimen for patients at risk

Adults. Amoxicillin, 3 g PO, 1 hour before procedure, followed by 1.5 g amoxicillin 6 hours later. For amoxicillin/penicillin-allergic patients, erythromycin ethylsuccinate, 800 mg PO or erythromycin stearate, 1 g PO, 2 hours before procedure, followed by half the dose 6 hours later. For amoxicillin/penicillin/erythromycin-sensitive patients, clindamycin, 300 mg PO, 1 hour before procedure, followed by 150 mg 6 hours later.

Children. Amoxicillin, 50 mg/kg; erythromycin ethylsuccinate or erythromycin stearate, 20 mg/kg; or clindamycin, 10 mg/kg; followed 6 hours later by half the dose. Total pediatric dose should not exceed total adult dose.

Alternative regimens

Patients unable to take oral medications. Ampicillin, 2 g IV or IM, 30 minutes before procedure, followed 6 hours later by ampicillin, 1 g IV or IM, or amoxicillin, 1.5 g PO.

Ampicillin/amoxicillin/penicillin-allergic patients unable to take oral medications. Clindamycin, 300 mg IV, 30 minutes before the procedure, followed by 150 mg IV or PO, 6 hours later.

Patients considered high risk and not candidates for standard regimen. Ampicillin, 2 g IV or IM, plus gentamycin, 1.5 mg/kg IV or IM (not to exceed 80 mg), 30 minutes before procedure, followed by amoxicillin, 1.5 g PO, 6 hours after the initial dose; alternatively, the parenteral regimen may be repeated 8 hours after initial dose.

Ampicillin/amoxicillin/penicillin-allergic patients considered at high risk. Vancomycin, 1 g IV, administered over 1 hour starting 1 hour before procedure; no repeat dose is necessary.

Children. Ampicillin, 50 mg/kg; clindamycin, 10 mg/kg; gentamycin, 2 mg/kg; vancomycin, 20 mg/kg; followed by half the dose 6 hours later; amoxicillin, 25 mg/kg, is follow-up dose in this regimen. Total pediatric dose should not exceed total adult dose.

Although chlorhexidine mouth rinses are recommended for all patients before treatment, use of these antimicrobial agents is *strongly* encouraged for all patients who require prophylactic antibiotic coverage.

Antianxiety Regimens

Because patients very often have been misinformed about root canal treatment, it is understandable that some may experience increased anxiety. Fortunately, however, the vast majority of patients are able to tolerate their anxiety, control their behavior, and allow treatment to proceed with few problems. Appropriate behavioral approaches can be used to manage the most anxious dental patients. Retrospective studies[15] concerning dental anxiety have clearly demonstrated that patients' anxiety states can be effectively reduced by explaining procedures before starting, by giving specific information during treatment, by warning about the possibility of mild discomfort that can be controlled, by verbal support and reassurance, and by showing personal warmth. Many of these measures can be taken during the case presentation.

Although the clinician's hope and desire may not cure a patient's fear of root canal treatment, each clinician should realize that anxious patients are not all alike and each should be managed individually. If behavioral solutions are not feasible or effective in a particular case, pharmacologic approaches to managing the patient may be exercised. Selection of such pharmacotherapeutic techniques must involve a careful assessment of the relative risks and benefits of the alternative approaches. All pharmacologic treatment regimens include the need for good local anesthetic technique, and range from nitrous oxide plus oxygen sedation, oral sedation, or intravenous or conscious sedation for the management of mild to moderate anxiety states. For further information on these issues, the reader is referred to Chapter 20.

Pain Control with Local Anesthesia

It is paramount to obtain a high level of pain control when performing root canal treatment, and in no other specialty is this task as challenging or as demanding. The clinician must strive for "painless" local anesthetic injection technique with relatively rapid onset of analgesia (see Chapter 20).

PREPARATION OF RADIOGRAPHS

Radiographs are essential to all phases of endodontic therapy. They inform the diagnosis and the various treatment phases and help evaluate the success or failure of treatment. Because root canal treatment relies on accurate radiographs, it is necessary to master radiographic techniques to achieve films of maximum diagnostic quality. Such mastery minimizes retaking of films and avoids additional exposure of patients. Expertise in radiographic interpretation is essential for recognizing deviations from the norm and for understanding the limitations associated with endodontic radiography.

Functions, Requirements, and Limitations of Radiographs in Endodontics

The primary radiograph used in endodontics is the periapical radiograph. In diagnosis this film is used to identify abnormal conditions in the pulp and periradicular tissues, and to determine the number of roots and canals, location of canals, and root curvatures. Because the radiograph is a two-dimensional image, which is a major limitation, it is often advantageous to take additional radiographs at different horizontal or vertical angulations when treating multicanaled or multirooted teeth and those with severe root curvature. These supplemental radiographs enhance visualization and evaluation of the three-dimensional structure of the tooth.

Technically, for endodontic purposes a radiograph should depict the tooth in the center of film. Consistent film placement in this manner will minimize errors of interpretation, as this is the area of the film where distortion is least. In addition, at least 3 mm of bone must be visible beyond the apex of the tooth. Failure to capture this bony area may result in misdiagnosis, improper interpretation of the apical extent of a root, or incorrect determination of file lengths for canal cleaning and shaping. Finally, the image on the film must be as anatomically correct as possible. Image shape distortion caused by elongation or foreshortening may lead to interpretative errors during diagnosis and treatment.[22,24]

The bitewing radiograph may be useful as a supplemental film. This film normally has less image distortion because of its parallel placement, and it provides critical information on the anatomic crown of the tooth. This includes the anatomic extent of the pulp chamber, the existence of pulp stones or calcifications, recurrent decay, the depth of existing restorations, and any evidence of previous pulp therapy.[23,49] The bitewing also indicates the relationship of remaining tooth structure to the crestal height of bone and thus can aid in determining the restorability of the tooth.

In addition to their diagnostic value, high-quality radiographs are mandatory during the treatment phase. Technique is even more critical, since working radiographs must be taken while the rubber dam system is in place. Visibility is reduced and the bows of the clamp often restrict precise film positioning. During treatment, periradicular radiographs are used to determine canal working lengths; the location of superimposed objects, canals, and anatomic landmarks (by altering cone angulations); biomechanical instrumentation; and master cone adaptation (Fig. 5-1, *C* to *F*). Following completion of the root canal procedure, a radiograph is taken to determine the quality of the root canal filling or obturation. Recall radiographs taken at similar angulations enhance assessment of the success or failure of treatment (Fig. 5-1, *I* and *J*).

The astute clinician can perceive that precise radiographic interpretation is undoubtedly one of the most valuable sources of information for endodontic diagnosis and treatment, but the radiograph is only an adjunctive tool and can be misleading. Information gleaned from proper inspection of the radiograph is not always absolute and must always be integrated with information gathered from a thorough medical and dental history, clinical examination, and various pulp-testing procedures as described in Chapter 1.

Use of the radiograph depends on an understanding of its limitations *and* its advantages. The advantages are obvious: the radiograph allows a privileged look inside the jaw. The information it furnishes is essential and cannot be obtained from

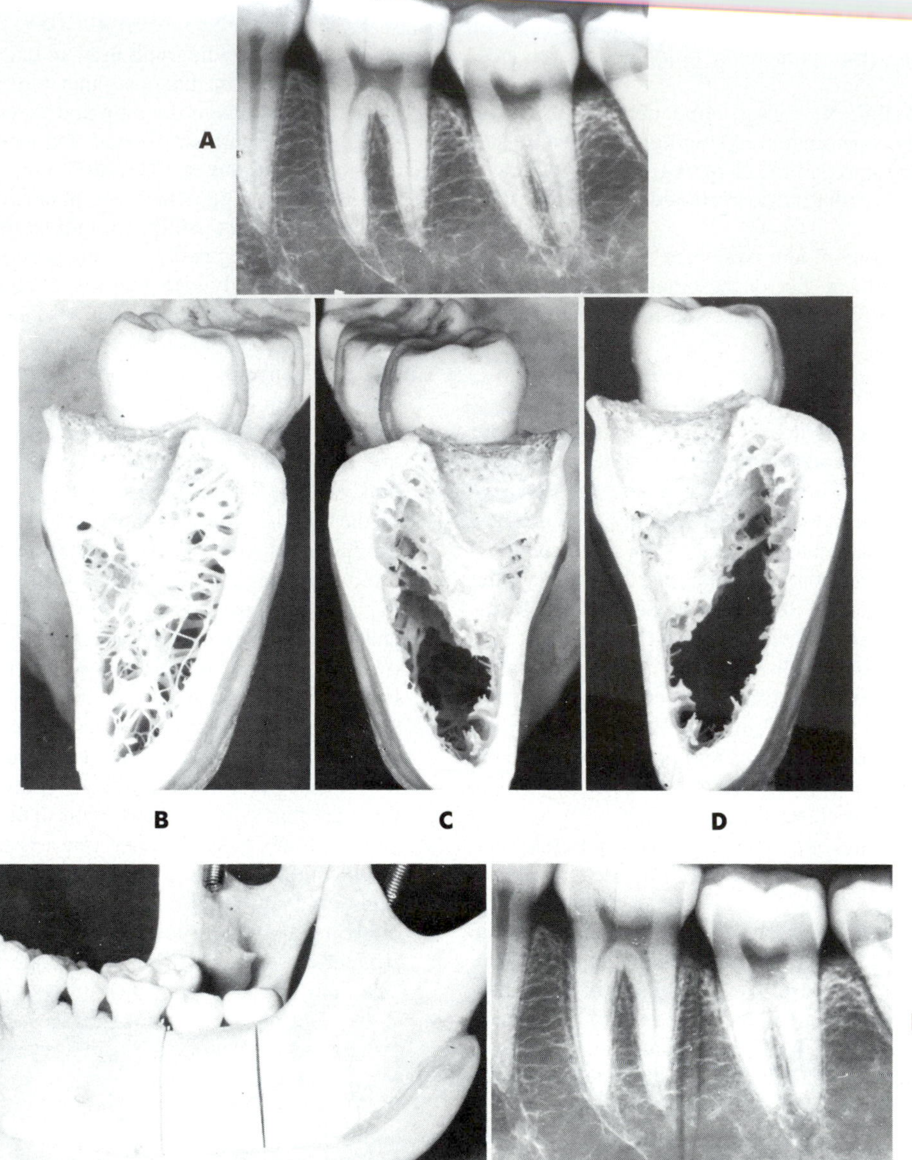

FIG. 5-5 A, Radiograph before any bone removal. **B,** Buccal-lingual section demonstrating cortical and cancellous bone. **C,** Removal of cancellous bone *without* infringement on the junctional trabeculae or cortical bone. **D,** Block section removed, demonstrating extent of destruction. **E,** Block section rearticulated to mandible with acrylic splint. **F,** Radiograph after removal of cancellous bone. Note there is no radiographic evidence of periradicular bone destruction.

any other source, yet its value is not diminished by a critical appraisal of its limitations.

One of the major limitations of radiographs is their inability to detect bone destruction or pathosis when it is limited to cancellous bone. Studies[45] have proven that radiolucencies usually do not appear unless there is external or internal erosion of the cortical plate (Fig. 5-5). This factor must be considered in evaluating teeth that become symptomatic but show no radiographic changes. In most cases, root structure anatomically approaches cortical bone, and if the plate is especially thin radiolucent lesions may be visible before there is significant destruction of the cortical plate. Nevertheless, inflammation and resorption affecting the cortical plates must still be sufficiently extensive before a lesion is visible radiographically.

Principles of Endodontic Radiography

Film placement and cone angulation

For endodontic purposes, the paralleling technique produces the most accurate periradicular radiograph. Also known as the *long-cone* or *right-angle* technique, it produces improved images; the film is placed parallel to the long axis of the teeth, and the central beam is directed at right angles to the film and aligned through the root apex (Fig. 5-6, *A* and *B*). To achieve

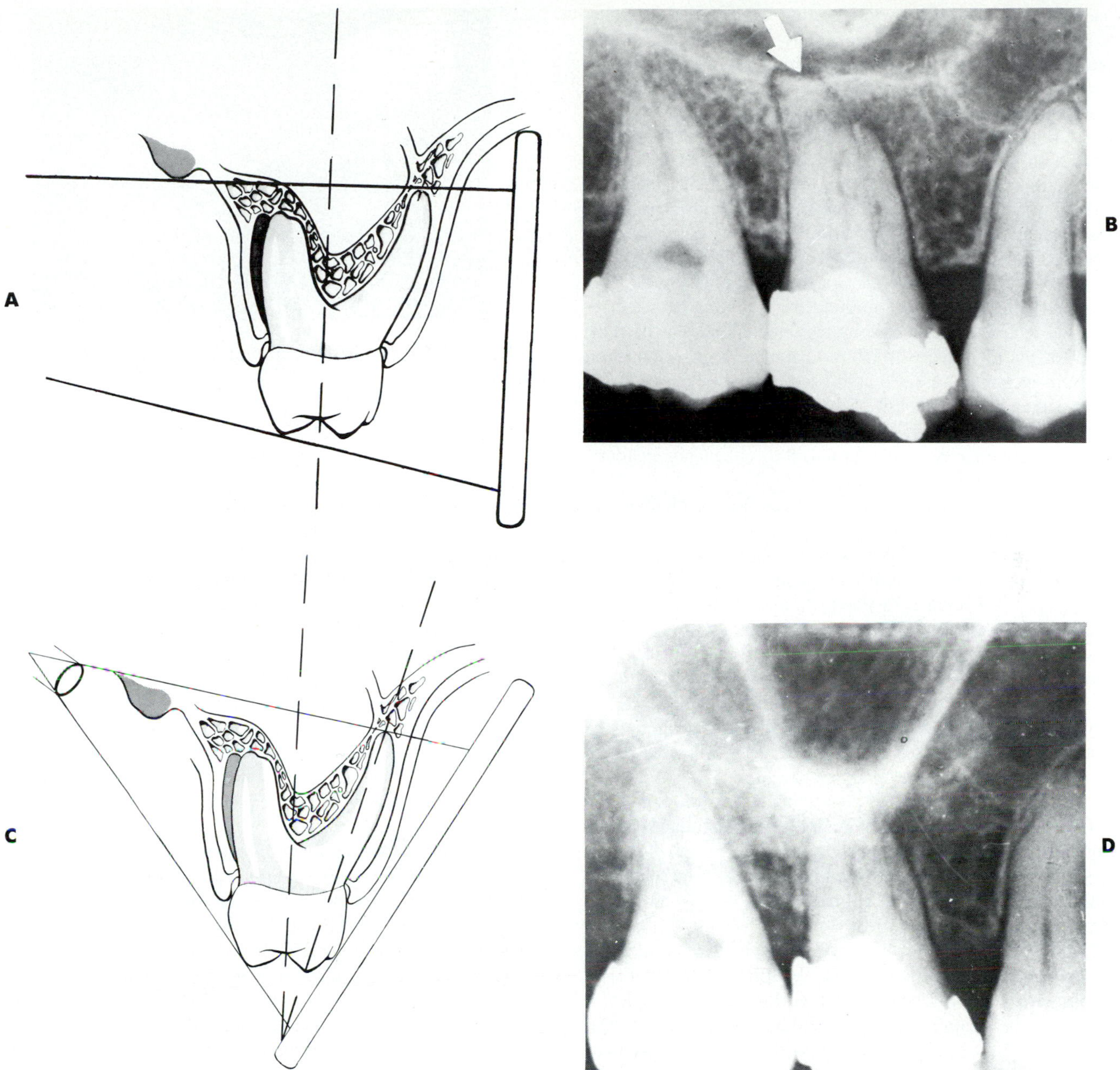

FIG. 5-6 A, Paralleling or right-angle technique. **B,** Projection of the zygomatic process above the root apices with the right angle technique allowing visualization of the periradicular pathosis *(arrow)*. **C,** Bisecting-angle technique. **D,** Superimposition of the zygomatic process over the root apices of the maxillary first molar with the bisecting-angle technique.

this parallel orientation it is often necessary to position the film away from the tooth, toward the middle of the oral cavity, especially when the rubber dam clamp is in position.[24] The long cone (16 to 20 inches) aiming device is used in the paralleling technique to increase the focal spot-to-object distance. This has the effect of directing only the most central and parallel rays of the beam to the film and teeth, thus reducing size distortion.[24,37,38] This technique permits more accurate reproduction of all of the tooth's dimensions, thus enhancing a determination of the tooth's length and relationship to surrounding anatomic structures.[22] In addition, the paralleling technique reduces the possibility of superimposing the zygomatic processes over the apices of maxillary molars, which often occurs with more angulated films, such as those produced by means of the bisecting-angle technique (Fig. 5-6, *C* and *D*). Thus, if properly used, the paralleling technique will provide the clinician with films with the least distortion, minimal superimposition, and utmost clarity.

Variations in size and shape of the oral structures (e.g., a shallow palatal vault, tori, and extremely long roots) or a patient's gagging often render absolutely true parallel placement of the film highly unlikely. To compensate for difficult placement, the film can be positioned so that it diverges as much as 20 degrees from the long axis of the tooth, with minimal longitudinal distortion. With maxillary molars, any increase in vertical angulation increases the chances of superimposing the zygomatic process over the buccal roots. A vertical angle of not more than 15 degrees should usually project the zygomatic process superiorly and away from the molar roots. To help achieve this, a modified paralleling technique[14] that increases vertical angulation by 10 to 20 degrees can be used. Though this orientation introduces a small degree of foreshortening, it increases periradicular definition in this troublesome maxillary posterior region. The Dunvale Snapex System (Dunvale Corporation, Gilberts, Ill.), a film holder and aiming device originally designed for the bisecting angle technique, has been altered for the modified paralleling technique.[14] In conjunction with this technique, a distal angulated radiograph, (i.e., a 10- to 20-degree horizontal shift of the cone from the distal (beam is directed toward the mesial) tends to project buccal roots and the zygomatic process to the mesial, thus enhancing anatomic clarity.[14]

The bisecting angle is not preferred for endodontic radiography; however, when a modified paralleling technique cannot be used there may be no choice because of difficult anatomic configurations or patient management problems.[14,24,37,38] The basis of this technique is to place the film directly against the teeth without deforming the film (Fig. 5-6, *C* and *D*). The structure of the teeth, however, is such that with the film in this position there is an obvious angle between the plane of the film and the long axis of the teeth. This causes distortion, because the tooth is not parallel to the film. If the x-ray beam is directed at a right angle to the film, the image on the film will be shorter than the actual tooth, or foreshortened; if the beam is directed perpendicularly to the long axis of the teeth, the image will be much longer than the tooth, or elongated. Thus, by directing the central beam perpendicular to an imaginary line that bisects the angle between tooth and film, the length of the tooth's image on the film should be the same as the actual length of the tooth.

Even though the projected length of the tooth is correct, the image will show distortion because the film and object are not parallel and the x-ray beam is not directed at right angles to both. This distortion increases along the image towards its apical extent. The technique produces additional error potential, as the clinician must imagine the line bisecting the angle, an angle that in itself is difficult to assess. Besides producing more frequent superimposition of the zygomatic arch over apices of maxillary molars, the bisecting angle technique causes greater image distortion than the paralleling technique and makes it difficult for the operator to reproduce radiographs at similar angulations to assess healing following root canal treatment (Fig. 5-6, *C* and *D*).[24]

Film holders and aiming devices

Film holders and aiming devices are required for the paralleling technique because they reduce geometric distortion caused by misorientation of the film, central beam, and tooth.* They also minimize cone cutting, improve diagnostic quality, and allow similarly angulated radiographs to be taken during treatment and at recall. By eliminating the patient's finger from the x-ray field and, thus the potential for displacing the film, these devices help minimize retakes and make it easier for the patient and clinician to properly position the film.

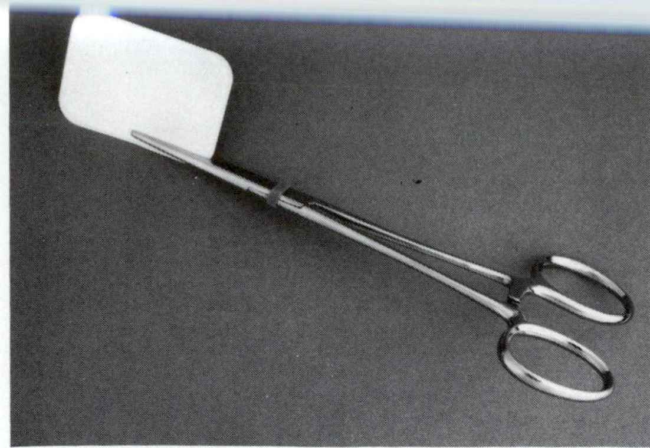

FIG. 5-7 Hemostat aids in film placement and in cone alignment.

A number of commercial devices are available that position the film parallel and at various distances from the teeth, but one of the most versatile film-holding devices is the hemostat (Fig. 5-7). A hemostat-held film is positioned by the operator, and the handle is used to align the cone vertically and horizontally. The patient then holds the hemostat in the same position and the cone is positioned at a 90-degree angle to the film. When taking working radiographs, a radiolucent plastic rubber dam frame, such as an Ostby or Young frame, should be used and not removed. To position the hemostat or other film-holding device, a corner of the rubber dam is released for visibility and to allow the subsequent placement of the device-held film.

Besides the Dunvale Snapex System that was mentioned earlier, the major commercial film holding and aiming devices include the XCP (cxtension cone paralleling) instruments, the EndoRay endodontic film holder, the Uni-Bite film holder, the EZ-Grip film holder, the EZ-Grip IIe film holder with aiming device, and the Crawford Film Holder System (Figs. 5-8 to 5-11). Variations in the use of the XCP system, for example, can prevent displacement of the rubber dam clamp and increase periradicular coverage during endodontic procedures. The film is placed off center in the bite block, and the cone is similarly placed off center with respect to the aiming ring. This allows for placement of the bite block adjacent to the rubber dam clamp without altering the parallel relation of the cone to the film (Fig. 5-12). A customized hemostat with rubber bite block attached can also be made to assist film placement during the taking of working radiographs. Other specialized film holders, such as the EndoRay and the Crawford Film Holder System, have been designed to help the dentist secure parallel working films with the rubber dam clamp in place. These holders generally have in common an x-ray beam-guiding device, for proper beam-film relationship, and a modified bite block and film holder, for proper positioning over or around the rubber dam clamp (Figs. 5-13 and 5-14).

Exposure and film qualities

The intricacies of proper kilovoltage, milliamperage, and time selection serve as examples of how the diagnostic quality of a film may be altered by changes in the film's density and

*References 14, 23, 24, 37, 38, 49.

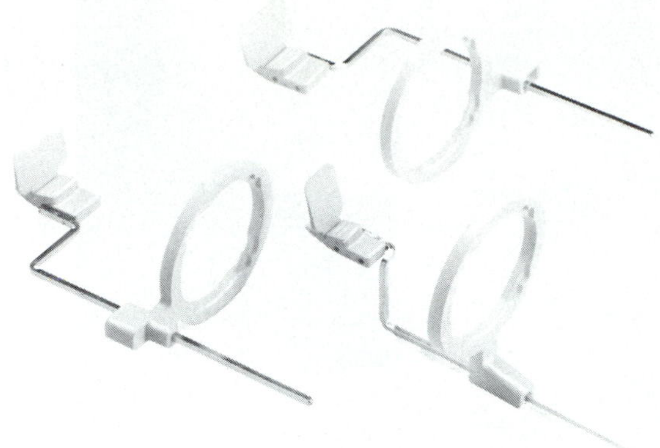

FIG. 5-8 XCP (extension cone paralleling) instruments hold the x-ray film packets and aid in cone alignment. Cone cutting is prevented and consistent angulation can be achieved. (Courtesy Rinn Corporation, Elgin, Ill.)

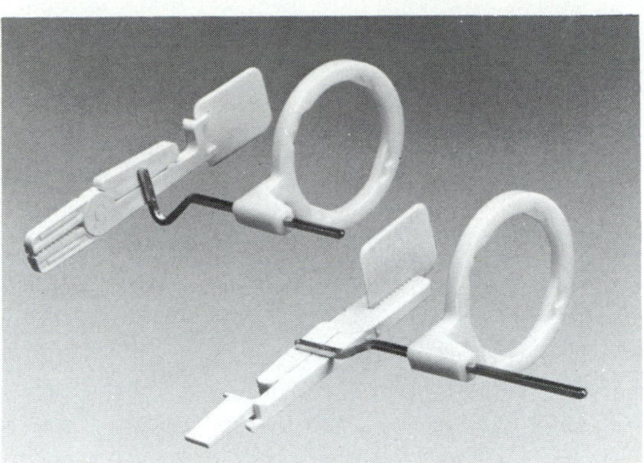

FIG. 5-10 EZ-Grip IIe film holder and aiming ring. The biting portion of the instrument is reduced to make it easier to place the instrument around the rubber dam. (Courtesy Rinn Corporation, Elgin, Ill.)

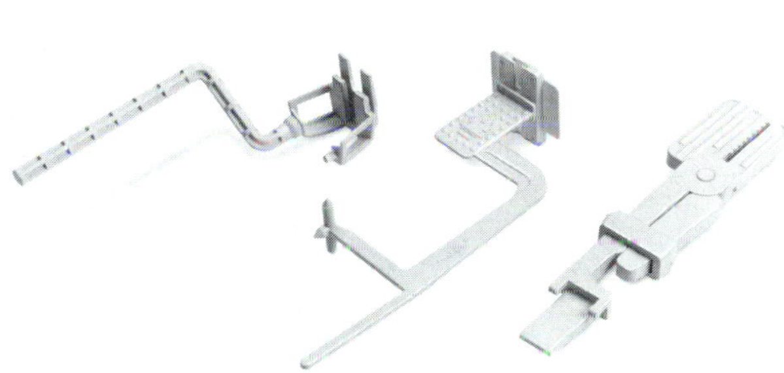

FIG. 5-9 Film-holding devices *(from left):* EndoRay, Uni-Bite, and EZ-Grip. (Courtesy Rinn Corporation, Elgin, Ill.)

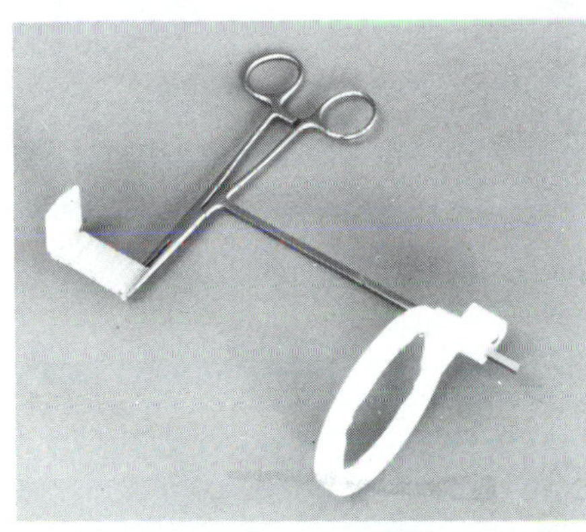

FIG. 5-11 Crawford Film Holder System. Components include Kelly hemostat with aiming rod attached, aiming ring, and bite block. (Courtesy Dr. Frank Crawford, Palm Desert, Calif.)

contrast.[24,38] Density is the degree of darkening of the film, whereas contrast is the difference between densities. The amount of darkening depends on the quantity and quality of radiation delivered to the film, the subject thickness, and the developing or processing conditions. Milliamperage controls the electron flow from cathode to anode; the greater the electron flow per unit of time, the greater will be the quantity of radiation produced. Proper density is primarily a function of milliamperage and time. Kilovoltage also affects film density by controlling the quality and penetrability of the rays. Higher kilovoltage settings produce shorter wavelengths that are more penetrating than the longer wavelengths produced at lower settings.[24,38] The ability to control the penetrability of the rays by alterations in kilovoltage affects the amount of radiation reaching the film and the degree of darkening or density. Variations in density can be controlled by altering exposure time or milliamperage for each respective unit.[24,38]

Contrast is defined as the difference between shades of gray or the difference between densities. Most of the variation observed in endodontic radiography is due to subject contrast, which depends on the thickness and density of the subject and the kilovoltage used. Thus, kilovoltage is really the only exposure parameter under the clinician's control that directly affects subject contrast.[23,24,38] Exposure time and milliamperage control the number of x-rays only and therefore have most of their impact on the density of the film image. A radiographic film may exhibit a long scale of contrast (low contrast) (i.e., more shades of gray or more useful densities); high-kilovoltage techniques (90 kVp) produce this long scale of contrast as a result of the increased penetrating power of the rays. This results in images with many more shades of gray and less distinct differences (Fig. 5-15). Films exposed at low kilovoltage settings (60 kVp) exhibit short-scale contrast (high contrast) with sharp differences between a few shades of gray, black, and white.[23,24,38] Although perhaps more difficult to read, films exposed at higher kilovoltage settings (90 kVp) make possible a greater degree of discrimination between images, often enhancing their diagnostic quality; films exposed at a

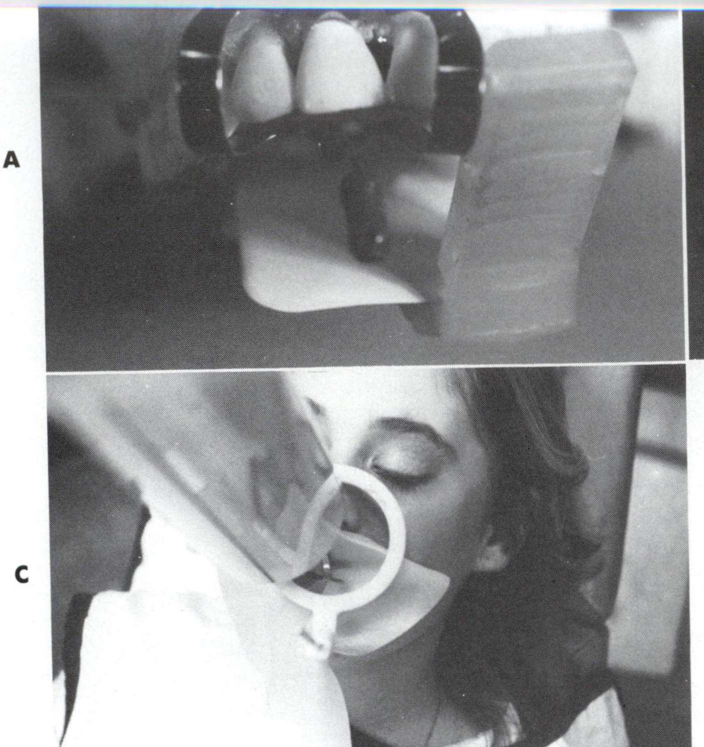

FIG. 5-12 **A,** Placement of a bite block on the tooth adjacent to the rubber dam clamp. **B,** Placement of the film off center in the bite block. **C,** Alignment of the x-ray cone.

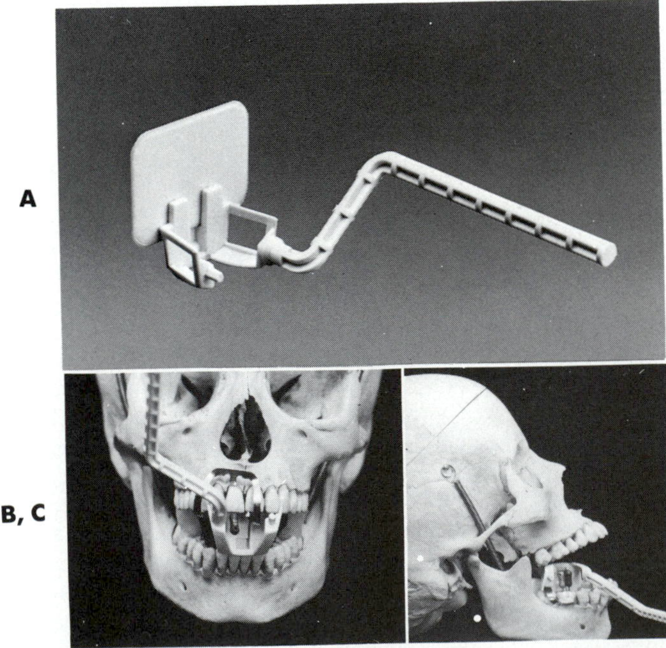

FIG. 5-13 A, EndoRay (posterior) film holder has a positioning arm to guide the cone to the center of the film. (Courtesy Rinn Corporation, Elgin, Ill.) **B** and **C,** Anterior and posterior EndoRay film holders in place over the rubber dam clamp. Handle aids in determining cone position and angulation.

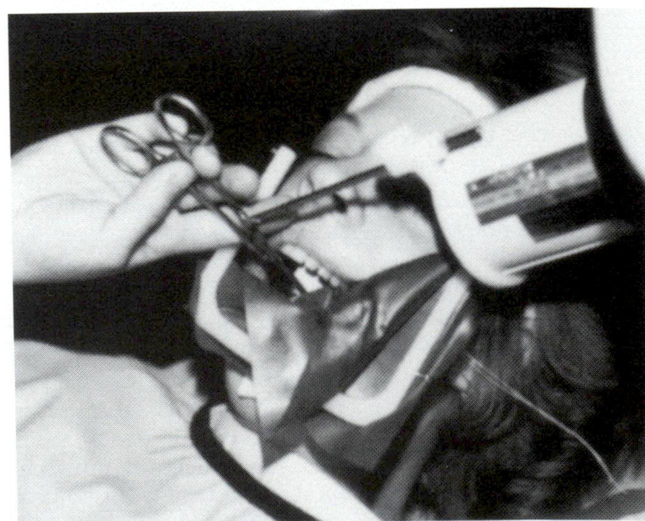

FIG. 5-14 Patient maintains position of film by holding handle of the hemostat of the Crawford Film Holder System. Note that the bite block is not used when rubber dam is in place.

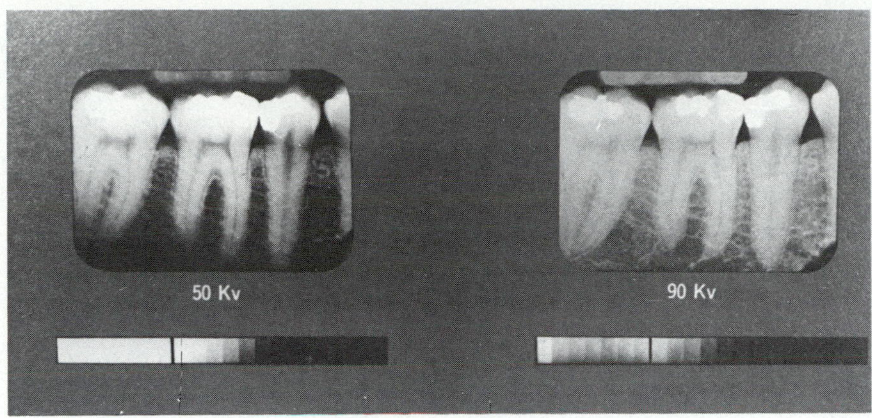

FIG. 5-15 Comparison of short-scale and long-scale contrast produced by altering the kilovoltage. Note the increased shades of gray in the film produced at 90 kVp. (Courtesy Rinn Corporation, Elgin, Ill.)

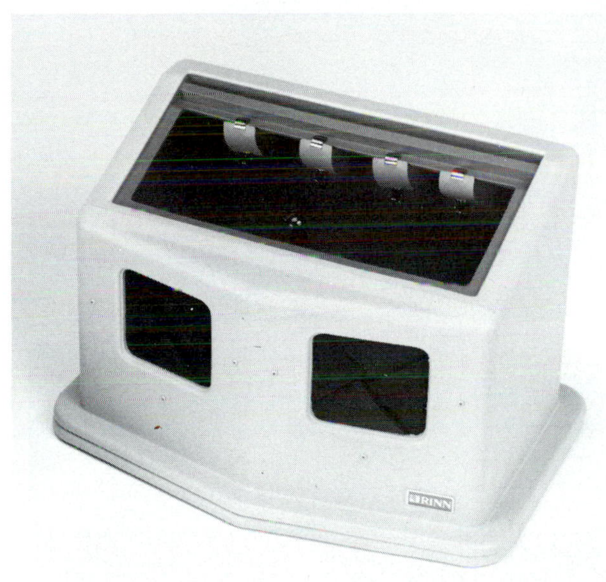

FIG. 5-16 Chairside darkroom allows rapid processing of endodontic working films. (Courtesy Rinn Corporation, Elgin, Ill.)

lower kilovoltage (70 kVp) have better clarity and contrast between radiopaque and radiolucent structures, such as endodontic instruments near the root apex. Nevertheless, the optimal kilovoltage and exposure time should be individualized for each x-ray unit and exposure requirement.

Processing

Proper darkroom organization, film handling, and adherence to the time-temperature method of film processing play important roles in producing films of high quality.[38] For the sake of expediency in the production of working films in endodontics, rapid processing methods are used to produce relatively good films in less than 1-2 minutes (Fig. 5-16).[23,24,38] Although the contrast in using rapid-processing chemicals is lower than that achieved by means of conventional techniques, the radiographs have sufficient diagnostic quality to be used for treatment films and are obtained in less time, and with less patient discomfort. Rapid-processing solutions are available commercially but tend to vary in shelf life and tank life and in the production of films of permanent quality. To maintain the radiographic image for documentation, it is recommended that after it has been evaluated it be returned to the fixer for 10 minutes more and then washed for 20 minutes and dried. An alternative is to reprocess the film by means of the conventional technique. Double film packets can also be used for working films: one can be processed rapidly and the other conventionally. Regardless of what method is used for working films, a controlled time-temperature method should be used for the diagnostic qualities desired in pretreatment, postreatment, and recall radiographs. All radiographs taken during the course of endodontic treatment should be preserved as a part of the patient's permanent record.

Radiographic Interpretation in Endodontics

Examination and differential interpretation

Radiographic interpretation is not strictly the identification of a problem and the establishment of a diagnosis. The dentist must read the film carefully, with an eye toward diagnosis and treatment. Frequently overlooked are small areas of resorption, invaginated enamel, minute fracture lines, extra canals or roots, calcified canals, and, in turn, the potential problems they may create during treatment (Fig. 5-17). Problems during treatment, additional time, and extra expense can be avoided, or at least anticipated, if a thorough radiographic examination is conducted. As mentioned earlier, additional exposures at various angulations may be necessary to gain a better insight into the three dimensional structure of a tooth.

Many anatomic structures and osteolytic lesions can be mistaken for pulpoperiradicular lesions. Among the more commonly misinterpreted anatomic structures are the mental foramen (Fig. 5-18) and the incisive foramen. These radiolucencies can be differentiated from pathologic conditions by exposures at different angulations and by pulp-testing procedures. Radiolucencies not associated with the root apex will move or be projected away from the apex by varying the angulation. Radiolucent areas resulting from sparse trabeculation can also

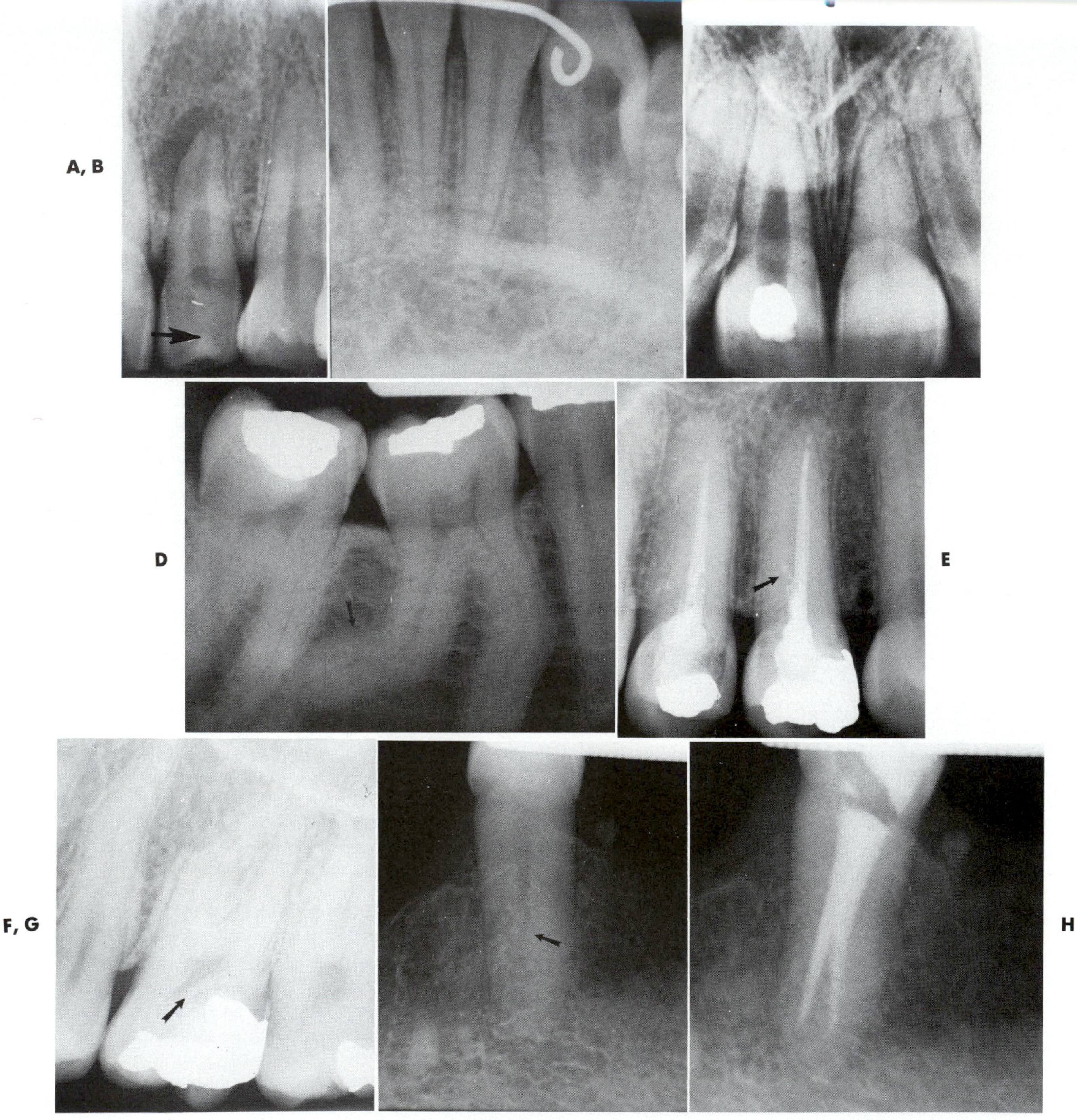

FIG. 5-17 Cases requiring careful interpretation. **A,** Enamel invagination on the incisal aspect of the maxillary lateral incisor *(arrow)*. This must be sealed following endodontic treatment to prevent coronal leakage through the invaginated channel. **B,** External root resorption on a mandibular canine. Note that the canal system can be followed through the resorptive defect. **C,** Opposite reactions to traumatic injury to the maxillary central incisors. The right central incisor exhibits almost complete calcification of the canal, whereas the left one exhibits an excessively large canal as a result of internal resorption in the coronal two thirds. **D,** Mandibular first molar with a dilacerated (sharply angled) root system. **E,** Evidence of another canal in an endodontically treated maxillary first premolar. Arrow indicates root canal sealer in this unprepared canal. **F,** Evidence of a previous pulp cap on a maxillary first molar. Arrow indicates bridge formation with reduction in size of the pulp chamber. **G,** Bifurcation *(arrow)* of the root canal in a mandibular first premolar. **H,** Completed endodontic treatment on tooth in **G** verifies presence of two canals.

simulate radiolucent lesions and in such cases must be differentiated from the lamina dura and periodontal ligament space.

A commonly misinterpreted osteolytic lesion is periapical cemental dysplasia or cementoma (Fig. 5-19). The use of pulp-testing procedures and follow-up radiographic examinations will prevent the mistake of diagnosing this as a pulpoperiradicular lesion. The development of this lesion can be followed radiographically from its osteolytic stage through its osteogenic stage.

Other anatomic radiolucencies that must be differentiated from pulpoperiradicular lesions are maxillary sinus, nutrient canals, nasal fossa, and the lateral or submandibular fossa. Many systemic conditions can mimic or affect the radiographic appearance of the alveolar process. A discussion of these conditions is beyond the scope of this chapter, but the reader is encouraged to read further in any oral pathology textbook.

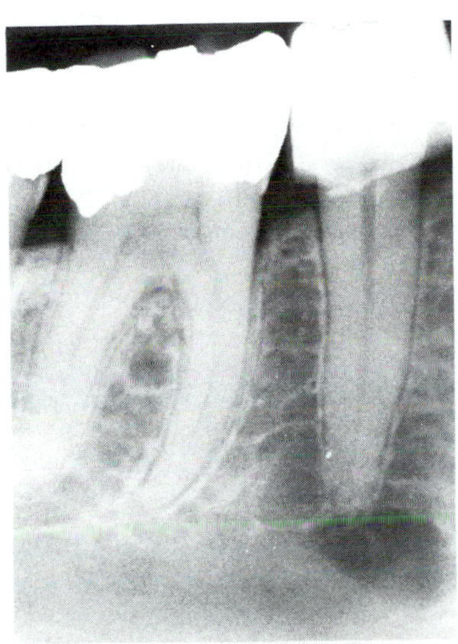

FIG. 5-18 A mandibular second premolar with an apparent periradicular radiolucency. Pulp-testing procedures indicated a normal response; the radiolucency is the mental foramen.

Lamina dura: a question of integrity

One of the key challenges in endodontic radiographic interpretation is understanding the integrity, or lack of integrity, of the lamina dura, especially in relation to the health of the pulp. Anatomically, the lamina dura[23,24] is a layer of compact bone (the cribriform plate or alveolar bone proper) that lines the tooth socket; noxious products emanating from the root canal system can effect a change in this structure that is visible radiographically. X-ray beams passing tangentially through the socket must pass through many times the width of the adjacent alveolus and are attenuated by this greater thickness of bone, producing the characteristic "white line" (Fig. 5-20). If, for example, the beam is directed more obliquely, so that it is not as attenuated, the lamina dura appears more diffuse, or may not be discernible at all. Therefore the presence or absence and integrity of the lamina dura are determined largely by the shape and position of the root, and, in turn, by its bony crypt, in relation to the x-ray beam. This explanation is consistent with the radiographic and clinical findings of teeth with normal pulps and no distinct lamina dura.[45]

Changes in the integrity of the periodontal ligament space, the lamina dura, and the surrounding periradicular bone certainly have diagnostic value, especially when recent radiographs are compared with previous ones. However, the significance of such changes must be tempered by a thorough understanding of the features that give rise to these images.

Buccal-object rule (cone shift)

In endodontic therapy, it is imperative that the clinician know the spatial or buccal-lingual relation of an object within the tooth or alveolus. The technique used to identify the spatial relation of an object is called the *cone* or *tube shift technique*. Other names for this procedure are the *buccal object rule, Clark's rule,* and the *SLOB* (same lingual, opposite buccal) rule.[24,25,38,44] Proper application of the technique allows the dentist to locate additional canals or roots, to distinguish between objects that have been superimposed and between various types of resorption, to determine the buccal-lingual position of fractures and perforative defects, to locate foreign bodies, and to locate anatomic landmarks in relation to the root apex, such as the mandibular canal.[23,49]

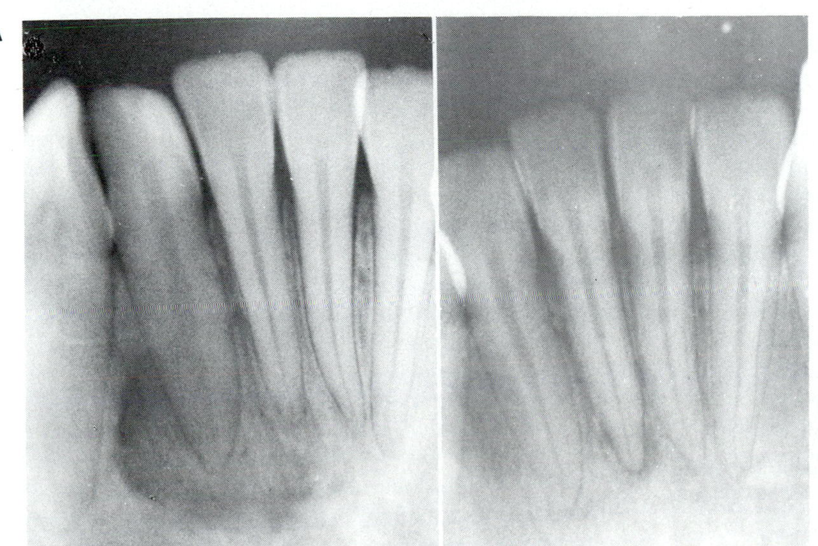

FIG. 5-19 Variations in appearance of periapical cemental dysplasia (cementoma). **A,** Osteolytic stage at apex of the mandibular lateral incisor. **B,** One year later: regeneration of bone around the apex of the lateral incisor and appearance of a radiolucency around the central incisor.

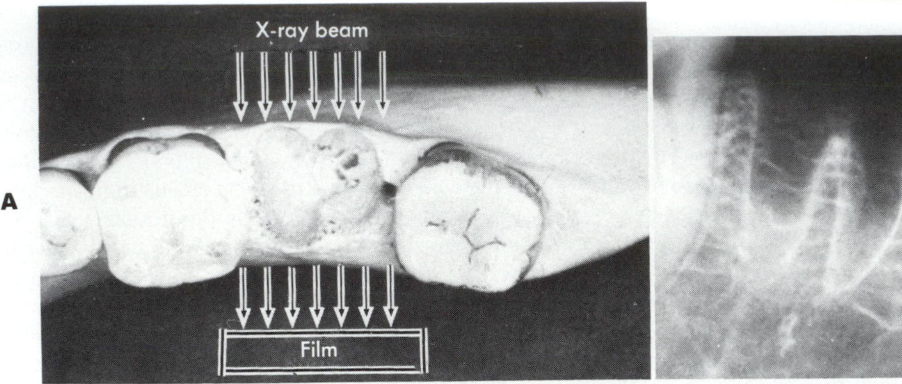

FIG. 5-20 A, Attenuation of x-rays passing tangentially through the socket by the greater thickness of bone on the periphery of the socket. This results in a greater radiopacity of the periphery as compared with the adjacent alveolar bone. **B,** White lines (lamina dura) produced by these attenuated rays.

The buccal object rule relates to the manner in which the relative position of radiographic images of two separate objects changes when the projection angle at which the images were made is changed. The principle states that the object closest to the buccal surface appears to move in the direction opposite the movement of the cone or tube head, when compared to a second film. Objects closest to the lingual surface appear to move in the same direction that the cone moved, thus "same lingual, opposite buccal" rule. Figure 5-21 shows three simulated radiographs of a buccal object (circle) and a lingual object (triangle) exposed at different horizontal angles. The position of the objects on each radiograph is compared with the reference structure (i.e., the mesial root apex of the mandibular first molar). The first radiograph (Fig. 5-21, *A* and *B*) shows superimposition of the two objects; in this case the tube head was positioned for a straight-on view. In the second radiograph (Fig. 5-21, *C* and *D*), the tube head shifted mesially and the beam was directed at the reference object from a more mesial angulation. In this case, the lingual object (triangle) moved mesially with respect to the reference object, and the buccal object (circle) moved distally with respect to the reference object. In the third radiograph (Fig. 5-21, *E* and *F*), the tube head shifted distally and the beam was directed at the reference object from a more distal angulation; here the triangle moved distally with respect to the mesial root of the mandibular first molar and the circle moved mesially. These radiographic relations confirm that the lingual object (triangle) moves in the same direction with respect to reference structures as the x-ray tube and that the buccal object (circle) moves in the opposite direction of the x-ray tube. Thus, according to the rule, the object farthest (most buccal) from the film moves farthest on the film with respect to a change in horizontal angulation of the x-ray cone. In an endodontically treated mandibular molar with four canals (Fig. 5-22), a straight-on view results in superimposition of the root-filled canals on the radiograph. If the cone is angled from mesial to distal, the mesiolingual and distolingual canals will move mesially and the mesiobuccal and distobuccal canals will move distally on the radiograph when compared with the straight-on view.

The examples cited above involve application of the buccal object rule using changes in horizontal angulation. The clinician should be aware that this rule applies to changes in vertical angulation as well (Fig. 5-23). To locate the position of the mandibular canal relative to mandibular molar root apices, one must take radiographs at different vertical angulations. If the canal moves with or in the same direction as the cone head, the canal is lingual to the root apices; if the mandibular canal moves opposite the direction of the cone head, the canal is buccal to the root apices. The clinician should recognize the wide range of applicability of the buccal object rule in determining the buccal-lingual relationship of structures not visible in a two-dimensional image.

Digitization of ionizing radiation

A new radiographic system called RadioVisioGraphy (RVG) digitizes ionizing radiation.[40,42] Developed in France by Dr. Francis Mouyen, the system provides an instantaneous image on a video monitor while reducing radiation exposure by 80%.[40,42]

The RVG device has three components. The "Radio" component consists of a hypersensitive intraoral sensor (Fig. 5-24, *A*) and a conventional x-ray unit. The small sensor (24 by 37 by 11 mm) contains a fluoroscopic sensor screen, a set of optic fibers, and a miniature charged coupling device that translates the image produced into an electronic signal that is subsequently transmitted to the display-processing unit. For infection control, disposable latex sheaths are used to cover the sensor when it is in use (Fig. 5-24, *B*); the sensor itself is cold-sterilized while the sensor positioners are autoclavable. An exposure time in the range of hundredths of a second is all that is needed to generate the image.[42]

The second component, the "Visio" portion, consists of a video monitor and display-processing unit (Fig. 5-24, *C*). As the image is transmitted to the processing unit, it is digitized and memorized by the computer. The unit magnifies the image four times for immediate display on the video monitor and has the additional capability of producing colored images. It can also display multiple images simultaneously, including a full-mouth series on one screen. Because the image is digitized, further manipulation of the image is possible; this includes enhancement, contrast stretching, and reversing. A zoom feature is also available to enlarge a portion of the im-

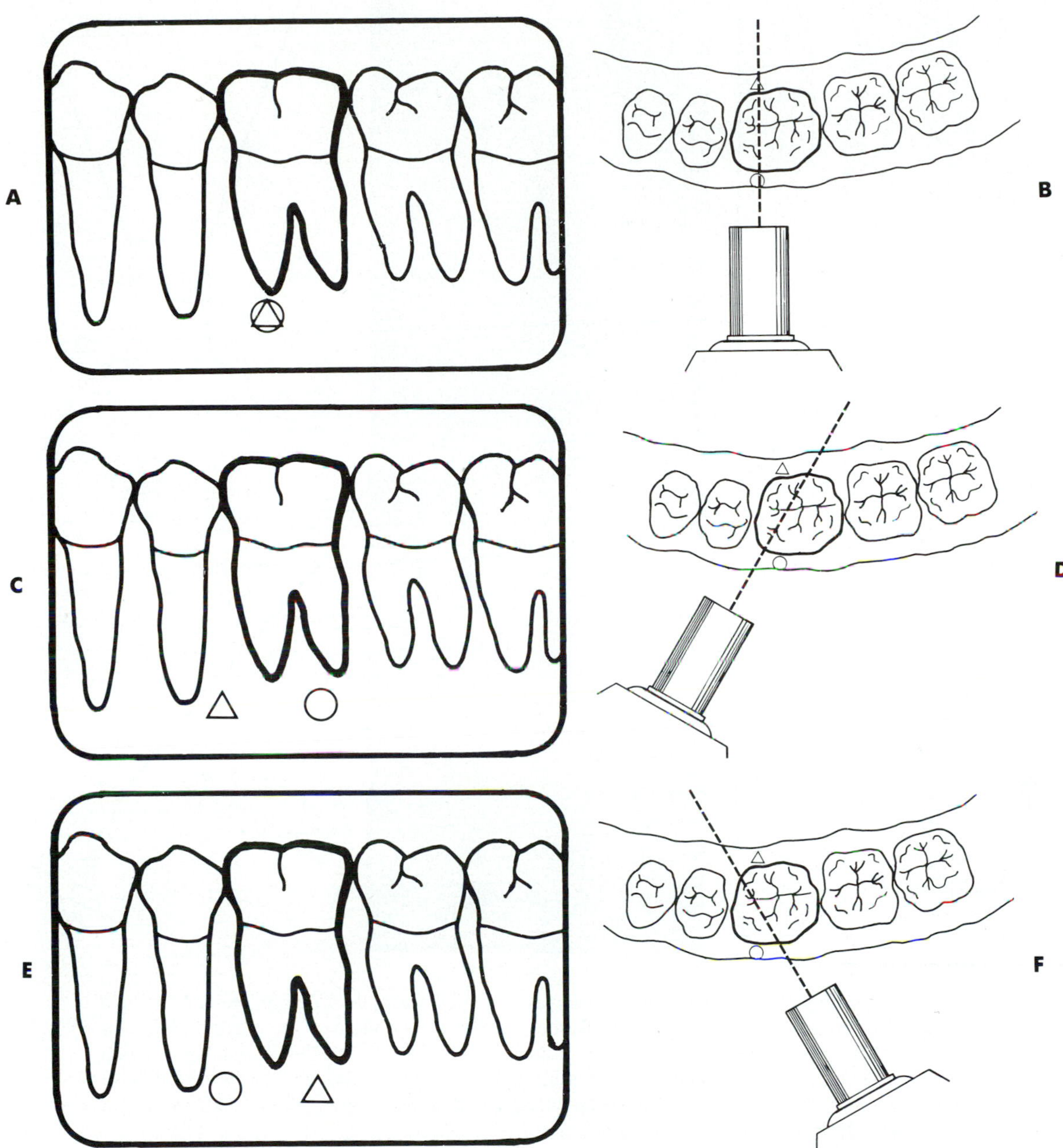

FIG. 5-21 Objects may be localized with respect to reference structures by using the buccal object rule (tube-shift technique). **A** and **B,** A straight-on view will cause superimposition of the buccal object *(circle)* with the lingual object *(triangle)*. **C** and **D,** Using the tube-shift technique, the lingual object *(triangle)* will appear more mesial with respect to the mesial root of the mandibular first molar, and the buccal object *(circle)* will appear more distal on a second view projected from the mesial. **E** and **F,** The object *(triangle)* on the lingual surface will appear more distal with respect to the mesial root of the mandibular first molar, and the object *(circle)* on the buccal surface will appear more mesial on a view projected from the distal aspect.

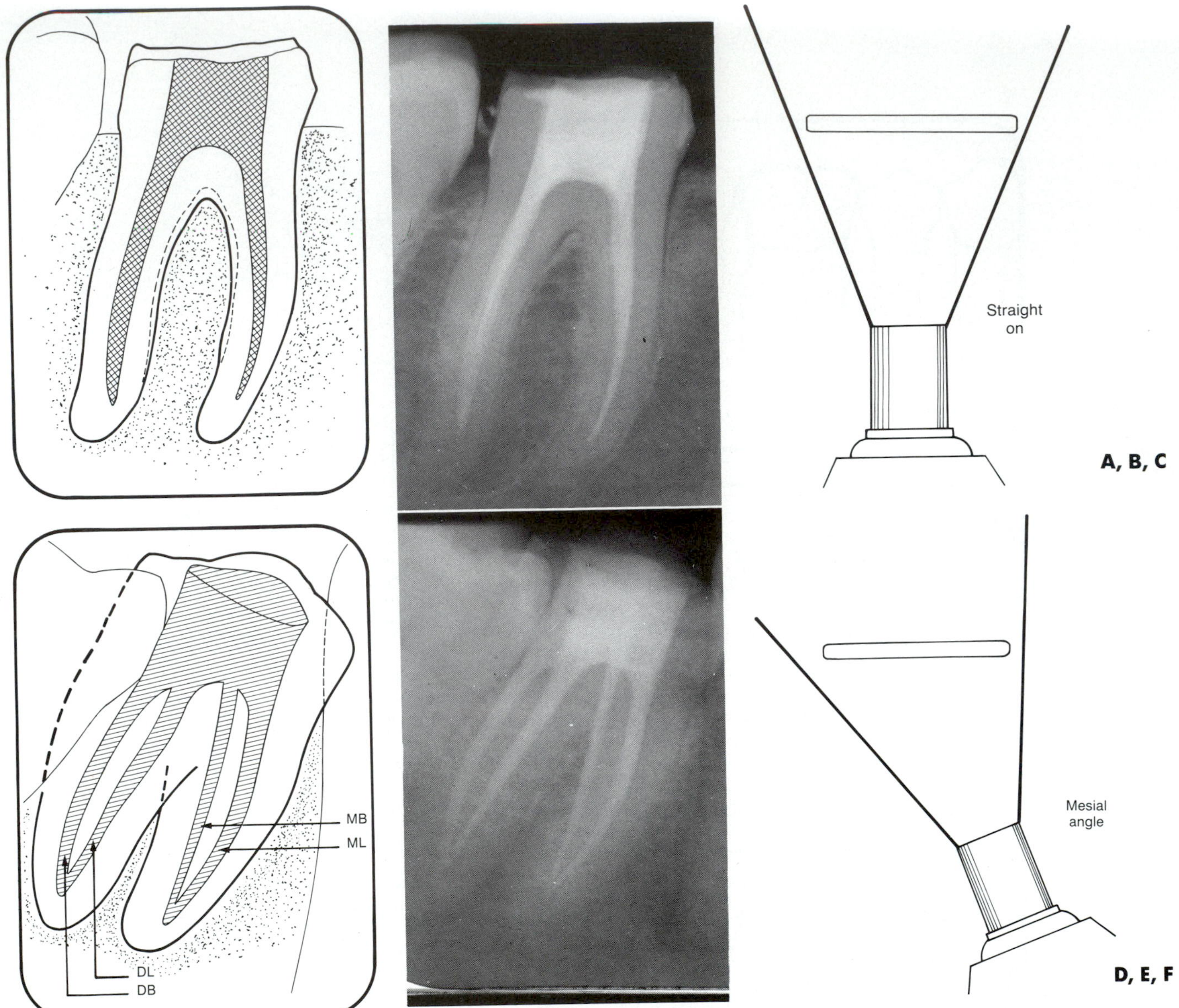

FIG. 5-22 Comparison of straight-on and mesial-angled views of an endodontically treated mandibular molar with four canals. **A, B,** and **C,** Straight-on view of the mandibular molar shows superimposition of the root canal fillings. **D, E,** and **F,** Mesial-to-distal angulation produces separation of the canals. The mesiolingual and distolingual root-filled canals move mesially (towards the cone), and the mesiobuccal and distobuccal root-filled canals move distally (away from the cone) on the radiograph.

age up to full screen size. The third component is "Graphy," a high-resolution videoprinter that instantly provides a hard copy of the screen image, using the same video signal.

The advantages of RVG seem numerous, but the primary ones include the elimination of x-ray film, significant reduction in exposure time, and instantaneous image display. A recent study showed that RVG resolution was slightly lower than that produced with silver halide film emulsions, but radiographic information can be increased with the electronic image treatment capabilities of the system.[40] The system appears to be very promising for endodontics.

PREPARATION FOR ACCESS: TOOTH ISOLATION

Principles and Rationale

The use of the rubber dam is mandatory in root canal treatment.[12,13] Developed in the nineteenth century by S. C. Barnum, the rubber dam has evolved over the years from a system that was designed to isolate teeth for placement of gold foil to one of sophistication for the ultimate protection of both patient and clinician.[49] The advantages[4,11,21,28] and absolute necessity of the rubber dam must always take precedence over convenience and expediency, a rationale often cited by clini-

A, B

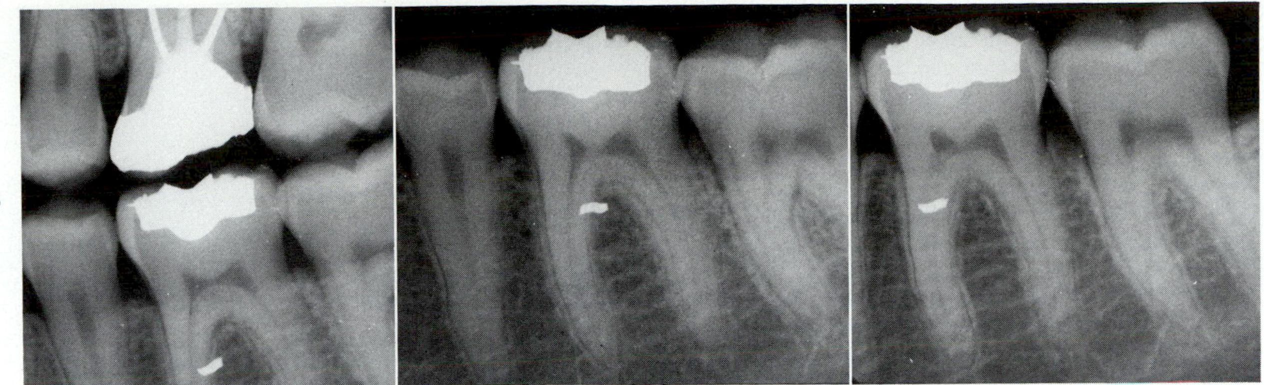

C

FIG. 5-23 Examples of the buccal object rule using shifts in vertical and horizontal angulations. **A,** Bite-wing radiograph (straight-on view with minimal horizontal and vertical angulation) depicts amalgam particle superimposed over the mesial root of the mandibular first molar. To determine the buccal/lingual location of the object, the tube-shift technique (buccal object rule) must be applied. **B,** The periapical radiograph was taken by shifting the vertical angulation of the cone (i.e., the x-ray beam was projected more steeply upward). Since the amalgam particle moved in the opposite direction to that of the cone compared with the bitewing radiograph, the amalgam particle lies on the buccal aspect of the tooth. **C,** The periapical radiograph was taken by shifting the horizontal angulation of the cone (the x-ray was taken from a distal angle). Compared to both **A** and **B,** each taken straight-on with minimal horizontal angulation, the amalgam particle moved opposite the direction of movement of the cone or tube head, confirming that the amalgam particle lies on the buccal aspect of the tooth.

A

B

C

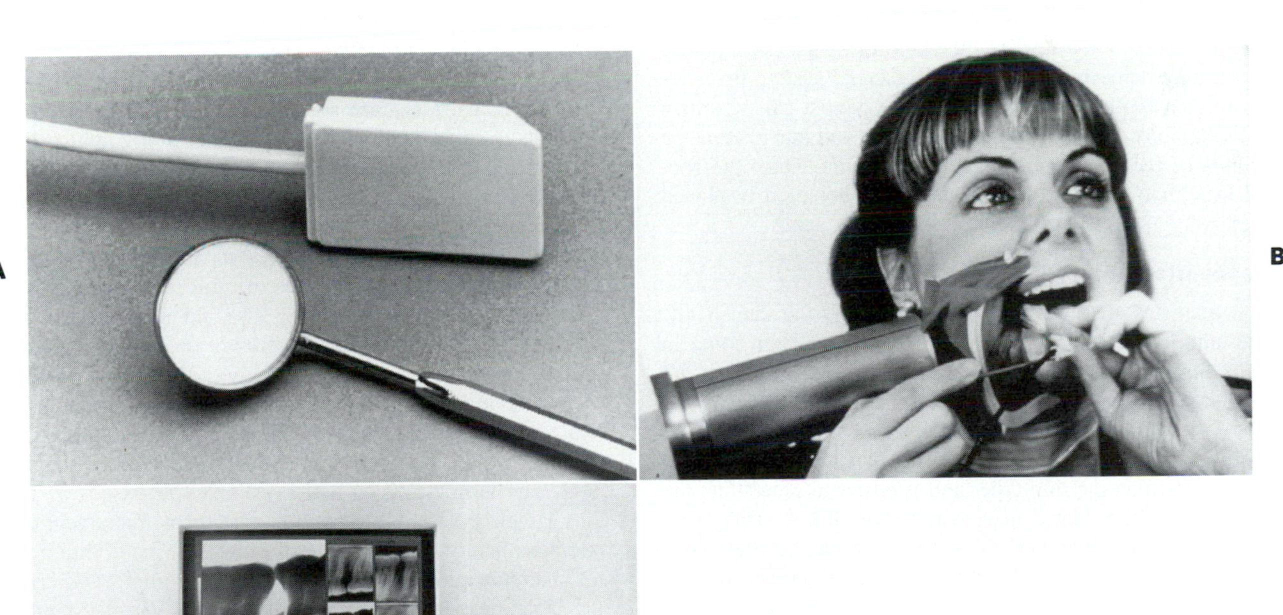

FIG. 5-24 RadioVisioGraphy system. **A,** Intraoral sensor with optic fiber attachment. **B,** Folding dam allows the sheathed sensor to be placed. **C,** Video monitor and display processing unit. (Courtesy Trophy USA, Marietta, Ga.)

cians who condemn its use. Properly placed, the rubber dam facilitates treatment by isolating the tooth from obstacles such as saliva and the tongue, which can disrupt any procedure. Proper rubber dam placement can be done quickly and will enhance the entire procedure.

The rationale for use of the rubber dam in endodontics is that it ensures the following[4,11,21,28,49]:

1. Patient protection from aspiration or the swallowing of instruments, tooth debris, medicaments, and irrigating solutions.
2. Clinician Protection—Today's litigious society certainly focuses on the negligent clinician who fails to use a rubber dam on a patient who subsequently swallows or aspirates an endodontic file. *Routine placement of the rubber dam is considered to be the standard of care.*[12,13]
3. A surgically clean operating field isolated from saliva, hemorrhage, and other tissue fluids. The dam reduces the risk of cross-contamination of the root canal system and provides an excellent barrier to the potential spread of infectious agents.[11,21] *It is a required component of any infection control program.**
4. Retraction and protection of the soft tissues.
5. Improved Visibility—The rubber dam provides a dry field and reduces mirror fogging.
6. Increased Efficiency—The rubber dam minimizes patient conversation during treatment and the need for frequent rinsing. It relaxes the patient and saves time.

The dentist should be aware that in some situations, especially in teeth with crowns, access into the pulp system may be difficult without first orienting root structure to the adjacent teeth and periodontal tissues. Radiographically, the coronal pulp system is often obscured by the restoration and, as a result, the dentist may misdirect the bur during access. In these cases, it may be necessary to locate the canal system first, before the dam is placed. In doing so, the dentist can visualize root topography, making it easier to orient the bur toward the long axis of the roots and prevent perforation. Once the root canal system is located, however, the rubber dam is placed immediately.

Armamentarium

The mainstay of the rubber dam system is the dam itself. These autoclavable sheets of thin, flat, latex rubber come in various thicknesses (thin, medium, heavy, extra heavy, and special heavy) and in two sizes (5 by 5 inches and 6 by 6 inches). For endodontic purposes, the medium thickness is probably best, because it tends to tear less easily, retracts soft tissues better than the thin type, and is easier to place than the heavier types. The dam is also manufactured in a variety colors ranging from light yellow to blue, green, or gray. The darker-colored dams may afford better visual contrast, thus reducing eye strain, but the lighter-colored ones, because of their translucency, have the advantage of naturally illuminating the operating field and allowing easier film placement underneath the dam. Depending upon individual preference and specific conditions associated with a tooth, the dentist may find it necessary to vary the color and/or thickness of the rubber dam used. Glare and eyestrain can be reduced and contrast enhanced by routinely placing the dull side of the dam toward the operator.

*References 2, 8-10, 16, 18, 32, 51.

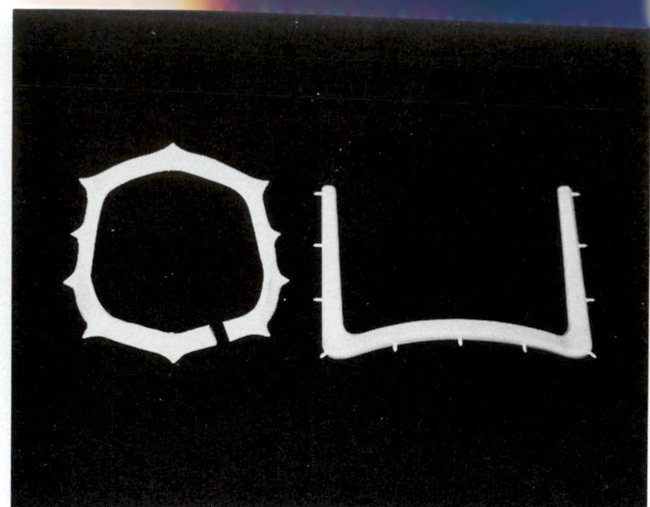

FIG. 5-25 Plastic rubber dam frames. *Left,* Nygaard-Ostby (N-O) frame. *Right,* Young's frame.

Another component of the rubber dam system is the rubber dam frame, which is designed to retract and stabilize the dam. Both metal and plastic frames are available, but plastic ones are recommended for endodontic procedures. They appear radiolucent, do not mask key areas on working films, and do not have to be removed before film placement. The Young rubber dam frame (plastic type), the Star Visi frame, and the Nygaard-Ostby (N-O) frame are examples of radiolucent frames used in endodontics (Fig. 5-25). The Handidam rubber dam system also provides a radiolucent plastic frame (Fig. 5-26). Metal frames are seldom used today; because of their radiopacity, they tend to block out the radiograph and, if removed, may result in destabilization of the dam and salivary contamination of the canal system, thus negating the "sterile" environment that was previously attained.

Rubber dam clamps or retainers anchor the dam to the tooth requiring treatment or, in cases of multiple tooth isolation, to the most posterior tooth. They also aid in soft tissue retraction. The clamps are made of shiny or dull stainless steel, and each consists of a bow and two jaws. Regardless of the type of jaw configuration, the prongs of the jaws should engage at least four points on the tooth. This clamp-to-tooth relationship stabilizes the retainer and prevents any rocking which, in itself, can be injurious to both hard and soft tissues.[29,36]

Clamps are available from a variety of manufacturers and are specifically designed for all classes of teeth with a variety of anatomic configurations. For most uncomplicated endodontic isolations, the dentist's basic armamentarium should consist of winged clamps; a butterfly type clamp for anterior teeth; a universal premolar clamp; a mandibular molar clamp; and a maxillary molar clamp (Fig. 5-27). The wings, which are extensions of the jaws, not only provide for additional soft tissue retraction but also facilitate placement of the rubber dam, frame, and retainer as a single unit (see the section on methods of rubber dam placement, which follows). Other retainers are designed for specific clinical situations in which clamp placement may be difficult. For example, when minimal coronal tooth structure remains, a clamp with apically inclined jaws

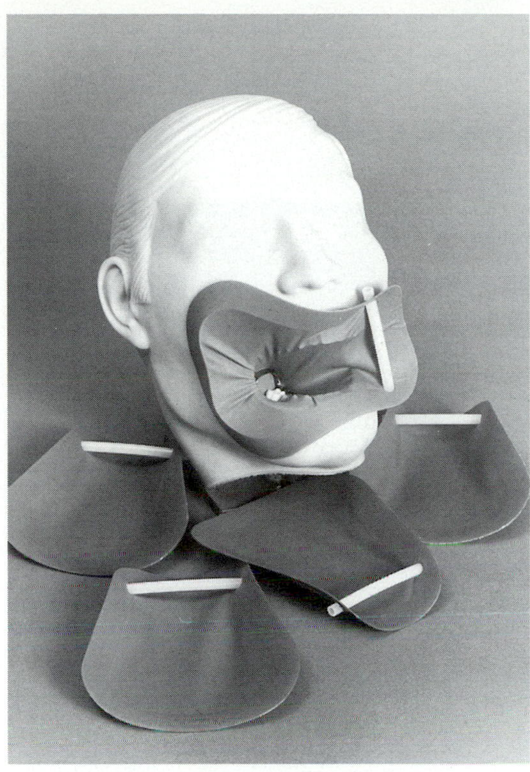

FIG. 5-26 The Handidam is a rubber dam system with built-in plastic frame. The disposable frame bends easily for film placement. (Courtesy Aseptico, Kirkland, Wash.)

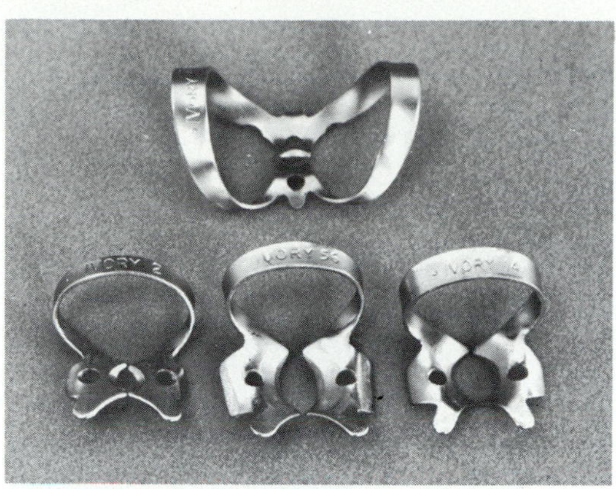

FIG. 5-27 Basic set of Ivory winged rubber dam clamps: on top, no. 9 butterfly clamp for anterior teeth; on bottom, from left, no. 2 premolar clamp, no. 56 mandibular molar clamp, and no. 14 maxillary molar clamp. (Courtesy Columbus Dental, Division of Miles Inc., St. Louis, Mo.)

may be used to engage tooth structure at or below the level of the free gingival margin (Fig. 5-28). Clamps with serrated jaws also may increase stabilization of broken-down teeth. Another type of retainer, the Ivory no. 21 clamp (Columbus Dental, Div. of Miles Inc., St. Louis, Mo.), should also be included in the dentist's armamentarium (Fig. 5-29). Its anterior extension allows for retraction of dam around a severely broken-down tooth while the clamp itself is placed on a tooth proximal to the one being treated (Fig. 5-30).

The Annoni Endo-Illuminator (Analytic Technology, Redmond, Wash.) system is new to the specialty of endodontics (Fig. 5-31). Through its fiberoptic attachment to specially designed autoclavable retainers, the high-intensity light generated by the Endo-Illuminator transilluminates pulp chambers and canal orifices so that pulp systems are easier to identify and locate.

The remaining components of the rubber dam system include the rubber dam punch and the rubber dam forceps. The punch has a series of holes on a rotating disc from which the dentist can select according to the size of tooth or teeth to be isolated. The forceps holds and carries the retainer during placement and removal.

Methods of Rubber Dam Placement

As mentioned earlier, an expedient method of dam placement is to position the bow of the clamp through the hole in the dam and place the rubber over the wings of the clamp (a winged clamp is required).[23,49] The clamp is stretched by the forceps to maintain the position of the clamp in the dam, and

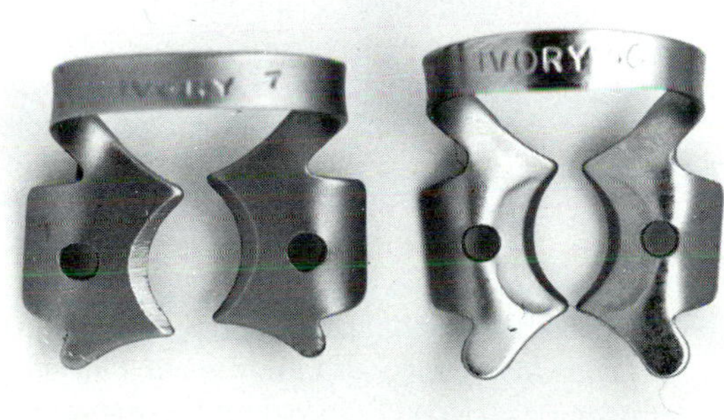

FIG. 5-28 Mandibular molar clamps. Clamp on right has jaws inclined apically to engage tooth with minimal tooth structure remaining. (Courtesy Columbus Dental, Division of Miles Inc., St. Louis, Mo.)

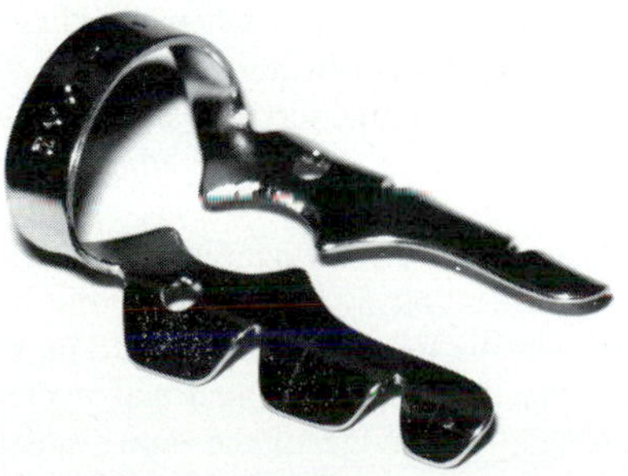

FIG. 5-29 Ivory no. 21 clamp for isolation of severely broken-down teeth. (Courtesy Columbus Dental, Division of Miles Inc., St. Louis, Mo.)

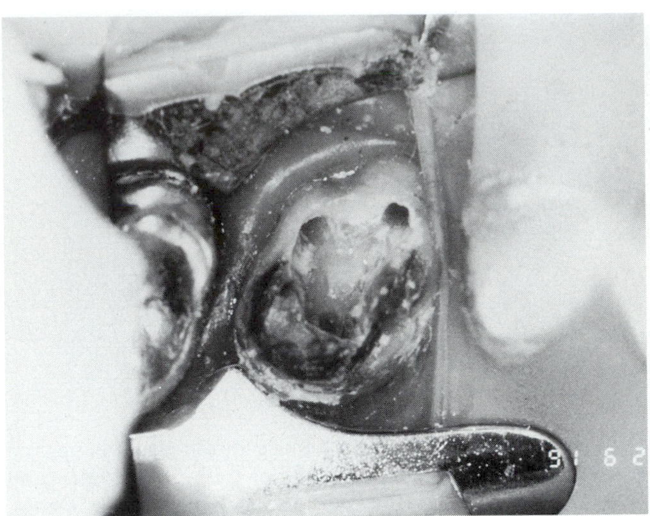

FIG. 5-30 Ivory no. 21 clamp is placed on the maxillary second molar to isolate a severely broken-down maxillary first molar.

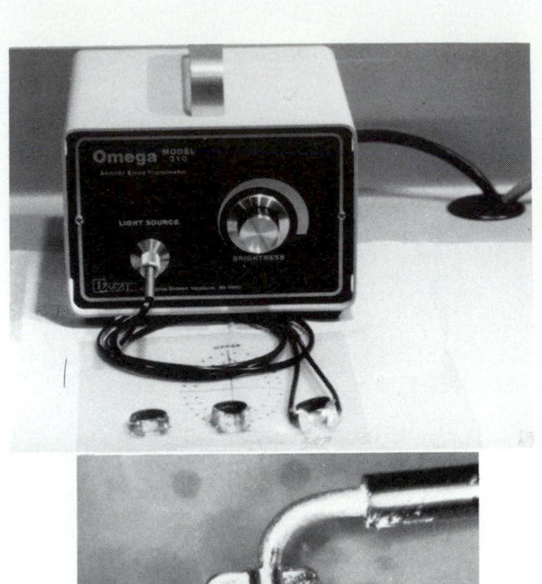

A

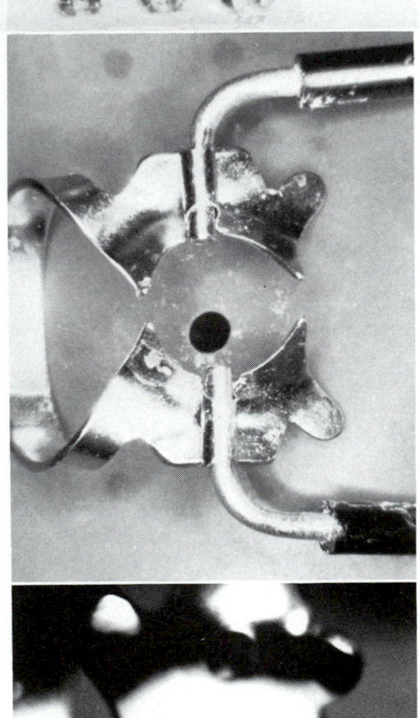

B

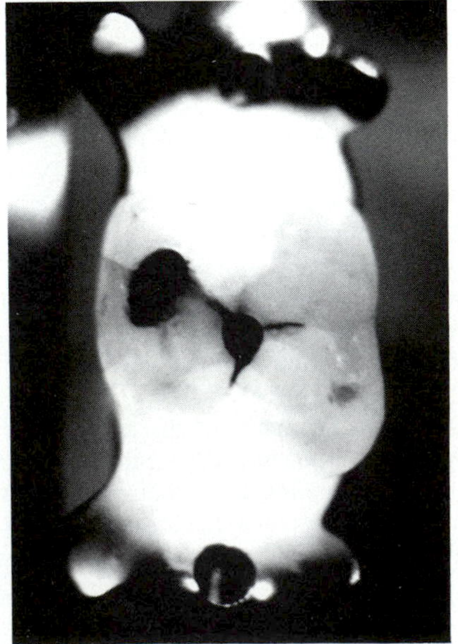

C

FIG. 5-31 The Annoni Endo-Illuminator System. **A,** Fiber-optic unit with attachments to clamp. **B,** Clamp specially designed for fiber-optic attachments. **C,** Maxillary molar "illuminated" via fiber optics. (Courtesy Analytic Technology, Redmond, Wash.)

the dam is attached to the plastic frame, allowing for placement of dam, clamp, and frame in one motion (Fig. 5-32). Once the clamp is secured on the tooth, the dam is teased under the wings of the clamp with a plastic instrument.

Another way is to place the clamp, usually wingless, on the tooth and then stretch the dam over the clamped tooth (Fig. 5-33).[23,49] This method offers the advantage of enabling the clinician to see exactly where the jaws of the clamp engage the tooth, thus avoiding possible impingement on the gingival tissues. Gentle finger pressure on the buccal and lingual apron of the clamp before the dam is placed can be used to test how securely the clamp fits. Variations of this method include placing the clamp and dam first, followed by the frame, or placing the rubber dam first, followed by the clamp and then the frame.[49]

A third method, the split-dam technique,[23] may be used to isolate anterior teeth without using a rubber dam clamp. Not only is this technique useful when there is insufficient crown structure, as in the case of horizontal fractures, but it also prevents the possibility of the jaws of the clamp chipping the margins of teeth restored with porcelain crowns or laminates. Studies[29,36] on the effects of retainers on porcelain-fused-to-metal restorations and tooth structure itself have demonstrated that there can be significant damage to cervical porcelain, as well as to dentin and cementum, even when the clamp is properly stabilized. Thus, for teeth with porcelain restorations ligation with dental floss is recommended as an alternate method to retract the dam and tissues, or the adjacent tooth can be clamped.

In the split-dam method, two overlapping holes are punched in the dam. A cotton roll is placed under the lip in the mucobuccal fold over the tooth to be treated. The rubber dam is stretched over the tooth to be treated and over one adjacent tooth on each side. The edge of the dam is carefully teased through the contacts on the distal sides of the two adjacent teeth. Dental floss helps carry the dam down around the gingiva. The tension produced by the stretched dam, aided by the rubber dam frame, secures the dam in place. The tight fit and

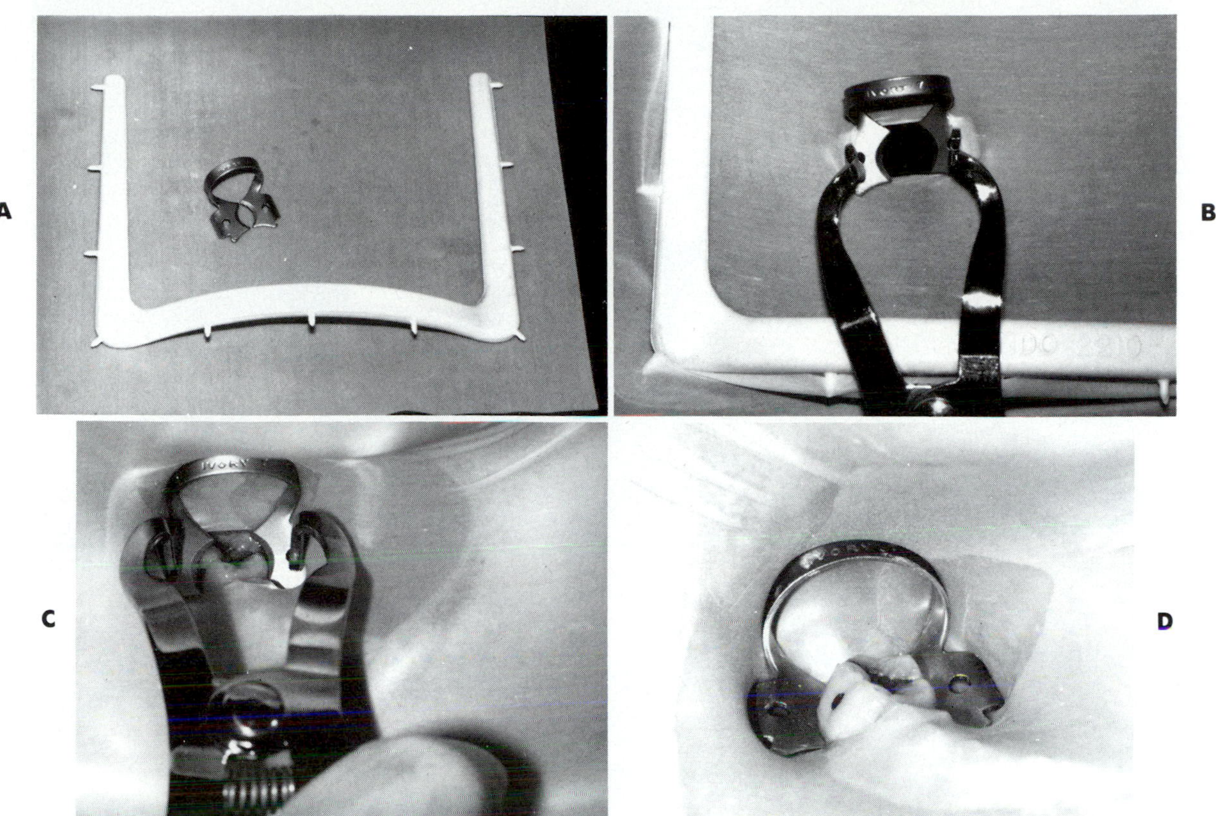

FIG. 5-32 **A,** Rubber dam, clamp, and frame. **B,** Clamp positioned in the dam with frame attached and held in position with rubber dam forceps. **C,** Dam, clamp, and frame carried to mouth as one unit and placed over the tooth. **D,** Clamp in place with four-point contact with rubber tucked under the wings.

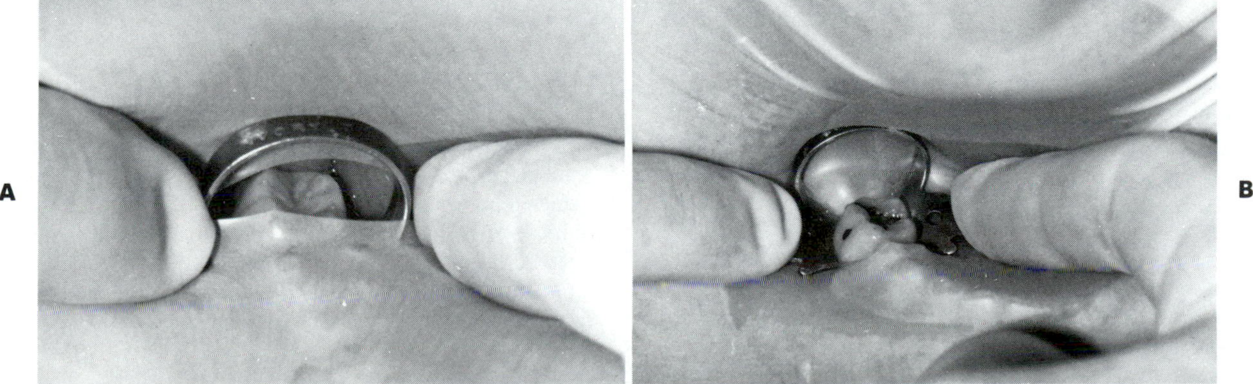

FIG. 5-33 **A,** After the clamp is placed, the dam is attached to the frame and gently stretched over the clamped tooth with the index finger of each hand. **B,** Clamp is tested for a secure fit with gentle finger pressure alternately on the buccal and lingual aspects of the clamp apron.

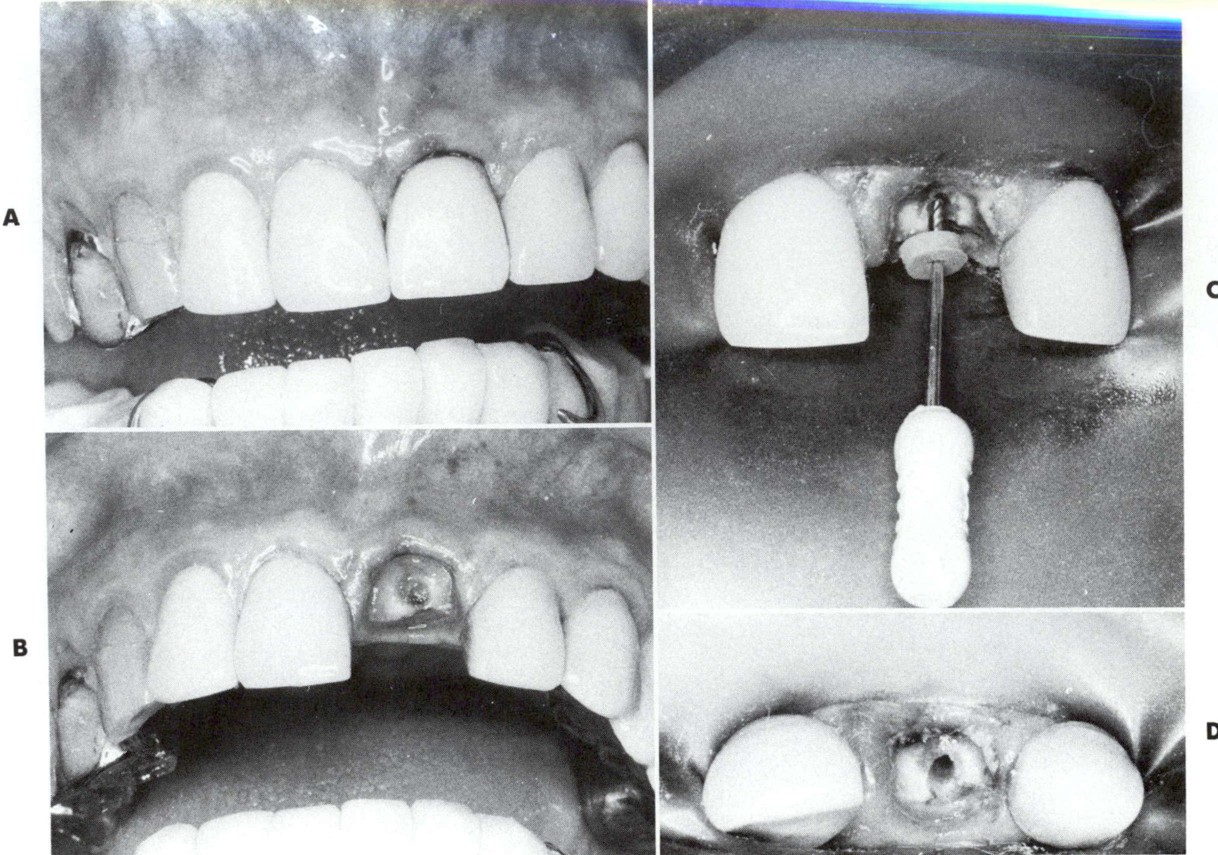

FIG. 5-34 Split-dam technique. **A,** Maxillary central incisor with a horizontal fracture at the cervical area. **B,** Appearance after removal of the coronal fragment. **C,** Cotton roll in place in the mucobuccal fold and rubber dam stretched over the two adjacent teeth. **D,** Appearance after pulp extirpation.

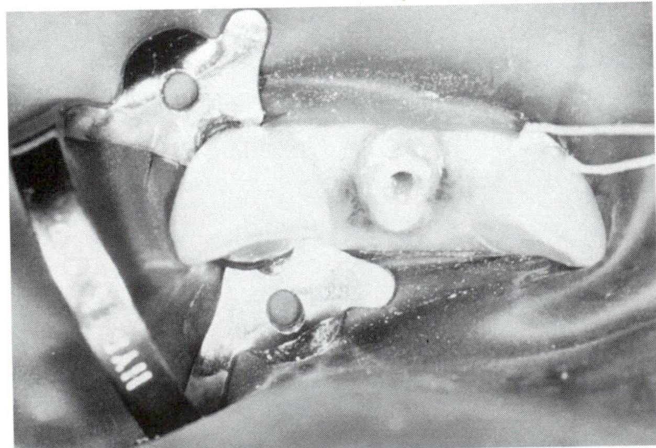

FIG. 5-35 Split-dam technique. Premolar clamp on maxillary central incisor along with ligation on the maxillary canine prevents dam slippage and aids in dam retraction during endodontic treatment on broken-down maxillary lateral incisor. (Courtesy Dr. James L. Gutmann.)

the cotton roll produce a relatively dry field (Fig. 5-34). If the dam has a tendency to slip, a premolar clamp may be used on a tooth distal to the three isolated teeth, or even on an adjacent tooth (Fig. 5-35). The clamp is placed over the rubber dam, which then acts as a cushion against the jaws of the clamp.

Aids in Rubber Dam Placement

Punching and positioning of holes

The rubber dam may be divided into four equal quadrants, and the proper place for the hole is estimated according to which tooth is undergoing treatment. The more distal the tooth, the closer to the center is the placement of the hole.[23] This method becomes easier as the clinician gains experience. The hole must be punched cleanly, without tags or tears. If the dam is torn, it may leak or permit continued tearing when stretched over the clamp and tooth.

Orientation of the dam and bunching

The rubber dam must be attached to the frame with enough tension to retract soft tissues and prevent bunching, without tearing the dam or displacing the clamp. The rubber dam should completely cover the patient's mouth without infringing on the patient's nose or eyes. To prevent bunching of the dam in the occlusal embrasure, only the edge of the interseptal portion of the dam is teased between the teeth. Dental floss is then used to carry the dam through the contacts. These contacts should always be tested with dental floss before the dam is placed. A plastic instrument is used to invert the edge of the dam around the tooth to provide a seal.

Problem-Solving in Tooth Isolation

Leakage

The best way to prevent seepage through the rubber dam is meticulous placement of the entire system. Proper selection and placement of the clamp, sharply punched, correctly positioned holes, use of a dam of adequate thickness, and inversion of the dam around the tooth all help reduce leakage through the dam and into the root canal system.[4,28,35,49] Nevertheless, there are clinical situations in which small tears, holes, or continuous minor leaks may occur. These often can be patched or blocked with Cavit, Orabase, rubber base adhesive,[7] "liquid" rubber dam, or periodontal packing. If leakage continues, the dam should be replaced with a new one.

Because salivary secretions can seep through even a well-placed rubber dam, persons who salivate excessively may require premedication to reduce saliva flow to a manageable level. Failure to control salivation may result in salivary contamination of the canal system and pooling of saliva beneath the dam as well as drooling and possible choking. Such occurrences can disrupt treatment and should be prevented. Excessive saliva flow can be reduced through the use of an anticholinergic drug such as atropine sulfate, propantheline bromide (Pro-Banthine), methantheline (Banthine), or the new drug, glycopyrrolate (Robinul).[27] Therapeutic doses of atropine sulfate for adults range from 0.3 to 1 mg PO, 1 to 2 hours before the procedure. The synthetic anticholinergic drug propantheline bromide (Pro-Banthine) reportedly has fewer side effects than Banthine.[27] The usual adult dose of Pro-Banthine for an adult is 7.5 to 15 mg PO, 30 to 45 minutes before the appointment. Because they can cause undesirable autonomic effects, especially through various drug interactions, the anticholinergics should be used only in specific cases and only as a last resort.

Unusual tooth shapes or positions that cause inadequate clamp placement

Some teeth do not conform to the variety of clamps available. These include partially erupted teeth, teeth prepared for crowns, and teeth fractured or broken down to the extent that their margins are subgingival. To handle these cases, rubber dam retainers may be customized by modifying the jaws to adapt to a particular tooth (Fig. 5-36).[50] In partially erupted teeth or cone-shaped teeth such as those prepared for full coverage, one technique[48] is to place spots of self-curing resin on the cervical surface of the tooth. These resin beads act as a scaffold for the retainer during treatment. Another method[26] is to place small acid-etched composite lips on the teeth; these resin lips serve as artificial undercuts and remain on the teeth between appointments. When the root canal treatment is complete, the resin beads are easily removed. In multiple-treatment cases involving misshapen teeth, a customized acrylic retainer[46] can be used in conjunction with a dam to isolate the operating field.

A

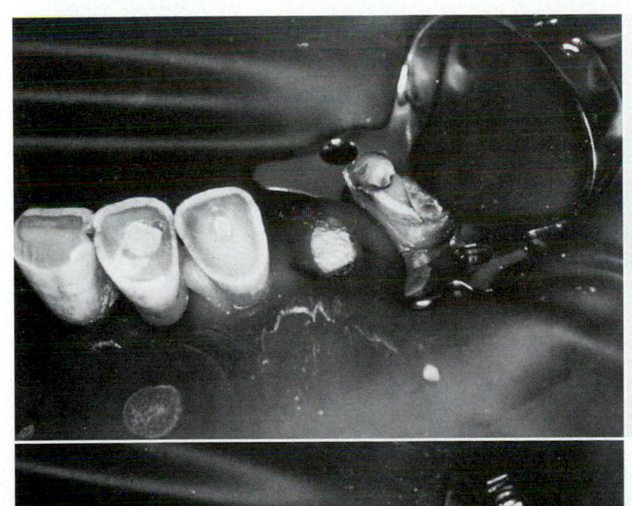

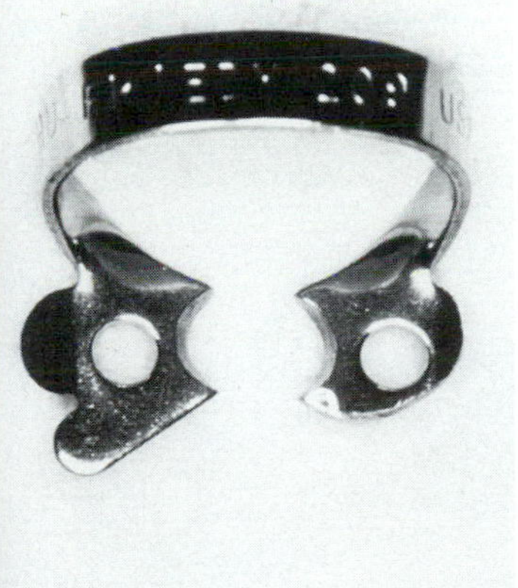

B

C

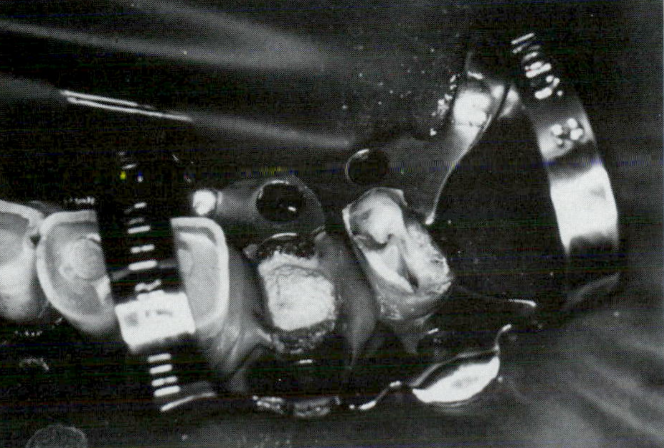

FIG. 5-36 A, Isolation rendered difficult by multiple, severely broken-down mandibular premolars. **B,** Modified premolar rubber dam clamp. **C,** Modified clamp in place on first premolar to accommodate wings of distal clamp. (Courtesy Dr. Robert Roda.)

Loss of tooth structure

If insufficient tooth structure prevents the placement of a clamp, the clinician must first determine whether the tooth is periodontally sound and restorable. Meticulous and thorough treatment planning often can prevent embarrassing situations for both doctor and patient. One example is the not uncommon case in which the endodontic treatment is completed before restorability is determined and it is then discovered that the tooth cannot be restored.

Once a tooth is deemed restorable but the margin of sound tooth structure is subgingival, a number of methods should be considered. As mentioned earlier, less invasive methods, such as using a clamp with prongs inclined apically or using an Ivory no. 21 clamp, should be attempted first (Fig. 5-30). If neither of these techniques effectively isolates the tooth, the dentist may consider the clamping of the attached gingiva and alveolar process. In this

soft tissue anesthesia be induced before the clamp is placed. Although the procedure may cause some minor postoperative discomfort, the periodontal tissues recover quickly with minimal postoperative care.

Restorative procedures

If none of the techniques mentioned above is desirable, a variety of restorative methods may be considered to build up the tooth so that a retainer can be placed properly.[34,35,49] A preformed copper band, a temporary crown, or an orthodontic band (Figs. 5-37 and 5-38) may be cemented over the remaining natural crown. This band or crown not only enables the clamp to be retained successfully; it also serves as a seal for the retention of intracanal medicaments and the temporary filling between appointments. These temporary bands or crowns

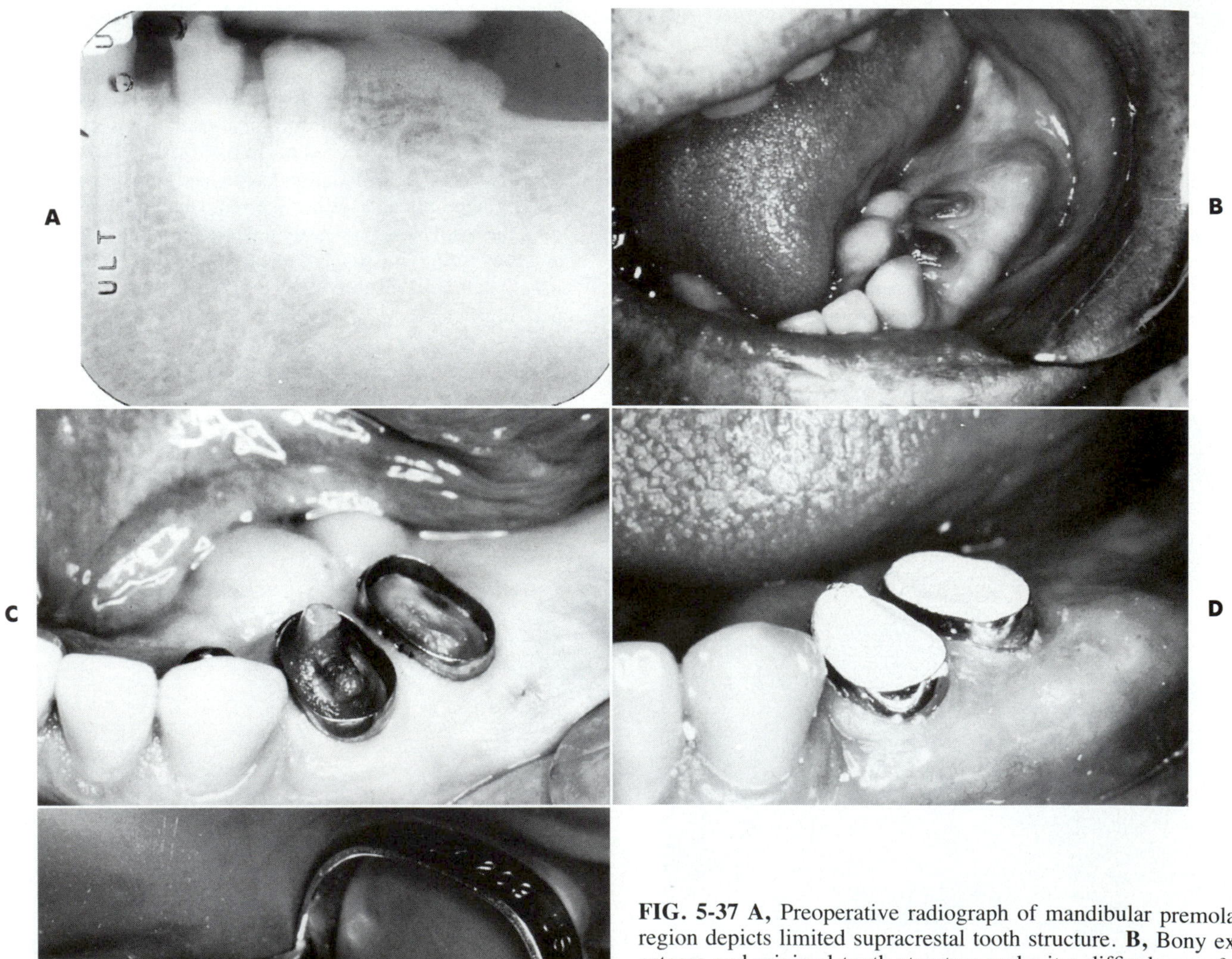

FIG. 5-37 A, Preoperative radiograph of mandibular premolar region depicts limited supracrestal tooth structure. **B,** Bony exostoses and minimal tooth structure make it a difficult case for tooth isolation. **C,** Fitted orthodontic bands on mandibular premolars. **D,** Orthodontic bands cemented in place with IRM (reinforced zinc oxide-eugenol cement). **E,** Effective isolation with rubber dam clamp placed on distal tooth. (Courtesy Dr. Robert Roda.)

have several disadvantages. One of the main problems is their inability to provide a superior seal. Another concern is that particles of these soft metals or cement can block canal systems during access opening and instrumentation. Third, these temporary crowns and bands, if they become displaced or are not properly contoured, can cause periodontal inflammation.

Occasionally so little tooth structure remains that even band or crown placement is not possible. In these cases it becomes necessary to replace the missing tooth structure to facilitate placement of the rubber dam clamp and prevent leakage into the pulp cavity during the course of treatment.[34,35,49] Replacement of missing tooth structure can be accomplished by means of pin-retained amalgam buildups, composites, glass ionomer cements such as Ketac-Silver or Fuji II (Fig. 5-39), or dentin-bonding systems such as Scotchbond 2, Tenure Bond, Gluma, or C&B Metabond.[49] Although these newer dentin-bonding systems form a very strong immediate bond and are generally simple to use, any restorative method for building up a broken-down tooth is time consuming, can impede endodontic procedures, and may duplicate restorative treatment. Many restorations that have been hollowed out by access cavities are weakened and require redoing.

Periodontal procedures

As a result of excessive crown destruction or incomplete eruption, the presence of gingival tissue may preclude the use of a clamp without severe gingival impingement. Various techniques of gingivectomy (Fig. 5-40) or electrosurgery have been suggested for cases in which the remaining tooth structure still lies above the crestal bone. With an inadequate zone of attached gingiva, osseous defects, or a poor anatomic form, an apically positioned flap with a reverse bevel incision is the technique of choice to "lengthen" the crown.[34,35]

Electrosurgery and the conventional gingivectomy are crown-lengthening procedures for teeth that have sufficient attached gingiva and no infrabony involvement.[34,35] The electrosurgery method offers the advantage of leaving a virtually bloodless site for immediate rubber dam placement. Electrosurgery units have become highly sophisticated and are capable of providing both cutting and coagulating currents that, when used properly, will not cause cellular coagulation. The wide variety of sizes and shapes of surgical electrodes enables the clinician to reach areas that are inaccessible to the scalpel. Furthermore, electrosurgery facilitates the removal of unwanted tissue in such a manner as to recreate normal gingival architecture. This feature, combined with controlled hemostasis, makes the instrument extremely useful in the preparation of some teeth for placement of the rubber dam clamp. The main drawback of electrosurgery is the potential for damage to the adjacent tissues; if the electrode contacts bone, significant destruction of bone can occur. As a result, this technique is not recommended when the distance between the crestal

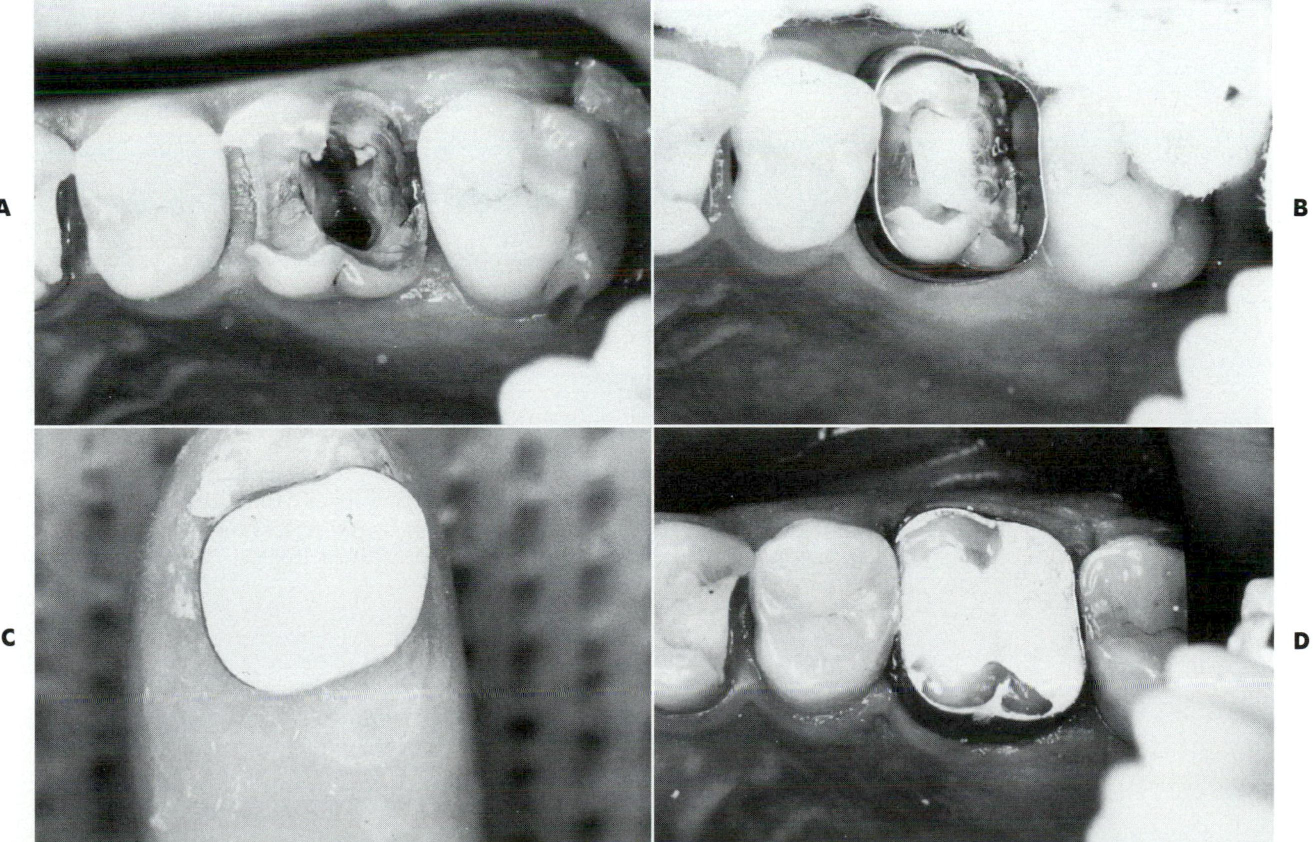

FIG. 5-38 A, Broken-down maxillary molar following removal of restoration, post, and caries. **B,** Fitted orthodontic band; cotton in access opening to protect orifices. **C,** IRM loaded into band prior to cementation. **D,** Completed temporary restoration prior to rubber dam placement. (Courtesy Dr. Robert Roda.)

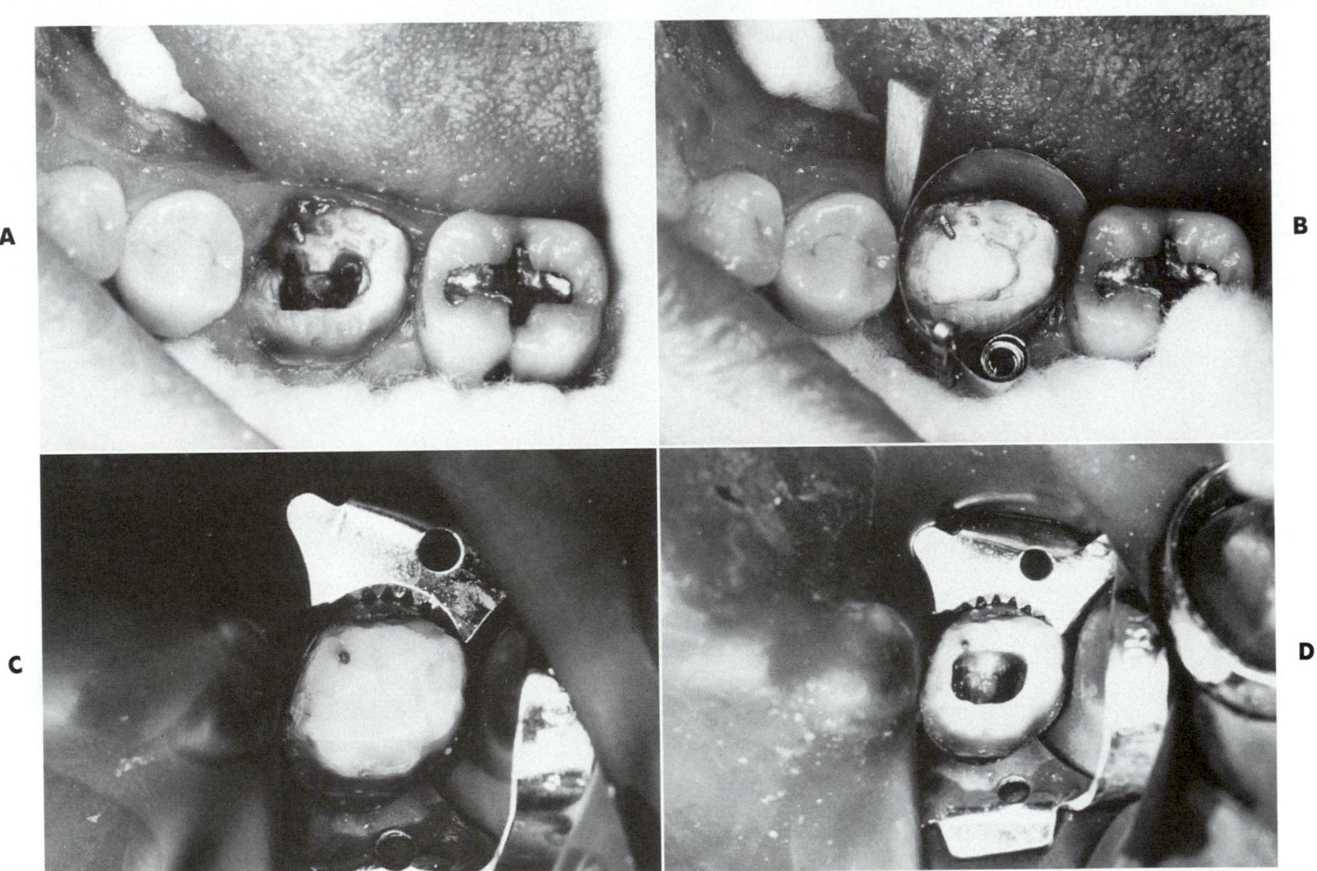

FIG. 5-39 A, Broken-down mandibular molar following crown and caries removal; preexisting pin will aid retention of restorative material. **B,** Isolation with wedged Automatrix. **C,** Completed temporary restoration using glass ionomer cement (Fuji II). **D,** Access through completed restoration following rubber dam placement. (Courtesy Dr. Robert Roda.)

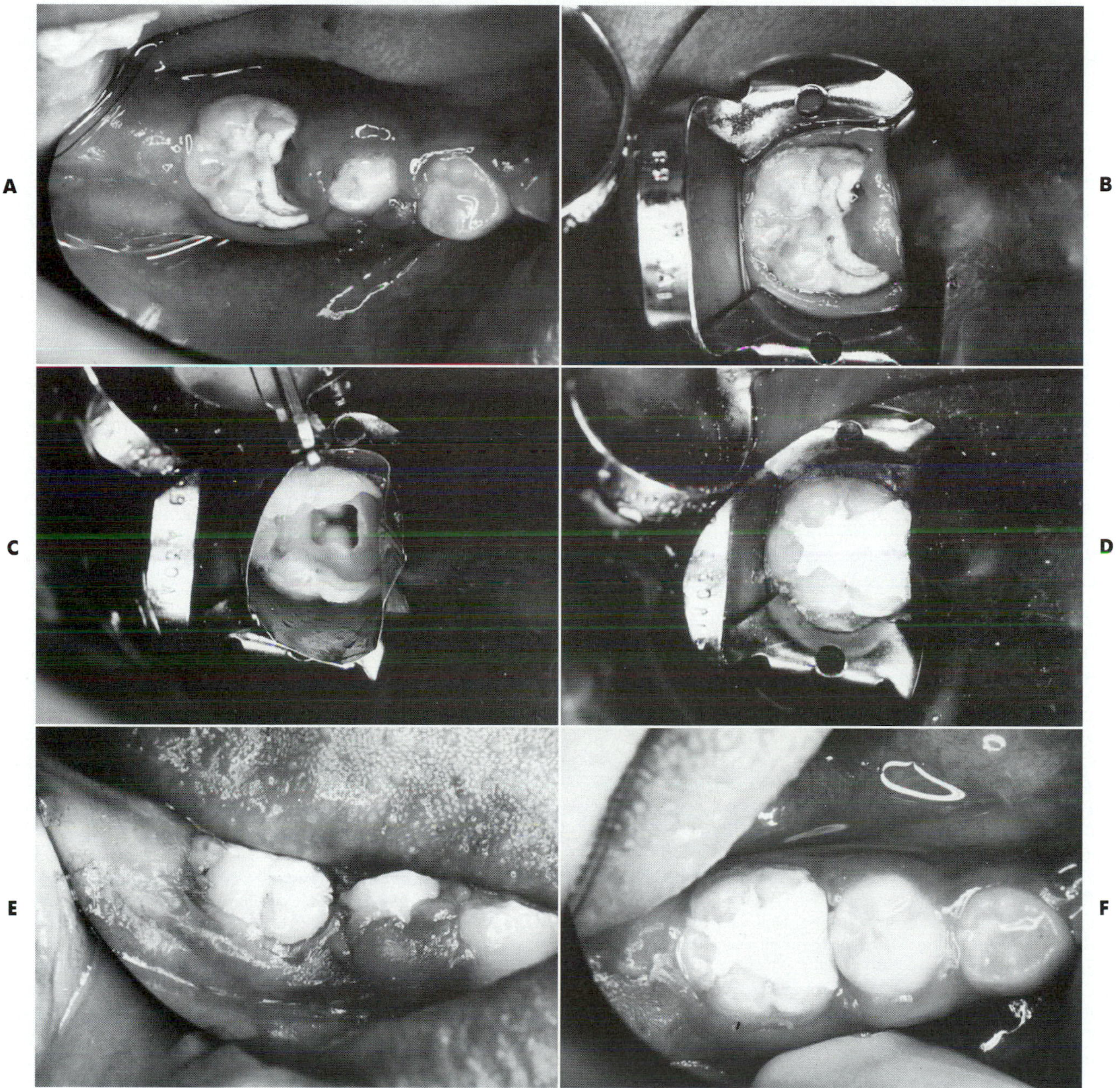

FIG. 5-40 A, Gingival hypertrophy on mandibular molar and erupting premolar of young patient, mandibular molar requires root canal treatment. **B,** Rubber dam clamp impinging on gingival tissues; tissue removed with scalpel. **C,** Automatrix placed immediately following tissue removal; bleeding was minimal. **D,** Placement of IRM temporary restoration following pulpectomy. **E,** Postoperative facial view immediately following gingivectomy; note hemostasis. **F,** Six-week postoperative occlusal view exhibits fully-exposed mandibular molar and recently erupted premolar. (Courtesy Dr. Robert Roda.)

level of bone and the remaining tooth structure is minimal. Compared to electrosurgery, conventional gingivectomy presents the major problem of hemorrhage following the procedure; this forces delay of endodontic treatment until tissues have healed.

The apically positioned flap[34,35] is a crown-lengthening technique for teeth with inadequate attached gingiva, infrabony pockets, or remaining tooth structure below the level of crestal bone. With this technique as well, endodontic treatment should be delayed until sufficient healing has taken place.

Orthodontic procedures

The most common indication for orthodontic extrusion is a fracture of the anterior tooth margin below the crestal bone.[34,35] The clinician should be aware that, because bone and soft tissue attachments follow the tooth during extrusion, crown-lengthening procedures after extrusion are often necessary to achieve the desired clinical crown length and restore the biologic and esthetic tissue relationships. Ultimately, the purpose of orthodontic extrusion is to erupt the tooth to provide 2 to 3 mm of root length above crestal bone level.

CONCLUSION

Success in endodontic therapy is predicated on a host of factors, many of which are controllable before the clinician ever initiates treatment. Proper and thorough preparation of both patient and tooth for endodontic treatment should lay the groundwork for a relatively trouble-free experience that will increase the chances for the ultimate success of the entire treatment.

REFERENCES

1. American Dental Association: Your teeth can be saved by endodontic (root canal) treatment, Chicago, 1985, The Association.
2. American Dental Association: OSHA: what you must know, Chicago, 1992, The Association.
3. American Dental Association: Statement regarding dental handpieces, Chicago, 1992, The Association.
4. Antrim DD: Endodontics and the rubber dam: a review of techniques, J Acad Gen Dent 31:294, 1983.
5. Baumgartner JC, Heggers JP, and Harrison JW: The incidence of bacteremias related to endodontic procedures. I. Nonsurgical endodontics, J Endod 2:135, 1976.
6. Bender IB, Seltzer S, and Yermish, M: The incidence of bacteremia in patients with rheumatic heart disease, Oral Surg 13:353, 1960.
7. Bramwell JD, and Hicks ML: Solving isolation problems with rubber base adhesive, J Endod 12:363, 1986.
8. Centers for Disease Control: Recommended infection control practices for dentistry, MMWR 35:237, 1986.
9. Centers for Disease Control: Recommendations for prevention of HIV transmission in health care settings, MMWR 36(suppl 2S):1987.
10. Centers for Disease Control: Recommendations for preventing transmission of human immunodeficiency virus and hepatitis B virus to patients during exposure-prone invasive procedures, MMWR 40:1, 1991.
11. Cochran MA, Miller CH, and Sheldrake MA: The efficacy of the rubber dam as a barrier to the spread of microorganisms during dental treatment, J Am Dent Assoc 119:141, 1989.
12. Cohen S: Endodontics and litigation: an American perspective, Int Dent J 39:13, 1989.
13. Cohen S, and Schwartz SF: Endodontic complications and the law, J Endod 13:191, 1987.
14. Cohn SA: Endodontic radiography: principles and clinical techniques, Gilberts, Ill, 1988, Dunvale Corp.
15. Corah NL, Gale EN, and Illig SJ: Assessment of a dental anxiety scale, J Am Dent Assoc 97:816, 1978.
16. Council on Dental Materials, Instruments, and Equipment, Council on Dental Practice, and Council on Dental Therapeutics: Infection control recommendations for the dental office and the dental laboratory, J Am Dent Assoc 116:241, 1988.
17. Dajani AS, et al: Prevention of bacterial endocarditis, recommendations by the American Heart Association, JAMA 264:2919, 1990.
18. Department of Labor, Occupational Safety and Health Administration, 29 CFR Part 1910.1030: Occupational exposure to bloodborne pathogens, final rule, Federal Register 56(235):64004, 1991.
19. Donnelly JC, Hartwell GR, and Johnson WB: Clinical evaluation of Ektaspeed x-ray film for use in endodontics, J Endod 11:90, 1985.
20. Farman AG, Mendel RW, and von Fraunhofer JA: Ultraspeed versus Ektaspeed x-ray film; endodontists' perceptions, J Endod 14:615, 1988.
21. Forrest W, and Perez RS: The rubber dam as a surgical drape: protection against AIDS and hepatitis, J Acad Gen Dentistry 37:236, 1989.
22. Forsberg J: Radiographic reproduction of endodontic "working length" comparing the paralleling and bisecting-angle techniques, Oral Surg 64:353, 1987.
23. Glickman GN, and Schwartz SF: Preparation for treatment. In Cohen S, and Burns RC, eds: Pathways of the pulp, ed 5, St. Louis, 1991, Times Mirror/Mosby College Publishing.
24. Goaz PW, and White SC: Oral radiology: principles and interpretation, ed 3, St. Louis, 1993, Times Mirror/Mosby College Publishing.
25. Goerig AC, and Neaverth EJ: A simplified look at the buccal object rule in endodontics, J Endod 13:570, 1987.
26. Greene RR, Sikora FA, and House JE: Rubber dam application to crownless and cone-shaped teeth, J Endod 10:82, 1984.
27. Holroyd SV, Wynn RL, and Requa-Clark B: Clinical pharmacology in the dental practice, ed 4, St. Louis, 1988, Times Mirror/Mosby College Publishing.
28. Janus CE: The rubber dam reviewed, Compend Contin Dent Ed 5:155, 1984.
29. Jeffrey IWM, and Woolford MJ: An investigation of possible iatrogenic damage caused by metal rubber dam clamps, Int Endod J 22:85, 1989.
30. Kantor ML, et al: Efficacy of dental radiographic practices: options for image receptors, examination selection, and patient selection, J Am Dent Assoc 119:259, 1989.
31. Kelly WH: Radiographic asepsis in endodontic practice, J Acad Gen Dent 37:302, 1989.
32. Kolstad RA: Biohazard control in dentistry, Dallas, Tex, 1993, Baylor College of Dentistry Press.
33. Little JW, and Falace DA: Dental management of the medically compromised patient, ed 3, St. Louis, 1988, Times Mirror/Mosby College Publishing.
34. Lovdahl PE, and Gutmann JL: Periodontal and restorative considerations prior to endodontic therapy, J Acad Gen Dent 28:38, 1980.
35. Lovdahl PE, and Wade CK: Problems in tooth isolation and postendodontic restoration. In Gutmann JL, et al, eds: Problem solving in endodontics: prevention, identification, and management, ed 2, Chicago, 1992, Times Mirror/Mosby College Publishing.
36. Madison S, Jordan RD, and Krell KV: The effects of rubber dam retainers on porcelain-fused-to-metal restorations, J Endod 12:183, 1986.
37. Messing JJ, and Stock CJR: Color atlas of endodontics, St. Louis, 1988, Times Mirror/Mosby College Publishing.
38. Miles DA, et al: Radiographic imaging for dental auxiliaries, Philadelphia, 1989, WB Saunders Co.
39. Montgomery EH, and Kroeger DC: Principles of anti-infective therapy, Dent Clin North Am 28:423, 1984.
40. Mouyen F, et al: Presentation and physical evaluation of RadioVisioGraphy, Oral Surg 68:238, 1989.
41. Pollack BR, ed: Handbook of dental jurisprudence and risk management, Littleton, Mass, 1987, PSG Publishing Co.
42. RadioVisioGraphy User's Manual, Marietta, Ga, 1992, Trophy USA.

43. Requa-Clark B, and Holroyd SV: Antiinfective agents. In Holroyd SV, Wynn RL, and Requa-Clark B, eds: Clinical pharmacology in dental practice, ed 4, St. Louis, 1988, Times Mirror/Mosby College Publishing.
44. Richards AG: The buccal object rule, Dent Radiogr Photogr 53:37, 1980.
45. Schwartz SF, and Foster JK: Roentgenographic interpretation of experimentally produced boney lesions. I, Oral Surg 32:606, 1971.
46. Teplitsky PE: Custom acrylic retainer for endodontic isolation, J Endod 14:150, 1988.
47. Torabinejad M, et al: Absorbed radiation by various tissues during simulated endodontic radiography, J Endod 15:249, 1989.
48. Wakabayashi H, et al: A clinical technique for the retention of a rubber dam clamp, J Endod 12:422, 1986.
49. Walton RE, and Torabinejad M: Principles and practice of endodontics, Philadelphia, 1989, WB Saunders Co.
50. Weisman M: A modification of the no. 3 rubber dam clamp, J Endod 9:30, 1983.
51. Wood PR: Cross-infection control in dentistry: a practical illustrated guide, London, 1992, Times Mirror/Mosby College Publishing.

Self-assessment questions

1. It has been established that
   a. exposure to HIV is more likely than exposure to hepatitis B virus.
   b. transmission of tuberculosis is primarily blood-borne.
   c. HIV is less fragile than the hepatitis B virus.
   d. each patient should be considered potentially infectious.
2. Endodontic files
   a. are disposed of after one use.
   b. are considered reusable sharps.
   c. may be picked up by hand before decontamination.
   d. may be disposed of in "generic refuse."
3. To prevent cross-contamination after exposure of the x-ray film
   a. gloves are superfluous.
   b. overgloves are placed over contaminated gloves.
   c. dispose of film packet in generic refuse.
   d. disinfect with sodium hypochlorite.
4. Informed consent information for endodontic therapy excludes
   a. alternatives to recommended treatment.
   b. procedure and prognosis.
   c. a description of OSHA regulations.
   d. foreseeable and material risks.
5. Radiographic exposure for purposes of endodontic therapy
   a. has no place for fast, sensitive speed film.
   b. is minimized with RadioVisioGraphy.
   c. is unnecessary.
   d. does not require informed consent.
6. X-ray units should be
   a. optimally capable of utilizing 70 kVp.
   b. pointed in shape.
   c. collimated to reduce exposure level, not to exceed 7 cm at the skin surface.
   d. collimated to reduce exposure level, not to exceed 9 cm at the skin surface.
7. The American Heart Association recommends for prophylactic antibiotic coverage
   a. penicillin V rather than amoxicillin.
   b. amoxicillin rather than penicillin V.
   c. Keflex rather than penicillin.
   d. cephalosporins rather than erythromycin.
8. Radiographic contrast can be directly affected by altering
   a. milliamperage.
   b. exposure time.
   c. kilovoltage.
   d. angulation.
9. An osteolytic lesion visualized on a radiograph could be mistaken for
   a. granuloma.
   b. cyst.
   c. cementoma.
   d. all of the above.
10. The buccal object rule states
    a. that the object farther from the buccal surface appears to move in the direction opposite the movement of the tube head.
    b. that the object closest to the buccal surface appears to move in the same direction as the tube head.
    c. that the object closest to the buccal surface appears to move in the direction opposite that of the tube head.
    d. that objects closest to the lingual surface appear on the film to move in the direction opposite the movement of the cone.
11. With the cone moved to the distal and facing towards the mesial, the mesiobuccal root of the first molar
    a. will be projected mesially on the film.
    b. will be projected distally on the film.
    c. will not move.
    d. appears to move lingually.
12. To enhance tooth isolation to prevent contamination
    a. isolation with cotton rolls is used.
    b. anticholinergic and systemic antibiotic drugs are used.
    c. isolation with rubber dam is used.
    d. direct access will achieve the goal.
13. To enhance crown preparation and retention, crown lengthening is completed by
    a. electrosurgery in the presence of infrabony defects.
    b. conventional gingivectomy in the presence of infrabony defects.
    c. laser surgery in the presence of infrabony defects.
    d. apically positioned flap, reverse bevel in the presence of infrabony defects.

Chapter 6

Armamentarium and Sterilization

Robert E. Averbach
Donald J. Kleier

Armamentarium

Robert E. Averbach

The number of endodontic cases treated each year continues to increase in quantum leaps as endodontic therapy becomes an integral part of general dental practice. The clinician is bombarded with an assortment of new products and techniques designed to make treatment faster and more effective. The age of high technology has arrived in endodontics, and in this chapter we provide an overview of contemporary trends, describing the most current components of the endodontist's armamentarium. The explosion of knowledge and concern in the area of clinical asepsis and infection control is detailed in the second part of the chapter. All the technological advances and manufacturers' marketing messages cannot replace careful attention to the basic biologic principles of high-quality endodontic treatment.

RADIOGRAPHY

A high-quality preoperative radiograph is critical before endodontic treatment is instituted. As described in Chapter 5, the paralleling technique, utilizing special film holders, produces radiographs with minimal image distortion. Tooth length measurements and diagnostic information from the radiograph tend to be more accurate when the paralleling technique is used.

The radiographs obtained during endodontic treatment pose a different set of problems. These views include root length determination, verification of filling cone placement, and other procedures performed with the rubber dam in place. The rubber dam may make the positioning of these "working" radiographs more difficult. A variety of film holders were recently introduced that are designed to overcome radiographic distortion problems (see Figs. 5-22 to 5-24). All these devices are specifically designed to aid in placing the film and tube head in proper relation to the tooth undergoing endodontic treatment. These devices are of considerable value in obtaining an accurate and distortion-free "working film" with files or filling points protruding from the tooth and with the rubber dam in place.

The choice of dental x-ray film for endodontic radiographs is shifting from Ultraspeed to Ektaspeed (both by Eastman Kodak Company, Rochester, N.Y.), since Ektaspeed is twice as fast and consequently requires half the x-ray exposure. Though Ektaspeed is reported to be more grainy and less sharp than Ultraspeed film, careful attention to exposure and processing variables produces an image of good diagnostic quality. A rapid, automated film processor is helpful for producing high-quality films (Fig. 6-1).

Variations in film processing for endodontics were described in Chapter 5. Once the film has been exposed and processed, the clinician's ability to discern subtle variations in the radiograph will be enhanced by two factors: magnification and peripheral light shielding. A high-quality magnifying system of 1.5 to 3 power will often clarify an extra canal or hard-to-visualize apex (Fig. 6-2). A cutout of black construction paper on the viewbox effectively masks peripheral light and permits perception of subtle differences in film density.

DIAGNOSIS

The armamentarium for diagnostic testing was described in Chapter 1. The technology of pulp testing continues to become more sophisticated and reliable. Examination techniques for

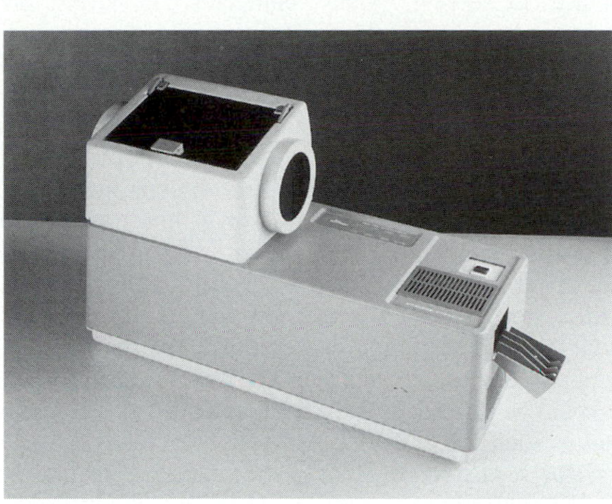

FIG. 6-1 Peri-Pro II film processor. (Courtesy of Air Techniques Inc., Hicksville, N.Y.)

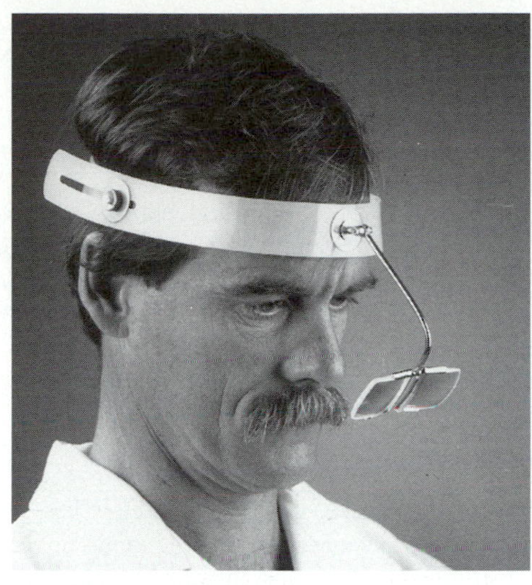

FIG. 6-2 Atwood magnifying loupes. (Courtesy of Atwood Industries, Cardiff by the Sea, Calif.)

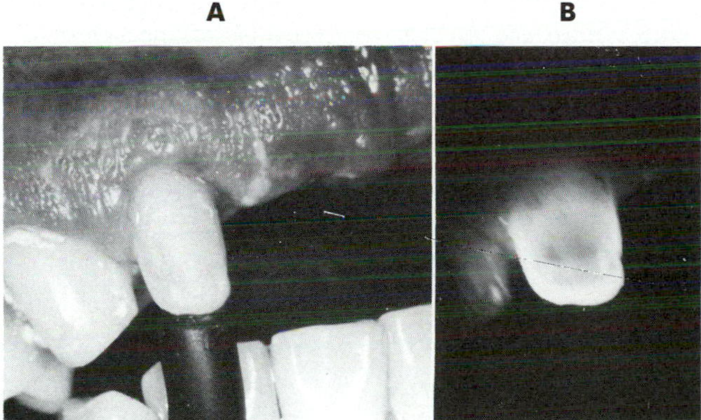

FIG. 6-3 Transillumination of pulpal "blush." **A,** Transillumination of lingual of full crown preparation. **B,** Operatory lights out, demonstration of "blush."

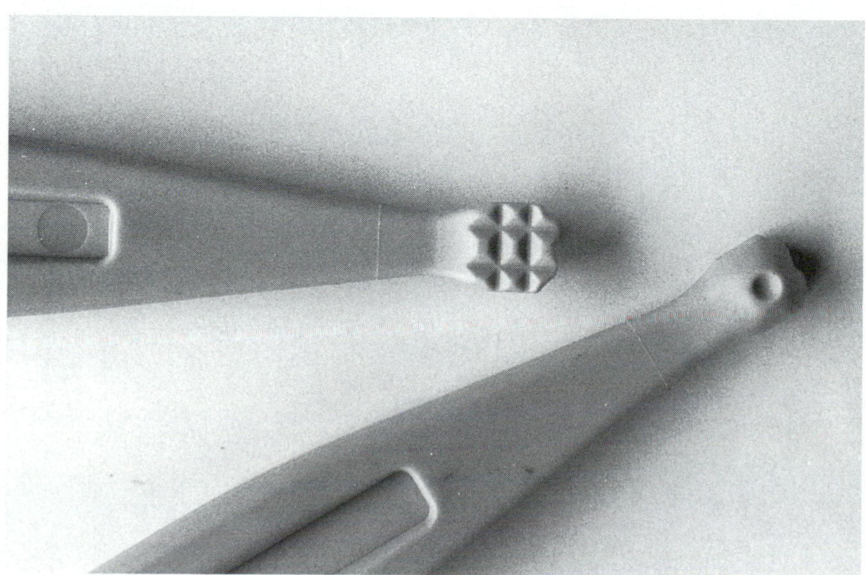

FIG. 6-4 Fracfinder tips. (Courtesy of Denbur Inc., Oakbrook, Ill.)

disclosing tooth fractures with a fiberoptic light source were shown in Chapter 1. This transillumination technique is also valuable for determining the extent of a pulpal "blush" following extensive tooth preparation. The operatory lights are dimmed and the transilluminator is placed on the lingual surface of the preparation (Fig. 6-3).

The technique of detecting a cracked tooth by wedging cusps was also described in Chapter 1. An additional wedging modality for the diagnosis of fractured teeth is the "Fracfinder" (Fracfinder, Denbur Corp.) (Fig. 6-4). This plastic device is used as a selective wedge on or between the cusps as the patient bites. Sharp pain on *release* of biting pressure often indicates a cracked tooth.

ORGANIZATION SYSTEMS

The trend toward preset trays and cassettes has simplified and streamlined the organization, storage, and delivery of endodontic instruments. Particular instruments and tray set-ups are the choice of the individual clinician, but certain basic principles are common to all systems. A basic set-up contains most of the commonly used long-handled instruments, such as mouth mirror, endodontic explorer, long spoon excavator, plastic instrument, and locking forceps. These are often supplemented by items such as irrigating syringe and needles, ruler, sterile paper points, burs, and rubber dam clamps. A sample cassette set-up is shown in Figure 6-5. A wide variety of file stands and file boxes are now available that facilitate organizational simplicity and sterility (Fig. 6-6). Whatever system is chosen, the emphasis is on keeping the set-up easy for the staff to restock and sterilize, and convenient for the clinician, whether the operator works alone or with a chairside assistant.

RUBBER DAM

Rubber dam material for endodontic therapy is currently available in a variety of colors and thicknesses—and, yes, even scents! Advocates of the heavy-weight dam prefer its close adaptation ... resistance to tearing. Many clinicians, however, prefer medium- or light-weight dam material, citing its increased resilience and ease of application. Color is also a matter of personal preference. Dark-colored dam material provides sharp contrast between the tooth and dam; light-colored material permits visualization of the x-ray filmholder's position when a working radiograph is being exposed. Options include green dam scented with wintergreen and royal blue, which yields good visual contrast plus "eye appeal." Regardless of which color, thickness, or fragrance is chosen, all dam material should be stored away from heat and light to prevent the latex from drying and becoming less flexible. Tearing of the dam upon application usually indicates that the material is dried out and should be discarded. Refrigerating dam material seems to extend its shelf life.

An almost endless array of rubber dam clamps are available to isolate special problem situations. The "tiger-jaw" clamps (Fig. 6-7) are especially useful for holding the dam on broken-down posterior teeth. The winged style of clamp is preferred, since it provides better tissue retraction and allows the use of the "unit" placement technique described in Chapter 5.

Any good-quality rubber dam punch will accomplish the goal of creating a clean hole for the tooth. Care must be taken to punch a hole without "nicks" in the rim, to prevent accidental tearing and leakage. The Ivory design clamp forceps are preferred in endodontics because they allow the dentist to apply gingival force when seating a clamp (Fig. 6-8). This pressure is sometimes needed to engage undercuts on a broken-down tooth, allowing the clamp to be stable. A radiolucent plastic rubber dam frame eliminates the need for removing the frame while exposing "working" radiographs.

ACCESS PREPARATION THROUGH A CROWN

Gaining access through a porcelain-fused-to-metal crown is more difficult than gaining access through natural tooth structure or other restorative materials. One approach is to use a

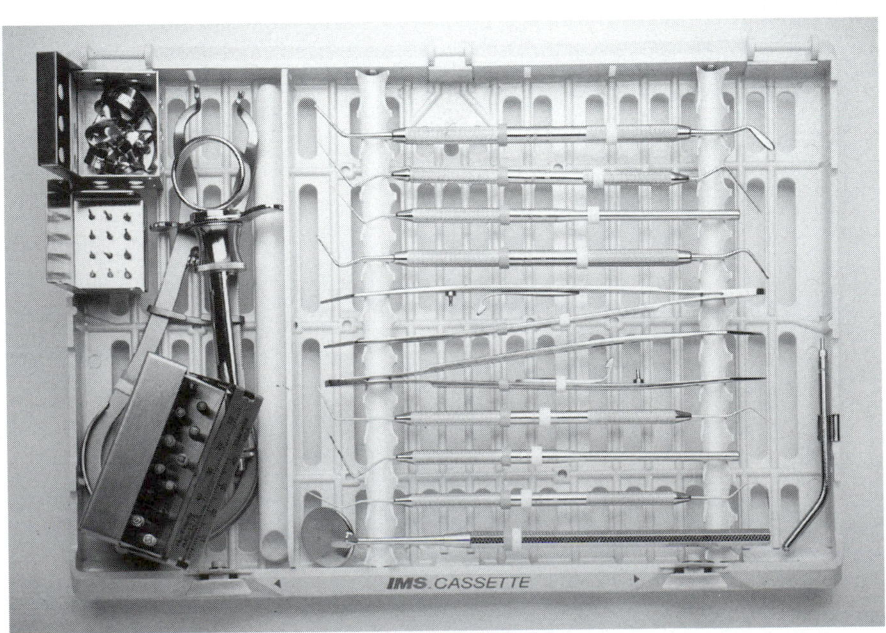

FIG. 6-5 IMS instrument cassette. (Courtesy of Hu-Friedy Co., Chicago, Ill.)

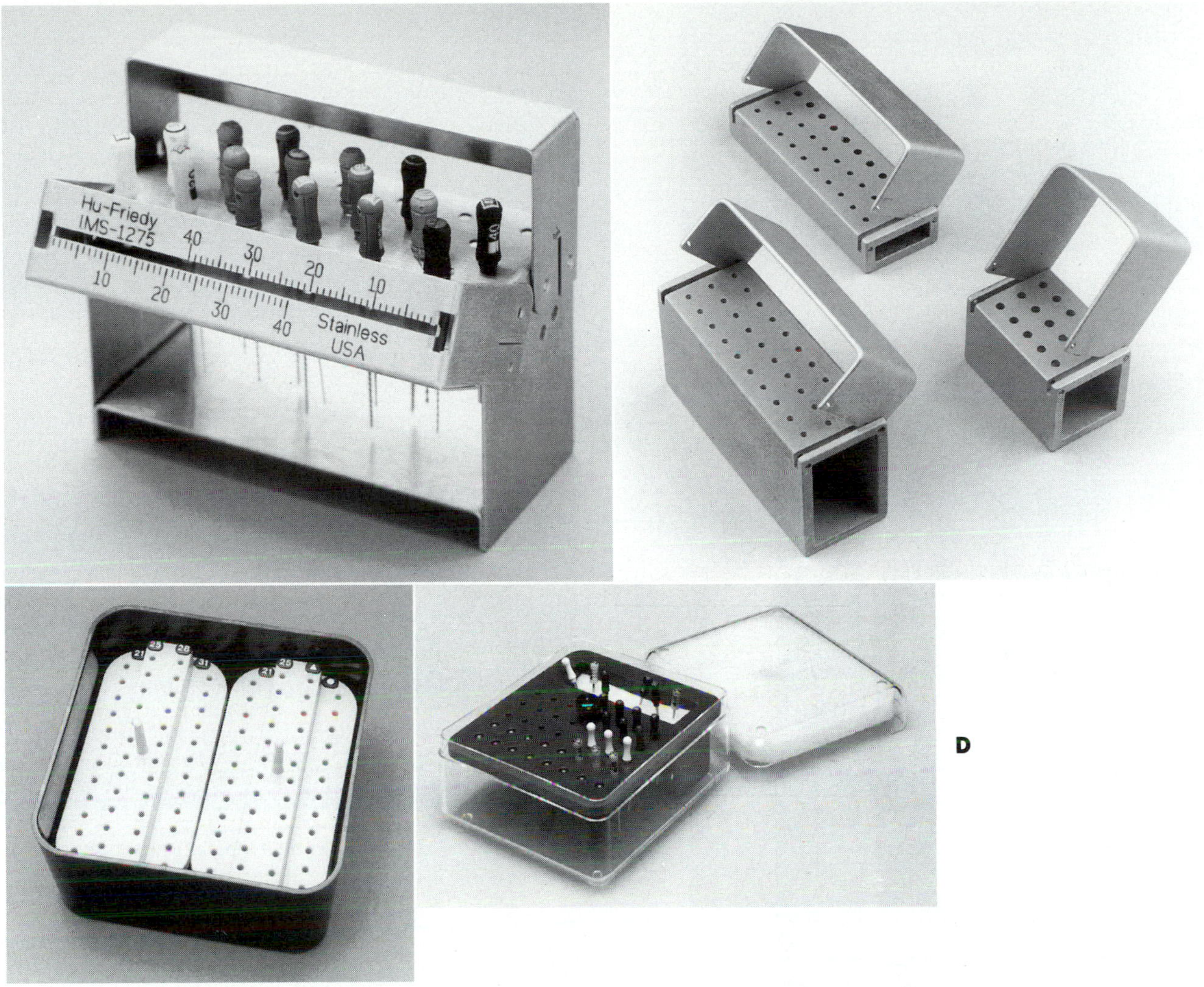

A

C

B

D

FIG. 6-6 A, File stand (Courtesy of Hu-Friedy Co., Chicago, Ill.). **B,** File stand (Courtesy of Premier Dental Products, Norristown, Pa.). **C,** File and bur stands (Courtesy of Brassler USA, Savannah, Ga.). **D,** File stand (Courtesy of Caulk/Dentsply, Milford, Del.).

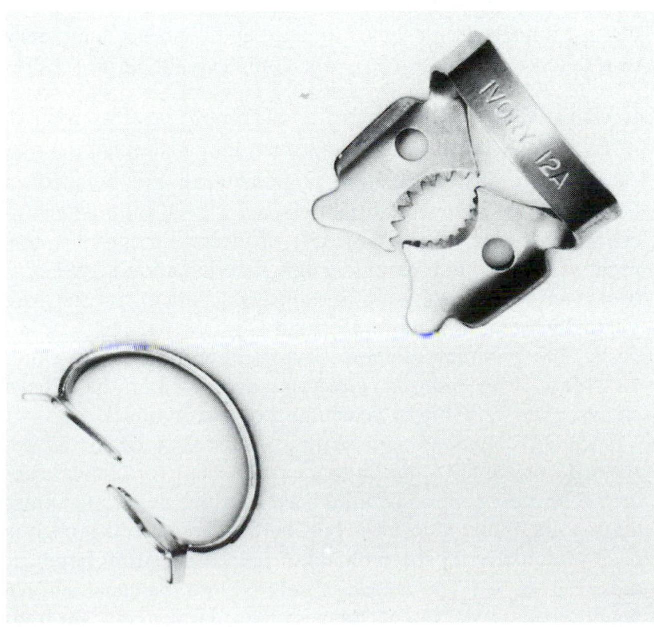

FIG. 6-7 Ivory "Tiger" serrated rubber dam clamp. (Courtesy of Miles Dental Products, South Bend, Ind.)

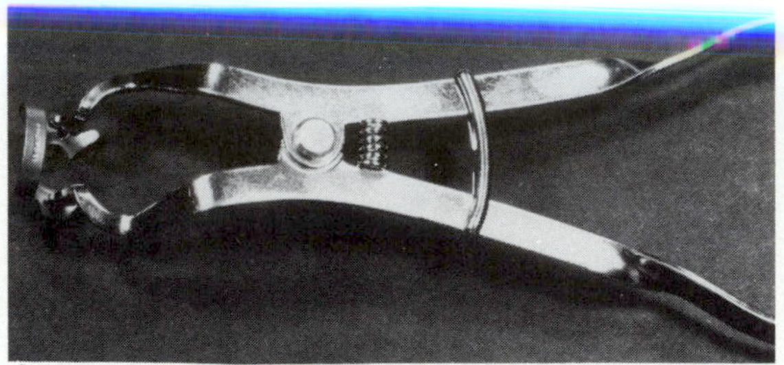

FIG. 6-8 Ivory clamp forceps.

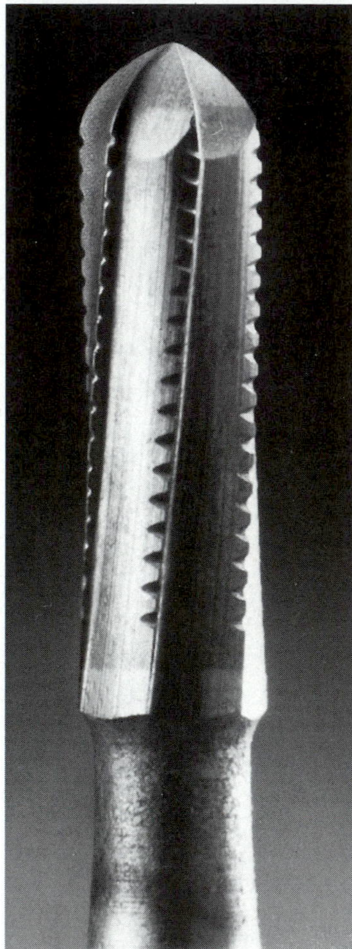

FIG. 6-9 Fine crosscut "Beaver" bur for reduced handpiece chatter when penetrating metal alloys. (Courtesy of Midwest Dental Products Corp., Des Plains, Ill.)

small round diamond with copious water spray to create the outline form in the porcelain. The metal substructure is then penetrated with either a tungsten-tipped or new carbide-end cutting bur (Fig. 6-9). This two-stage technique reduces the possibility of porcelain fracture or chipping.

HAND INSTRUMENTS

A sample cassette for endodontics was shown in Figure 6-5. The long, double-ended spoon excavator is specifically designed for endodontic therapy. It allows the clinician to remove coronal pulp tissue, caries, or cotton pellets that may be deep in the tooth's crown (Fig. 6-10). The double-ended endodontic explorer is used to locate and probe the orifice of the root canal as it joins the pulp chamber (Fig. 6-11). Locking endodontic forceps facilitate the transfer of paper points and gutta-percha cones from assistant to dentist (Fig. 6-12). Plastic filling instruments are designed to place and condense temporary restorations. A periodontal probe completes the basic set-up.

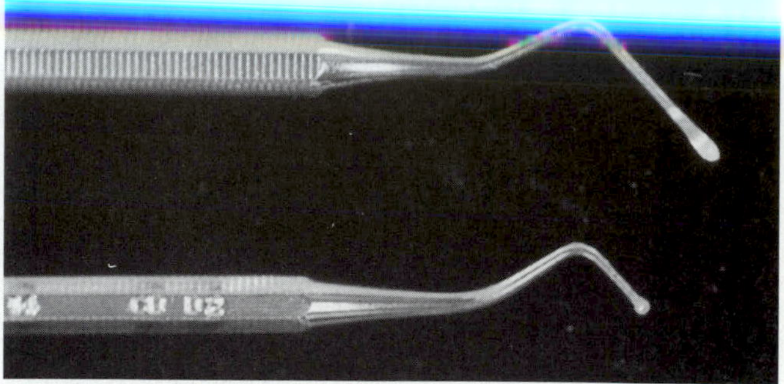

FIG. 6-10 Endo spoon *(top)* vs. operative spoon excavator *(bottom)*.

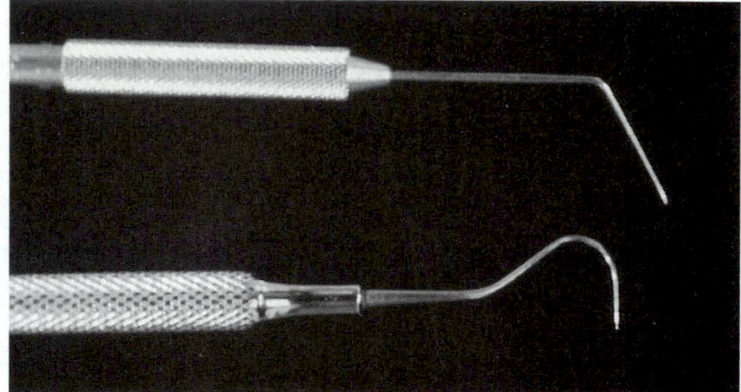

FIG. 6-11 Endo explorer *(top)* vs. operative explorer *(bottom)*.

CANAL PREPARATION

Techniques for determining the "working length" of the root canal before instrumentation is undertaken are detailed in Chapter 8. Silicone stop dispensers and special millimeter rulers are available (Fig. 6-13). Use of electronic apex locators as an adjunct to radiographic length determination is still controversial because they are not always accurate, but they are gradually becoming more accepted (Fig. 6-14). As they improve, the accuracy of these devices is becoming more predictable.[21,41] In addition, electronic apex locators have been shown to be valuable in detecting root perforation.[29]

Cleaning, shaping, and sealing of the root canal, as described in Chapter 8, are primary components of clinical success. The most commonly used hand instruments in canal preparation are endodontic files (Fig. 6-15). The barbed broach is used principally for the removal of pulp tissue from large canals (Fig. 6-16). The broach is inserted into the canal and rotated to engage the tissue. Because these instruments are frag-

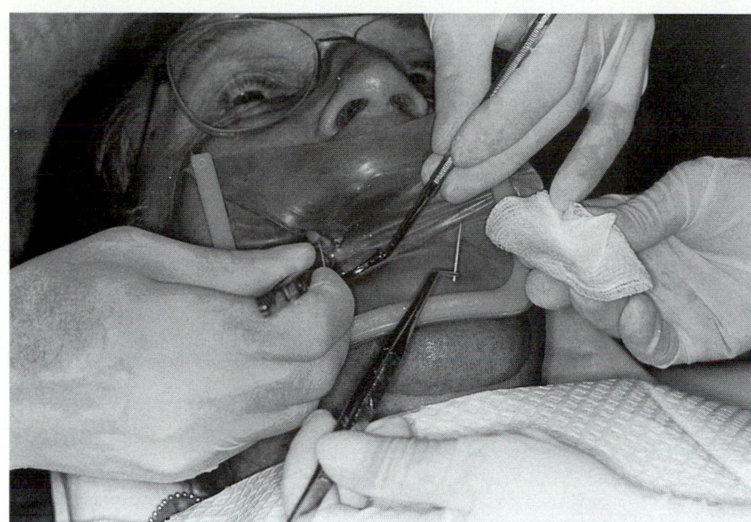

FIG. 6-12 Locking forceps transfer of paper points.

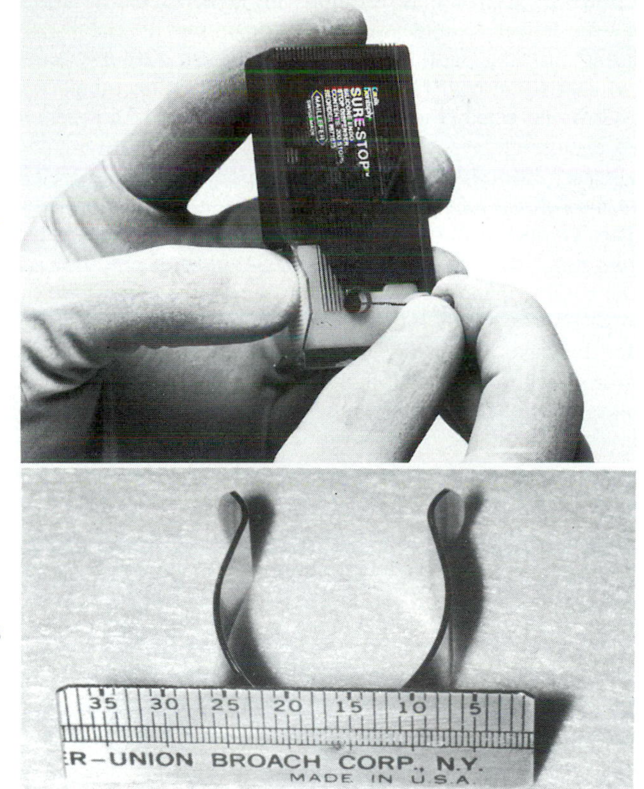

FIG. 6-13 A, Silicone stop dispenser. (Courtesy of Caulk-Dentsply, Milford, Del.) **B,** Millimeter thumb ruler.

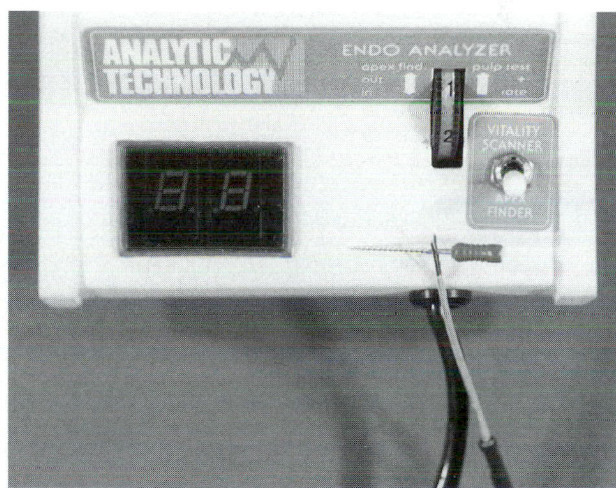

FIG. 6-14 Electronic apex locator plus pulp tester.

ile and prone to breakage, great care must be exercised in their use! Introduction of new file designs has increased dramatically during the past few years. Triangular, square, and rhomboid blanks are usually used in the manufacturing of these hand instruments. Variations in metallurgy, cutting blade angle, degree of twist, flute spacing, and cutting or noncutting tip have complicated the clinician's choice of instruments (Fig. 6-17).[26,39,42] In addition, recent evidence suggests that rounded-tipped files, when manipulated with a specific motion, may produce more consistent root canal preparations.[8,22,31] A detailed description of these file variations is found in Chapter 14.

The introduction of automated systems for canal preparation is also progressing at a dizzying rate. Mechanical systems such as the Giromatic handpiece have been available for many years (see Chapter 8).

The introduction of sonic and ultrasonic systems as adjuncts to canal preparation seems to be a very promising development in the endodontic armamentarium. All these devices, to a greater or lesser degree, share certain basic principles that allow the instrument to flush and clean the canal while maintaining much of the natural root curvature (see Chapter 8). The devices oscillate or vibrate at various frequencies when energized. The energy is then transferred to the intracanal instruments used in the cleaning and shaping process. No actual rotation of the instrument is used, so, theoretically, the canal shape and natural anatomic constriction are preserved, as de-

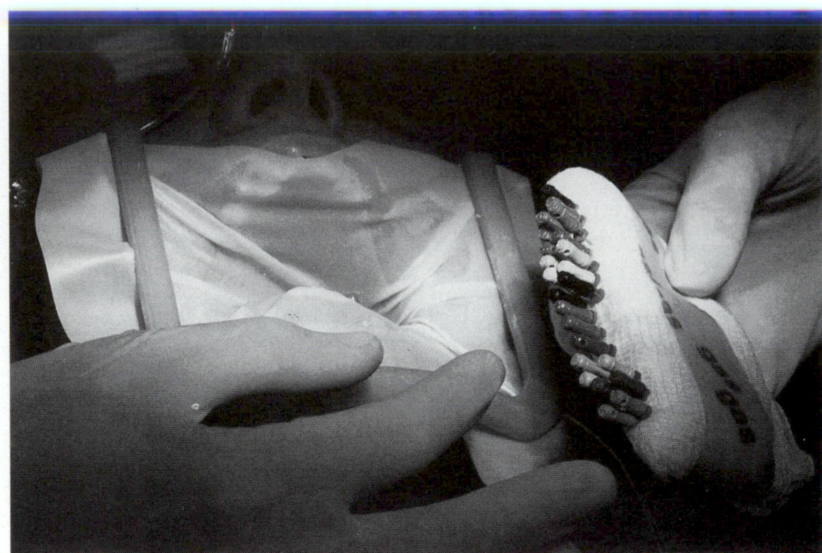

FIG. 6-15 Four-handed transfer of files in sterile gauze pack.

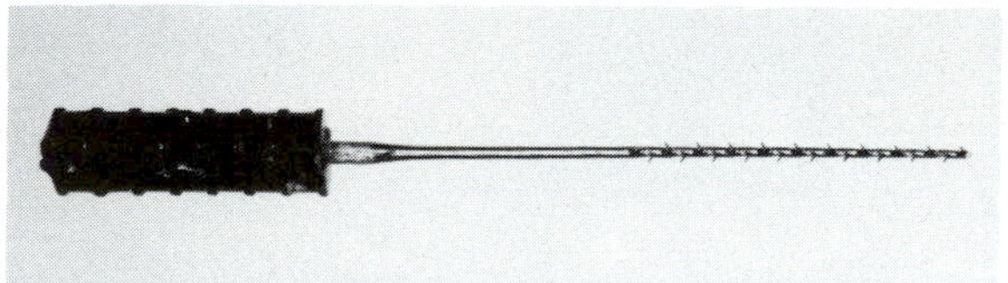

FIG. 6-16 Barbed broach.

scribed in Chapter 8. In addition, all the sonic and ultrasonic devices deliver copious streams of irrigant into the canal space during instrumentation, providing enhanced flushing action and debris removal. Controversy still exists concerning these devices and whether or not they are living up to their marketing claims.[7,33]

Rotary instruments are used principally as flaring devices for the coronal portion of the canal. The most common is the Gates-Glidden drill (Fig. 6-18). Sized in increasing diameters from no. 1 through no. 6, the Gates-Glidden should be used in a passive manner to enlarge the canal orifice and flare the prepared root canal. Using excessive force may either perforate the canal or fracture the instrument. The Gates-Glidden drill is designed to break high on the shaft if excessive resistance is encountered, allowing the clinician to easily remove the fragment.[32]

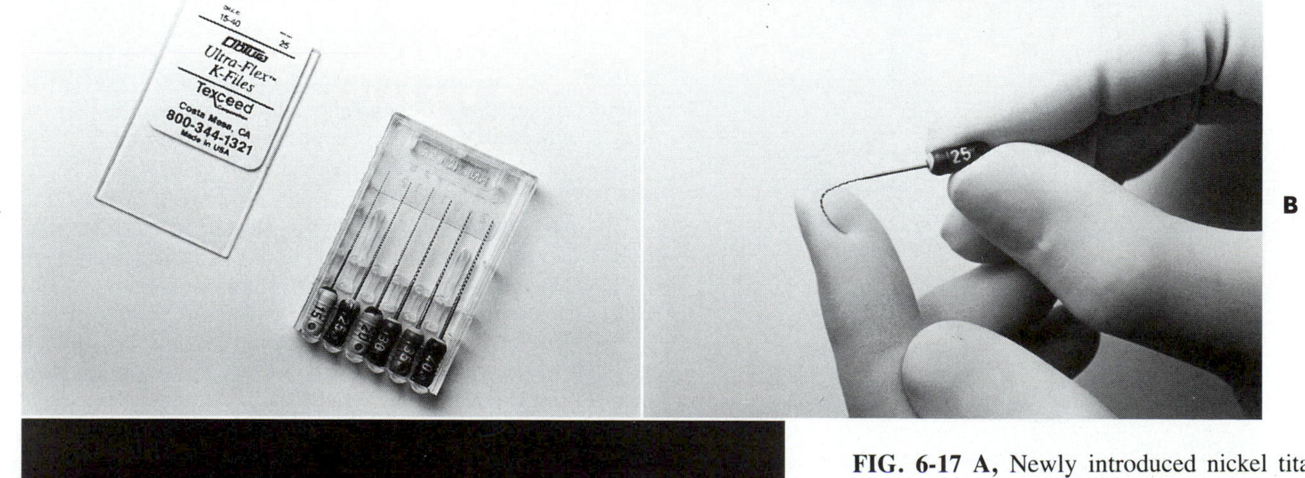

FIG. 6-17 A, Newly introduced nickel titanium files. (Courtesy of Texceed Corp., Costa Mesa, Calif.) **B,** Demonstration of flexibility of nickel-titanium file. (Courtesy of Texceed Corp., Costa Mesa, Calif.) **C,** Rounded "pilot" tip of Canal Master instrument. (Courtesy of Brassler USA, Savannah, Ga.)

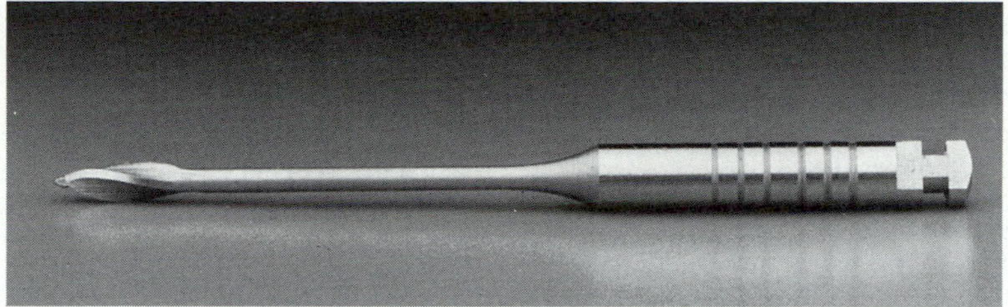

FIG. 6-18 Gates-Glidden drill. (Courtesy of Brassler USA, Savannah, Ga.)

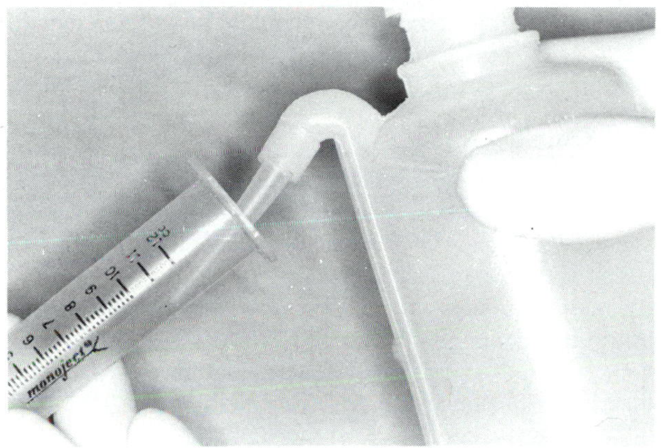

FIG. 6-19 Back-filling of irrigation syringe from wash bottle.

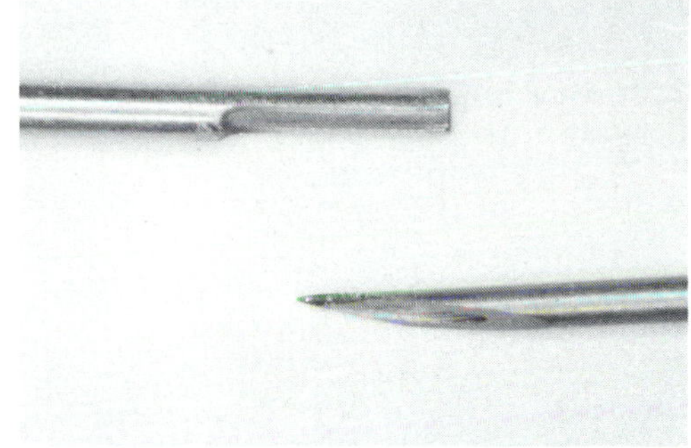

FIG. 6-20 Irrigating needles. *(Top)* Notched tip. *(Bottom)* Standard hypodermic.

IRRIGATION

Irrigation of the canal during instrumentation is described in Chapter 8. Systems for the delivery of irrigating solution into the root canal range from simple disposable syringes to complex devices capable of simultaneously irrigating and aspirating. The choice for the clinician is one of convenience and cost. The smaller syringe barrels (less than 10 ml) require frequent refilling during the instrumentation phase of therapy. Plastic syringes in the 10 to 20 ml range may offer the best combination of sufficient solution volume and ease of handling. "Back-filling" of the syringe from a 500-ml plastic laboratory wash bottle filled with the irrigant of choice saves time and effort over aspirating the solution into the barrel from a container (Fig. 6-19). The barrel tip should be a Luer-Lok design rather than friction fit, to prevent accidental needle dislodgement during irrigation.

Two basic types of needle tip designs are shown in Figure 6-20: the standard beveled hypodermic tip and the notched tip. The latter design helps prevent the accidental forcing of irrigating solution into the periapical tissues should the needle bind in the canal. Severe reactions have been reported if this occurs.[9]

Paper points of various sizes are available to dry the canal following irrigation. Paper points are used sequentially in the locking forceps until no moisture is evident on the paper point. Presterilized "cell" packaging is preferred over bulk packaging to maintain asepsis (Fig. 6-21).

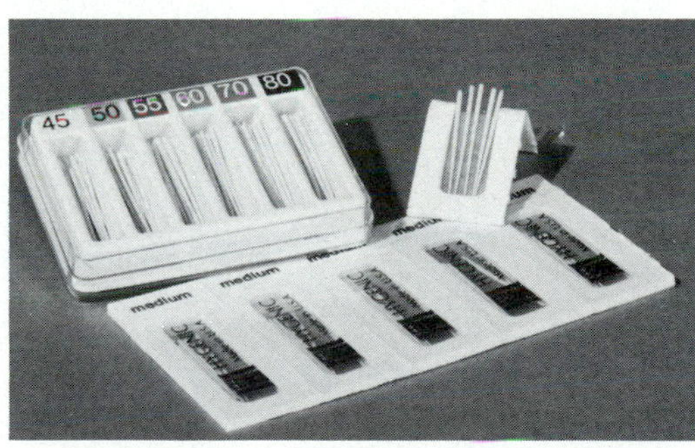

FIG. 6-21 Paper point—bulk versus "cell" packaging. (Courtesy of Hygienic Corp., Akron, Ohio)

OBTURATION

Most root canal filling methods employ root canal sealer as an integral part of the obturation technique. The most popular class of sealer cements used in endodontics are based on zinc oxide–eugenol formulations. These products require a glass slab and cement spatula for mixing to the desired consistency. Sealers containing calcium hydroxide are also available. Reports detailing the biologic response and physical characteristics of these products are now in the scientific literature.[1,40] Root canal obturation materials and techniques are discussed

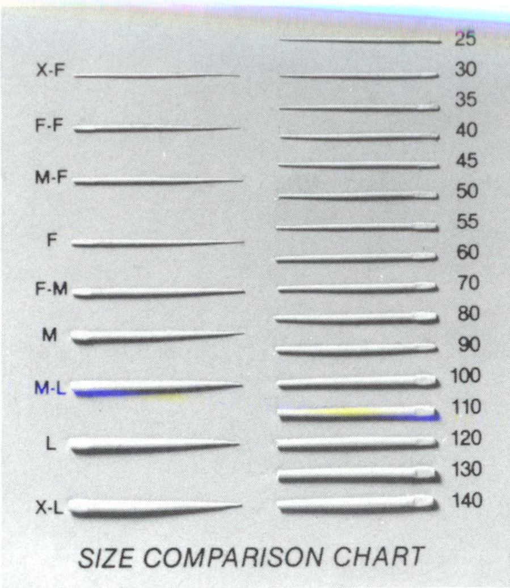

FIG. 6-22 Nonstandardized versus standardized gutta-percha cones. (Courtesy of Hygienic Corp., Akron, Ohio)

commonly used in contemporary ... available as standardized cones corresponding to the approximate size of root canal instruments (no. 15 to 140). Nonstandardized cones are more tapered, and are sized from extra fine through extra large. The two styles are compared in Figure 6-22.

Specialized instruments used in obturating the root canal with gutta-percha include spreaders and pluggers (Fig. 6-23). Spreaders are available in a wide variety of lengths and tapers and are used primarily in the lateral condensation technique to compact gutta-percha filling material. Pluggers, also called condensers, are flat-ended rather than pointed and are used primarily to compact filling materials in a vertical fashion. A rotary instrument for the removal of compacted gutta-percha has recently been introduced (Fig. 6-24). This device breaks up and removes gutta-percha from the canal, facilitating retreatment procedures.

On the "high-tech" front, devices for the heating, delivery, and compaction of gutta-percha into the prepared root canal are now available. A detailed description of these devices is presented in Chapter 9; they include the Obtura II system by Texceed (Fig. 6-25) and the Ultrafil system by Hygienic. In addition, new systems for the placement and compaction of warm gutta-percha on filelike carrier cores have been introduced (Fig. 6-26). The endodontic literature is replete with controversy about many of these new systems.[12,24,30]

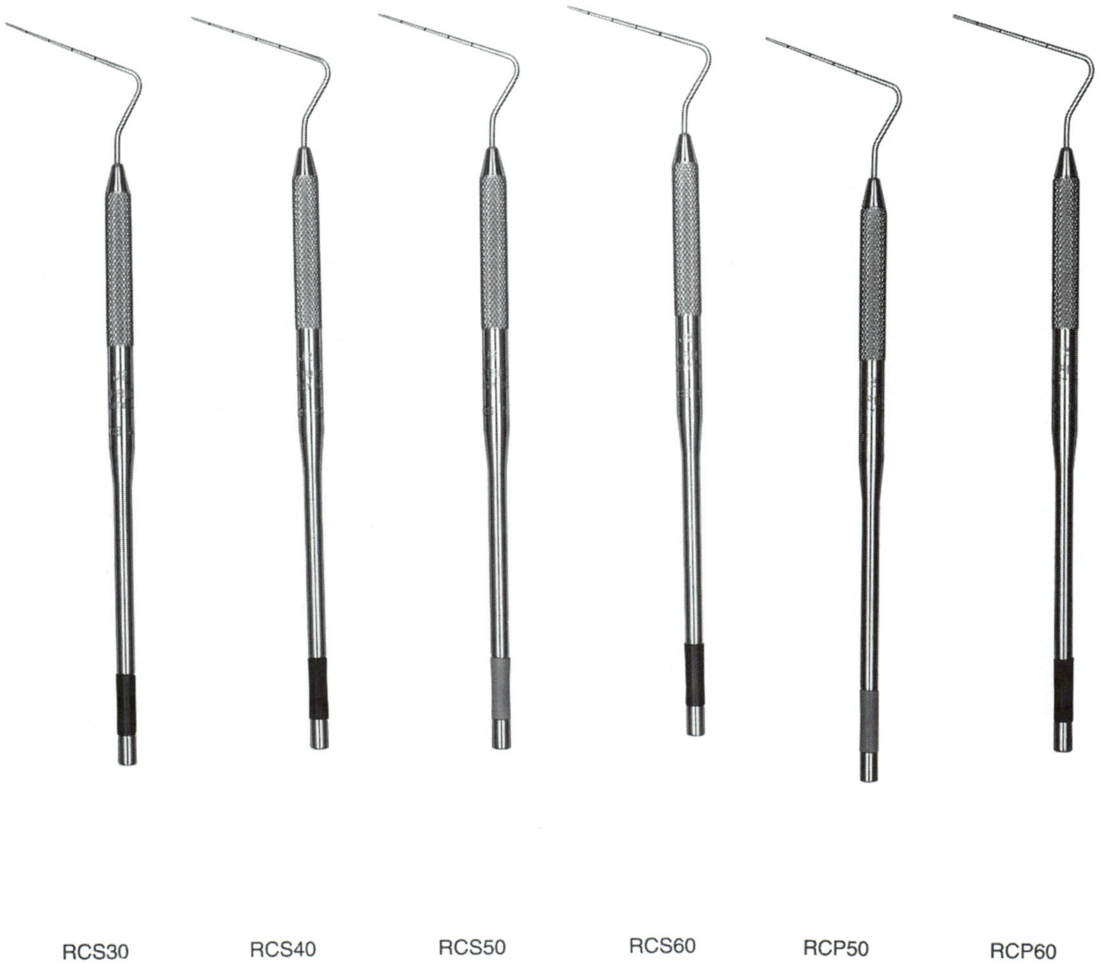

FIG. 6-23 ISO sized spreaders and pluggers. (Courtesy of Hu-Friedy Co., Chicago, Ill.)

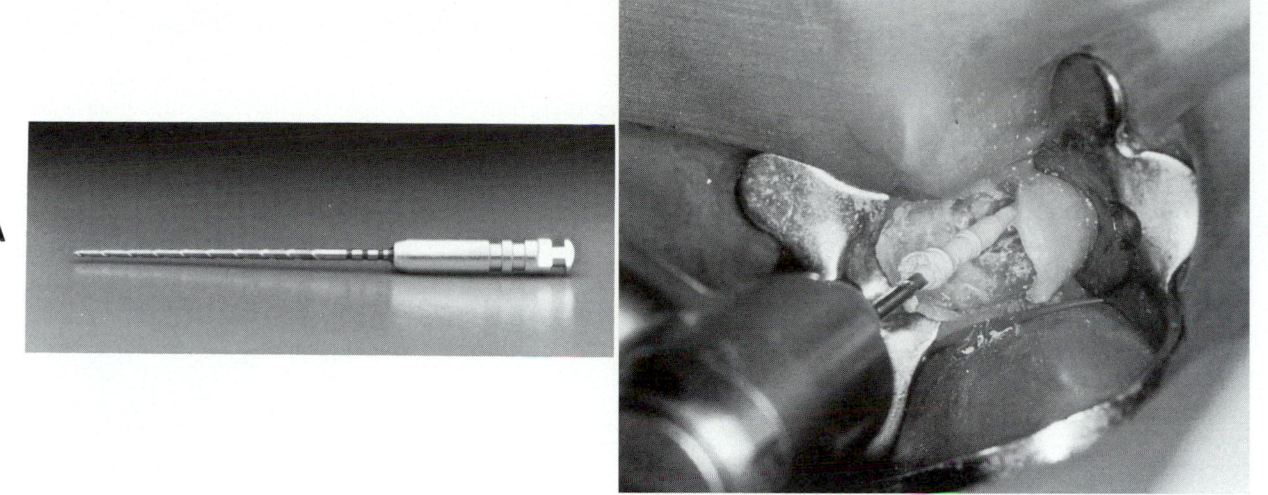

FIG. 6-24 A, GPX gutta-percha remover. (Courtesy of Brassler USA, Savannah, Ga.) **B,** Gutta-percha being removed by GPX.

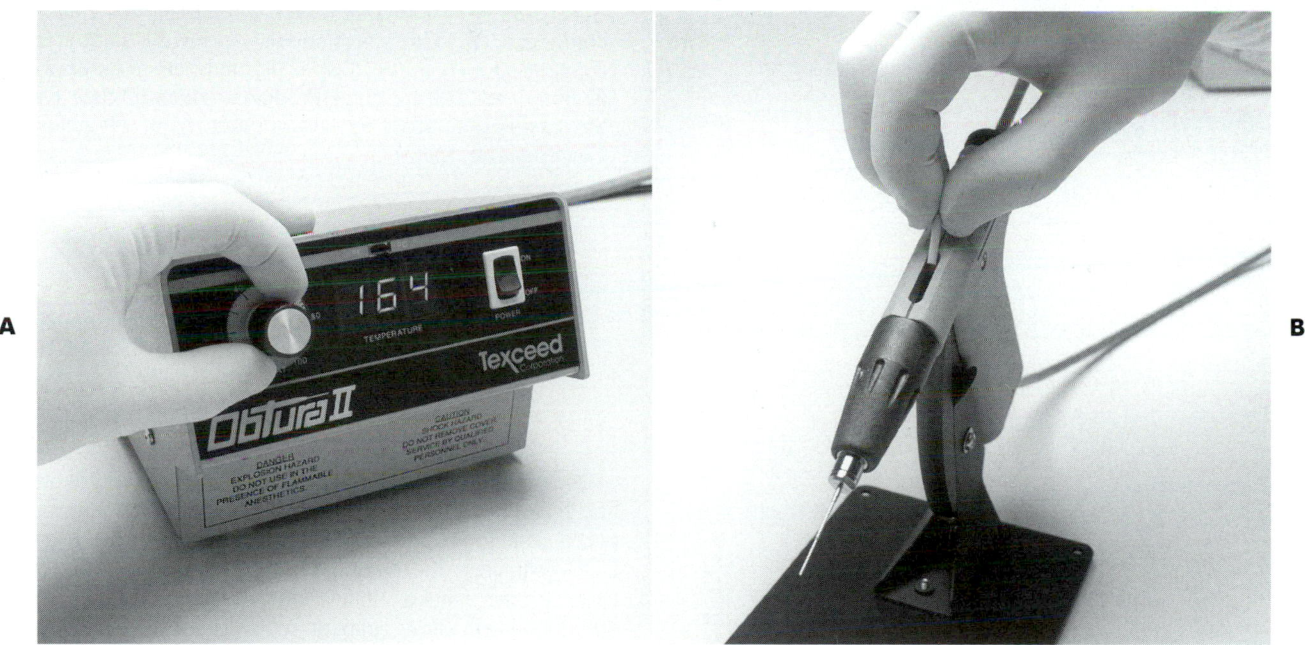

FIG. 6-25 A, Obtura II showing the digital temperature display. **B,** Loading gutta-percha into Obtura II chamber. (Courtesy of Texceed Corp., Costa Mesa, Calif.)

Temporary restorative materials used in endodontics must provide a high-quality seal of the access preparation to prevent microbial contamination of the root canal. Premixed products such as Cavit and TERM have become popular for temporary-access cavity sealing. Cavit (Fig. 6-27) is a moisture-initiated, autopolymerized, premixed calcium sulfate–polyvinyl chloride acetate, whereas TERM is a visible light–initiated, composite-like product whose main component is urethane dimethacrylate polymer. Both products are characterized by ease of insertion and removal, plus demonstrated resistance to marginal leakage.[19,43]

Sterilization

Donald J. Kleier

Infection control recommendations from the American Dental Association (ADA), Centers for Disease Control (CDC), Occupational Safety and Health Administration (OSHA), and other government agencies have permanently changed the way dentists deliver care.[4,13,18] The dentist has a significant responsibility for the health of patients, employees, and co-workers. In this section we examine some of the basics of infection control as it relates to the practice of endodontics.

A

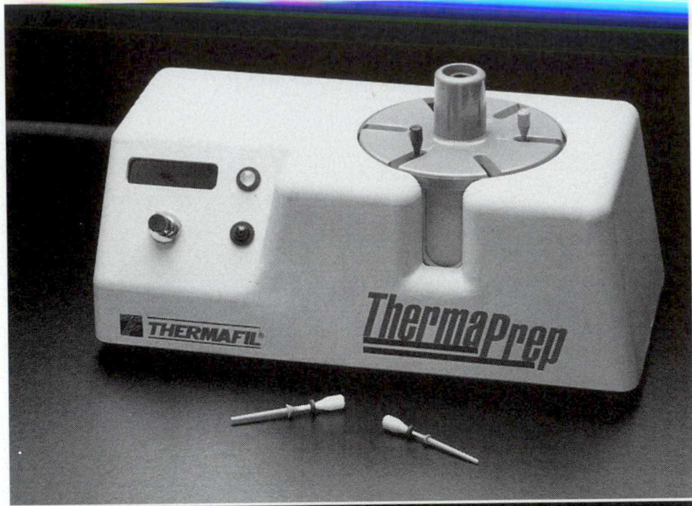

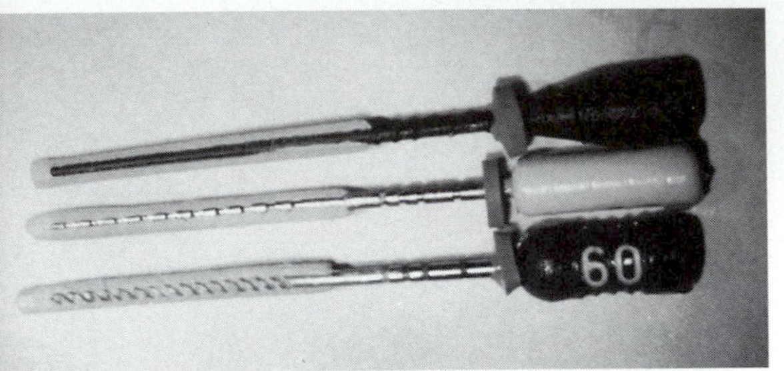

C

B

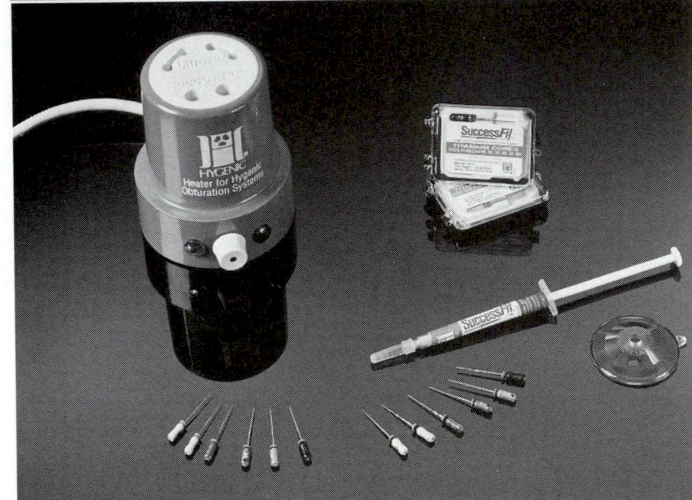

FIG. 6-26 A, Thermaprep oven for heating Thermafil obturators. **B,** Cross-section of Thermafil obturator cores. *(Top to bottom)* Plastic, titanium, stainless steel. (Courtesy of Tulsa Dental Products, Tulsa, Okla.) **C,** SuccessFil obturation system. (Courtesy of Hygienic Corp., Akron, Ohio)

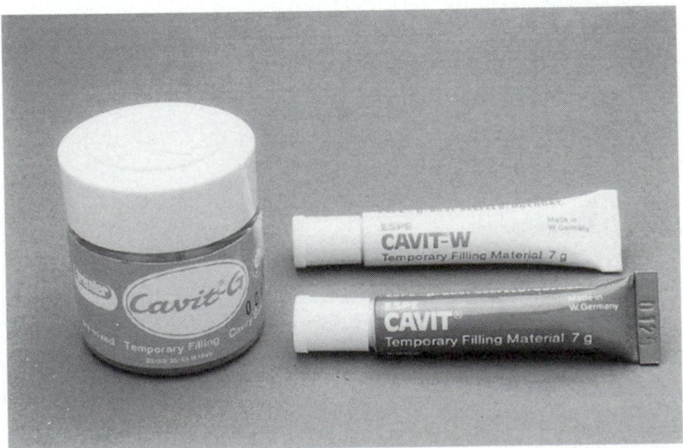

FIG. 6-27 Cavit-G, Cavit-W, and Cavit temporary filling materials. (Courtesy of Premier Dental Products Co., Norristown, Pa.)

The concept of universal precautions is being adopted by health care facilities because of the *inability* to distinguish between contagious and noncontagious patients. By 1993, the CDC estimates, the cumulative number of diagnosed AIDS cases in the United States will be between 330,000 and 405,000. Fortunately, patient transmission to dental professionals has never been reported. The seroprevalence rate among dentists is lower than that in the general population. Use of universal precautions in the management of all patients significantly reduces the risk of occupational exposure to infection with human immunodeficiency virus (HIV) and other blood-borne pathogens.[6]

Since HIV appears to be more difficult to transmit than hepatitis B virus (HBV), practices that prevent transmission of HBV can serve as models for preventing transmission of other contagious diseases.[16] Infection control procedures that protect against HBV should protect against HIV.

VACCINATION

Although AIDS is of concern to dental health care workers, their risk of contracting hepatitis B is far greater.[14] All dentists and staff who have patient contact should be vaccinated against HBV.

BARRIER TECHNIQUES

The most effective method of preventing cross-contamination is personal barrier techniques. Latex treatment gloves must be worn by all dental health care workers involved with direct patient care. Surgical masks or chin-length plastic face shields protect the face and oral and nasal mucosa from splattered blood and saliva and from aerosols. Protective eyewear should be worn, together with a surgical mask, as an alternative to a plastic face shield. Protective clothing must be worn when there is risk of exposure to body fluids. Clothing must be changed when visibly soiled by fluids.[4,18]

The dentist has the responsibility for understanding disease transmission thoroughly and possessing the knowledge to prevent cross-infection. Knowing how to safely handle and sterilize contaminated endodontic instruments is an essential part of this responsibility. All instruments that come into contact with blood or saliva must be sterilized or discarded.

DEFINITION OF TERMS

The purpose of this section is to help clarify certain terms that are used in discussing office infection control.

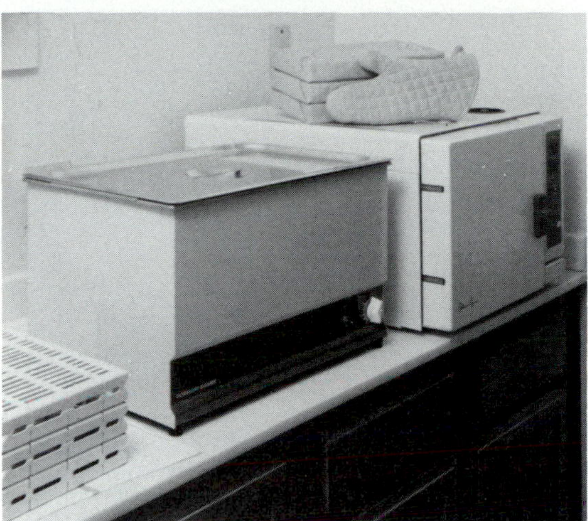

FIG. 6-28 Office sterilization area showing instrument cassettes, ultrasonic cleaner, and autoclave. (Courtesy of Dr. Elizabeth S. Barr.)

sterilization A physical or chemical procedure that *destroys all microbial life,* including highly resistant bacterial endospores. Sterilization is a verifiable procedure.

disinfection A less lethal process than sterilization, it eliminates virtually all pathogenic vegetative microorganisms, but not necessarily all microbial forms (spores). Disinfection usually is reserved for large environmental surfaces that cannot be sterilized (e.g., a dental chair). Disinfection lacks the margin of safety afforded by sterilization procedures. Disinfection is nonverifiable.

bacterial vegetative form Active, multiplying microorganisms.

bacterial spore form (endospore) A more complex structure than the vegetative cell from which it forms. Spores form in response to environmental conditions and are more resistant to sterilization methods than vegetative forms.

virus An extremely *small agent that grows and reproduces only in living host cells.* The virus particle consists of a central core of nucleic acid and an outer coat of protein. It is generally agreed that virus particles are much *less* resistant to thermal inactivation than bacterial spores.[11]

pathogenic microorganism A microorganism that causes or is associated with disease.

cross-infection Transmission of infectious material from one person to another.

biological indicator A preparation of microorganisms, usually bacterial spores, that serves as a challenge to the efficiency of a given sterilization process or cycle. Negative bacterial growth from a biologic indicator verifies sterilization.

process indicator Strip, tape, or tab applied to or packaged in a sterilizer load. Special inks or chemicals within the indicator change color when subjected to heat, steam, or chemical vapor and indicate that the load has been cycled through the sterilizer. Process indicators *do not* verify sterilization.

universal precautions Routine use of the same infection control procedures for all patients, regardless of medical history.

INSTRUMENT PREPARATION

The preoperative handling, cleaning, and packaging of contaminated instruments are frequently sources of injury and possible infection. Dental staff performing such procedures should wear reusable heavy rubber work gloves similar to household cleaning gloves.[4] Contaminated instruments that will not be cleaned immediately should be placed in a holding solution so that blood, saliva, and tissue will not dry on the surfaces. Ultrasonic cleaner detergent or *iodophor* solution, placed in a basin, is an effective holding solution.

An ultrasonic cleaner, which is many times more effective and safer than hand scrubbing, should be the choice for definitive instrument cleaning. Instruments cleaned in an ultrasonic device should be suspended in a perforated basket. When an ultrasonic cleaner is on, nothing should come into contact with the tank's bottom, and its lid should be in place.[20] The cleaner should run at least 5 minutes per load. Once the cycle is complete, the clean instruments are rinsed under a high volume of cool water, placed on a clean dry towel and rolled or patted, and then air dried. The ultrasonic solution should be discarded daily and the tub of the ultrasonic machine disinfected. The instruments are now very clean, but not sterile. Continued precautions are necessary until the instruments have been sterilized. Cassettes have been developed that allow health care workers to use, clean, package, and sterilize dental instruments with a minimum of handling (Fig. 6-28). Instruments packaged in a cassette system may require additional time in an ultrasonic cleaner. The manufacturer recommendations regarding time should be strictly followed.[34]

Clean instruments ready for sterilization should be packaged in containers designed for the specific sterilization process to be employed (Fig. 6-29). The sterilizing agent must be able to penetrate the instrument package and come into intimate contact with microorganisms. The package and sterilizer must be compatible.

METHOD OF STERILIZATION

The oldest and most reliable agent for destroying microorganisms is heat. The most commonly used means of sterilization in endodontic practice include steam under pressure, chemical vapor, prolonged dry heat, intense dry heat, and glutaraldehyde solutions. Ethylene oxide gas is discussed here briefly, but it is not practical for most dental office environments.

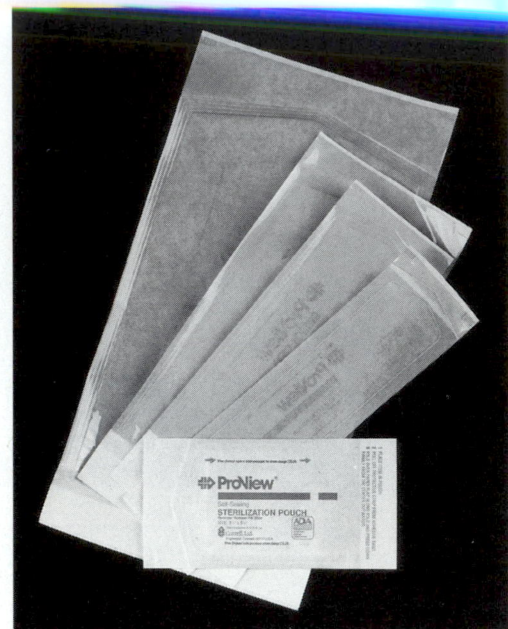

FIG. 6-29 Self-sealing sterilization pouches. (Courtesy of Cottrell, Ltd., Englewood, Colo.)

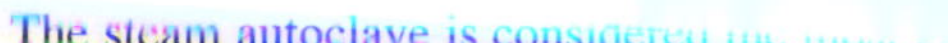

The steam autoclave is considered the most [illegible] of sterilization, except when penetration is limited or heat and moisture damage is a problem. Moist heat kills microorganisms through protein coagulation, RNA and DNA breakdown, and release of low-molecular-weight intracellular constituents.[11] The autoclave sterilizes in 15 to 40 minutes at 121° C (249.8° F), at a pressure of 15 pounds per square inch. The time required depends on the type of load placed in the autoclave and its permeability. Once the entire load has reached temperature (121° C/249.8° F), it will be rendered sterile in 15 minutes. An adequate margin of safety for load warm-up and steam penetration requires an autoclave time of at least 30 minutes. The clinician should always allow more time for load warm-up if there is any doubt. Existing chamber air is the most detrimental factor to efficient steam sterilization. Modern autoclaves use a gravity displacement method to evacuate this air, thus providing a fully saturated chamber with no cold or hot spots. Instruments and packages placed in an autoclave must be properly arranged so that the pressurized steam may circulate freely around and through the load. Since recirculation of water tends to concentrate contaminants in an autoclave, only fresh deionized (distilled) water should be used for each cycle.[15] When instruments are heated in a steam autoclave, rust and corrosion can occur. Chemical corrosion inhibitors, which are commercially available, will protect sharp instruments.[28]

A

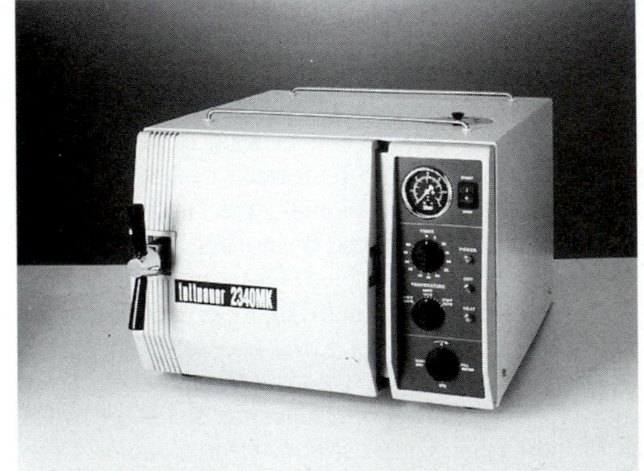

B

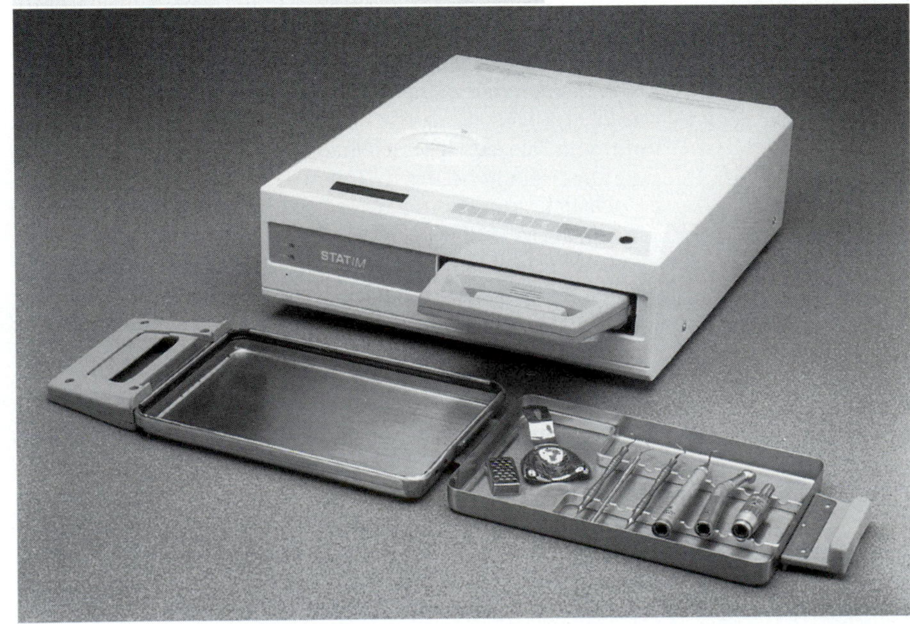

FIG. 6-30 Rapid-cycle autoclaves. **A,** Kwiklave. (Courtesy of Tuttnauer USA Co. Ltd., Ronkonkoma, N.Y.) **B,** Statim cassette autoclave. (Courtesy of SciCan, Pittsburgh, Pa.)

Several rapid-speed autoclaves have been developed primarily for use in dentistry. Some of these devices may limit the chamber load size but have a sterilization cycle much shorter than the traditional steam autoclave (Fig. 6-30).

Advantages:

1. Relatively quick turnaround time for instruments.
2. Excellent penetration of packages.
3. Does not destroy cotton or cloth products.
4. Sterilization is verifiable.

Disadvantages:

1. Materials must be air dried at completion of the cycle.
2. Because certain metals may corrode or dull, antirust pretreatment may be required Most stainless steels are resistant to autoclave damage.
3. Heat-sensitive materials can be destroyed.

Unsaturated Chemical Vapor

The 1928 patent of Dr. George Hollenback and the work of Hollenback and Harvey in the 1940s culminated in the development of an unsaturated chemical vapor sterilization system. This system, using a device similar to an autoclave, is called *Harvey Chemiclave* or chemical vapor sterilizer (Fig. 6-31). The principle of Chemiclave sterilization is that although some water is necessary to catalyze the destruction of all microorganisms in a relatively short time, water saturation is not necessary. Like autoclave sterilization, chemical vapor sterilization kills microorganisms by destroying vital protein systems. Unsaturated chemical vapor sterilization uses a solution containing specific amounts of various alcohols, acetone, ketone, and formaldehyde, and its water content is well below the 15% level that causes rust and corrosion. When the Chemiclave is heated to 132° C (270° F) and pressurized to at least 20 pounds per square inch, sterilization occurs in 20 minutes. As in the autoclave, sterilization in the Chemiclave requires careful arrangement of the load to be sterilized. The vapor must be allowed to circulate freely within the Chemiclave and to penetrate instrument wrapping material. Chemiclave solution is not recirculated; a fresh mixture of the solution is used for each cycle. The Chemiclave loses more than half its solution to ambient air as vapor. Although it has been shown that this vapor does not contain formaldehyde and is environmentally safe, the vapor has a definite characteristic odor. Adequate ventilation is a necessity when a chemical vapor sterilizer is being used. New models have a built-in filter unit that removes the odor of the residual vapors.

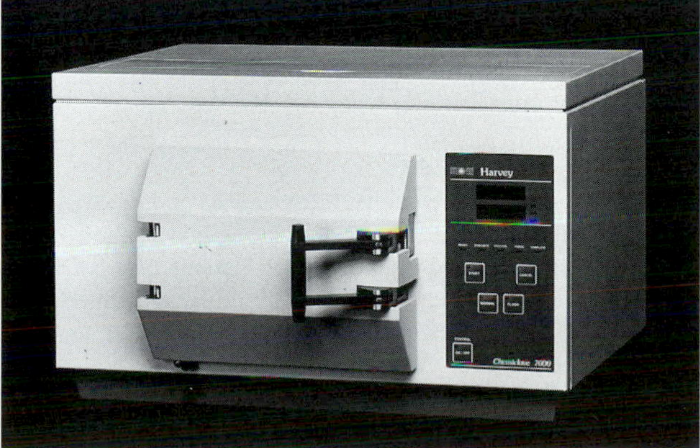

FIG. 6-31 Chemical vapor sterilizer. (Courtesy of MDT Co., Gardena, Calif.)

Advantages:

1. Not corrosive to metals.
2. Relatively quick turnaround time for instruments.
3. Load comes out dry.
4. Sterilization is verifiable.

Disadvantages:

1. Vapor odor may be offensive, requiring increased ventilation.
2. Special chemicals must be purchased and inventoried.
3. Heat-sensitive materials can be destroyed.

Prolonged Dry Heat

There are complicating factors associated with sterilization by dry heat. The time and temperature factors may vary considerably, according to heat diffusion, amount of heat available from the heating medium, amount of available moisture, and heat loss through the heating container's walls. Dry heat kills microorganisms primarily through an oxidation process. Protein coagulation also takes place, depending on the water content of the protein and the temperature of sterilization. Dry heat sterilization, like chemical vapor and autoclave sterilization, is verifiable. Dry heat is very slow to penetrate instrument loads. It sterilizes at 160° C (320° F) in 30 minutes, but instrument loads may take 30 to 90 minutes to reach that temperature.[17] To provide a margin of safety, instruments must be sterilized at 160° C (320° F) for 2 hours. An internal means of determining and calibrating temperature is an essential component of any dry heat sterilizer. If the sterilizer has multiple heating elements on different surfaces, together with an internal fan to circulate air, heat transfer becomes much more efficient. It is important that loads be positioned within the dry heat sterilizer so that they do not touch each other. Instrument cases must not be stacked one upon the other. The hot air must be allowed to circulate freely within the sterilizer.

High concentrations of mercury vapor can develop in a dry heat sterilizer that has been used to sterilize amalgam instruments. Great care must be exercised to keep scrap amalgam out of any sterilizing device. Once contaminated with mercury or amalgam, a sterilizer continues to produce mercury vapor for many cycles.[15]

Advantages:

1. Large load capability.
2. Complete corrosion protection for dry instruments.
3. Low initial cost of equipment.
4. Sterilization is verifiable.

Disadvantages:

1. Slow instrument turnaround because of poor heat exchange.
2. Sterilization cycles not as exact as in moist heat sterilization.
3. Dry heat sterilizer must be calibrated and monitored.
4. If sterilizer temperature is too high, instruments may be damaged.

Rapid Dry Heat Sterilization

Small chamber, high-speed dry heat sterilizers have been developed primarily for use in dentistry. Load limitations exist, but these devices are much faster than prolonged dry heat (Fig. 6-32).

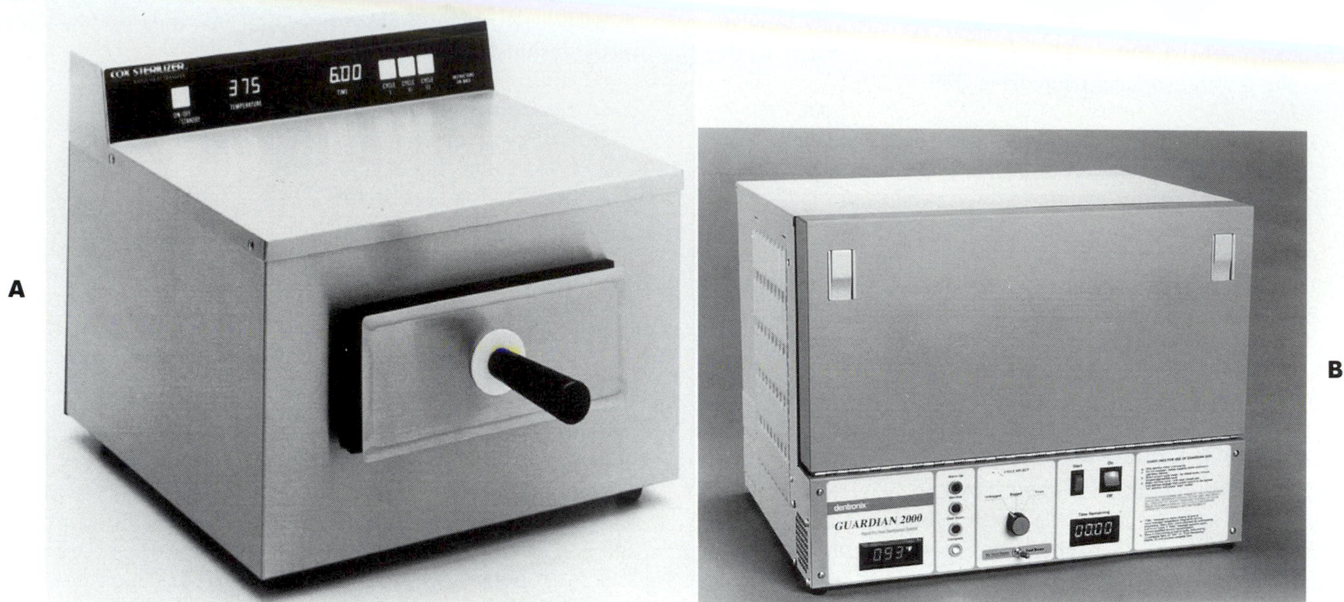

FIG. 6-32 Rapid-dry heat sterilizers. **A,** Rapid heat transfer sterilizer. (Courtesy of Cox Sterile Products, Inc., Dallas, Tex.) **B,** Rapid-dry heat sterilizer. (Courtesy of Dentronix, Pa.)

Intense Dry Heat

Chairside sterilization of endodontic files can be accomplished by using a glass bead or salt sterilizer (Fig. 6-33). This device is a metal crucible that heats a transfer medium of glass beads or salt. Clean endodontic instruments of small mass are positioned in the transfer medium and allowed to remain for a prescribed time. The transfer medium heats the endodontic instrument through heat convection and kills any adherent microorganisms. At a temperature of 220° C (428° F), contaminated endodontic instruments require 15 seconds to be sterilized. Endodontic chairside sterilizers often need extensive warm-up times; some require 3 hours to reach full operating temperature. The sterilizers often need calibration adjustment to reach a specific desired temperature. A wide range of temperature gradients may exist within the transfer medium. This process should be used *only as a backup* to the previously described methods of bulk sterilization.

Advantages:

1. Small and convenient to use.
2. Serves as an emergency backup to other methods of sterilization.

Disadvantages:

1. Only instruments of small mass can be sterilized.
2. Only a few instruments can be sterilized at one time.
3. Sterilization is nonverifiable.

Ethylene Oxide Gas

Ethylene oxide (ETO) was first used as a sterilizing agent in the late 1940s by the Army Chemical Corps. Since then, ETO has become an increasingly popular means of sterilization, especially in hospitals. The extreme penetrability of the ETO molecule, together with its effectiveness at low temperatures (70° F to 140° F), make it ideal for sterilizing heat-sensitive materials. ETO kills microorganisms by reacting chemically with nucleic acids.[11] The basic reaction is alkylation of hydroxyl groups. Sterilization requires several hours and extended aeration time for soft goods.

Even though ETO sterilization seems an ideal solution for some dental instruments, such as handpieces, it is best used in hospitals or other strictly controlled environments. ETO is thought to be potentially mutagenic and carcinogenic. Use of such a potentially dangerous substance must be weighed against its possible benefits.

Advantages:

1. Operates effectively at low temperature.
2. Gas is extremely penetrative.
3. Can be used to sterilize sensitive equipment such as dental handpieces.
4. Sterilization is verifiable.

Disadvantages:

1. Gas is potentially mutagenic and carcinogenic.
2. Requires an aeration chamber.
3. Cycle time lasts many hours (often overnight).
4. Usually only hospital based.

Handpiece Sterilization

The Food and Drug Administration (FDA) and the ADA recommend that reusable dental handpieces and related instruments be heat sterilized between each patient use.[5,10] Handpieces that cannot be heat sterilized should be retrofitted to attain heat tolerance. Handpieces that cannot be heat sterilized should not be used. Chemical disinfection is not recommended. Handpieces can be sterilized by steam, chemical vapor, and ETO. They should not be sterilized with dry heat. Strict adherence to manufacturers' maintenance recommendations is necessary to ensure handpiece longevity.

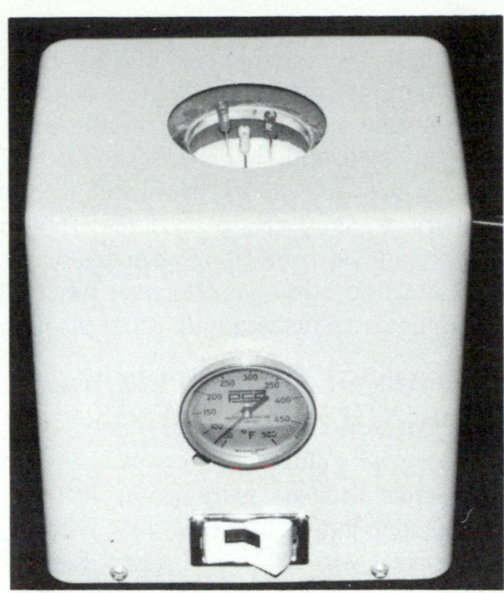

FIG. 6-33 High-temperature endodontic sterilizer. (Courtesy of Pulpdent Co. of America, Brookline, Mass.)

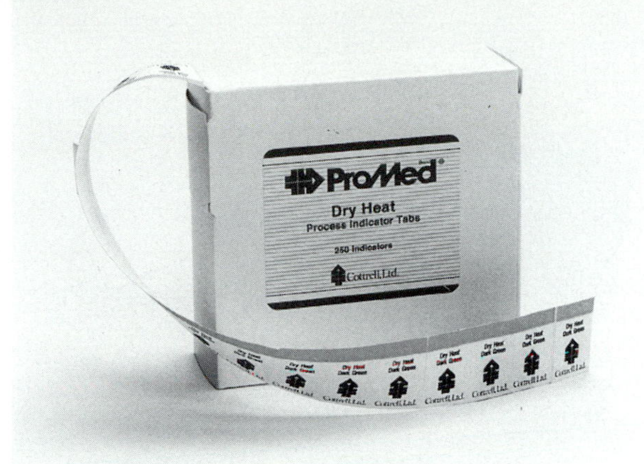

FIG. 6-34 Dry heat process indicator tabs. (Courtesy Cottrell, Ltd., Englewood, Colo.)

Glutaraldehyde Solutions

For endodontic instruments sterilization by heat is the method of choice; however, the use of glutaraldehyde preparations for the chemical sterilization of heat-sensitive equipment has become a widespread practice. Glutaraldehyde kills microorganisms by altering essential protein components.[11] The glutaraldehyde molecule has two active carbonyl groups, which react with proteins through cross-linking reactions. Many aqueous glutaraldehyde solutions are mildly acidic. In the acidic state the glutaraldehyde molecule is stable but not sporicidal. When the glutaraldehyde solution is "activated" by a suitable alkaline buffer, full antimicrobial activity occurs. Unfortunately, when the glutaraldehyde solution is rendered alkaline, a slow polymerization reaction takes place and the glutaraldehyde loses its biocidal capability with time. Because of this polymerization reaction, in normal clinical practice activated glutaraldehyde solutions usually have a shelf life of 14 days. Some new preparations have been formulated at less alkaline pH values or at an acid pH to lower the rate of polymerization and therefore extend the useful life of the solution. In these extended-life products, the addition of a surfactant maintains a biocidal activity.

The biocidal activity of glutaraldehyde may be adversely affected by substandard preparation of "activated" glutaraldehyde, contamination of the solution by protein debris, failure to change the solution at proper intervals, water dilution of residual glutaraldehyde by washed instruments that have not been dried, and the slow but continuous polymerization of the glutaraldehyde molecule. Instruments contaminated with blood or saliva must remain submerged in glutaraldehyde long enough for spore forms to be killed. Sterilization may take 6 to 10 hours, depending on what product is used.

Advantages:

1. Sterilizes heat-sensitive equipment.
2. Is relatively noncorrosive and nontoxic.

Disadvantages:

1. Requires long immersion time.
2. Has some odor, which may be objectionable, especially if solution is heated.
3. Sterilization is nonverifiable.
4. Is irritating to mucous membranes (e.g., eyes).

Monitoring Sterilization

Two methods are commonly used to monitor in-office sterilization: *process* indicators and *biologic* indicators. Both are necessary parts of infection control.

Process indicators are usually strips, tape, or paper products marked with special ink that changes color on exposure to heat, steam, chemical vapor, or ETO (Fig. 6-34). The ink changes color when the items being processed have been subjected to sterilizing conditions, but a process indicator usually does not monitor how long such conditions were present. There are specific process indicators for different methods of sterilization. The process indicator's main role in infection control is to prevent accidental use of materials that have not been circulated through the sterilizer. A color change in a process indicator does not ensure proper function of the equipment or that sterilization has been achieved.

Biologic indicators are usually preparations of nonpathogenic bacterial spores that serve as a challenge to a specific method of sterilization. If a sterilization method destroys spore forms that are highly resistant to that method, it is logical to assume that all other life forms have also been destroyed. The bacterial spores are usually attached to a paper strip within a biologically protected packet. The spore packet is placed between instrument packages or within an instrument package itself. After the sterilizer has cycled, the spore strip is cultured for a specific time. Lack of culture growth indicates sterility.

Every sterilizer load should contain at least one process indicator. A safer method is to attach a process indicator to each sterilized item. Each sterilizer should be checked weekly with a biologic indicator to ensure proper functioning of sterilizer equipment and proper loading technique.[2,3,16] Records should be maintained, especially of the biologic indicator results. Without periodic biologic monitoring, the clinician cannot be positive that sterilization failures are not occurring. Several studies have shown that sterilization failures can occur in pri-

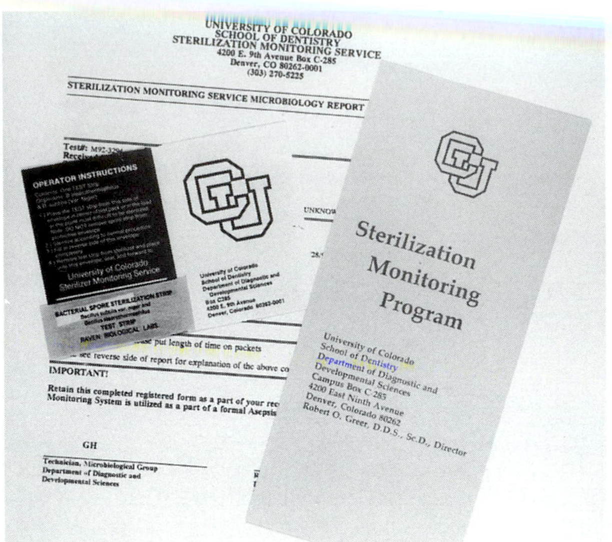

FIG. 6-35 Sterilization monitoring program: instructions, spore test strips, and microbiology report. (Courtesy of University of Colorado School of Dentistry.)

vate dental offices.[23,37] An increasing number of universities and private companies provide mail-in biologic monitoring services (Fig. 6-35).

Causes of Sterilization Failure:

1. Improper instrument preparation.
2. Improper packaging of instruments.
3. Improper loading of the sterilizer chamber.
4. Improper temperature in the sterilization chamber.
5. Improper timing of the sterilization cycle.
6. Equipment malfunction.

METHODS OF DISINFECTION

Surface disinfectants should have an Environmental Protection Agency (EPA) registration number and should be capable of killing *Mycobacterium tuberculosis* (TB).[16] These products should be used in strict accordance with the manufacturer's instructions. Disinfection, which does not kill spore forms, should be reserved for wiping large surfaces such as cart tops and dental chairs. Solutions of sodium hypochlorite and iodophors are two broad-spectrum disinfectants that are capable of killing many microorganisms. These disinfectants are superior to alcohols, phenolics, and quaternary ammonium compounds.

Sodium hypochlorite or household bleach in a dilute solution (¼ cup bleach to 1 gallon tap water) can be used to wipe down environmental surfaces. The surfaces to be disinfected should be kept moist for a minimum of 10 minutes; 30 minutes is ideal.[11,16] The free chlorine in sodium hypochlorite solutions is thought to inactivate sulfhydryl enzymes and nucleic acids and to denature proteins. Sodium hypochlorite is very biocidal against bacterial vegetative forms, viruses, and some spore forms. Unfortunately, hypochlorite is corrosive to metals, irritating to skin and eyes, and has a strong odor.

Iodophors are combinations of iodine and a solubilizing agent. When diluted with water, this combination continuously releases a small amount of free iodine. The manufacturer's recommendations for dilution must be strictly followed to achieve [illegible] by hard water, heat, and organic contamination. [illegible] lutions have a built-in color indicator that changes when the free iodine molecules have been exhausted. Areas or equipment to be disinfected with iodophors should be kept moist for 10 to 30 minutes. Iodophors are biocidal against vegetative bacteria, viruses, and some spore forms. They are less corrosive to metals and less irritating than hypochlorites. This method of disinfecting offers an effective, practical approach without the problems associated with other disinfectants.[11,16]

STERILIZATION OF GUTTA-PERCHA AND ENDODONTIC INSTRUMENTS

The sterilization of gutta-percha cones is of importance in endodontic practice because gutta-percha is the material of choice for root canal obturation. Since this material may come into intimate contact with periapical tissue during obturation, it should not be allowed to serve as a vehicle for pathogenic microorganisms. In one study, 8% of commercially available gutta-percha cones, when removed from their package, were found to be contaminated with pathogens.[35] Another study, however, showed that gutta-percha cones were sterile when removed from the manufacturer's package. This study also concluded that storing gutta-percha cones in paraformaldehyde-containing jars was an ineffective sterilizing method when gutta-percha cones were contaminated with bacterial endospores.[25] Immersing gutta-percha cones in 5.25% sodium hypochlorite (full-strength household bleach) for 1 minute is very effective in killing vegetative microorganisms and spore forms.[38]

EFFECT OF REPEATED STERILIZATION ON INSTRUMENTS

The effect of repeated sterilization on the physical characteristics of endodontic files has been studied.[27,36] Repeated sterilization of stainless steel endodontic files, using any heat method described in this chapter, will not cause corrosion, weakness, or an increased rate of rotational failure.

REFERENCES

1. Al-Khatib ZZ, et al: The antimicrobial effect of various endodontic sealers, Oral Surg 70:784, 1990.
2. American Dental Association Council on Dental Materials, Instruments and Equipment, and Dental Therapeutics: Biological indicators for verifying sterilization, J Am Dent Assoc 117:653, 1988.
3. American Dental Association Council on Dental Materials, Instruments and Equipment: Sterilization required for infection control, J Am Dent Assoc 122:80, 1991.
4. American Dental Association Council on Dental Materials, Instruments and Equipment, Dental Practice, and Dental Therapeutics: Infection control recommendations for the dental office and the dental laboratory, J Am Dent Assoc 123:1, 1992.
5. American Dental Association: Five states move quickly on handpiece sterilization, J Am Dent Assoc 123:119, 1992.
6. American Dental Association Division of Scientific Affairs: Facts about AIDS for the dental team, J Am Dent Assoc 123(Suppl 7):1, 1992.
7. Archer R, et al: An in vivo evaluation of the efficacy of ultrasound after step-back preparation in mandibular molars, J Endod 18:549, 1992.
8. Backman CA, Oswald RJ, and Pitts DL: A radiographic comparison of two root canal instrumentation techniques, J Endod 18:19, 1992.
9. Becking AG: Complications in the use of sodium hypochlorite during endodontic treatment, Oral Surg 71:346, 1991.

10. Benson J: Dental handpiece sterilization, FDA Lett 9/28/92.
11. Block S, et al: Disinfection, sterilization and preservation, ed 4, Philadelphia, 1991, Lea & Febiger.
12. Budd CS, Weller RN, and Kulild JC: A comparison of thermoplasticized injectable gutta-percha obturation techniques, J Endod 17:260, 1991.
13. Centers for Disease Control: Recommended infection-control practices for dentistry, MMWR 35:238, 1986.
14. Centers for Disease Control: Protection against viral hepatitis, MMWR 39:1, 1990.
15. Cooley RL, Stilley J, and Lubow RM: Mercury vapor produced during sterilization of amalgam-contaminated instruments, J Prosthet Dent 53:304, 1985.
16. Cottone J, Terezhalmy G, and Molinari J: Practical infection control in dentistry, Philadelphia, 1991, Lea & Febiger.
17. Crawford J: Clinical asepsis in dentistry, Dallas, Tex, 1987, R.A. Kolstad.
18. Department of Labor, Occupational Safety and Health Administration: 29 CRF Part 1910.1030, Occupational exposure to bloodborne pathogens, final rule, Fed Reg 56(235):64004-64182, 1991.
19. Deveau E, et al: Bacterial microleakage of Cavit, IRM and TERM, Oral Surg 74:634, 1992.
20. Eames WB, Bryington SQ, and Neal SB: A comparison of eight ultrasonic cleaners, Gen Dent 30:242, 1985.
21. Fouad AF, et al: A clinical evaluation of five electronic root canal measuring instruments, J Endod 16:446, 1990.
22. Gilles JA, and del Rio CE: A comparison of the Canal Master endodontic instrument and K-type files for enlargement of curved root canals, J Endod 16:561, 1990.
23. Hastreiter R, et al: Effectiveness of dental office instrument sterilization procedures, J Am Dent Assoc 122:51, 1991.
24. Hata G, et al: Sealing ability of Thermafil with and without sealer, J Endod 18:322, 1992.
25. Higgins JR, Newton CW, and Palenik CJ: The use of paraformaldehyde powder for the sterile storage of gutta-percha cones, J Endod 12:242, 1988.
26. Hudson DA, Remeikis NA, and Van Cura JE: Instrumentation of curved root canals: a comparison study, J Endod 18:448, 1992.
27. Iverson GW, von Fraunhofer JA, and Herrmann JW: The effects of various sterilization methods on the torsional strength of endodontic files, J Endod 11:266, 1985.
28. Johnson GK, et al: Effect of four anticorrosive dips on the cutting efficiency of dental carbide burs, J Am Dent Assoc 114:648, 1987.
29. Kaufman AY, and Senia K: Conservative treatment of root perforations using apex locator and thermatic compactor. J Endod 15:267, 1989.
30. Lares C, and El Deeb ME: The sealing ability of the Thermafil obturation technique. J Endod 16:474, 1990.
31. Leseberg DA, and Montgomery S: The effects of Canal Master, Flex-R and K-Flex instrumentation on root canal configuration, J Endod 17:59, 1991.
32. Luebke NH, and Brantley WA: Torsional and metallurgical properties of rotary endodontic instruments. II. Stainless steel Gates-Glidden drills, J Endod 17:319, 1991.
33. Mandel E, Machtou P, and Friedman S: Scanning electron microscope observation of canal cleanliness, J Endod 16:279, 1990.
34. Miller C: Cleaning, sterilization and disinfection: basics of microbial killing for infection control, J Am Dent Assoc 124:48-56, 1993.
35. Montgomery S: Chemical decontamination of gutta-percha cones with polyvinyl pyrrolidone-iodine, Oral Surg 31:258, 1971.
36. Morrison SW, Newton CW, and Brown CE: The effects of steam sterilization and usage on cutting efficiency of endodontic instruments, J Endod 15:427, 1989.
37. Palenik MS, et al: A survey of sterilization practices in selected endodontic offices, J Endod 12:206, 1988.
38. Senia SE, et al: Rapid sterilization of gutta-percha cones with 5.25% sodium hypochlorite, J Endod 1:136, 1975.
39. Seto BG, Nicholls JI, and Harrington GW: Torsional properties of twisted and machined endodontic files, J Endod 16:355, 1990.
40. Sleder FS, Ludlow MO, and Bohacek JR: Long-term sealing ability of a calcium hydroxide sealer, J Endod 17:541, 1991.
41. Stein TJ, and Corcoran JF: Nonionizing method of locating the apical constriction in root canals, Oral Surg 71:96, 1991.
42. Stenman E, and Spangberg LSW: Machining efficiency of Flex-R, K-Flex, Trio-Cut and S files, J Endod 16:575, 1990.
43. Turner JE, et al: Microleakage of temporary endodontic restorations in teeth restored with amalgam, J Endod 16:1, 1990.

Self-assessment questions

1. Infection control procedures
   a. that protect against monilial infection protect against HBV.
   b. that protect against HBV should protect against HIV.
   c. that protect against HIV should protect against HBV.
   d. are controlled with the use of the rubber dam.
2. Color change in a process indicator strip indicates
   a. verification of sterilization.
   b. verification of completed sterilization cycle.
   c. a change in pH.
   d. a need to reprocess.
3. The organism least resistant to thermal inactivation is
   a. bacterial spores.
   b. virus.
   c. *Streptococcus mutans*.
   d. spirochete.
4. Rapid-speed autoclaves
   a. require at least 30 minutes for sterilization.
   b. require no antirust pretreatment.
   c. destroy cloth products.
   d. produce verifiable sterilization.
5. Chemiclave
   a. corrodes instruments.
   b. solution can be recirculated.
   c. sterilization is verifiable.
   d. does not affect heat-sensitive materials.
6. Dry heat
   a. provides corrosion protection for dry instruments.
   b. requires only 30 minutes.
   c. has no mercury vapor effect.
   d. does not destroy heat-sensitive materials.
7. Chairside dry heat glass bead or salt sterilization
   a. is verifiable.
   b. serves as an emergency backup.
   c. requires a brief time to warm up.
   d. can sterilize a large number of instruments.
8. Glutaraldehyde
   a. requires a short period of sterilization.
   b. is relatively noncorrosive.
   c. results in verifiable sterilization.
   d. is nonirritating and nontoxic.
9. The sterilizer
   a. is effective if the process indicator changes color.
   b. should be checked weekly with a biologic indicator.
   c. should be checked daily with a biologic indicator.
   d. should be checked for sterilization of bacteria rather than spores.
10. Gutta-percha is best sterilized in
    a. an autoclave.
    b. dry heat.
    c. 5.5% sodium hypochlorite for 1 minute.
    d. paraformaldehyde for 1 minute.

Chapter 7

Tooth Morphology and Access Openings

Richard C. Burns
L. Stephen Buchanan

The hard tissue repository of the dental pulp takes on many configurations that must be understood before treatment starts

RELATIONSHIP OF TOOTH MORPHOLOGY AND ACCESS CAVITY PREPARATION

Endodontics textbooks have tended to concentrate on the preparation of access cavities in ideal anatomic crowns in teeth with ideal root canals. The thrust of this chapter is to emphasize the practical world of canal morphology with the proved complexities that exist.

From the early work of Hess[11] to the recent studies demonstrating anatomic complexities of the root canal system, it has been established that the root with a graceful tapering canal and a single apical foramen is the exception rather than the rule. Investigators have shown multiple foramina, fins, deltas, loops, furcation accessory canals, etc., in most teeth. The student and the clinician must approach the tooth to be treated assuming that these "aberrations" occur so often that they must be considered normal anatomy.

Access preparations can be divided into the visual and the assumed. The coronal anatomy, in whatever state it exists, is the first indication of the assumed and is the first key to the root position and root canal system.

A thorough investigation of the sulcus, coronal clefts, restorations, tooth angulation, cusp position, occlusion, and contacts is mandatory before access is begun. Palpation of buccal or labial soft tissue will help determine root position (see Fig. 7-9, *E*). Some clinicians advocate access cavity preparation prior to rubber dam placement as a visual aid to prevent disorientation.

Before entry the clinician must visualize the expected location of the coronal pulp chamber and canal orifice position. Unnecessary tooth removal may compromise the final restoration. It is important at this time to call upon one's knowledge of tooth morphology.

It is humbling to be aware of the complexity of the spaces we are expected to clean and fill. We can take comfort, however, in knowing that our modern methods of treating root canals result in a very high rate of success.

Kasahara and associates[12] studied transparent specimens of 510 extracted maxillary central incisors for anatomic detail. More than 60% of the specimens showed accessory canals that were impossible to clean mechanically. Most lateral branches were small; 80% were the size of a no. 10 reamer or smaller, and only 3% were thicker than a no. 40 reamer. Apical foramina located away from the apex were observed in 45% of the teeth.

COMPLEX ANATOMY

A sagittal section of the mandibular first premolar (Fig. 7-1) reveals one of the truly difficult situations facing the clinician. Instead of distinct individual canals, this tooth presents a fine ribbon-shaped canal system that is almost impossible to clean and shape thoroughly, much less to obturate. The section shown in Figure 7-2 was located 8 mm apical to the cementum-enamel junction. The root was 14 mm long.[5] This example of anatomic complexity illustrates that internal morphology is far from predictable.

The teeth shown in Figure 7-3 may be the longest on record. The maxillary cuspid measures 41 mm (Fig. 7-3, *A*) from incisal to apex. It was one of six maxillary teeth that were re-

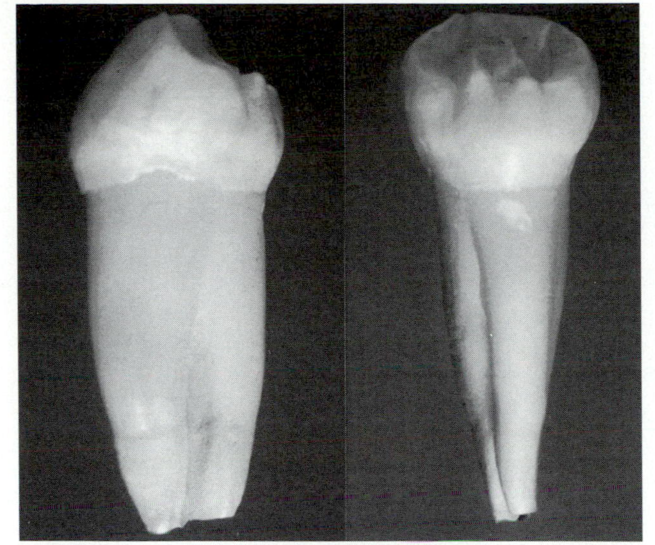

FIG. 7-1 Mandibular first premolar. **A,** Distal view. **B,** Lingual view.

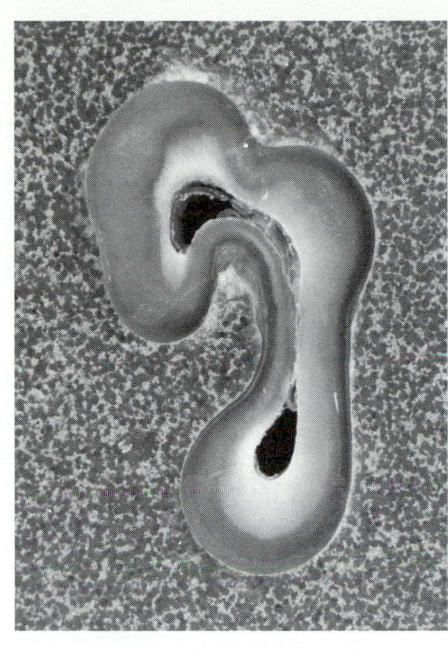

FIG. 7-2 Root section of the premolar shown in Fig. 7-1.

FIG. 7-3 A, Maxillary cuspid measures 41 mm from incisal to apex. **B,** Note that the central incisor is 30 mm long. (From Booth JM: The longest tooth? Aust Endod News 13(3), 1988.)

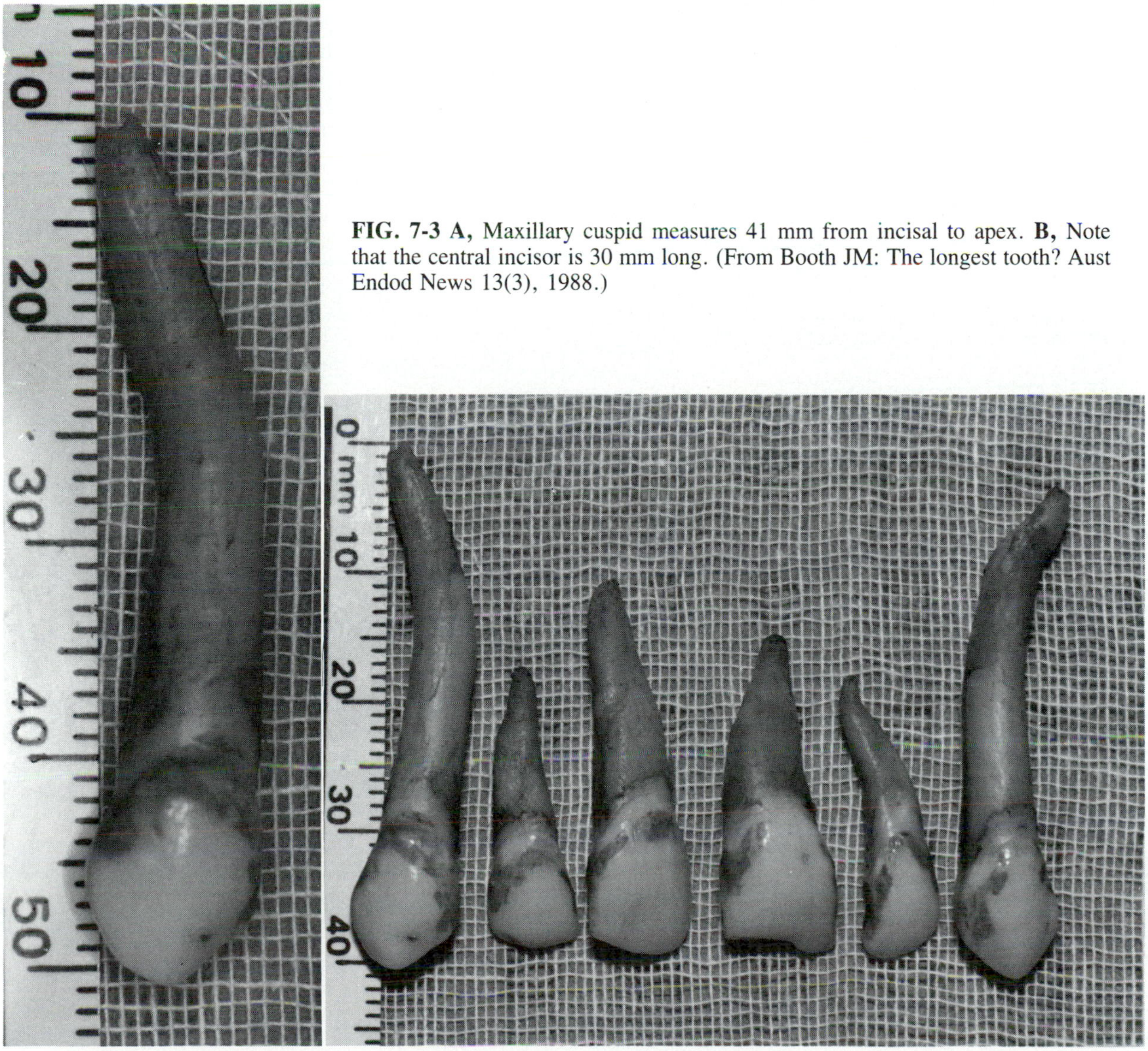

TABLE 7-1. Tooth length determination

Maxillary	Length (mm)	Mandibular	Length (mm)
Central incisor		Central incisor	
Average	22.5	Average	20.7
Greatest	27.0	Greatest	24.0
Least	18.0	Least	16.0
Lateral incisor		Lateral incisor	
Average	22.0	Average	21.1
Greatest	26.0	Greatest	27.0
Least	17.0	Least	18.0
Canine		Canine	
Average	26.5	Average	25.6
Greatest	32.0	Greatest	32.5
Least	20.0	Least	18.0
First premolar		First premolar	
Average	20.6	Average	21.6
Greatest	22.5	Greatest	26.0
Least	17.0	Least	18.0
Second premolar		Second premolar	
Average	21.5	Average	22.3
Greatest	27.0	Greatest	26.0
Least	16.0	Least	18.0
First molar		First molar	
Average	20.8	Average	21.0
Greatest	24.0	Greatest	24.0
Least	17.0	Least	18.0
Second molar		Second molar	
Average	20.0	Average	19.8
Greatest	24.0	Greatest	22.0
Least	16.0	Least	18.0
Third molar		Third molar	
Average	17.1	Average	18.5
Greatest	22.0	Greatest	20.0
Least	14.0	Least	16.0

Modified from Black GV: Descriptive anatomy of the human teeth, ed 4, Philadelphia, 1897, SS White Dental Manufacturing Co.

moved prior to placement of immediate dentures. The central incisor is 30 mm long (Fig. 7-3, *B*). These teeth were discovered by Dr. Gary Wilkie of Korumburra, Victoria, Australia. The patient is a 31-year-old female, 5 feet 2 inches tall, from the Netherlands.[2] The woman in 1993 received her second full denture. The reason for removing these teeth, which were situated in normal bone, was a common decision arrived at by the patient and her dentist.[23] Average tooth lengths are shown in Table 7-1.

ENTERING THE PULP CHAMBER

Initial entry is best made through enamel or restorative materials with a fissure bur or inverted cone bur (Fig. 7-4, *A*). A proper outline form, as shown on pages 135 to 167, is prepared well into the dentin. If doubt exists as to the location of the pulp chamber and canal orifice(s), the outline form may be made conservatively until the chamber is unroofed.

The next step is done with a no. 4 or 6 surgical-length round bur. When the bur has dropped through the roof of the chamber (Fig. 7-4, *B*), no further cutting in an apical direction should be attempted. All action must be in a "sweeping-out motion" until clear access is gained to the canal orifice(s) with no impairment of future instrumentation (Fig. 7-4, *C*).

Any pulp stones, loose calcifications, restorative materials, and/or debris must be removed at this time.

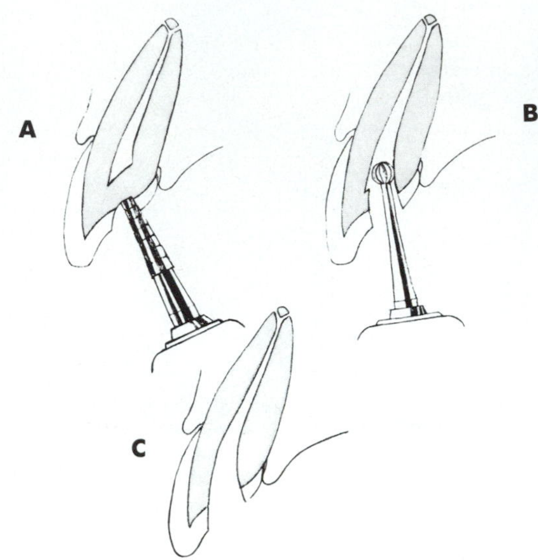

FIG. 7-4 A, Fissure bur in a high-speed handpiece. **B,** After "dropping through" the roof of the chamber, the clinician switches to a long-shanked no. 2 or 4 round bur. With a "sweeping outward motion" the clinician cleans and shapes the wall of the upper chamber. **C,** Completed shaping of the upper pulp chamber.

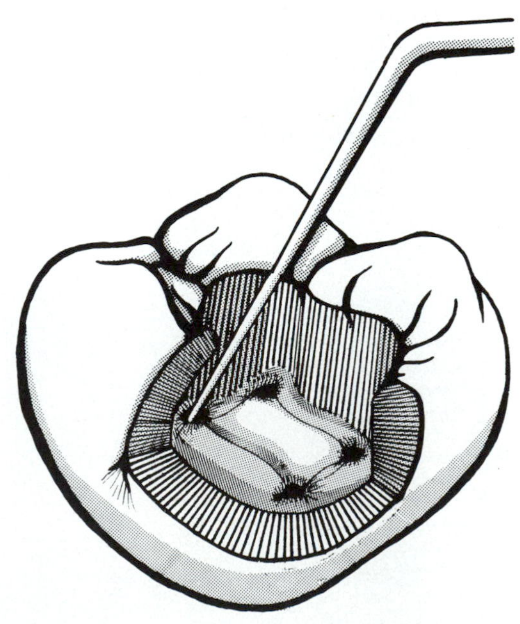

FIG. 7-5 Indispensable in endodontic treatment, the endodontic pathfinder serves as an explorer to locate orifices, as an indicator of canal angulation, and often as a chipping tool to remove calcification.

USE OF THE PATHFINDER FOR LOCATING ORIFICES

After the pulp chamber is opened, the canal orifices are located with the endodontic pathfinder (Fig. 7-5). This instrument is to the endodontist what a probe is to the periodontist. Reaching, feeling, often digging at the hard tissue, it is the extension of the clinician's fingers. Natural anatomy dictates the usual places for orifices; but restorations, dentinal protrusions, and dystrophic calcifications can alter the actual configuration encountered. While probing the chamber floor, the pathfinder often penetrates or dislodges calcific deposits blocking an orifice.

Positioning the instrument in the orifice enables the clinician to check the shaft for clearance of the orifice walls. Additionally, the pathfinder is used to determine the angle at which the canals depart the main chamber.

The endodontic pathfinder is preferred over the rotating bur as the instrument for locating canal orifices. The double-ended design offers two angles of approach.

High-speed Handpieces

True-running high-rpm turbine handpieces are mandatory for gaining access into the endodontically involved tooth. The addition of fiberoptics improves the visibility during probing of the deeper reaches of the pulp chambers. The placement of a rubber dam clamp containing fiberoptic lights gives additional illumination.

ACCESS CAVITY PREPARATION IN INCISORS (Fig. 7-6)

Incisors, particularly mandibular incisors, are often weakened coronally by excessive removal of tooth structure. The mesiodistal width of the pulp chamber is often narrower than the bur used to make the initial access. Because of the ease of visibility and clear definition of external anatomy, lateral perforations (toward the cervical or root surface) are rare.

Labial perforations (cervical or root surface), however, are common, especially with calcifications. To prevent this occurrence, the clinician must consider the relationship between the incisal edge and the location of the pulp chamber. If the incisal edge is intact, it is almost impossible to perforate *lingually*. Therefore, in calcified cases when the bur does not drop easily into the chamber, the clinician should change to smaller-diameter burs and, keeping the long axis in mind, direct the cutting action in apical-lingual version. If the canal orifice still does not materialize after cutting in an apical direction, the clinician should remove the bur, place it in the access cavity, and expose a radiograph; the resultant film will reveal the depth of cutting and the angulation of cutting from mesial to distal.

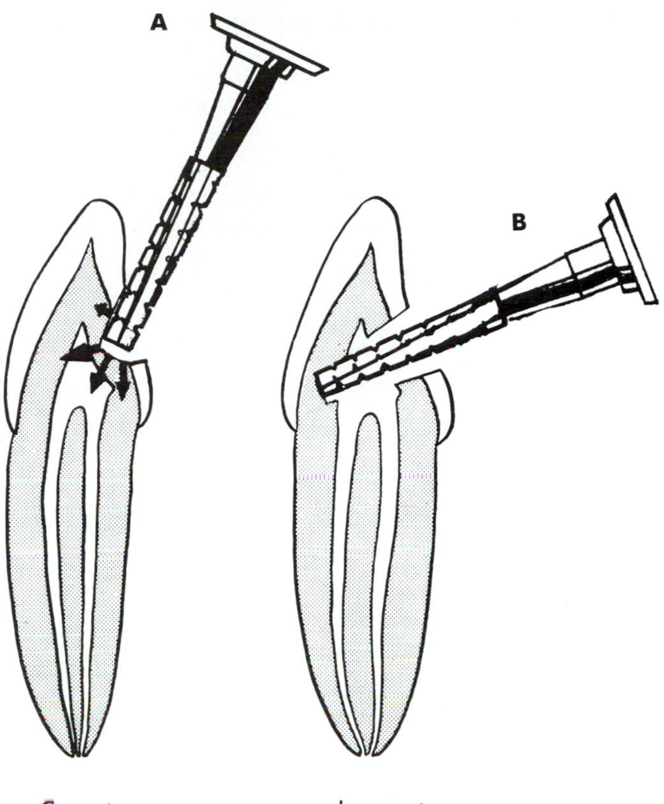

FIG. 7-6 A, Sweeping motion in a slightly downward lingual-to-labial direction *(arrows),* until the chamber is engaged, to obtain the best access to the lingual canal. **B,** Incorrect approach: directing the end-cutting bur in a straight lingual-to-labial direction. Mutilation of tooth structure and perforation will be the result in this small and narrow incisor.

ACCESS THROUGH FULL VENEER CROWNS

Properly made crowns are constructed with the occlusal relationship of the opposing tooth as a primary consideration. A cast crown may be made in any shape, diameter, height, or angle; this cast crown alteration can destroy the visual relationship to the true long axis. Careful study of the preoperative radiograph will identify most of these situations.

Achieving access through crowns should be done with coolants, even when the rubber dam is used. Friction-generated heat can damage adjacent soft tissue, including the periodontal ligament; and with an anesthetized or nonvital tooth the patient will not be aware of pain. Once penetration of the metal is accomplished, the clinician can change to a sharp round bur and move toward the central pulp chamber. Metal filings and debris from the access cavity should be removed frequently because small slivers can cause large obstructions in the fine canal system.

When sufficient access has been gained, the clinician should search margins and internal spaces for caries and leaks and the pulpal floor for signs of fracture or perforation. Occasionally caries can be removed through the occlusal access cavity and the tooth can be properly restored. The interior of a crown can be a surprise package, containing everything from total caries to intact dentin (as seen in periodontally induced pulp death).

METHODS OF DETERMINING ANATOMIC DETAIL

Beyond the visual perception is the often complex root canal system. The clinician must use every available means to determine the anatomic configuration before commencing instrumentation. Figure 7-7 illustrates several techniques and methods:

1. When the radiograph shows that the canal suddenly stops in the radicular region *(A_1)*, the assumption is that it has bifurcated (or trifurcated) into much finer diameters. To confirm this division, a second radiograph is exposed from a mesial angulation of 10 to 30 degrees. The resultant film will show either more roots or multiple ver-

tical lines indicating the peripheries of additional root surfaces (A_2).

2. A radiograph also reveals many clues to anatomic "aberrations": lateral radiolucencies indicating the presence of lateral or accessory canals (B_1); an abrupt ending of a large canal signifying a bifurcation (B_1 and B_2); a knoblike image indicating an apex that curves toward or away from the beam of the x-ray machine (B_3); multiple vertical lines, as shown in this curved mesial root (B_4), indicating the possibility of a thin root, which may be hourglass shaped in cross section and susceptible to perforation.
3. The endodontic pathfinder inserted into the orifice openings will reveal the direction that the canals take in leaving the main chamber (*C*).
4. Digital perception with a hand instrument can identify

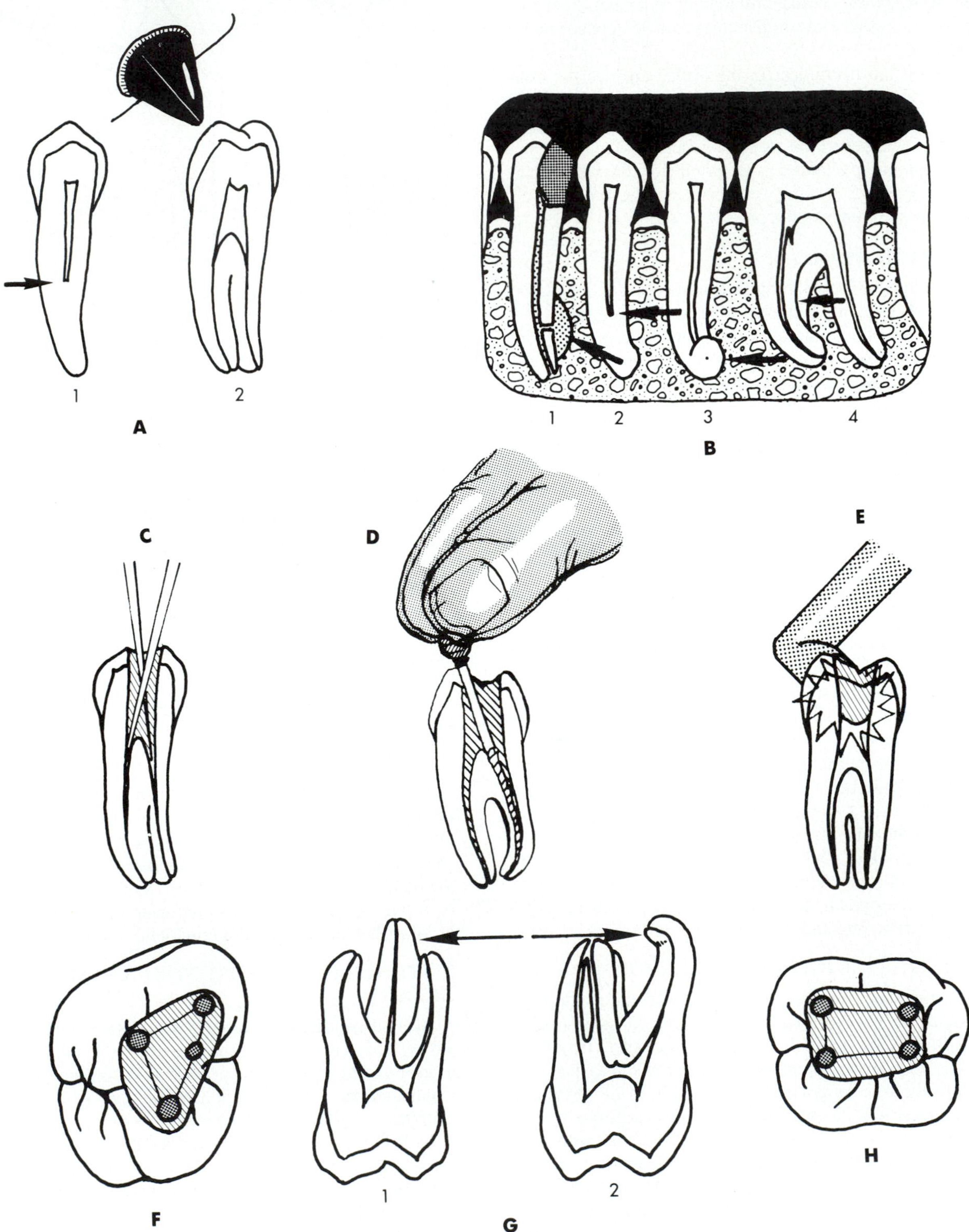

FIG. 7-7 Techniques for determining anatomic configuration.

curvatures, obstruction, root division, and additional canal orifices *(D)*.

5. Fiberoptic illumination can reveal calcifications, orifice location, and fractures *(E)*.
6. Knowledge of root canal anatomy will prompt the clinician always to search for additional canal orifices where they are known to occur—for instance, the usual location of a fourth canal in the maxillary first permanent molar between the mesiobuccal and palatal canals along the developmental groove *(F)*.
7. Further knowledge of root formation can save the clinician difficulties with instrumentation—for example, in what appears radiographically to be a normal palatal root of a maxillary first permanent molar (G_1) but is actually a root with a sharp apical curvature toward the buccal (G_2).
8. Ethnic characteristics as well as other physical differences can be manifested in tooth morphology, for example, the common occurrence of four canals in Asian peoples *(H)*.

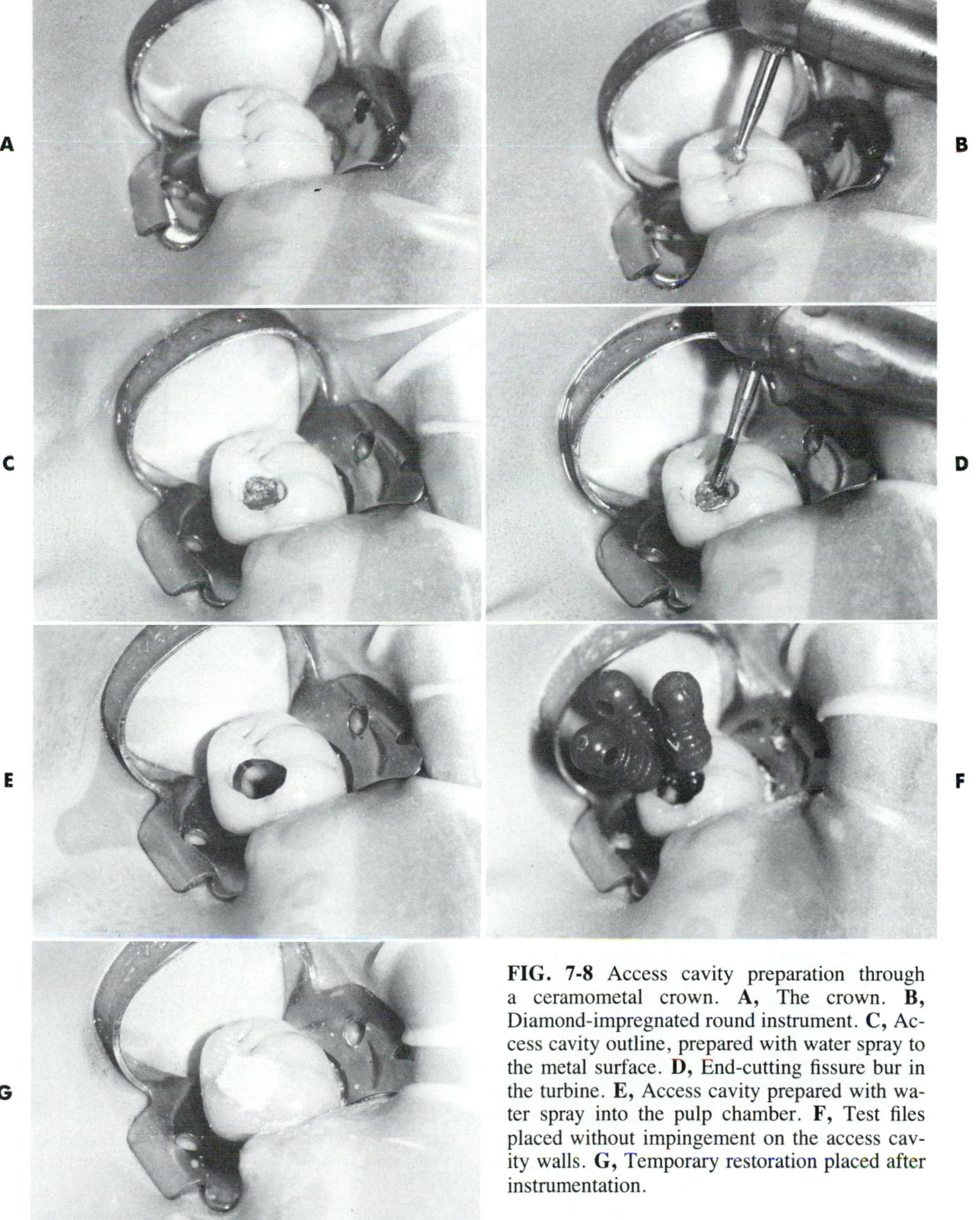

FIG. 7-8 Access cavity preparation through a ceramometal crown. **A,** The crown. **B,** Diamond-impregnated round instrument. **C,** Access cavity outline, prepared with water spray to the metal surface. **D,** End-cutting fissure bur in the turbine. **E,** Access cavity prepared with water spray into the pulp chamber. **F,** Test files placed without impingement on the access cavity walls. **G,** Temporary restoration placed after instrumentation.

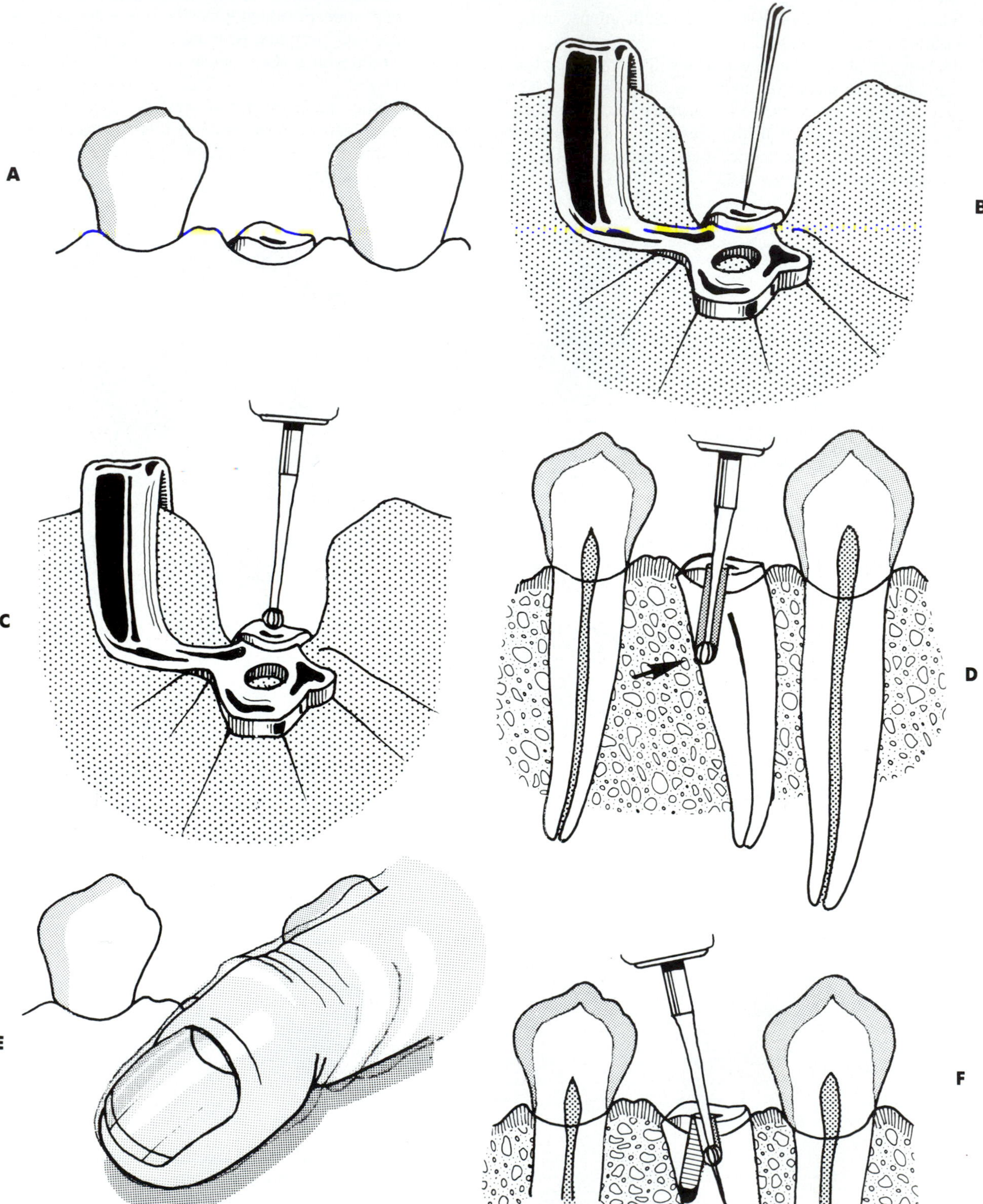

FIG. 7-9 Errors in access cavity when the anatomic crown is missing. **A,** Mandibular first premolar with the crown missing. **B,** An endodontic explorer fails to penetrate the calcified pulp chamber. **C,** Long-shank round bur directed in the assumed long axis of the root. **D,** Perforation of the root wall *(arrow)* because of the clinician's failure to consider root angulation. **E,** Palpation of the buccal root anatomy to determine root angulation. **F,** Correct bur angulation following repair of the perforation.

INTRODUCTION TO PLATES I TO XVI

The anatomy presented in the following plates is a combination of examples of human teeth, illustrations representing ideal morphology,* and radiographs of completed endodontic procedures demonstrating unusual pulpal configuration.

Experienced clinicians will note that the access openings herein described are slightly larger than those described in other textbooks. This size represents the composite opinion of several leading endodontists in the United States.

The average time of eruption and average age of calcification are from *Anatomy of Orofacial Structures* by Brand and Isselhard.[4]

*Contained in this series are many classic illustrations from Zeisz and Nuckolls. These extremely accurate and excellent drawings are reproductions of the work of these authors, aided by the artistic talents of Mr. Walter B. Schwarz.

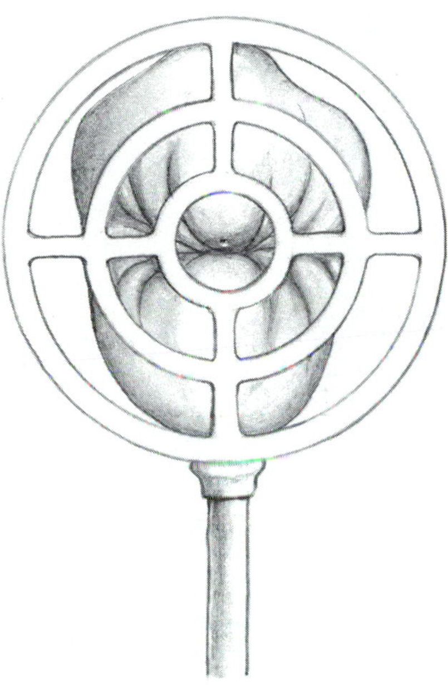

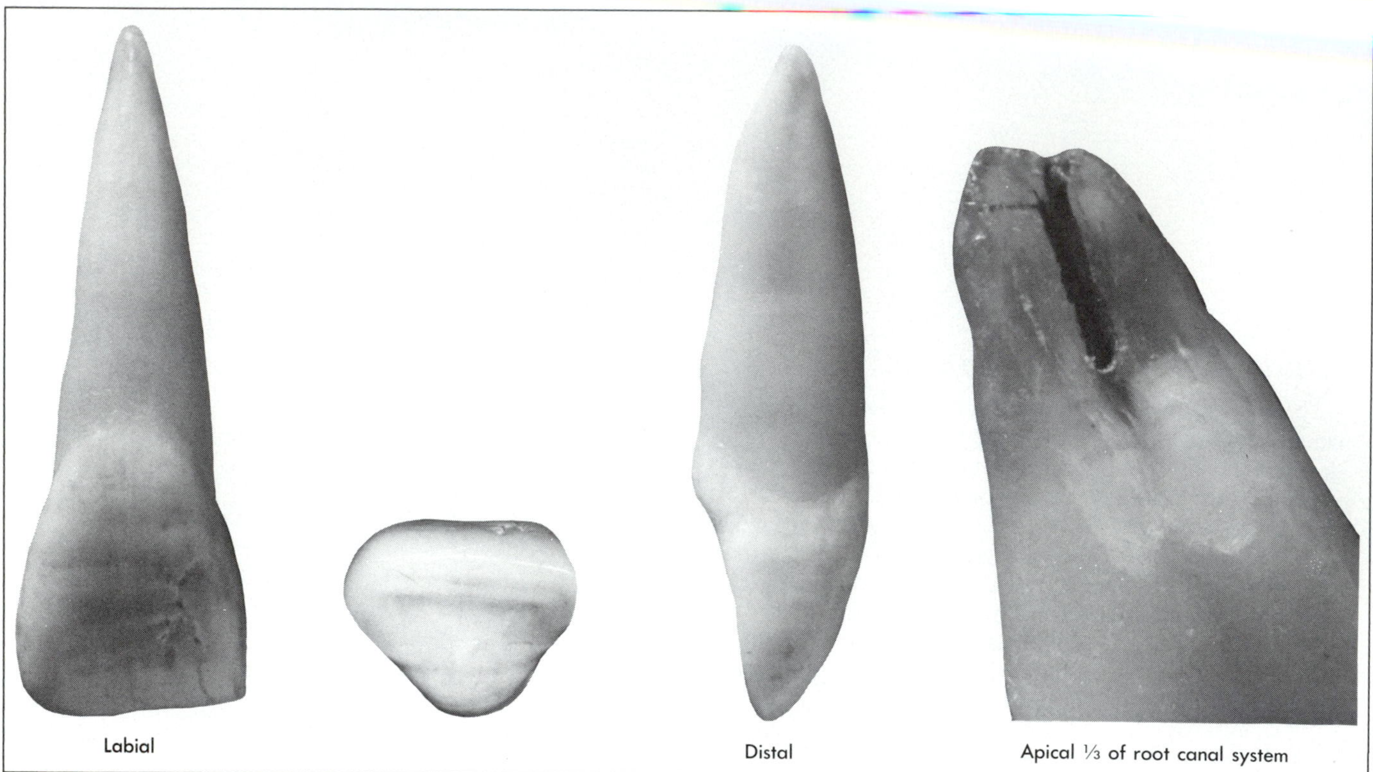

Average time of eruption: 7 to 8 years
Average age of calcification: 10 years
Average length: 22.5 mm

Somewhat rectangular from the labial aspect and shovel-shaped from the proximal, the crown of the maxillary central is more than adequate for endodontic access and is positioned ideally for direct mirror visualization. This tooth is especially suitable for a first clinical experience because more than a third of its canal is directly visible. Visualization of the canal proper may be enhanced with fiberoptic illumination.

The first entry point, with the end-cutting fissure bur, is made just above the cingulum (Fig. 7-4, *A*). The direction should be in the long axis of the root. A roughly triangular opening is made in anticipation of the final shape of the access cavity. Often, penetration of the shallow pulp chamber occurs during initial entry. When the sensation of "dropping through the roof" of the pulp chamber has been felt, the long-shanked no. 4 or 6 round bur replaces the fissure bur (Fig. 7-4, *B*).

The "belly" of the round bur is utilized to sweep out toward the incisal; one must be certain to expose the entire chamber completely (Fig. 7-4, *C*). It may be necessary to return to the fissure bur to extend and refine the final shape of the access cavity. All caries, grossly discolored dentin, and pulp calcifications are removed at this time. Leaking restorations or proximal caries should be removed and an adequate temporary restoration placed.

Conical and rapidly tapering toward the apex, the root morphology is quite distinctive. Cross-sectionally the radicular canal is slightly triangular at the cervical aspect, gradually becoming round as it approaches the apical foramen.

Multiple canals are rare, but accessory and lateral canals are common. Kasahara and others[12] studied 510 maxillary central incisors to determine thickness and curvature of the root canal, condition of any accessory canals, and location of the apical foramen. Data revealed that the thickness and curvature of canals showed adequate preparation at approximately a size 60 instrument at the apical constriction, that over 60% of the specimens showed accessory canals, and that the apical foramen was located apart from the apex in 45% of the teeth.

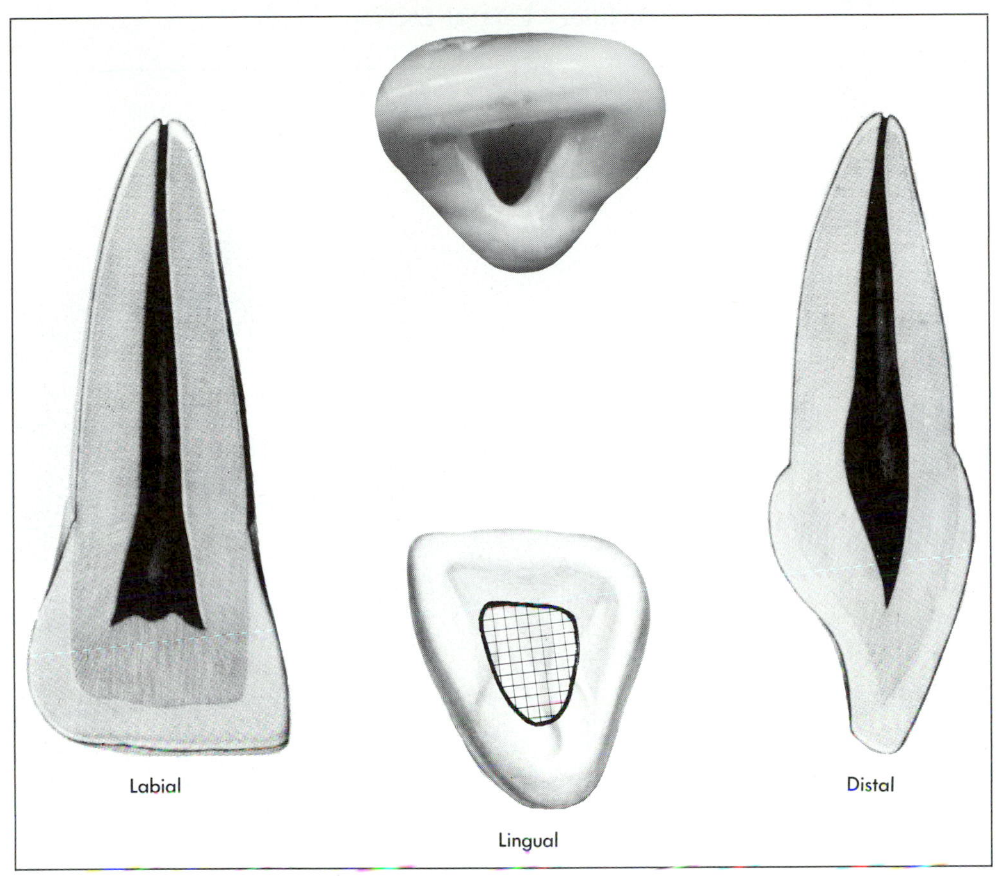

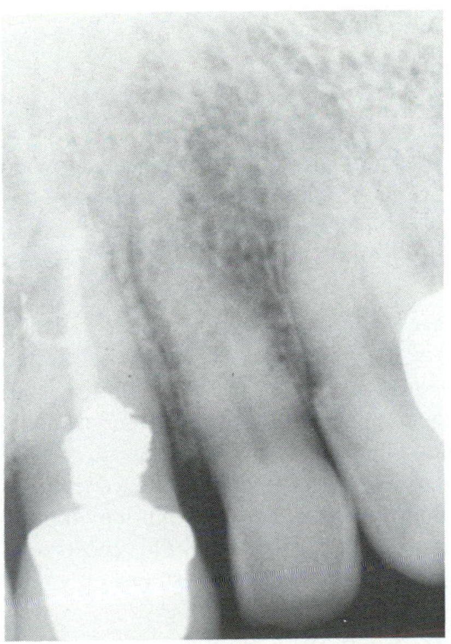

PLATE 7-I-5. Curved accessory canal with straight lateral canal intersecting.

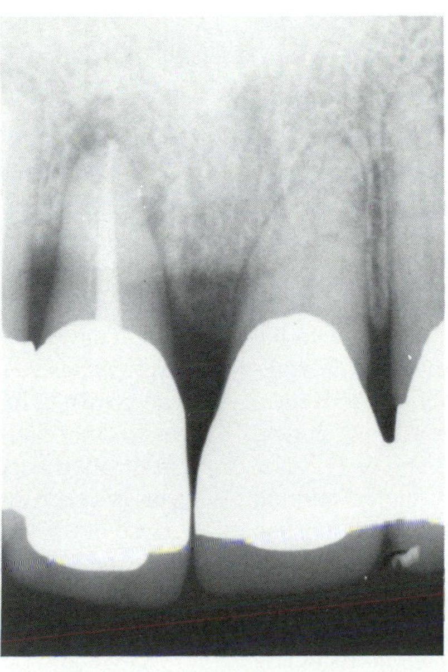

PLATE 7-I-6. Parallel accessory canal to main canal with simple lateral canal.

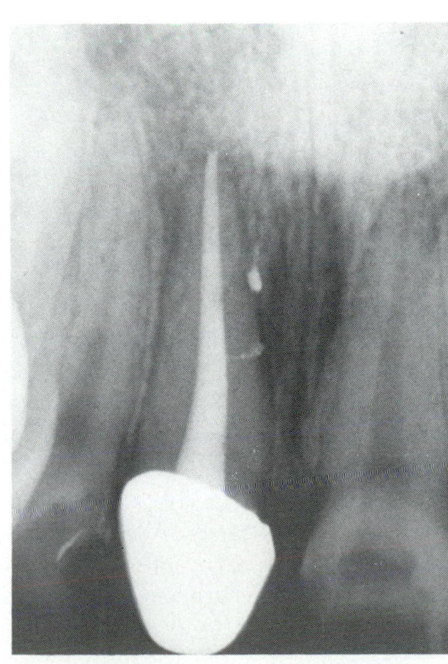

PLATE 7-I-7. Double lateral canals.

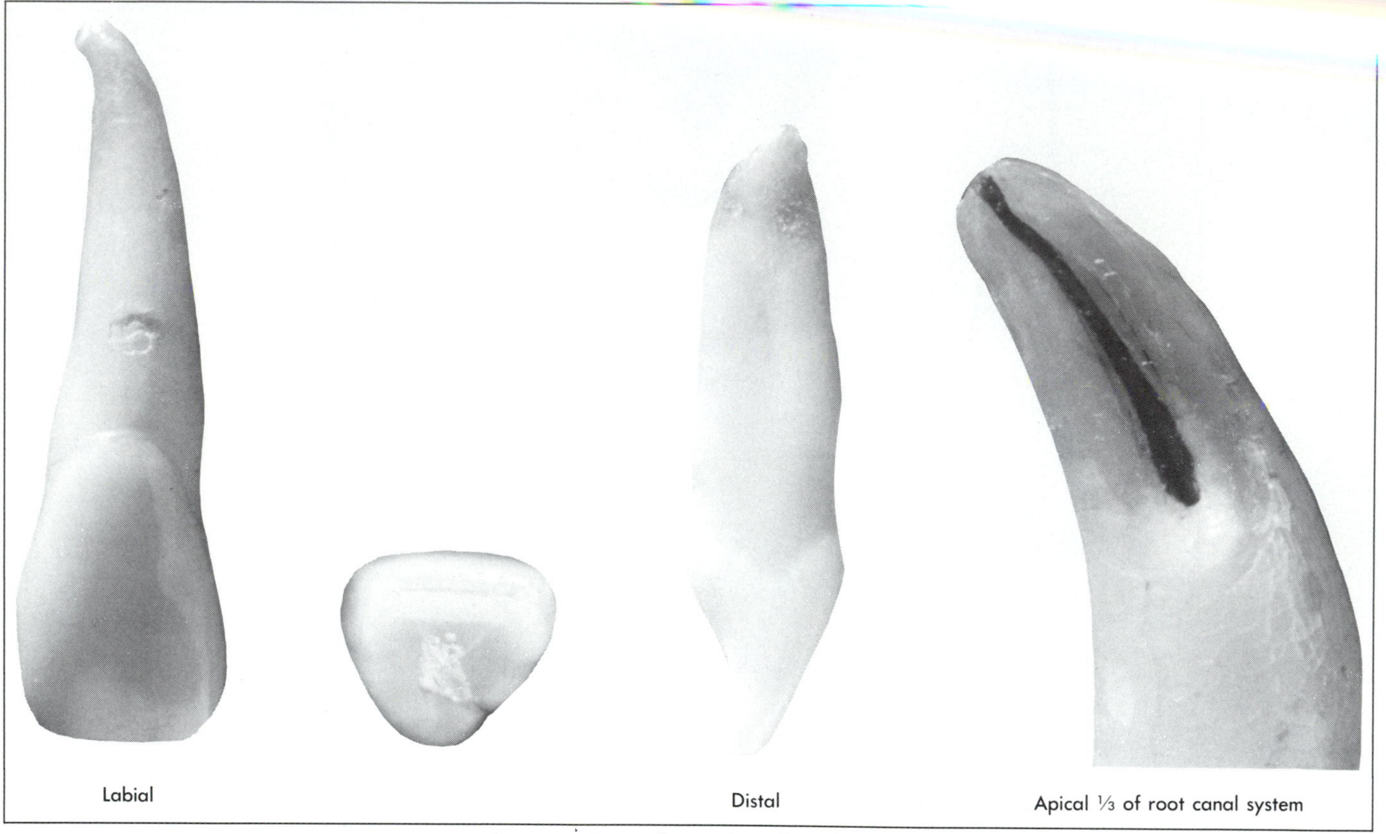

Average time of eruption: 8 to 9 years
Average age of calcification: 11 years
Average length: 22.0 mm

Tending toward an oval shape, the crown of the maxillary lateral incisor is as near to ideal for endodontic access as that of the central incisor. Fiber-optic illumination may, likewise, be helpful during access to this tooth.

The initial entry, with the end-cutting fissure bur, is made just above the cingulum. The access cavity is ovoid. Often the fissure bur will engage the shallow pulp chamber while making the initial opening. When the chamber roof is removed, a no. 4 or 6 round bur is used to sweep out all remaining caries, discoloration, and pulp calcifications.

It may be necessary to return to the fissure bur in refining the ovoid access cavity. Adequate flaring is then accomplished with round burs. Care must be exercised that explorers, endodontic cutting instruments, and packing instruments do not contact the access cavity walls.

To ensure that the canals remain clean and hermetically sealed, all caries and leaking restorations must be removed and replaced with temporary sealing materials.

The radicular cross-sectional pulp chamber varies from ovoid at the cervical to round at the apical foramen. The root is slightly conical and tends toward curvature, usually toward the distal, in its apical portion. The apical foramen is generally closer to the anatomic apex than in the maxillary central but may be found on the lateral aspect within 1 or 2 mm of the apex.

On rare occasions, access is complicated by a dens-in-dente, an invagination of part of the lingual surface of the tooth into the crown. This creates a space within the tooth that is lined by enamel and communicates with the mouth. Dens in dente most often occurs in maxillary lateral incisors, but it can occur in other teeth. These teeth are predisposed to decay because of the anatomic malformation, and the pulp may die before the root apex is completely developed.[10] This mostly coronal mass should be dealt with mechanically and either removed or bypassed.

Goon and others reported the first case of complex involvement of the entire facial aspect of a tooth root. An alveolar crest to apex facial root defect led to early pulpal necrosis and periapical rarefaction.[8]

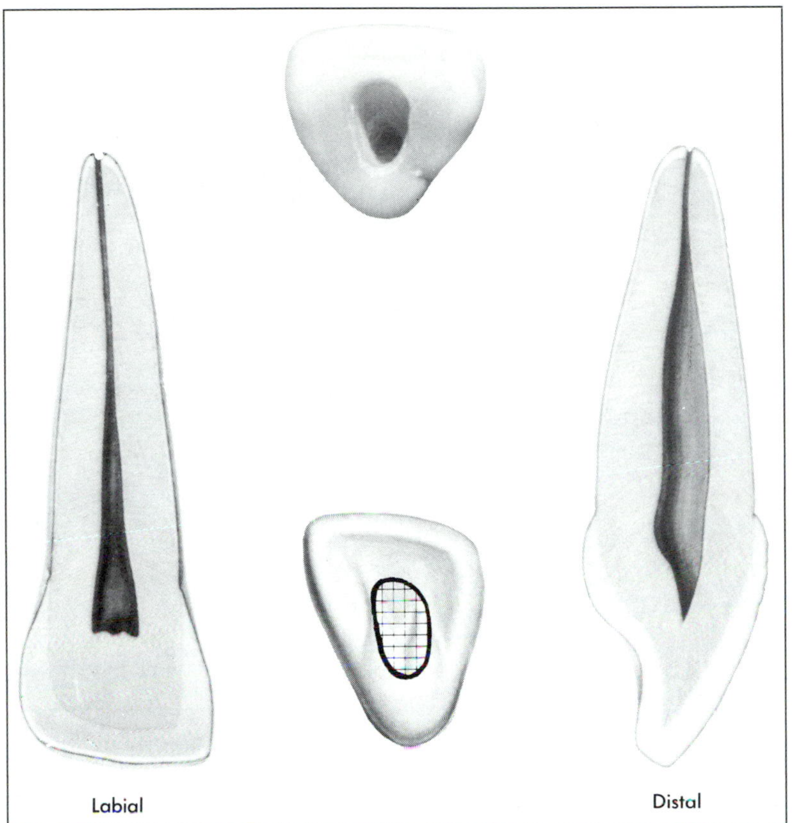

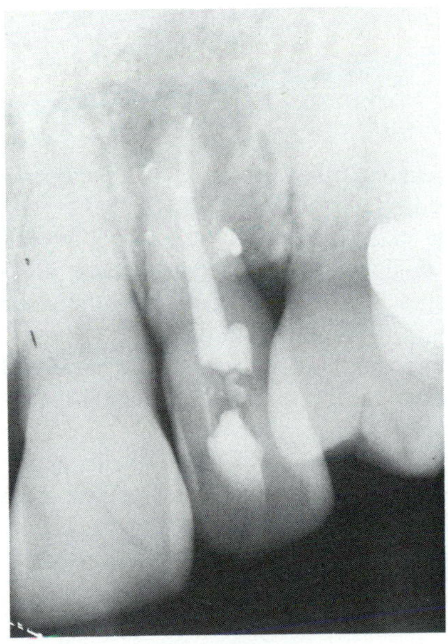

PLATE 7-II-5. Lateral incisor with a canal loop and multiple canals with associated lesions.

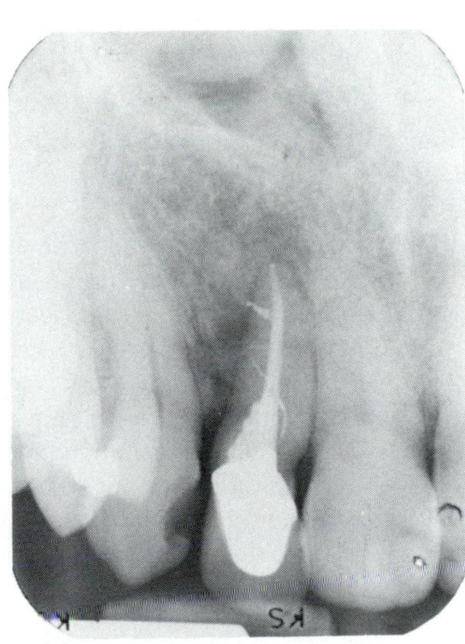

PLATE 7-II-6. Multiple portals of exit.

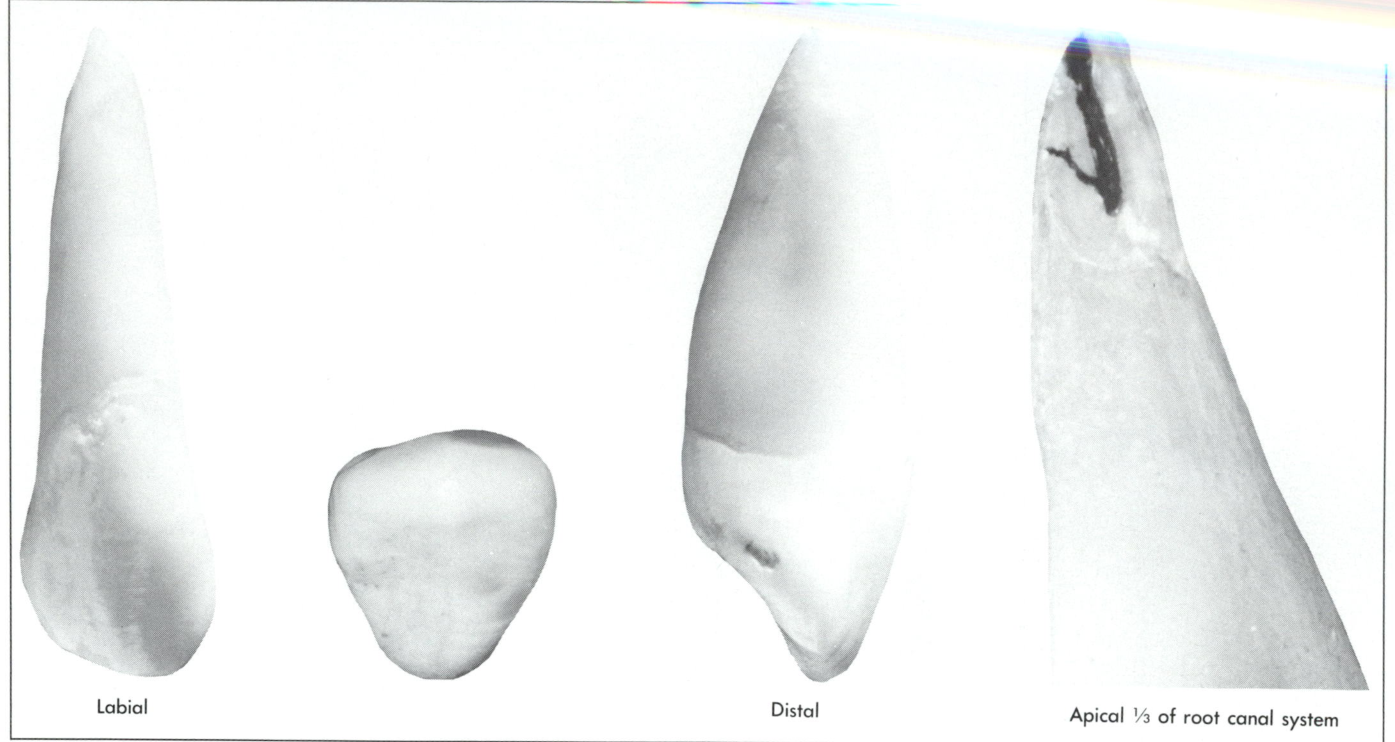

Average time of eruption: 10 to 12 years
Average age of calcification: 13 to 15 years
Average length: 26.5 mm

The longest tooth in the dental arch, the canine has a formidable shape designed to withstand heavy occlusal stress. Its long, thickly enameled crown sustains heavy incisal wear but often displays deep cervical erosion with aging.

The access cavity corresponds to the lingual crown shape and is ovoid. To achieve straight-line access, one often must extend the cavity incisally, but not so far as to weaken the heavily functioning cusp. Initial access is made slightly below midcrown on the palatal side. If the pulp chamber is located deeper, a no. 4 or 6 long-shanked round bur may be required. The sweeping-out motion of this bur will reveal an ovoid pulp chamber. The chamber remains ovoid as it continues apically through the cervical region and below. Attention must be given to directional filing so this ovoid chamber will be thoroughly cleaned.

The radicular canal is reasonably straight and quite long. Most canines require instruments that are 25 mm or longer. The apex will often curve — in any direction — in the last 2 or 3 mm.

Canine morphology seldom varies radically, and lateral and accessory canals occur less frequently than in the maxillary incisors.

This buccal bone over the eminence often disintegrates, and fenestration is a common finding. The apical foramen is usually close to the anatomic apex but may be laterally positioned, especially when apical curvature is present.

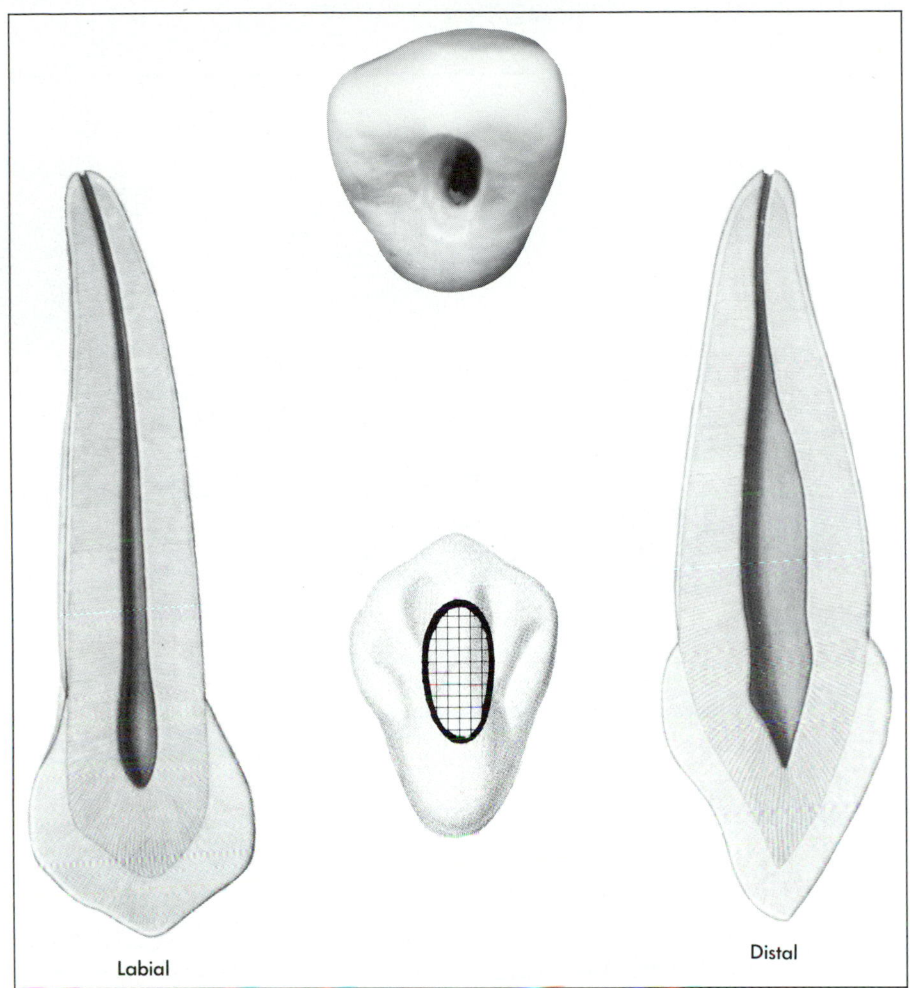

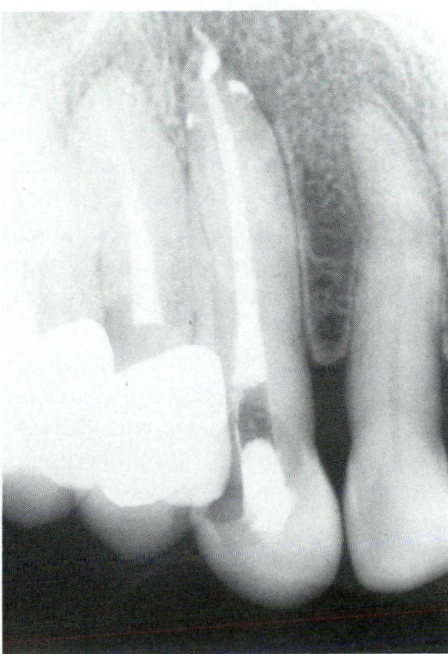

PLATE 7-III-5. Canine with multiple accessory foramina.

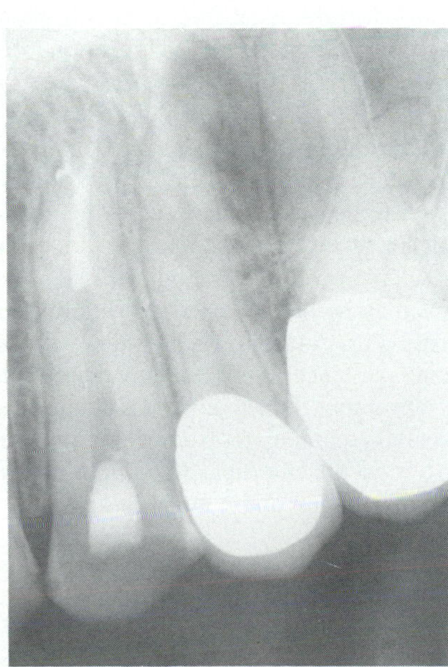

PLATE 7-III-6. Maxillary canine with lateral canal dividing into two additional canals.

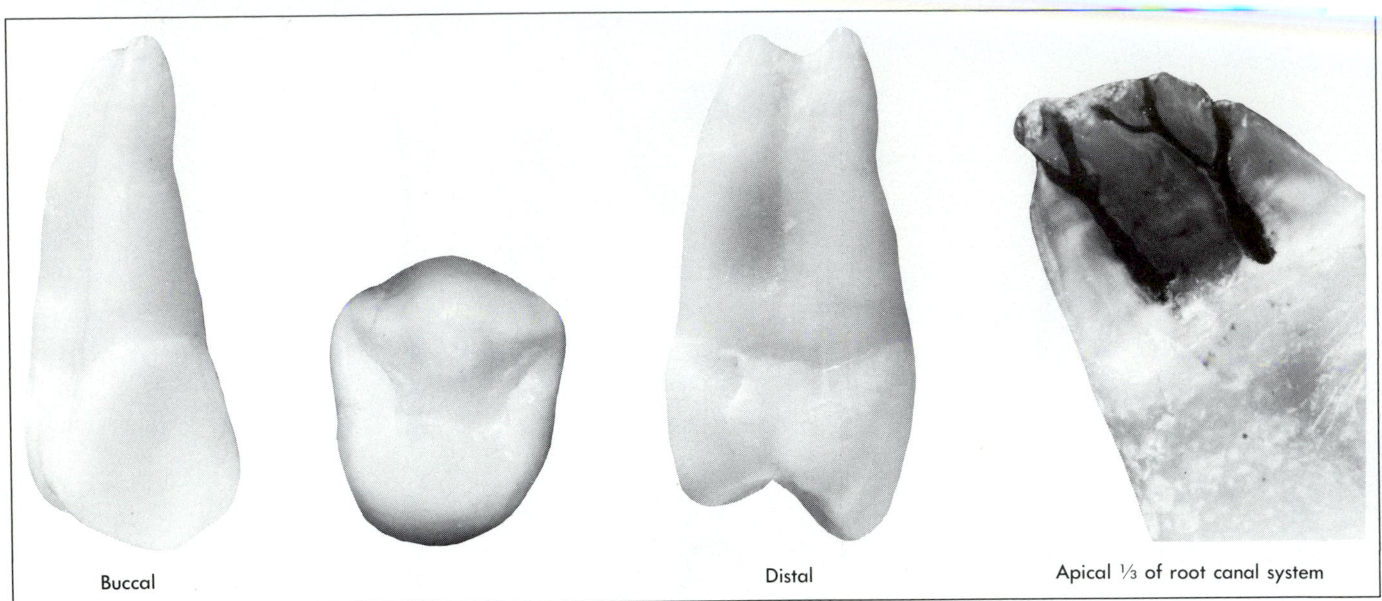

Average time of eruption: 10 to 11 years
Average age of calcification: 12 to 13 years
Average length: 20.6 mm

Most commonly birooted, the maxillary first premolar is a transitional tooth between incisor and molar. Loss of the posterior molars subjects the premolars to heavy occlusal loads. Removable appliances increase torque on these frequently clasped teeth, and the additional forces, in concert with deep carious lesions, can induce heavy calcification of the pulp chambers. Early posterior tooth loss often causes rotation, which can complicate the locating of pulp chambers.

The canal orifices lie below and slightly central to the cusp tips. The initial opening is in the central fossa and is ovoid in the buccal-palatal dimension. When one orifice has been located, the clinician should look carefully for a developmental groove leading to the opening of another canal. The angulation of the roots may be determined by positioning of the endodontic explorer (Fig. 7-12, *C*). Radiographic division of the roots on a routine periapical film often indicates tooth rotation (Fig. 7-12, *A*). Divergent roots require less occlusal access extension. Conversely, parallel roots may require removal of tooth structure toward the cusp tips. All caries and leaking restorations must be removed and a suitable temporary restoration placed.

Radicular irregularities consist of fused roots with separate canals, fused roots with interconnections or "webbing," fused roots with a common apical foramen, and the unusual but always to be considered three-rooted tooth. In the last situation the buccal orifices are not clearly visible with a mouth mirror. Directional positioning of the endodontic explorer or a small file will identify the anatomy. Carns and Skidmore[5] reported that the incidence of maxillary first premolars with three roots, three canals, and three foramina was 6% of the cases studied. The root is considerably shorter than in the canine, and distal curvature is not uncommon. The apical foramen is usually close to the anatomic apex. Root lengths, if the cusps are intact and used as reference points, are usually the same. The apical portion of the roots often tapers rapidly, ending in extremely narrow and curved root tips.

The prevalence of mesial-distal vertical crown or root fracture of the first premolar requires that the clinician remove all restorations at the inception of endodontic therapy and carefully inspect the coronal anatomy with a fiberoptic light.

After endodontic treatment, full occlusal coverage is mandatory to ensure against vertical or crown or root fracture.

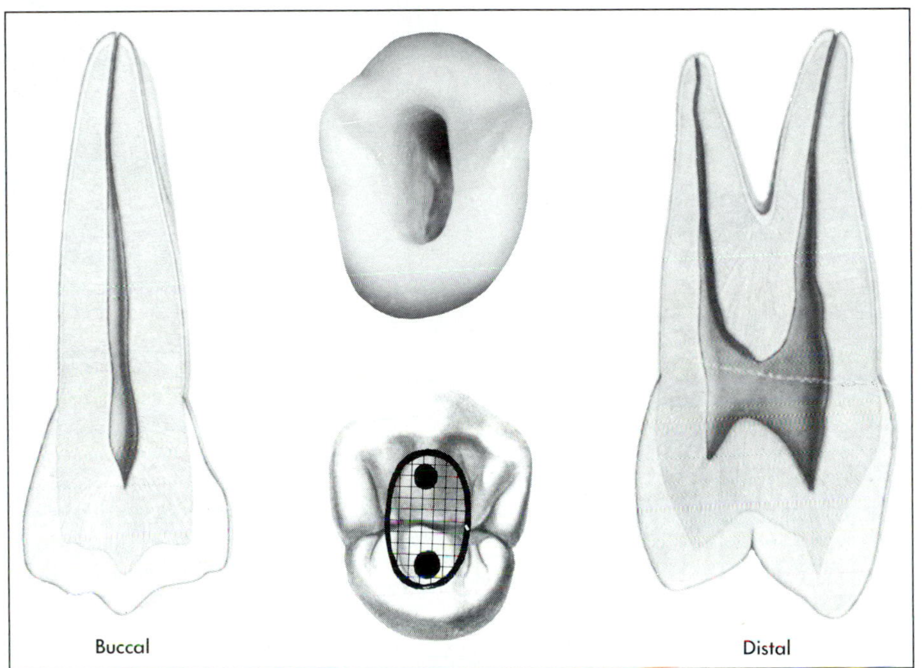

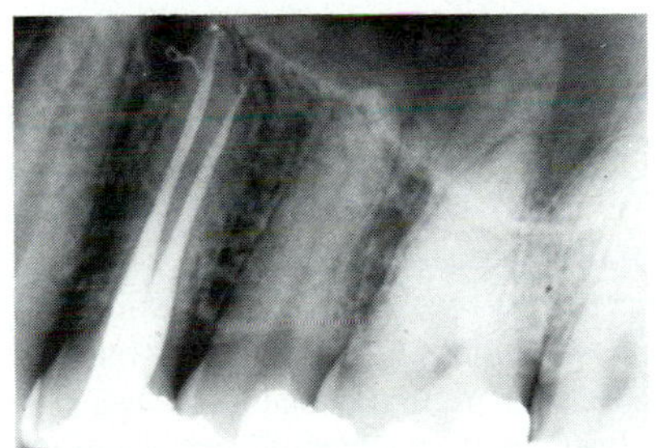

PLATE 7-IV-5. Lateral bony lesion associated with filled lateral canal.

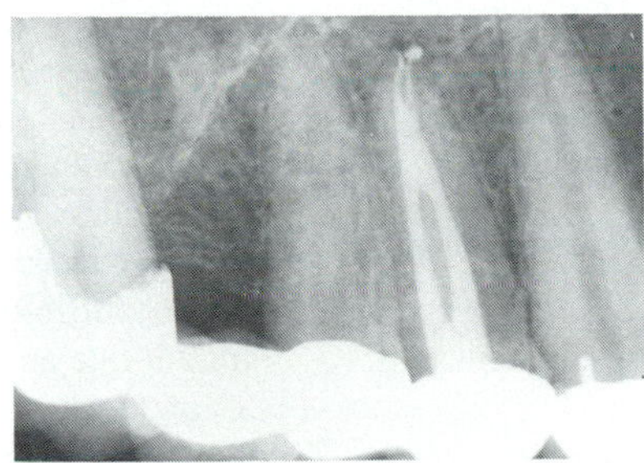

PLATE 7-IV-6. Two canals fusing and redividing.

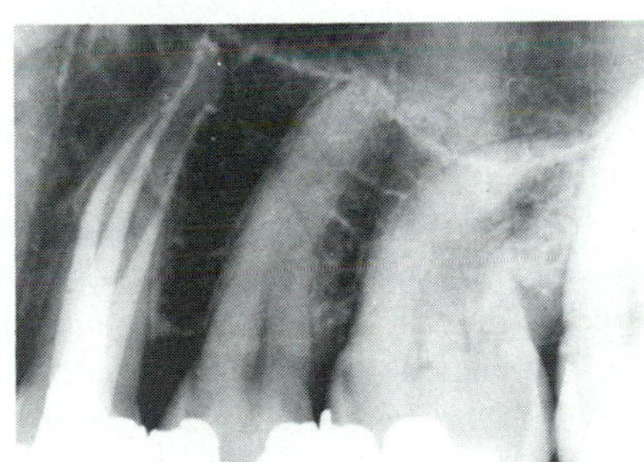

PLATE 7-IV-7. Three canals in a maxillary first bicuspid.

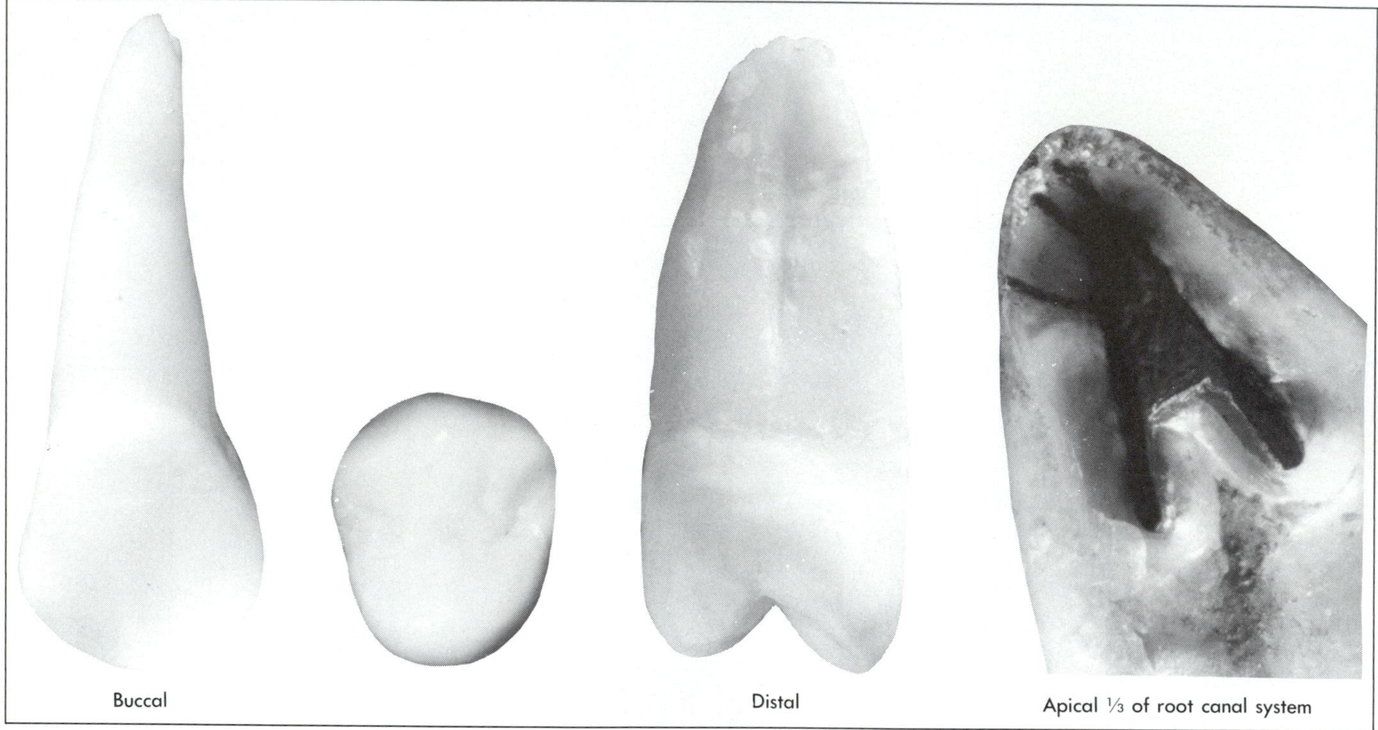

Average time of eruption: 10 to 12 years
Average age of calcification: 12 to 14 years
Average length: 21.5 mm

Similar to the first premolar in coronal morphology, the second premolar varies mainly in root form. Its crown is narrower in the buccal-palatal dimension and slightly wider in the mesial-distal. The canal orifice is centrally located but often appears more as a slot than as a single ovoid opening. When the slot-shaped opening appears, the clinician must assume that the tooth has two canals until proved otherwise.

The basic outline of the tooth is slightly ovoid but wider from mesial to distal than the outline of the first premolar. All caries and leaking restorations must be removed and replaced with a suitable temporary restoration.

Radicular morphology may present two separate canals, two canals anastomosing to a single canal, or two canals with interconnections or "webbing." Accessory and lateral canals may be present, but less often than in incisors. Vertucci and associates[21] stated that 75% of maxillary second premolars in their study had one canal at the apex, 24% had two foramina, and 1% had three foramina. Of the teeth studied, 59.5% had accessory canals. These clinicians also reported that when two canals join into one, the *palatal* canal frequently exhibits a straight-line access to the apex. They further pointed out that "if, on the direct periapical exposure, a root canal shows a sudden narrowing, or even disappears, it means that at this point the canal divides into two parts, which either remain separate (type V) or merge (type II) before reaching the apex."

The root length of the maxillary second molar is much like that of the first premolar; and apical curvature is not uncommon, particularly with large sinus cavities.

After endodontic treatment, full occlusal coverage is mandatory to ensure against vertical cuspal or crown-root fracture.

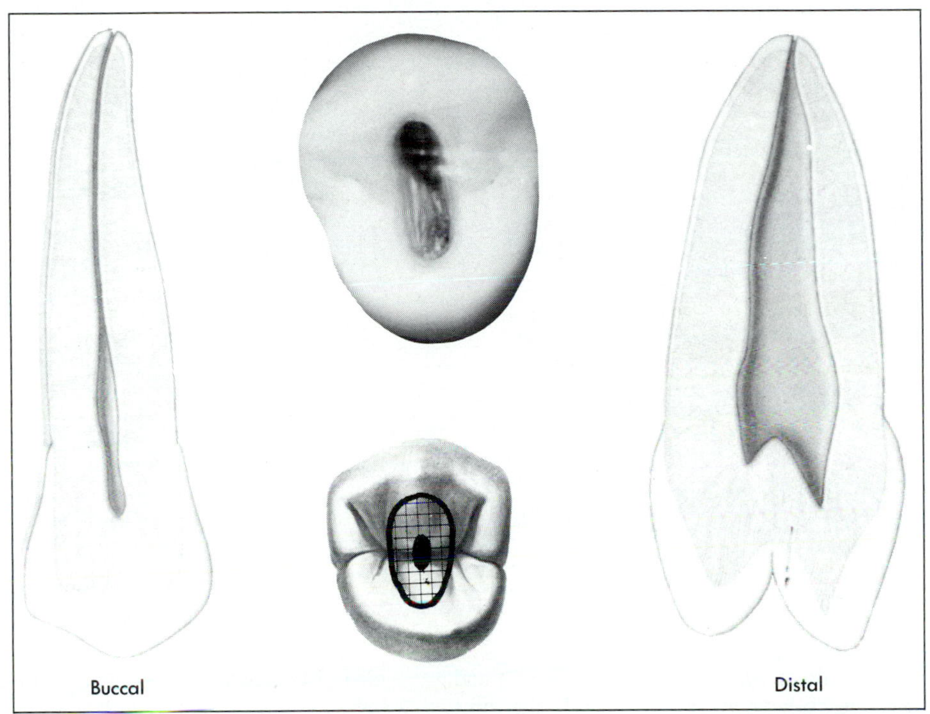

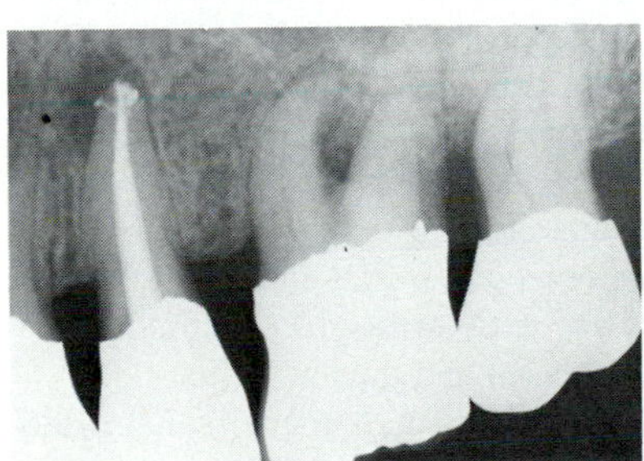

PLATE 7-V-5. Multiple foramina.

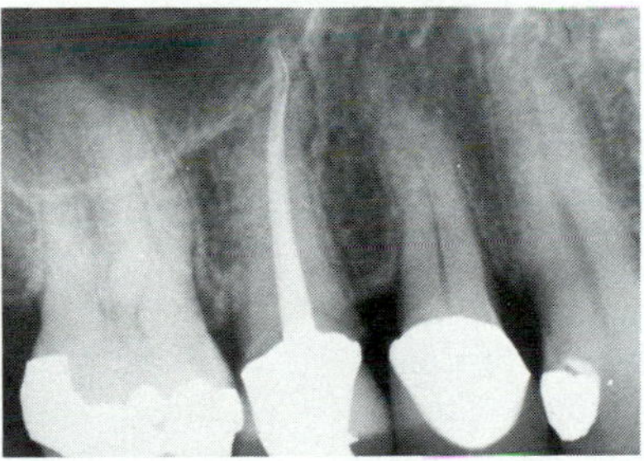

PLATE 7-V-6. Single canal dividing into two canals.

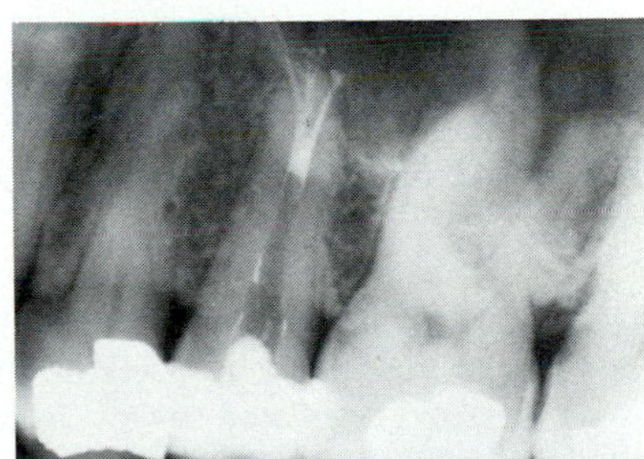

PLATE 7-V-7. Single canal splitting into three canals.

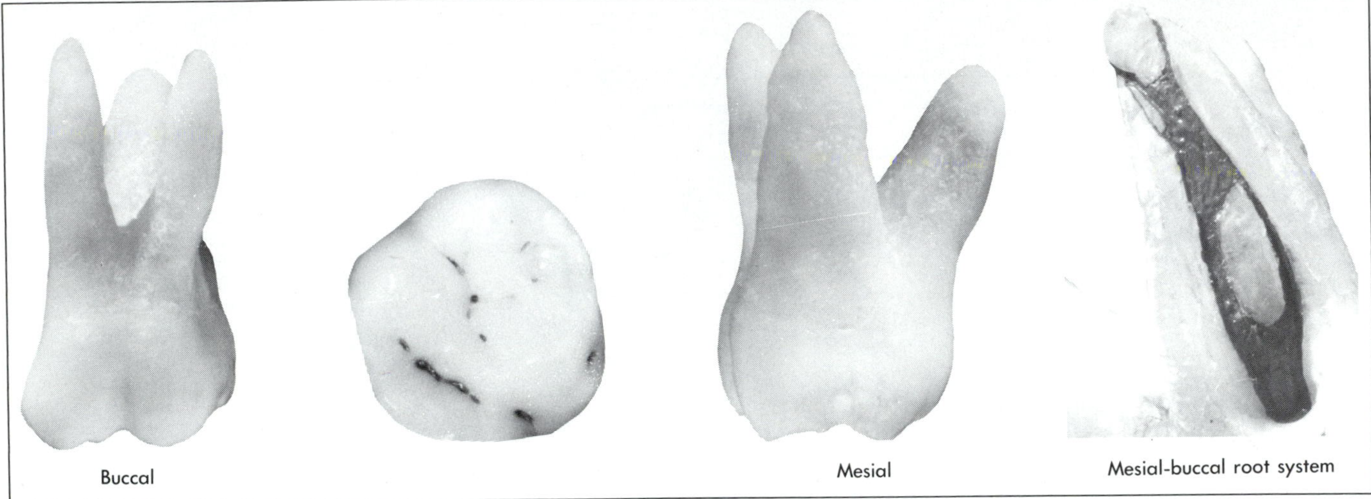

Average time of eruption: 6 to 7 years
Average age of calcification: 9 to 10 years
Average length: 20.8 mm

The tooth largest in volume and most complex in root and root canal anatomy, the "6-year molar" is possibly the most treated, least understood, posterior tooth. It is the posterior tooth with the highest endodontic failure rate and unquestionably one of the most important teeth.

Three individual roots of the maxillary first molar provide a tripod: the palatal root, which is the longest, and the distal-buccal and mesial-buccal roots, which are about the same length.

The palatal root is often curved buccally in its apical third. Of the three canals, it offers the easiest access and has the largest diameter. Its orifice lies well toward the palatal surface and it is sharply angulated away from the midline. Cross-sectionally it is flat and ribbonlike, requiring close attention to débridement and instrumentation; fortunately there is rarely more than one apical foramen.

The distal-buccal root is conical and usually straight. It invariably has a single canal.

The mesial-buccal root of the first molar has generated more research, clinical investigation, and pure frustration than has probably any other root in the mouth. Green[9] stated that two foramina were present in 14% of mesial-buccal roots of the maxillary first molars studied and two orifices were noted in 36%. Pineda[17] reported that 42% of these roots manifested two canals and two apical foramina. Slowey[19] supported Pineda's conclusions within a few percentage points. Kulild, in a recent study, indicated that a second ML canal was contained in the coronal half of 95.2% of the mesial-buccal roots examined. The canals were located with hand instruments (54.2%), bur (31.3%), and microscope (9.6%). Each tooth was sectioned in 1-mm increments and although not all canals reached the apex, this study revealed that 71.1% had two patent canals at the apex. It is the author's opinion that the spaces located beyond true canals were finlike extensions found commonly in the broad buccolingual root of the maxillary first molar. The fact that almost half of these roots bear two canals, whether they join into a single foramen or not, is enough reason *always to assume that two canals exist* until careful examination proves otherwise. The extra orifice lies centrally somewhere between the mesial-buccal and palatal orifices.

Kulild[14] also reported that the mesial-lingual canal orifice averaged 1.82 mm lingual to the mesial-buccal canal orifice. Searching for the extra orifice is aided by using the fiberoptic light and by locating the developmental line between the mesial-buccal and palatal orifices. The second canal within the mesial-buccal root is always smaller than the other canals and, so, is often more difficult to clean and shape. Gaining access to the primary canal within the mesial-buccal root can be made easier by improving the angle of approach.

All caries, leaking restorations, and pulpal calcifications must be removed prior to initiating endodontic treatment. After treatment it is mandatory to institute full coverage to ensure against vertical cuspal or crown-root fracture. It is also advisable to place internal metal reinforcement whenever there is a significant loss of coronal tooth structures.

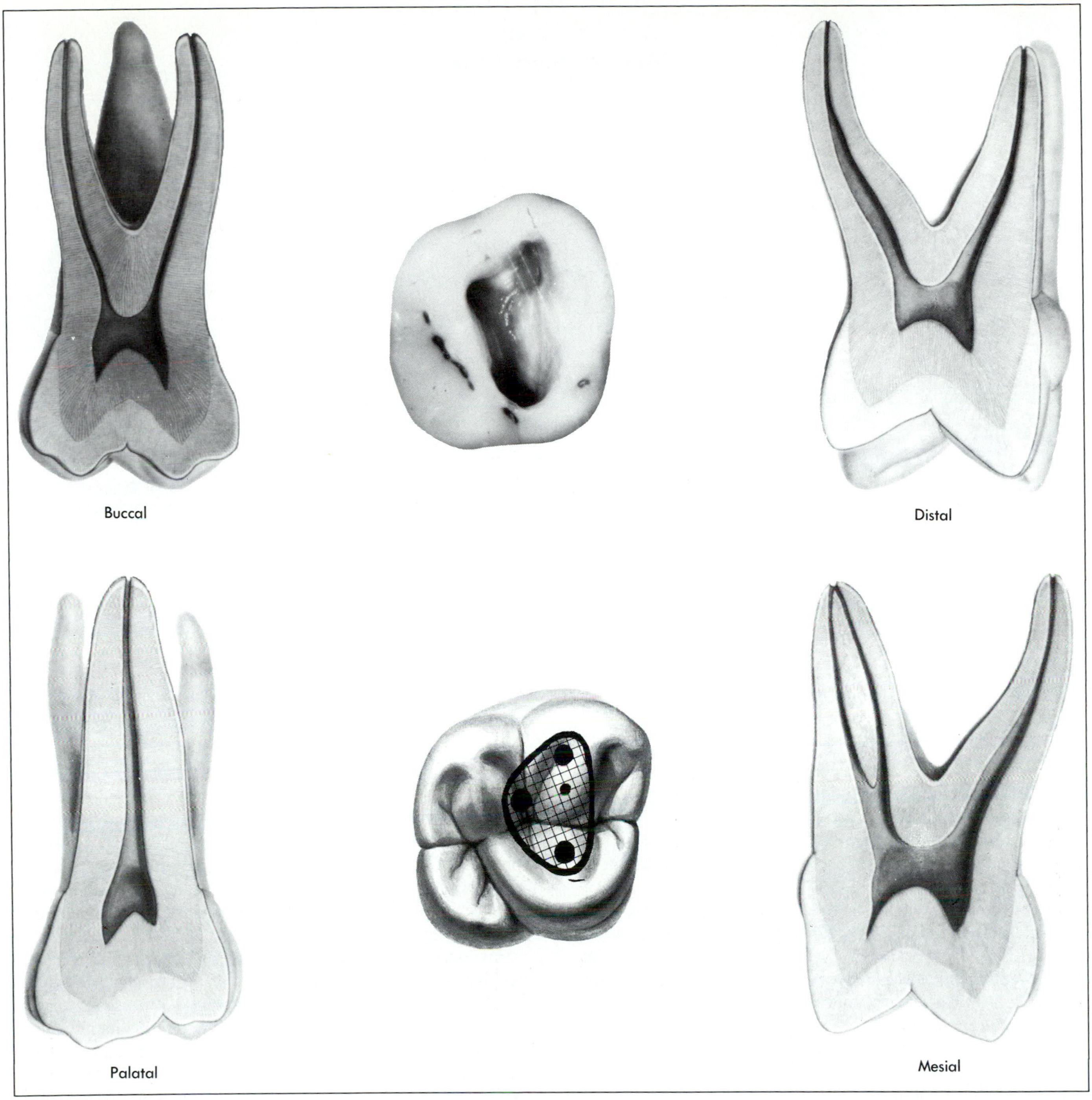

Buccal

Distal

Palatal

Mesial

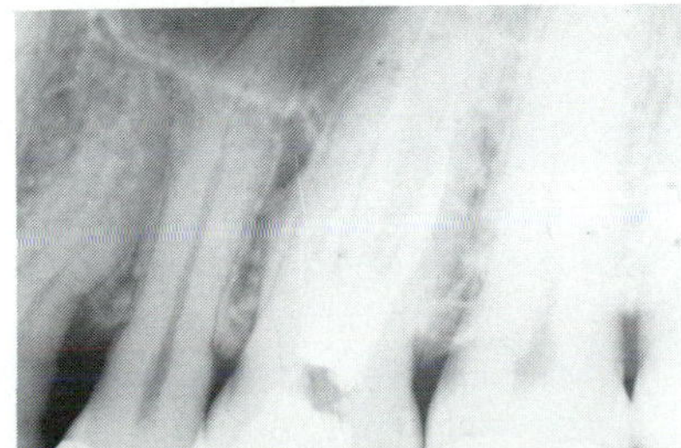

PLATE 7-VI-7. Fourth canal in mesiobuccal root; loops and accessory canals.

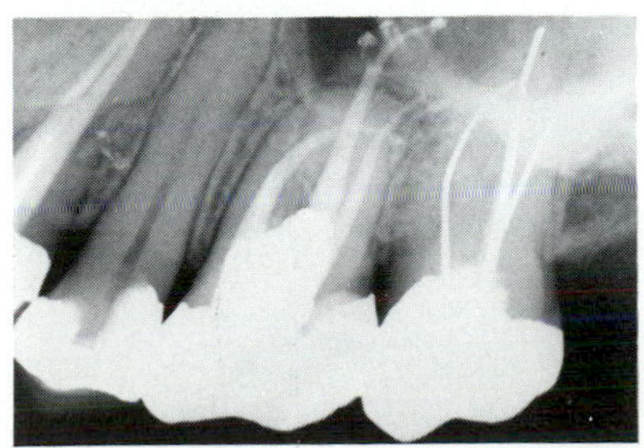

PLATE 7-VI-8. Sharp curvature and multiple accessory canals in palatal root (contrast to silver cones in second molar).

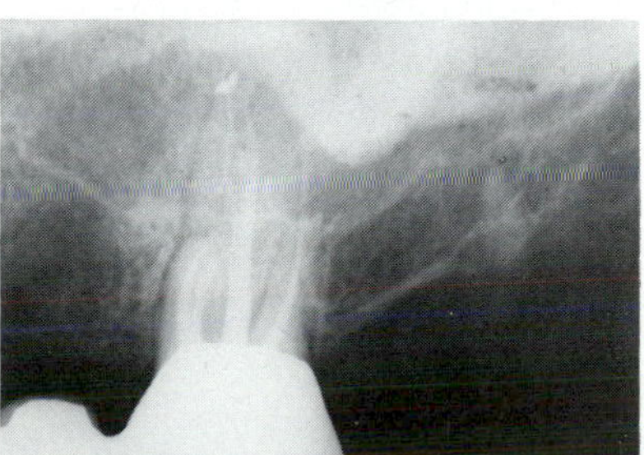

PLATE 7-VI-9. Second canals in both mesiobuccal and lingual canals.

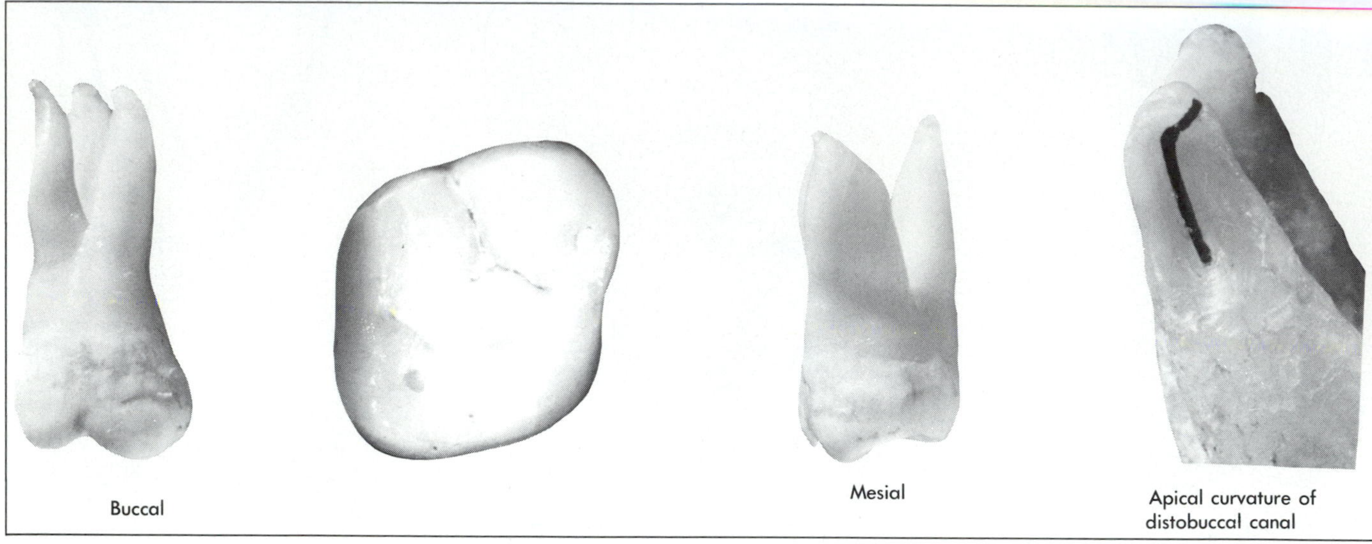

Average time of eruption: 11 to 13 years
Average age of calcification: 14 to 16 years
Average length: 20.0 mm

Coronally, the maxillary second molar closely resembles the maxillary first molar, although it is not as square and massive. Access in both teeth can usually be adequately prepared without disturbing the transverse ridge. The second molar is often easier to prepare because of the straight-line access to the orifices.

The distinguishing morphologic feature of the maxillary second molar is its three roots grouped close together, and sometimes fused. The parallel root canals are frequently superimposed radiographically. They are usually shorter than the roots of the first molar and not as curved. The three orifices may form a flat triangle, sometimes almost a straight line. The floor of the chamber is markedly convex, giving a slightly funnel shape to the canal orifices. Occasionally the canals curve into the chamber at a sharp angle to the floor, making it necessary to remove a lip of dentin so the canal can be entered more in a direct line with the canal axis.[9]

Complications in access occur when the molar is tipped in distal version. Initial opening with an end-cutting fissure bur is followed by a short-shanked round bur, which is best suited to uncover the pulp chamber and shape the access cavity. Then small hand instruments are used to establish canal continuity and working length. The bulk of the cleaning and shaping may now be accomplished with engine-mounted files on reciprocating handpieces.

To enhance radiographic visibility, especially when there is interference with the malar process, a more perpendicular and distal-angular radiograph may be exposed.

All caries, leaking restorations, and pulpal calcifications must be removed prior to initiating endodontic treatment. Full occlusal coverage is mandatory to ensure against vertical cuspal or crown-root fracture. Internal reinforcement, when indicated, should be incorporated immediately after endodontic treatment.

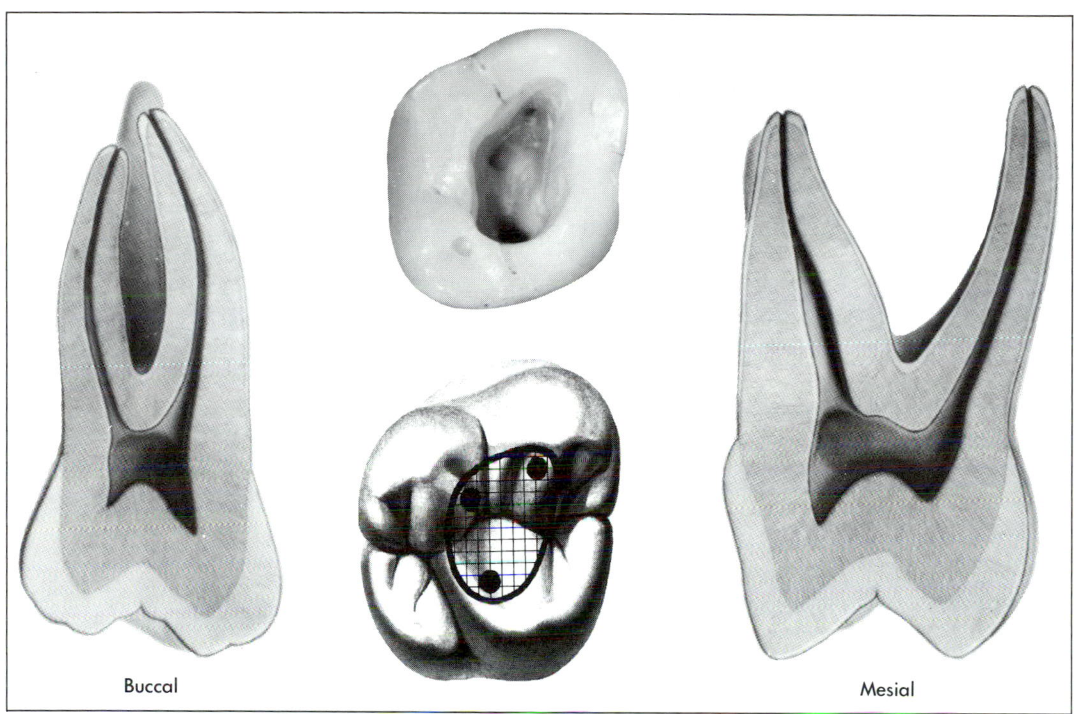

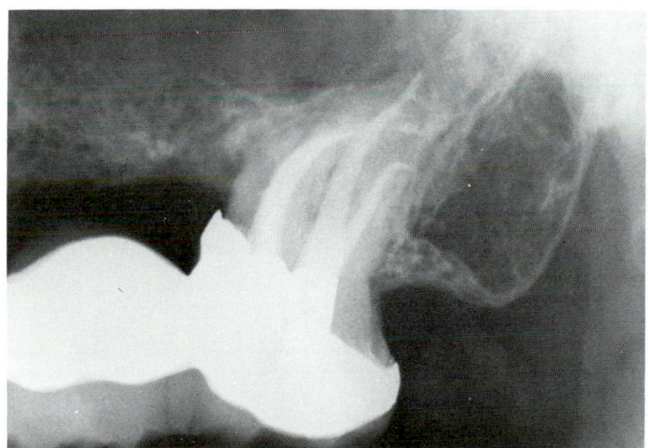

PLATE 7-VII-5. Severely curved mesiobuccal root with right angle curve in distobuccal root.

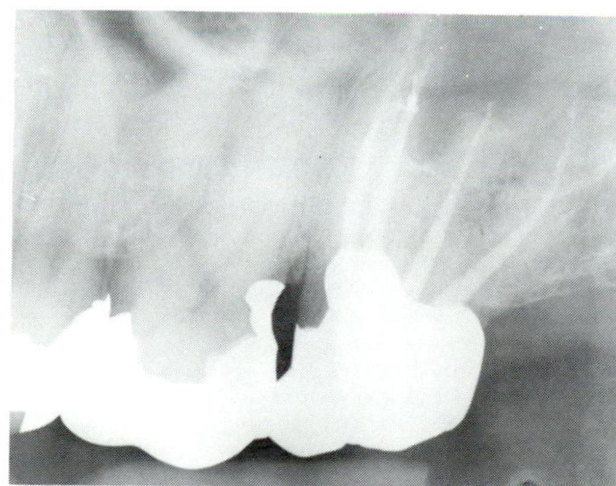

PLATE 7-VII-6. Four-rooted maxillary second molar.

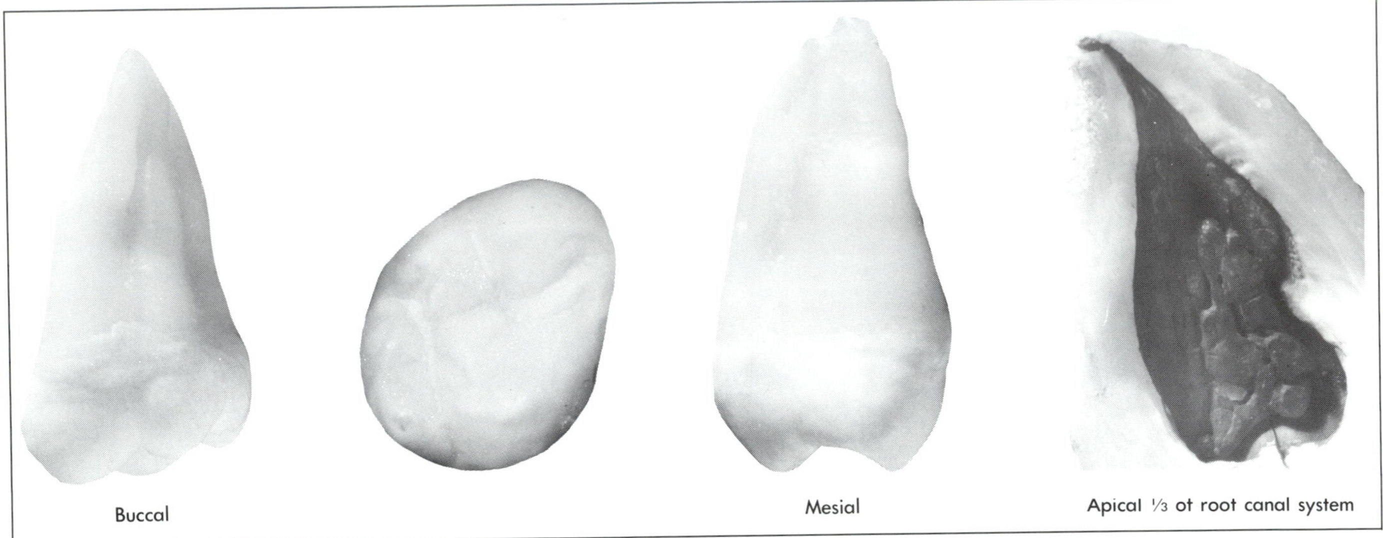

Average time of eruption: 17 to 22 years
Average age of calcification: 18 to 25 years
Average length: 17.0 mm

Loss of the maxillary first and second molars is often the reason for considering the third molar as a strategic abutment. The other indication for endodontic treatment and full coverage is a fully functioning mandibular third molar.

Careful examination of root morphology is important before recommending treatment. Many third molars present adequate root formation; and given reasonable accessibility, there is no reason why they cannot remain as functioning dentition after endodontic therapy.

The radicular anatomy of the third molar is completely unpredictable, and it may be advisable to explore the root canal morphology before promising success.

As an alternative to conventional hand instrumentation, the use of engine-mounted files in reciprocating handpieces may simplify the problem of accessibility. Precurving instruments helps guide them through tortuous canals.

For visual and mechanical convenience the access may be overextended slightly with the knowledge that full coverage is mandatory. All caries, leaking restorations, and pulpal calcifications must be removed prior to instituting treatment.

Some third molars will have only a single canal, some two, and most three. The orifice openings may be made in either a triangular arrangement or a nearly straight-line.

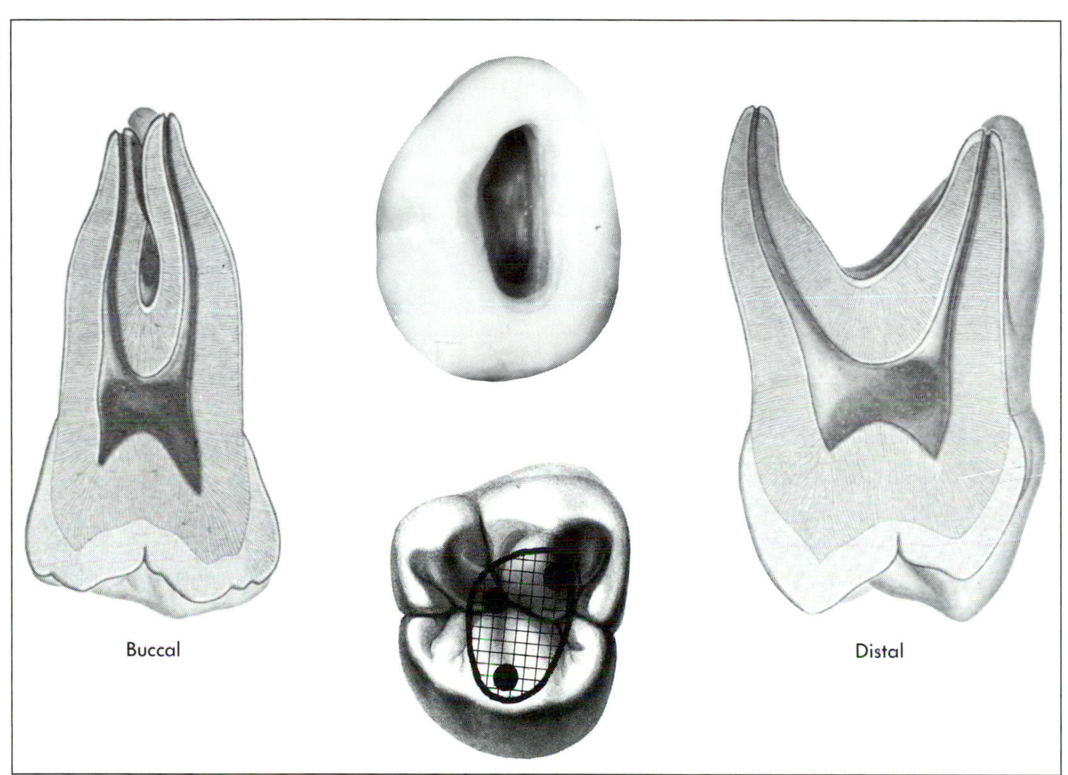

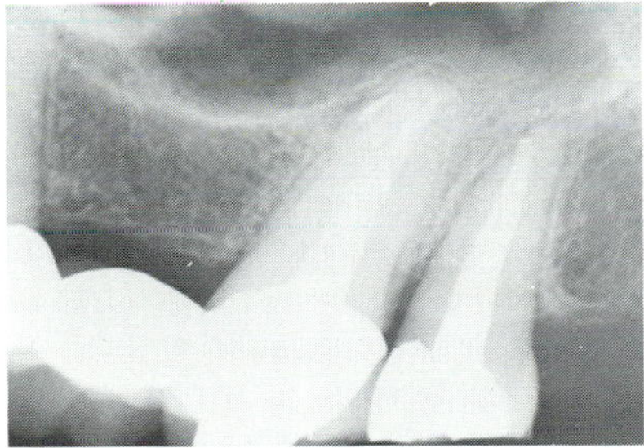

PLATE 7-VIII-5. Showing canals fuses into single canal. (Note multiple accessories in second molar.)

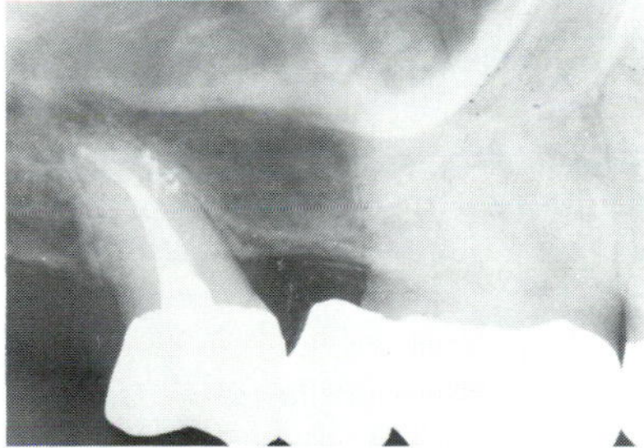

PLATE 7-VIII-6. Distal bridge abutment with major accessory canal.

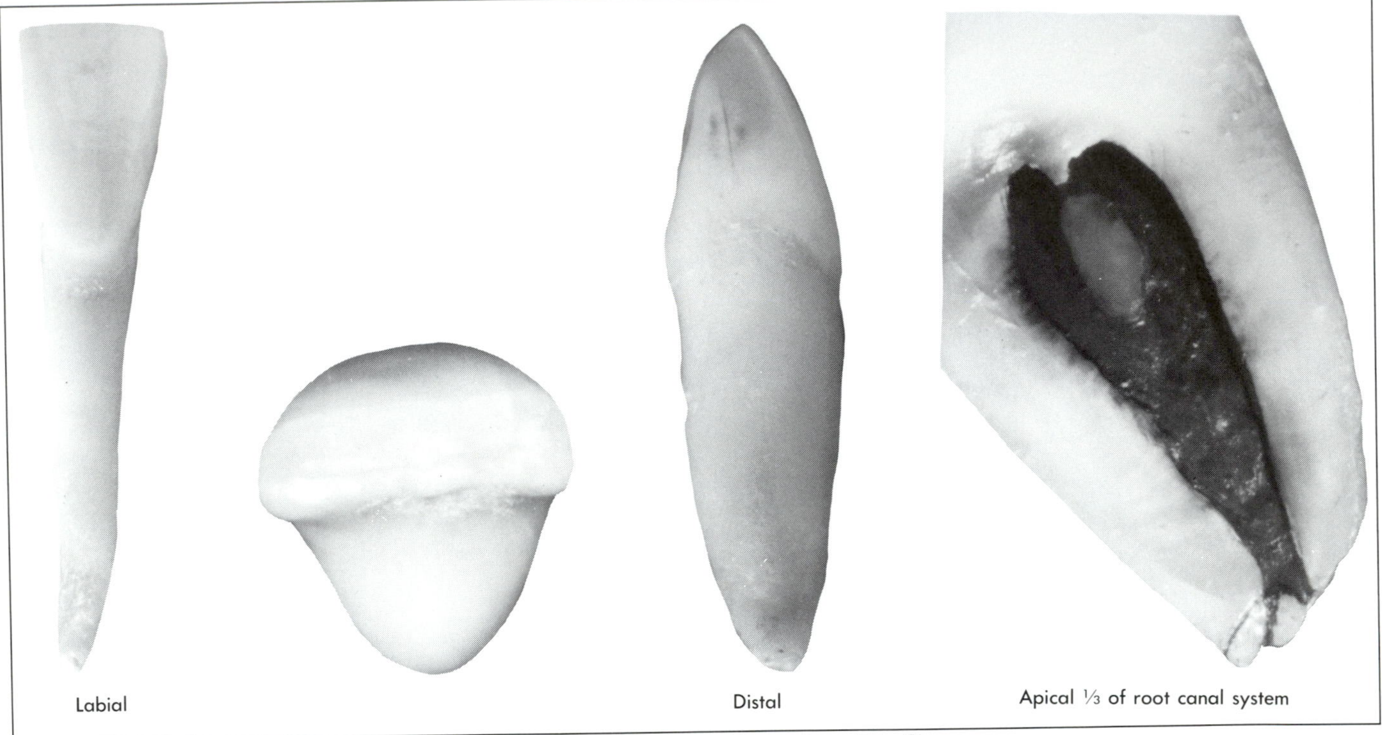

Average time of eruption: 6 to 8 years
Average age of calcification: 9 to 10 years
Average length: 20.7 mm

Narrow and flat in the labial-lingual dimension, the mandibular incisors are the smallest human adult teeth. Visible radiographically from only one plane, they often appear more accessible than they really are. The narrow lingual crown offers a limited area for access. Smaller fissure burs and no. 2 round burs cause less mutilation of coronal dentition. The access cavity should be ovoid, with attention given to a lingual approach (Fig. 7-6).

Frequently the mandibular incisors have two canals. One study[1] reported that 41.4% of mandibular incisors studied had two separate canals; of these, only 1.3% had two separate foramina. The clinician should search for the second canal immediately upon completing the access cavity. Endodontic failures in mandibular incisors usually arise from uncleaned canals, most commonly toward the lingual. Access may be extended incisally when indicated to permit maximum labial-lingual freedom.

Although labial perforations are common, they may be avoided if the clinician remembers that it is nearly impossible to perforate in a lingual direction because of the bur shank's contacting the incisal edge. The ribbon-shaped canal (Fig. 7-2) is common enough to be considered normal and demands special attention in cleaning and shaping.

Ribbon-shaped canals in narrow hourglass cross-sectional anatomy invite lateral perforation by endodontic files and Gates-Glidden drills. Minimal flaring and dowel space preparation are indicated to ensure against ripping through proximal root walls.

Apical curvatures and accessory canals are common in mandibular incisors.

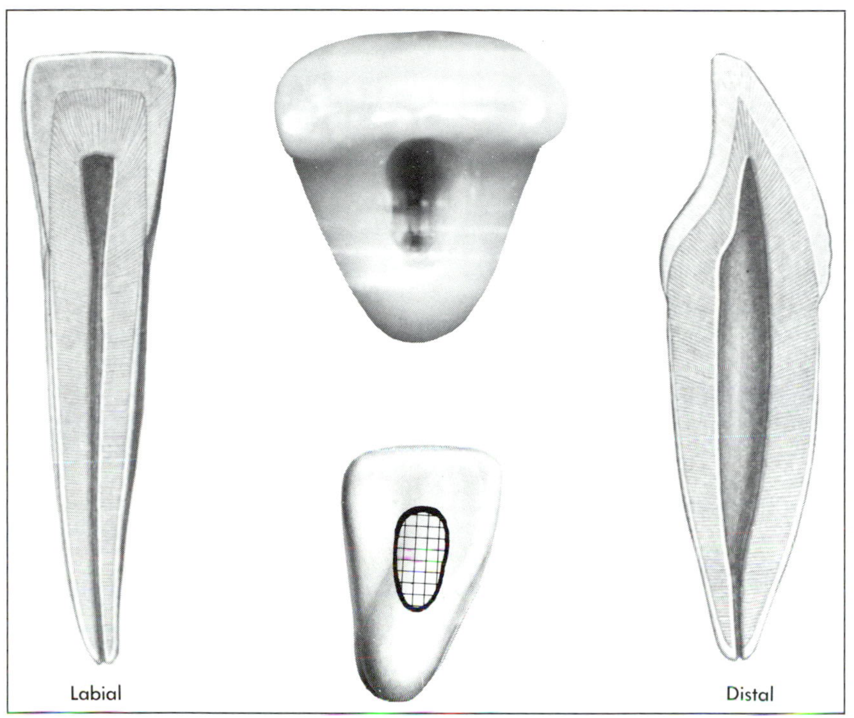

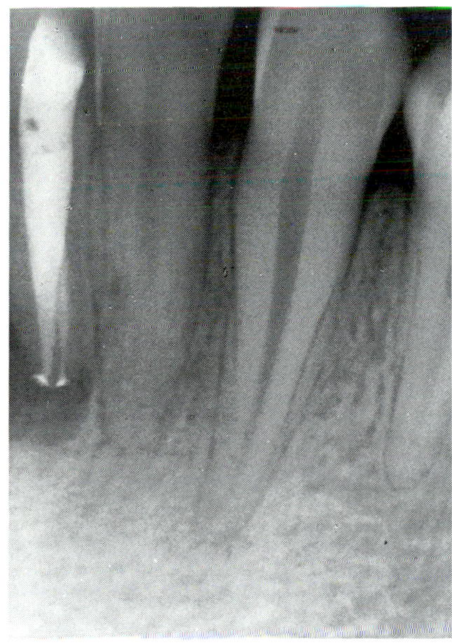

PLATE 7-IX-5. Two-rooted mandibular lateral incisor.

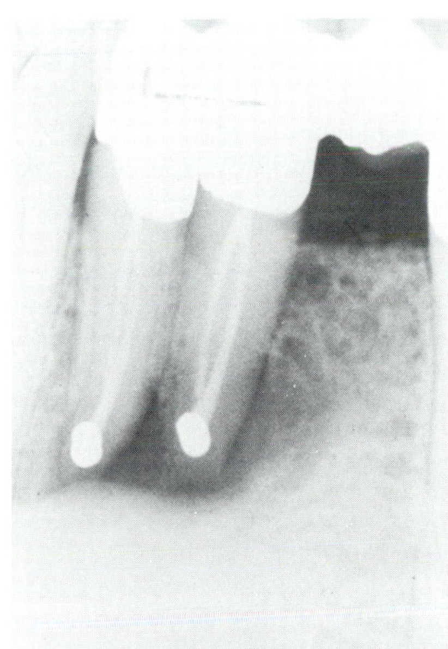

PLATE 7-IX-6. Mandibular lateral and central, both with two canals.

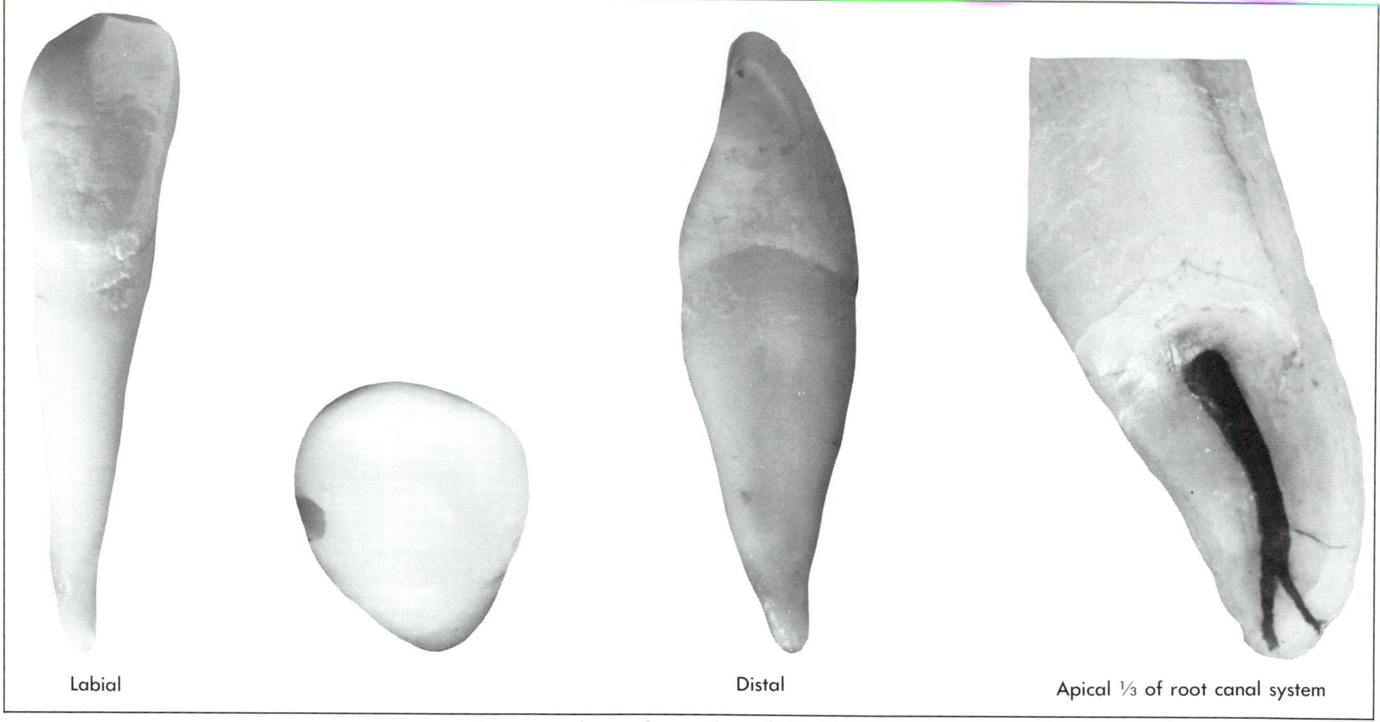

Average time of eruption: 9 to 10 years
Average age of calcification: 13 years
Average length: 25.6 mm

Sturdy and considerably wider mesial-distally than the incisors, the mandibular canines seldom present endodontic problems. The unusual occurrence of two roots can create difficulty, but this is rare.

The access cavity is ovoid and may be extended incisally for labial-lingual accessibility. The canal is somewhat ovoid at the cervical, becoming round at midroot. Directional instrumentation is necessary to débride the canal walls completely.

If there are two roots, one is always easier to instrument. The other must be opened and funneled in concert with the first to prevent packing of dentin debris and loss of access (Fig. 7-33). Precurving of instruments at initial access will enable the clinician to trace down the buccal or lingual root wall until the tip engages the orifice. When the difficult canal is located, every effort should be made to shape and funnel the opening to maintain continued access.

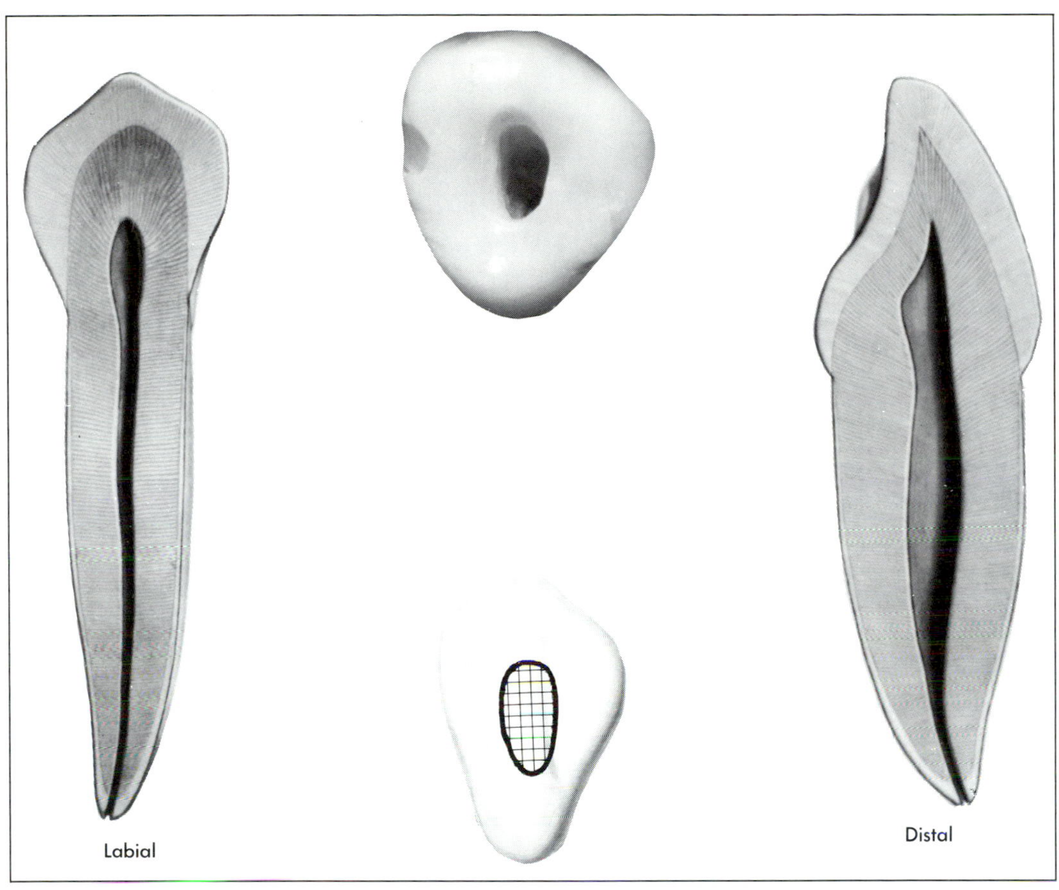

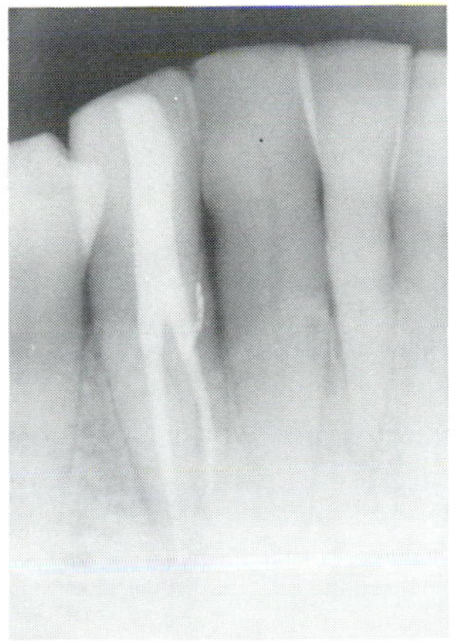

PLATE 7-X-5. Two-rooted mandibular canine.

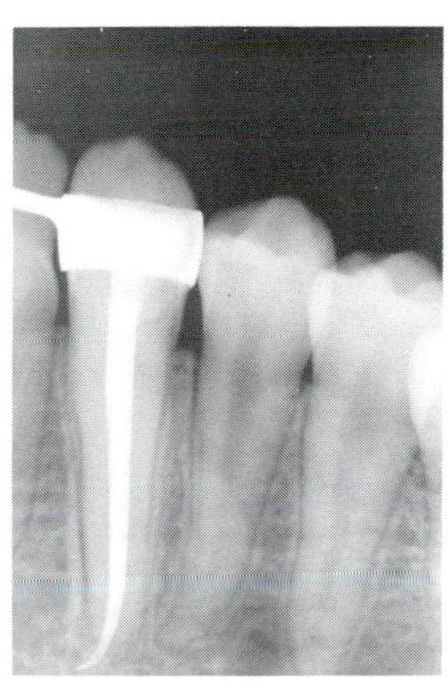

PLATE 7-X-6. Sharp distal curvature at apex.

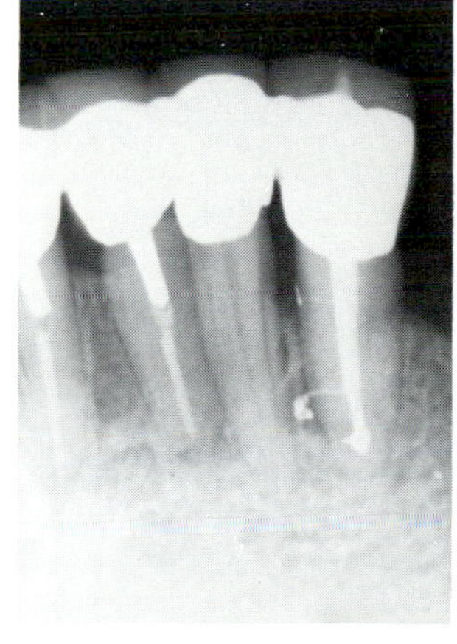

PLATE 7-X-7. Two lateral canals. The incisal canal is above the crest of bone and was probably responsible for pocket depth.

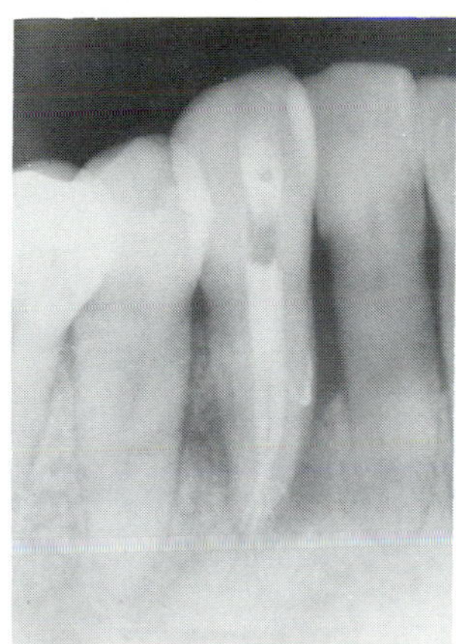

PLATE 7-X-8. Twin-canaled mandibular canine with significant lateral canals feeding a periodontal defect.

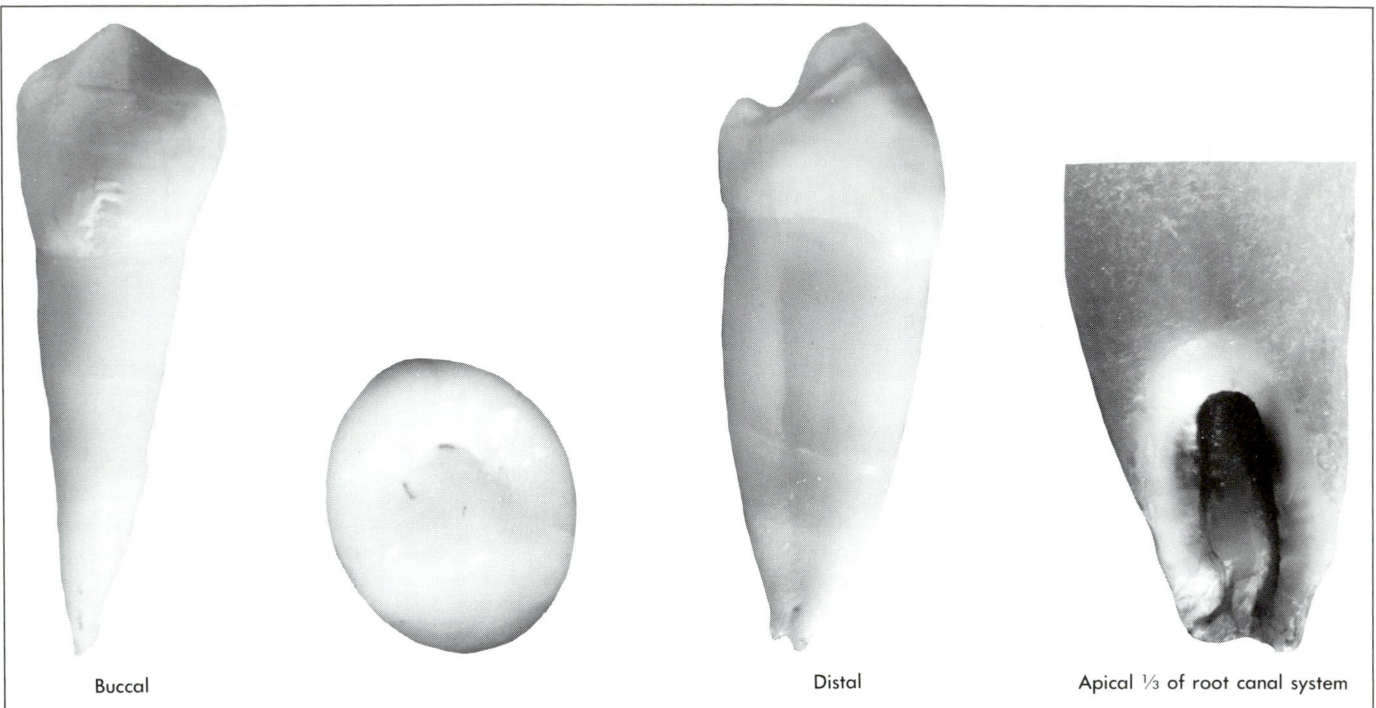

Average time of eruption: 10 to 12 years
Average age of calcification: 12 to 13 years
Average length: 21.6 mm

Often considered an enigma to the endodontist, the mandibular first premolar with dual canals dividing at various levels of the root can generate complex mechanical problems.

The coronal anatomy consists of a well-developed buccal cusp and a small or almost nonexistent lingual outgrowth of enamel. Access is made slightly buccal to the central groove and is directed in the long axis of the root toward the central cervical area. The ovoid pulp chamber is reached with end-cutting fissure burs and long-shanked no. 4 or 6 round burs. The cross section of the cervical pulp chamber is almost round in a single-canal tooth and is ovoid in two-canal teeth.

Another investigation[26] reported that "a second or third canal exists in at least 23% of first mandibular bicuspids." The canals may divide almost anywhere down the root. Because of the absence of direct access, cleaning, shaping, and filling of these teeth can be extremely difficult.

A recent study by Vertucci[20] revealed that the mandibular first premolar had one canal at the apex in 74.0% of the teeth studied, two canals at the apex in 25.5%, and three canals at the apex in the remaining 0.5% (Table 7-2).

TABLE 7-2. Classification and percentage of canal types found in mandibular first and second premolars

Classification	In first premolars (%)	In second premolars (%)
One canal at apex		
Type 1	70.0	97.5
Type 2	4.0	0.0
Of total	74.0	97.5
Two canals at apex		
Type 3	1.5	0.0
Type 4	24.0	2.5
Of total	25.5	2.5
Three canals at apex		
Type 5	0.5	0.0
Of total	0.5	0.0

From Vertucci FJ: J Am Dent Assoc 97:47, 1978.

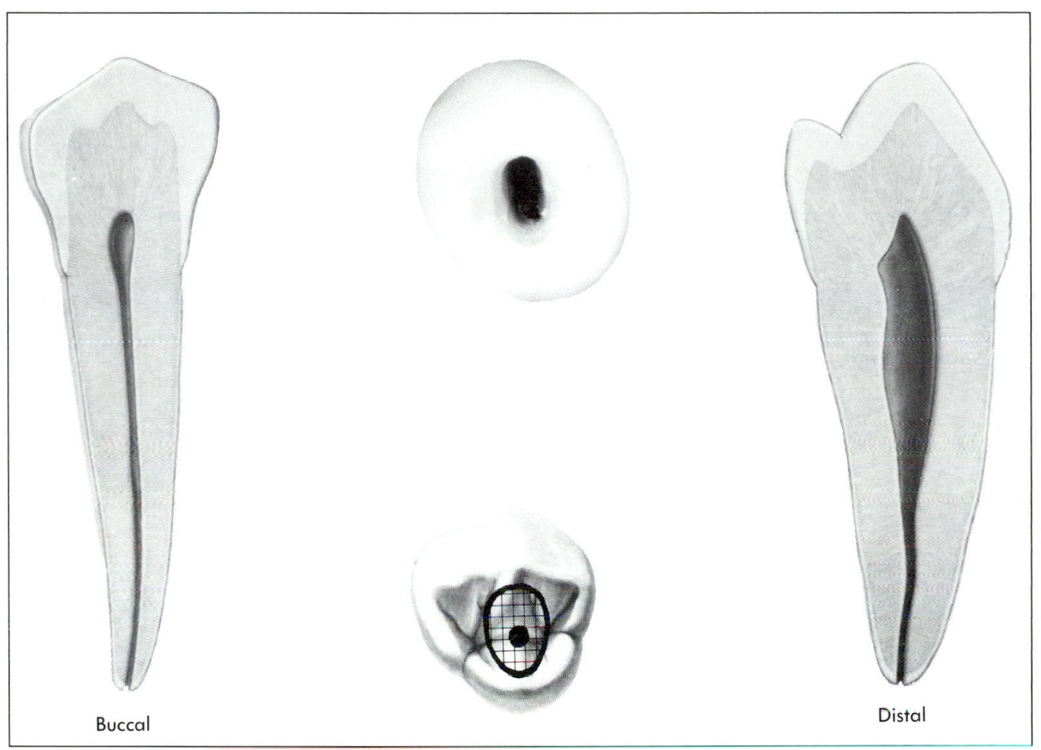

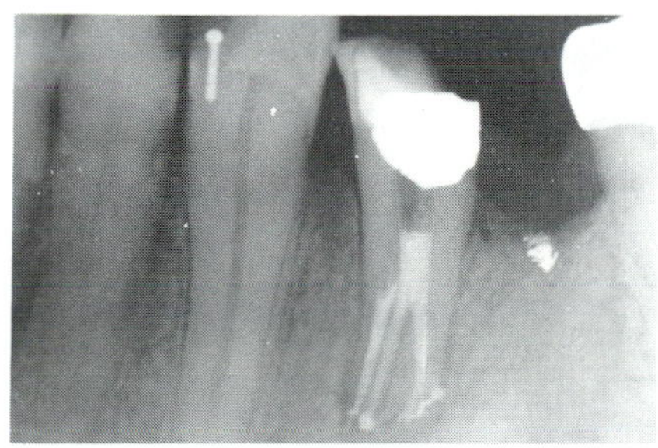

PLATE 7-XI-5. Three-rooted mandibular first bicuspid.

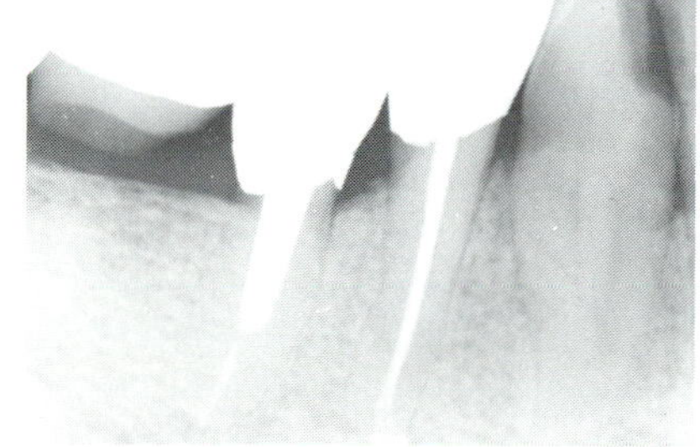

PLATE 7-XI-6. Single canal dividing at apex.

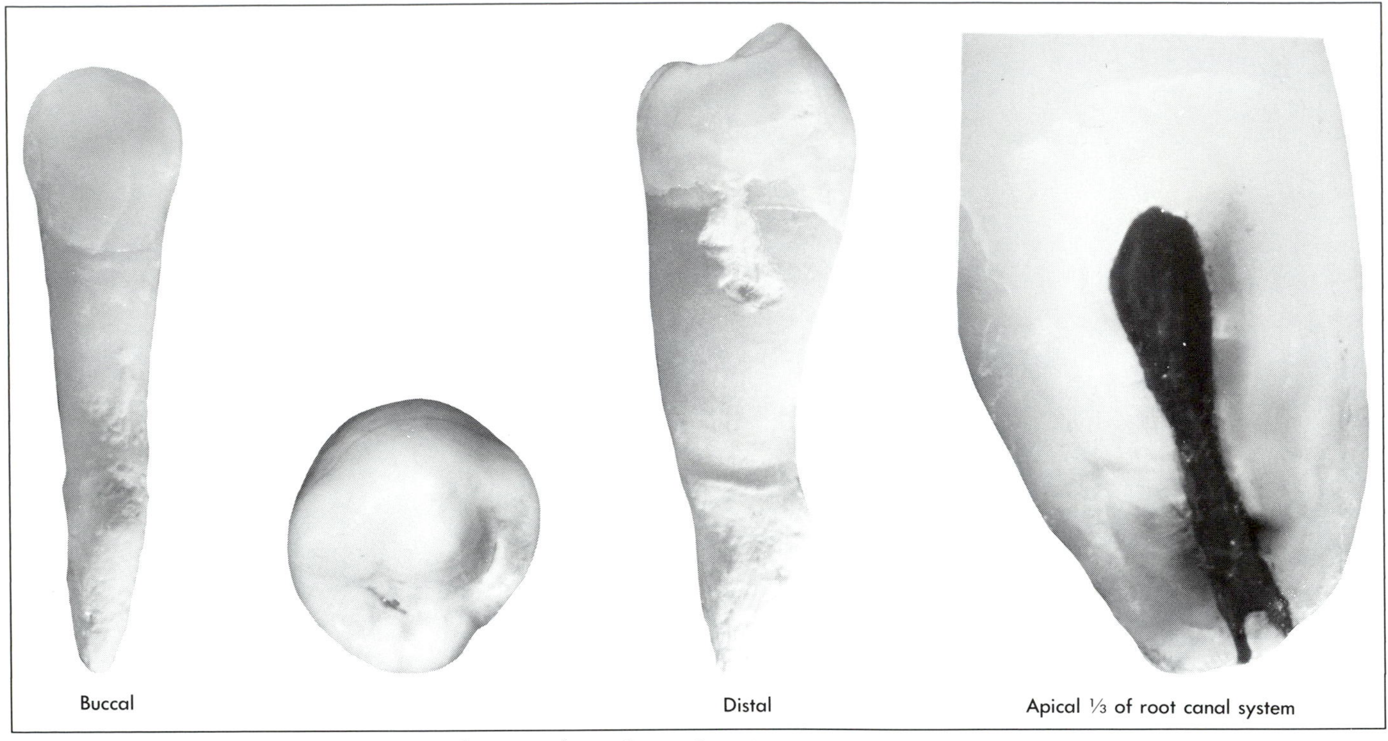

Average time of eruption: 11 to 12 years
Average age of calcification: 13 to 14 years
Average length: 22.3 mm

Very similar coronally to the first premolar, the mandibular second premolar presents less of a radicular problem.

Its crown has a well-developed buccal cusp and a much better-formed lingual cusp than in the first premolar. Access is made slightly ovoid, wider in the mesial-distal dimension. The first opening, with the end-cutting fissure bur, is made approximately in the central groove and is extended and refined with no. 4 and 6 round burs.

Investigators[26] reported that only 12% of mandibular second molars studied had a second or third canal. Vertucci[20] also showed that the second premolar had one canal at the apex in 97.5% and two canals at the apex in only 2.5% of the teeth studied. In 1991, Bram and Fleisher[3] reported a case of four distinct canals.

An important consideration that must not be overlooked is the anatomic position of the mental foramen and the neurovascular structures that pass through it. The proximity of these nerves and blood vessels when acute exacerbation of the mandibular premolars occurs can result in temporary paresthesia from the fulminating inflammatory process. Exacerbations in this region seem to be intense and more resistant to nonsurgical therapy than in other parts of the mouth.

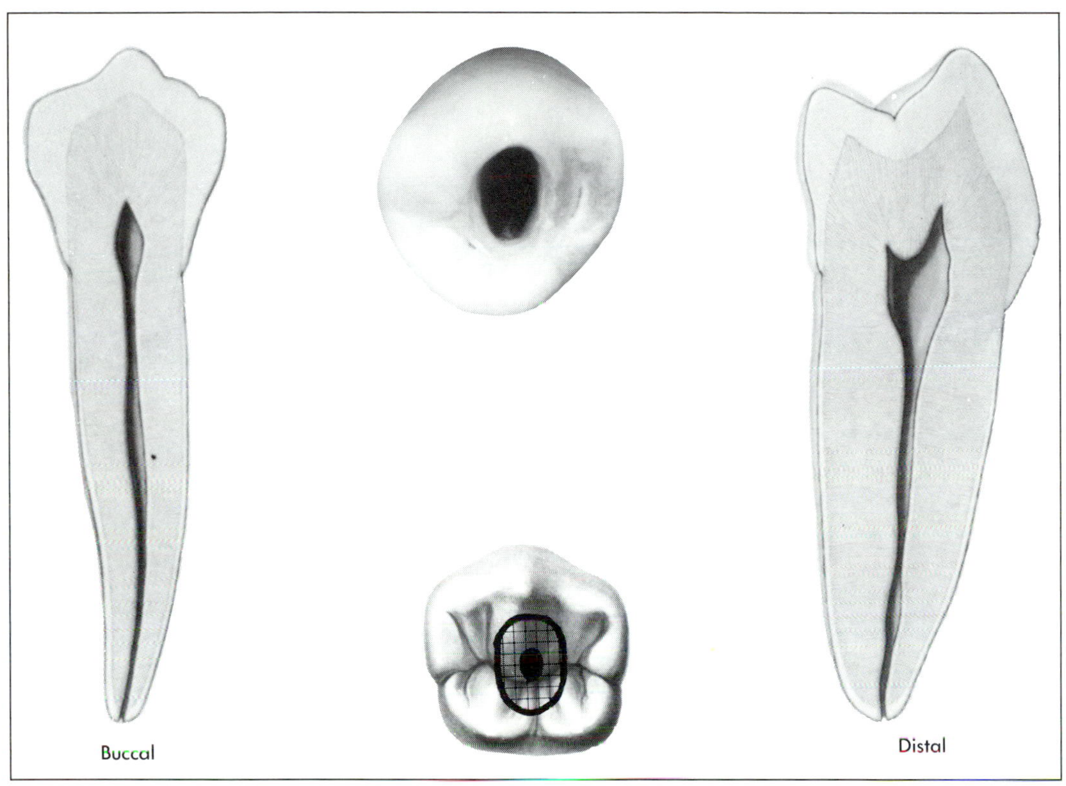

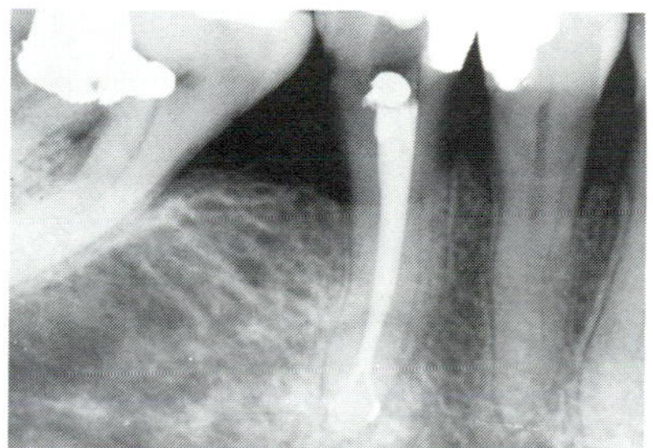

PLATE 7-XII-5. Single canal dividing at apex.

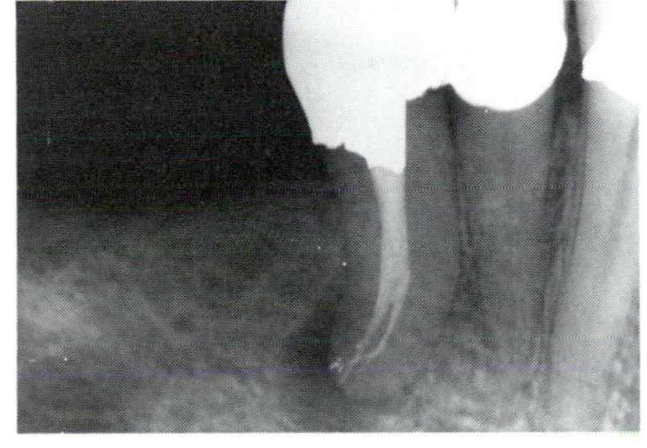

PLATE 7-XII-6. Single canal dividing and crossing over at apex.

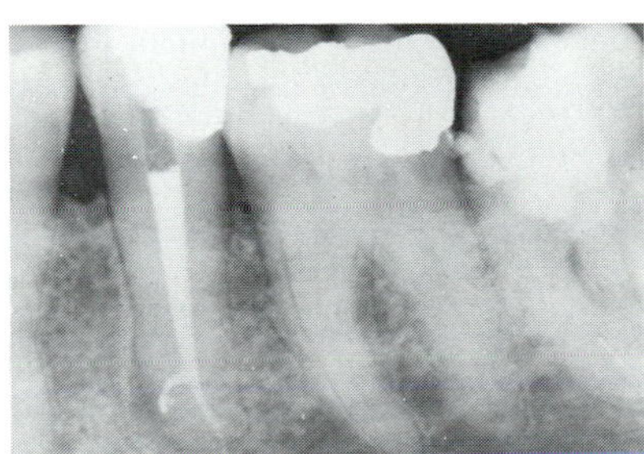

PLATE 7-XII-7. Single canal with lateral accessory canal.

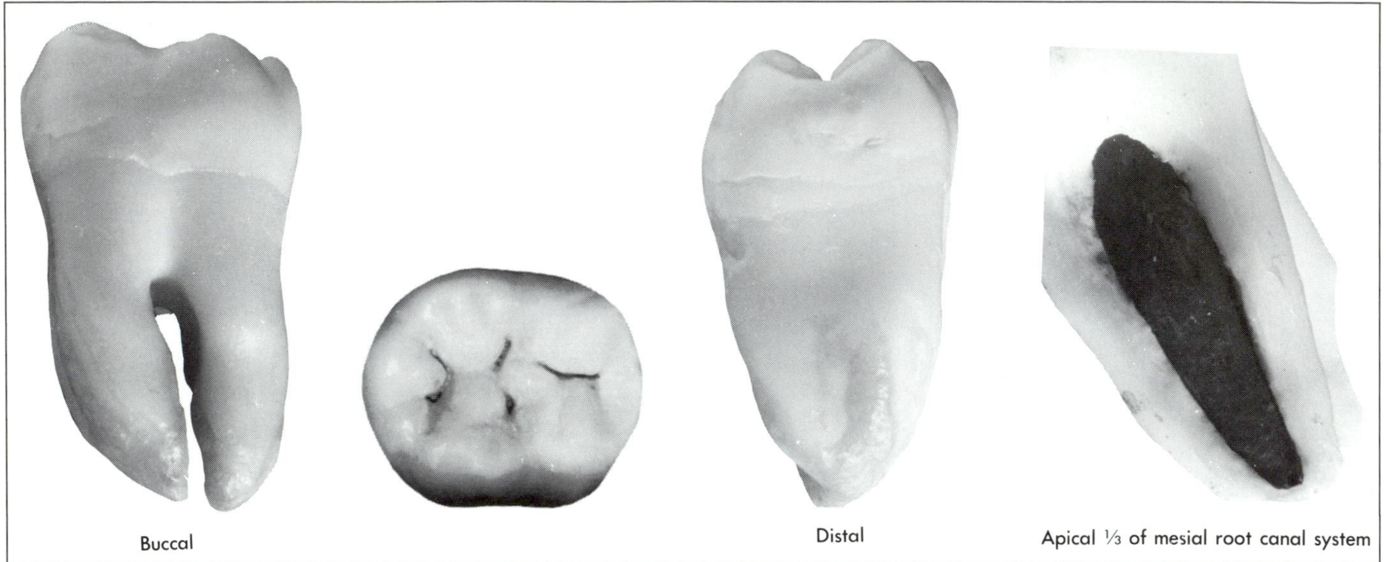

Average time of eruption: 6 years
Average age of calcification: 9 to 10 years
Average length: 21.0 mm

The earliest permanent posterior tooth to erupt, the mandibular first molar seems to be the most frequently in need of endodontic treatment. It usually has two roots but occasionally three, with two canals in the mesial and one or two canals in the distal root.

The distal root is readily accessible to endodontic cavity preparation and mechanical instrumentation, and the clinician can frequently see directly into the orifice(s). The canals of the distal root are larger than those of the mesial root. Occasionally the orifice is wide from buccal to lingual. This anatomy indicates the possibility of a second canal or a ribbonlike canal with a complex webbing that can complicate cleaning and shaping.

The mesial roots are usually curved, with the greatest curvature in the mesial-buccal canal. The orifices are usually well separated within the main pulp chamber and occur in the buccal and lingual under the cusp tips.

This tooth is often extensively restored. It is almost always under heavy occlusal stress; thus the coronal pulp chambers are frequently calcified. The distal canals are easiest to locate; once these locations are positively identified, the mesial canals will be found in the aforementioned locations in the same horizontal plane.

Because the mesial canal openings lie under the mesial cusps, they may be impossible to locate with conventional cavity preparations. It will then be necessary to remove cuspal hard tissue or restoration to locate the orifice. As part of the access preparation, the unsupported cusps of posterior teeth must be reduced.[22] Remember, this tooth, like all posterior teeth, should always receive full occlusal coverage after endodontic therapy (see Chapter 22). Therefore a wider access cavity to locate landmarks and orifices is better than ignoring one or more canals for the sake of a "conservative" preparation, which may lead to failure.

Skidmore and Bjorndal[18] stated that approximately one third of the mandibular first molars studied had four root canals. When a tooth contained two canals, "they either remained two distinct canals with separate apical foramina, united and formed a common apical foramen, or communicated with each other partially or completely by transverse anastomoses. . . . If the traditional triangular outline were changed to a more rectangular one, it would permit better visualization and exploration of a possible fourth canal in the distal root."

Multiple accessory foramina are located in the furcation areas of mandibular molars.[13] They are usually impossible to clean and shape directly and are rarely seen, except occasionally on postoperative radiographs if they have been filled with root canal sealer or warmed gutta-percha. It would be proper to assume that if irrigating solutions have the property of "seeking out" and disposing of protein degeneration products, then the furcation area of the pulp chamber should be thoroughly exposed (calcific adhesions removed, etc.) to allow the solutions to reach the tiny openings.

All caries, leaking restorations, and pulpal calcifications must be removed prior to endodontic treatment, and full cuspal protection and internal reinforcement are recommended.

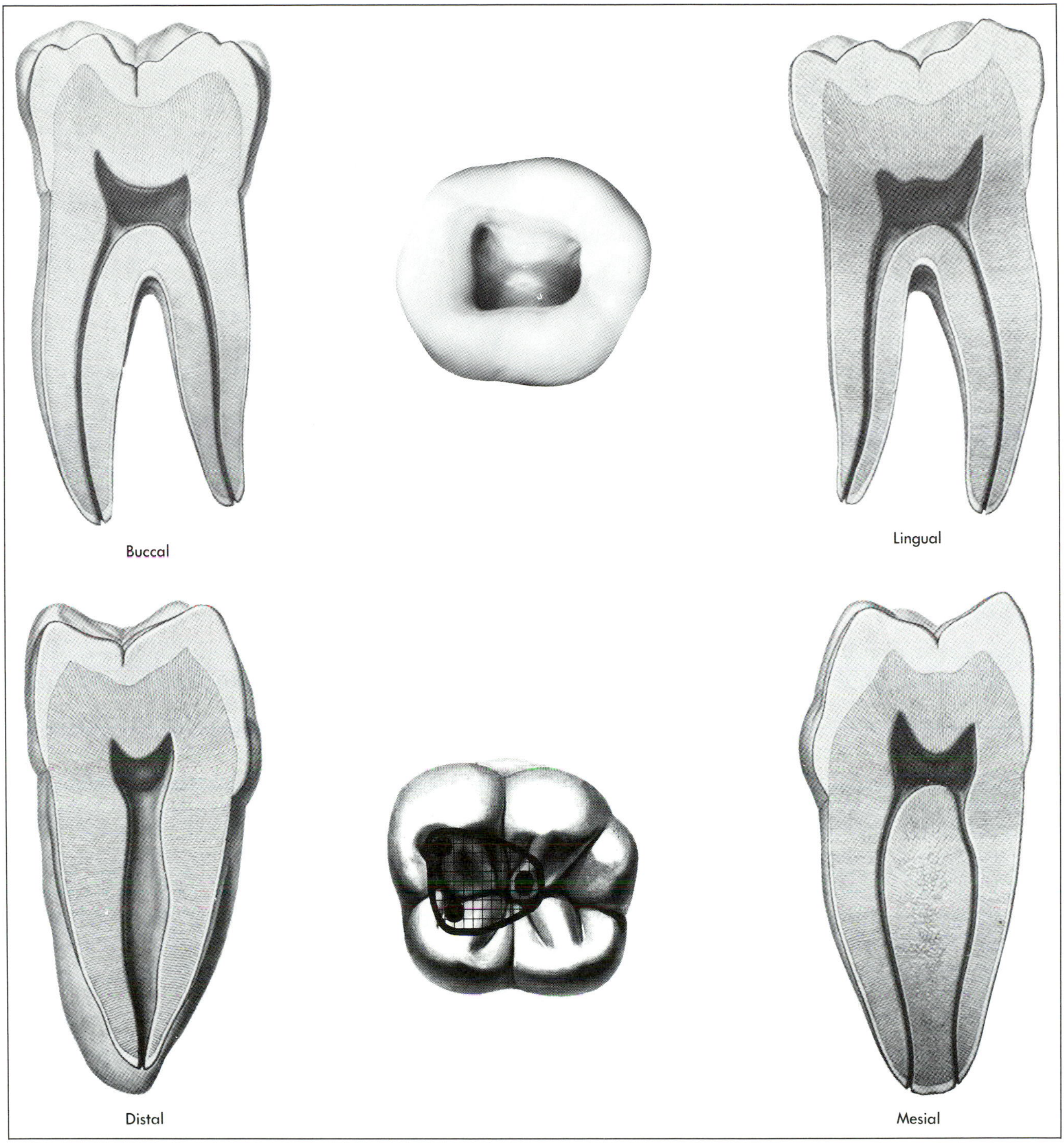

Buccal

Lingual

Distal

Mesial

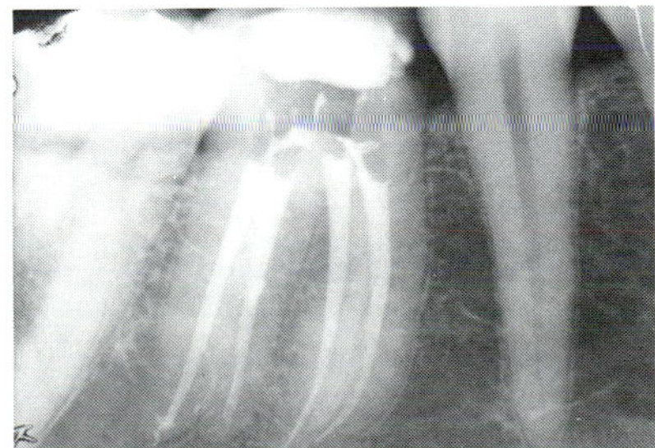

PLATE 7-XIII-7. Mandibular first molar with four roots.

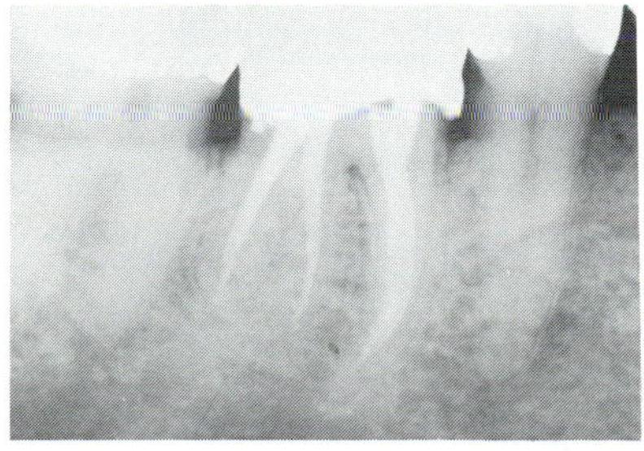

PLATE 7-XIII-8. Mandibular first molar with four roots with wide division of the distal roots.

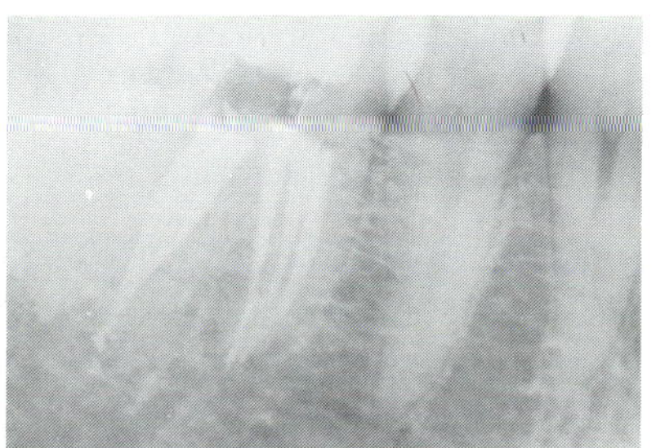

PLATE 7-XIII-9. Mandibular first molar with three mesial canals.

Mandibular Second Molar

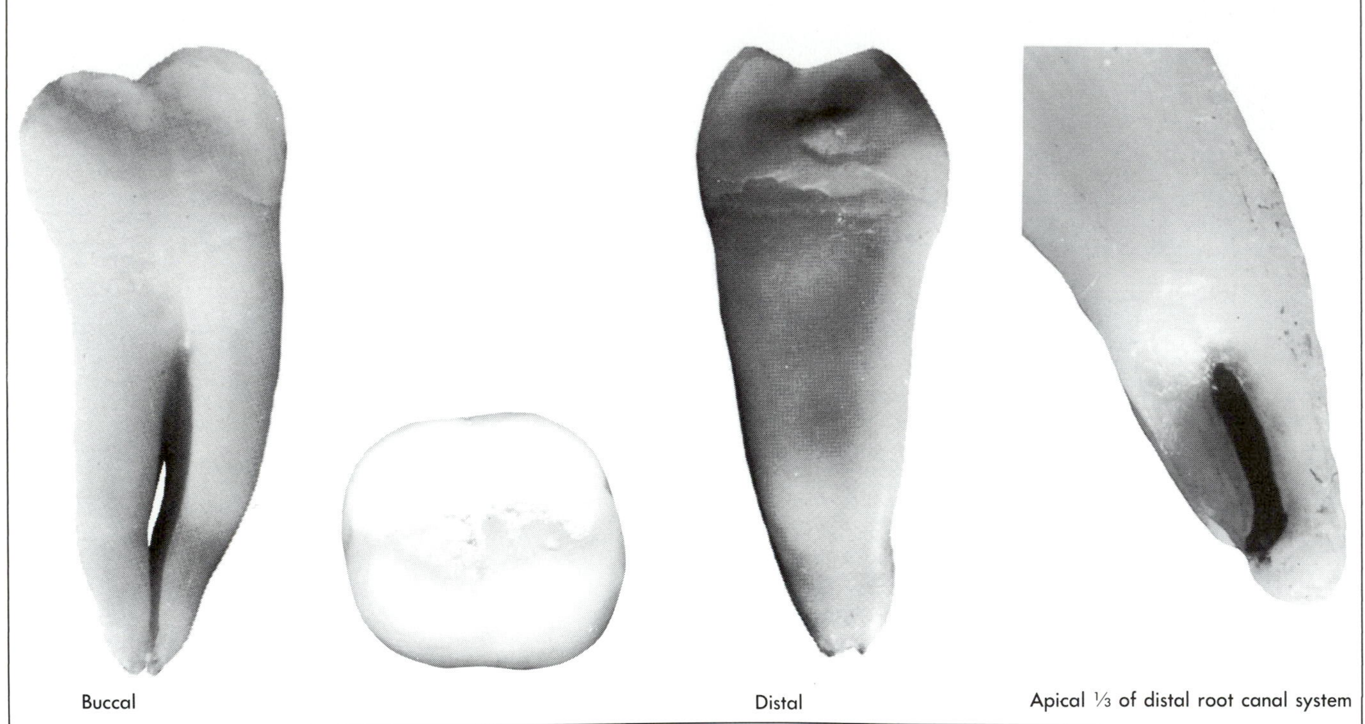

Average time of eruption: 11 to 13 years
Average age of calcification: 14 to 15 years
Average length: 19.8 mm

Somewhat smaller coronally than the mandibular first molar and tending toward more symmetry, the mandibular second molar is identified by the proximity of its roots. The roots often sweep distally in a gradual curve with the apices close together. The degree and configuration of canal curvature were studied in the mesial roots of 100 randomly selected mandibular first and second molars. One hundred percent of the specimens demonstrated curvature in both buccal-lingual and mesial-distal views.[6]

Access is made in the mesial aspect of the crown, with the opening extending only slightly distal to the central groove. After penetration with the end-cutting fissure bur, the long-shanked round bur is used to sweep outwardly until unobstructed access is achieved. The distal angulation of the roots often permits less extension of the opening than in the mandibular first molar.

Close attention should be given to the shape of the distal orifice. A narrow, ovoid opening indicates a ribbon-shaped distal canal, requiring more directional-type filing.

All caries, leaking fillings, and pulpal calcifications must be removed and replaced with a suitable temporary restoration prior to endodontic therapy.

The mandibular second molar is the most susceptible to vertical fracture. After access preparation the clinician should utilize the fiberoptic light to search the floor of the chamber prior to endodontic treatment. The prognosis of mesial-distal crown-root fractures is very poor.

Full occlusal coverage after endodontic therapy is mandatory to ensure against future problems with vertical fracture.

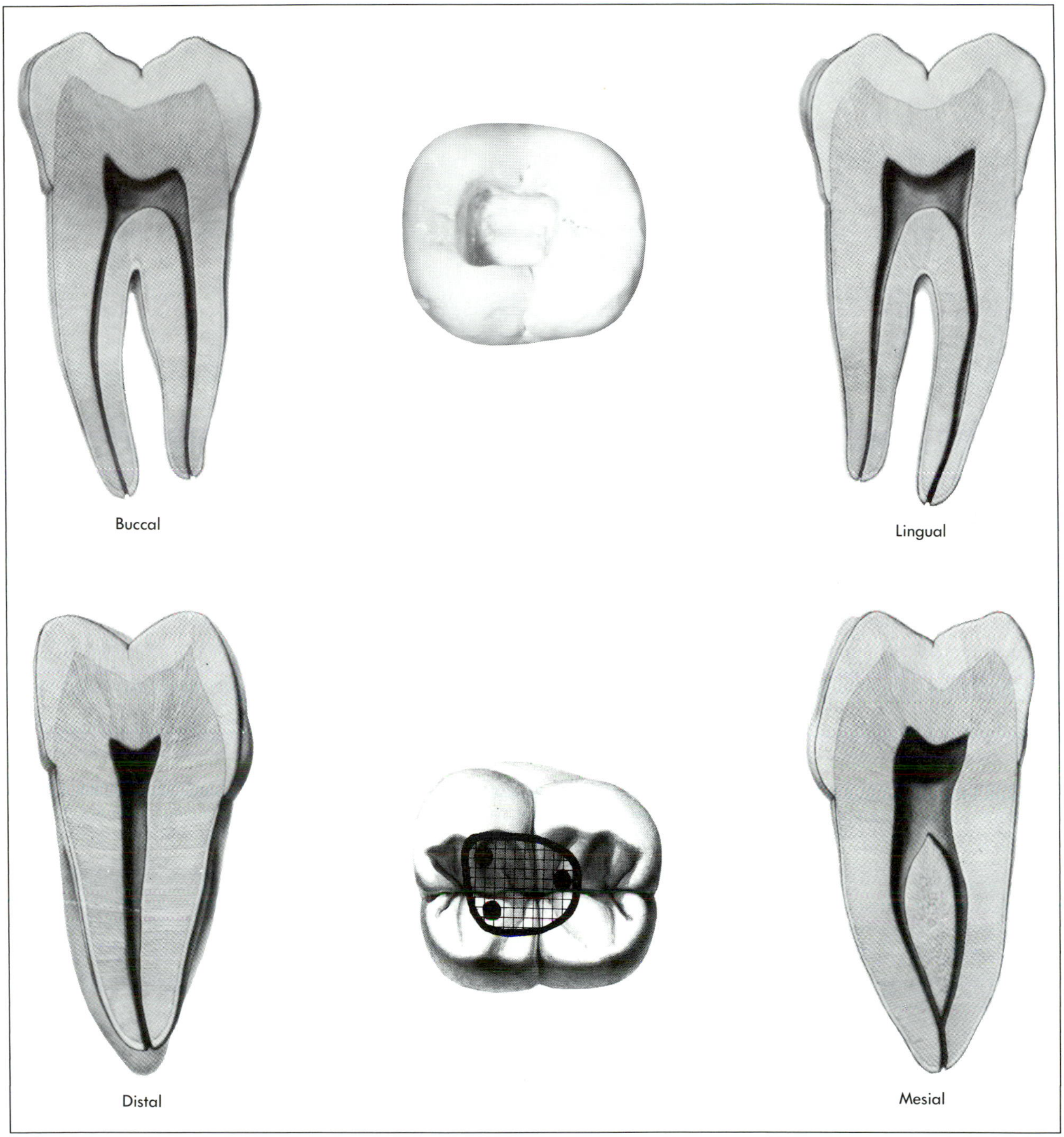

Buccal

Lingual

Distal

Mesial

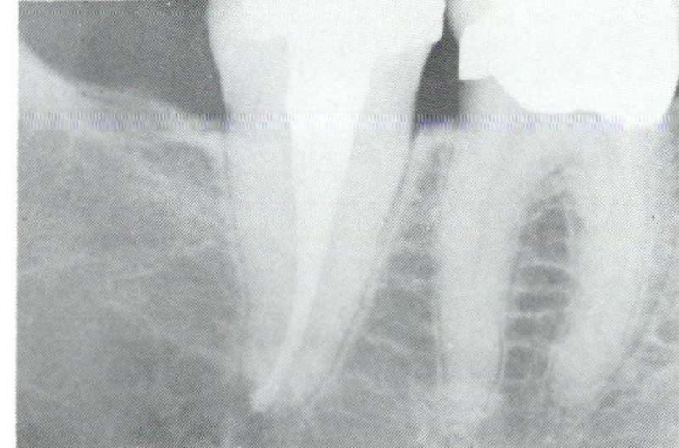

PLATE 7-XIV-8. Mandibular second molar with anastamosis of all canals into one.

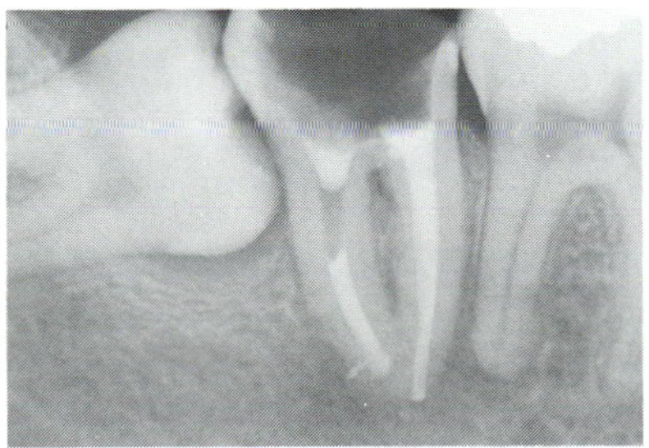

PLATE 7-XIV-9. Accessory canal at distal root apex.

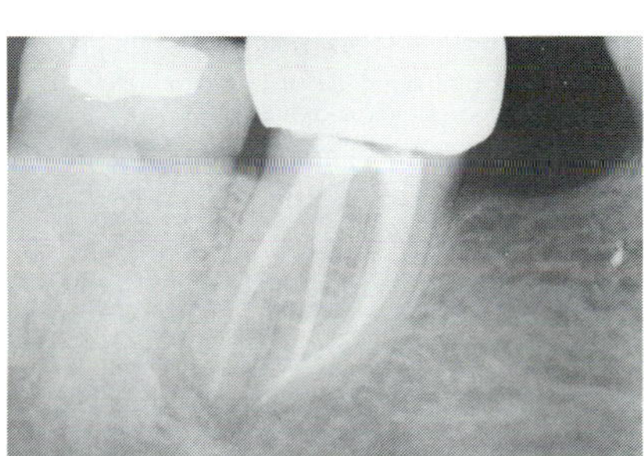

PLATE 7-XIV-10. Fusion of mesial canals at mesial root apex.

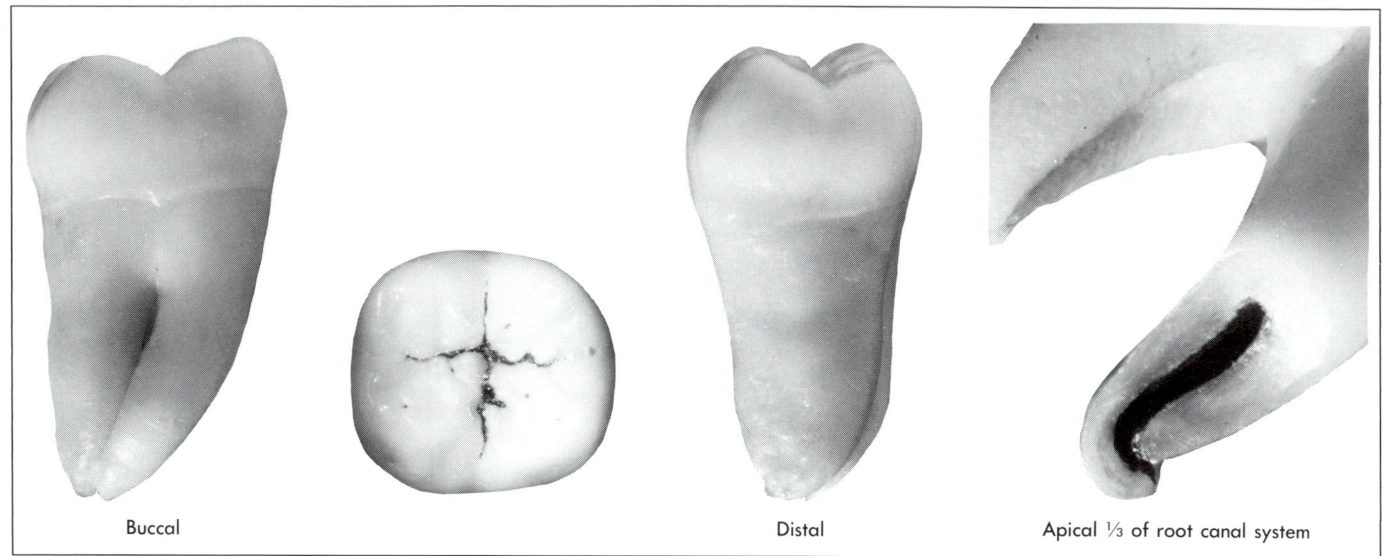

Average time of eruption: 17 to 21 years
Average age of calcification: 18 to 25 years
Average length: 18.5 mm

Anatomically unpredictable, the mandibular third molar must be evaluated on the basis of its root formation. Well-formed crowns are often supported by fused, short, severely curved, or malformed roots. Most teeth can be successfully treated endodontically, regardless of anatomic irregularities, but root surface volume in contact with bone is what determines long-term prognosis.

The clinician may find a single canal that is wide at the neck and tapers to a single apical foramen. Access is gained through the mesial aspect of the crown. Distally angulated roots often permit less extension of the access cavity. Difficult accessibility in the arch occasionally can be simplified by the use of engine-mounted files on reciprocal handpieces.

All caries, leaking restorations, and pulpal calcifications should be removed and replaced with adequate temporary restoration. If the tooth is in heavy occlusal function, full cuspal protection is indicated postendodontically.

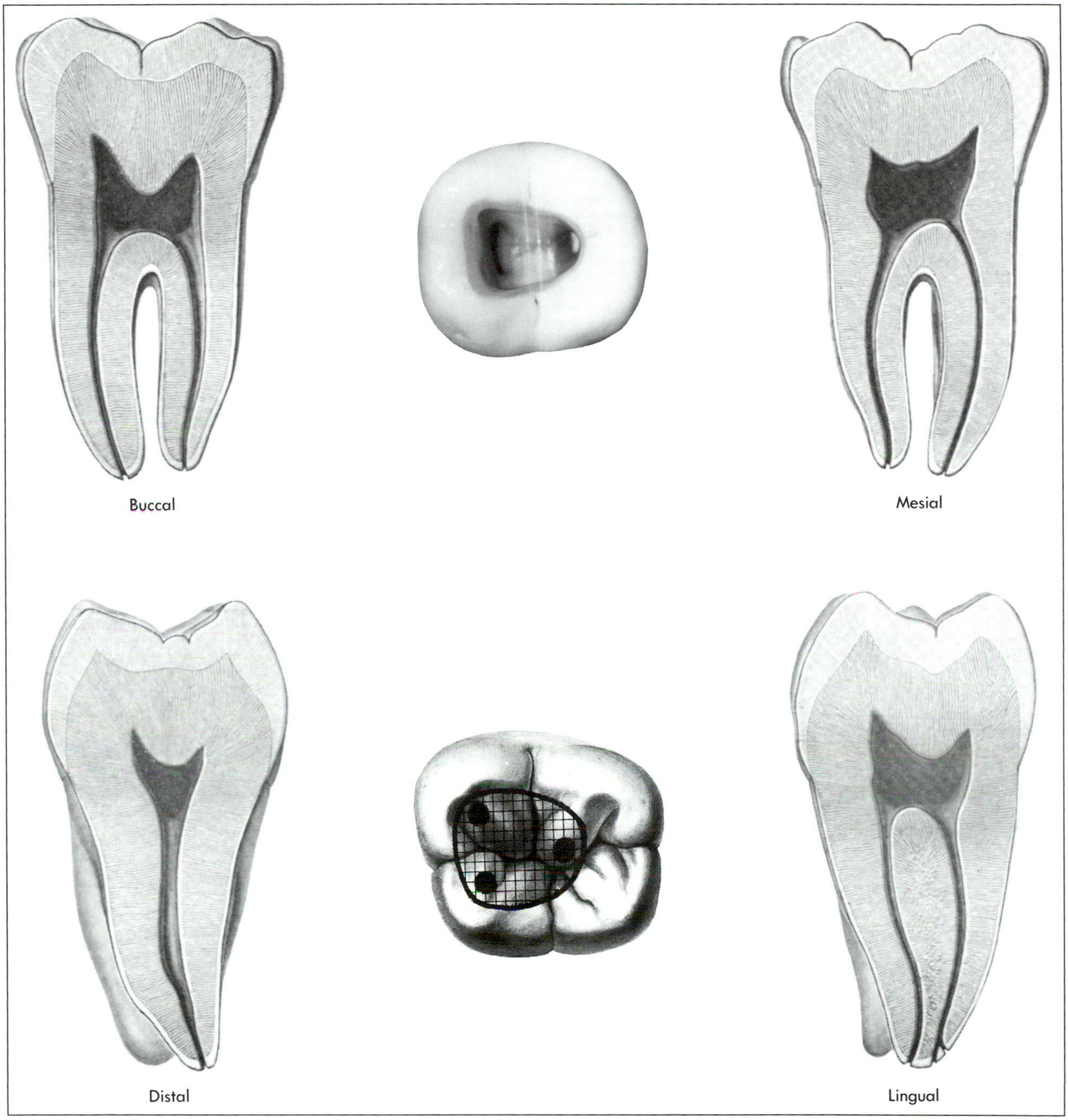

Buccal

Mesial

Distal

Lingual

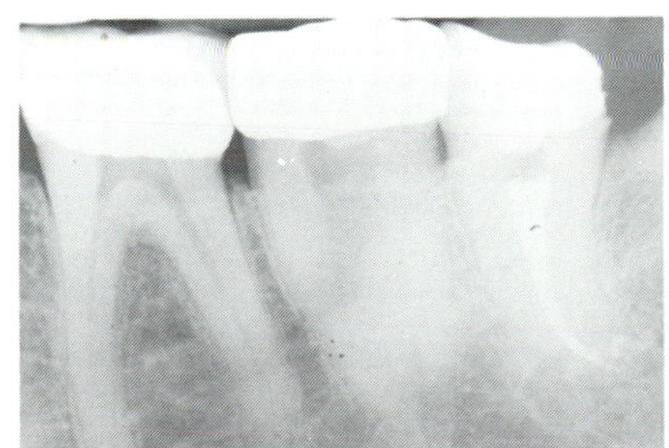

PLATE 7-XV-7. Third molar with accessory foramina at apex.

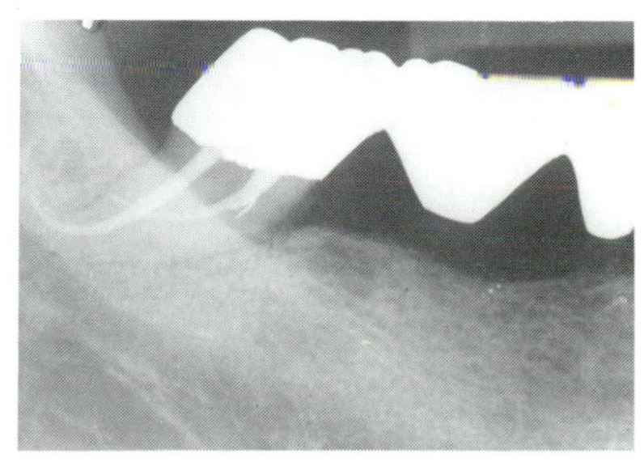

PLATE 7-XV-8. Complex curved root anatomy.

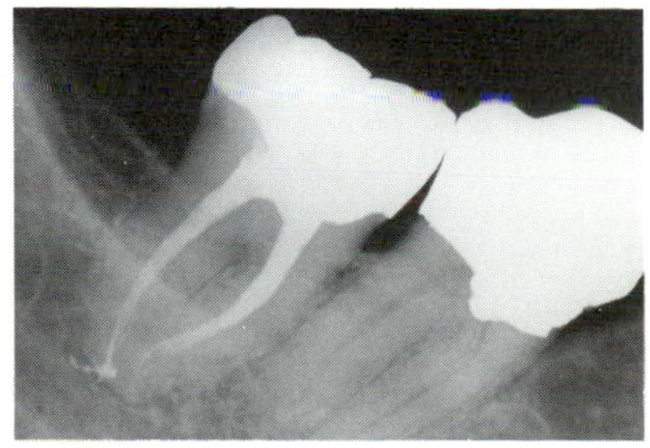

PLATE 7-XV-9. Complex apical anatomy.

The C-Shaped Mandibular Molar

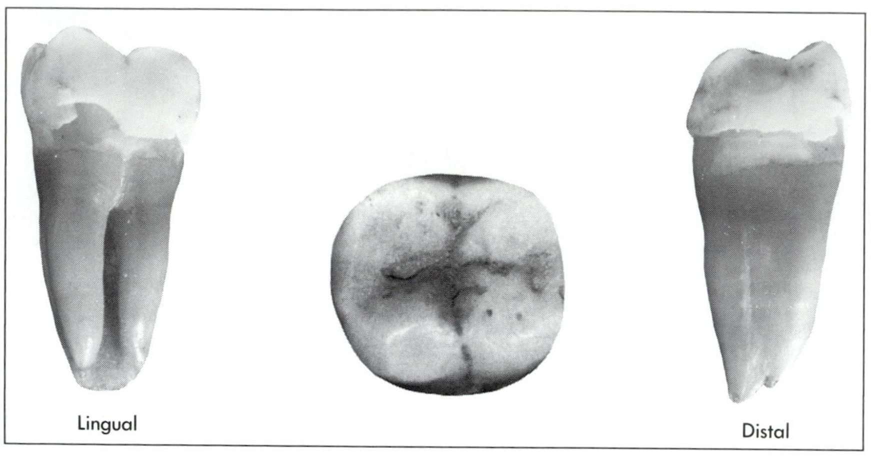

The C-shaped molar is so named for the cross-sectional morphology of the root and root canal. Instead of having several discrete orifices, the pulp chamber of the C-shaped molar has a single ribbon-shaped orifice with a 180-degree arc, starting at the mesial-lingual line angle, sweeping around the buccal to end at the distal aspect of the pulp chamber (Plate 7-XVI-2).

Below the orifice level, the root structure of C-shaped molars can harbor a wide range of anatomic variations. These can be classified into two basic groups: (1) those with a single ribbonlike C-shaped canal from orifice to apex and (2) those with three distinct canals below the usual C-shaped orifice.

Fortunately, C-shaped molars with a single swath of canal are the exception rather than the rule. Melton and others[15] found that the C-shaped canals can vary in number and shape along the length of the root, with the result that débridement, obturation, and restoration in this group may be unusually difficult (Plate 7-XVI-6 and 7-XVI-7). More common is the second type of C-shaped molar, with its discrete canals having an unusual form. The mesial-lingual canal is separate and distinct from the apex, although it may be significantly shorter than mesial-buccal and distal canals (Plate 7-XVI-4). These canals are easily overinstrumented in C-shaped molars with a single apex (Plate 7-XVI-5) as they may end 2 to 4 mm short of the apex.

In these molars the mesial-buccal canal swings back and merges with the distal canal, and these exit onto the root surface through a single foramen. A few of these molars with C-shaped orifices have mesial-buccal and distal canals which do not merge, but have separate portals of exit.

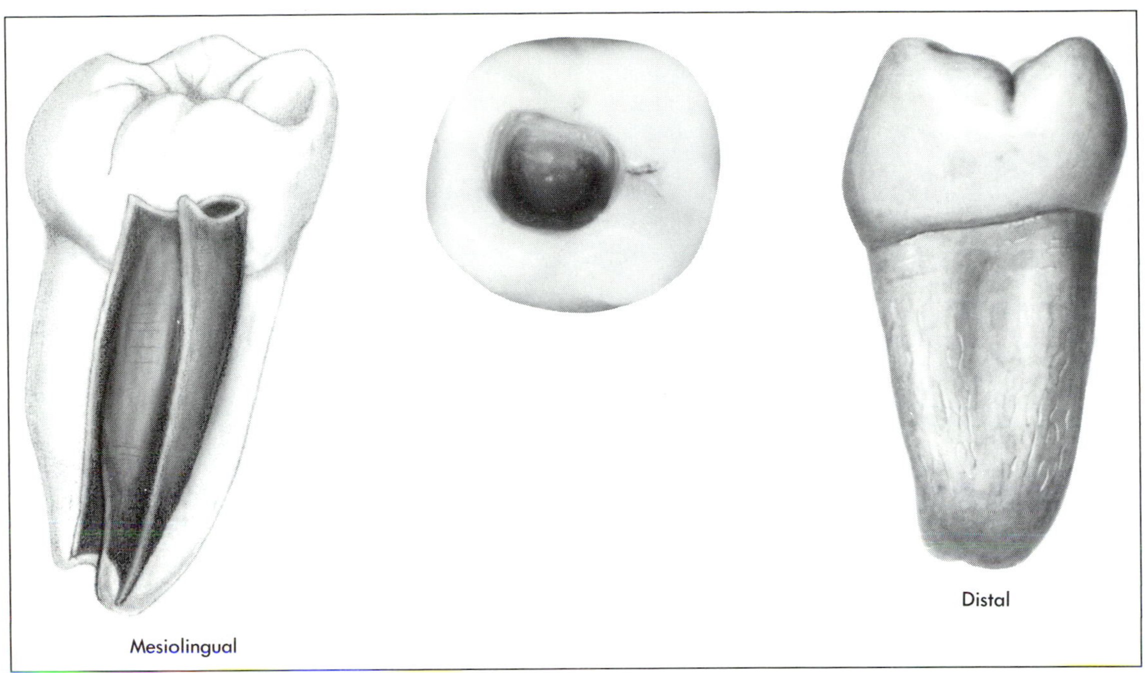

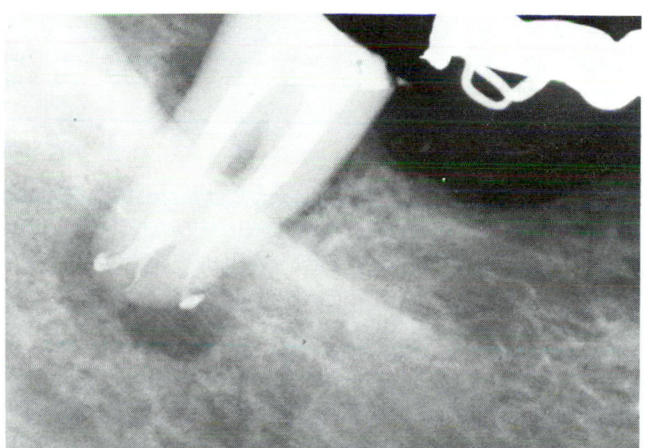

PLATE 7-XVI-4. Mandibular second molar with multiple foramina.

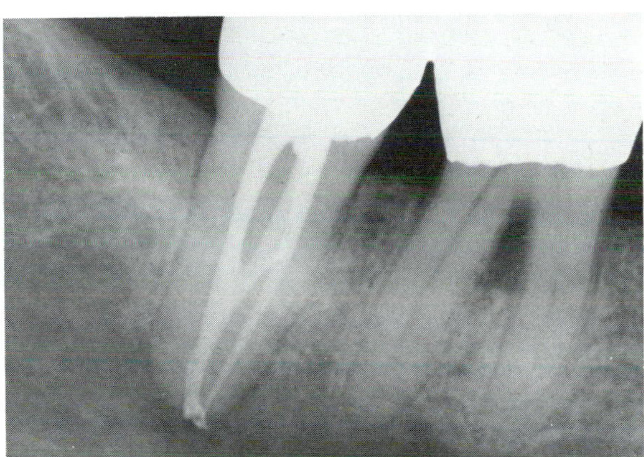

PLATE 7-XVI-5. Mandibular second molar with interconnecting canal anatomy.

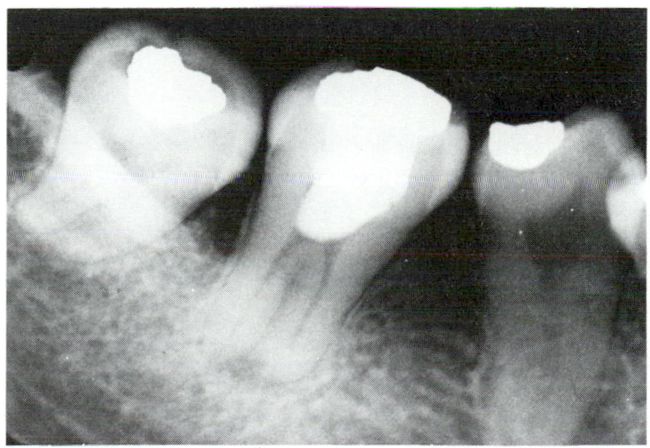

PLATE 7-XVI-6. Preop of mandibular first molar with C-shaped canal.

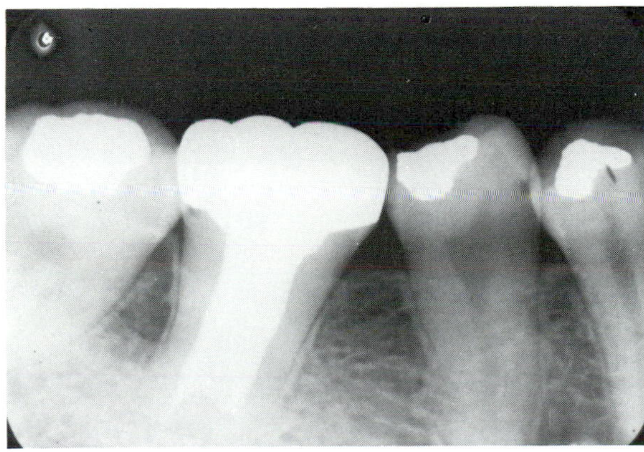

PLATE 7-XVI-7. Finished endodontics showing complete obturation of the ribbon-like canal spaces.

METHODS OF LOCATING CALCIFIED CANALS

Preoperative radiographs (Fig. 7-10) often appear to reveal total, or nearly total, calcification of the main pulp chamber and radicular canal spaces. Unfortunately, the spaces have adequate room to allow passage of millions of microorganisms. The narrowing of these pulpal pathways is often caused by chronic inflammatory processes such as caries, medications, occlusal trauma, and aging.

Despite severe coronal calcification, the clinician must assume that all canals exist and must be cleaned, shaped, and filled to the canal terminus. It has been demonstrated that canals become less calcified as they approach the root apex. There are many methods of locating these spaces (Figs. 7-11 to 7-29). It is recommended that the illustrated sequences be followed to achieve the most successful result.

In the event of inability to locate the canal orifice(s), the prudent clinician will stop excavating dentin lest the tooth structure be weakened. Retrograde procedures become conservative when compared with perforations or root fractures. There is no rapid technique for dealing with calcified cases. Painstaking removal of small amounts of dentin has proven to be the safest approach.

Text continued on p. 173.

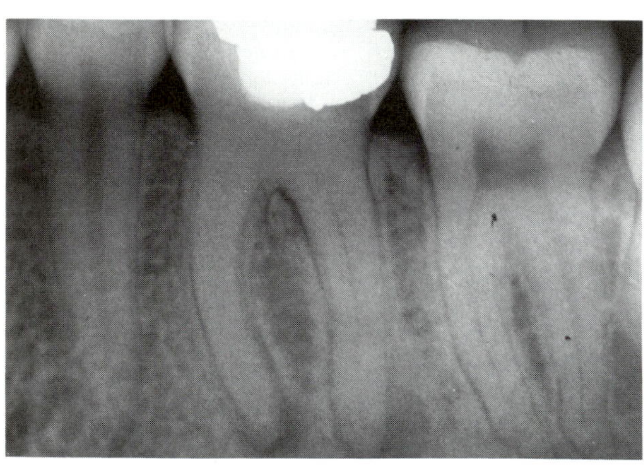

FIG. 7-10 Radiograph of a nonvital mandibular molar with calcified canals.

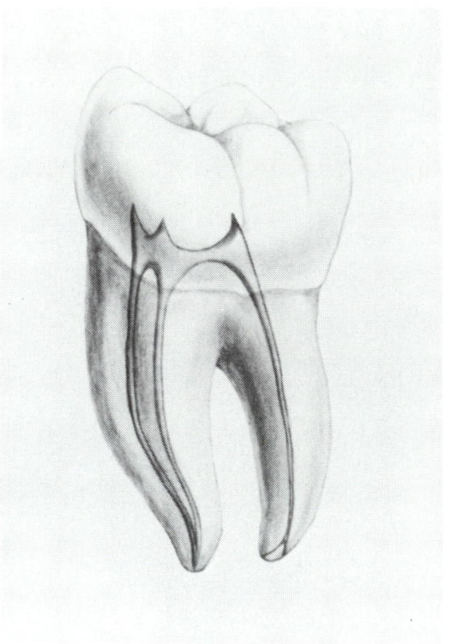

FIG. 7-12 Mandibular first molar with normal pulp chambers.

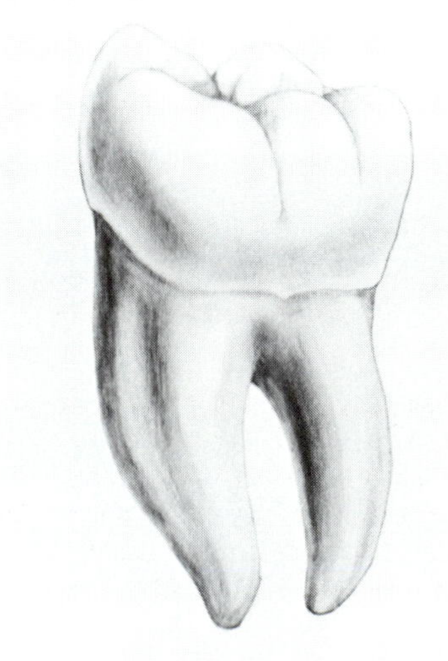

FIG. 7-11 Exterior view of mandibular first permanent molar.

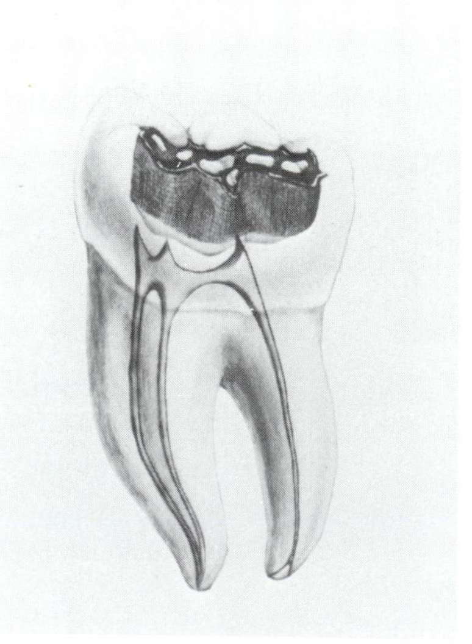

FIG. 7-13 Mandibular first molar with class I amalgam restoration and normal pulp chambers.

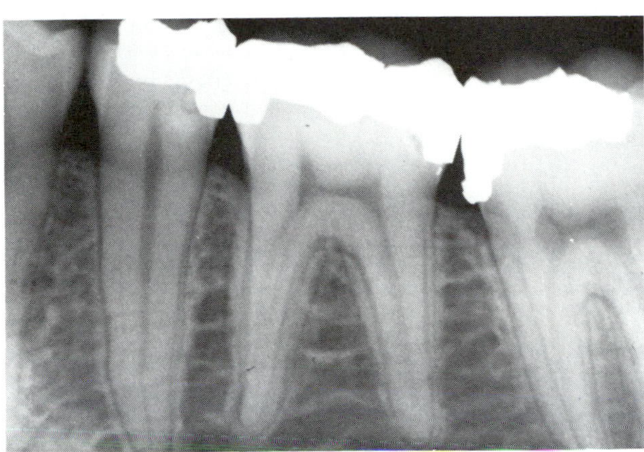

FIG. 7-14 Radiograph of actual case taken in 1976 at the time of first symptoms. The tooth was not treated endodontically because tests showed it to be vital. Caries was removed from under mesial amalgam, calcium hydroxide was placed.

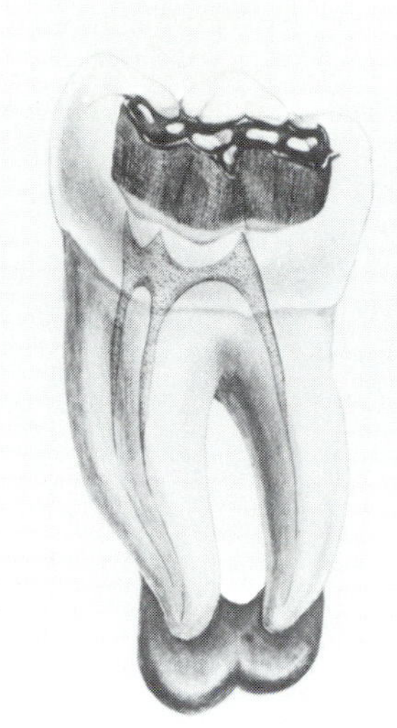

FIG. 7-16 Mandibular first molar with a class I amalgam, calcified canals, and periapical radiolucency. The assumption is that a pulpal exposure has occurred, causing calcification and, ultimately, necrosis of the pulp tissue.

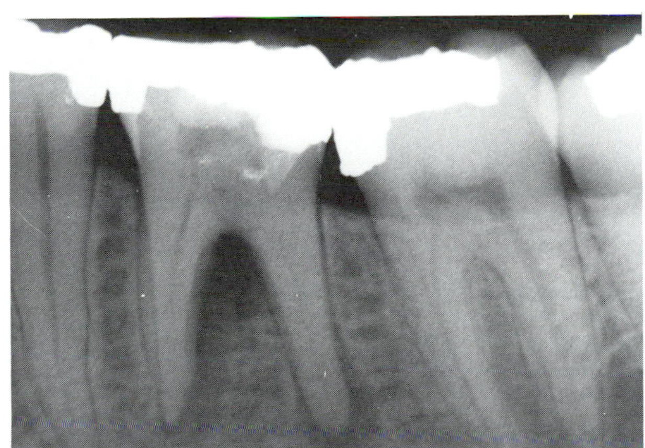

FIG. 7-15 Radiograph of tooth in Figure 7-14 taken in 1989 reveals severe calcification of the pulp chambers and periapical and furcal radiolucencies.

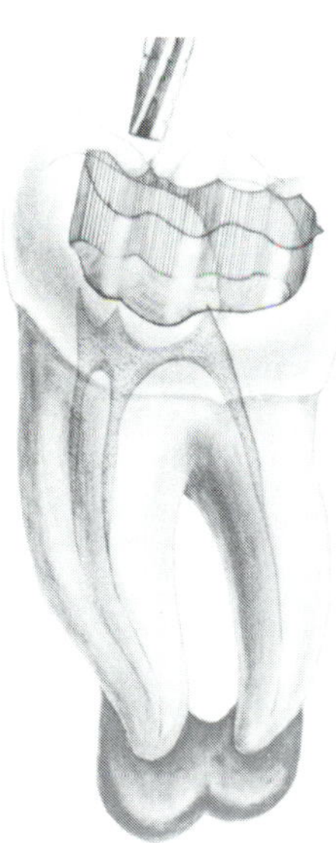

FIG. 7-17 Illustration showing excavation of amalgam and base material. The cavity preparation should be extended toward the assumed location of the pulp chamber. At this phase of treatment the clinician must attempt to provide maximum visibility of the roof of the main chamber. All caries, cements, and discolored dentin should be removed.

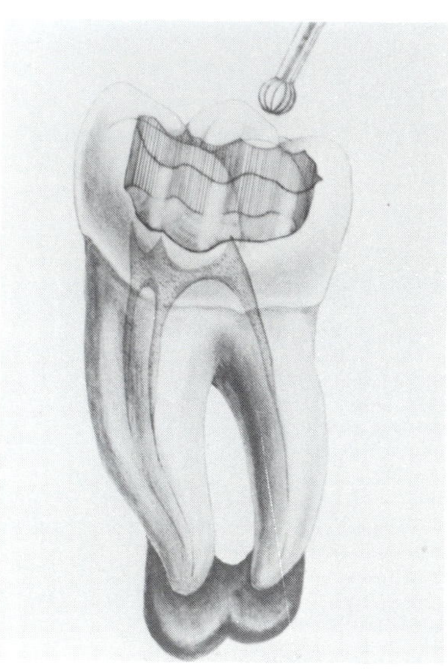

FIG. 7-18 Using a long-shank no. 4 or 6 round bur, the assumed location of the main pulp chamber is explored.

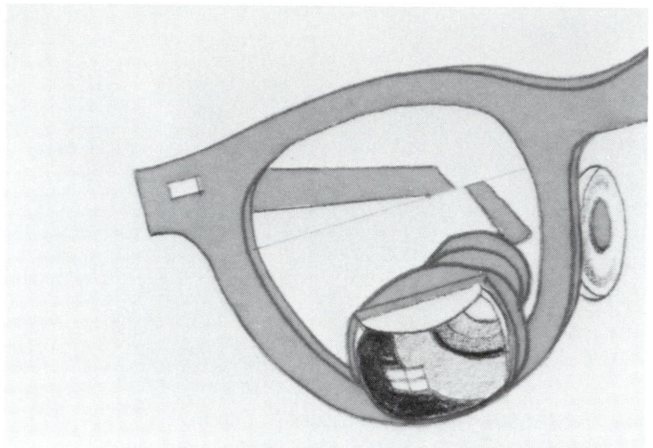

FIG. 7-20 High-magnification eyeglasses, loupes, or the operating microscope are helpful in searching for anatomic landmarks. Even apparently totally calcified main pulp chambers leave a "tattoo," or a retained outline, in the dentin. The shape of the pulp chamber in the mandibular first molar will be roughly triangular or rectangular. The canal orifices are usually found closest to the points of the triangle or the corners of the rectangle. Other landmarks are the cusp tips (if they remain). The orifices often lie directly beneath them.

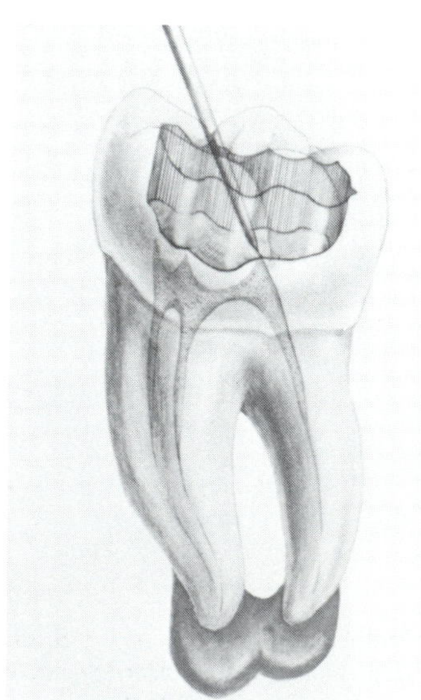

FIG. 7-19 The endodontic explorer, DG 16 (HU-Friedy), is used to explore the region of the pulpal floor. It is as important to the clinician doing endodontics as the periodontal probe is to the dentist performing periodontal diagnosis. It is an examining instrument and a chipping tool, often being called upon to "flake away" calcified dentin. Reparative dentin is slightly softer than normal dentin. A slight "tug back" in the area of the canal orifice often signals the presence of a canal.

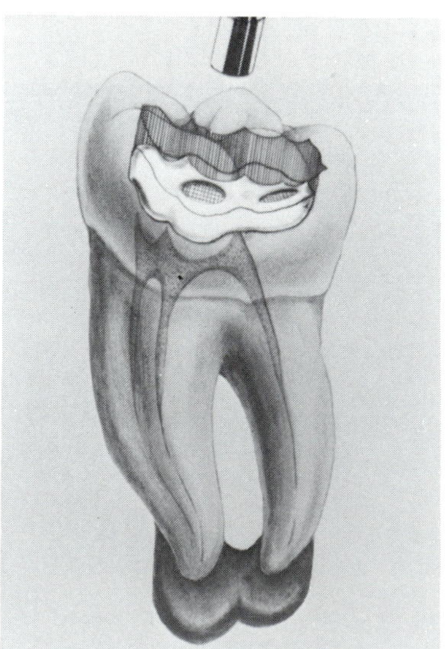

FIG. 7-21 As excavation proceeds apically, it is advisable to check the proximity of the furcation. One technique is to place warmed baseplate gutta-percha in the chamber floor with an amalgam plugger. An angled bitewing radiograph reveals the amount of dentin remaining.

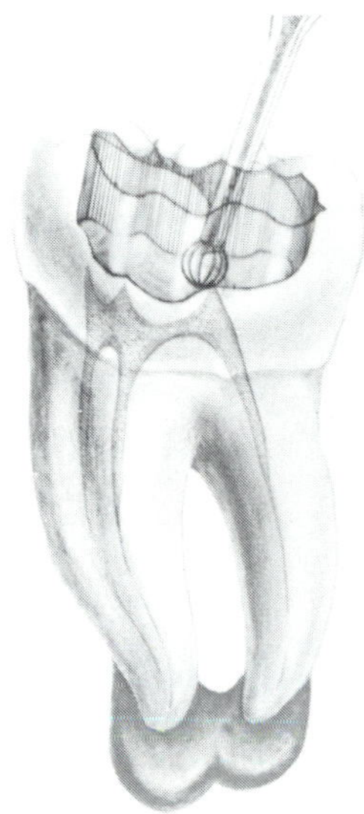

FIG. 7-22 Deeper excavation with no. 4 and 2 round burs, following landmarks (removal of the rubber dam can often assist), will usually produce a small orifice.

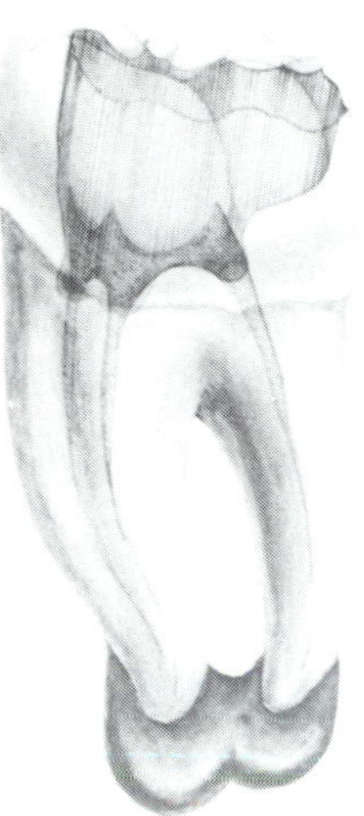

FIG. 7-24 Excavation extended apically in the direction of the root apices.

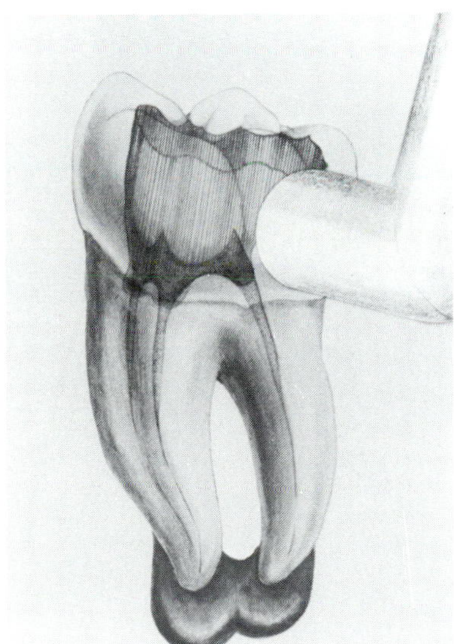

FIG. 7-23 As an adjunct to maximum visibility with magnification, the fiberoptic light can be applied to the buccal or lingual aspect of the crown. Transillumination often reveals landmarks otherwise invisible to the naked eye.

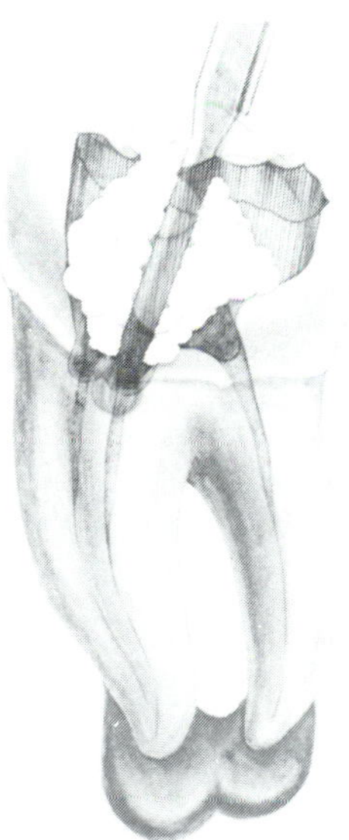

FIG. 7-25 At this point in the search, the clinician should begin to feel concern about the loss of important tooth structure, which could lead to vertical root fracture. The bur may be removed from the handpiece and placed in the excavation site. Packing cotton pellets around the shaft maintains the position and angulation of the bur. The radiograph taken at right angles through the tooth will reveal the depth and the angulation of the search.

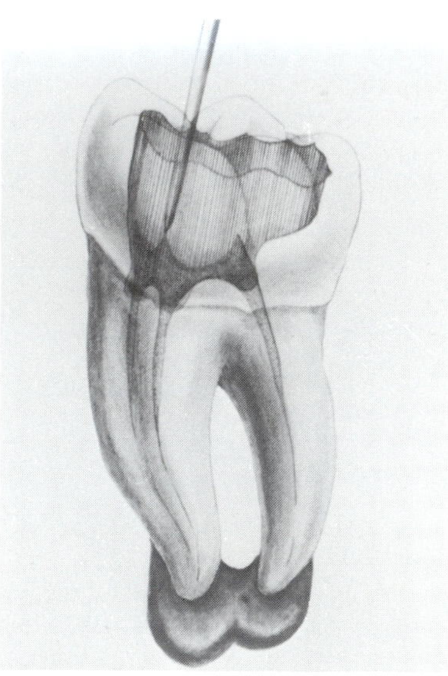

FIG. 7-26 Further excavation apically with a long-shank no. 2 round bur helps to locate the orifice. The endodontic explorer is the first instrument to identify a pinpoint opening.

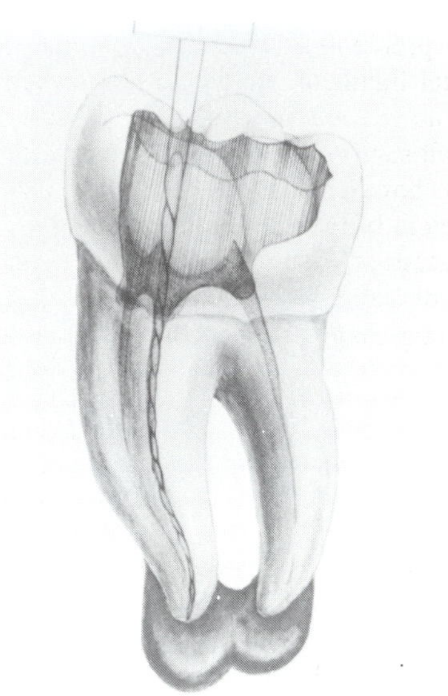

FIG. 7-28 A larger instrument is shown passing two curvatures to the apex by locating one canal in a multicanal tooth. It is usually possible to locate the second, third, or fourth canal once the first one has been located.

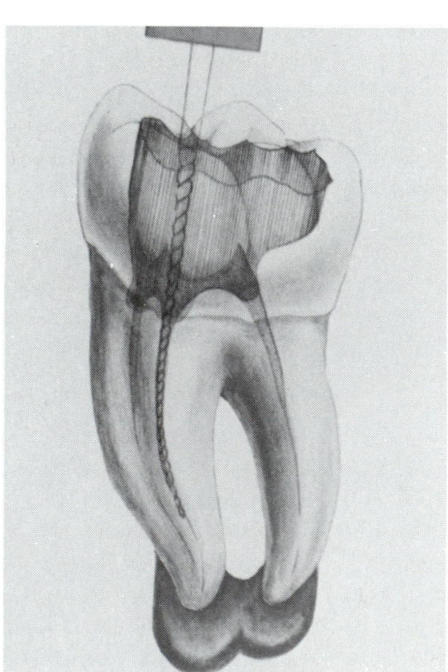

FIG. 7-27 At the first indication of a space, the smallest instrument (a no. 06 or 08 file) should be introduced. Gentle passive movement, both apical and rotational, often produces some penetration. A slight pull, signaling resistance, is usually an indication that one has located the canal. Careful file manipulation, frequent recapitulation, and canal lubricants (e.g., Calcinase, Glyoxide, R-C Prep) will assist in gaining access to the apical terminus. It is suggested that the access to the canal orifice be widened until the clinician can readily relocate the orifice.

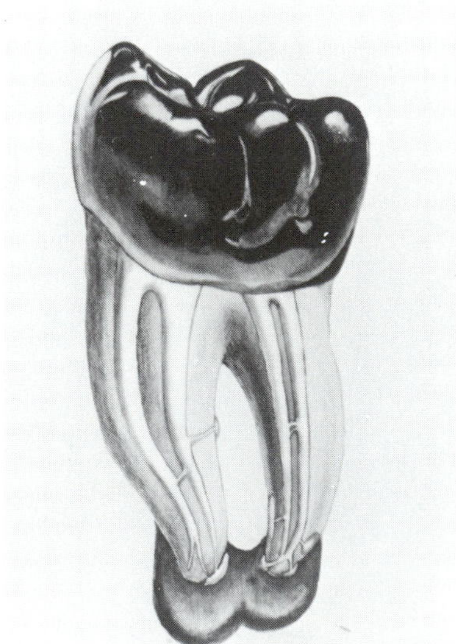

FIG. 7-29 Final canal obturation and restoration revealing anatomic complexities. This drawing appeared on the cover of the fifth edition of *Pathways of the Pulp*. (The simulations of the prepared and filled canals are courtesy of Dr. Clifford Ruddle.)

PERIODONTAL-ENDODONTIC SITUATION

Complications of aging alone make locating canal orifices difficult. The problems of bone loss, chronic inflammation of the periodontal ligament, mobility, and leakage into the root canal system are a combined periodontal-endodontic situation. The gradual closure of the internal spaces may be observed as the protective bone enclosure melts away from the root surfaces. The height of the pulp space now moves apically, making occlusal access difficult. Perforations of root walls and furcations are most common as the clinician reaches deeper and deeper with long-shanked burs. One means of locating the position of the bur tip and proper angle of approach is to stop, remove the bur from the handpiece, and replace it in the cavity, pack the cavity around the bur with cotton (Fig. 7-25), and take a periapical film.

Periodontal patients may suffer caries on exposed root surfaces and thus require extensive class V restorations. These restorations and the calcification often accompanying them can make gaining occlusal access to some canals impossible. It may become necessary in unusual cases to remove the restorative material and then locate, clean, and shape the canals from the buccal aspect (Fig. 7-34).

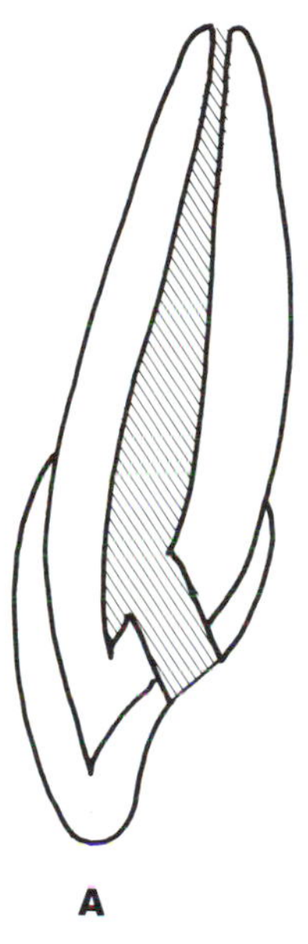

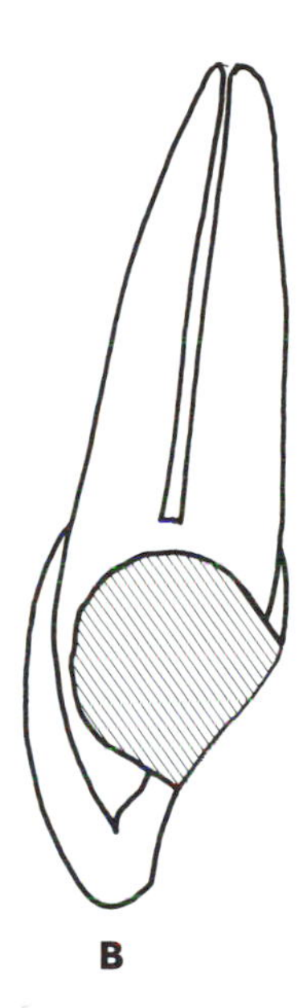

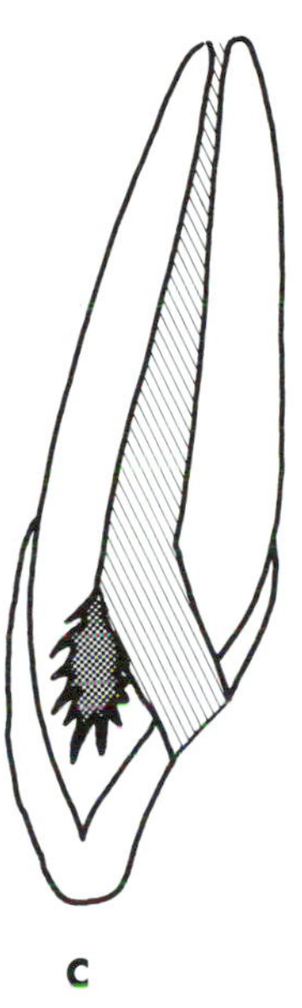

D

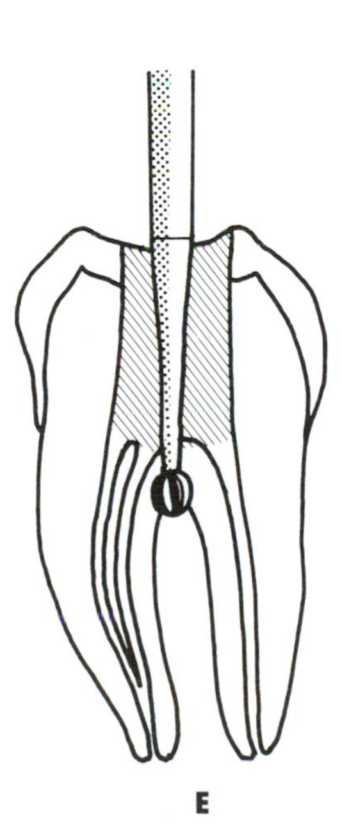

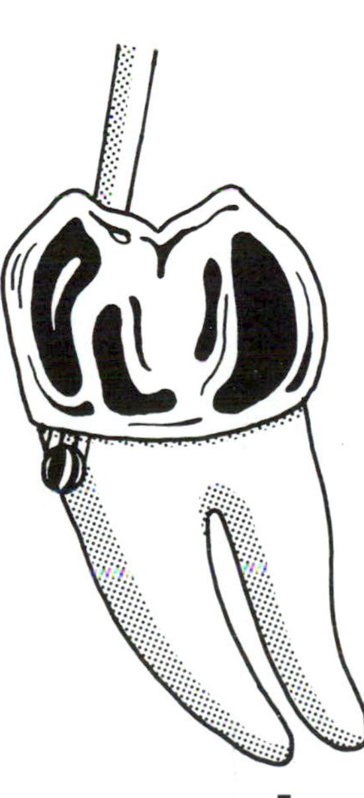

FIG. 7-30 Difficulties created by poor access preparation. **A,** Inadequate opening, which compromises instrumentation, invites coronal discoloration, and prevents good obturation. **B,** Overzealous tooth removal, resulting in mutilation of coronal tooth structure and weakening leading to coronal fracture. **C,** Inadequate caries removal, resulting in future carious destruction and discoloration. **D,** Labial perforation (lingual perforation with intact crowns is all but impossible in incisors). Surgical repair is possible, but permanent disfigurement and periodontal destruction will result. **E,** Furcal perforation of any magnitude, which (1) is difficult to repair, (2) causes periodontal destruction, and (3) weakens tooth structure, invites fracture. **F,** Misinterpretation of angulation (particularly common with full crowns) and subsequent root perforation. This is extremely difficult to repair; and even when it is repaired correctly, because it occurred in a difficult maintenance area the result is a permanent periodontal problem.

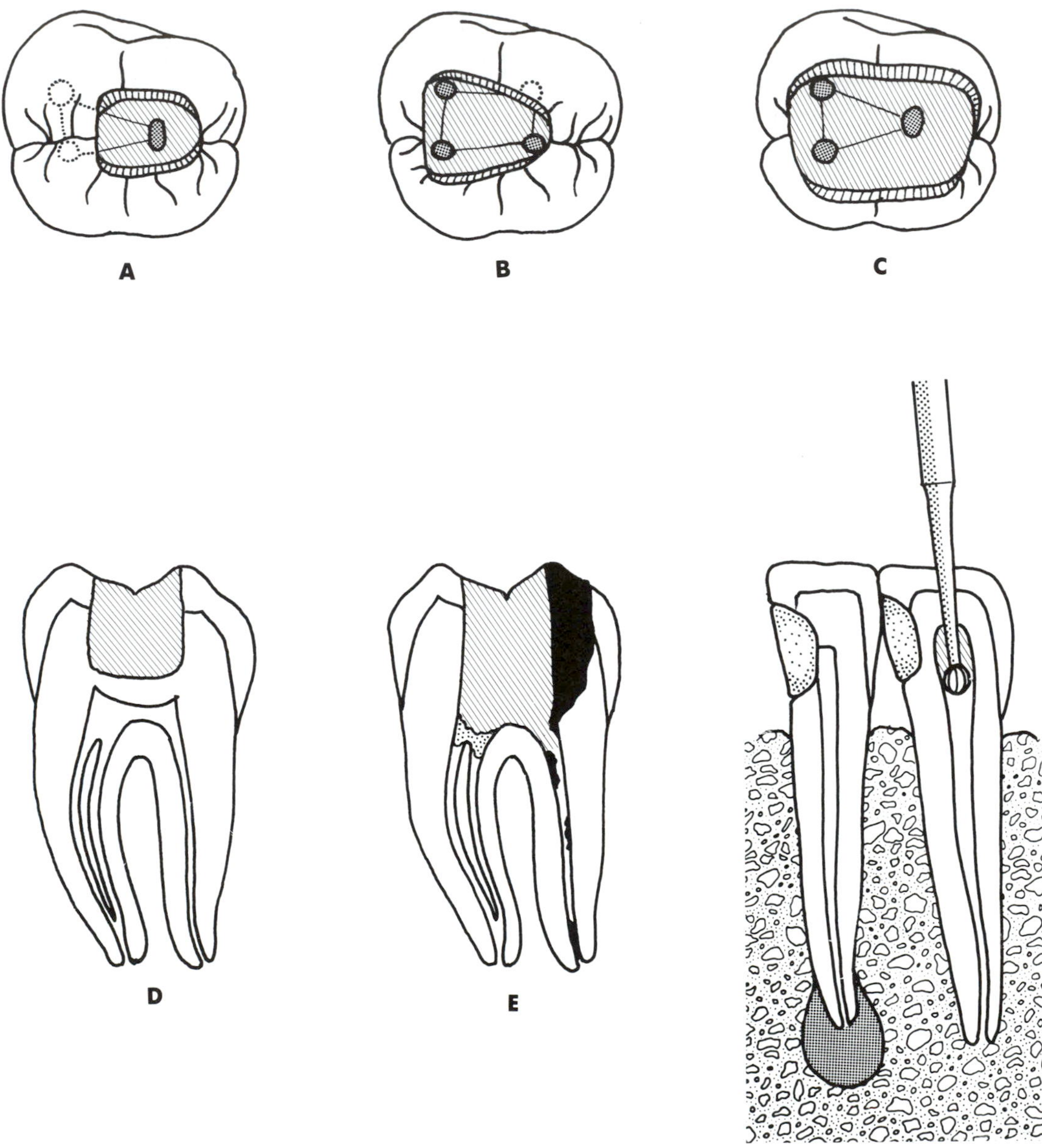

FIG. 7-31 Common errors in access preparation. **A,** Poor access placement and inadequate extension, leaving orifices unexposed. **B,** Better extension but not including the fourth canal orifice. **C,** Overextension, which weakens coronal tooth structure and compromises final restoration. **D,** Failure to reach the main pulp chamber is a serious error unless the space is heavily calcified. Bitewing radiographs are excellent aids in determining vertical depth. **E,** An iatrogenic problem is allowing debris to fall into the orifices. Amalgam filings and dentin debris can block access and result in endodontic failure. **F,** The most embarrassing error, and the one with the most damaging medical-legal potential, is entering the wrong tooth. A common site of this mishap is teeth that appear identical coronally, and the simple mistake is placing the rubber dam on the wrong tooth. Beginning the access cavity *before* placement of the rubber dam helps avoid this problem.

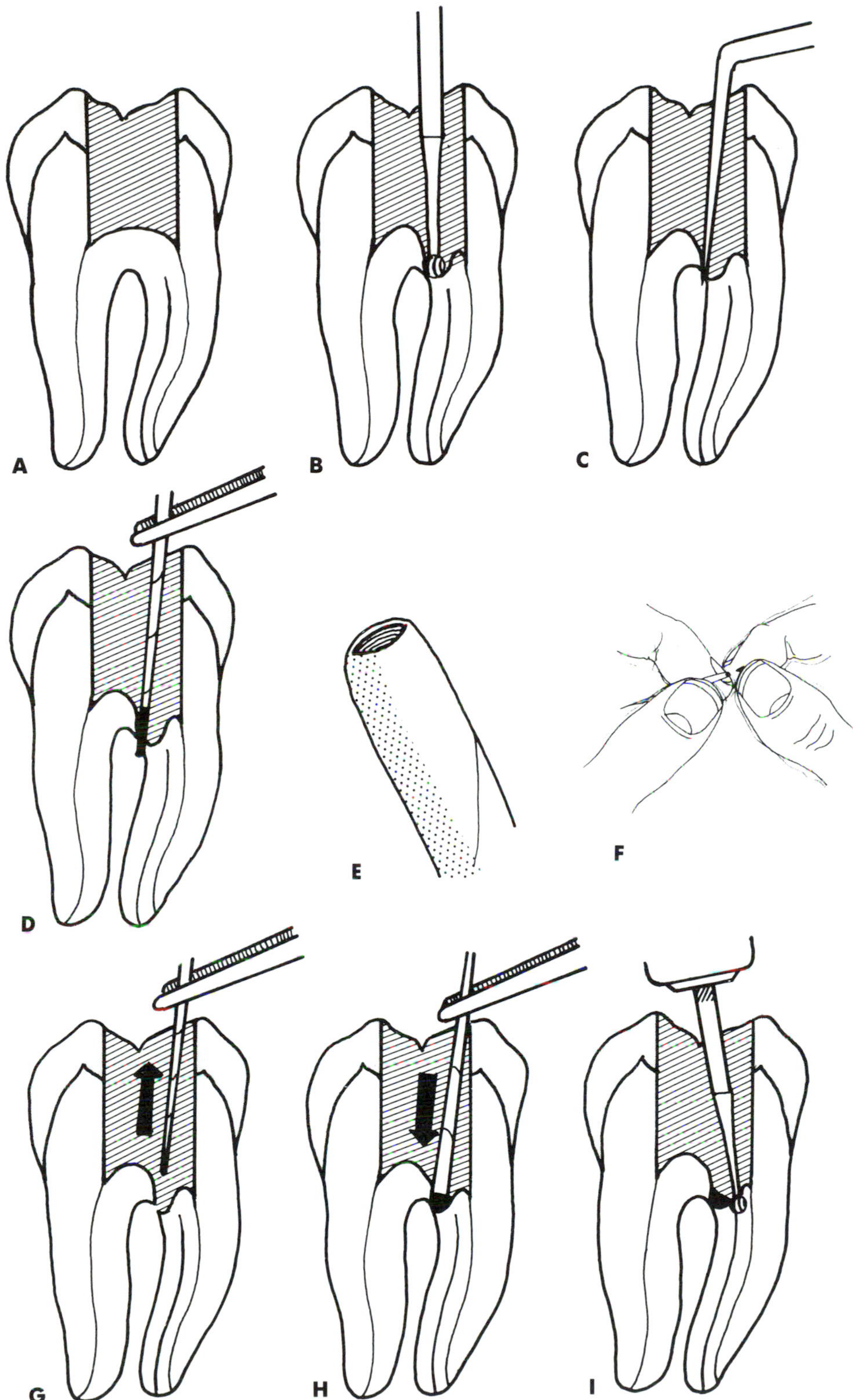

FIG. 7-32 Perforation repair. **A,** Access achieved in two canals but not in the calcified third canal. **B,** Minute furcal perforation during search for the elusive canal. **C,** Probing the perforation site with an endodontic pathfinder. **D,** Using absorbent point for hemorrhage control. **E,** Butt end of a paper point illustrating the recess in the tip created by the manufacturer's rolling thin paper to form the absorbent point. **F,** Placing a small bullet of fresh amalgam in the recess of the absorbent point. **G,** Removing the paper absorbent point. **H,** Inverting the point and depositing amalgam into the perforation (minimal tamping action). **I,** Adjusting the direction of the small round bur to locate the canal.

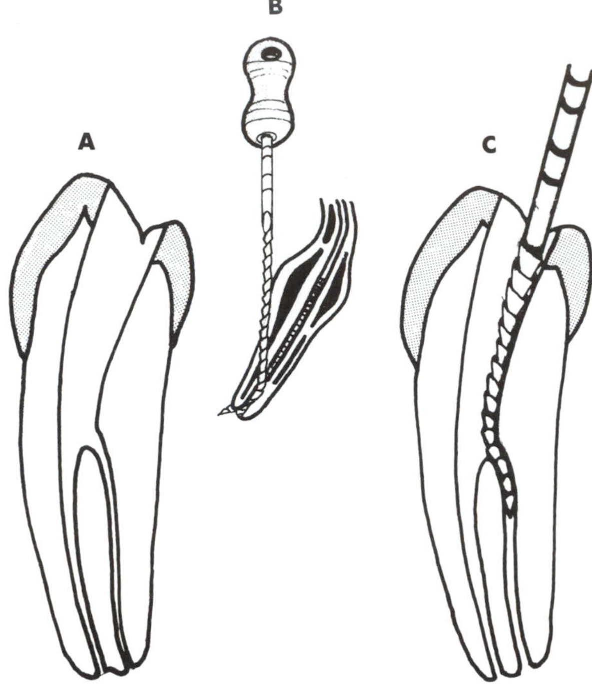

FIG. 7-33 A, Mandibular first premolar with division of the root canal system in the radicular portion of the tooth. **B,** Prebend endodontic file to facilitate access. **C,** Sliding the precurved instrument down the root wall until the tip engages the point of bifurcation.

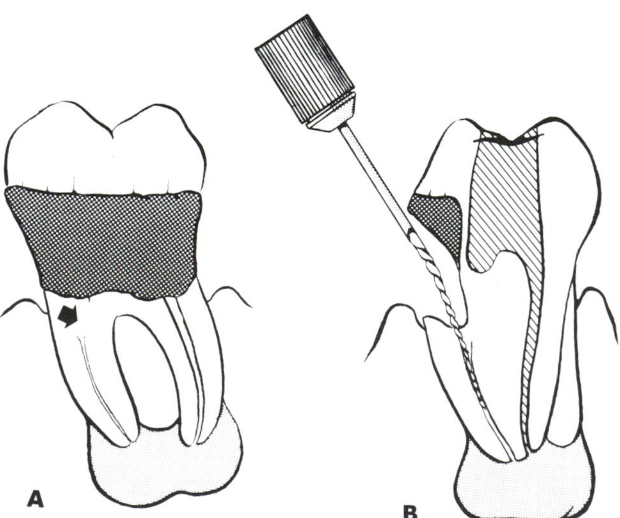

FIG. 7-34 A, Extensive class V restoration necessitated by root caries and periodontal disease leading to canal calcification *(arrow)*. **B,** Gaining access to these canals occluded by calcification may require removing the facial restoration and obtaining access from the buccal surface.

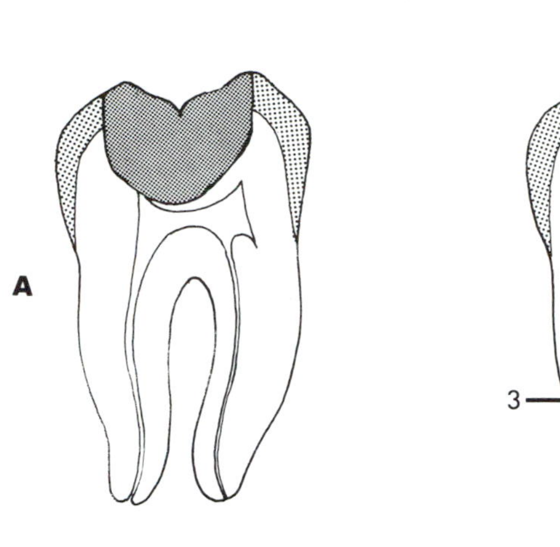

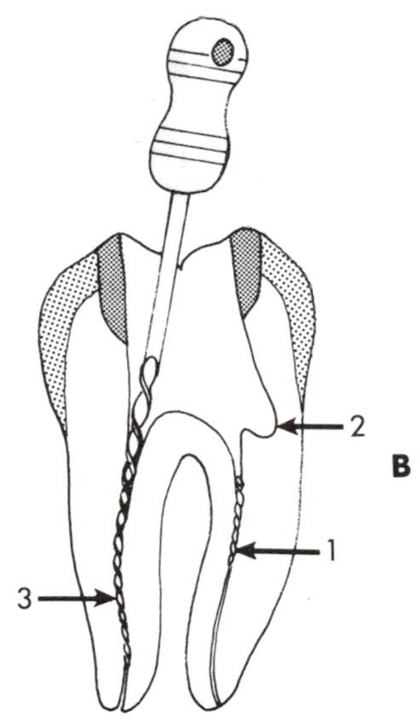

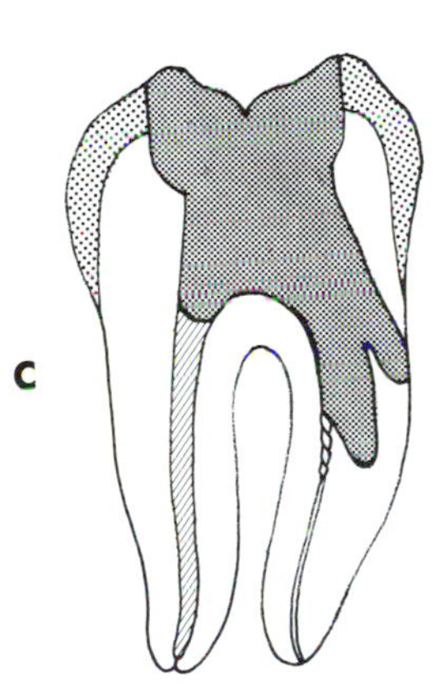

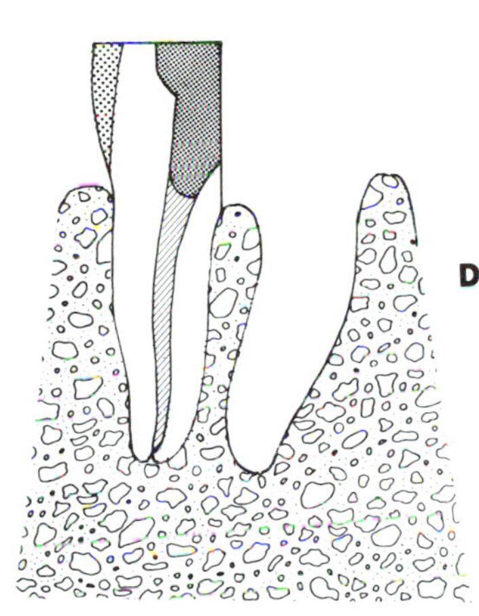

FIG. 7-35 Hemisection as an alternative when mutilation occurs during access preparation. **A,** Calcification after advanced caries and the application of calcium hydroxide can result in serious difficulties in making access. **B,** *1,* An instrument has fractured in the mesial canal; *2,* a second mesial canal seems totally calcified; and, *3,* the third canal, in the distal root, is navigable. **C,** Searching for canals and instrument fragments can result in mutilation of tooth structure. **D,** Obturation of one root and placement of amalgam in access areas will restore the intracanal spaces **(C)** in preparation for routine hemisection. Reinforcement with a dowel and core may be performed prior to final restoration.

REFERENCES

1. Benjamin KA, and Dowson J: Incidence of two-root canals in human mandibular incisor teeth, Oral Surg 38:122, 1974.
2. Booth JM: The longest tooth? Austral Endod News 13(3):17, 1988.
3. Bram SM, and Fleisher R: Endodontic therapy in a mandibular second bicuspid with four canals, J Endod 17:513, 1991.
4. Brand RW, and Isselhard DE: Anatomy of orofacial structures, ed 5, St. Louis, 1994, Times Mirror/Mosby College Publishing.
5. Carns EJ, and Skidmore AE: Configurations and deviations of root canals of maxillary first premolars, Oral Surg 36:880, 1973.
6. Cunningham CJ, and Senia ES: A three dimensional study of canal curvatures in the mesial roots of mandibular molars, J Endod 18:294, 1992.
7. Gher ME, and Vernino AR: Root anatomy: a local factor in inflammatory periodontal disease, Int J Periodont Restor Dent 1:53, 1981.
8. Goon WW, et al: Complex facial radicular groove in a maxillary lateral incisor, J Endod 17:244, 1991.
9. Green D: Double canals in single roots, Oral Surg 35:689, 1973.
10. Grossman LI: Endodontic practice, ed 10, Philadelphia, 1981, Lea & Febiger.
11. Hess W, and Zürcher E: The anatomy of the root canals of the teeth of the permanent and deciduous dentitions, New York, 1925, William Wood & Co.
12. Kasahara E, et al: Root canal system of the maxillary central incisor, J Endod 16(4):158, 1990.
13. Koenigs JF, Brilliant JD, and Foreman DW Jr: Preliminary scanning electron microscope investigation of accessory foramina in the furcation areas of human molar teeth, Oral Surg 38:773, 1974.
14. Kulild JC, and Peters DD: Incidence and configuration of canal systems in the mesiobuccal root of maxillary first and second molars, J Endod 16:311, 1990.
15. Melton DC, Krell KV, and Fuller MW: Anatomical and histological features of C-shaped canals in mandibular second molars, J Endod 1991.
16. Meyer VW: Die anatomie der Wurzelkanäle, dargestellt an mikroskopischen Rekonstruktionsmodellen, Dtsch Zahnärztl Z 25:1064, 1970.
17. Pineda F: Roentgenographic investigations of the mesiobuccal root of the maxillary first molar, Oral Surg 36:253, 1973.
18. Skidmore AE, and Bjorndal AM: Root canal morphology of the human mandibular first molar, Oral Surg 32:778, 1971.
19. Slowey RR: Radiographic aids in the detection of extra root canals, Oral Surg 37:762, 1974.
20. Vertucci FJ: Root canal morphology of mandibular premolars, J Am Dent Assoc 97:47, 1978.
21. Vertucci F, Seelig A, and Gillis R: Root canal morphology of the human maxillary second premolar, Oral Surg 38:456, 1974.

28:419, 1969.
23. Wilkie G, Personal communication, Melbourne, Australia,

and second premolars,

Self-assessment questions

1. Kasahara and colleagues reported that
   a. accessory canals are capable of being cleaned mechanically at least 60% of the time.
   b. over 60% of teeth examined showed accessory canals that were impossible to clean mechanically.
   c. apical foramina were located at the apex 80% of the time.
   d. canals terminate in the shape of a delta 45% of the time.
2. Once the pulp chamber has been opened, canal orifices are located with
   a. a periodontal curette.
   b. a spoon excavator.
   c. an inverted cone bur.
   d. an endodontic pathfinder.
3. Access cavity preparation of anterior teeth
   a. is completed using a K-type file.
   b. often can result in lateral cervical or root surface perforations.
   c. often can result in labial cervical or root surface perforations.
   d. are initiated using a no. 6 or 8 round bur.
4. Fourth canals are usually found in
   a. maxillary first premolars.
   b. maxillary second premolars.
   c. maxillary first molars.
   d. mandibular premolars.
5. The fourth canal is often found in
   a. the mesiobuccal root of the maxillary first molar.
   b. the mesial root of the maxillary first premolar.
   c. the palatal root of the maxillary first molar.
   d. the distobuccal root of the maxillary first molar.
6. Entry into a maxillary central incisor is made
   a. below (apical to) the cingulum in the direction of the long axis of the tooth.
   b. just coronal to the cingulum in the direction of the long axis of the tooth.
   c. to include the marginal ridges.
   d. with a slow-speed bur.
7. Maxillary canines
   a. are usually less than 25 mm long.
   b. are 25 mm or longer.
   c. possess extremely curved canals.
   d. have an anatomic apex distant from the apical foramen.
8. Vertucci and colleagues describe that
   a. 50% of the maxillary second premolars have one canal at the apex.
   b. maxillary second premolars that have two canals have two distinct apical foramina.
   c. 75% of maxillary second premolars have one canal at the apex.
   d. accessory canals are more prevalent in maxillary second premolars than in incisors.
9. The maxillary first molar
   a. has a palatal root that curves lingually.
   b. has a distobuccal root with two canals ending in a common orifice.
   c. should be approached for endodontic treatment with the assumption that two canals exist in the mesiobuccal root.
   d. should be approached for endodontic treatment with the assumption that one canal exists in the mesiobuccal root.
10. Mandibular incisors
    a. often have two separate apical foramina.
    b. two of five can have two separate canals.
    c. average 19 mm in length.
    d. are less likely to be perforated labially than lingually during access preparation.
11. Mandibular premolars
    a. can have more than one canal 12% to 23% of the time.
    b. are less prone to acute exacerbations.
    c. rarely present complex mechanical problems.
    d. are, on average, 19 mm long.
12. Multiple accessory foramina
    a. are more often present at the apex of the mandibular incisor.
    b. are more often present in the furcation of the maxillary premolar.
    c. are more often present in the furcation of the mandibular first molar.
    d. are accessible for mechanical instrumentation.
13. The mandibular first molar
    a. has a fourth canal two-thirds of the time.
    b. has a fourth canal half the time.
    c. is the most difficult to treat.
    d. has a fourth canal one-third of the time.
14. When a calcified root canal cannot be located or instrumented
    a. extraction is the treatment of choice.
    b. retrograde and replantation procedures should be considered.
    c. the dentist must proceed with the understanding that an unexplored or unfilled canal is worse than a perforation.
    d. it is no longer accessible to bacterial infection.

Chapter 8

Cleaning and Shaping the Root Canal System

John D. West
James B. Roane
Albert C. Goerig

INTRODUCTION

Techniques for cleaning and shaping root canals differ in accordance with clinical observations, research discoveries, and traditionally accepted values. For example, there is universal agreement that one should irrigate, but the proper type and strength of irrigant remain in dispute. There is universal agreement that the canal system should be cleaned and shaped, but differences remain over the extent of enlargement. There are different views on the terminal point for cleaning and shaping the root canal system. There is no consensus about the clinical importance of chelating agents used during cleaning. These examples illustrate a simple truth: the best procedure for all conditions has not been described. The astute clinician needs to be very familiar with the three major cleaning and shaping techniques, in order to provide the best patient care for all clinical conditions. In this chapter we discuss principles and applications of three current cleaning and shaping techniques. Each technique reflects its author's application of basic science and research knowledge into the clinical practice of endodontics. The format provides a broad view of endodontic principles and the clinical incorporation of current basic science knowledge. Each is written by a clinician experienced with its concepts and implementation.

THE ESSENCE OF ENDODONTICS

Clinical evidence demonstrates that root canal systems can be cleaned and shaped in three dimensions and can be obturated in three dimensions with a high degree of predictability, approaching 100% success. Three major elements determine the predictability of successful endodontics. The first is knowledge, the second is skill, and the third is desire. For endodontics in the mid-1990s these three critical elements are in complete balance. The endodontic disease process has been identified, and treatment has been developed. Discipline and skills need to be developed, but the critical factor is *desire*. It can be done if we *want* to do it. Successful endodontics is a decision.

ANATOMICALLY GENERATED ENDODONTICS

There is now general consensus about what makes endodontic therapy work so predictably. Every portal of exit is important, because every portal of exit is *potentially* significant.[74] Lesions of endodontic origin may exist anywhere along the surface of the root, including bifurcations, trifurcations, and the base of infrabony pockets.[72] With this awareness, endodontists began to think of endodontics in a different way. The rationale of endodontic treatment is based on simple biologic principles. Because the pulp is surrounded by dentin it cannot benefit fully from the body's natural inflammatory response. First, the microcirculatory system of the pulp *lacks* a significant collateral circulation. Second, the pulp consists of a relatively *large* volume of tissue for a relatively small blood supply. And finally, the pulp of the root canal system is *locked* into the unyielding walls of surrounding dentin. Because of

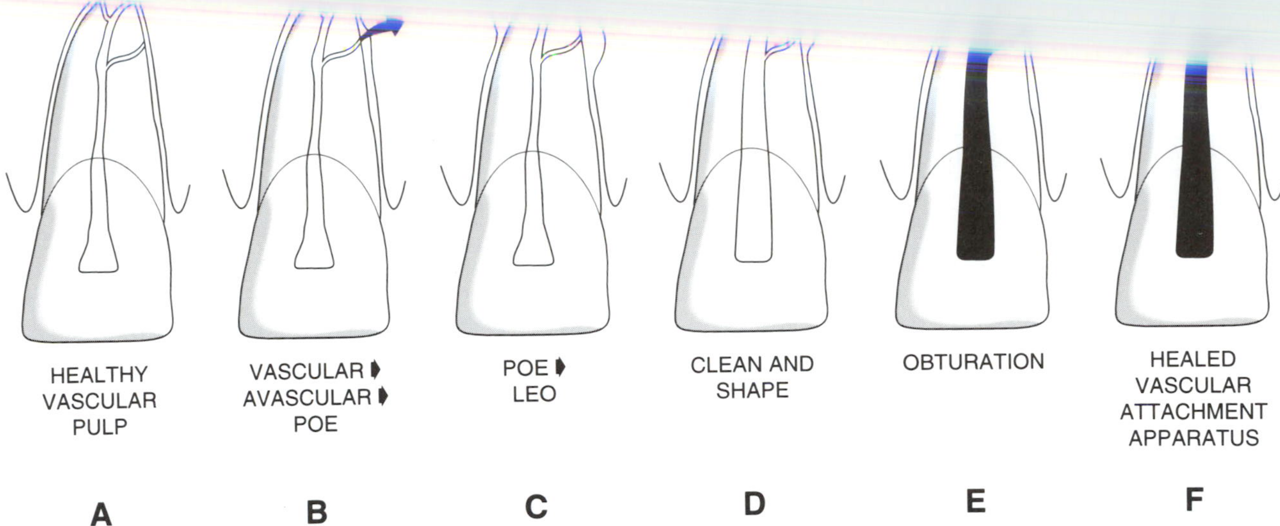

FIG. 8-1 Rationale of endodontics. **A,** Healthy, vascular pulp, having the disadvantage of lack of significant collateral circulation, a large volume of tissue to a relatively small blood supply, and locked into unyielding walls of dentin. **B,** When the pulp becomes necrotic, viable and nonviable irritants spill through the portals of exit (POE) into the vascular attachment apparatus. **C,** Lesions of endodontic origin (LEO) are produced. **D,** Healing commences with cleaning and shaping. **E,** Three-dimensional obturation eliminates the source of the LEO. The attachment apparatus is cured. **F,** The LEO has healed.

caries, restorative procedures, or trauma, a vascular pulp may degenerate into avascular necrosis. The necrotic material then seeps out of the portals of exit of the root canal system and into the supporting vascular attachment apparatus, generating lesions of endodontic origin (LEO, Fig. 8-1). If the root canal system is sealed permanently in three dimensions, then resolution can be expected. Virtually any endodontically diseased tooth can be treated successfully, if the root canal system is sealed in three dimensions and if the periodontal condition is healthy or can be made so. Longevity of a tooth is based not on the pulp, but on healthy attachment apparatus. Therefore, treatment must be based on the effectiveness of cleaning, shaping, and packing the root canal system with a permanent, biologically inert root canal filling.

THE ROOT CANAL SYSTEM

The root canal system is our road map to success (Fig. 8-11, *J*). In the past, we have been thinking only vertically. Many students were taught that the first concern in root canal preparation was "working length." We understand now that the critical issue is three-dimensionality.

Root canals exist as multiple interrelationships. Root canal systems are not cylinders but ribbons, sheets, and banners. They can be more than six times wider in a buccolingual direction than in a mesiodistal direction. Eccentricity and abnormality are "normal." Maxillary first and second molars have four canal systems more than 90% of the time.[50] A quarter or more of mandibular molars have two distal canals (Fig. 8-15, *F*).

CLEANING AND SHAPING: THE MASTER SKILL

Almost 30 years ago, Schilder introduced the concept (and the expression phrase) "cleaning and shaping."[73] Endodontics of the future will be better distinguished by the cleaning and shaping technique. In fact, most obturation problems are really problems of cleaning and shaping. The two concepts, cleaning and shaping *and* three-dimensional obturation, are *inseparable*. The secret to successful clinical endodontics is proper shaping.

What is the modern meaning of cleaning and shaping? *Cleaning* refers to the removal of *all* contents of the root canal system before and during shaping: organic substrates, microflora, bacterial byproducts, food, caries, denticles, pulp stones, dense collagen, previous root canal filling material, and dentinal filings resulting from root canal preparation (see Fig. 8-11, *L*). *Shaping* refers to a specific cavity form with five design objectives. The shape permits vertical pluggers to fit freely within the root canal system and to generate the hydraulics required to transform and capture a maximum cushion of gutta-percha and a microfilm of sealer into all foramina. Equally important, shaping facilitates three-dimensional cleaning by allowing easy access to files and irrigants during the shaping process.

Cleaning and shaping skills separate *predictability* from *hope*, *mastery* from *mediocrity*, *design* from *default*, and *choice* from *chance*. Cleaning and shaping has two special distinctions. The first is that endodontic therapy is the *only* dental procedure that relies so much on "feel". The tactile sense is extremely important in endodontic treatment. A lighter touch, more delicate use of instruments, and greater restraint by the practitioner will produce better results. Endodontic treatment is performed primarily through the sense of touch.

The second distinction of cleaning and shaping is accountability. In periodontics, orthodontics, and restorative dentistry, compliance of the patient, their healing capacity, laboratory quality, home care, and susceptibility to disease play significant roles in success. In endodontics, the *clinician* is the major clinical variable. Our ability and willingness to deal with root canal anatomy is the formula for success.

Three major concepts of cleaning and shaping have been integrated into endodontics. These three technique distinctions can be used in combination with each other or exclusively.

THE SCHILDER METHOD

Herbert Schilder taught endodontists to think and operate in the third dimension.[73,74] Schilder's five mechanical objectives for successful cleaning and shaping were first introduced to the endodontic literature 20 years ago.[74] Since their introduction, the design objectives have become accepted widely, understood and appreciated more thoroughly, and have given the clinician a specific and intelligent goal during root canal preparation. The use of each instrument has a specific purpose in achieving permanent three-dimensional obturation.

Schilder's Mechanical Objectives

1. *Develop a continuously tapering conical form in the root canal preparation*. This shape mimics the natural shape of canals before they undergo calcification and formation of secondary dentin. The goal is to create a conical form from access cavity to foramen (Fig. 8-2, *A-F*). When this vision is imprinted in the clinician's mind during cleaning and shaping procedures, instrument selection is simplified. In addition, the preparation should be smooth and appropriate for the length, shape, and size of the root that surrounds it. The funnel must merge into the access cavity so that instruments will slide into the canal. The access cavity and the root canal preparation are continuous. The narrowest part of the continuously tapering cone is located apically, and the widest is found coronally. Irrigation and instruments can now clean and shape all the walls of the root canal preparation. The continuously tapering cone allows hydraulic principles to operate by the restricted flow principle. As flow is restricted during the compaction procedures, it causes the gutta-percha and sealer to take the path of least resistance; namely the apical and lateral foramina.
2. *Make the canal narrower apically, with the narrowest cross-sectional diameter at its terminus*. The second objective is a corollary of the first. The diameter becomes narrower as the preparation extends apically (Fig. 8-2, *G–J*). The only exception is a tooth with internal resorption or an unusual bulge in the natural shape of the root canal (Fig. 8-2, *I* and *J*). This objective creates control and compaction at *every* level of the preparation. The second objective focuses on harmonizing cavity form with the thermomechanical properties of gutta-percha to achieve a hermetic seal.[31,32,77,78] To obturate all foramina, the preparation must be shaped serially in a decreasing taper. To preserve apical patency, the dentin mud must be suspended in sodium hypochlorite and the radiographic terminus used as the reference (Fig. 8-15, *E*). The cementodentinal junction is not clinically meaningful and may vary histologically up to several millimeters. To use it as *the guide* could jeopardize mechanical objectives 3, 4, and 5. The operator may clean to the apex, the anatomic apex, the radiographic apex, the apical constriction, the apical foramen, the cementodentinal junction, or the radiographic terminus (Fig. 8-15, *D* and *E*). The only landmark that can be identified consistently is the radiographic terminus.
3. *Make the preparation in multiple planes*. It is often valuable for learning to analyze the root canals of extracted teeth. The root canals *within* curved roots are similarly curved. The third objective preserves this natural curve or "flow" (Fig. 8-2).
4. *Never transport the foramen*. If we examine the root canals of extracted teeth, few of the exit foramina are located at the apex of the root. They usually are located to the side of the apex.[51] In addition, many root tips have several foramina with root tips that curve significantly at the apical third or occasionally in the middle third. Delicate foramina can be lost during root canal preparation by improper sequencing of instruments, insufficient irrigation, not enough tactile finesse, or not enough delicacy. This objective facilitates the achievement of objective no. 3, *flow*. Maintaining patency to the radiographic terminus and carefully shaping, sculpting, and shaving the inside of the canal are essential to mastering shaping.

   Often the angle of access and angle of incidence differ. The angle of access refers to the orientation of the instrument as it slides down the body of the root canal. The angle of incidence refers to the turn required to *follow* the path of the root canal (see Fig. 8-14).

   Foramina may be transported externally or internally (Fig. 8-3). *External* transportation is caused by failing to precurve files, using large instruments, or being too heavy handed. The original apical foramen is torn. Instruments should be used only a few seconds at a time. When an instrument is overused, the elastic memory of the instrument may create the teardrop and tearing of the apical foramen. This "hourglass" shape makes it more difficult to properly obturate the foramen. Many endodontic failures result from external transportation (Fig. 8-4, *A* and *B*).

   The second form of external transportation is direct perforation. This destructive error usually begins with a ledge or apical blockage. The deflected instrument continues its misdirection until it perforates the root surface (Fig. 8-3). This external perforation also can become an external teardrop tear.

   Internal transportation occurs when the foramen becomes clogged with dentin mud or denticles (Fig. 8-4, *C–L*). These particles may irritate the attachment apparatus after root canal filling or the particles may prevent obturation of other apical foramina that branch off the "main" canal. Finally, this internally transported foramen may perforate the external root surface through a false path.
5. *Keep the apical foramen as small as is practical*. The final foramen size will vary, depending on the canal (Fig. 8-5). Some foramina are small and some are large; some are round, some are oval, and some have unusual shapes. The goal of objective 4 is to preserve foraminal size and shape at the apical constricture. This can be achieved only by carefully maintaining patency to the radiographic terminus by constantly reconfirming patency *through* the foramen with a loose-fitting instrument. Since patency is so important to success, the clinician discovers a sense of security. The operator cleans the foramen but does not

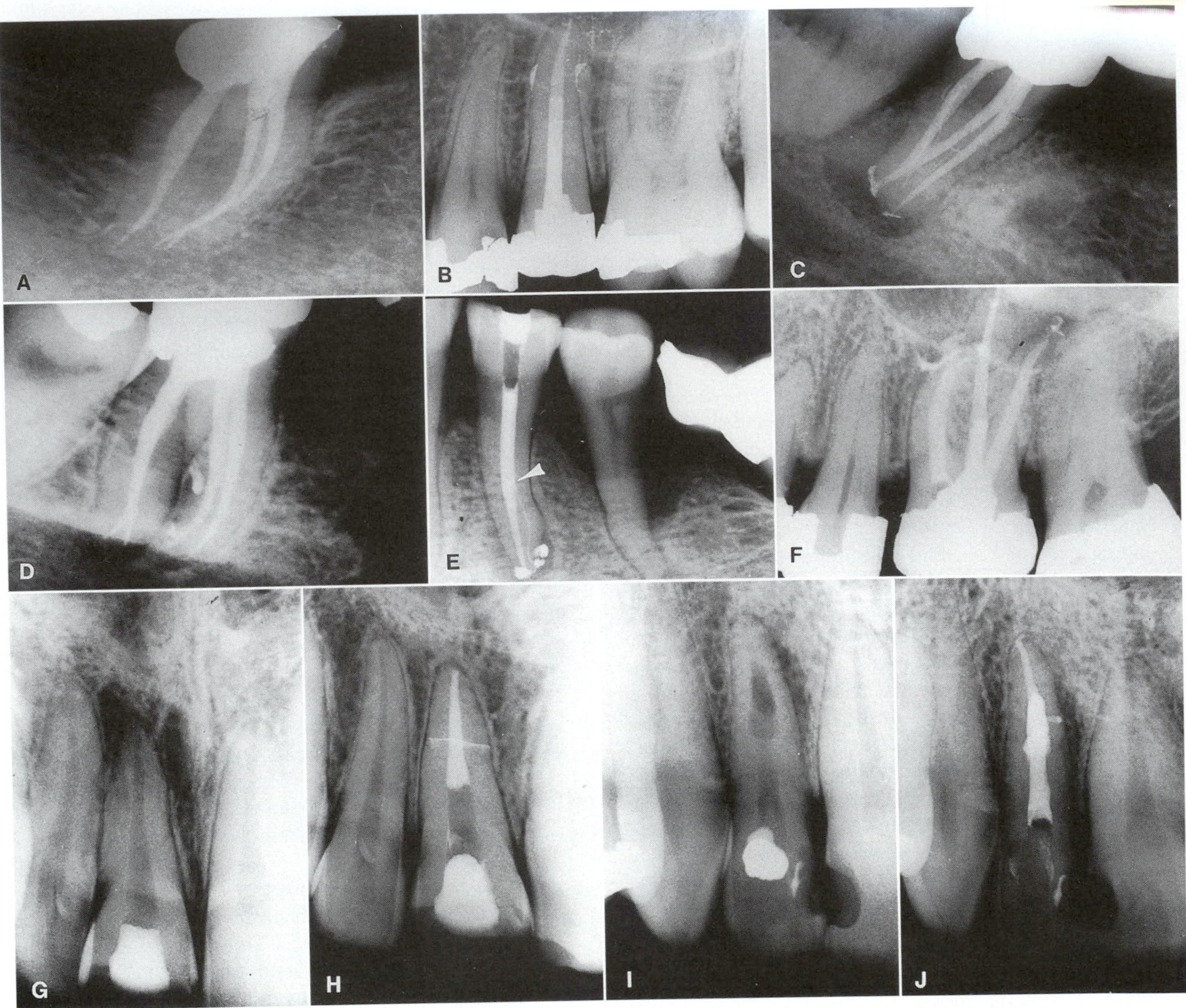

FIG. 8-2 Schilder mechanical objectives no. 1, 2, and 3. **A,** Radiographic obturation demonstrates *flow* where the root canal preparation exists in the same multiple planes as the original root canal. **B,** The apical third continuously tapering cone provides restricted flow so that gutta-percha and sealer extrude into all foramina. **C,** Delicate shaping creates obturation of the spaces previously occupied by microcirculatory systems. **D,** Proper shaping allows for obturation of two apical foramina in the distal network as well as furcal lateral portals of exit. **E,** Even previously *undiscovered* root canal system branches are filled simply because shaping provides appropriate internal hydraulics in packing *(arrow)*. **F,** Every shaped canal has more than one portal of exit. Because of mechanical objectives being met, all foramina are filled. **G,** Pretreatment radiograph of maxillary central incisor as it was referred. **H,** Mechanical objective no. 2 results in predictable obturation of previously undiscovered horizontal fracture. **I,** Pretreatment radiograph of maxillary lateral incisor. **J,** Single exception to mechanical objective no. 2 means that the resorptive site is not contained within the continuously tapering cone per se; otherwise the structural integrity of the tooth would be jeopardized.

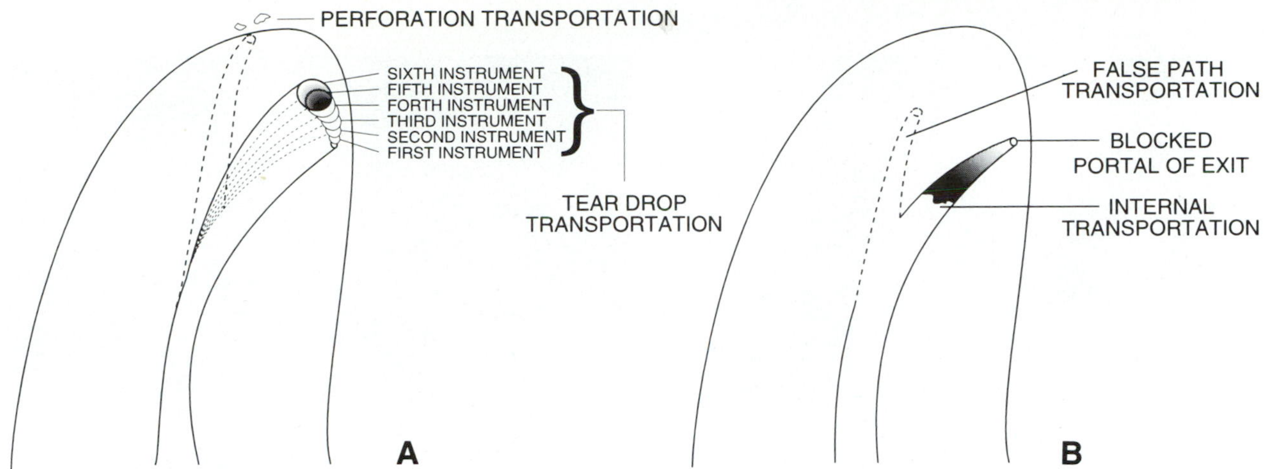

FIG. 8-3 Portal of exit transportation. **A,** External transportation occurs when same instrument or progressively larger instruments tear the portal of exit into a teardrop shape on the external root surface. External transportation can occur in two forms: a teardrop shape or a direct perforation, which can become a tangential tear. **B,** Internal transportation occurs when the portal of exit is moved internal to its external position by blocking the canal with dentin mud. A new false path begins.

enlarge or distort it. After careful probing to the radiographic terminus, the canal is shaped inside.

To clean and predictably seal the foramen, the size of the file used at the *end* of the cleaning and shaping should be at least a No. 20 or 25. Correct shaping and observance of objectives 1 through 4 will produce an apical constriction of minimal diameter. By creating a continuously tapering cone, precurving instruments, and maximizing irrigation, the flow of the root canal preparation is preserved. There is no advantage to creating a wider foramen unless the canal is too small to predictably compact gutta-percha and sealer (no. 10 or 15).

The goal is to clean but not enlarge the foramen. If the diameter of a foramen is increased from an ISO no. 20 to an ISO no. 40 instrument, the *area* of the foramen has increased four times! Not only does this increase the risk of tearing, but it increases the potential for microleakage (Fig. 8-6) around the margin.

In summary, the goal is to produce a three-dimensional, continuously tapering, multiplaned cone from access cavity to radiographic terminus while preserving foraminal position and size (Fig. 8-7).

"The Look"

Schilder refers to *the look* as the radiographic appearance of three-dimensional obturation, when all five mechanical objectives have been achieved. The mechanical concepts are in harmony with the natural root canal anatomy. The look is unmistakable (Figs. 8-7 to 8-10).

Irrigation

The success of cleaning and shaping is enhanced by sodium hypochlorite. Three percent sodium hypochlorite dissolves detached organic material during cleaning and shaping (Fig. 8-11). Some research suggests that sodium hypochlorite even reaches the apex of the root. Sodium hypochlorite chemically dissolves soft tissue, lubricates, and creates a suspension in which the dentin mud can be washed away gently through irrigation and instrument manipulation.

If gravity pulls dentin mud away from the apical area, sodium hypochlorite is very effective; however, when the patient is oriented so that dentin mud tends to fall toward the apical area (as in most mandibular teeth), alternating with 3% hydrogen peroxide allows for effervescence and flotation of the dentin mud (Fig. 8-11, *I*). This is often overlooked in cleaning and shaping techniques. When patients are reclined significantly, the maxillary teeth can sometimes benefit from alternating with peroxide compounds.

Irrigation should be performed gently with the irrigating syringe constantly moving to avoid locking the needle in the canal. Several drops of irrigant are left in the access opening (Fig. 8-11, *G* and *H*).

Clinical Technique for Cleaning and Shaping

The following description is a simulation for a "generic" tooth (Fig. 8-12, *A*). Just as an artist would never use the exact order of brush strokes to paint, this sequence should not be memorized; rather, it serves as a guide to understanding the concept of cleaning and shaping. The reader should get a sense of the dynamics and sequence of root canal cleaning and of how the sculpted form develops during the *shaping*. In this example, four recapitulations will be necessary to achieve the proper shape for the *cone fit,* which is the *last* step of successful cleaning and shaping.

With a good access cavity gently irrigated with sodium hypochlorite, the precurved no. 10 file is guided gently into the access cavity. The position of the rubber stop and the length of the tooth are not significant at this time. The clinician must tactilely feel and "see" with the instrument tip. The next step is to follow the path to the radiographic terminus. The path is always present, but occasionally the instrument suddenly stops. However, with a gentle turn of the precurved number

Text continued on p. 190.

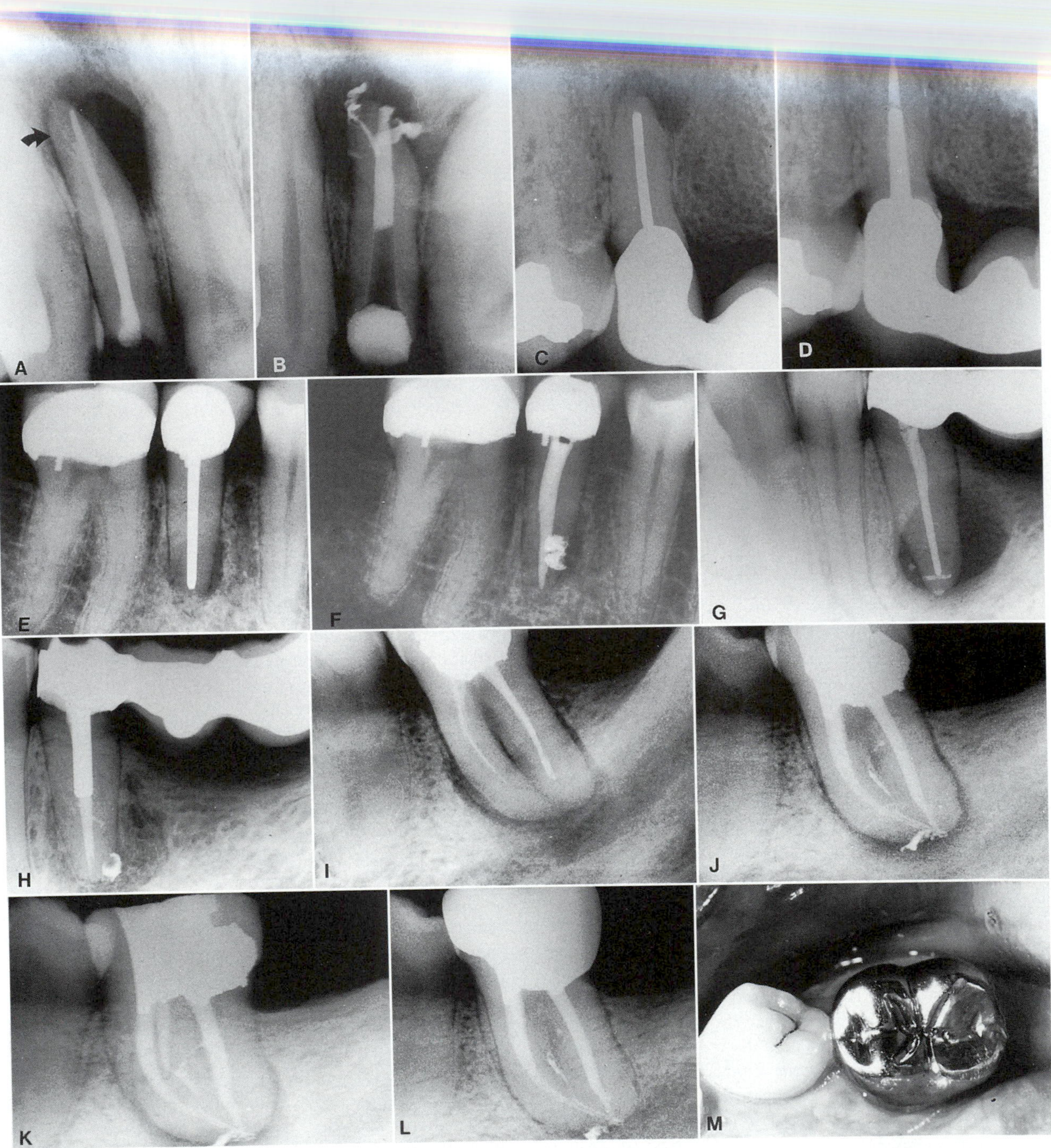

FIG. 8-4 Mechanical objective no. 4. **A,** Original root canal system portal of exit remains underfilled *(arrow),* and a significant LEO has developed adjacent to the externally transported portal of exit. **B,** After proper shaping, original and transported foramina are sealed. **C,** Internally transported portal of exit. **D,** Retreatment allows for cleaning and obturation of the original foramen with subsequent healing. **E,** Internal transportation prevents obturation of major lateral foramen as well as the apical foramen. **F,** By regaining the apical portal of exit, the obturation is possible for the lateral foramen as well. **G,** Multiple internally transported foramina. **H,** Predictable healing progressing well after obturation at 6-month recall. **I,** Internal transportation of important lone distal molar. **J,** Retreatment creates the possibility for healing. **K,** Oblique radiograph indicates previously underfilled internal anatomy. **L,** Seven-month recall demonstrates radiographic healing of the attachment apparatus and symptoms subside. **M,** Final restoration after healing of the attachment apparatus.

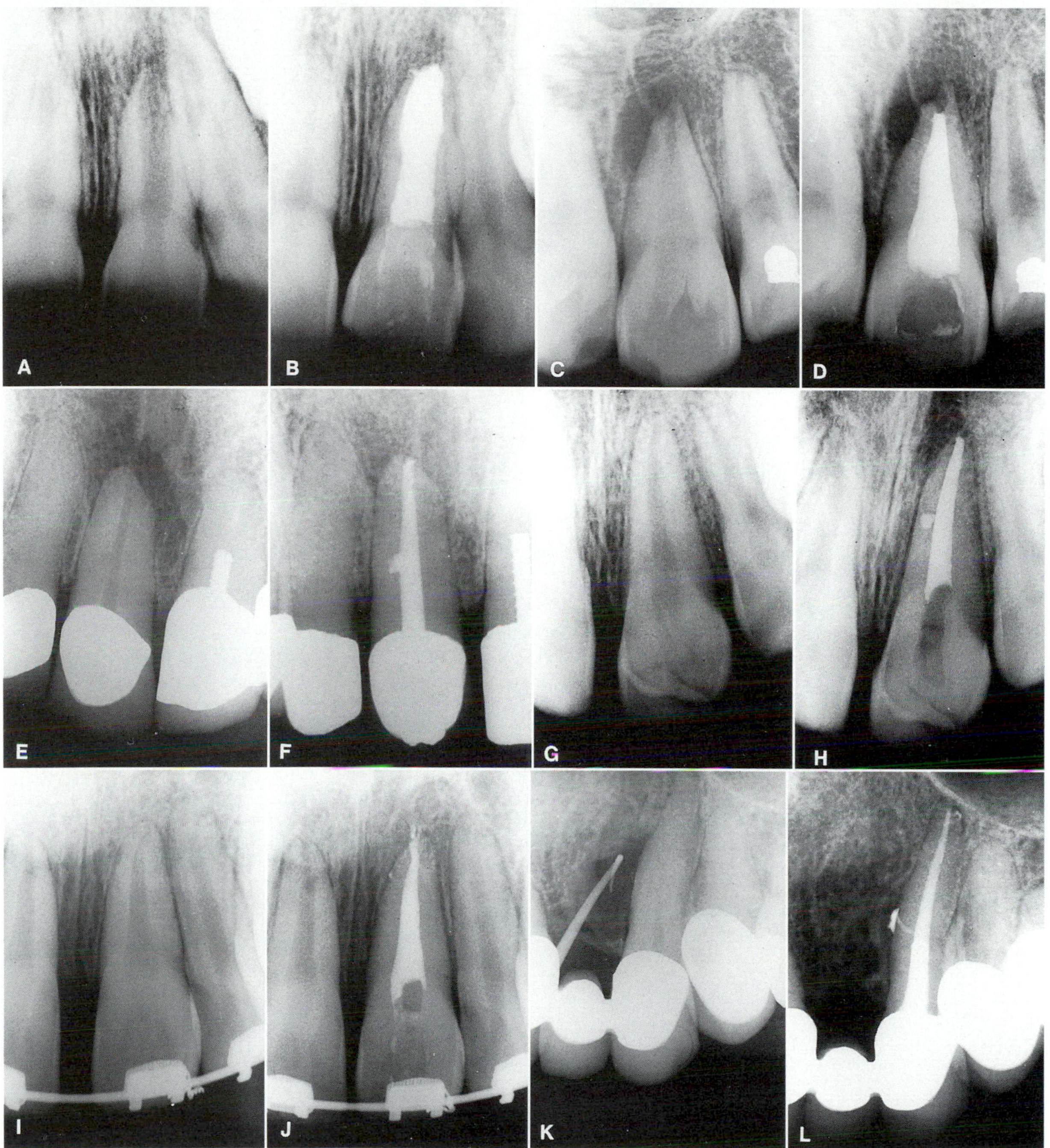

FIG. 8-5 Mechanical objective no. 5. **A,** Central incisor with large foramen. **B,** Obturation is complete with filling of an apical portal of exit emanating toward the mesial. **C,** Lateral and apical radiolucency of central incisor. **D,** Preserving the size and shape of the apical foramen, the canal is shaped inside, still generating enough internal pressure to obturate two lateral portals of exit. **E,** Internal resorption is suggested in the pretreatment radiograph. **F,** Foramen size is preserved and, even with relatively large apical opening, sufficient internal obturation pressure is generated to fill the resorptive defect. **G,** Pretreatment radiograph of a central incisor. **H,** Final foramen size is appropriate for this tooth. **I,** Pretreatment radiograph. **J,** Root canal system is shaped inside the portal of exit size with subsequent obturation to the radiographic terminus. **K,** Smaller apical canal size with the gutta-percha cone tracing the lateral sinus tract. **L,** The smaller apical foramen size is retained with appropriate internal shaping followed by subsequent obturation of the root canal system.

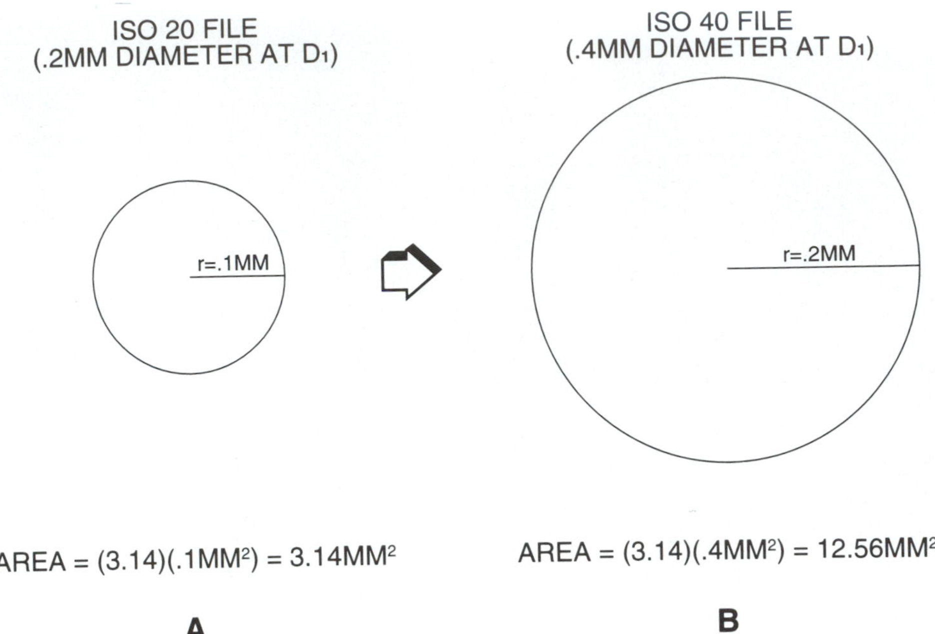

FIG. 8-6 Enlarging the foramen results in a significant increase in surface area and circumference, increasing the potential for microleakage. **A,** Radius of 0.1 mm. **B,** When the radius is increased to 0.2 mm, the area of the circle is increased four times.

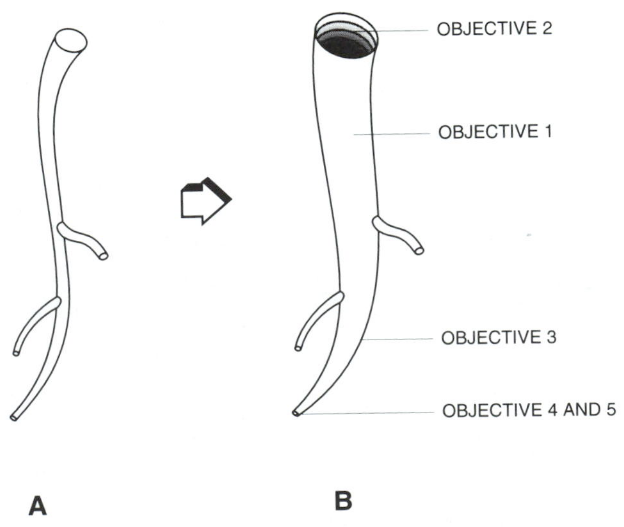

FIG. 8-7 Line drawing demonstrates all five Schilder mechanical objectives. **A,** Example of a root canal network consisting of an orifice and three foramina. **B,** Cleaning and shaping is a concept that produces a three-dimensional, continuously tapering, multiplaned cone from access cavity to radiographic terminus while preserving foraminal position and size.

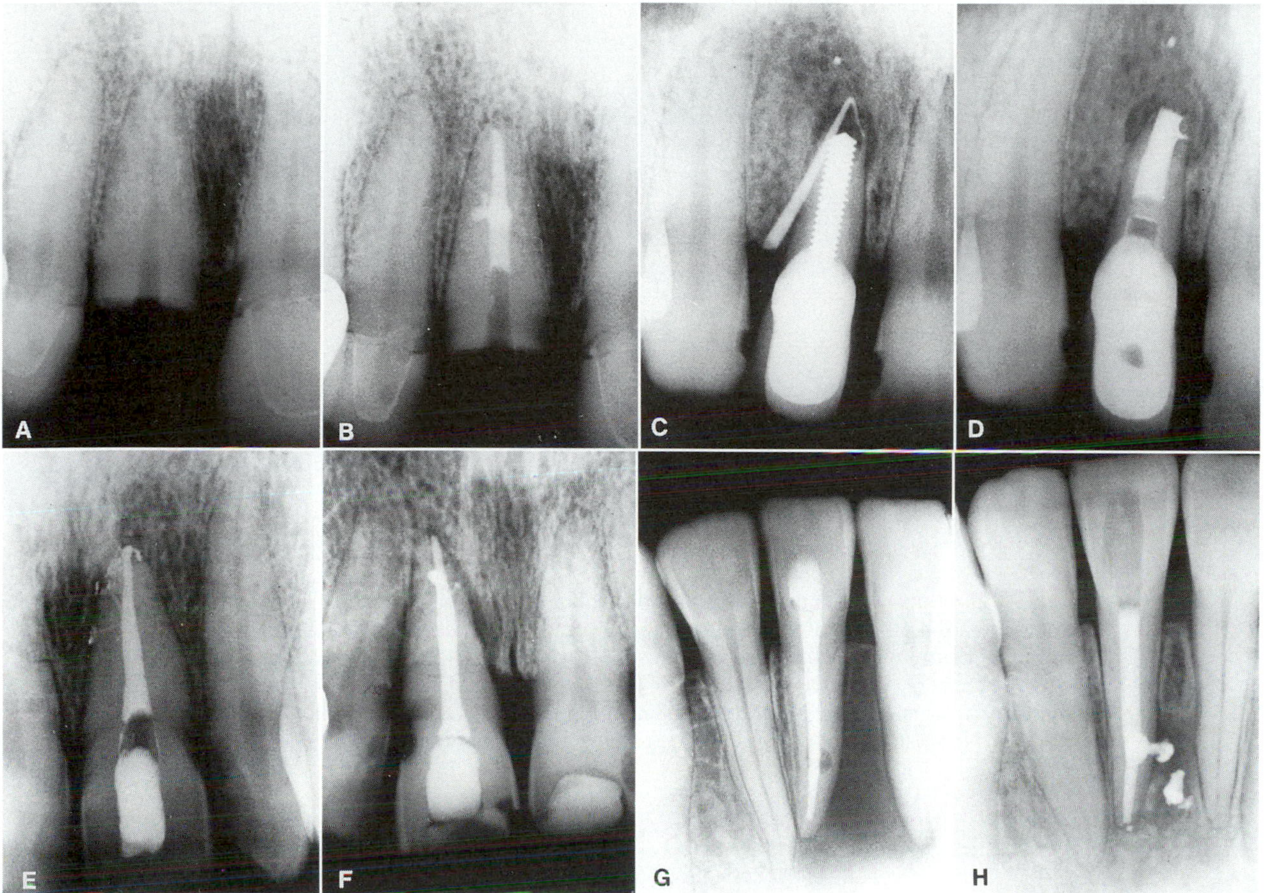

FIG. 8-8 "The Look" in anterior teeth. **A,** Apparently simple anatomy exists in fractured central incisor. **B,** However, the packed root canal system reveals more complex anatomy. Often the more complex anatomy is discovered when the root canal system is obturated. There is no distinction between resorptive portals of exit and lateral canals. All are considered portals of exit of the root canal system. **C,** Pretreatment radiograph demonstrates external transportation of the apical foramen during post preparation and placement. A gutta-percha cone traces the sinus tract. **D,** After nonsurgical post removal the root canal system is cleaned, shaped, and packed. By developing a precise and gradual taper, enough compaction pressure is developed to seal a lateral portal and to maintain apical control. The fifth mechanical cleaning and shaping objective of keeping the foramen as small as practical is still achieved by shaping inside the given foramen dimension while maintaining patency. **E** and **F,** Well-shaped maxillary central incisors create automatic lateral components in the packing process. This measurable lateral force results in elimination of anatomy that exists throughout the entire surface of the root. **G,** Internal transportation of the apical portal of exit prevents three-dimensional obturation and a subsequent LEO. Resorptive site in apical third is also underfilled because of inappropriate shaping and compaction technique. **H,** The successful retreatment of this incisor results directly from a logical and scientific root canal cavity design.

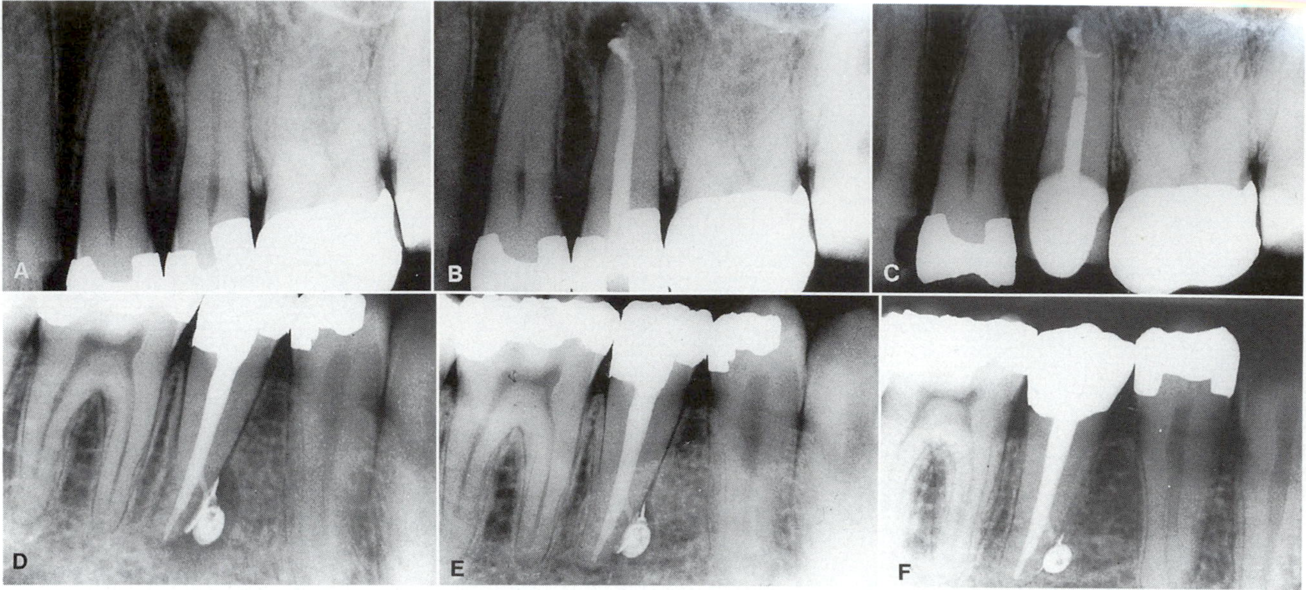

FIG. 8-9 "The Look" in single-rooted posterior teeth. **A,** Pretreatment. **B,** The development of a shape that has its narrowest diameter apically and widest diameter coronally makes the apical third sealing of the root canal system simple, predictable, and controllable. **C,** Three-months' healing. **D,** Complete apical control of the apical foramen and with expected surplus filling material from cleaned but not shaped lateral foramen. **E,** One-year recall. **F,** Seventeen-year recall. Notice the lateral portal of exit remains visibly obturated.

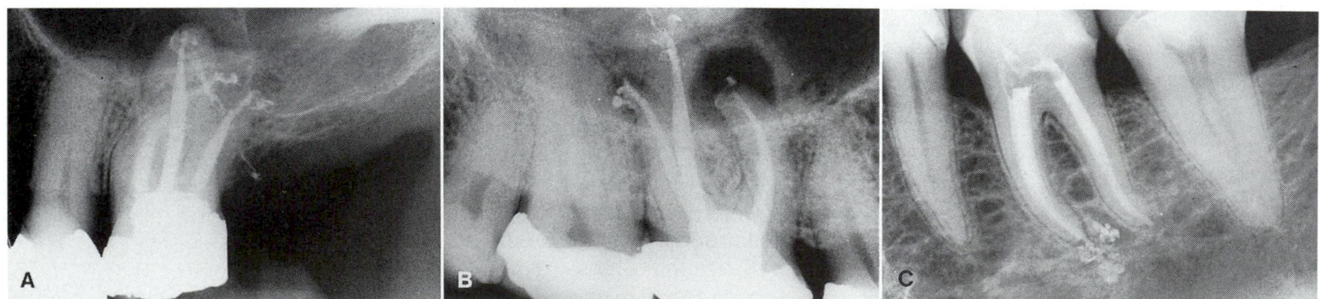

FIG. 8-10 "The Look" in multirooted posterior teeth. **A,** Proper shaping allows for *flow* in the root canal system. Flow, the third mechanical objective, refers to a prepared conical shape occurring in the same multiple planes as the original curvatures of the root canal system. **B,** Numerous foramina are naturally obturated by proper shaping. **C,** Mandibular molar gives the sense that the root canal packing takes on the same multiple planes as the original root canal.

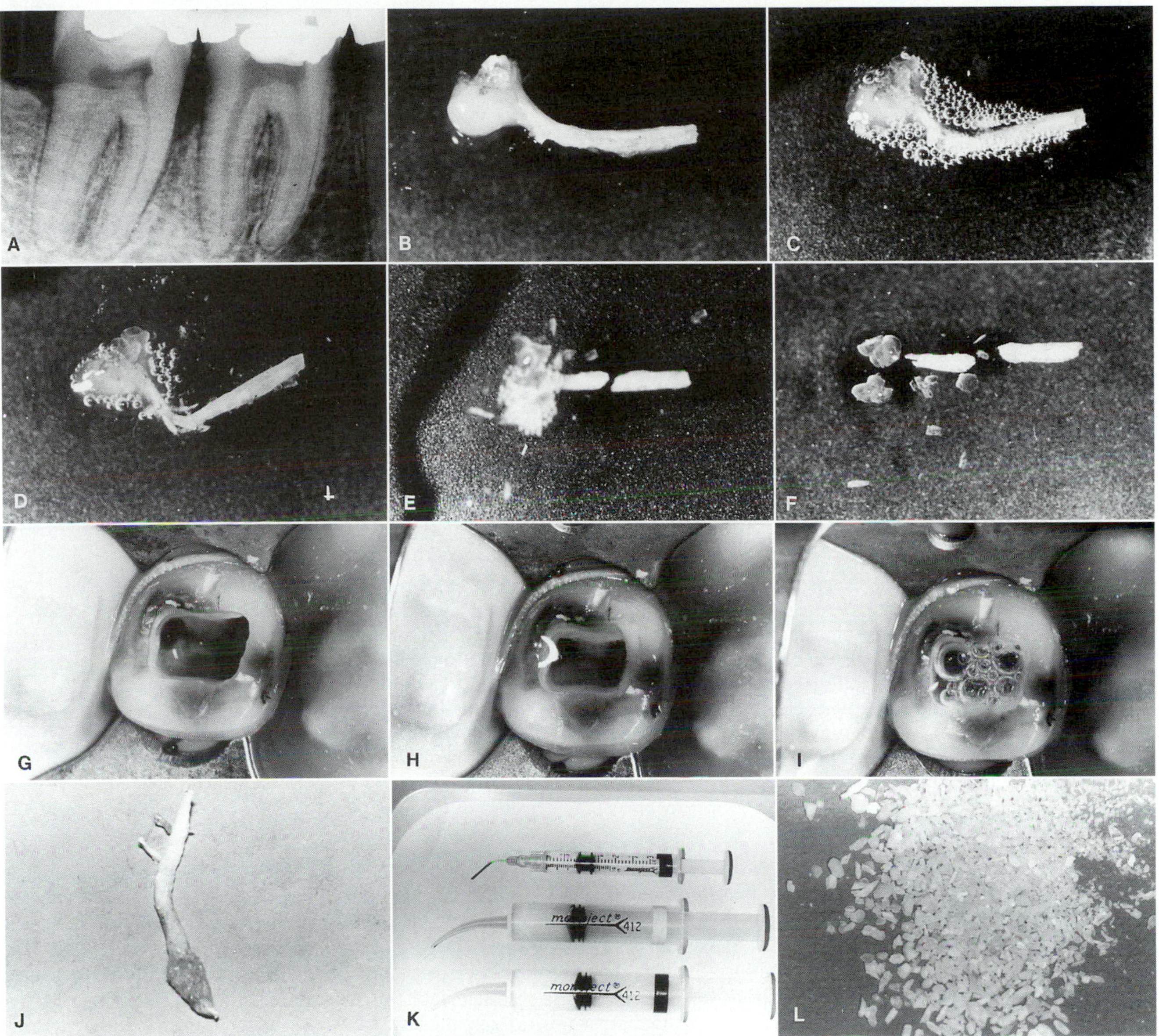

FIG. 8-11 Irrigation. **A,** Pretreatment radiograph of a mandibular first molar. **B,** Extirpated pulp. **C,** A drop of 3% sodium hypochlorite is placed on the pulp and photographed. **D,** Ten minutes later, digestion of the organic matrix is evident. **E,** At 30 minutes, organic material is essentially in solution. **F,** After 45 minutes, all organic material is dissolved, leaving remaining denticles and calcifications. Remember these potential calcifications in all cleaning and shaping. **G,** Mandibular molar with sodium hypochlorite only at the base of the access cavity. **H,** Sodium hypochlorite filled to the top of the cavity surface, as it should be. **I,** Combination of 3% hydrogen peroxide with sodium hypochlorite creates effervescence and elevates dentin mud away from the apical third and toward the chamber where it can be easily turned over and aspirated with subsequent irrigation. **J,** Extirpated pulp with foraminal appendages, revealing the true three dimensional nature of the root canal system. **K,** Irrigating syringes for 3% sodium hypochlorite and hydrogen peroxide. Larger syringes are for chamber irrigation, and sodium hypochlorite is in a smaller syringe for delicate irrigation slightly deeper into the cervical third of the canal. **L,** A dissolved pulp collection of 50 pulps showing numerous denticles, calcifications, and small pulp stones. Their presence is a major reason that endodontics requires such a light touch.

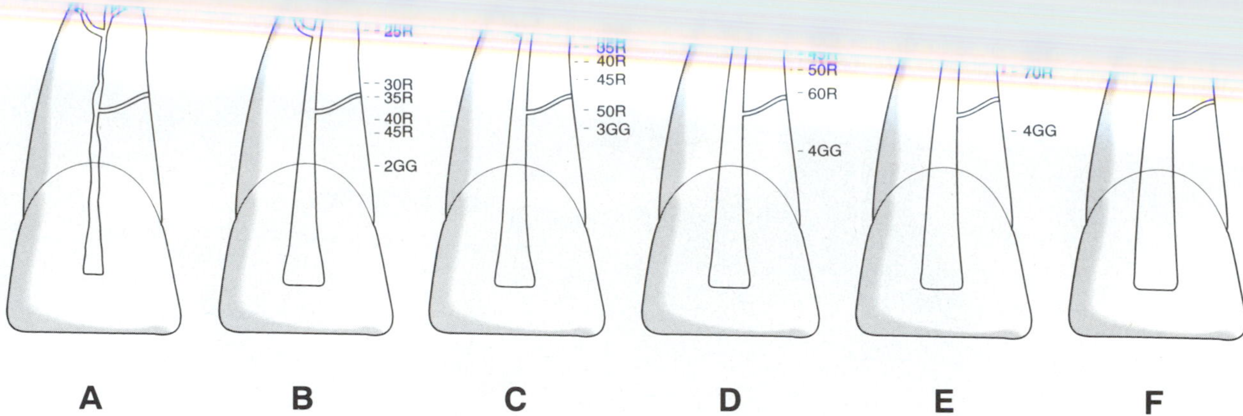

FIG. 8-12 Proper root canal preparation through serial shaping and recapitulation. **A,** A canal requiring cleaning and shaping. **B,** Developing shape after the first series of files and reamers. Notice that the larger reamers are never placed to their maximum physical depth but, rather, short of the radiographic terminus. **C,** Position of instrument depth after the *first recapitulation*. The no. 20 file now falls to the radiographic terminus where previously it did not extend. The no. 25, 30, 35, 40, and 45 reamers are now easily advanced apically. The Gates-Glidden drills are shimmied only in the cervical third. **D,** After the *second recapitulation,* the root canal begins to take on the correct shape. The position of the instruments is dictated by the developing shape of the canal and not by the preconceived instrument level dictated by the operator. Notice how the apical and middle thirds of the shape begin to blend now with the access cavity. **E,** After the *third recapitulation,* the shaping is almost complete with larger instruments progressing apically. **F,** After the *final recapitulation,* it is discovered that the foramen minimal size is a no. 30 file, and the continuously tapering cone shape of the last few millimeters is verified by each subsequent-sized instrument sliding short of the radiographic terminus. Each subsequent instrument should fall easily to its position and then meet resistance from the remaining tapering cone. The cone fit is then the final evidence that all five mechanical objectives have been achieved and that the root canal system is ready for three-dimensional obturation.

10 file, the instrument usually will progress apically through or around the necrotic debris, dense collagen, or small pulp stones and denticles. If the instrument does not bypass the obstacle, the file is withdrawn (Fig. 8-13). Again the file is precurved with a slightly different curvature and the chamber is gently irrigated. This sequence is repeated until the radiographic terminus is reached.

Why are we spending so much time on the first instrument? Because the first instrument is the key. Once the radiographic terminus has been reached, success depends solely on the cleaning and shaping mechanics. The fundamental techniques are *patency confirmation and serial carving,* which was previously described as *serial filing, reaming,* and *recapitulation.*[18,74,76] *Recapitulation is sequential reentry and reuse of each previous instrument.* Recapitulation does not merely confirm patency; it involves careful, rhythmic sequencing of the series of files and reamers in order to create the shape that achieves the five mechanical objectives. Most of excellent endodontics depends on cleaning and shaping, and most successful cleaning and shaping depends on the first instrument that reaches the radiographic terminus. At some point, we have weaved and threaded our way to the radiographic terminus. This must be verified by an accurate radiograph and with an electronic apex locator. The operator must not manipulate the instrument while waiting for the radiograph—for two reasons: If the foramen has been passed, it could be inadvertently torn. If the instrument is positioned coronal to the foramen, dentin mud could be packed into the foraminal opening. *There is one chance in three that the instrument is in the correct position.* Patience is paramount. Sodium hypochlorite is used to irrigate. If the radiograph indicates that the instrument is long, the dentist must pull back, adjust the rubber stop to the reference, and expose another radiograph, or advance immediately to the no. 15 file and repeat all the maneuvers described above. If the instrument is coronal to the radiographic terminus, the operator carefully slides it apically by continuing to follow the curvature of the canal and exposes a new radiograph. If the instrument does not advance, it is slid back out, the canal is irrigated, and the instrument is recurved before another try is made (Fig. 8-13).

Once the first instrument has reached the radiographic terminus, the rubber stop is set against the closest access reference and the file is moved in vertical strokes of a half millimeter to a 1- or 2-mm amplitude: the tighter the canal, the less the amplitude (Fig. 8-14, *D*). Sometimes when the first instrument is snug, flexing the fingers produces enough movement of the instrument (Fig. 8-16, *F* and *G*). At some point the instrument will begin to release as the dentin is worn away and the instrument is freed. It is essential to recognize that these are vertical strokes and no attempt is made to circumferentially create shape with the small instrument. The purpose is to navigate and establish the path to the foramen using the

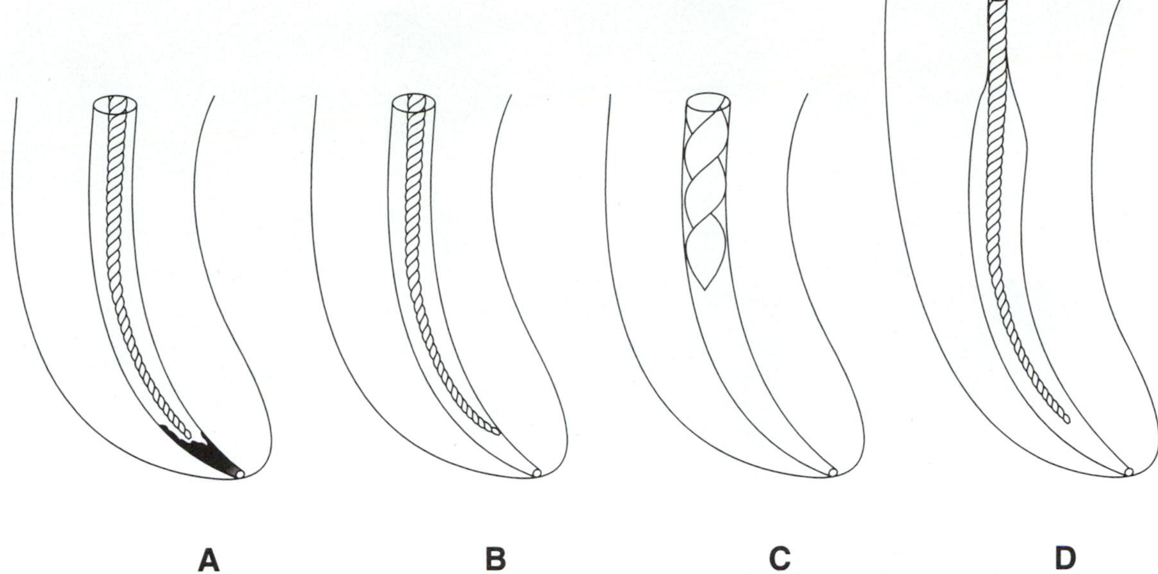

FIG. 8-13 There are four possible causes for canal blockage. **A,** The canal is blocked with dentin mud. Irrigate with sodium hypochlorite, place a significant apical curve on the file or reamer as shown in Fig. 8-14, *C,* and slide the instrument back into the root canal system. Before the instrument reaches maximum resistance, slide it out of the root canal and irrigate again. Do this enough times that the dentin mud is disrupted and each instrument will slip apically toward the radiographic terminus until finally patency is again achieved. **B,** The angle of access is divergent from the angle of incidence. The solution is to remove the instrument, recurve it, and slide it back into place. As soon as the curvature matches the original curvature of the root canal, the instrument will extend to the radiographic terminus, and cleaning and shaping can continue. **C,** The tip of the instrument is too wide for the existing shape. Remove the instrument and return to a narrower one. Do not proceed until that instrument fits loosely. **D,** The instrument experiences restriction somewhere short of the apical third. The correction is to lightly and serially shape the restrictive area, so that the file easily falls to the radiographic terminus.

long axis of the precurved file with a short in-and-out motion. The file is loosening dense collagen, dentin mud, and dentinal filings from the canal walls. When this material surrounds the file, the file is withdrawn and the root canal is irrigated with sodium hypochlorite.

Now the pace quickens, but the light touch is maintained. The rubber stop of a no. 15 file is set the same length as a no. 10 file. The clinician follows the no. 15 file in the same fashion as the no. 10 file, and the sequence is repeated. Once the no. 15 file is loose through gentle vertical strokes, the canal is irrigated and the precurved no. 20 reamer will slide short of the radiographic terminus. Random sculpting occurs on withdrawal of the reamer. Any dentin shavings or debris that have accumulated will be drawn away. The rubber stops are set by comparing the length of the two instruments. A ruler is an unnecessary step, a step that can add error to the measurement.

In the past, files were for filing, reamers were for reaming, and Gates-Glidden drills were for drilling (Fig. 8-14). The distinction now is that files are for following and maintaining patency and discovering a pathway to the foramen. Reamers are for carrying away dentin shavings and debris and for carving. The envelope of motion of the precurved reamer randomly shaves the dentinal walls.[76] This sculpting occurs exclusively on *withdrawal*. This is how to avoid ledges. Reamers are for carving in relatively straight canals and the relatively straight portion of curved canals. Many dentists and endodontists have avoided the use of reamers, and this is unfortunate. It is difficult to carve delicately with files without forcing dentin into apical foramina (Fig. 8-16). The Gates-Glidden drill is used simply as a brush, to shape the coronal third (sometimes half) of the root canal so that it blends smoothly with the access cavity. The operator always shapes away from the furca with the Gates-Glidden drill.

The precurved no. 25 reamer shaves the dentinal walls to the point of maximum resistance and is withdrawn in a light carving fashion. The no. 30, 35, 40, and 45 reamers are used in the same way (Fig. 8-12, *B*). If the no. 50 reamer barely fits into the orifice, it is removed. The access cavity flows to the coronal third of the root canal with the no. 2 Gates-Glidden drill. This essential step removes restrictive dentin and allows larger reamers to fall freely and deeper into the evolving shape. Confirm patency with a no. 15 file and the *first recapitulation* begins by reintroducing the initial series of files and reamers (Fig. 8-12, *C*).

In the first recapitulation, the no. 20 file should advance to the foramen. The no. 20 precurved reamer carries away dentin debris. At least 2 ml of sodium hypochlorite is used to irrigate between *every* instrument use. Now that the no. 25 reamer is not restricted, it should advance deeper into the root

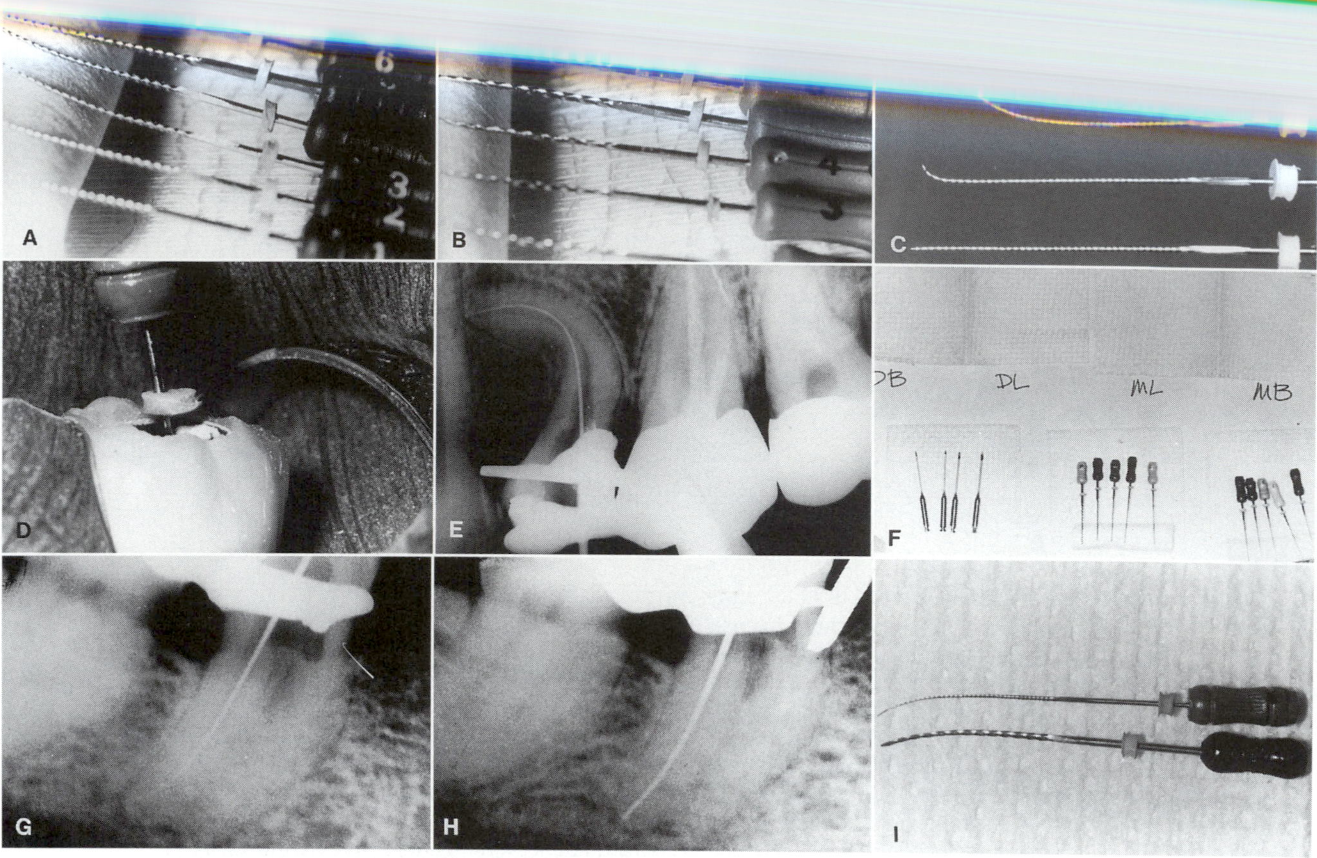

FIG. 8-14 A and **B,** Demonstrate the eventual rubber stop position of the final shaping. Note that the instruments are progressively set short of the full length of the root canal system. Cleaning and shaping is achieved through serial reaming, filing, and recapitulation. **C,** The lower straight instrument can be transformed into multiple curves, including abrupt apical turns, gentle curvatures, and finally curves in multiple planes to randomize the directional possibilities of instruments as they advance apically. **D,** Rubber stop reference is essential to successful cleaning and shaping. **E,** The radiographic terminus is the only reproducible guideline for successful cleaning and shaping. **F,** Anticipate four canals in all molars by identifying them with their own 2 by 2 gauze. At completion of cleaning and shaping, each gauze square will store the first and last instrument to the radiographic terminus as well as the gutta-percha cone. **G,** First instrument to the radiograph terminus. **H,** Last instrument to the radiographic terminus. **I,** Notice the length difference between the first and last instrument of this molar, demonstrating the shortening of canal length after several recapitulations. It is important to expose a treatment film after several recapitulations, in order to prevent external transportation.

canal. The clinician should use the envelope of motion to gently carve the walls of the root canal. The precurved no. 30 and 35 reamers are gently advanced into the root canal but not to the maximum physical depth. The technique is to slip in and allow the withdrawing envelope of motion of the precurved reamer to carve the internal shape.

Now the no. 40 and 45 reamers should easily advance deeper into the root canal. For the first time, the no. 50 reamer should fit into the middle region of the root canal, and a slight amount of sculpting and carving can be accomplished. The no. 50 reamer is followed by a no. 3 Gates-Glidden drill, which is shimmied against the walls in the coronal one third of the root canal. Again, the canal is irrigated between files, reamers, and Gates-Glidden drills. In a mandibular tooth, RC-prep or hydrogen peroxide is alternated with sodium hypochlorite to create effervescence and elevate the dentin mud into the chamber. Then it can be aspirated easily and new irrigation is introduced. Confirm patency with a small file and begin a *second* recapitulation (Fig. 8-12, *D*).

It is unlikely that the canal could be blocked at this point if this step-by-step procedure is followed. However, it is still possible that some dentin mud has accumulated (Fig. 8-15). After irrigating, the smallest instrument that reached the foramen is retrieved and an abrupt apical curve is created (not a bend) so the last half millimeter is not straight (Fig. 8-14, *C*). This instrument will dislodge the dentin mud (Fig. 8-15). The technique should be careful and light; sliding and irrigating, sliding and irrigating, slipping and irrigating, sliding and irri-

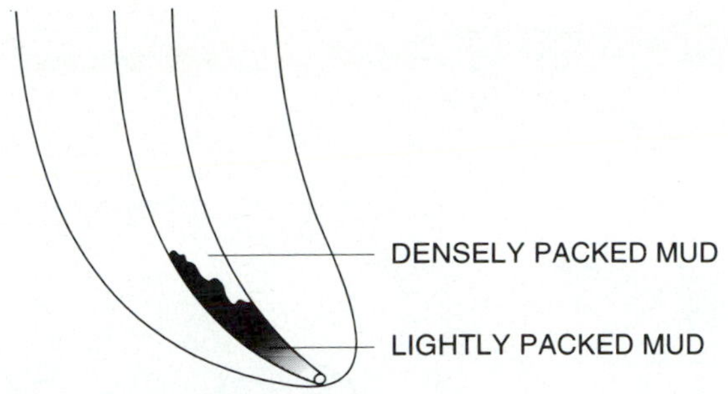

FIG. 8-15 The densest dentin mud is usually most coronal. Disrupt the dentin mud in this area and then the instruments will easily slide through the lightly packed dentin mud to the radiographic terminus.

gating. The canal is still there (Fig. 8-13, *A–D*). With time the foramen *will* be reached.

Now the no. 25 file should reach to the foramen and suddenly and *gently* hug the dentinal walls (Fig. 8-12, *D*). The instruments are loose until the canal narrows to their diameter; then they fit loosely against the dentinal walls. The no. 30 reamer should be 1 to 2 mm from the foramen when it is advanced into the canal. The no. 35, 40, 45, and 50 reamers provide further shaping after the second recapitulation. The no. 60 reamer should now extend into the middle third of the root. One or two carvings with the no. 60 reamer selectively enlarges the midportion of the root canal. The no. 4 Gates-Glidden drill is used to brush the walls in the cervical third and to continue to blend the shape of the apical third with the coronal third.

Patency is confirmed before the *third* recapitulation is begun. If recapitulation is done properly, no instrument goes to the same place twice. They automatically extend deeper into the canal. In our example, the no. 30 file nearly reaches the foramen, while the no. 35, 40, 45, 50, 60, and 70 reamers are shaping and sculpting close behind (Fig. 8-12, *E*). A progress radiograph (Fig. 8-14, *G–I*) is exposed. The no. 4 Gates-Glidden drill is used for final blending of the coronal third and the access cavity. After irrigation and confirmation of patency, the *fourth* and final recapitulation begins. Actually, the operator cannot know that this is the final recapitulation (Fig. 8-12, *F*). If the desired shape has not been achieved, another recapitulation is necessary (Fig. 8-14, *A* and *B*). At times one or two recapitulations make the difference between an adequate and an excellent result.

When are cleaning and shaping complete? They are complete when the cone fits. If the conventional gutta-percha cone fits to the radiographic terminus, the shape is conducive to compaction of gutta-percha and sealer into the foramina.

Motions of Cleaning and Shaping

Cleaning and shaping are dynamically delicate motions, flowing, rhythmic, and energetic. In order to use files and reamers efficiently, the movements require distinction. There are six distinctive motions of files and reamers.

Follow. Follow (Fig. 8-16, *A–F*) is usually performed with files. They are used initially during cleaning and shaping, or any time an obstruction blocks the foramen. Irrigating, precurving, different kinds of curves, curving all the way to the tip of the instrument, and multiple curves in multiple directions of the instrument are all part of follow.

Follow-withdraw. For follow and withdrawal (Fig. 8-16, *G* and *H*), again, the file is the most useful instrument. The motion is used when the foramen is reached, and the next step is to create the path from access cavity to foramen. The motion is follow and then withdraw, or "follow and pull," or "follow and remove." It is, simply, an in-and-out, passive motion that makes no attempt to shape the canal.

Cart. Carting (Fig. 8-16, *I*) refers to the extension of a reamer to or near the radiographic terminus. The precurved reamer should gently and randomly touch the dentinal walls and "cart" away debris.

Carve. Carving (Fig. 8-16, *J–L*) is for shaping. Reamers are the best instruments for carving and sculpting. The key is not to press the instrument apically but simply to touch the dentin with a precurved reamer and shape on withdrawal, thinking *gentleness*. The operator never forces an instrument by penetrating to the maximum physical depth.

Smooth. Smoothing (Fig. 8-16, *M*) is usually accomplished with files. In the past most endodontic procedures were performed with a smoothing or circumferential filing motion. If the previous four motions are followed, smoothing is rarely required.

Patency. Patency (Fig. 8-16, *M*) is achieved with files or reamers. It means simply that the portal of exit has been cleared of any debris in its path. Again, if the clinician has been diligent with the other motions, confirming patency is simplified.

THE BALANCED-FORCE TECHNIQUE

Fundamentals of Cleaning and Shaping

Purpose

Cleaning and shaping are the basics of endodontic therapy. Cleaning is a combined chemical and mechanical process, while shaping is purely a mechanical one. Cleaning removes affected, infected, antigenic, and substrate material from the canal system (Fig. 8-17). Shaping enlarges the canal's diameter and smoothes the walls as it removes crevices, fissures, and irregularities from the system. Thorough cleaning and shaping allow the clinician to completely seal the canal system. Once the root canal system is properly sealed, periapical healing or repair almost always follows.

Cleaning

Cleaning must eliminate tissue remnants, antigenic materials, inflammatory chemicals, and bacteria from the canal space.[4,5,10] Inadequate cleaning generates short-term treatment failure and allows periradicular inflammation and/or infection to persist (Fig. 8-18). Cleaning entails both mechanical removal of contents and chemical dissolution, detoxification, and removal of inflammatory and potentially inflammatory substances. Cleaning requires the use of instruments to physically remove substances, irrigating systems to flush loosened materials away, and chemicals to dissolve contents from inaccessible regions (Fig. 8-19).

Shaping

Shaping the canal system facilitates obturation. During this process, instrumentation must give the system a form that will ensure tissue removal and a shape that will enhance total filling of the root canal system in three dimensions.[6,26] Inadequate

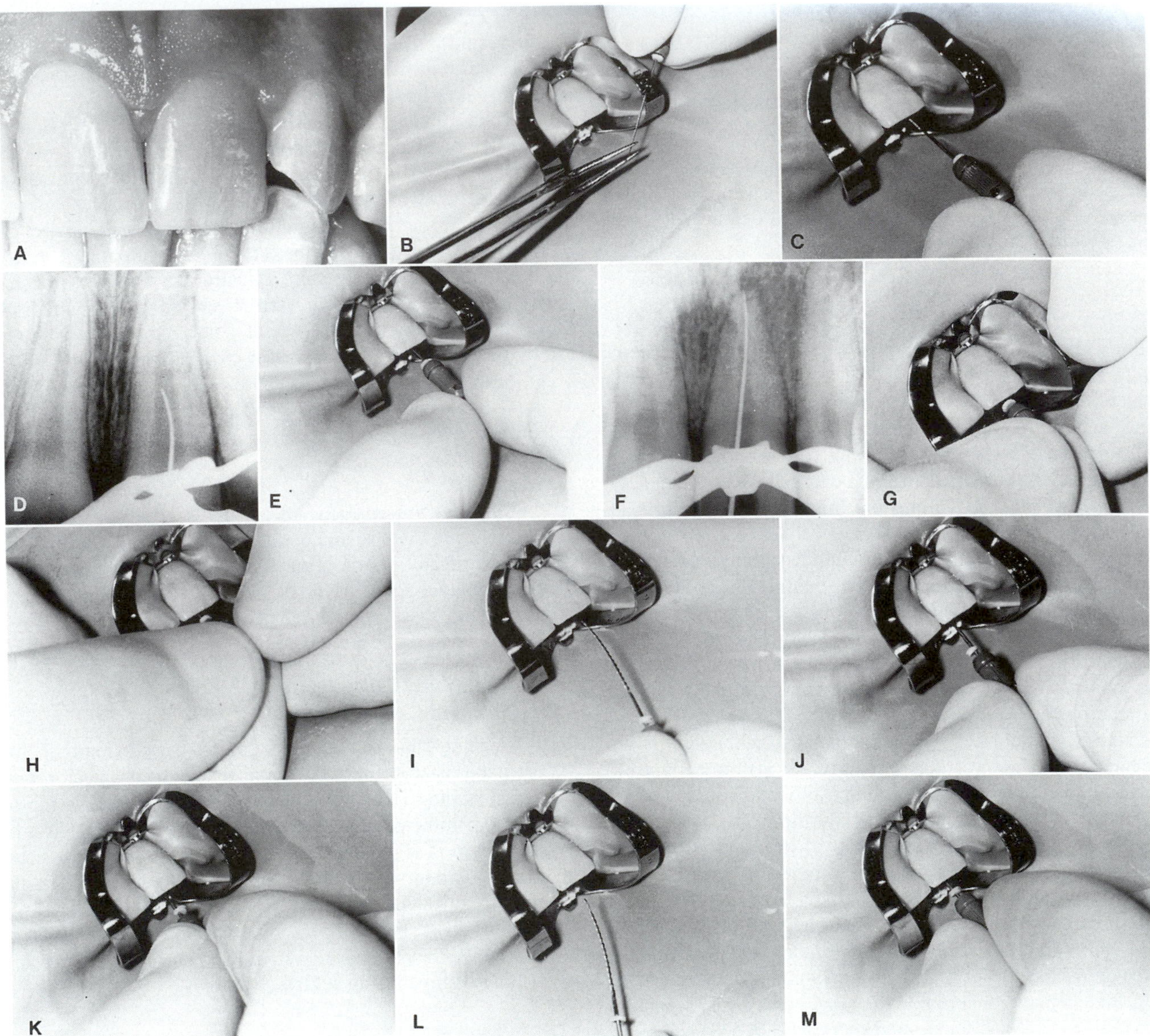

FIG. 8-16 Motions of cleaning and shaping. **A,** Pretreatment photograph of the central incisor. **B,** Careful curving of the apical portion of the file with appropriate cotton pliers. **C,** *Follow* the #10 file into the root canal system. **D,** Radiograph of advancing file. **E,** Continue to *follow* the instrument with almost no finger contact until the radiographic terminus is reached. **F,** Radiograph, verifying first instrument. **G** and **H,** Demonstrate the *follow/withdraw* reproduction of the path to the portal of exit. Notice small amplitude. Unlike *following,* this motion requires stable finger rest positions. **I,** File is followed by the same size reamer to *cart* away any dentin mud. **J** to **L,** *Carving* using the envelope of motion of the precurved reamer, randomly shaving the dentinal walls. **M,** A similar motion is needed to *smooth* the walls and also to confirm *patency*. All six motions are not static, but are rhythmic and in combination. However, their distinctions allow the operator greater mastery in producing proper shapes.

shaping causes inadequate obturation. As a result, safe harbors in the avascular root canal space remain open and allow for the persistence of noxious irritants. Slow dissemination of these bioactive substances through unsealed portals of exit is reported to be our most common cause of long-term endodontic failure (Fig. 8-20).[43] It is important to properly and completely shape all canals during the treatment process, to obtain a maximum therapeutic response for the patient. Nearly all obturation difficulties encountered by clinicians are in fact related to poor shaping results achieved early in treatment. Even simple canals that are poorly shaped are difficult if not impossible to obturate properly, whereas extremely complex root canal systems can be sealed by a novice if the shaping has been accomplished skillfully.

Shaping contributes significantly to the cleaning process because it establishes the necessary canal diameter to allow delivery of irrigation fluids to the entire canal space. It is a mechanical process accomplished with files, reamers, drills, sonic, ultrasonic powered instruments, and other mechanical devices. Shaping imparts a gradual taper to the smoothed canal walls as they converge toward the apex.

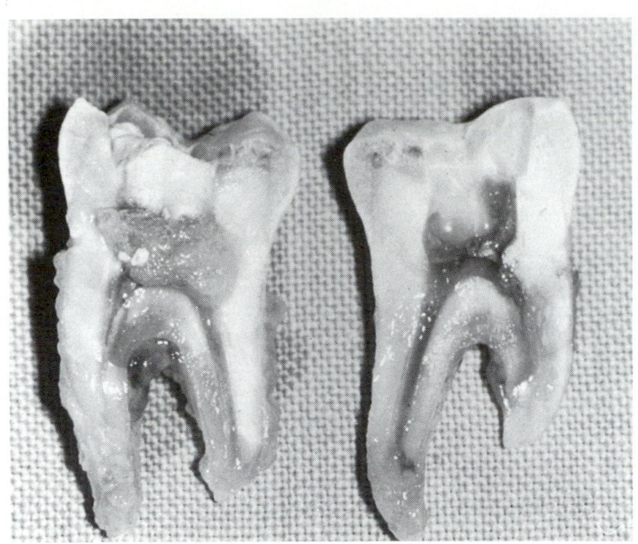

FIG. 8-17 This fractured mandibular molar reveals the canal contents of an endodontically involved tooth. Note the gross discoloration, débris, and contaminated appearance of the canal passages. Treatment must shape and cleanse these canals to ensure periapical healing.

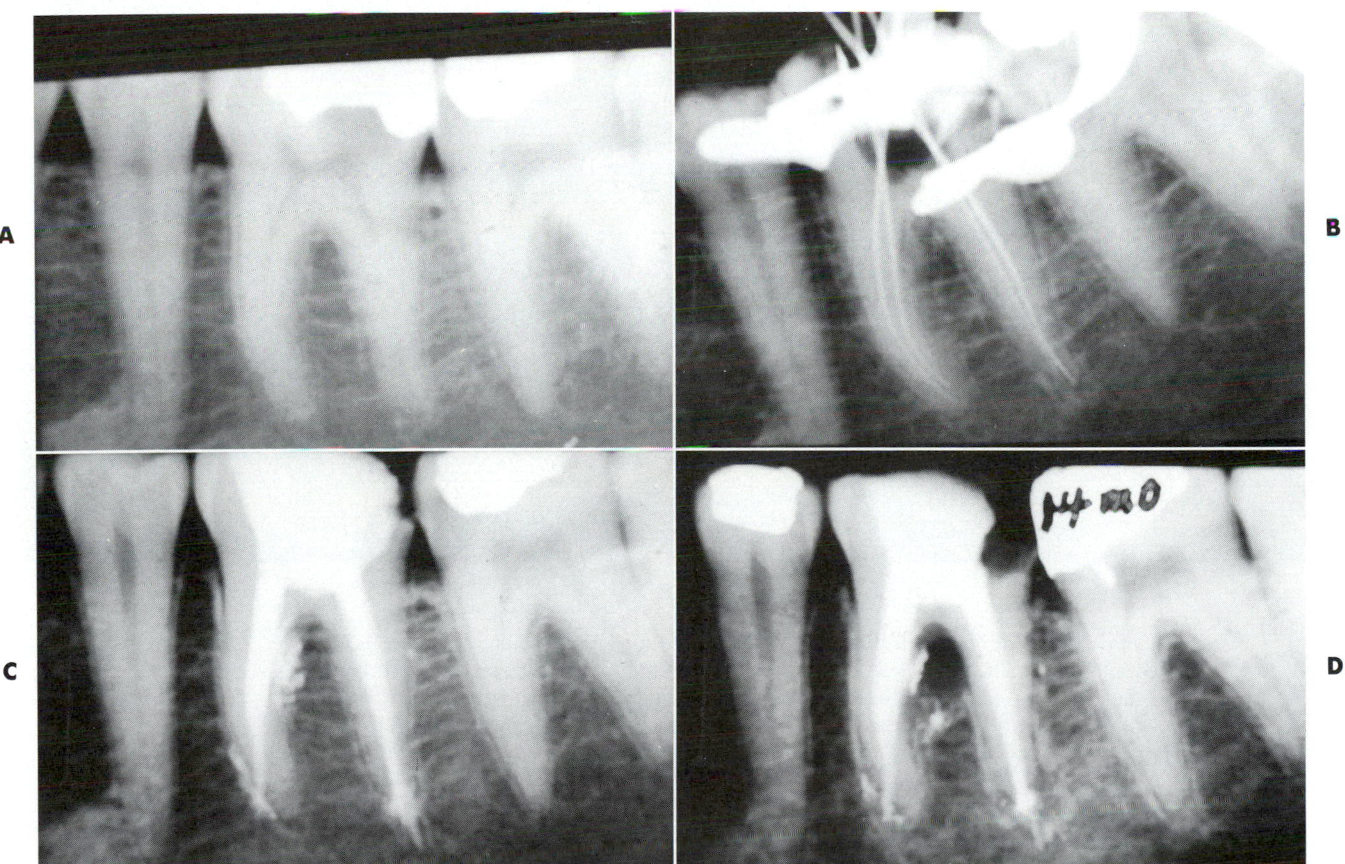

FIG. 8-18 A, Preoperative radiograph of a mandibular molar. The M root is curved throughout its entire length. **B,** Working files placed to the apex in four canals. **C,** Obturation film discloses a M furcal perforation from excessive GG depths, a M apical perforation, and a short M fill. The D foramen has been zipped and the fill overextended. **D,** A 14-month recall discloses the osseous damage that resulted. This tooth was lost as a result of improper treatment.

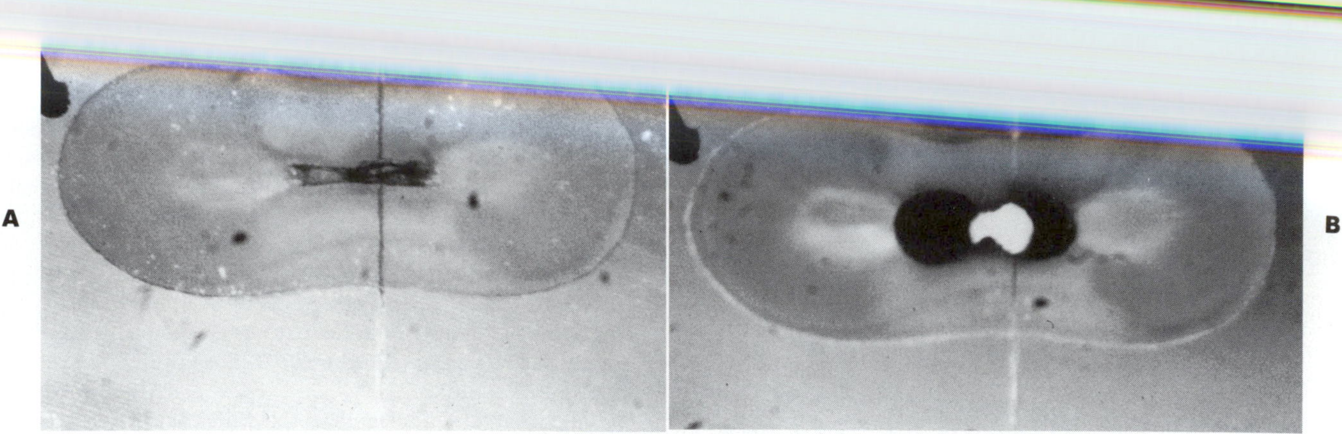

FIG. 8-19 A, This cross section was made about 5 mm coronal to the foramen in a maxillary premolar. Note how the canal space is oval and narrow. Treatment needs to clear this space of all debris and shape the walls. **B,** This posttreatment view of the same section reveals that instrumentation has cleaned the canal completely and shaped the entire perimeter. There is a confluence of two preparations, each proceeding from opposite ends of the oval space.

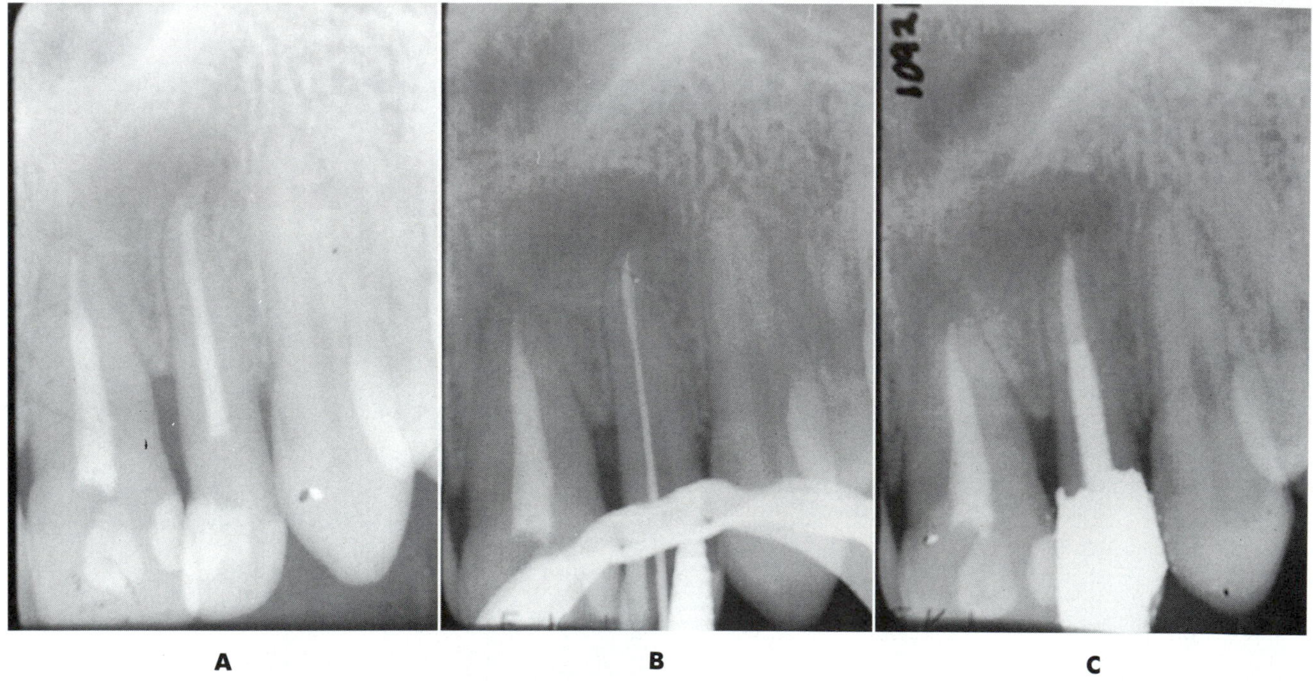

FIG. 8-20 An endodontic failure. **A,** Obturation is short of the apex and the tooth is symptomatic. **B,** The canal was blocked at the obturation point; however, that was bypassed and the canal was negotiated to the periodontal ligament. **C,** The posttreatment film shows a three-dimensional fill to the periodontal ligament; healing is expected.

Principles of Irrigation

Canal irrigation should always precede canal probing. Irrigation with just water simply flushes away loose, necrotic, contaminated materials before they are inadvertently pushed deeper into the canal (Fig. 8-21)[10]; however, irrigation with chemicals that have additional actions is strongly recommended. The benefits of irrigating with sodium hypochlorite include: (1) gross débridement, (2) lubrication, (3) elimination of microbes, (4) dissolution of soft tissues, and (5) removal of the smear layer. Accomplishing all five ends requires a combination of at least two fluids: (1) a lavage, lubricant, tissue solvent, and microbicide, and (2) a chelator or a dilute acid.

Types of Irrigation Solutions

Isotonic saline

Isotonic saline solution has been advocated by some as an irrigation fluid. In isotonic concentration, it produces no recognized tissue damage and was demonstrated in one study to

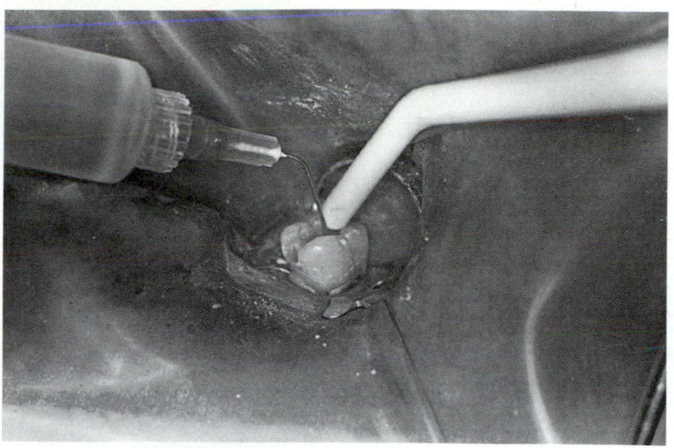

FIG. 8-21 Irrigation is easily accomplished with a 25- to 28-gauge needle and a disposable Luer-Lok syringe. The needle should be bent near the hub to facilitate access into the canals. Suction must accompany irrigation to prevent accidental leakage into the oral cavity.

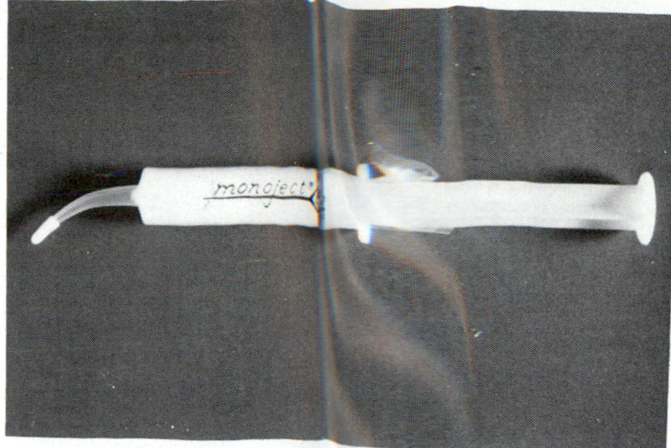

FIG. 8-22 RC Prep loaded into a large disposable syringe to allow filling of access cavity during initial preparation. Files working through this lubricant will carry it into the canal, thereby decreasing the chance of fibrous apical blockage early in treatment.

flush debris from the canals as thoroughly as sodium hypochlorite.[10] Saline accomplishes gross débridement and lubrication. Sterile isotonic saline may be obtained in 1-L IV containers for parceling out and use in individual treatments. Caution should be used in storage, loading and handling. This solution must not be contaminated with foreign biologic materials before or during use. Irrigation with saline sacrifices chemical destruction of microbiologic matter and dissolution of mechanically inaccessible tissues (e.g., in accessory canals and intercanal tissue bridges). Isotonic saline is too mild to thoroughly clean canals.

Sodium hypochlorite

Sodium hypochlorite (NaOCl) is by far the most commonly used irrigant in endodontic therapy. It can fulfill the first four actions. Such products as Clorox and Purex bleach are common sources of concentrated sodium hypochlorite (5.25%). Many clinicians prefer diluted concentrations to reduce the irritation potential of NaOCl. A 2.5% solution is commonly recommended, although full-strength and 1.25% solutions may also be used. One should be aware that dilution reduces the dissolution power. NaOCl is an inorganic solution that is consumed in the dissolution process.[9,12] The rate and extent of dissolution are related to the concentration of the NaOCl solution.[39]

Chelating agents

Disodium ethylenediamine-tetraacetate (EDTA), and an EDTA, sodium hydroxide, cetyl-trimethylammonium bromide and water mixture (REDTA), are chelating agents that may be used to irrigate the canal.[64] They remove the smear layer and may be used to soften obstructing dentin. These agents are not used in all situations, and a specific indication should exist when they are employed. They can soften the dentin throughout the canal system if they are sealed into the canal between visits or if they are used for an extended time during cleaning and shaping.[28]

Lubricants

RC Prep, Glyoxide, and surgical jelly may be useful during initial canal negotiation procedures (Fig. 8-22). These agents

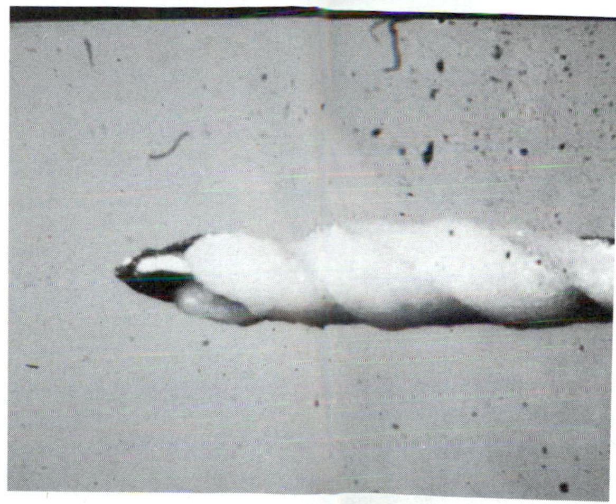

FIG. 8-23 Dentin debris is created by the cutting action of files and other shaping instruments. A portion of that débris may be packed against the blades and removed with the file, some débris is compacted into the dentin surface forming a smear layer, and the remainder is removed by irrigation.

have lubricating properties and facilitate instrument movement within the canal. They are used primarily during the early stages of preparation to eliminate soft tissue blockage.[12]

Effects of Irrigation

Gross débridement

Generally speaking, infected root canal systems are filled with materials that have an inflammatory potential. The physical act of shaping generates additional debris, which can elicit additional inflammatory response (Fig. 8-23). An irrigant can simply wash away such materials. Gross débridement is analogous to the simple washing of an open and contaminated wound. It is a most important process of treatment.

Frequency of irrigation and volume of the irrigant used are important factors in the removal of debris.[10,17,67] The frequency of irrigation should increase as instrumentation approaches the apical constricture.[12] An appropriate volume of

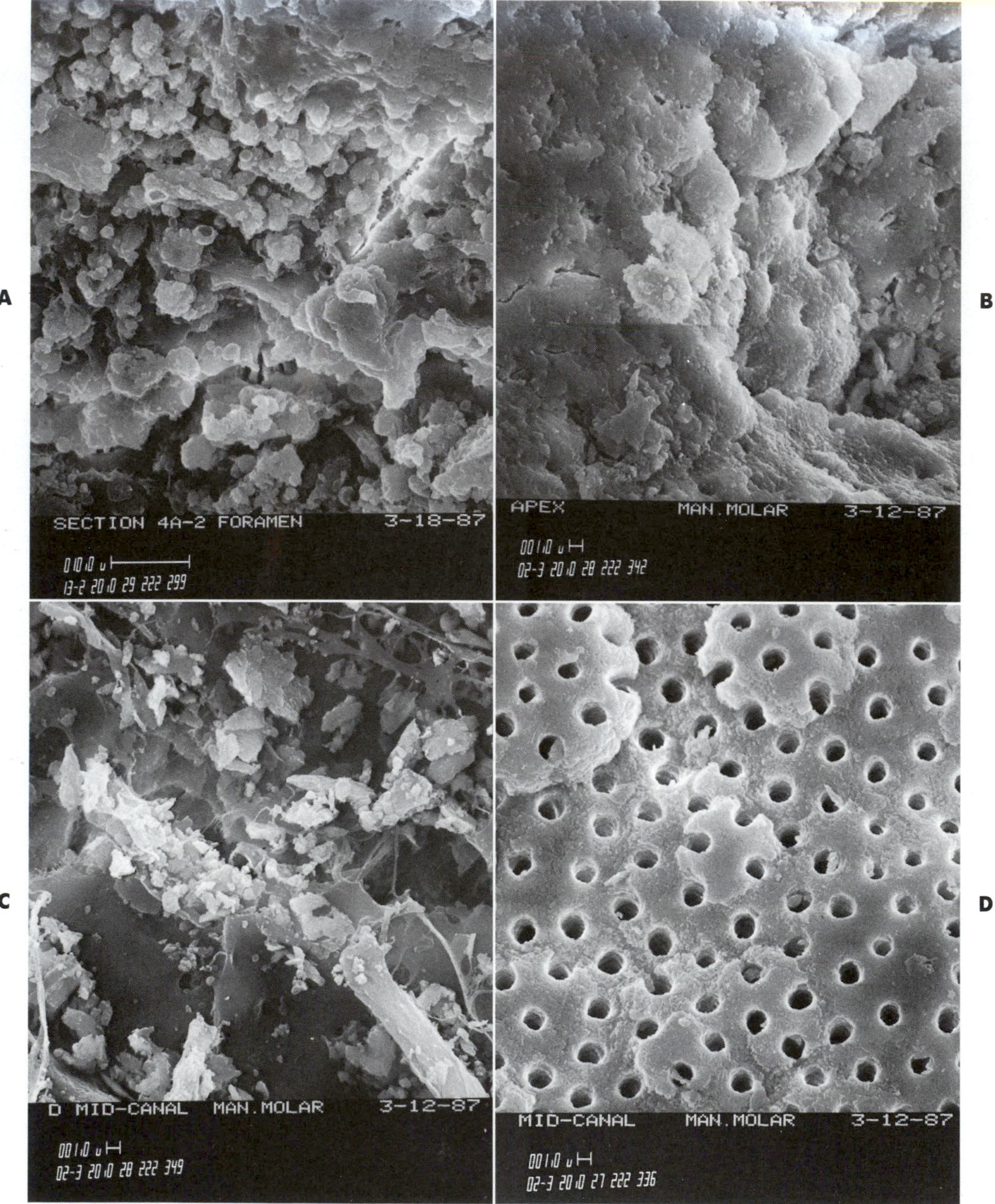

FIG. 8-24 SEMs from the canal system of a mandibular molar. **A,** This is from an area near the foramen. It has an irregular surface and may retain cellular debris. **B,** This view is from the control zone and displays tubules coated with the smear layer. **C,** This view is from a narrow crevice region in the midcanal area. Cellular fragment and a small vessel-like structure remain. **D,** This view is from another open but still uninstrumented region in the midcanal area. All cellular debris has been removed by the action of 5.25% NaOCl. The tubules are clean and open. No smear was formed.

irrigant is at least 1 to 2 ml each time the canal is flushed.[11,74] A key to improving the apical efficacy of irrigants is to use a patency file before each irrigation.[11] This small procedural nuance—patency confirmation before irrigation—works significantly better than irrigating without recapitulation. The reason is easy to appreciate. The patency file simply moves debris, compacted into the apex, back into solution. Loosened in this manner, apical debris is more likely to be flushed out by the irrigant. While the preparation diameter is small, placing a file into the apical third is the best way to move irrigant to that region. The instrument displaces canal contents, and when it is removed irrigant is allowed to flow to the vacated space. This action alone is not sufficient to remove pulpal tissues in small-caliber canal preparations.[79]

Elimination of microbes

Sodium hypochlorite (NaOCl) has proven the most effective antimicrobial irrigant.[87] It can kill all microbes in root canals, including spore-forming bacteria and viruses. Microbicidal effect can be accomplished even with diluted concentrations of NaOCl.[21,40] Clinicians should insist on using only irrigants with antimicrobicidal properties.

Dissolution of pulp remnants

Using NaOCl in low concentration (below 2.5%) predictably eliminates infection but does not consistently dissolve pulpal remnants[89] unless excessive time is spent in treatment. Baumgartner and Mader[8] confirmed that 2.5% NaOCl is extremely effective in removing vital pulp tissue from dentinal walls.[11] They also noted that walls untouched by files (Fig. 8-24) were cleaned when adequate concentrations of NaOCl were used. Cunningham and colleagues[19,20] have demonstrated a relationship between temperature and the activity of sodium hypochlorite.

The dissolving efficacy of sodium hypochlorite is influenced by the structural integrity of the connective tissue components of the pulp.[2] If the pulp is already decomposed, it won't take long to dissolve the remaining soft tissue remnants. If the pulp is vital and little structural degeneration has occurred, it will take longer for NaOCl to dissolve the remnants. In this respect, cleaning procedures should not be hurried, especially when the pulpal tissues are still supported by circulation.

Removal of the smear layer

The smear layer is composed of débris compacted into the surface of dentinal tubules by the action of instruments. It is burnished into the surfaces as the edges of instruments slide by. It is composed of fractured bits of dentin and soft tissue from the canal. These materials are released into the flute space of preparation instruments (Figs. 8-23, 8-24) and smeared over the canal surface by passage of trailing cutting edges. Since the smear layer is primarily calcific it is most effectively removed by the action of mild acids and chelating agents (e.g., EDTA and REDTA).

Exceptional cleaning efficacy has been demonstrated for a combination of sodium hypochlorite and REDTA solutions during cleaning procedures.[30] This combination removes soft tissue remnants as well as the organic/inorganic smear layer. Baumgartner and Mader[8] demonstrated that all canal walls that are planed with cutting instruments develop a smear layer. The instrumented regions require a chelating agent to remove the smear and reopen the tubules. Canal walls not touched by files did not develop a smear layer and therefore needed only NaOCl to be cleaned (Fig. 8-24).[3]

There is no clinical consensus as to whether the smear layer should be removed. Those in favor of leaving the smear intact argue that it may be a clinical factor that actually enhances endodontic success. It appears to plug the dentinal tubules, microbes and tissue included. This plugging may help prevent bacterial egress from the tubules after treatment. Williams and Goldman have shown that the smear layer will slow bacterial movement, but it does not prevent eventual egress.[93] Kennedy et al[47] indicate from their experimentation that teeth obturated with gutta-percha are more completely sealed when the smear layer is removed. This finding is also supported by Wade's group.[85] For these reasons it appears prudent to create the cleanest dentinal surface possible by using chelating agents.

Ultrasonics Irrigation

Ultrasonic handpieces have not performed as well as expected in apical shaping efficiency;[21,56,65,83,94] however, ultrasonics vibration is unparalleled in its ability to enhance cleaning with irrigants.[2-4,12,48,55] Used with a small file held free of the canal walls, the ultrasonics energy warms the solutions in the canal and the resonant vibrations cause movement of aqueous irrigants, an effect called *acoustic streaming* (Fig. 8-25). Used as irrigating instruments ultrasonics handpieces must be handled with care to avoid roughness and ledging in the apical third of canals.[13,14]

Ultrasonic activation of NaOCl has been shown to be most effective in the apical third of the canal, owing to the greater amplitudes of vibratory movement at the file tip.[3,46] Because the cleaning effects of ultrasonic energy are most ideal when the energized instrument is loose in the canal, it is probably best to use ultrasonics after shaping is completed.[33,41,49]

Ultrasonic irrigation adds significantly to the cost and complexity of the clinical irrigation system. This factor must be weighed against its potential value,[33,38] especially considering

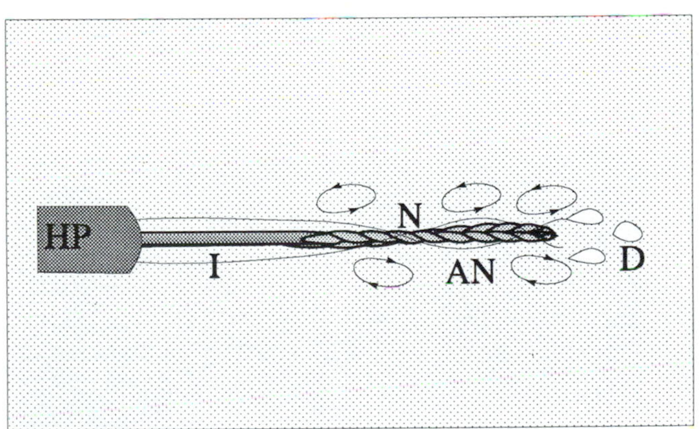

FIG. 8-25 This illustration depicts fluid flow about an instrument activated by ultrasonic energy waves. *HP* is the ultrasonic handpiece; —I—represents fluid flow, *N* is a nodal region of the file movement. Little or no movement occurs in these areas. *AN* is antinode. Oscillating file displacement occurs at these points. The maximum displacement occurs at the instrument tip. The elliptical flow patterns are eddies of acoustic streaming. *D* are droplets of water that are expelled from the end of an instrument operated free in space.

that mixtures of chemicals placed with inexpensive syringes are also effective in removing tissues and smear layer from the canal wall.[8,29] Exposure is a limiting factor to all cleaning, including ultrasonics irrigation. Exposure is significantly influenced by the shaping[46] because space must be created and contents removed before any irrigation fluid can enter an area.[16,42] Acoustic streaming causes flow along the outside of an instrument and a small instrument of 0.15 mm diameter can be used to deliver the irrigant. This would be an ideal solution, but acoustic streaming is limited by the amplitude of the sonic vibration and requires a minimum canal diameter of about 0.25 mm for the no. 15 file.[3,5,87] If the canal is narrower, the instrument will suffer a damping effect and no flow will occur. Curvature may also damp the oscillations and stop acoustic streaming, especially without precurving of the file.[2] On the other hand, syringes are limited by the diameter of their delivery needle, both internal bore and external diameter. The smallest practical irrigation needle size is 27 gauge. Its external diameter is 0.39 mm. When it is used, the canal diameter must be greater than the area of the needle lumen, if fluids are to escape freely past the needle and return into the access cavity.[17,67]

Length Determination

Every part of endodontic treatment is controlled by a measurement of the instrument's penetration depth into the canal. This length is typically determined in millimeters. It is measured from a point on the tooth's coronal surface that is within the clinician's field of view. It varies from the complete canal length to some arbitrarily determined point near the termination of the canal space (Fig. 8-26).

Biologic rationale for working length

Working length determines the extent of canal cleaning and shaping that will be accomplished. This measurement limits the penetration depth of subsequent instruments and determines the ultimate form of the shaping process. Cleaning and shaping can have no greater precision than the working length. It is extremely important to make an accurate determination. The most clinically relevant working length landmark is the apical constricture, regardless of whether it is in dentin or cementum.[22] The constricture is the narrowest point of the canal,[52] and therefore the narrowest diameter of the blood supply. Beyond the constricture, the canal widens and develops a broad vascular supply. Therefore, from a biologic perspective, the constricture is the most rational point at which to end the canal preparation, since the existence of a functional blood supply controls the inflammatory process. Intraradicular termination of the cleansing process leaves a canal content interface equal in area to the total inflammatory process (1:1). Termination beyond the constricture provides a greater area of blood supply than of irritant interface. Extraradicular termination of the working length can theoretically provide a hemisphere of vascular support to the inflammatory process. That gives a numerically superior advantage to the inflammatory process. The surrounding vital tissues have more capacity to destroy irritants and restore the area to a biologically functional state. Thus, cleaning and shaping to the apical constricture most completely eliminates pathogenic canal contents and allows the inflammatory healing mechanisms to complete.

Optimal length

From a procedural perspective, it is advantageous to treat to the constricture because it is a morphologic landmark[34–36] that can be felt by the experienced clinician. As the canal is shaped, coronal to the apical constricture, it becomes progressively easier to locate the constricture with a small-patency file and tactile sense. The experienced hand can detect an abrupt increase in resistance followed by a rapid decline as the instrument tip passes beyond the constricture.

Using the apical constricture as the working length landmark is very desirable because it means that the preparation will terminate at the narrowest canal diameter. This preparation shape helps to optimize the apical seal when the canal is subsequently filled.[6,26,74] Only the diameter of the constricture is exposed to the apical tissues.

Clinicians are ill-advised to treat root canals short of this endpoint, because lateral and accessory canals are more com-

A

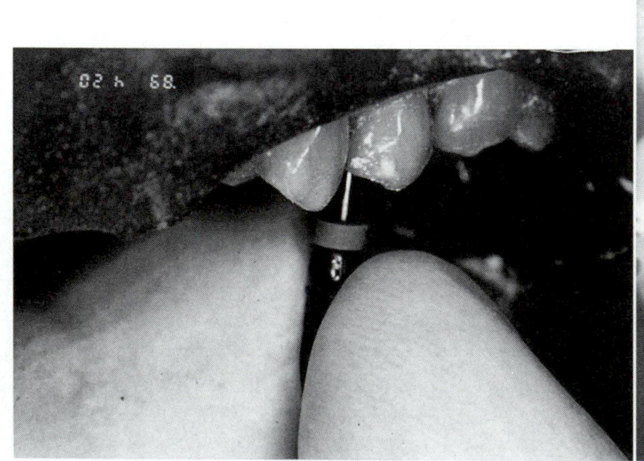

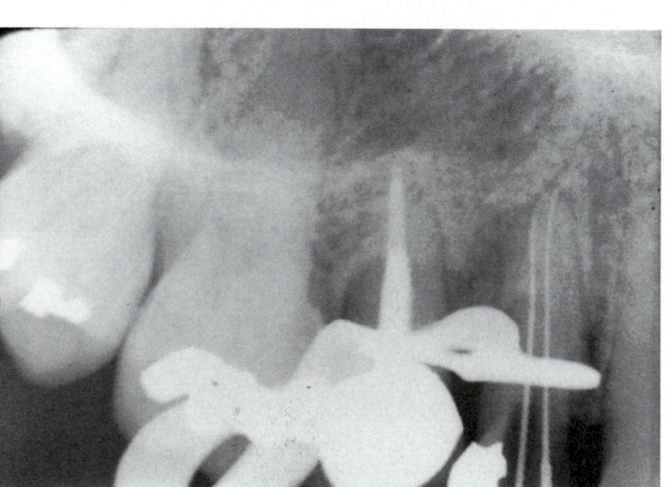

B

FIG. 8-26 A, The file is being oscillated right and left to place it to the estimated radiographic length. When it stops or the marker reaches the cusp tip, a working length radiograph is exposed. **B,** This radiograph indicates the desired file position has been achieved in both canals. These lengths are carefully measured and recorded.

mon near the apex. Considering the possibility of an accessory canal, treating just 1 to 2 mm short of the apical constricture can leave 2 to 4 mm of untreated canal. Such a length could significantly increase the chances for persistent periapical infection or inflammation. A region of canal that is 0.25 mm in diameter and 1 mm long can contain approximately 80,000 streptococci. This is surely a sufficient number to produce at least a moderate inflammation (Fig. 8-20).

Methods of determining canal length

Because we cannot directly visualize the ends of root canals in vivo, length determination requires careful clinical assessment. Only by correlating many confirming pieces of evidence can clinicians indirectly discern the true terminus of root canals.

Radiographic. The most commonly used method of determining the length of a canal is radiography. The clinician starts by placing a file to a preestimated length and then exposes a film. The location of the instrument tip is read from this film and any necessary changes in length are made. Changes greater than 0.5 mm should be verified by an additional radiograph. The exact canal preparation depth depends on the technique and philosophy of the operator. The periodontal ligament space typically is used to identify the apical termination of the canal.* This point includes the expanding portion of the canal beyond the constricture; consequently, techniques routinely make an allowance. The preparation length is shortened from the full length to the periodontal ligament space by at least 0.5 mm initially. Greater adjustments are recommended in some techniques.

Electronic. Apex locators may be used to determine the canal length (see Fig. 6-14). The unit is connected to a file that can be inserted to the canal terminus, and a second lead is attached to the oral mucosa. The pulp is extirpated, the canal is irrigated and dried, then the attached file is inserted to the apex. This precaution eliminates ionic conduction, which can give a premature indication that the apex has been reached. The more recent impedance models apparently are not as sensitive to ionic solutions as the older resistance-based units. The dryness is perhaps not as important in that case.[59]

Apex locators are most helpful in placing the first length-determination file. At that time the working length must be estimated from a preoperative radiograph. This method requires some clinical experience to be used successfully; controlling the first file into the canal with an apex locator reduces guesswork. Over time use of an apex locator can guide the clinician as he or she develops tactile sense.

The clinician must be careful to avoid contaminating the file while connecting the electrical lead and inserting the measurement instrument. The file can be placed into the canal some distance before the lead is attached, to reduce the chance of accidental contamination. From there the file is carefully oscillated and gently pressed toward the apex. As it approaches the foramen, the electrical resistance or impedance gradually increases and reaches the calibrated level as it contacts vital tissues. The location is verified by slow withdrawal and reinsertion. The indicator is carefully observed during this action to ensure the same apical indication is given. If the point repeats several times, it is typically a reliable measurement. Some clinicians recommend leaving the file at this indicated depth and exposing a radiograph to verify the position. Used in conjunction with a radiograph, the locator is an effective adjunct.[25] Accidental passage through an accessory canal would indicate contact with the periodontal ligament space; however, the length would be inappropriate (Fig. 8-27). A radiograph would illustrate the need for additional adjustment. Electronic apex locators are especially useful when treating teeth with calcified pulp chambers, as a minute perforation can be discerned before it is enlarged.

Tactile. The experienced clinician develops a keen tactile sense and can gain considerable information from passing an instrument through a canal. This ability must be developed, and for clinicians beginning a career certain bits of information may speed the development of such ability. Following access, when interferences in the coronal third of the canal are removed, the observant clinician can detect a sudden increase in resistance as a small file approaches the apex.[12] Careful study of the apical anatomy discloses two facts that make tactile identification possible: (1) the unresorbed canal commonly constricts just before exiting the root, and (2) it frequently changes course in the last 2 to 3 mm.[52] Both structures apply pressure to the file. A narrowing presses more tightly against the instrument, whereas curvature deflects the instrument from a straight path. Both consume energy, and the sensitive hand can detect a sudden change in pressure required to accomplish insertion. The awareness of this change may be enhanced by the use of a file that is larger than the expected constricture.[68]

When the coronal two-thirds of the canal is constricted, clinicians cannot discern with accuracy what they feel because the file may be binding coronally rather than apically. As preparation develops space in the coronal two-thirds (i.e., radicular access), the quality of tactile information improves. At that point files bind only in the apical area, and resistance must lie in that region. When only the tip of the file binds in the canal it becomes a sensitive instrument with which the experienced clinician can accurately determine passage through the foramen. At this point, it also has access to pass through apical accessory canals.

Paper point evaluation. Once the preparation is complete, a paper point may yield more than a dry canal.[12] After the moisture has been removed, the point may be used to detect apical moisture and/or bleeding. A bloody or moist tip suggests an overextended preparation. Further assessment of the apical preparation and working length should be made in this event. The point of wetness often gives an approximate location to the actual canal end point. A wet and/or bloody point may also indicate that the foramen has been zipped or the apex perforated during preparation. These conditions would require additional canal shaping in addition to adjustment of the working length.

Radiographs, electronic apex locators, tactile sense, and paper point evaluation used in harmony ensure that the final shaping and obturation will extend the full length of the canal.

Instrument Selection

Before the canal is shaped files must be chosen. This used to be a simple matter; however, today it has become complex. Many canal preparation instruments are available, all of which are capable of cleaning canals, but each requires different manipulation. An understanding of these differences is essential before progressing into the clinical preparation techniques.

The choice must be made between K-type, H-type, and

*References 7, 12, 27, 59, 61, 68, 75, 84.

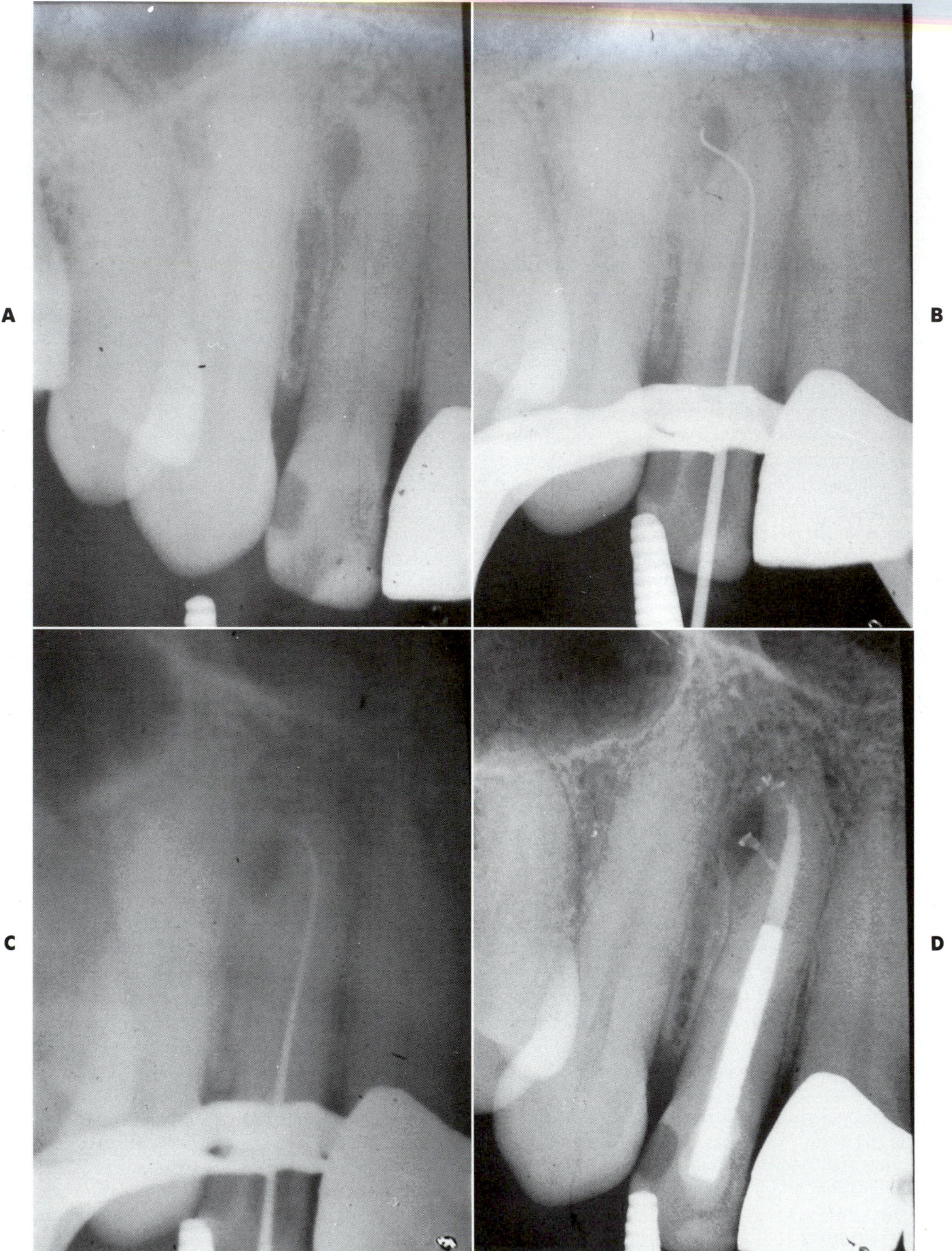

FIG. 8-27 A, Preoperative radiograph of a lateral incisor. **B,** File has passed through an accessory canal. The radiograph identifies this condition, while relying solely on an apex locator would result in a short preparation. **C,** This working view discloses the primary canal and its radiographic terminus. **D,** The final radiograph demonstrates that both portals of exit have been sealed.

B-type (R type in Chapter 13) hand instruments. For engine-driven cutting, the selection of a Gates-Glidden or Peezo type drill is necessary. For sonic and ultrasonic applications a decision of application (i.e., irrigation or preparation) must be made in order to select the proper instrument. For more information on all of these instruments, the reader is referred to Chapter 14.

Motions of Instrumentation

Several motions of manipulation are useful for generating or controlling the cutting activity of an endodontic file. These may be referred to as *envelopes of motion,* historically (1) file, (2) ream, (3) watch winding, and (4) balanced force instrumentation.

Filing

The term *filing* indicates a push-pull action with the instrument (Fig. 8-28). These two motions are the most limited of all those used for preparation. The inward passage of a K-type file under working loads is capable of damaging the canal wall very quickly, even when the slightest curvature is encountered. During the inward stroke, the cutting force is a combination of both resistance to bending and the apically directed hand pressure (Fig. 8-29). These two combine at the junctional angle of the instrument tip and gouge the curving canal wall very quickly. The gouge imparts a shape that does not allow even a small instrument to pass beyond it. This procedural error can occur anywhere beyond the point where a canal begins to curve. It does not occur before the curvature because the canal is straight. Without deflection there is no force that will hold the instrument tip against the canal wall. Canal ledging is responsible for more short endodontic obturations than any other procedural errors. The withdrawal or pull portion of this action produces very little potential for canal wall damage. Most current techniques use a passive insertion or a quarter turn insertion, precurving of the instrument, and a pulling withdrawal from the canal. Such techniques can reliably enlarge canals to appropriate diameters.

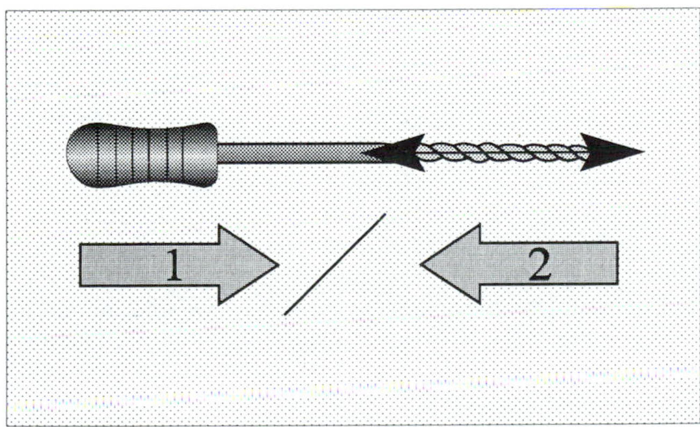

FIG. 8-28 The motion of filing is illustrated. The arrow indicates pushing into (1) and pulling straight back (2) from the canal. The inward motion is powered by the hand and the rigidity of the file. A canal wall can be damaged very quickly by this motion. Damage can occur with very small-diameter files.

Filing is an effective technique with Hedström type instruments since they do not engage during the insertion action and cut efficiently during the withdrawal motion. A major limitation of filing with a conventional Hedström is that it can easily cut through the middle of a curvature and cause strip perforation of the root. Precurving the file and anticurvature directing of the stroke must be used in order to avoid a mishap. The Unifile and S file designs are less efficient with filing motions than a conventional Hedström file. The blades of these instruments spiral around the file with a steeper inclination, more like a reamer of the K-type design. This blade configuration allows the cutting edges to slip more during a withdrawal stroke, so these instruments are more effective with the ream-and-file technique described later.

Reaming

The term *ream* indicates clockwise or right-hand rotation of an instrument (Fig. 8-30). Rotating any endodontic hand instrument to the right may be risky, though this risk is subtle and goes unnoticed until an instrument fractures under the load. The cutting edges of all endodontic files and reamers spiral about the shaft of the instrument. This configuration causes them to slide into the canal as the edges rotate to the right. As

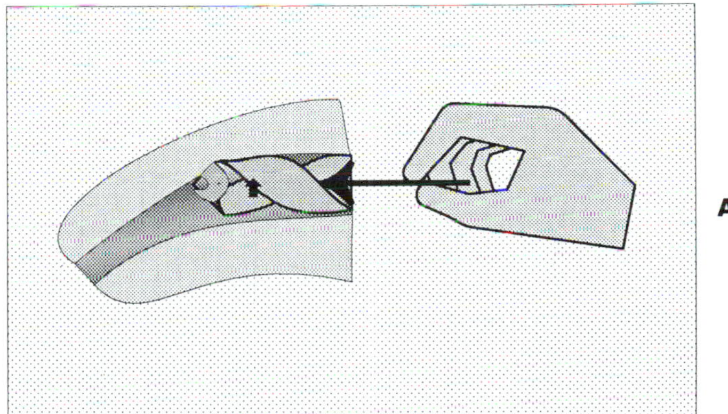

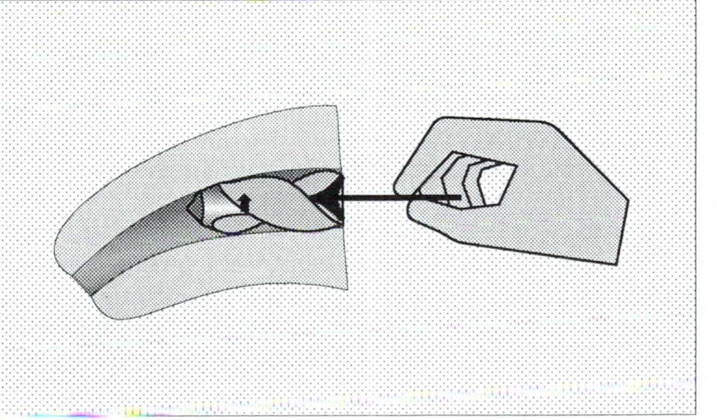

FIG. 8-29 A, If a standard K-type file is pushed into a curved canal the junctional angles gouge the wall rather than reorient to the curvature. This action can form a ledge very rapidly (i.e., with five or six strokes). **B,** The same motion with a modified tip produces little alteration of the canal wall since most of the cutting ability has been removed. This is not a desirable motion for most canals. It is useful only to smooth a previously roughened area.

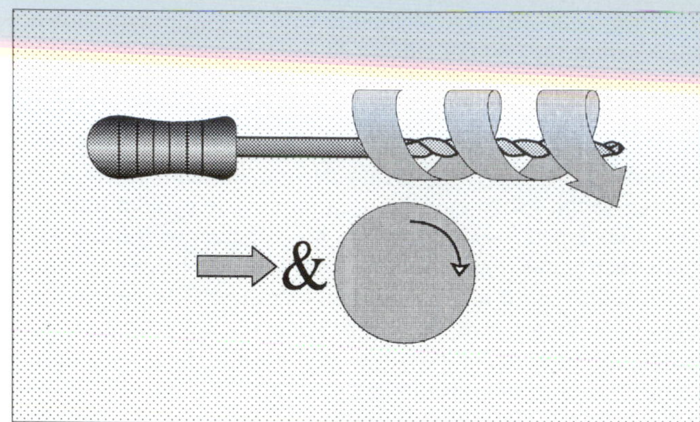

FIG. 8-30 The motion of reaming is a simple clockwise or right-hand rotation of the preparation instrument. The instrument must be restrained from insertion to generate a cutting effect. Instrument fracture is increased when this motion is employed.

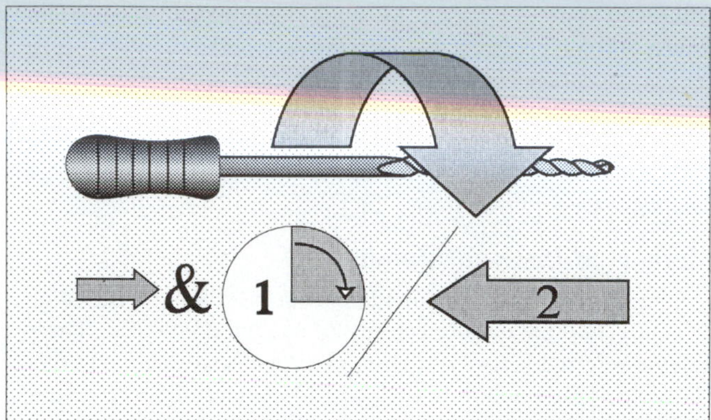

FIG. 8-31 A turn-and-pull motion is illustrated. A quarter turn to the right is followed by a straight outward pull. The arrow indicates a light inward force, which engages the file before rotation. The pull motion strips out treads started by the one fourth turn to the right motion. Angles up to a half turn have been advocated. This can be an effective motion if the instrument is not forcefully pushed toward the apex and the preparation depths are allowed to diminish with each subsequent instrument.

they slide into the canal more and more of the length of the instrument engages the canal. This in turn increases the strain or working load against the instrument. That strain continues to rise until the instrument ceases to move and the rotation force bends it *or* the clinician ceases rotation. If the instrument overinserts and bends, further rotation will break it. Unfortunately, forcefully pulling it from the canal may also fracture it. Specialized instruments (i.e., reamers) evolved from efforts to manage the complexity and consequences of this motion. They have a nearly axial orientation of the cutting edges and feed themselves into the canal with less force when rotated to the right than K-type or H-type files. This altered reaction may decrease a reamer's potential to cause apical ledging and reduces their tendency to aggressively thread into the canal as the instrument is rotated. Reamers can be used in a counter-clockwise balanced force motion, just as other K-type instruments can.

Turn-and-pull

The turn-and-pull cutting motion is a combination of a reaming and filing motion previously described (Fig. 8-31). The file is inserted with a quarter turn clockwise and inwardly directed hand pressure (i.e., reaming). Positioned into the canal by this action the file is subsequently withdrawn (i.e., filing). The rotation during placement sets the cutting edges of the file into dentin and the nonrotating withdrawal breaks loose the dentin that has been engaged. The resulting shaping is a spiraling groove along the canal wall, a groove that duplicates the spiraling axis of the instrument's cutting edges. Repeated placement with additional quarter turns and straight withdrawal gradually enlarges the canal's diameter to that of the file. In this process the instrument is allowed to cut actively without guidance, and a ledge can be generated with rather small-diameter files. Weine and coworkers demonstrated a tendency toward "hourglass" canal shapes when quarter turn-and-pull techniques were used to create apical stop preparations.[89] It may be concluded that a one-fourth turn-and-pull cutting motion is detrimental when used to create an apical stop preparation. On the other hand, clinical experience has demonstrated that it is relatively safe when step-back instrumentation is employed.[60]

Schilder[72] recommends clockwise rotation of a half revolution followed by withdrawal. Unlike the preceding description, he does not encourage insertion toward the apex; rather, he gradually allows the preparation to progress out of the canal. Each time a file is withdrawn it is followed by the next in the series. Each is inserted once and withdrawn. After the series, the canal is recapitulated with a patency file and the process is repeated. Each time the instrumentation series is repeated each file penetrates deeper into the canal. The process is continued until the canal is shaped adequately to ensure complete cleansing. Accomplished in this manner, turn-and-pull can be used very effectively and can produce excellent clinical results; however, the process is tedious and time consuming.

Watch-winding

Watch-winding is the back-and-forth oscillation of a file (30 to 60 degrees) right and (30 to 60 degrees) left as the instrument is pushed forward into the canal (Fig. 8-32). It is an expanded use of the insertion technique described by Ingle as *vaivén* in his first text edition.[7] It is a definite advancement in file motion and is very effective. The back-and-forth movement of K-type files and reamers causes them to plane dentinal walls rather efficiently. This motion is very useful during shaping procedures. It is less aggressive than quarter turn-and-pull motions, as the tip is not pushed as far into the apical regions of the canal with each motion and the chances for apical ledging are reduced. In a way, watch-winding is a predecessor to the balanced force technique (see below), as the 30 to 60 degrees of clockwise rotation pushes the file tip and working edges into the canal, and the 30 to 60 degrees of counterclockwise turn partially cuts away the engaged dentin. Each cut opens space and frees the instrument for deeper insertion with the next clockwise motion. The watch-winding technique is effective with all K-type files; the oscillating movement will easily insert small instruments through canals.

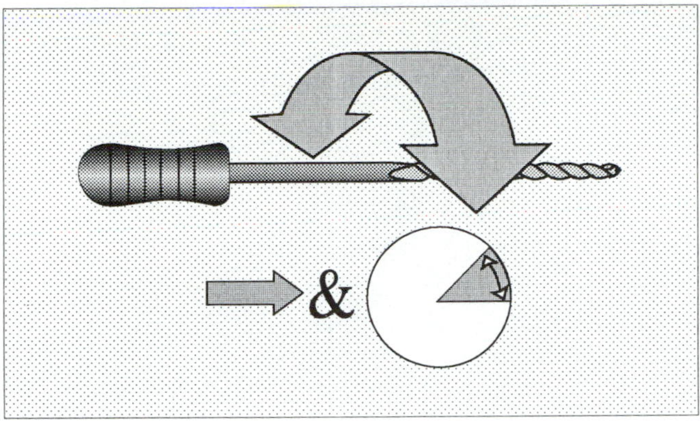

FIG. 8-32 A watch-winding motion is illustrated. The arched arrow indicates a gentle right and left rocking motion that causes the instrument to cut while light inward pressure *(straight arrow)* keeps the file engaged and progressing towards the apex. The arc of rotation is indicated by the shaded region in the circle.

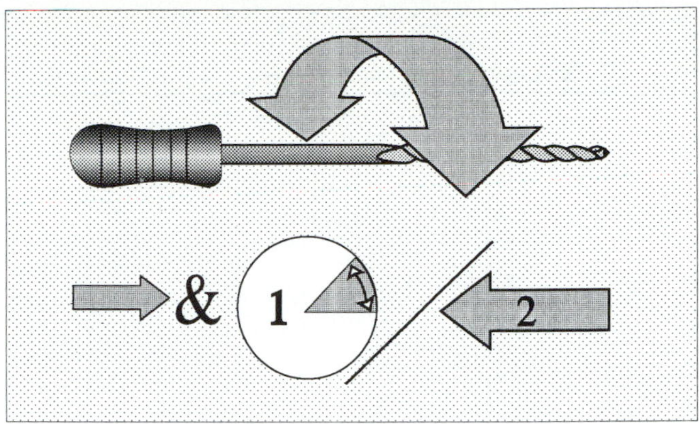

FIG. 8-33 A watch-wind and pull motion is illustrated. This is used primarily with Hedström files. (1) An inward pressure is maintained *(straight arrow),* while the file is gently rocked right and left, through the arc indicated by the shaded region of the circle. (2) When insertion stops, all rotation is ceased and the instrument is withdrawn from the canal.

Watch-winding and pull

When used with Hedström files, watch-winding cannot cut dentin with the backstroke. It can only wiggle and wedge the nearly horizontal unidirectional edges tightly into opposing canal walls. Thus positioned, the engaged dentin is removal during a subsequent pull stroke. With Hedström files the technique is watch-winding and pull (Fig. 8-33). With each clockwise rotation the instrument moves apically until it meets resistance and must be freed by a pull stroke. When further apical placement ceases, it is time to change the file size. The succeeding size will be larger if the proper working depth was achieved and smaller if it was not.

Balanced force technique

The balanced force technique[68,69] is a most efficient way to cut dentin. This technique calls for oscillation of the preparation instruments right and left with different arcs in either direction (Fig. 8-34). To insert an instrument, it is rotated to the right (clockwise) a quarter turn as gentle inward pressure is exerted by the clinician's hand. This action pulls the instrument into the canal and positions the cutting edges "equally" into the surrounding walls. Next, the instrument is rotated left (counterclockwise) at least one-third of a revolution. Rotation of one or two revolutions is preferred, but it may be utilized only when no curvature or a generalized curvature is present. Left-hand rotation attempts to unthread the instrument and drives it from the canal, so the clinician must press inward to prevent outward movement and to obtain a cutting action. The inward pressure and rotation are the complete cutting load, and both are under the clinician's direct sensory control. File fracture is unlikely unless pressures are applied that exceed the torque resistance of the instrument (Table 8-1).

As described in the preceding section on reaming, clockwise rotation must be applied cautiously. The insertion forces exerted press an instrument into the tooth structure, and if excessive insertion occurs, the file may lock and become distorted. When so placed, it may not be able to move when counterclockwise rotation begins. If it does not rotate to the left, it can fracture very quickly in that direction of rotation (i.e., usually less than one revolution). *Very light pressure* should be

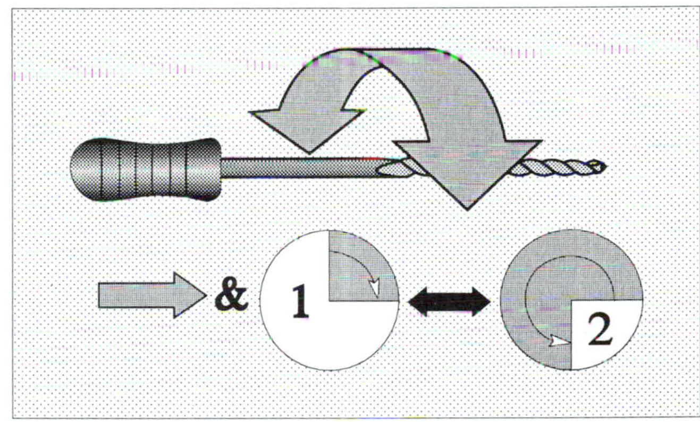

FIG. 8-34 Balanced force motions are illustrated. The small straight arrow indicates a sustained light inward pressure. (1) indicates the initiating quarter turn to the right. (2) indicates the larger arc used when the file is rotated to the left to drill the canal open. The black arrow indicates that one should alternate these two directions until the working depth is reached. The inward pressure and the rotating force should always be very light.

used with balanced force instrumentation. The instruments should feed into the canal in very shallow increments, and the canal should be drilled open to the file diameter at each depth before further insertion is attempted. Gentle, patient oscillation of the instruments will gradually carry them to the working depth. Once at that depth, they must undergo one final motion. Positioned at this deepest point of insertion, the instrument should be rotated to the right, with insertion prevented, for about half to one entire revolution. This action sweeps the walls and loads debris from the canal space against the coronal side of the cutting edges. Thus located, the file will remove much of the fractured dentinal material and other contents from the canal as it is withdrawn (Fig. 8-7). Balanced force instrumentation has been demonstrated to extrude no

TABLE 8-1. *

Size	K reamer (g/cm)	K file (g/cm)	Finger load (g/cm)
08	5	5	25
10	6	6	30
15	8	8	40
20	12	18	60–90
25	20	30	100–150
30	35	45	175–225
35	50	65	250–325
40	70	100	325–500
45	95	120	450–600
50	120	170	600–850

*The file handle gives us approximately 2 mm leverage; therefore the pressure exerted between the fingertips and the file handle may be five times greater than the torque values given. A 25-g load is comparable to the weight of four quarters setting on the fingertip. If instruments are turned with forces smaller than that listed they are not likely to be broken. Exceeding the given values can easily result in damage and separation from rotation. Triangular instruments should be considered the same as reamers. Torque values are from ISO/DIS 3630.2.

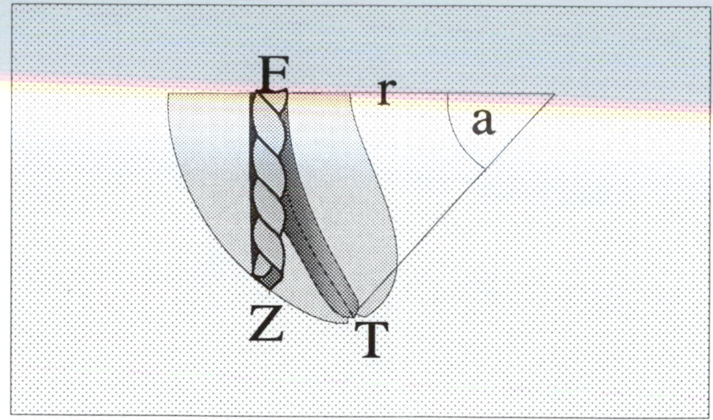

FIG. 8-35 This illustration depicts the interaction between an instrument and a curved canal. The arc *a* describes the angle of canal curvature, *r* describes the radius of that arc, *FT* is the curvature, and *FZ* is the passive position of the instrument. As the canal pulls the file to *FT* a restoring force is developed within the file. That force attempts to move the file to *FZ*. The greater the angle *a*, the shorter the radius *r*, and the larger the file *FZ*, the more likely it is that the preparation will progress to the path *FZ*. This is one of two forces that activate the junctional angles of K-type files.

more debris through the apex than other techniques of canal preparation.[23,60] *Balanced force instrumentation is specifically designed to operate K-type endodontic instruments* and should not be used with Broach type or Hedström type instruments, since neither possesses left-hand cutting capacity.

Simultaneous apical pressure and counter-clockwise rotation of the file strikes a balance between tooth structure and instrument elastic memory. This balance locates the instrument very near the canal axis, even in severely curved canals; so this technique avoids recognizable transportation of the original canal path,[7,54,66,69–71,80] when used with files that have a modified tip configuration (Flex-R, Canal Master). The technique has been shown to work effectively without precurving.[82] While this is true in the body of curved canals, an apical bend is frequently required before a file will pass through a sharply deviated apical foramen. The more the canal curves the less balanced force follows its true central axis. The more extensive the curve, the more important file bending becomes. An instrument triangular in cross section is preferred, since such a cross section is associated with the least metal mass, and the smaller the mass the more flexible is the instrument. This means less force is required to bend the instrument into the shape of the canal, and the preparation result is less canal transportation during cleaning and shaping. Triangular instruments *must* be used with lightened working loads, as they are not as strong as diamond-shaped or square configurations.[68]

Clinicians should be aware when using this technique that files can be broken.[70] When a rotational cutting technique is used, one must constantly monitor file integrity and throw out files that show winding or unwinding of the blade spirals. Additionally, files should be replaced following each curved case, as many of the characteristics of instrument fatigue and impending file breakage are invisible to the human eye.[81]

Curvature: The Engine of Complications

An engine is a power source for an action. Any instrument action requires an engine. An endodontic file preparation has two: the operator's hand and the instrument shaft. The hand force engine is obvious, but the instrument engine is not. As an instrument is curved, elastic forces develop internally. These forces attempt to return the instrument to its original shape and are responsible for straightening of the final canal shape and location (Fig. 8-35). If it were not for these forces, the final shaping would have the same linear axis as the original canal. These internal elastic forces (i.e., restoring forces) act on the canal wall during preparation and influence the amount of dentin removed. They are particularly influential at the junction of the instrument tip and its cutting edges. This region is the most efficient cutting surface along an instrument,[62] and when activated by the restoring forces it removes more tissue than at any other region. This phenomenon is responsible for apical transportation and its consequences. The restoring forces are what power the changes in canal shape as they act through the sharp surfaces of the instrument. The strength of the engine is directly related to the metal composition of the instrument, the cross-sectional area of the instrument, and the angle of deflection. The greater the angle of deflection, the greater the power developed. The larger the instrument, the larger the cross section and the greater the power. The more rigid the material the instrument is manufactured from, the greater the power it produces. Evaluation of these relationships gives guidance in the following ways:

1. Radicular access minimizes the deflection of larger instruments.
2. A triangular cross section is preferred, especially as instrument size increases above 0.25 mm cutting diameter.
3. Less rigid metals may be advantageous, provided they do not introduce some undesirable characteristic like unpredictable fracture.

Nickel titanium instruments are presently being investigated and offer promise of improved preparation accuracy as a result of reduced engine force. They do, however, suffer from unpredictable fracture. Specialized designs, like Canal Master,[91] also reduce the power of the instrument engine.

These instruments do not cut over most of the canal length and have a small-diameter shaft that reduces its total cross-sectional area.[92] Canal Master instruments have suffered from increased risk of fracture, and they require an altered preparation strategy in order to obtain a shape that will accept a tapered gutta-percha cone.

Precurving instruments

A precurved file is a valuable tool for feeling canal passages and for moving around calcification, ledges and through curved foramina. It is used also in an attempt to alleviate the adverse effects of canal curvature. A properly shaped file is curved smoothly to its tip. Its shape should accurately replicate the expected canal curvature. Sharp kinks should be avoided, as they predispose the instrument to fracture (see Fig. 8-14, *C*).[12]

The primary difficulty of precurving is limited canal access coronal to the curvature. In order to insert a curved instrument and maintain the shape, there must be adequate width in the coronal region to allow undisturbed passage of the curved region. If the canal is not curved the same as the file or is not as wide as the file curvature, then the canal will reshape the file and straighten the curvature. Early radicular access solves much of this dilemma in that it widens the coronal regions and establishes clearance to pass the precurved instrument into the canal undisturbed. If the canal is arched through its entire length, then precurving may be accomplished very easily. Precurving is not a condition required by the balanced force technique, but it is common in others.

Anticurvature filing

Anticurvature is a method of applying instrument pressure so that shaping will occur away from the inside of the root curvature in the coronal and middle third of a canal (Fig. 8-36). Abou-Rass, Frank, and Glick[1] described the anticurvature filing concept for curved canals, emphasizing that during shaping procedures files should be pulled from canals as pressure is applied to the outside canal wall. This directionally applied pressure, they suggest, prevents dangerous midcurvature straightening in curved canals and associated laceration of a furcal area during preparation. Anticurvature pressure application is effective until the canal contacts the file at three points within the canal. Beyond there, the canal curvature, not the clinician, determines the cutting pressure.

Radicular access

Radicular access[27] of some type is employed in all cleaning and shaping techniques today. The concept was first promoted by Dr. Schilder[72] as body shaping in his cleaning and shaping technique, and it has many different conceptualizations today.[24,27,53] It is a most important step in the cleaning and shaping strategy of every case. Radicular access creates space in the more coronal regions of the canal. This space enhances placing and manipulating subsequent files as it increases the depth and effectiveness of irrigation (Fig. 8-37). Radicular access may be accomplished with rotary instruments or by circumferential filing. Circumferential filing may be accomplished with hand-held K-type or H-type files, sonically or ultrasonically activated files, shapers, or diamond-coated instruments.

The more adequate coronal shapes developed with radicular access provide important advantages in irrigation efficacy,[67] apical control,[27] cone fit, and condensation procedures, regardless of the filling technique used.[24,74] Subsequent smaller apical preparation size allows more consistent avoidance of apical ledging, ripping, and perforation.[11,73] The rapid change of diameter leading to the foramen provides a reliable apical resistance form and helps to contain the filling material within the root.[26]

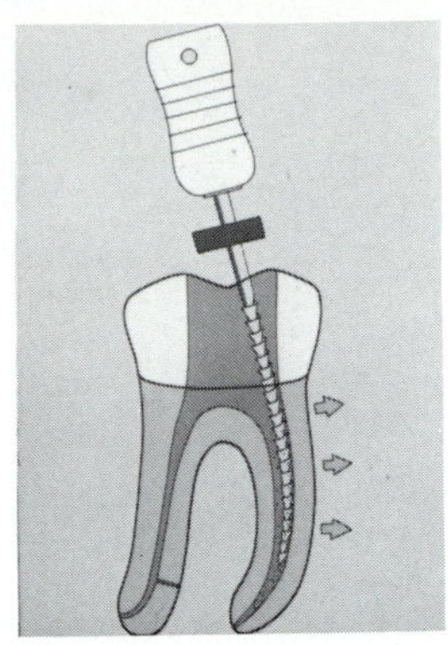

FIG. 8-36 Hedström file used in an anticurvature direction. The top of the handle is pulled into the curvature while the shank end of the handle is pushed away (anticurvature) from the inside of the curve, thereby balancing the cutting flutes only against the safer part of the root canal.

Engine-driven enlargement

The preferred method of developing a radicular access is to use Gates-Glidden drills[12,27,68,75] mounted in the right-angled low-speed handpiece. Different sequences may be employed. The more conventional method is to begin after the canal length has been determined and the space has been increased to that of a size 25 to 35 file (Fig. 8-38). The access cavity is flooded with sodium hypochlorite, and the radicular access is enlarged with a rotating no. 2 Gates-Glidden drill into the canal. This drill will pull inwardly as a result of rotation but may require slight encouragement from the clinician. The drill should be backed out of the canal after penetrating 1 to 2 mm and cleaned of debris before allowing it to pass deeper. Irrigating fluids within the chamber area wash debris from the rotating instrument as it is withdrawn into the coronal access cavity. The drill can then return to the previous depth unloaded. From there it again advances apically. In-and-out movement is repeated until the no. 2 drill reaches its intended depth or until the clinician determines that a curvature is preventing it from penetrating further. These instruments are not intended to drill around curvatures, and any attempt to do so can cause egregious procedural errors. Situations range from a canal blocked by a broken Gates-Glidden drill (Fig. 8-39) to a root perforated by a preparation of too large diameter (Fig. 8-2).

Once the no. 2 Gates-Glidden drill has completed its work, the canal is thoroughly irrigated. A no. 3 Gates-Glidden drill is gradually introduced into the canal. The clinician must be alert and ready to stop sudden apical movement of this and any subsequent drill. The preceding drill opened the canal wide enough so that it now offers little resistance against inward force. Also, the length of cutting surface has increased and the drill will generate greater inward force. Together, these

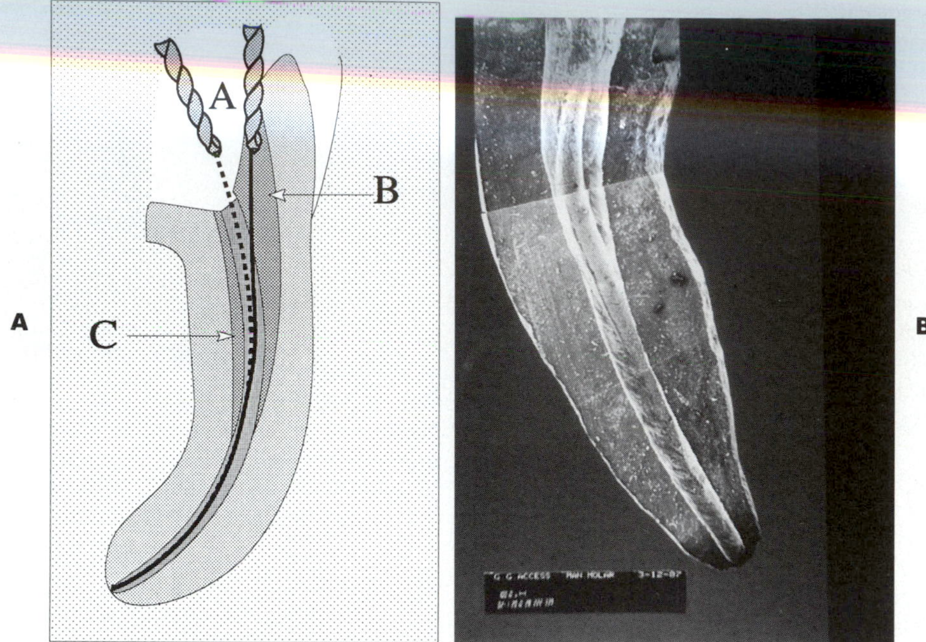

FIG. 8-37 A, Changes of instrument passage resulting from a radicular access key: solid line is the initial path of the file, dashed line is the resultant path of the file, *A* is the effective angle reduction of file curvature, *B* is the dentin intentionally removed to facilitate the angle change, and *C* is dentin lost as a result of canal enlarging. Reduction in region *C* must be kept to a minimum. **B,** This SEM reconstructs the M root of a mandibular molar. The wide coronal space is that of the radicular access. The original canal channel can be seen in the coronal and middle thirds, and the changed angle is obvious. The apical half of this canal exhibits completely planed walls. A file passes through this canal in a nearly straight path, allowing large-diameter preparations. The apical prep is that of a no. 45 file.

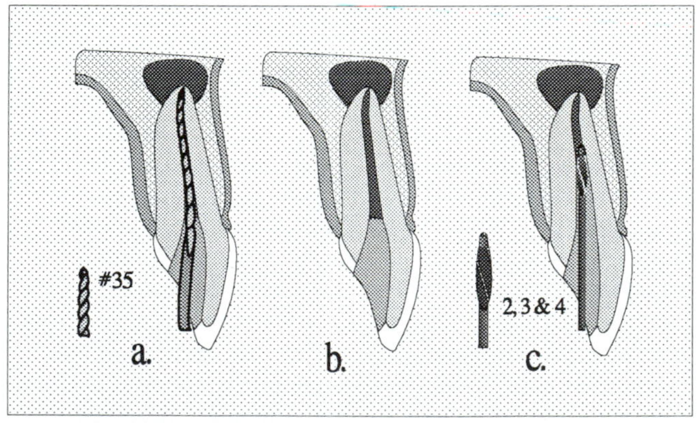

FIG. 8-38 Illustration of the canal when a typical radicular access is enlarged with a GG drill. **a,** The canal is enlarged apically through files no. 35. **b,** The file is removed and the canal is flooded with NaOCl. **c,** The GG is gradually worked in and out of the canal until it reaches the desired depth.

facts mean that each subsequent Gates-Glidden drill will pass more freely and rapidly into the canal than its predecessor. Generally, only small-diameter Gates-Gliddens drills are used in molars, because of the risk of perforation.

The "crown-down" preparation concept advocates beginning the radicular access with the larger instruments first (Fig. 8-40).[57,63] Each instrument is allowed to penetrate a short distance into the canal, generally 2 mm. In this method each drill is pressing against approximately the same canal resistance and there is no tendency for large instruments to overinsert. Small instruments may do so, but the consequences of excessive penetration are managed far more easily than those of a perforated root. Generally, this sequence allows the greater radicular access preparation depth.

While a radicular access is being made the clinician must follow the shape of each canal. If the canal is oval or oblong, that shape should be enhanced by preparing from both ends of the oval (Fig. 8-41). The entire wall of the canal is planned with an outward-directed stroke. The exception is the inward side of curved and concave roots (i.e., the mesial roots of molars), where the preparation is always directed away from the curvature (i.e., anticurvature). Round canals should finish round but larger, oval canals finish oval, and separate figure-of-eight canals end as two separate round to oval spaces (Fig. 8-3). Canals of this shape should flare away from the interconnecting groove. Each drill is withdrawn outward in an active manner, so as to slightly flare its opening to meet that of

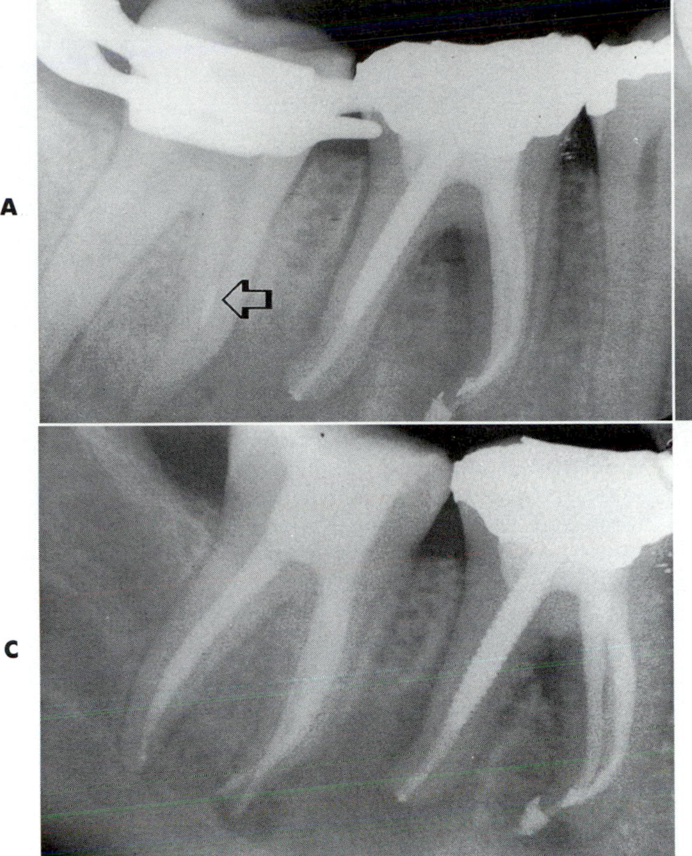

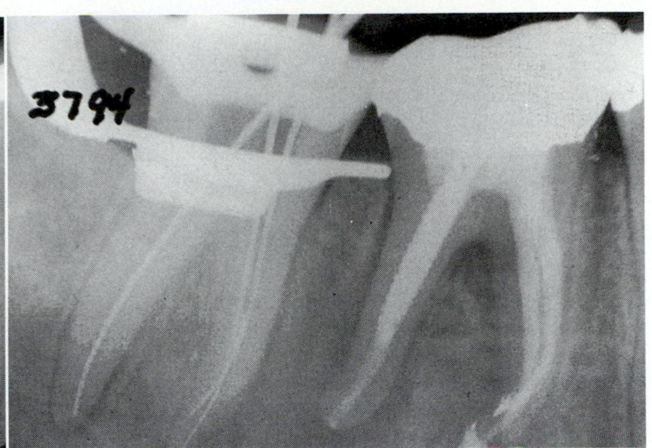

FIG. 8-39 A, The M canal of this molar is blocked by the cutting head of a GG ⇐ **B,** Careful manipulation of a small file reestablishes a passage through the flute space of the drill head. **C,** Following the bypass and final instrumentation the canal system was successfully obturated and can be expected to repair normally.

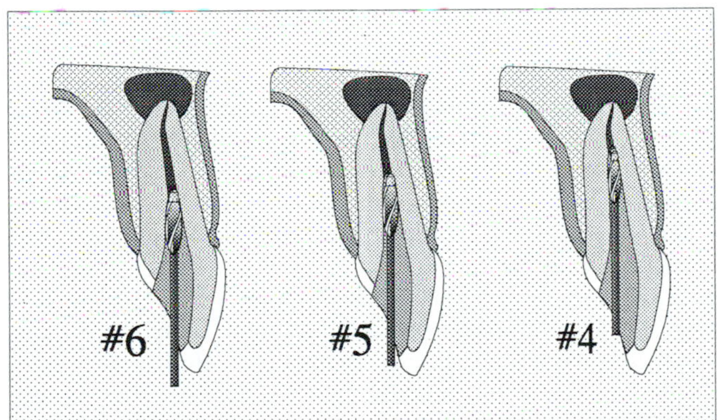

FIG. 8-40 The crown-down approach begins with the larger GG first. In the depicted maxillary incisor the no. 6 GG starts the procedure and enlarges to its specified depth, usually 2 to 4 mm beyond where it first engaged the canal walls. The no. 5 penetrates an additional 2 mm and the no. 4 another 2 mm. The no. 3 and 2 Gates-Glidden drills may be used to extend the depth.

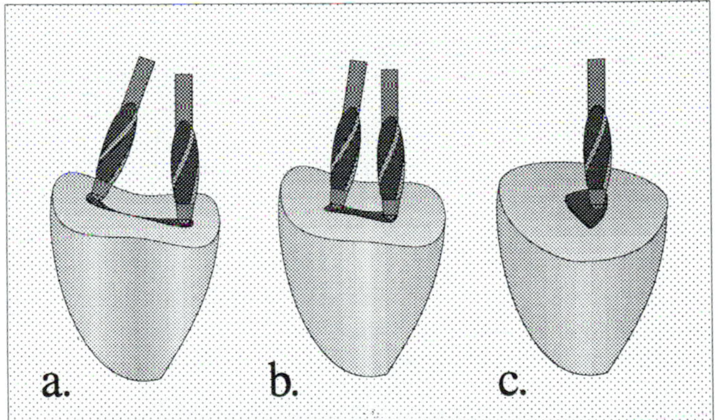

FIG. 8-41 Illustration of GG positioning for radicular access preparations in different shapes of canals. **a,** Figure-8 canal typical of M roots of molars and some single-rooted premolars. Each canal receives a single pass with pressure applied away from the curvature. **b,** Oval canal typical of the larger roots of molars and single-rooted premolars. The joining areas can be cleaned with the smaller GGs. Passage is made down both ends of the oval shape as if two canals existed. **c,** Irregular round typical of maxillary incisors, two-rooted premolars, and DF roots of maxillary molars. A single pass is usually sufficient.

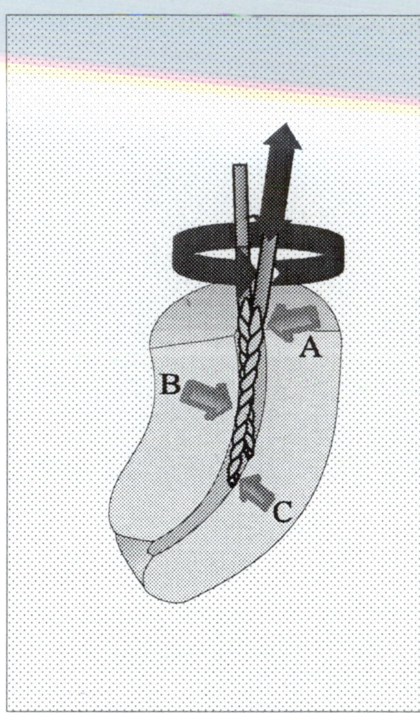

FIG. 8-42 Illustration of circumferential filing used to establish a radicular access. This may be accomplished effectively, provided the files are not pushed into the canal deep enough to cause bending of the instruments (i.e., past point *C*).

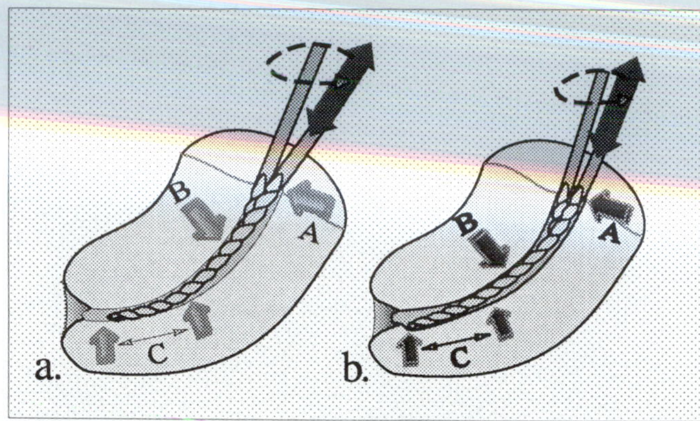

FIG. 8-43 Reaction of an instrument after it passes into a curve (i.e., past point *C*). **a,** The instrument remains in the same apical location, regardless of how the clinician moves the upper shaft and handle. **b,** Continued filing beyond the most coronal arrow *(C)* will cause transportation of the canal in regions *A*, *B*, and *C*. Changes will be most apparent in the regions of *C*, since the instrument tip functions in that area.

the next larger drill. This requires a flare of 0.20 mm over the 2 mm of prepared space. This flaring prevents the creation of parallel walls, a condition that adversely affects the dissipation of condensing pressures during obturation.

Manual enlargement

Techniques for manually shaping the coronal two thirds of the canal with a circumferential filing action are well-established.[88] The body of the canal is repeatedly filed about its diameter in an effort to grossly flare that portion and to create space to better reach the apical regions (Fig. 8-42). This process works only when there is no curvature in the portion of the canal being flared. If a curvature is present the file will consistently press against the same wall, regardless of the direction the operator moves his/her hand (Fig. 8-43). This process is slow with K-type files but may be accomplished rapidly with H-type files. Even the speed of H-type files is no match for that of rotary instruments, but speed is not our only concern, and some clinicians still prefer to flare by hand.

Iatrogenic Complications Arising from Cleaning and Shaping

Iatrogenic changes in the canal wall occur rapidly, and frequently unbeknownst to the clinician. The majority of cleaning and shaping complications are a result of improper control over the preparation instruments. Resulting damage is therefore a mechanical injury to the canal system. Blockage, laceration, and foraminal damage are the most common results. Each alters the reliability of the procedure and *must* be prevented if one is to obtain the best possible prognosis for the patient.

Blockage

The canal may suddenly loose patency during a cleaning and shaping process. This can be a result of tissue compression, debris accumulation, wall damage, or instrument separation. Any of these conditions blocks access into the deeper regions of the canal. Early detection and incorporation of the proper corrective action can prevent secondary damage, damage that can cause the situation to become so adverse that cleaning cannot be completed internally. Correcting a blockage requires preparation comprehension gained through experience. Without extensive experience one may not recognize signs and make timely and appropriate decisions. Therefore, an inexperienced clinician should request assistance when a blockage persists.

Soft tissues

When pulp tissue is intact, the clinician must be cognizant that it can be packed into the apex by insertion of instruments. Extirpation of tissue is an important factor in reducing this potential problem. Generally, placing an instrument into the foramen and carefully rotating it there cuts the tissues loose and facilitates their removal.

Clinical experience has shown that lubricants such as RC Prep or Glyoxide tend to emulsify the pulp stump and so prevent cohesion of collagenous debris. They are best used only during the initial "negotiation" phase of cleaning and shaping (i.e., until enough coronal enlargement is created to allow the effective use of irrigants).[8]

Hard tissues

Dentin chips generated by the cutting action of files and drills settle into the apical regions and if not removed by recapitulation and irrigation can obstruct that region. Filing near the canal terminus exaggerates apical blockage by packing debris into the smaller apical regions (Figs. 8-13, *A*, and 8-15). Once the canal is blocked by chips, continued generation extends the depth of blockage and causes obturation to fall short

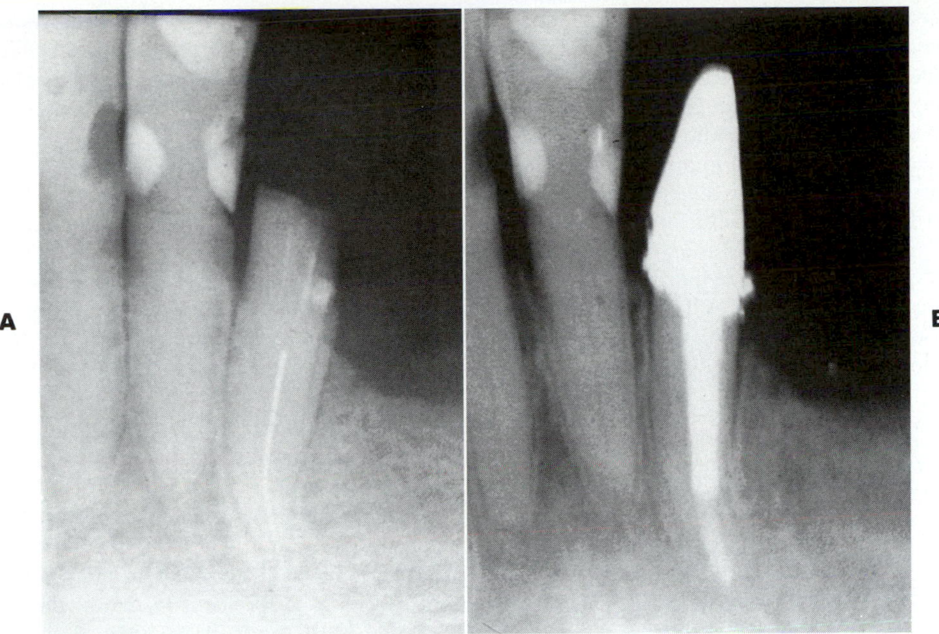

FIG. 8-44 A, This canal is blocked by a fractured instrument. **B,** Ultrasonic instrumentation opened space enough to allow retrieval and completion of treatment. A post retained core has been fabricated. Critical teeth must be approached cautiously and deserve the attention of an extremely skilled clinician.

of the canal terminus. Accumulation of debris contributes to the formation of ledges.

Some blockages are present in the canal before instrumentation. These are natural calcifications that have accumulated along the vascular channels and on canal walls (Fig. 8-11, *L*). Pulp stones and secondary calcifications that project from the canal wall may be moved down the canal and become lodged by insertion of an instrument. These can on occasion be bypassed by precurving the tip of preparation instruments. Loose pulp stones, which are wedged into the small diameter of deep apical canal spaces, are very difficult to remove or to instrument past. Once bypassed the particle is often reoriented to again obstruct the canal. Frequent, generous irrigation and early radicular access help reduce the risk of accidental blockage with particles. Teeth with a diminished pulp chamber, narrowed canals, long-standing periodontal involvement, and/or multiple previous restorations are more likely to contain calcifications and manifest hard tissue blockage.

Broken instruments

During the cleaning and shaping of a canal system overstressing of an instrument can cause it to break in the canal. The fragment blocks the canal system and prevents routine cleaning and shaping (Figs. 8-27, 8-39, 8-44). Clinical recall evaluation has shown that broken instruments whose tip rests in the apical constriction are not as likely to fail as those that lie more coronally. In all situations blockage compromises cleaning, shaping, and sealing. This type of blockage is preventable and requires constant attention to the force used to manipulate instruments. Frequent and close instrument examination and instrument disposal are the best preventives. Absolute awareness of the minute stress that each instrument can withstand without suffering irreversible structural damage is essential before prevention of separated instruments is possible. Minimal torque resistance and angle to fracture for standardized instruments provide a valuable relative measure of the strength of instruments in relation to their cutting diameter (see Table 8-1).

Furcal perforations

A furcal perforation is a midcurvature opening into the periodontal ligament space and is the worst possible outcome of any cleaning and shaping procedure. Its location is close to the clinical crown and consequently is very likely to develop or continue microleakage from the coronal restorations into the space. Iatrogenic damage in this region must be prevented in order to give a tooth a reasonable chance for long-term functional stability and freedom from endodontic infections.

Furcal perforations result from improper file manipulation or oversized radicular access preparations. The risk of occurrence can be minimized by incorporating anticurvature pressure when cutting instruments are pushed or pulled in a curved canal system. Anticurvature pressure is extremely effective when used with Gates-Glidden drills in early radicular access preparations. Anticurvature technique is commonly advocated by clinicians who employ conventional Hedström files for the preparation of curved canals, since conventional Hedströms are very capable of creating a midcanal perforation and must be carefully used in curved roots. Anticurvature principles provide little protection against perforation in the apical regions of a canal, but that is not a region in which a Hedström file is prone to perforate.

Another most important consideration in preventing furcal perforations is developing the discipline to *never* take large

Gates-Glidden or Peezo drills deeply into root canals. Deep insertion generally is not the operator's intention but rather a result of self-propelled inward motion of the drill. New drills of the larger sizes (no. 3 to 6) often grab the canal walls and pull themselves deeply into the canal before the clinician can stop the handpiece. A helpful technique *to prevent this sometimes disastrous occurrence is to run the handpiece in reverse direction with new drills.* Run thus, the drills tend to back out of the canal. By applying more apical pressure the drill can be moved into the canal and made to cut dentin. It will go only to the intended depth, since it does not self-propel when rotated counterclockwise, and the applied pressure can be terminated as the desired depth is obtained. A reverse order of drill sizes is also very reliable in reducing furcal lacerations from excessive penetration depths. This technique seems more demanding and is difficult for many clinicians to master (see Fig. 8-40).

Apical perforations

When the apical region of a canal is curved, conditions exists that can result in an apical communication other than the foramen. Here the communication is most often a result of uncontrolled transportation and subsequent ledge formation. Attempts to reestablish canal length past the ledge finally result in the file tip cutting straight through the root structure and into the periodontal ligament space (Fig. 8-45).

Altered foramina: rip/zip

When instruments are passed through a foramen they can change the shape of that region very rapidly and irreversibly. Placed through the foramen, an instrument receives its support primarily from that region of the canal. This relationship means a file will concentrate its internal forces against the structure of the foramen. In return, that delicate region must provide resistance to those forces and to the abrasive effects of instrument movements. In a nutshell, a few in-and-out movements can open a single side of the foramen several millimeters (Figs. 8-3, *A,* and 8-46).

When the foramen is zipped it can not be cleansed of tissue over most of its surfaces. Transportation of this type has a most serious effect on the prognosis for a treatment and is therefore recognized with special terminology (i.e., rip or zip). Opening of the foramen should be kept relatively small and a minimal number of passes made through it. If an enlargement of the foraminal diameter is desired, that enlargement should be the last and final step of the instrumentation procedure.

Foramina are delicate. At the interface between a canal system and the attachment apparatus, foramina must be maintained in their original position if complete removal of pulpal tissues and elimination of periapical stimuli is to occur. Instruments that pass through the foramina are routinely kept rather small (i.e. no. 10 or 15). They are precurved to mini-

A

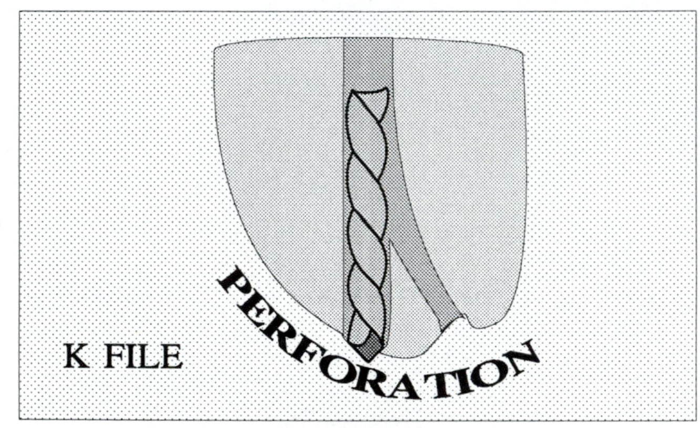

B

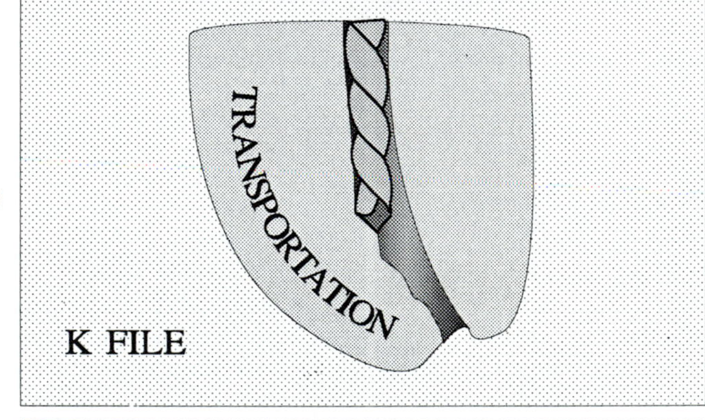

C

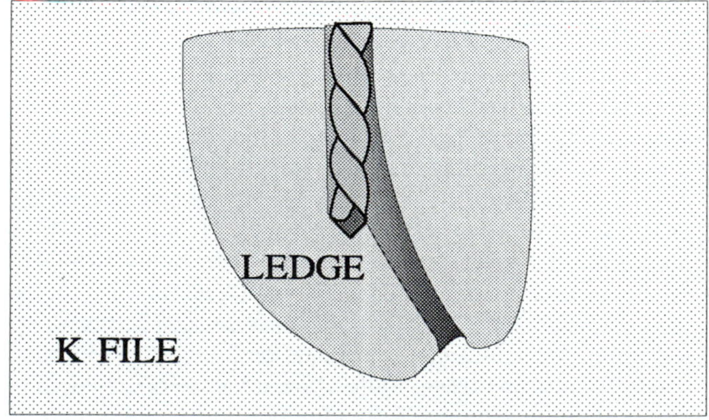

FIG. 8-45 A, An apical perforation. This event is always preceded by transportation **(B)** and ledge formation **(C)**. It becomes a perforation when forceful attempts to bypass the ledge cause the instrument to penetrate from the ledge to the periodontal ligament.

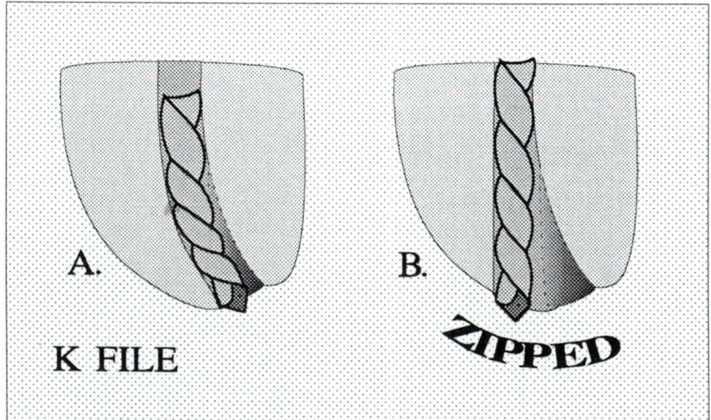

FIG. 8-46 A, When a small file is placed through the foramen it rests on the outer side of the curvature. **B,** Filing with the instrument through the foramen will zip the foramen rapidly. The shaded area retains tissues, dentin debris, and other canal contents, and the obturation point cannot seal the resulting shape. Apical failure is very likely.

mize elastic forces that would be generated should the foramen have to alter their path. If the foramen is to be prepared to a specified diameter, that alteration is accomplished as the final step of cleaning and shaping and with a piloted (safe tip) file. The final shape must be round in order to not change the relationship between the canal and the supportive structures. For obturation the foramen must be smaller than the apical shaping diameter, free of tissue, and contoured so that a gutta-percha cone will adapt tightly into the patent space (round is optimal; Fig. 8-47).

Cleaning and Shaping Techniques

Few dentists would dispute the importance of cleaning root canal systems, but when it comes to describing the specific, practical steps by which to achieve this objective there is considerable diversity. Researchers, educators and clinicians have agonized for decades over working length and irrigation concept.[74,90] In spite of our obviously incomplete knowledge, we must strive to use concepts and techniques that fill the voids and yet provide predictable positive clinical responses.

THE STEP-DOWN TECHNIQUE

The fundamental importance of cleaning, shaping, débris removal, irrigation, tactile sense, and common sense were described earlier in this chapter. The authors are in complete accord about the goals of cleaning and shaping the root canal system. We differ only on how these goals are best attained. The two techniques previously described have much merit and wide support. However, in the last few years a third technique for cleaning and shaping has gained considerable support from experienced endodontists. This latest technique, called *step-down,* involves cleaning and shaping the canal from the coronal third down to the apical third. The apical third of the canal is approached only after the coronal two thirds is sculpted and disinfected. See Figs. 8-48 to 8-57.

The benefits of this technique include the following:

1. It eliminates cervical dentin constrictures and reduces canal curvatures, thereby giving the clinician full tactile awareness in the apical third.
2. It allows deeper and earlier penetration of the disinfecting irrigating solution into the inner recesses of the canal, thereby effectively cleaning the coronal two thirds of the canal before the apical third is approached.
3. It removes the major portion of the pulp and infecting microbes before the apical third is approached, thereby minimizing the risk of pushing pulpal or microbial irritants into the periapical region.
4. The working length is less likely to change during apical instrumentation because canal curvature has been reduced before working length is actually established.

Procedures to assure apical patency, as described earlier in this chapter, are not used while the coronal two thirds of the canal system is cleaned and shaped. However, after the coronal two thirds is prepared, passive instrumentation, recapitulation, and apical patency are used to clean and shape the apical third of the canal.

Once the access opening is established, RC-Prep is placed in the pulp chamber and the length of the canal is established radiographically or electronically to approximately 2 mm short of the apex. To make room for enlargement with Gates-

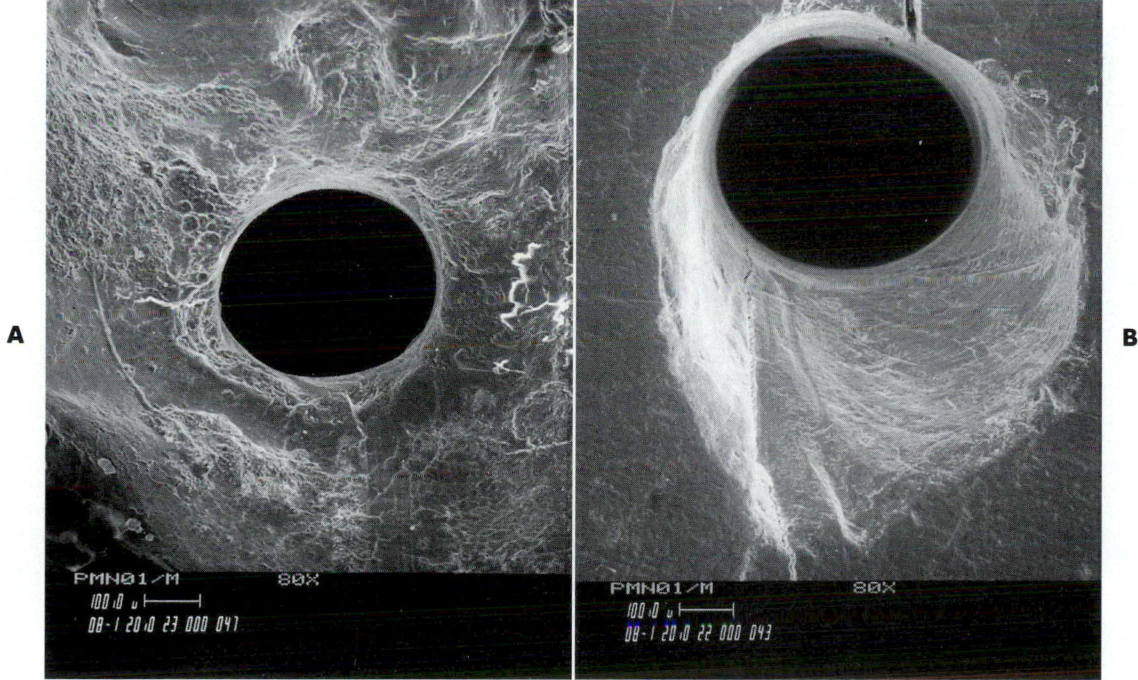

FIG. 8-47 Scanning electron micrograph of a prepared mesial apex from a mandibular molar. It was prepared using balanced force technique and Flex-R files (Moyco/Union Broach, York, Pa.). **A,** This external view of the foramen discloses a round and clear status; patency was made with a no. 25 file. **B,** This internal view of the control zone region reveals the clean machined and tapering form developed. The outer white elliptical diameter is that created by a no. 45 file, and the black opening is the patency of a no. 25 file.

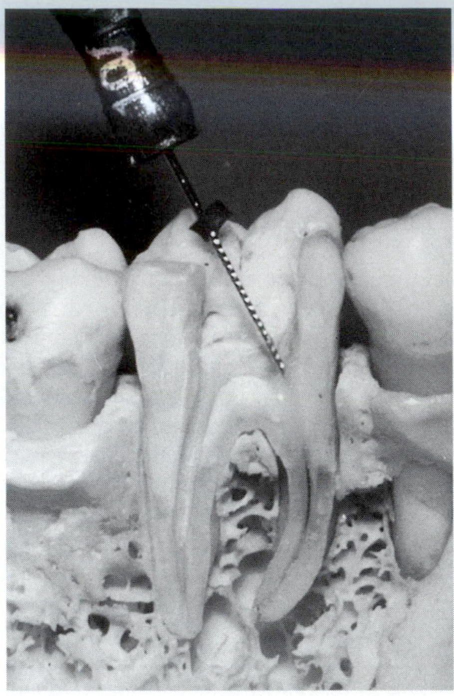

FIG. 8-48 A no. 10 file is used to establish the canal length 2 to 3 mm short of the apex. Each file is coated with RC-Prep before it enters the canal.

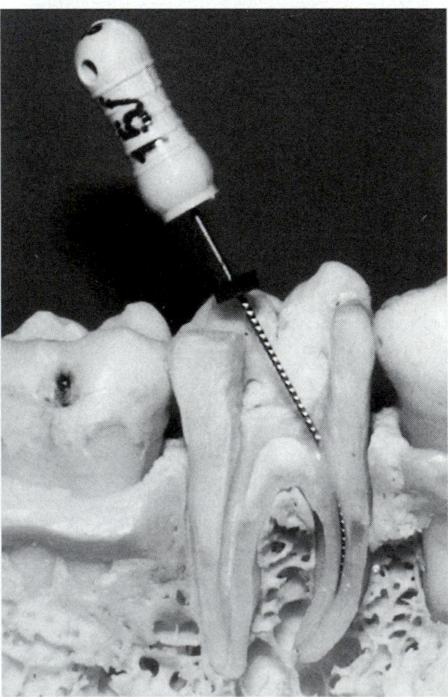

FIG. 8-49 Following copious irrigation with NaOCl, a no. 15 file is used with circumferential filing to start enlarging the coronal two thirds of the canal.

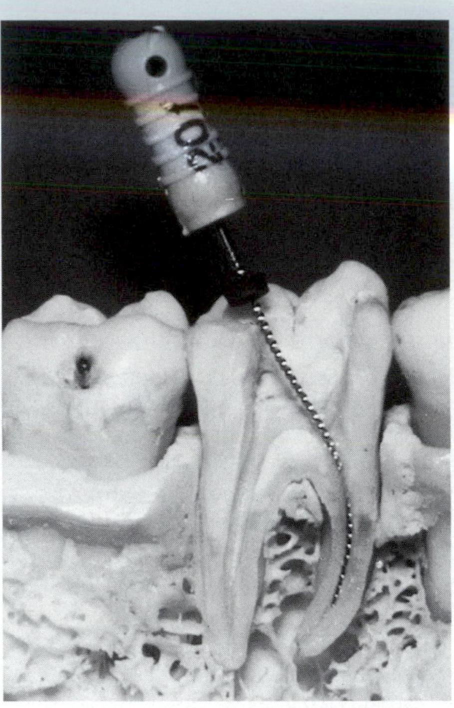

FIG. 8-50 As shown in Fig. 8-11, the canal chamber remains filled with NaOCl after each irrigation, then the next size enlarging file, coated with RC-Prep, continues the enlargement.

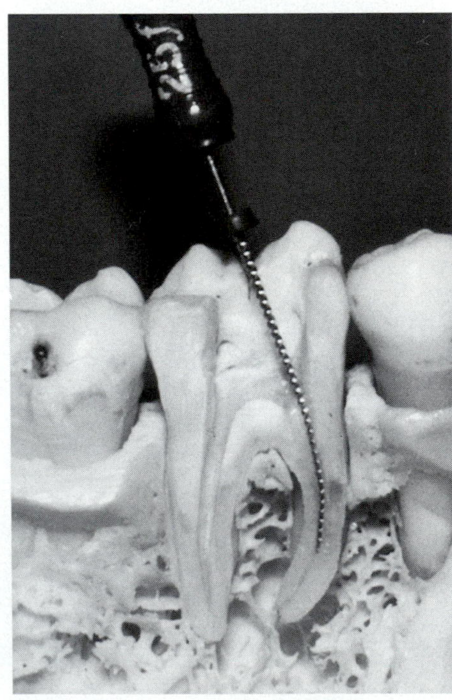

FIG. 8-51 As the larger files are used, they do not extend as far into the root canal. Although K files are shown here, Hedström files will more efficiently enlarge the canal with circumferential filing.

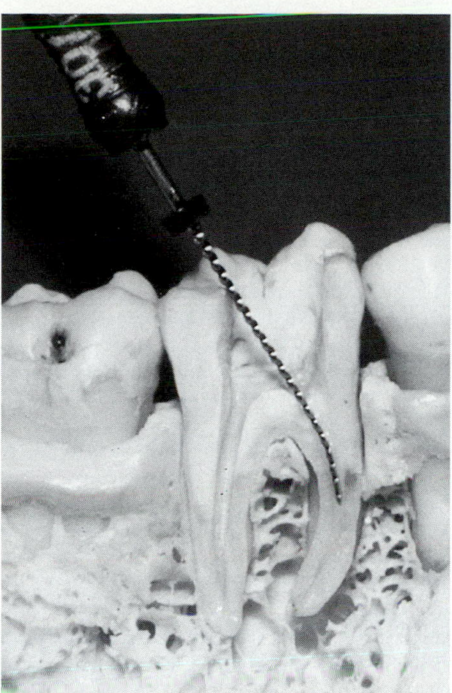

FIG. 8-52 The coronal half of the canal can be circumferentially filed to approximately the same depth with the stiffer files.

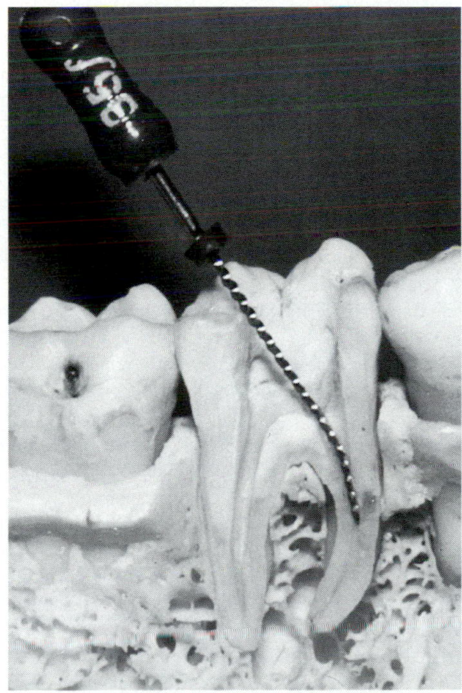

FIG. 8-53 By the time a no. 35 file is employed, at least 10 ml of NaOCl should have been used for irrigation. The canal has now been prepared for the GG burs.

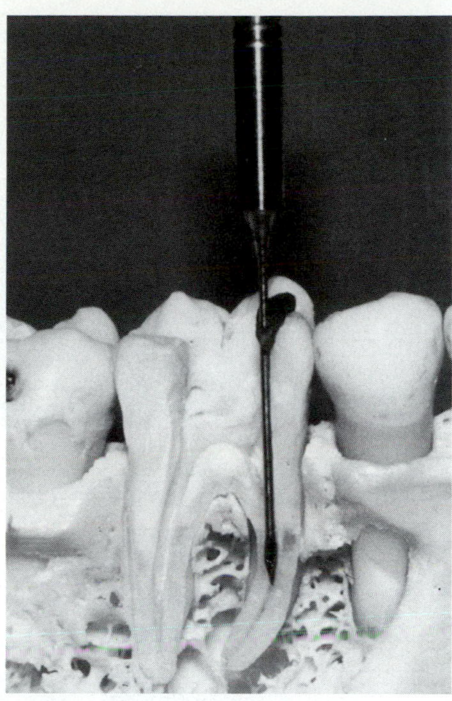

FIG. 8-54 A no. 2 GG bur enlarges the coronal half of the canal. Fine tactile sense is essential. If the GG bur contracts more than one wall of the canal, there is a risk of instrument fracture. With more curved or calcified canals, the no. 2 GG bur would not extend this far into the canal.

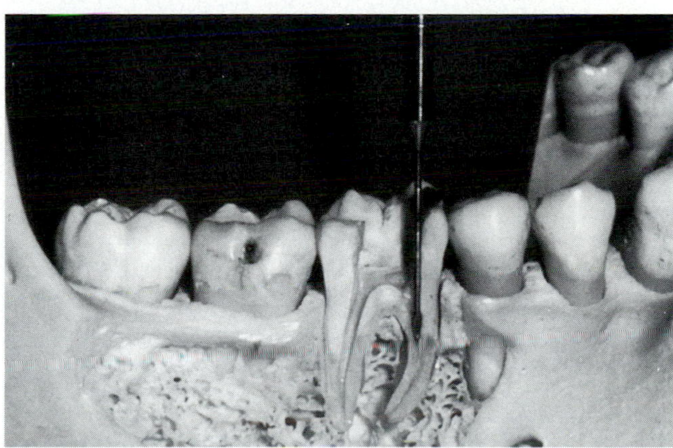

FIG. 8-55 A no. 3 GG bur should not extend beyond the coronal third of the canal.

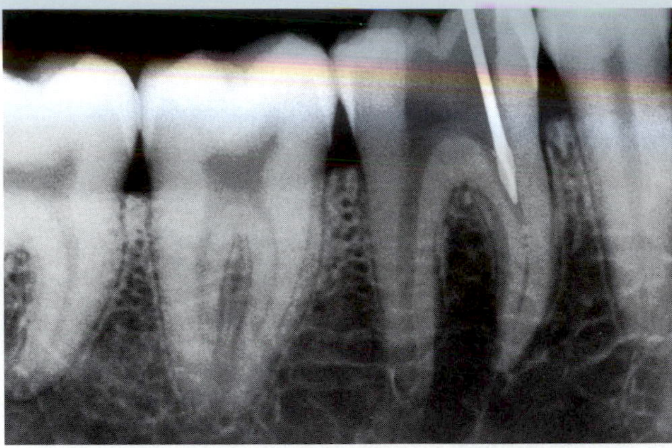

FIG. 8-56 In canals that are initially large, a no. 4 GG bur may be used to finish shaping the coronal 2 to 3 mm of the canal.

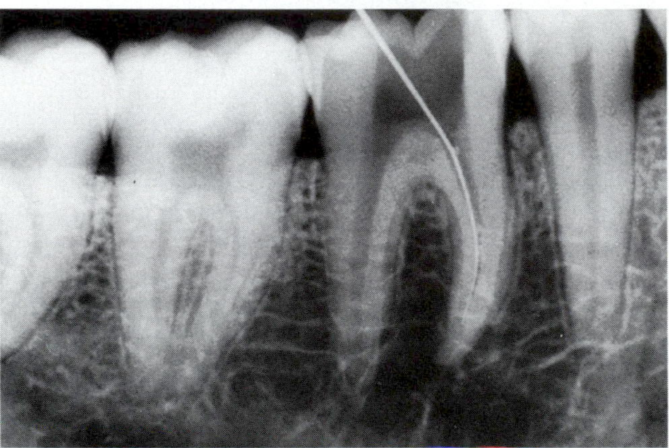

FIG. 8-57 Once the coronal two-thirds of the canal has been shaped and disinfected, the apical 2 to 3 mm of the canal may be approached for cleaning and shaping.

Glidden (GG) burs, K-type files no. 15 to 35 are sequentially placed in the canal. Circumferential filing with each instrument followed by copious irrigation with NaOCl (at least 2 ml after each file) establishes the pathway for the use of no. 2 and 3 GG burs. Once the coronal two thirds of the canal is sculpted and disinfected, the apical portion is cleaned and shaped, as described in the first portion of this chapter.

Good judgment and common sense must prevail in this technique, too. If the canal is initially large, larger instruments should be used. If the canal is excessively curved and calcified, the Schilder technique would be a more prudent option than the step-down.

CONCLUSION

We have presented three methods for cleaning and shaping root canals. Each has its advantages and limitations. Clinicians are best served by familiarizing themselves with each technique. Because each case has certain unique features, a clinician who has mastered each technique can thoughtfully and wisely choose the best one for cleaning and shaping the root canal to attain the common goals of excellence we all share with each other and with you, the reader.

REFERENCES

1. Abou-Rass M, Frank AL, and Glick DH: The anticurvature method to prepare the curved root canal, J Am Dent Assoc 101:792, 1980.
2. Abou-Rass M, Oglesby SW: Effects of temperature, concentration and tissue type on the solvent ability of sodium hypochlorite, J Endod 7:376-7, 1981.
3. Ahmad M, Pitt Ford TR, and Crum LA: Ultrasonic debridement of root canals: an insight into the mechanisms involved, J Endod 13:93, 1987.
4. Ahmad M, Pitt Ford TR, and Crum LA: Acoustic cavitation and its implications in ultrasonic root canal debridement [Abstract 14], J Endod 13:131, 1987.
5. Ahmad M, Pitt Ford TR, and Crum LA: Ultrasonic debridement of root canals: acoustic streaming and its possible role, J Endod 13:490, 1987.
6. Allison CA, Weber CR, and Walton RE: The influence of the method of canal preparation on the quality of apical and coronal seal, J Endod 5:298, 1979.
7. Backman CA, Oswald RJ, Pitts DL: A radiographic comparison of two root canal instrumentation techniques, J Endod 18:19, 1992.
8. Baumgartner JC, and Mader CL: A scanning electron microscopic evaluation of four root canal irrigation regimens, J Endod 13:147, 1987.
9. Baumgartner JC, et al: Histomorphometric comparison of canals prepared by four techniques, J Endod 18:530, 1992.
10. Becker GL, Cohen S, and Borer R: The sequelae of accidentally injecting sodium hypochlorite beyond the root apex, Oral Surg 38:633, 1974.
11. Buchanan LS: Management of the curved root canal: predictably treating the most common endodontic complexity, J Calif Dent Assoc 17:40, 1989.
12. Buchanan LS: Paradigm shifts in cleaning and shaping. J Calif Dent Assoc 23:24, 1991.
13. Cameron JA: The use of ultrasound in the cleaning of root canals: a clinical report, J Endod 8:472, 1982.
14. Cameron JA: The use of ultrasonics in the removal of smear layer: a scanning electron microscope study, J Endod 9:289, 1983.
15. Chenail BL, and Teplitsky PE: Endosonics in curved root canals, J Endod 11:369, 1985.
16. Chenail BL, and Teplitsky PE: Endosonics in curved root canals, part II, J Endod 14:214, 1988.
17. Chow TW: Mechanical effectiveness of root canal irrigation, J Endod 9:475, 1983.
18. Cohen S, Burns RC: Pathways of the pulp, ed 2, St. Louis, 1980, CV Mosby, p 111.
19. Cunningham W, and Balekjion A: Effect of temperature on collagen-dissolving ability of sodium hypochlorite irrigating solution, Oral Surg 49:175, 1980.
20. Cunningham W, and Joseph S: Effect of temperature on the bactericidal action of sodium hypochlorite endodontic irrigant, Oral Surg 50:569, 1980.
21. Cunningham W, et al: A comparison of antibacterial effectiveness of endosonic and hand root canal therapy, Oral Surg 54:238, 1982.
22. Dummer PMH, McGinn JH, and Rees DG: The position and topography of the apical canal constriction and apical foramen, Int Endod J 17:192, 1984.
23. Fairbourn DR, McWalter GM, and Montgomery S: The effect of four preparation techniques on the amount of apically extruded debris, J Endod 13:102, 1987.
24. Fava LRG: The double-flared technique: an alternative for biomechanical preparation, J Endod 9:76, 1983.
25. Fouad AF, et al: A clinical evaluation of five electronic root canal measuring instruments, J Endod 16:446, 1990.
26. George JW, Michanowicz AE, and Michanowicz JP: A method of

canal preparation to control apical extrusion of low-temperature thermoplasticized gutta-percha, J Endod 13:18, 1987.
27. Goerig AC, Michelich RJ, and Schultz HH: Instrumentation of root canals in molars using the step-down technique, J Endod 8:550, 1982.
28. Goldberg F, and Speilberg C: The effect of EDTAC and the variations of its working time analyzed with scanning electron microscopy, Oral Surg 53:74, 1982.
29. Goldman LB, et al: Scanning electron microscope study of a new irrigation method in endodontic treatment, Oral Surg 48:79, 1979.
30. Goldman M, et al: The efficacy of several endodontic irrigating solutions: a scanning electron microscope study, J Endod 8:487, 1982.
31. Goodman A, Schilder H, and Aldrich W: The thermomechanical properties of gutta-percha: II—The history of molecular chemistry of gutta-percha, Oral Surg 37:954, 1974.
32. Goodman A, Schilder H, and Aldrich W: The thermomechanical properties of gutta-percha: IV—A thermal profile of the warm gutta-percha packing procedure, Oral Surg 51:544, 1981.
33. Goodman A, et al: An in vitro comparison of the efficacy of the step-back technique versus the step-back/ultrasonic technique in human mandibular molars, J Endod 11:249, 1985.
34. Green D: A stereomicroscopic study of the root apices of 400 maxillary and mandibular anterior teeth, Oral Surg 9:249, 1956.
35. Green D: Stereomicroscopic study of 700 root apices of maxillary and mandibular posterior teeth, Oral Surg 13:728, 1960.
36. Green EN: Microscopic investigation of root canal diameters, J Am Dent Assoc 57:636, 1958.
37. Grossman LI, and Melman B: Solution of pulp tissue by chemical agents, J Am Dent Assoc 28:223, 1941.
38. Haidet J, et al: An in vivo comparison of the step-back technique versus a step-back/ultrasonic technique in human mandibular molars, J Endod 15:195, 1989.
39. Hand RE, Smith ML, and Harrison JW: Analysis of the effect of dilution on the necrotic tissue dissolution property of sodium hypochlorite, J Endod 4:60, 1978.
40. Harrison JW, and Hand RE: The effect of dilution and organic matter on the antibacterial property of 5.25% sodium hypochlorite, J Endod 7:128, 1981.
41. Huang L: The principle of electronic root canal measurement, Bull 4th Milit Med Coll 8:32, 1959.
42. Huang L: An experimental study of the principle of electronic root canal measurement, J Endod 13:60, 1987.
43. Ingle JI, and Taintor JF: Endodontics, ed 3, Philadelphia, 1985, Lea & Febiger.
44. Inoue N: An audiometric method for determining the length of root canals, J Can Dent Assoc 50:544, 1955.
45. Inoue N: A clinico-anatomical study for the determining of root canal length by use of a novelty low frequency oscillation device, Bull Tokyo Dent Coll 18:71, 1977.
46. Jackson FJ, and Nyborg WL: Small scale acoustic streaming near a locally excited membrane, J Acoust Soc Am 30:614, 1958.
47. Kennedy WA, Walker WA III, and Gough RW: Smear layer removal effects on apical leakage, J Endod 12:21, 1986.
48. Kerekes K, and Tronstad L: Morphometric observations on root canals of human teeth, J Endod 3:24, 74, 114, 1977.
49. Krell KV, Johnson RJ, and Madison S: Irrigation patterns during ultrasonic canal instrumentation: Part I—K-type files, J Endod 14:65, 1988.
50. Kulilid JC, and Peters DD: Incidence and configuration of canal systems in the mesiobuccal root of maxillary first and second molars, J Endod 7:311, 1990.
51. Duplicate reference deleted in proof; same as Ref 52.
52. Kuttler Y: Microscopic investigation of root apexes, J Am Dent Assoc 50:544, 1955.
53. Leeb J: Canal orifice enlargement as related to biomechanical preparation, J Endod 9:463, 1983.
54. Leseberg DA, and Montgomery S: The effects of Canal Master, Flex-R, and K-Flex instruments on root canal configuration, J Endod 17:59, 1991.
55. Lev R, et al: An in vitro comparison of the step-back technique versus a step-back/ultrasonic technique for 1 and 3 minutes, J Endod 13:523, 1987.
56. Loushine RJ, Weller RN, and Hartwell GR: Stereomicroscopic evaluation of canal shape following hand, sonic and ultrasonic instrumentation, J Endod 15:417, 1989.
57. Marshall FJ, and Pappin J: A crown-down pressureless preparation root canal enlargement technique, technique manual, Portland, Ore., 1980, Oregon Health Sciences University.
58. McDonald NJ, and Hovland EJ: An evaluation of the apex locator Endocater, J Endod 16:5, 1990.
59. McDonald NJ: The electronic determination of working length, Dent Clin North Am 36:293, 1992.
60. McKendry DJ: Comparison of balanced forces, endosonic, and step-back filling instrumentation techniques: quantification of extruded apical debris, J Endod 16:24, 1990.
61. Mullaney TP: Instrumentation of finely curved canals, Dent Clin North Am 23:575, 1979.
62. Miserendino LJ, et al: Cutting efficiency of endodontic hand instruments: Part 4—comparison of hybrid and traditional instrument designs, J Endod 14:451, 1989.
63. Morgan LF, and Montgomery S: An evaluation of the crown-down pressureless technique, J Endod 10:491, 1984.
64. Nygaard-Ostby L: Chelation in root canal therapy, Odont Tidskr 65:3, 1957.
65. Pedicord D, ElDeeb ME, and Messer HH: Hand versus ultrasonic instrumentation: its effect on canal shape and intrumentation time, J Endod 12:375, 1986.
66. Powell SE, Wong PD, Simon JHS: A comparison of the effect of modified and nonmodified instrument tips on apical canal configuration—part II, J Endod 14:224, 1988.
67. Ram Z: Effectiveness of root canal irrigation, Oral Surg 44:306, 1977.
68. Roane JB: Principles of preparation using the balanced force technique. In Hardin J, ed: Clark's clinical dentistry, Philadelphia, 1991, JB Lippincott Co.
69. Roane JB, Sabala CL, and Duncanson MG Jr: The "balanced force" concept for instrumentation of curved canals, J Endod 11:203, 1985.
70. Sabala CL, Roane JB, and Southard LZ: Instrumentation of curved canals using a modified tipped instrument: a comparison study, J Endod 14:59, 1988.
71. Saunders WP, and Saunders EM: Effect of noncutting tipped instruments on the quality of root canal preparation using a modified double flared technique, J Endod 18:32, 1992.
72. Schilder H: Periodontically-endodontically involved teeth. In Grossman LI, ed: Transactions of the Third International Conference on Endodontics, Philadelphia, 1963.
73. Schilder H: Filling root canals in three dimensions, Dent Clin North Am 11:723, 1967.
74. Schilder H: Cleaning and shaping the root canal, Dent Clin North Am 18:269, 1974.
75. Schilder H: Canal debridement and disinfection. In Cohen S, and Burns RC, eds: Pathways of the pulp, St. Louis, 1976, Mosby–Year Book, p 111.
76. Schilder H: Vertical compaction of warm gutta-percha. In Gerstein H, ed: Techniques in clinical endodontics. Philadelphia, 1983, WB Saunders.
77. Schilder H, Goodman A, and Aldrich W: The thermomechanical properties of gutta-percha: I—The compressibility of gutta-percha, Oral Surg 37:946, 1974.
78. Schilder H, Goodman A, and Aldrich W: The thermomechanical properties of gutta-percha: III—Determination of phase transition temperatures for gutta-percha, Oral Surg 38:109, 1974.
79. Senia ES, Marshall FJ, and Rosen S: The solvent action of sodium hypochlorite on pulp tissue of extracted teeth, Oral Surg 31:96, 1971.
80. Sepic AO, et al: A comparison of Flex-R files and K-type files for enlargement of severely curved molar root canals, J Endod 15:240, 1989.

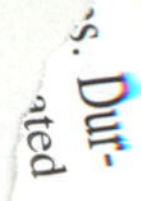

molar root canals with the Roane technique, J Endod 13:479, 1987.

83. Stamos DG, et al: An in vitro comparison study to quantitate the debridement ability of hand, sonic, and ultrasonic intrumentation, J Endod 13:434, 1987.
84. Von der Lehr WN, and Marsh RA: A radiographic study of the point of endodontic egress. Oral Surg 35:105, 1953.
85. Wade AK, Walker WA, and Gough RW: Smear layer removal effects on apical leakage, J Endod 12:21, 1986.
86. Walker A: Definite and dependable therapy for pulpless teeth, J Am Dent Assoc 23:1418, 1936.
87. Walmsley AD, and Williams AR: Effects of constraint on the oscillatory pattern of endosonic files, J Endod 15:189, 1989.

dures on original canal shape and on apical foramen shape, J Endod 1:255, 1975.

90. Weine FS: Endodontic therapy, ed 3, St Louis, 1982, Mosby–Year Book.
91. Wildey, WL, and Senia ES: A new root canal instrument and instrumentation technique: a preliminary report, Oral Surg 67:198, 1989.
92. Wildey WL, Senia ES, and Montgomery S: Another look at root canal instrumentation, Oral Surg 74:499, 1992.
93. Williams S, and Goldman M: Penetrability of the smeared layer by a strain of *Proteus vulgaris,* J Endod 11:385, 1985.
94. Yahya AS, and ElDeeb ME: Effect of sonic versus ultrasonic instrumentation on canal preparation, J Endod 15:235, 1989.

Self-assessment questions

1. Root canal morphology should be
   a. conical.
   b. cylindrical.
   c. three dimensional.
   d. predictable.
2. To achieve the objectives of vertical condensation, it is necessary to produce
   a. a cylindrical canal.
   b. a conical canal.
   c. a tapering conical canal.
   d. a straight canal.
3. To contain gutta-percha within the canal, instrumentation should result in
   a. cleaning beyond the anatomic apex.
   b. cleaning beyond the radiographic apex.
   c. a cylindrical canal shape.
   d. the narrowest cross-sectional diameter at the terminus.
4. To avoid external transportation of the root canal
   a. precurve instruments.
   b. use large instruments.
   c. avoid the use of sodium hypochlorite.
   d. use vigorous instrumentation.
5. According to the precepts of vertical condensation technology, the apical foramen should be
   a. as large as practicable.
   b. as small as practicable.
   c. oval.
   d. circular.
6. The projected success of creating patency relies principally on
   a. the choice of file type.
   b. irrigation.
   c. the first instrument to reach the apical terminus.
   d. the second instrument to reach the apical terminus.
7. Reentry and/or reuse of previously utilized instruments is
   a. capitulation.
   b. recapitulation.
   c. cleaning and shaping.
   d. reworking.
8. Irrigation of the root canal achieves
   a. débridement.
   b. dissolution of tissues.
   c. elimination of microbes.
   d. all of the above.
9. Each time the canal is flushed an appropriate volume of irrigant is
   a. 3 ml.
   b. 1 ml.
   c. 1 to 2 ml.
   d. 4 ml.
10. Débridement is most effective
    a. in large quantities.
    b. when used with recapitulation.
    c. when it remains in the canal between appointments.
    d. just prior to filling.
11. Removal of the smear layer
    a. is accomplished with irrigation.
    b. effectively reduces the microbial population.
    c. is unnecessary for effective cementation during root canal filling.
    d. is necessary for success.
12. Biologic rationale dictates
    a. overinstrumentation.
    b. underinstrumentation.
    c. that the working length stop at the apical constriction.
    d. partial pulp removal.
13. Blood at the tip of a paper point removed from the root canal indicates
    a. possible hematoma.
    b. possible incomplete irrigation.
    c. possible incomplete instrumentation.
    d. possible root perforation.
14. Filing with a Hedström file results in
    a. effective cutting on insertion.
    b. effective cutting on withdrawal.
    c. a lack of tactile sensation.
    d. narrower canal preparations.
15. The crown-down preparation advocates beginning radicular access with
    a. a smaller instrument first.
    b. precurvature of a smaller instrument.
    c. a larger instrument first.
    d. removal of the clinical crown.
16. To improve accuracy, negotiate curved canals, and reduce force of instrumentation, the following tools are recommended:
    a. carbon steel files.
    b. nickel titanium instruments.
    c. reamers.
    d. Hedström files.
17. Radicular access can be achieved by
    a. first using a Gates-Glidden drill throughout half the canal length.
    b. after instrumentation to no. 10, employ the Gates-Glidden drill.
    c. after instrumentation to no. 25, employ the Gates-Glidden drill.
    d. avoid Gates-Glidden drills when possible.
18. Furcal perforation is often the result of
    a. oversized radicular access preparations.
    b. use of Hedström files.
    c. natural occurrence.
    d. use of K-type files.

Chapter 9

Obturation of the Root Canal System

Nguyen Thanh Nguyen

OBJECTIVES OF CANAL OBTURATION

The final stage of endodontic treatment is to fill the entire root canal system and all its complex anatomic pathways completely and densely with nonirritating hermetic sealing agents. Total obliteration of the canal space and perfect sealing of the apical foramen at the dentin-cementum junction and accessory canals at locations other than the root apex with an inert, dimensionally stable, and biologically compatible material are the goals for consistently successful endodontic treatment (Fig. 9-1). Endodontic lesions positioned laterally to a root or asymmetrically about the root apex and periodontal sulcular defects of endodontic origin are vivid reminders of the complexity of the root canal system, with its numerous and infinite variety and location of canal ramifications described by many investigators (Figs. 9-2 to 9-4).

To become accomplished and versatile, it behooves a clinician to master several sound methods of obturating the root canal system. To be confined to only one obturation technique or material is to limit one's ability to undertake a diversity of complex cases. Not infrequently a combination of several materials and filling techniques proves most beneficial in sealing unusually complicated endodontic cases. The use of solvents, together with vertical condensation, heat, sealer hydraulic pressure, and/or mechanical compaction, improves the chance of success in sealing the complex root canal system three-dimensionally (Fig. 9-3). Nearly 60% of endodontic failure is apparently caused by incomplete obliteration of the canal space.[20] Unless a dense, well-adapted root canal filling is achieved, the prognosis may be jeopardized regardless of how well other phases of the treatment are carried out. Although cement sealers enhance the sealing ability of the root canal filling, a serious effort should be made to maximize the volume of the core material and minimize the amount of sealer between the inert core and the dentinal wall. An excellently compacted and tightly adapted endodontic filling should result in the complete closure of the dentinal wall–core material interface, achieving the best apical seal.

The success of the canal obturation is dependent on the excellence of the endodontic cavity design and on thorough canal shaping and cleaning. Regardless of the method employed to obturate the canal, the intensive efforts made toward obtaining total débridement and complete patency of the complex root canal system will facilitate its successful sealing three-dimensionally (Fig. 9-5).

Current studies[2,7,118] have shown that a flare-type preparation, as described in Chapter 7, which allows for more thorough débridement and deeper penetration of obturating instruments closer to the apex, will result in more effective condensation and better sealing of all the pathways of the root canal system.

A three-dimensionally well-filled root canal system does the following:

1. Prevents percolation and microleakage of periapical exudate into the root canal space. (An incompletely filled canal allows percolation of tissue exudate into the unfilled portion of the root canal, where it would stagnate. Subsequent breakdown of tissue fluids diffusing out into the periapical tissues would act as a physiochemical irritant to produce periapical inflammation [Fig. 9-6, *A*].)
2. Prevents reinfection. (Thorough sealing of the apical foramina prevents microorganisms from reinfecting the root canal during transient bacteremia. Bacteria trans-

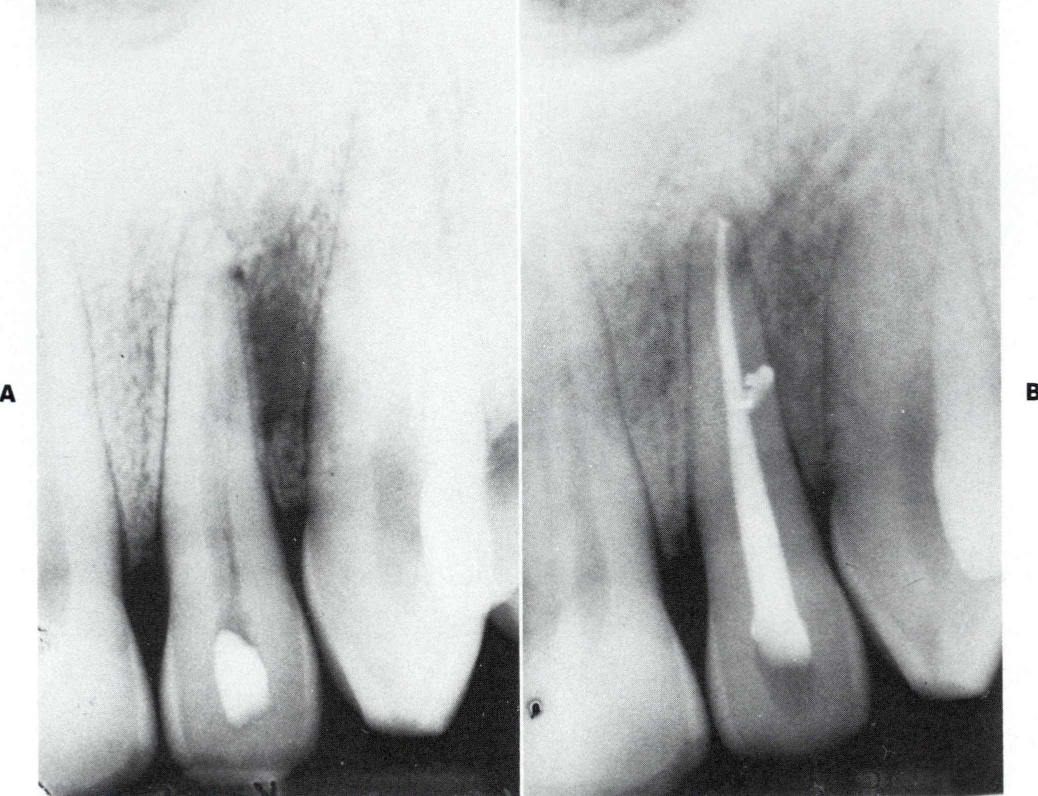

FIG. 9-1 A, Lateral incisor with a large endodontic lesion along the distal root surface. **B,** Six-month recall showing good healing. (Courtesy Dr. L. Stephen Buchanan.)

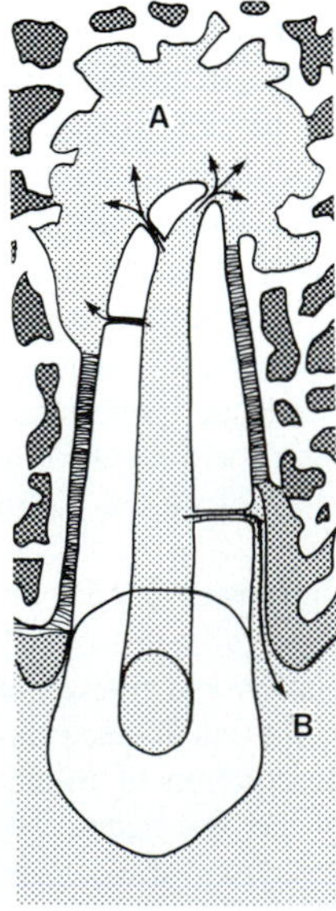

FIG. 9-2 A, Multiple portals of exit allowing egress of irritants contributing to the asymmetric lesions. **B,** Periodontal lesion of endodontic origin. (Courtesy Drs. L. Stephen Buchanan and Clifford J. Ruddle.)

ported to the periapical area may lodge, reenter, and reinfect the root canal and subsequently affect the periapical tissues.)

3. Creates a favorable biologic environment for the process of tissue healing to take place (Fig. 9-6, *B, C*).

APPROPRIATE TIME FOR OBTURATION

After the completion of root canal cleaning and shaping, the root canal is ready to be filled when the following criteria have been met:

1. The tooth is asymptomatic. There is no pain, tenderness, or apical periodontitis; the tooth is comfortable.
2. The canal is dry. There is no excessive exudate or seepage: excessive seepage of exudate is observed in wide-open canals and in cases of cysts.
3. There is no sinus tract. The tract (if one was previously present) should have closed.
4. There is no foul odor. A foul odor suggests the possibility of residual infection or leakage.
5. The temporary filling is intact. A broken or leaking filling causes recontamination of the canal. It is imperative that the tooth restoration be adequately prepared before endodontic treatment. The temporary filling material must seal hermetically to prevent contamination and must be strong enough to withstand the forces of mastication. Zinc oxide–eugenol cements provide the most effective seal against marginal leakage when no particular stress is present. Commercial preparations such as

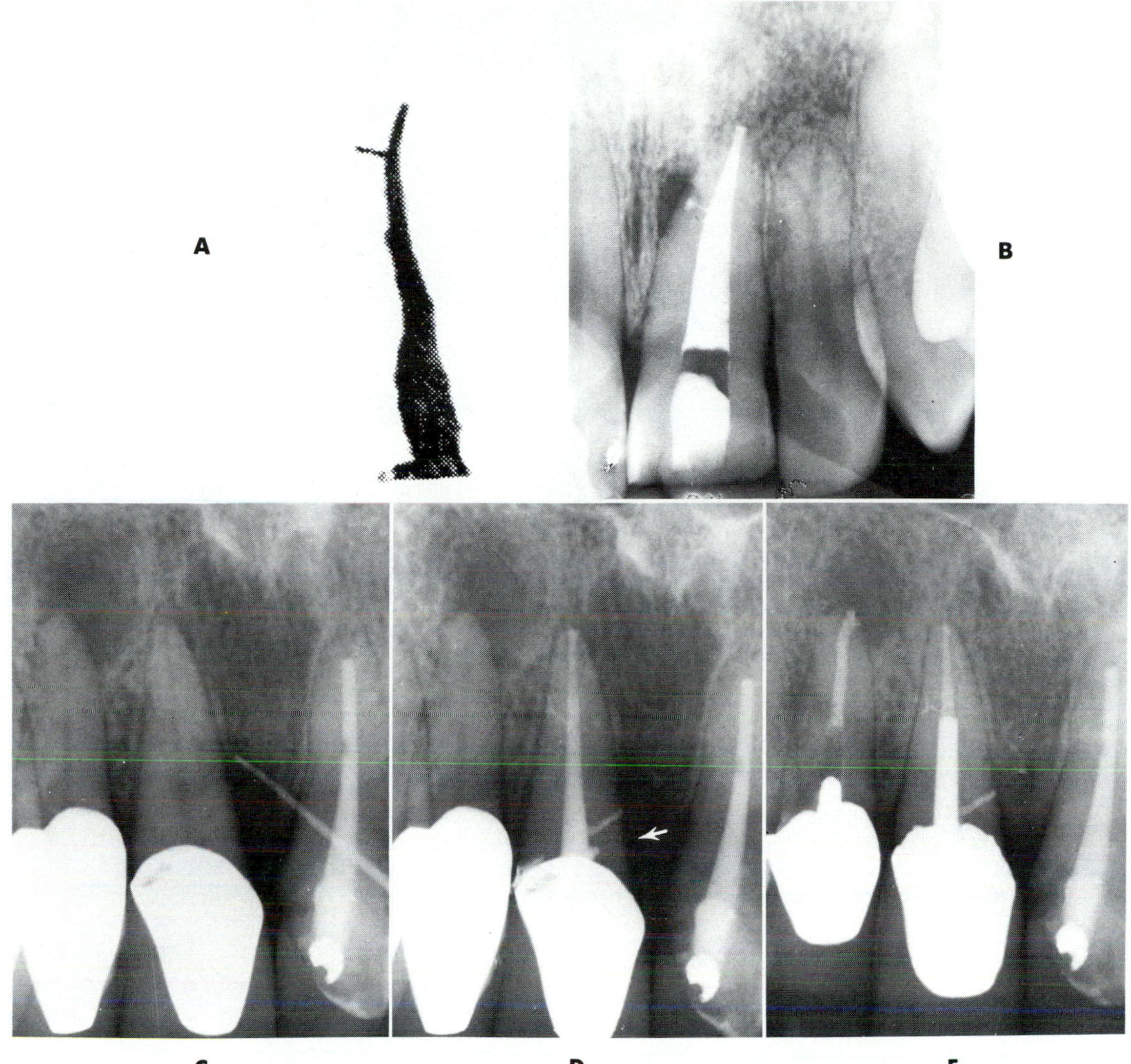

FIG. 9-3 A, Vulcanite rubber impression of a root canal system with a large lateral canal. (Walter Hess, 1925.) **B,** Similar clinical case. Note the absence of periapical pathosis and a significant lateral canal exiting to a lateral root lesion. Note also the bifurcated root canal system of the lateral incisor. **C,** Preoperative radiograph of a central incisor with a gutta-percha cone tracing the sinus tract to a large mesial crestal bone lesion. The intersulcular tissues were, fortunately, still intact. **D,** Postfilling radiograph demonstrating a well-obturated canal space with sealer filling the lateral canals and oozing out along the distal margin of the defective crown *(arrow)*. **E,** Six-month recall radiograph showing the new crown and post and significant healing laterally and apically. (Courtesy Dr. Clifford J. Ruddle.)

Cavit or IRM are satisfactory zinc oxide resin temporary fillings. Because of their slow setting time, the patient should be cautioned not to chew on the tooth for about 45 minutes after treatment. IRM is used in cases of heavy occlusal stress.

ROOT CANAL–FILLING MATERIALS

Types

A large variety of root canal–filling materials has been advocated throughout the years. The gamut runs from materials such as plaster of Paris, asbestos, and bamboo to precious metals such as gold and iridioplatinum. Many materials used have been rejected by the profession as impractical, irrational, or biologically unacceptable. Root canal–filling materials currently in use or under clinical investigation may be grouped into two categories.

Pastes

Paste-type filling materials include zinc oxide–eugenol cements with various additives, zinc oxide and synthetic resins (Cavit), epoxy resins (AH-26), acrylic, polyethylene, and polyvinyl resins (Diaket), polycarboxylate cements, and sili-

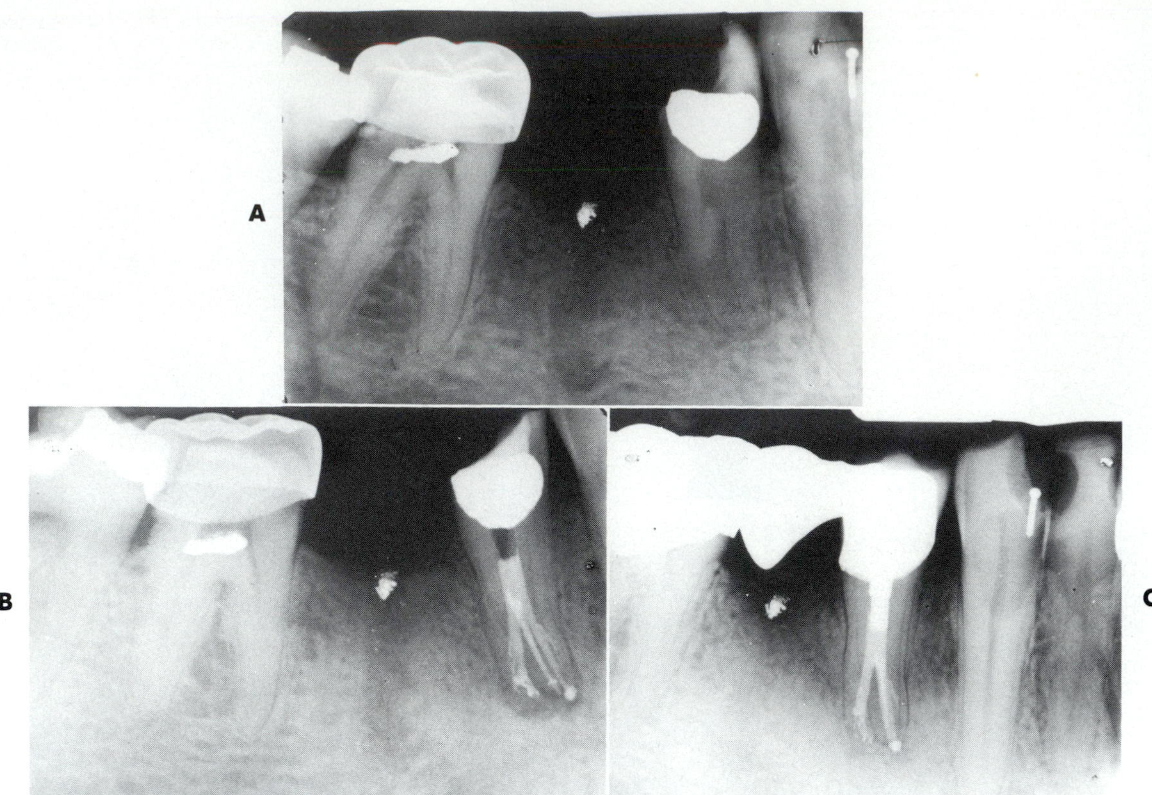

FIG. 9-4 A, Preoperative radiograph showing atypical root morphology of the mandibular first premolar. **B,** Postobturation radiograph. Note the three separate canals with multiple ramifications. **C,** One-year recall, good osseous repair. Warm gutta-percha with vertical condensation. (Courtesy Dr. L. Stephen Buchanan.)

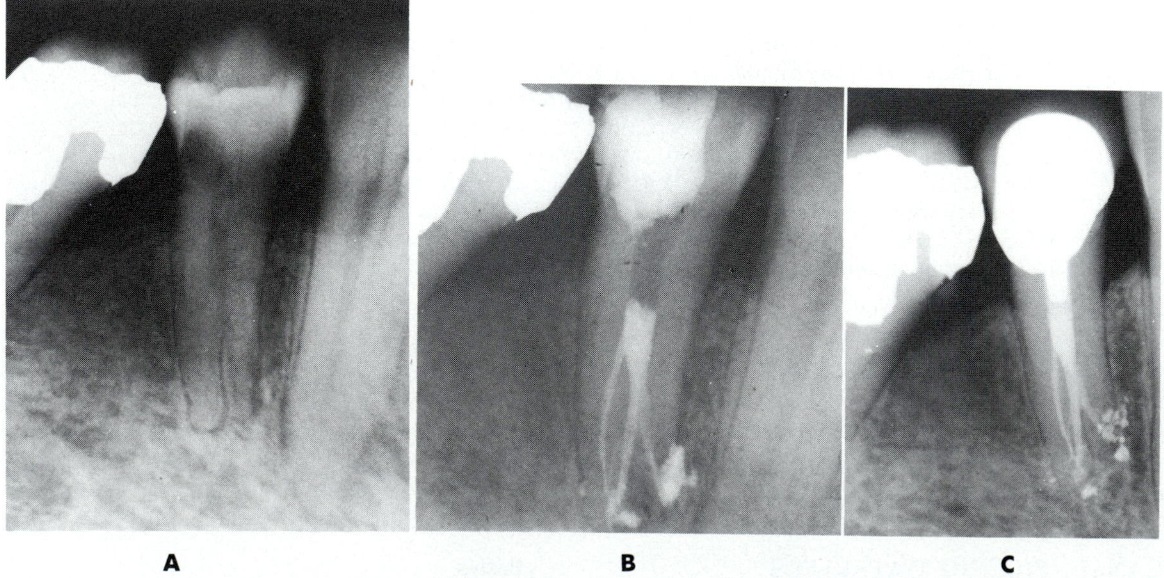

FIG. 9-5 A, Preoperative radiograph. Mandibular first premolar with two roots. Note the radiolucent area along the mesial aspect of mesial root. **B,** Postobturation radiograph. Note the ramifications and complexity of the filled system. Warm gutta-percha with vertical condensation. **C,** Good healing after 18 months. (Courtesy Dr. Robert J. Rosenberg.)

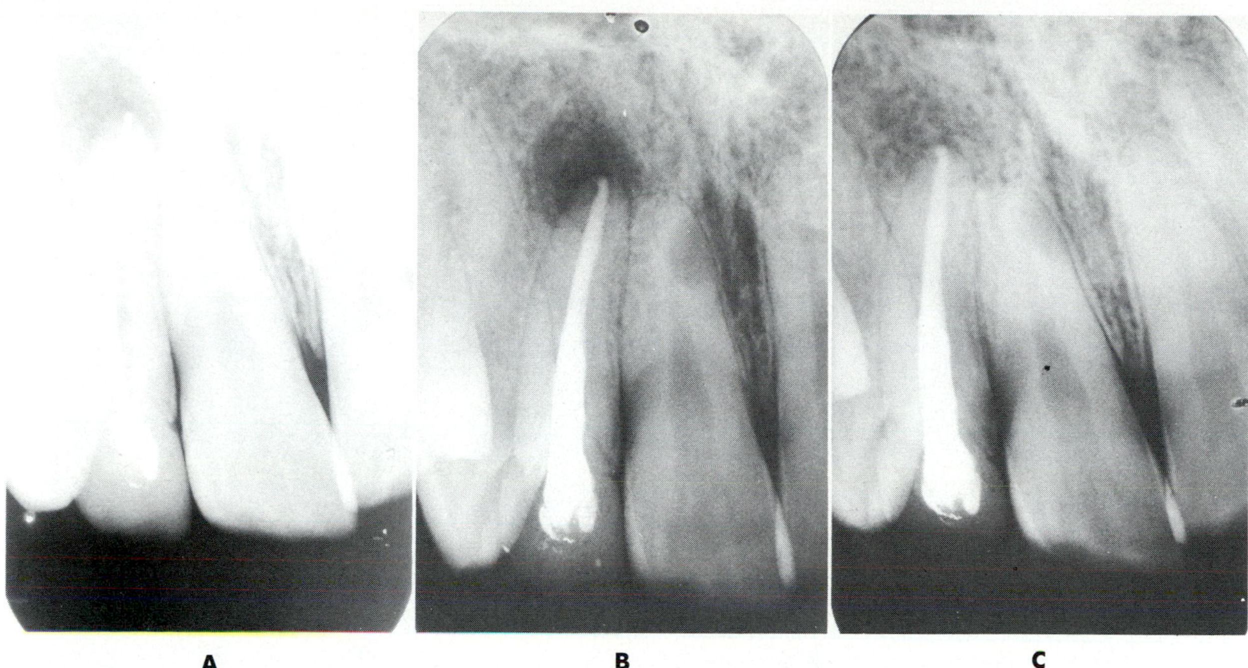

FIG. 9-6 Failure related to an incompletely filled canal. **A,** Percolation into the poorly filled portion, causing a persistent periapical lesion. **B,** After nonsurgical retreatment. The canal has been densely filled with gutta-percha. **C,** One year later, good repair.

cone rubber. Sometimes a solvent-altered gutta-percha paste has been used as the sole canal-filling material.

Semisolid materials

Gutta-percha (Fig. 9-7), acrylic, and gutta-percha composition cones are classified in the category of semisolid materials.

Role of Cement Sealers

The current methods most frequently used in canal obturation employ a semisolid, solid, or rigid cone cemented in the canal with a root canal cement sealer used as a binding agent. The sealer is needed to fill in irregularities and minor discrepancies between the filling and the canal walls. It acts as a lubricant and aids in the seating of the cones. It also fills the patent accessory canals and multiple foramina. (For a discussion of the various types of sealers available, see pp 230 to 232.)

Requirements for an Ideal Root Canal–Filling Material

According to Grossman,[34] an ideal root canal–filling material should:

1. Provide for easy manipulation with ample working time
2. Have dimensional stability; not shrink or change form after being inserted
3. Be able to seal the canal laterally and apically, conforming and adapting to the various shapes and contours of the individual canal
4. Not irritate periapical tissues
5. Be impervious to moisture and nonporous
6. Be unaffected by tissue fluids and insoluble in tissue fluids: not corrode or oxidize
7. Be bacteriostatic; at least, not encourage bacterial growth
8. Be radiopaque, easily discernible on radiographs
9. Not discolor the tooth structure
10. Be sterile or easily and quickly sterilizable immediately before insertion
11. Be easily removed from the canal, if necessary.

Requirements for an Ideal Root Canal Cement Sealer

An ideal root canal sealer should:[34]

1. Be tacky when mixed and have good adhesion to the canal wall
2. Have ample setting time, giving the clinician sufficient time to make necessary adjustments to the filling material
3. Be capable of producing a hermetic seal
4. Have very fine powder particles that mix easily with the cement liquid
5. Be radiopaque, often revealing the existence of accessory canals, multiple foramina, resorptive areas, fracture lines, and other unusual morphologic characteristics
6. Expand while setting
7. Be bacteriostatic
8. Be biologically acceptable; not irritate periapical tissues
9. Be insoluble in tissue fluids
10. Not stain the tooth structure
11. Be soluble in common solvents if removal becomes necessary

To these requirements one might add that an ideal root canal sealer:

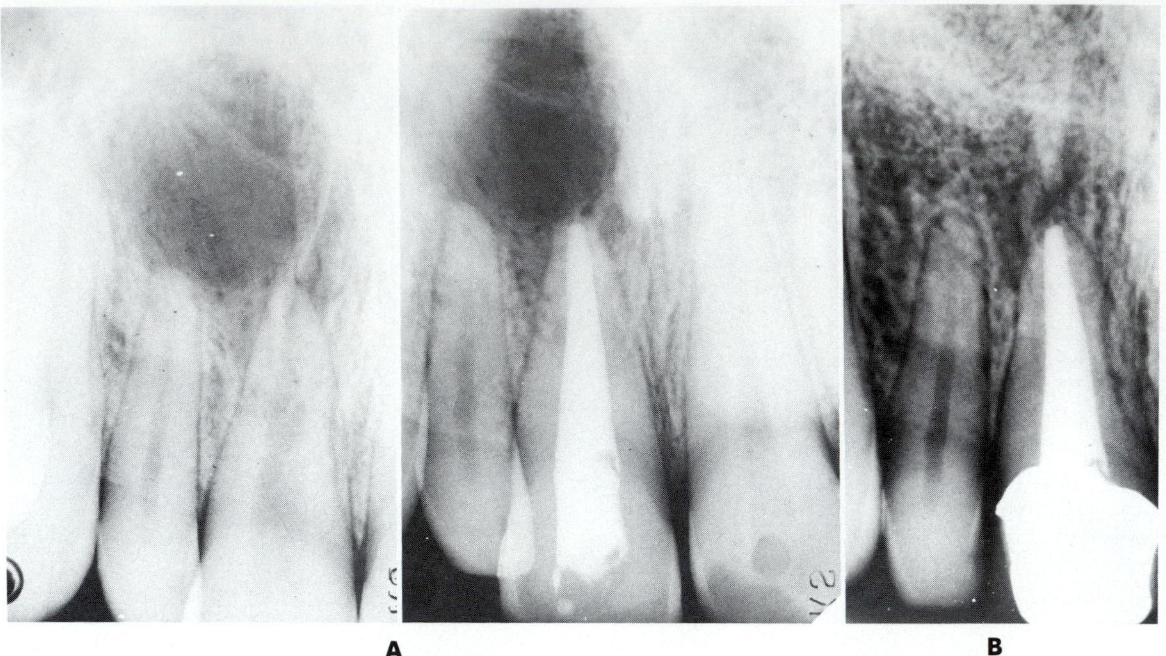

FIG. 9-7 A, Preoperative *(left)* and postoperative *(right)* views of the left central incisor. A large periapical lesion extends over the apex of the adjacent lateral incisor. No surgery was performed. The incisor was filled with gutta-percha. **B,** Eighteen-month recall, good osseous repair. The white appearance of the filling is indicative of its density.

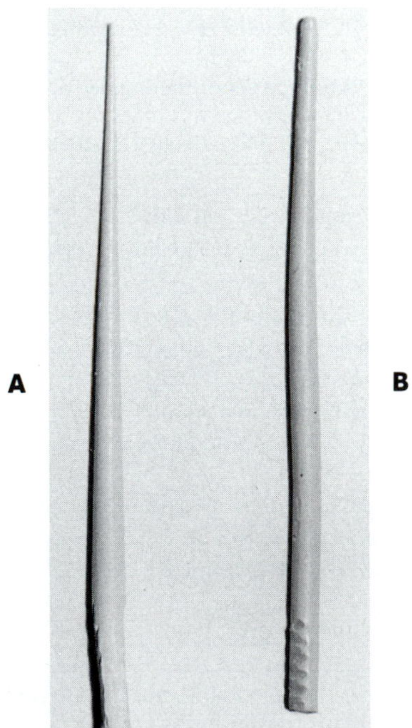

FIG. 9-8 Comparison of nonstandardized and standardized gutta-percha. **A,** Nonstandardized cones have greater taper. They may be used as auxiliary cones or as primary cones in some unusually shaped canals. **B,** Standardized cone with taper similar to that of root canal instruments.

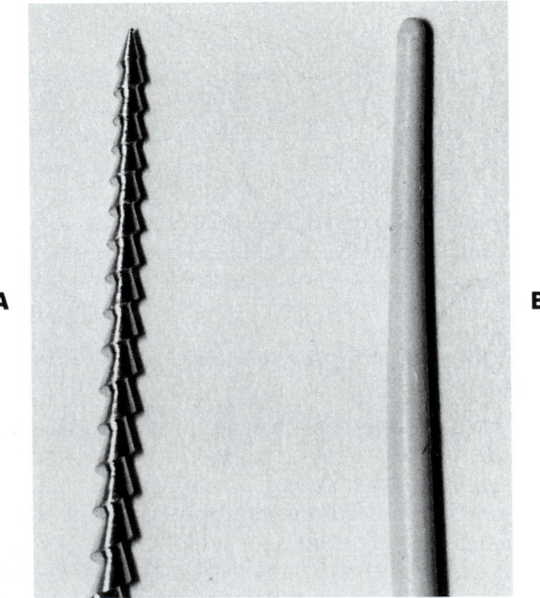

FIG. 9-9 Standardized gutta-percha cone with a taper similar to that of a Hedström file. **A,** File (largest-sized instrument, carried to working length). **B,** Corresponding size of a standardized gutta-percha cone.

12. Should not provoke an immune response in periapical tissues[8,9,109]
13. Should not be mutagenic or carcinogenic.[46,79]

Primary Cone Selection

The selection of cone material depends on the condition of the tooth, the type and size of the canals, the necessity for partial removal of such materials, and the philosophy of the clinician.

CANAL OBTURATION WITH A SEMISOLID MATERIAL: GUTTA-PERCHA

Gutta-percha, popularized by Bowman in 1867,[11] is the most widely used and accepted root canal–filling material. It seems to be the least toxic, least tissue-irritating, and least allergenic root canal–filling material available. The composition of gutta-percha cones varies according to brand. The clinician should be aware of the possible toxicity of the additives in each brand. Gutta-percha is a rubberlike substance manufactured in two different shapes: standardized and nonstandardized (or conventional) cones (Fig. 9-8).

Because they approximate the diameter and taper of root canal instruments (Fig. 9-9), standardized cones (no. 15 to 140) are normally used as *primary* cones.

Nonstandardized (or conventional) cones, more tapered in shape, are useful as *secondary* or *auxiliary* cones in lateral and vertical condensation (Figs. 9-10 and 9-11). Because of their greater flare, conventional cones in sizes *XX fine, X fine,* and *fine* make sturdier and more rigid primary cones in smaller-sized canals than do the small standardized cones. In an effort to standardize endodontic materials, recently made gutta-percha cones and paper points are color coded (Fig. 9-12).

Gutta-percha is slightly soluble in eucalyptol and freely soluble in turpentine, chloroform, ether, or xylol. Gutta-percha cones may be purchased in sterilized containers and should be refrigerated for longer shelf life. When gutta-percha becomes brittle from age and oxidation, it should be discarded, though it has been shown that it can be rejuvenated by alternating heating and cooling.[102]

Advantages

The advantages of gutta-percha as a filling material are these:

1. It is compactible and adapts excellently to the irregularities and contour of the canal by the lateral and vertical condensation method.
2. It can be softened and made plastic by heat or by organic solvents (eucalyptol, chloroform, xylol, turpentine).
3. It is inert.
4. It has dimensional stability; when unaltered by organic solvents, it will not shrink.
5. It is tissue tolerant (nonallergenic).
6. It will not discolor the tooth structure.
7. It is radiopaque.
8. It can be easily removed from the canal when necessary.

Disadvantages

The disadvantages of gutta-percha as a filling material are as follows:

1. It lacks rigidity. The smallest, standardized gutta-percha cones are relatively more difficult to use unless canals are enlarged above size no. 25. Because of their greater taper, nonstandardized cones of smaller sizes are more rigid than small standardized cones and often are used to better advantage as primary cones in small canals.
2. It lacks adhesive quality. Gutta-percha does not adhere to the canal walls; consequently, sealer is required. The necessary use of a cementing agent introduces the risk of using tissue-irritating sealers.

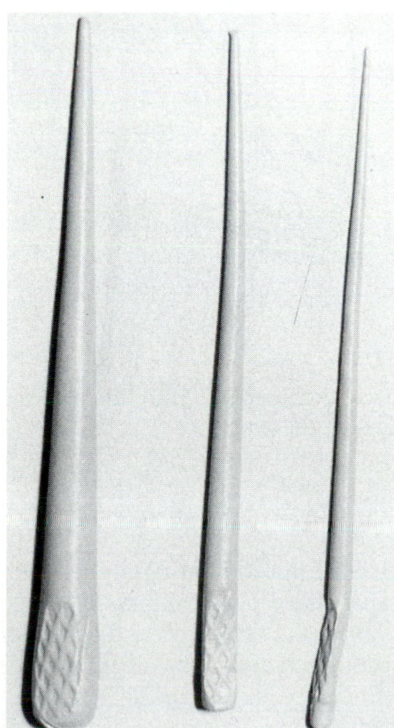

FIG. 9-10 Nonstandardized cones of different sizes.

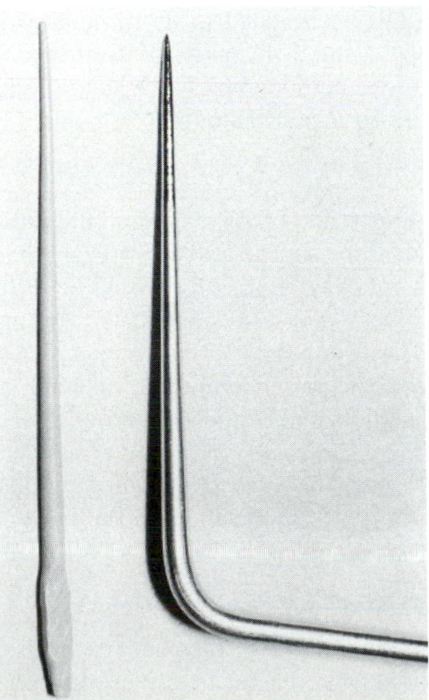

FIG. 9-11 Nonstandardized (old style) cone with the same taper as a root canal spreader. This type is used in lateral and vertical condensation.

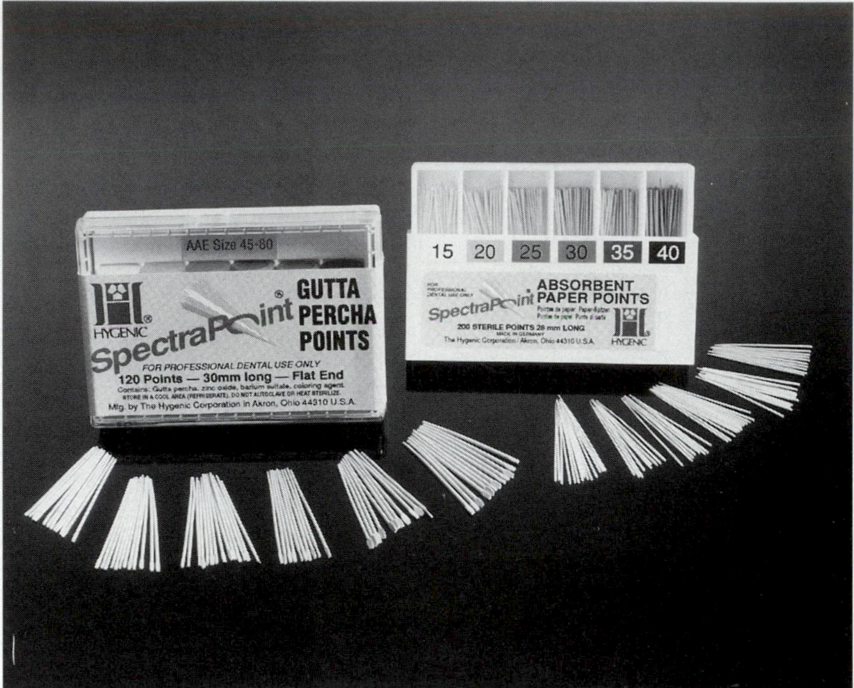

FIG. 9-12 Color-coded gutta-percha and paper points.

3. It can be easily displaced by pressure. Gutta-percha permits vertical distortion by stretching. This characteristic may tend to induce overextension during the condensing process. Unless it meets an obstruction or is packed against a definite apical constriction, it can be easily pushed beyond the apical foramen. To ensure against overextension with gutta-percha, a meticulous endodontic preparation with a constriction in the apical portion at the dentin-cementum junction is required, as described in Chapter 7.

In an effort to improve the working qualities of gutta-percha, acrylic resin has been added to its formula to increase rigidity. A group at the University of California reported that acrylic-reinforced gutta-percha has essentially the same irritational qualities as regular gutta-percha points.[82]

Procedure

The most important objective is to fill the canal system completely and densely and to seal the apical foramina hermetically. To fill the canal efficiently would be difficult if it were not designed and prepared specifically for use with gutta-percha cones. An endodontic preparation with a slight flare and a definite constriction or minimal opening at the dentin-cementum junction makes the task of condensing the gutta-percha into the canal easier and more effective. The presence of accessory canals and multiple apical foramina increases the difficulty of complete sanitization and filling of the root canal system.

Fitting of the primary gutta-percha cone

In determining the size of the primary cone, the clinician is guided by the largest reamer or file used in the final preparation of the root canal (Fig. 9-9).

The selected standardized cone is held with operating pliers at a length equivalent to the measured tooth length or working length. It is inserted into the canal until the beaks of the operating pliers touch the edge of the tooth or reference cusp (Fig. 9-13).

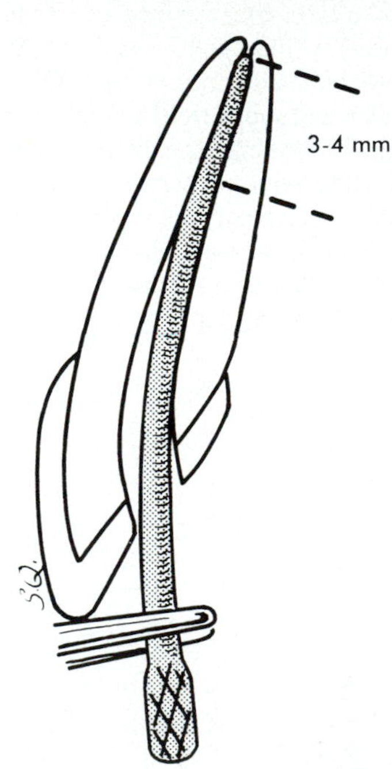

FIG. 9-13 Gutta-percha cone tightly fitted in the apical 3 to 4 mm (apical seat) of the canal.

The primary cone must (1) fit tightly laterally in the apical third of the canal (have good "tug-back"), (2) fit to the full length of the canal (i.e., to the dentin-cementum junction or about 1 mm from the radiographic apex), and (3) be impossible to force farther beyond the apical foramen.

A small indentation mark is made on the gutta-percha cone on the incisal edge of the tooth or reference cusp with the beaks of the operating pliers, the tip of a file, or the tip of an ex-

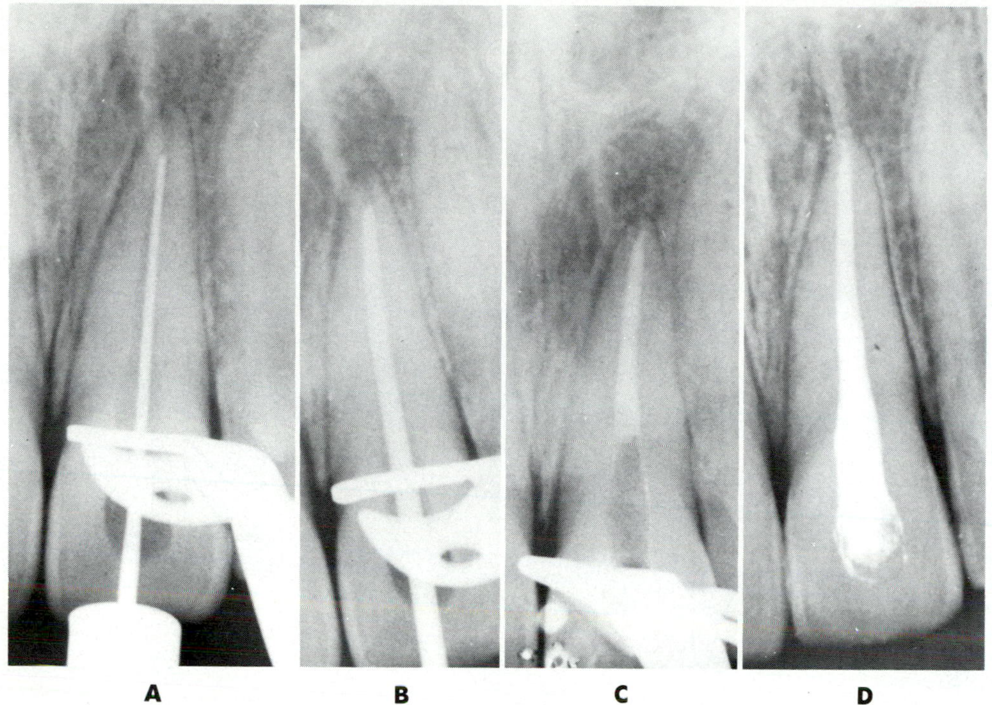

A B C D

FIG. 9-14 Maxillary central incisor filled with gutta-percha. **A,** Obtaining tooth length. **B,** Primary cone with good tug-back fitted 1 mm short of the apical foramen. **C,** Complete seating of the cone with condensation pressure and lubrication by sealer. Gutta-percha was removed to the apical two thirds of the apex in preparation for a dowell and core. **D,** Dowel-core reinforcement cemented.

plorer slightly warmed over a Bunsen burner. The tip of the file or explorer is positioned at a right angle to the incisal or occlusal edge of the tooth.

A radiograph is exposed when the cone is well-stabilized with sterile cotton pellets in the canal.

If the radiograph shows the cone to be within 0.5 to 1 mm of the apex, the cone is an acceptable length. A perfect coincidence of the image of the cone with the radiographic apex will produce a cone probably protruding beyond the apical foramen. When the cone is slightly short of the radiographic apex (1 to 1.5 mm), the added pressure of condensation plus the increased lubrication provided by the sealer will be sufficient to produce complete seating (Fig. 9-14).

If the radiograph shows the cone to be too short, a correct cone fit may be obtained in one of the following ways:

1. Rechecking the working length for precise tooth length measurement and preparing the canal again accordingly
2. Enlarging the canal by filing and then trying the cone again
3. Thinning out the cone by rolling it between two sterile glass slabs or with a sterile spatula on a sterile slab or by selecting a slightly smaller cone
4. Using the solvent dip technique in filling the canal (see next section)
5. Checking for the presence of debris clogging the canal near the apex. (Debris is removed best with a reamer or a Hedström file and copious irrigation.)

If the cone is too long, it is reduced proportionally from the small or apical end (Fig. 9-15). It is reinserted tightly into the canal, and a radiograph is exposed to verify the fit.

A radiolucent line appearing between the gutta-percha cone and the wall of the canal indicates that the cone may be too small (Fig. 9-16), that the canal preparation is not round, or that an extra canal is present (Fig. 9-17).

Chloroform dip technique.* The chloroform dip technique, as a cone-fitting method, is used in large canals requiring custom-made gutta-percha cones or when it is desired to further seat a cone size 50 or larger that is 2 or 3 mm short of the radiographic apex (Figs. 9-18 and 9-19). This technique may be used at the time of cone fitting or during obturation.

At trial fit stage. An imprint of the apical portion of the prepared canal can be obtained by using a solvent to superficially soften a gutta-percha cone.

The canal should be kept moist by irrigation; otherwise, some of the softened gutta-percha might stick to the dried dentinal walls. Occasionally the softened apical section of the cone detaches from the body of the cone and adheres to the canal. The detached segment can be easily removed with a Hedström file one size smaller than the last size used in the preparation of the canal.

The cone is held with the pliers at the correct operating length. The apical 4 to 5 mm of the cone is then dipped for a period of 4 to 6 seconds into a Dappen dish containing a solvent.

The softened cone is inserted into the canal with slight apical pressure until the beaks of the pliers touch the referring

*The reader is urged to use alternative organic solvents (e.g., xylol, turpentine, or eucalyptol) because of the FDA's identification of chloroform as a carcinogen.

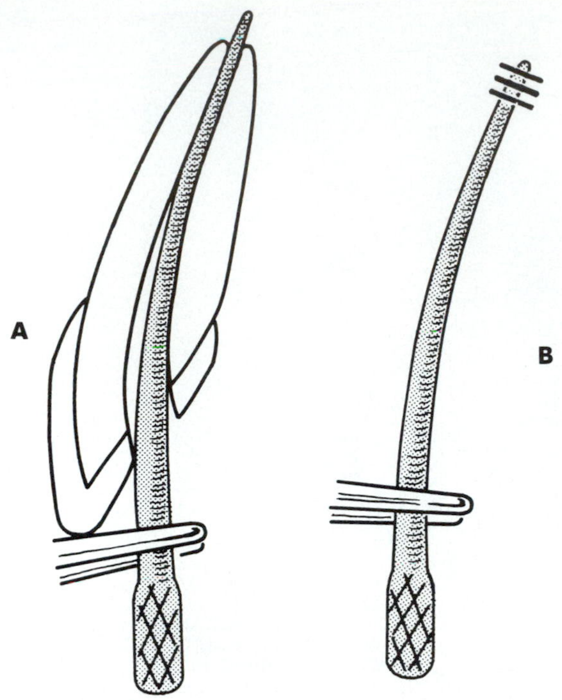

FIG. 9-15 **A,** Gutta-percha cone extending beyond the apex. **B,** Cone shortened a corresponding amount to improve its fit.

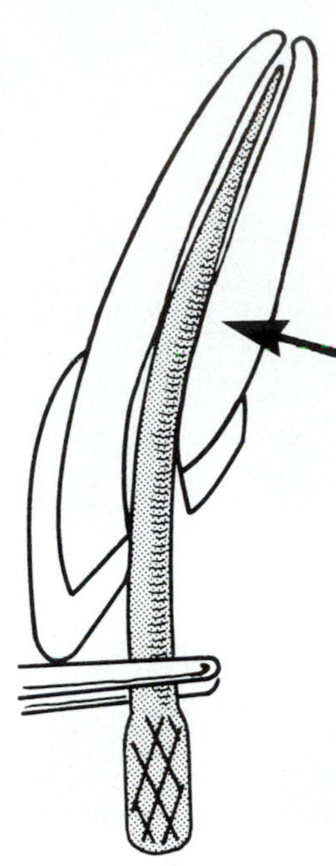

FIG. 9-16 Gutta-percha cone binding in the coronal half *(arrow)* but loosely fitted in the apical half, giving a false sense of a tight fit (tug-back).

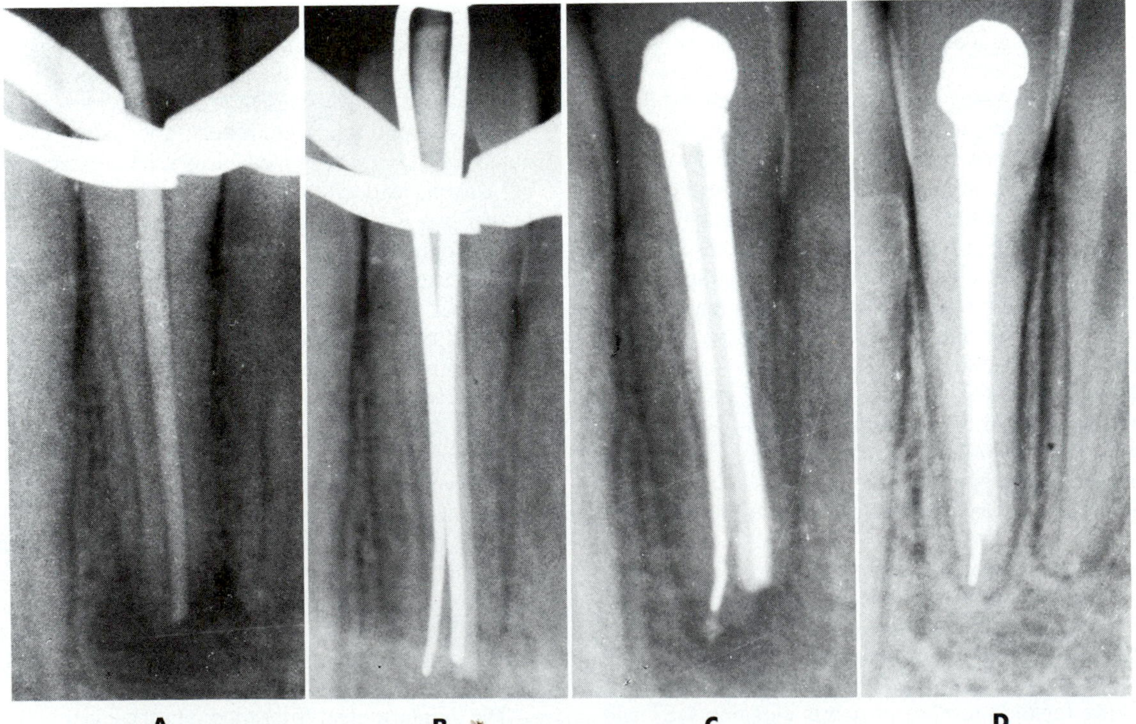

FIG. 9-17 Triple-rooted mandibular central incisor (quite rare). **A,** Tightly fitted gutta-percha cone (good tug-back). Radiolucent lines on both sides reveal the presence of two extra canals. **B,** Main canal fitted with a gutta-percha cone, two smaller canals fitted with silver cones. **C,** After filling. Note the three definite canals. **D,** Complete healing 1 year later.

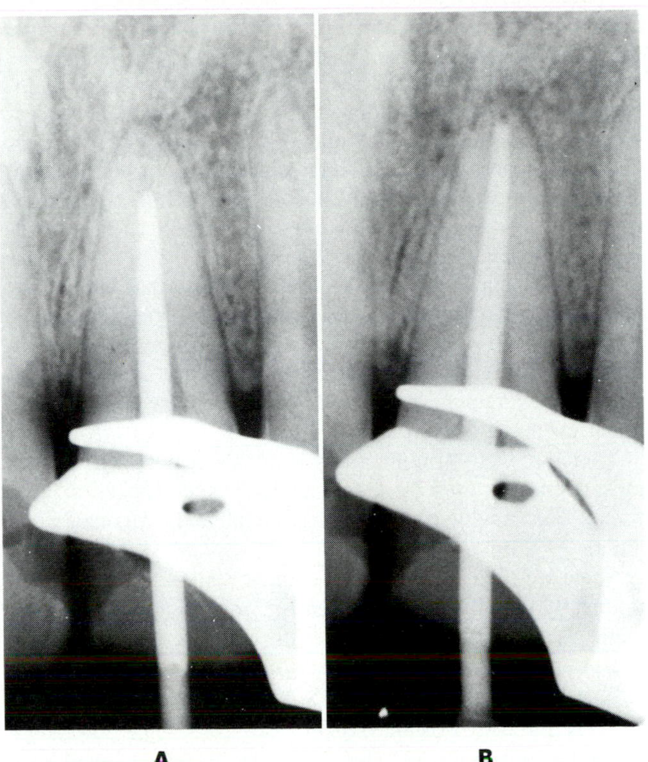

FIG. 9-18 A, Cone fitted quite short of the prepared canal length. **B,** Well-fitted cone obtained by dipping for a few seconds into a solvent and reinserting into the canal. (Note: The canal must be kept moist with irrigant to prevent the softened cone from sticking to the canal wall.)

landmark. It is then withdrawn slightly and reinserted a few times until a satisfactory imprint is obtained.

An indentation mark is placed on the cone at a level corresponding to the incisal edge of the crown, and a radiograph is used to verify correctness of fit.

While the radiograph is being developed, the cone should be removed from the canal and submerged in 99% isopropyl alcohol. This cone will be used later, when the canal is ready to be filled.

The canal is irrigated again to remove traces of the solvent.

At obturation stage. A tight-fitting gutta-percha cone about 2 to 3 mm short of the prepared canal length may be completely seated in the following manner:

1. The canal is coated with cement sealer.
2. The cone (uncoated) is held with pliers at the correct operating length, and the apical 4 to 5 mm of the cone is dipped into chloroform for 3 to 5 seconds. The dipping time depends on the amount of softening desired and on how far the cone must travel to reach the apical foramen.
3. The softened cone is inserted into the canal with steady pressure until the pliers touch the operating landmark (Fig. 9-20).

Wong and coworkers,[118] in an investigation of replication properties and volumetric change of three chloroform gutta-percha filling techniques, found that the chloroform dip technique produced fillings with significantly less shrinkage than

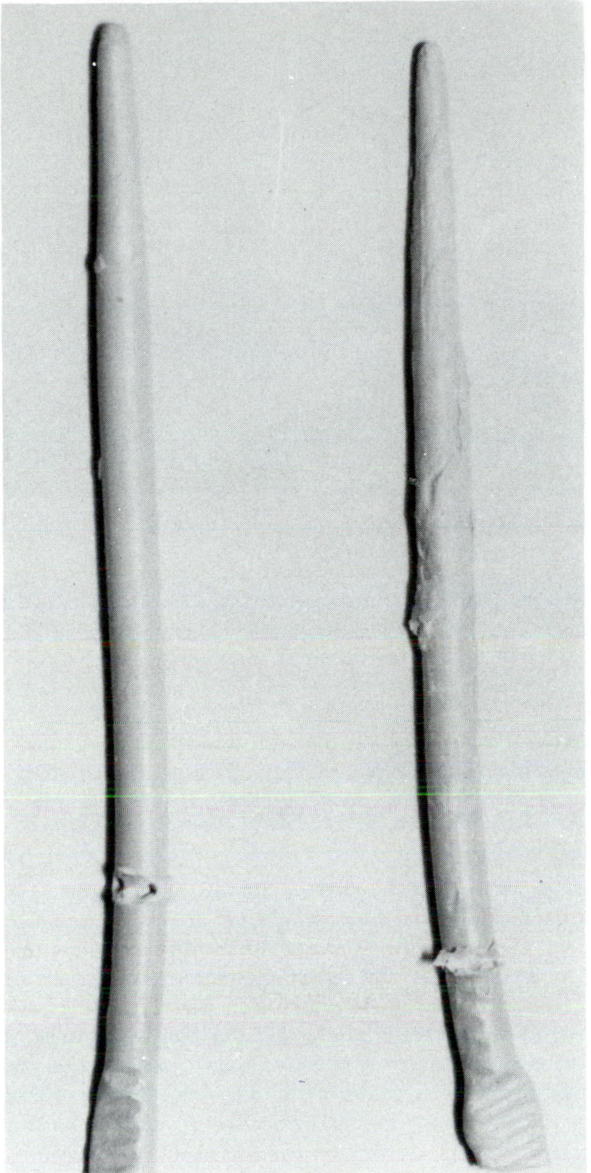

FIG. 9-19 Effect of solvent on the gutta-percha cone in Figure 9-18. *Left,* Before dipping. *Right,* After dipping. Note the impression of the canal space on the softened cone.

did the chloropercha and Kloroperka, N-Ø techniques. The chloroform dip fillings showed the least volume change—an average shrinkage of 1.40% in 2 weeks versus 12.42% for chloropercha and 4.86% for Kloroperka N-Ø fillings. If a chloroform technique is to be used, the chloroform dip filling technique is recommended because of its low shrinkage and excellent replication qualities.

Other investigations[56,88,93] on apical leakage reported that very brief softening of the master cone with chloroform produced poor sealing results. One group of investigators[57] suggested that chloroform may affect the gutta-percha dye absorption. Also, the gutta-percha shrinkage and the physical or chemical alteration of the sealer may be responsible for the leakage. Another group of investigators[88] thought, "the surface layer of the chloroform dissolved the sealer." Although

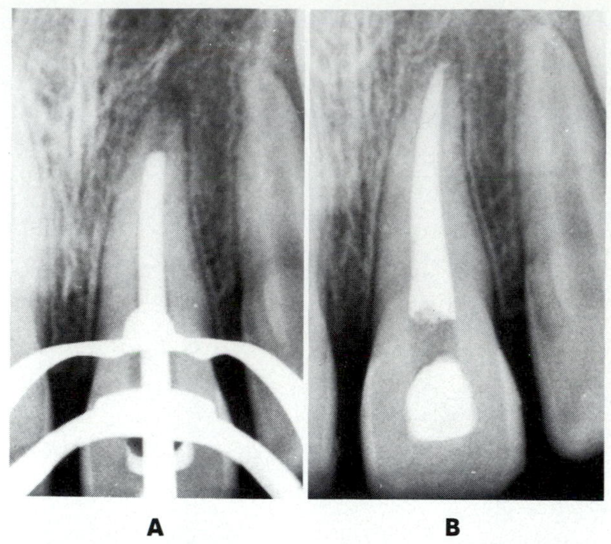

FIG. 9-20 Solvent technique at filling time. **A,** Primary cone fitted tightly about 2 mm short of the apex. **B,** Softened by solvent, the cone is completely seated apically.

"clinical" success of the chloroform-softened gutta-percha cone technique is accepted, it certainly bears further study.

ROOT CANAL CEMENT SEALERS AND THEIR PROPERTIES

Cements used in endodontics are often referred to as root canal cement sealers. Most sealers are composed of zinc oxide and eugenol with various additives to render them radiopaque, antibacterial, and adhesive. Some cements contain epoxy resins (AH-26) or polyvinyl resins (Diaket).

The root canal sealer acts as (1) a *binding agent* to cement the well-fitted primary cone into a canal, much as zinc phosphate cement binds a well-fitted inlay into a cavity preparation, (2) a *filler* for the discrepancies between the cone and the canal walls, and (3) a *lubricant* to facilitate the seating of the primary cone into the canal.

Before setting, the root canal cement can be made to flow and fill the accessory canals and multiple apical foramina by the lateral and vertical condensation method.

A good sealer should be biologically compatible and well tolerated by the periapical tissues.[103,104] *All* sealers are highly toxic when freshly prepared; however, their toxicity is greatly reduced after setting takes place. A few days after cementation, practically all root canal sealers produce varying degrees of periapical inflammation (usually temporary); this usually does not appear to prevent tissue healing and repair.

A root canal sealer should not provoke an immune response in periapical tissues.[8,9,109] Sealers of zinc oxide–eugenol type pastes modified with paraformaldehyde have been reported to alter dog pulp tissue, making it antigenically active.[8,9] In regard to mutagenicity or carcinogenicity, investigators[41] found that eugenol and its metabolites, although suspect, were uniformly negative in a bacterial mutagenicity test. The probability of eugenol acting as a carcinogen is therefore relatively low. However, formaldehyde- and paraformaldehyde-containing sealers are highly suspect. Following a study on the subject by the National Academy of Sciences,[28] the U.S. Consumer Product Safety Commission issued warnings about the hazards of formaldehyde.[42]

In their studies of tissue reactions to root canal cements investigators[22,23] reported that although most cement sealers were highly irritating to periapical tissues, the most severe alveolar and bone destruction was caused by poor débridement and poor filling of the root canal system. Minimal tissue reaction was found when the canal was not overfilled. Their findings were confirmed by other researchers,[100] who found, using human beings and monkeys as subjects, that overinstrumentation and overfilling caused immediate periapical inflammation, which tended to persist and to cause epithelial proliferation and cyst formation. In the group of teeth filled short of the foramen, the reaction was temporary and complete repair eventually took place.

There are many commercially available sealers. The sealers most commonly used by American dentists are Rickert's, Tubliseal, Wach's, chloropercha, eucapercha, and Grossman's formula.

Some well-known root canal cement sealers, which are less frequently used by American dentists, are zinc oxide and synthetic resins (Cavit), epoxy resins (AH-26; DeTrey, Ltd., U.S.A. distributor Dentsply), acrylic polyethylene and polyvinyl resins (Diaket; ESPE, U.S.A. distributor Premier Dental) and polycarboxylate cements. Other recently advocated root canal sealers include zinc oxide–noneugenol cement (Nogenol; COE Mfg. Co.), calcium hydroxide–containing cement (Dycal; Hygienic Rubber Co., Akron, Oh.; and Calciobiotic; Lee Pharmaceutical, South El Monte, Calif.),[29] plastics-containing cements such as Silastic medical adhesive type A, silicone rubber for syringe injection (Endo-Fill; Fuji G.C., Japan), and Fuji type I glass ionomer luting cement (L.D. Caulk Co.).[94,124] Researchers[92,121] have experimented with silicone rubber material sealed in the canals with cyanoacrylate, polycarboxylate or silicone adhesive, or Silastic.[54]

Rickert's sealer

Rickert's sealer contains powder—zinc oxide (41.2 parts), precipitated silver (30 parts), white resin (16 parts), and thymol iodide (12.8 parts); and liquid—oil of clove (78 parts) and Canada balsam (22 parts). It is germicidal, has excellent lubricating and adhesive qualities, and sets in about half an hour. Because of its silver content, Rickert's sealer may cause discoloration of tooth structure and must be removed meticulously from the crown and pulp chamber with xylol.

Tubliseal

Tubliseal contains zinc oxide (57.4%), bismuth trioxide (7.5%), oleoresins (21.25%), thymol iodide (3.75%), oils (7.5%), and a modifier (2.6%). This sealer is packaged in two collapsible tubes containing a base and an accelerator, which when mixed together in equal amounts form a creamy mix. Tubliseal mixes well, has excellent lubricating properties, and does not stain the tooth structure; however, it sets rather rapidly, especially in the presence of moisture.

Wach's sealer

Wach's sealer[74] contains powder—zinc oxide (10 g), calcium phosphate (2 g), bismuth subnitrate (3.5 g), bismuth subiodide (0.3 g), and heavy magnesium oxide (0.5 g); and liquid—Canada balsam (20 ml) and oil of clove (6 ml). This sealer is germicidal, has relatively low tissue irritation, and has

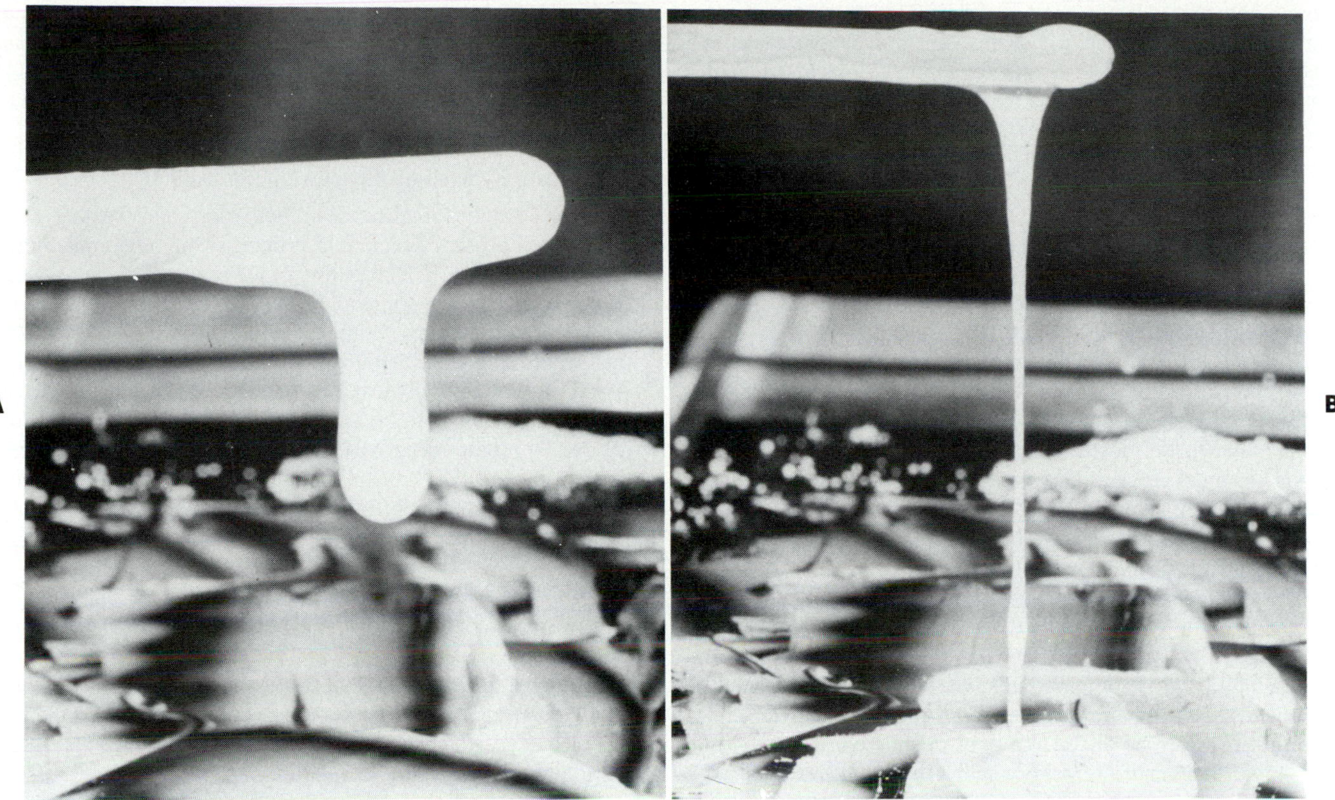

FIG. 9-21 Mixing Grossman's cement to a thick and creamy consistency. **A,** Drop test. The cement should drop off the spatula edge in 10 to 15 seconds. **B,** String-out test. The cement should string out for at least 1 inch when the spatula is raised slowly from the glass slab.

an adequate setting time; its lubricating qualities are limited, however. It should be mixed to a smooth, creamy consistency and should string out at least 1 inch when the spatula is raised from the glass slab. Because of its low level of tissue irritation and limited lubricating characteristics, this sealer is desirable when there is the possibility of overextension beyond the confines of the root canal.

Chloropercha and eucapercha

Chloropercha and eucapercha are made by dissolving gutta-percha in chloroform and eucalyptol, respectively. These are used by a few clinicians as the sole canal filling material, but more often they are used in combination with gutta-percha cones. Shrinkage after the evaporation of the solvent and irritation of the periapical tissue by the chloroform are definite disadvantages. The chloropercha filling method (pp. 247-248) can produce excellent results in the filling of unusual curvatures or in cases of perforation or ledge formation.

Grossman's sealer

Grossman's sealer is used widely and meets most of Grossman's own requirements for an ideal sealer; it presents a minimal degree of irritation and a high level of antimicrobial activity. It contains powder—zinc oxide reagent (42 parts), staybelite resin (27 parts), bismuth subcarbonate (15 parts), barium sulfate (15 parts), and sodium borate, anhydrous (1 part); and liquid—eugenol.

A sterile glass slab and spatula are used to mix a small amount of powder to a creamy consistency (Fig. 9-21). *No more than three drops of liquid should be used at a time.* Excessive time and effort would be required to spatulate a larger amount.

Tests for proper consistency include the "drop" test and the "string-out" test. With the *drop test,* the mass of cement is gathered onto the spatula held edgewise. The cement should not drop off of the spatula's edge in less than 10 to 12 seconds (Fig. 9-21, *A*). A root canal instrument may also be used for this test. After a no. 25 file is rotated in the gathered mass of cement, it is withdrawn and held in a vertical position. A correctly mixed cement should remain, with very little movement, on the blade of the instrument for 5 to 10 seconds. If a teardrop forms, the mix is too thin and more powder should be added.

With the *string-out* test the mass of cement is returned to the slab. After touching the mass of cement with its flat surface, the spatula is raised up *slowly* from the glass slab. The cement should string out at least 1 inch without breaking (Fig. 9-21, *B*).

Grossman's cement will not set hard on a glass slab for 6 to 8 hours. A mixed batch of cement can therefore be used for several hours. If it thickens, respatulation will break up any crystals formed and will restore the mix to proper consistency. In the canal, because of moisture in the dentinal tubules, the cement will begin to set in about half an hour.

The popularity of this cement results from its plasticity and its slow setting time, which is due to the presence of sodium borate anhydrate. It has good sealing potential and small volumetric change upon setting. However, zinc eugenate can be decomposed by water through a continuous loss of eugenol, making zinc oxide–eugenol a weak, unstable material. On the other hand, this ability to be absorbed is an advantage in case of apical extrusion of the sealer during canal obturation.

The cement is soluble in chloroform, carbon tetrachloride, xylol, or ether. It is easily removed from the glass slab and spatula with alcohol or a solvent.

Diaket

Diaket cement, a resin-reinforced chelate formed between zinc oxide and diketone, is known for its high resistance to absorption. First reported in 1952, Diaket was found in one study[120] to be less effective as a sealer than Tubliseal, but both were found to be more effective than paraformaldehyde zinc oxide–eugenol cement. Other studies on root canal sealing cements found Diaket and AH-26 to be satisfactory as sealers.[24,55] These cements have been used frequently to cement endoserous implants.

AH-26

AH-26, first reported about 1957, is an epoxy resin with low solubility. It is composed of silver powder (10%), bismuth trioxide (60%), titanium dioxide (5%), and hexamethylene tetramine (25%), to be mixed to a thick creamy consistency with the liquid bisphenol diglycidyl ether (100%). It has good adhesive property, antibacterial activity, and low toxicity and is tolerated well by periapical tissue.[22,25,87]

Two early studies[38,91] tested several root canal sealers, including N-2, by implanting them into the subcutaneous connective tissue of rats. They found that AH-26 elicited no response at 35 days, while N-2 provoked the "most severe inflammation elicited by any of the test materials."[91] Paresthesia following the overextension of AH-26 beyond the apex has been reported.[105,108] There was a case report[4] of paresthesia of the mental nerve resulting from gross overfilling with AH-26, but nerve function was completely restored 14 weeks after removal of the offending overfilled mandibular second premolar.

Like Rickert's cement, AH-26 contains silver powder; therefore, all traces of the sealer must be removed below the free gingiva level to prevent tooth discoloration.

Polycarboxylate cement

Some studies[75,101] have advocated the use of polycarboxylate cement as root canal cement. Composed of zinc oxide with polyacrylic as a liquid, polycarboxylate cement will bond to enamel and dentin. Polycarboxylates will set in a moist environment and are insoluble in water. Unfortunately, their rapid setting does not allow for ample working time. Other studies[5,99,116] have reported unfavorable results and have found that polycarboxylates are unsatisfactory and difficult to manipulate for endodontic use.

Nogenol

The zinc oxide–noneugenol cement Nogenol has been advocated as a less irritating sealer. One study[18] tested Nogenol subcutaneously against two eugenol-containing cements—Tubliseal and Rickert's cement—and found, "after 24 hours all sealers caused considerable inflammation." At 96 hours Nogenol was considerably less irritating than the other two sealers, even better than the polyethylene tubing control. At 6 months Tubliseal remained significantly more of an irritant than Rickert's cement, Nogenol, or the polyethylene control. Another study[113] found that Nogenol expands on setting and may improve its sealing efficacy with time.

Calcium hydroxide–based cement sealers

Several calcium hydroxide–based root canal sealers were reported to possess acceptable properties of biocompatibility and sealing ability. Calcium hydroxide material has an advantage over zinc oxide–eugenol because of its ability to preserve the vitality of the pulp stump. Several studies,[1,50,89a] reported that when compared with zinc oxide–eugenol sealer, Seal-Apex, a calcium hydroxide–based cement sealer (Kerr Sybron, Romulus, Mich.) and a new German calcium hydroxide sealer (base No. 081285 and catalyst No. 081385; Dentsply, Konstanz, West Germany) showed good sealing ability and biocompatibility.

Filling Techniques

Single-cone method

The single-cone method may be used when (1) the canal walls are reasonably parallel and the primary cone fits snugly in the apical third of the canal or (2) the canal is too wide and commercially available gutta-percha cones will not fit the canal adequately. A customized cone is then fashioned and fitted with the organic solvent technique.

Fabrication of a customized gutta-percha cone. Three or more gutta-percha cones are warmed together over a flame and are pressed and twisted together into a bundle (Fig. 9-22, *A* and *B*). The slightly warmed cones are rolled between two ster-

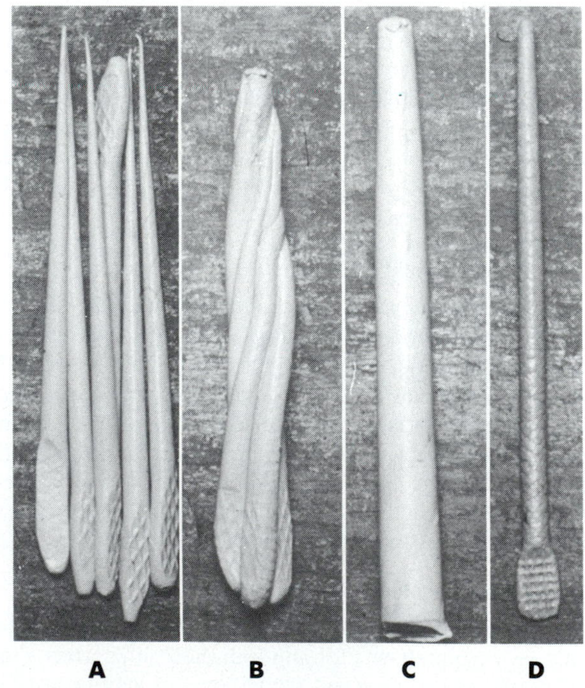

FIG. 9-22 Fabrication of a customized gutta-percha cone. **A** and **B,** Several gutta-percha points are warmed over a Bunsen burner and the tips are rolled together. **C,** Large fabricated cone. **D,** Largest-sized gutta-percha cone (no. 140) available commercially.

ile glass slabs held at an angle to make a cone with a diameter approximately the size of the canal (Fig. 9-22, *C*). If the angle of the slabs is too large for the canal, the cone is rewarmed and rerolled to a smaller diameter.

After the cone is allowed to cool and harden or is chilled with a spray of ethyl chloride, the apical end is softened superficially in a solvent. The softened cone is inserted with a few gentle pumping motions until it reaches the working length.

The customized cone is a replica of the internal shape of the canal (Fig. 9-23) and should be inserted in the same path and position when cemented.

When a customized cone is being cemented in the single-cone technique, it should be inserted very *slowly;* otherwise it will act as a plunger to force the cement sealer beyond the apical foramen (Fig. 9-24, *C*). Slow insertion of the customized cone will allow time for the cement to flow back coronally (Fig. 9-25). Often, the single-cone method leaves some space in the occlusal half of the canal not densely filled. Lateral condensation with the addition of several fine gutta-percha cones may at times be required to obtain a densely filled canal.

Lateral condensation method

The lateral condensation method is preferred to the single-cone method because most teeth present wide canals or flares that cannot be densely filled with a single gutta-percha or silver cone. Additional auxiliary cones inserted and condensed laterally around the primary cone can effectively fill irregularly shaped canals.

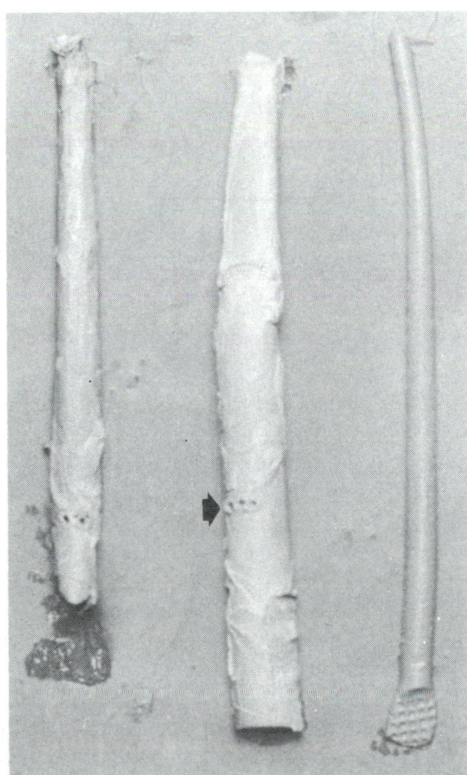

FIG. 9-23 *Left,* Customized, chloroform-fitted gutta-percha cone. *Center,* Dot marks *(arrow)* on the labial surface of the cone made by an explorer tip at the incisal edge to facilitate proper reinsertion at cementation time. *Right,* Largest-sized (no. 140) commercial cone for comparison.

However, overzealous lateral spreading to add more auxiliary cones, particularly with spreaders designed with too great a taper, may result in vertical root fractures.

To enhance the effectiveness and ease in canal obturation with the lateral condensation technique, Martin has designed a very efficient set of six color-coded, calibrated plugger-spreaders with both taper and size matching the ISO standardization of root canal files (L.D. Caulk/Dentsply). The calibrated instruments minimize the need to overflare the canal preparation to provide better access for condensing instruments to reach deeper into the apical area. One end of the instrument is a spreader, the other a plugger, thus allowing the operator to combine lateral and vertical condensation into one instrument procedure (Fig. 9-26). Length control is provided by markings on the shaft or by silicone rubber stops.

The lateral condensation technique, unlike the vertical compaction of warm gutta-percha, does not create the merging of the gutta-percha cones into a homogeneous mass. The added auxiliary cones are compressed laterally against each other and the canal walls. They tend to entrap undesirably large pools of cement-sealer in the filling mass. The lateral condensation tends to be concentrated more in the middle and occlusal third of the root canal space than in the apical third. Allison and colleagues[2] observed in vitro, "the group in which the spreader tip could be inserted to within 1 mm of the prepared length had considerably less microleakage than did the group in which the distance between the spreader tip and prepared length was great."

Innovative clinicians seek to improve this condition by designing spreaders that can reach very close to the apex. The use of finger pluggers (Figs. 9-30 and 9-31), the newly designed Martin set of spreader-pluggers (Fig. 9-26), the Endotec lateral heat condenser (L.D. Caulk Co./Dentsply, Milford, Del.; Fig. 9-37), and the Thermopact[96] (Degussa, France PB 125, 92203 Neuilly sur Seine; Fig. 9-40) are some of the more recent attempts to provide clinicians with instruments and devices to improve the compactness of gutta-percha in the apical third of the canal in order to obtain a denser and more effective three-dimensional seal of the root canal space (see Warm Lateral Condensation).

Wong and coworkers[117] in an in vitro study found that with lateral condensation the shape of a cast gold artificial root canal was replicated notably less well than with the warm gutta-percha vertical condensation, which placed a larger mass of gutta-percha into the canal. The mechanical compaction technique was judged better than lateral condensation in its ability to replicate the shape of the standard cast gold artificial root canal.

Lateral and vertical condensation method (Figs. 9-34 and 9-35)

The endodontic cavity should be designed and prepared specifically for the efficient use of gutta-percha cones as filling material. It should be so shaped that a continuously tapering funnel is created with the narrowest diameter at the dentin-cementum junction (about 0.5 to 1 mm from the radiographic apex) and the widest diameter at the access to the cavity. This constriction, with minimal apical opening, acts almost like a matrix, against which the mass of gutta-percha is forcibly condensed. The narrow apical opening at the dentin-cementum

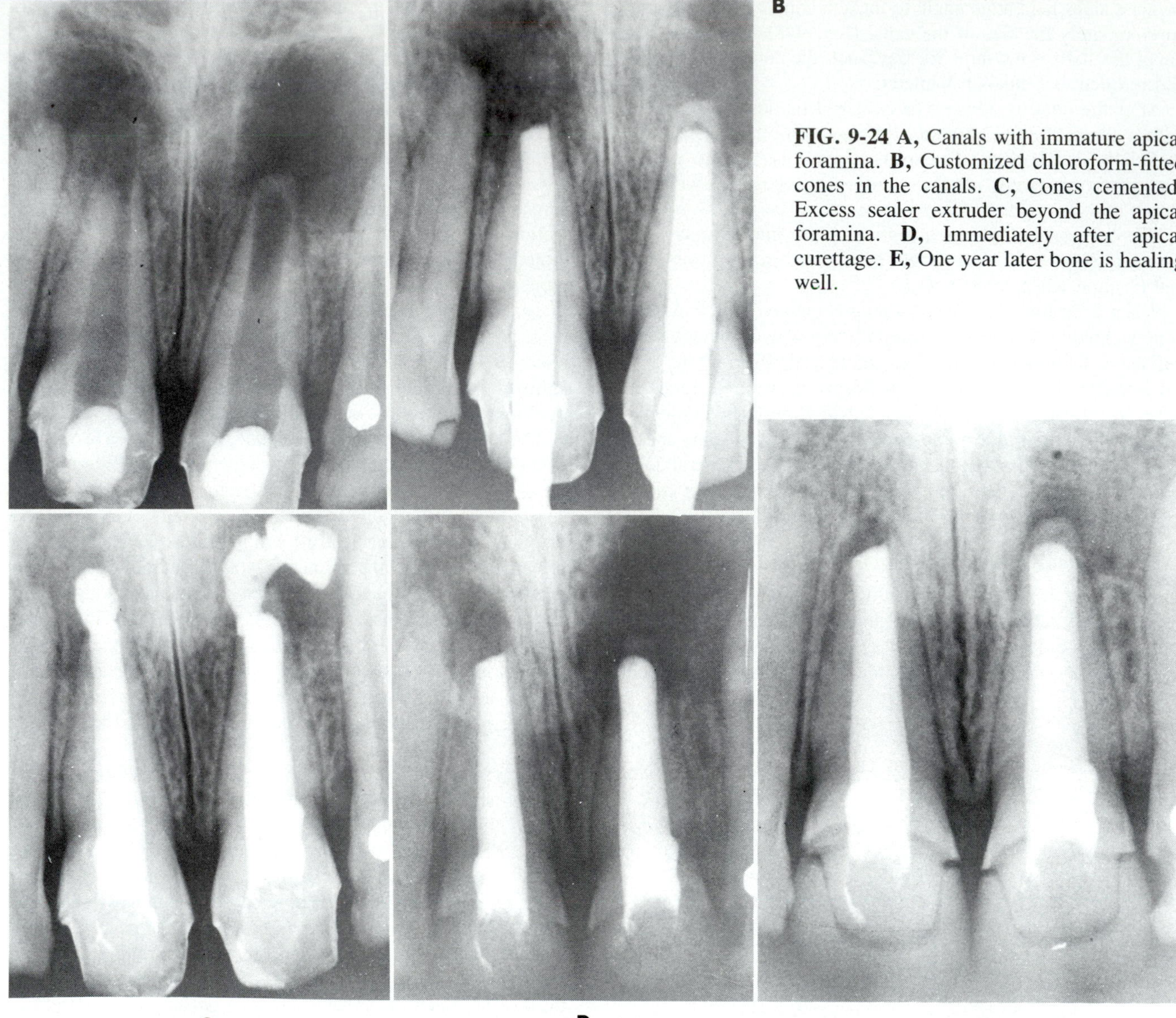

FIG. 9-24 A, Canals with immature apical foramina. **B,** Customized chloroform-fitted cones in the canals. **C,** Cones cemented. Excess sealer extruder beyond the apical foramina. **D,** Immediately after apical curettage. **E,** One year later bone is healing well.

junction prevents excess filling material from being forced beyond the apical foramen.

Overextension of files destroys the apical constriction by creating an apical "zip" and making it extremely difficult to prevent overextension of the filling material during the condensing process. The result is a poorly compacted filling with a doubtful apical seal. Invasion of periapical space by any filling material will cause periapical inflammation.

Preparation for obturation. The canal is sanitized again with irrigant solution as described in Chapter 7. With a no. 15 or 20 file the clinician rechecks the canal for patency to its full working length and to ascertain that there are no pulpal remnants or debris left at the apical terminus.

The tightly fitted primary cone with the apical tip 1 mm short of the radiographic apex is rechecked for correct fit, withdrawn, and placed into the 70% isopropyl alcohol.

To ensure the *removal of residual moisture* from the canal, it is necessary to dehydrate the canal walls before filling. This can be accomplished by flushing the canal with a solution of either 95% ethyl alcohol or 99% isopropyl alcohol placed in an irrigating syringe. To be effective, the alcohol should remain 2 to 3 minutes in the canal. The canal is then dried with sterile absorbent points inserted to a depth 1 mm short of the working length. An absorbent point is placed in the canal to absorb exudate until the clinician is ready to obturate.

Sterile spreaders and pluggers (Fig. 9-27) are prepared for lateral and vertical condensation. *Spreaders* are long, tapered, pointed instruments used to condense the filling material laterally against the canal walls, making room for insertion of additional auxiliary cones. *Pluggers,* or condensers, regardless of their width, have flat apical tips and are used to pack the gutta-percha mass vertically (Figs. 9-28 and 9-29). Like spreaders, pluggers come in different sizes, have depth markings on the shaft, and are either long- or shorthandled (Figs. 9-28 to 9-32).

Selection of pluggers. Three or four pluggers (Fig. 9-29) to be used in the coronal, middle, and apical thirds of the canal must be preselected to ensure loose fit. During the vertical

FIG. 9-25 **A,** Multiple absorbent points used to dry a large canal. **B** to **D,** Very slow insertion of a well-fitted customized cone, allowing ample time (1 to 2 minutes) for the sealer to flow out coronally.

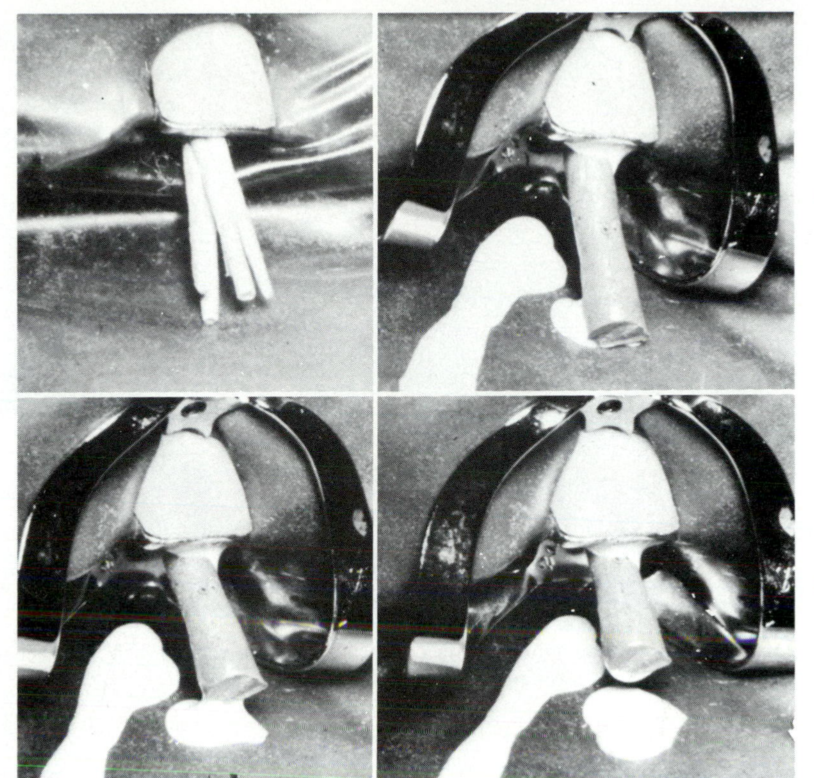

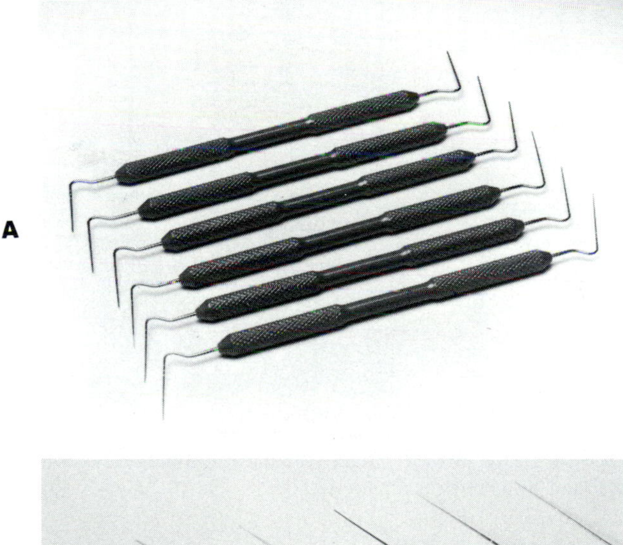

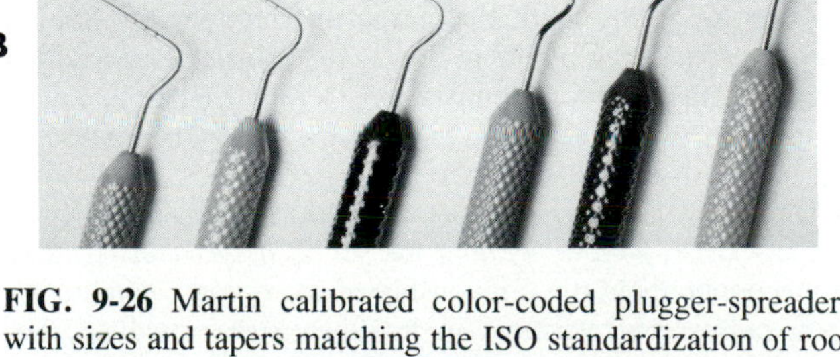

FIG. 9-26 Martin calibrated color-coded plugger-spreaders with sizes and tapers matching the ISO standardization of root canal files. **A,** Sizes no. 20, 25, 30, 40, 50, and 60. One end is a spreader for lateral condensation; the other end is a spreader for vertical condensation. **B,** Close-up of the spreaders' ends. (Courtesy Caulk/Dentsply, Milford, Del.)

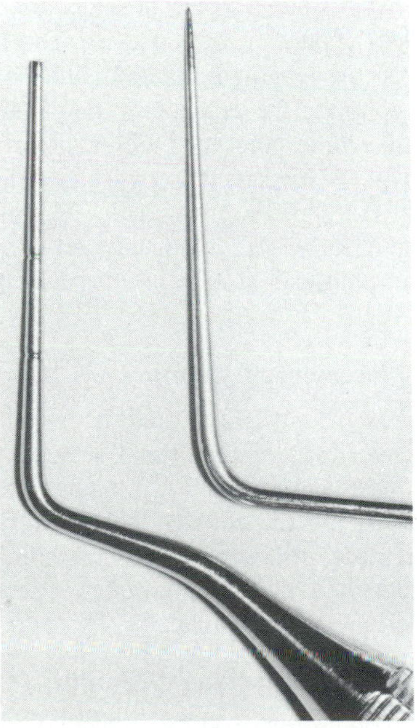

FIG. 9-27 *Left,* Root canal plugger with a flat tip and depth markings at 10 and 15 mm. *Right,* Spreader with a pointed tip.

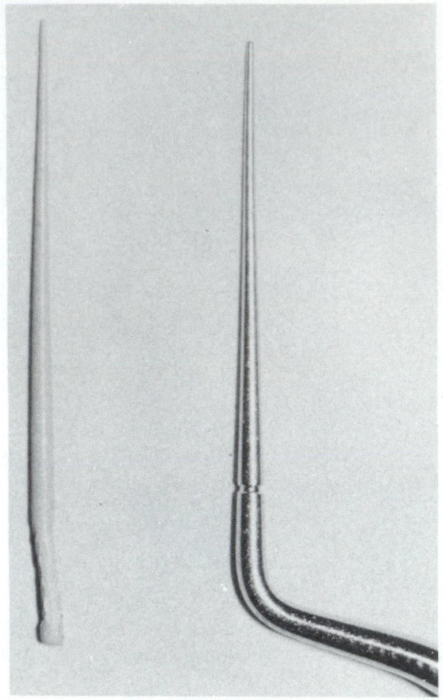

FIG. 9-28 *Left,* Fine gutta-percha cone (nonstandardized or regular type). *Right,* Fine plugger of similar size.

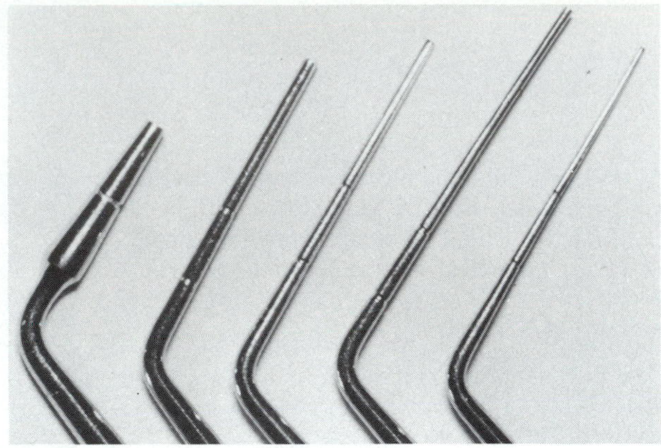

FIG. 9-29 University of California (Nguyen T. Nguyen) double-ended pluggers.

condensation phase the prefitted plugger will be compressing the gutta-percha mass apically, unimpeded by the walls of the canal.

Application of cement. The absorbent point is removed to check the moisture in the canal. If necessary the canal is dried again with additional absorbent points.

The cement is carried to the canal in small amounts on a sterile file one size smaller than the last instrument used for enlargement. If very small portions of sealer are carried in first, there will be less chance of trapping air. The file, set 1 mm short of the working length, is rotated *counterclockwise* as it is withdrawn, spinning the sealer into the canal; then a slow, gentle, pumping action, combined with a lateral rotary motion of the instrument, is used to thoroughly coat the canal walls and disperse air entrapped in the cement. The procedure is repeated until the canal walls are coated well with sealer.

An absorbent point can also be used to coat the canal walls with sealer.

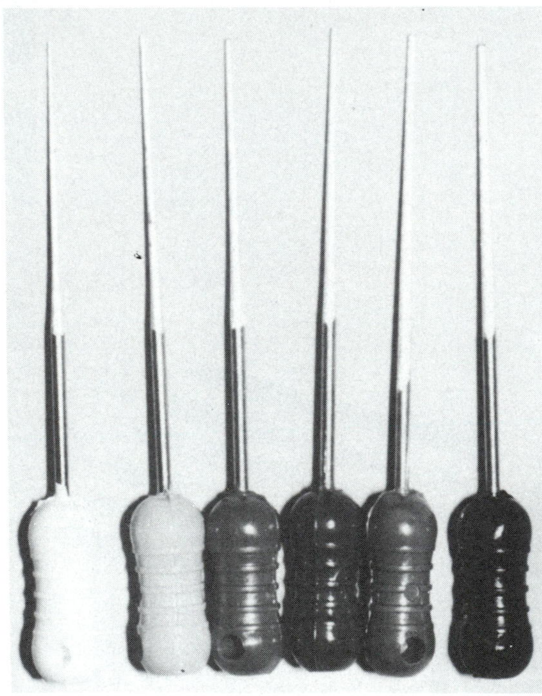

FIG. 9-30 Union Broach finger spreaders and pluggers, color-coded and mounted on plastic handles.

Ultrasonic placement of sealers

Several studies[45,66] have advocated the use of ultrasonic devices for the placement of root canal sealers. One recent in vitro study by West and associates,[115] using the mesial root of human mandibular molars, showed that the ultrasonic method of sealer placement, followed by lateral condensation with gutta-percha, resulted in more thorough coverage of canal walls than when the sealer was placed by hand instruments.

Lateral and vertical packing technique

The primary cone is removed from the alcohol and air dried. Its apical half is coated with sealer (Fig. 9-33, *B*) and inserted *slowly* and *gently* into the canal to the measured length (until the mark on the cone coincides with the incisal or occlusal edge; Fig. 9-33, *C*). Slow insertion of the cone permits the excess sealer to be dispersed toward the coronal end of the tooth (Fig. 9-25).

Note: When the tooth is not anesthetized, some sensation may be experienced by the patient as the cone is being inserted apically. This slight pain may be due to entrapped air that must be given time to be absorbed or to excess cement being pushed out beyond the apical foramen.

One or two auxiliary cones can be inserted alongside the primary cone, *with or without the use of a spreader*. If there is any doubt about the relationship of the primary cone to the apex, radiographic verification should be done immediately before more auxiliary cones are added with the aid of a spreader. If overextension occurs, usually because of improper apical preparation, the cones can be easily removed, the primary cone shortened, and the process repeated while the sealer is still

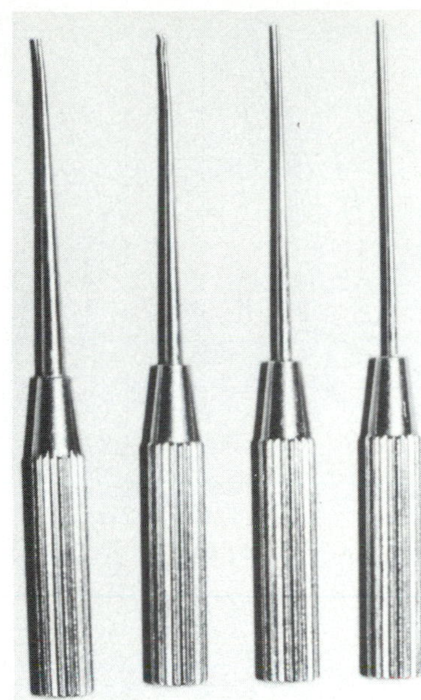

FIG. 9-31 Set of four Luks finger pluggers.

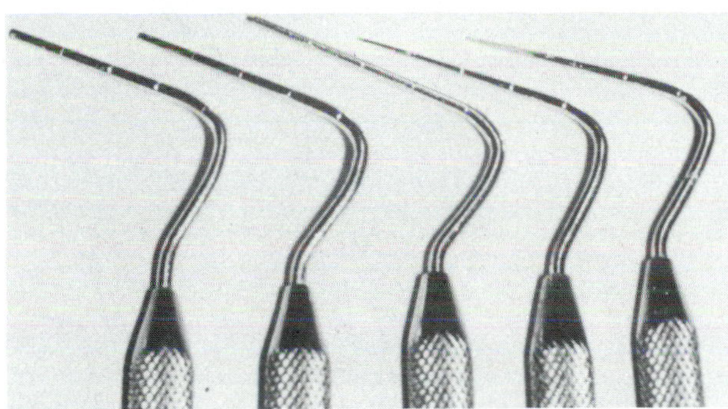

FIG. 9-32 Set of long-handled Kerr pluggers.

plastic. If the filling is short, the gutta-percha mass can be vertically packed farther apically.

A spreader is then inserted apically alongside the primary cone, wedging it against the canal wall and creating space for an additional cone. Lateral and apical pressure is applied by revolving the spreader through half an arc (Fig. 9-33, *D*).

The spreader is removed with one hand while a gutta-percha cone of corresponding size is inserted with the other hand in exactly the space just vacated by the spreader (Fig. 9-33, *E*).

Coating the auxiliary cone with sealer before insertion is optional. Some clinicians dip auxiliary cones into sealer or eucalyptol to give the cones sufficient lubrication to reach the space prepared for them.

The spreader is inserted again with apical pressure, making room for another cone. The spreading process is repeated several times until the wedged cones block further access to the canal (Figs. 9-33, *F*, and 9-34, *C*).

Vertical condensation is now combined with *lateral condensation* to obtain greater density and compactness and to force the filling material into the complex configuration and ramifications of the root canal system.

With the blade end of the spreader instrument heated *red-hot,* the butt ends of the cones are cut flush with the coronal opening (Fig. 9-33, *G*).

While the gutta-percha mass is still soft, because of the heat transmitted by the instrument, vertical compaction is done without delay. The gutta-percha mass is forcibly packed apically with a preselected *cold* plugger dipped into cement powder to prevent the still warm gutta-percha from sticking to it and being pulled out when the instrument is removed.

With a suitable-size plugger heated red-hot, the gutta-percha mass is removed to a level 3 or 4 mm beyond the canal orifice (Fig. 9-33, *H*). While the gutta-percha is still warm, a prefit smaller plugger is used with vertical pressure to condense it further apically (Fig. 9-33, *I*).

To be effective, the pluggers selected must fit loosely and work at all times within the gutta-percha mass, unimpeded by the walls of the canal. This vertical packing deep in the apical third of the canal forces the gutta-percha and sealer into the irregular configurations of the canal system and improves the chances of filling patent accessory canals and foramina (Fig. 9-33, *J*).

The whole canal is then filled by continuation of the spreading process followed by the insertion of auxiliary cones. When the spreader cannot be inserted more than 3 or 4 mm beyond the canal orifice, the spreading process is terminated (Fig. 9-33, *K*).

The protruding butt ends of the cones are removed with the blade end of the spreader instrument heated red-hot, and the gutta-percha mass is firmly condensed vertically (Fig. 9-33, *L, M*).

A radiograph is exposed to ascertain that there is an opaque, homogeneous filling to within 1 to 0.5 mm of the radiographic apex and that there are no radiolucent or fuzzy gray areas (voids) present in the canal. If the filling is short or shows voids, the gutta-percha mass is removed as far apically as needed with a red-hot plugger or a heat-carrier instrument. A smaller-width cold plugger is used to condense the softened gutta-percha apically. The process of vertical condensation combined with lateral condensation is repeated until the canal is filled to the desired height.

The filling procedure is completed as follows: When the canal is densely and completely filled, as verified by the radiograph, the coronal gutta-percha is removed to the canal orifice with a red-hot instrument. With a cold plugger the gutta-percha mass is condensed farther apically, forming a clean flat surface slightly below the cervical line (Fig. 9-33, *O*). The cement is cleaned from the pulp horns and the chamber wiped with alcohol or xylol (Fig. 9-33, *N*).

The crown is filled with a light shade of cement (the final restoration is placed at a later date). The rubber dam is now removed, the occlusion is checked, and two radiographs are exposed at different horizontal angles for future comparison.

If a *dowel* will be needed, the gutta-percha is removed a little deeper apically with a red-hot calibrated plugger or suitable rotating instruments, the chamber is packed with cotton pellets, and the access cavity is closed with a temporary cement. If circumstances allow, the dowel can also be made as soon as the root canal is sealed.

The combination of lateral and vertical condensation when used well can produce filling of great density and can effectively fill the complex root canal system three-dimensionally and in its entirety (Figs. 9-35 and 9-36).

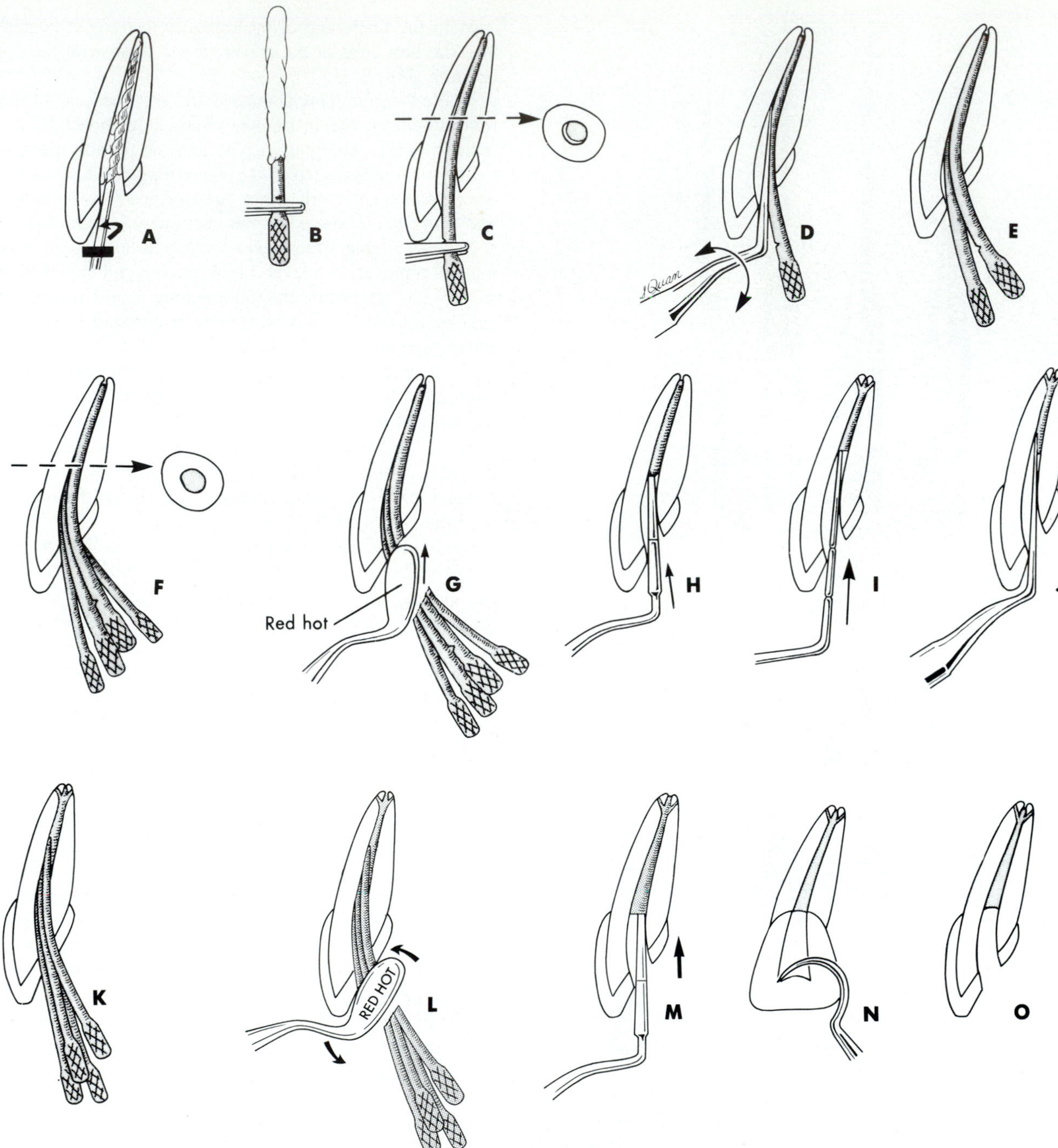

FIG. 9-33 Step-by-step procedure for lateral and vertical condensation. **A,** Cement carried into the canal with a reamer set 1 mm short of the working length. The file is rotated counterclockwise, spinning sealer into the canal. Note the constriction at the apex of the endodontic cavity preparation. **B,** Primary gutta-percha cone coated with cement sealer. **C,** Cone inserted into the canal until the mark on the cone coincides with the incisal edge. Arrow points to a cross section of the middle third of the canal. **D,** Spreading to create space for an additional cone. **E,** Auxiliary cone inserted into the space created by the spreader. **F,** Spreading process with several secondary cones added. Arrow points to a cross section of the middle third of the canal. **G,** Butt ends of the cones removed with a hot instrument. **H,** Vertical condensation packing the still-warm gutta-percha mass apically. **I,** After removal of the gutta-percha to the apical third of the canal, prefitted pluggers are used to vertically pack the gutta-percha mass farther apically. **J** and **K,** Continuation of spreading and cone addition until the remainder of the canal is densely filled. **L,** Butt ends of the additional accessory cones removed with an instrument heated red hot. **M,** The still-warm plasticized gutta-percha mass is packed vertically with a prefitted cold plugger to the canal orifice's level. **N,** Filling materials removed from the pulp chamber and pulpal horns. **O,** Final fill after condensation.

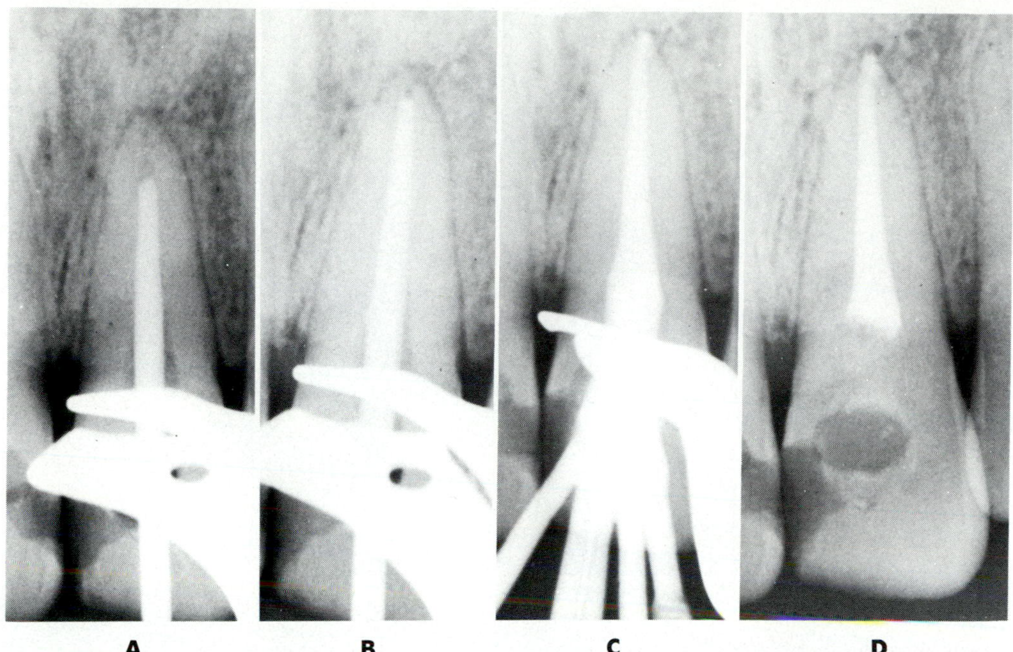

FIG. 9-34 Lateral and vertical condensation. **A,** Selected primary cone too short. **B,** Correct apical fit obtained by using the same cone dipped a few seconds into a solvent and reinserted to the working length. **C,** Cone cemented with several secondary cones inserted between the primary cone and the canal wall. **D,** Completed canal obturation after lateral and vertical condensation has been carried out.

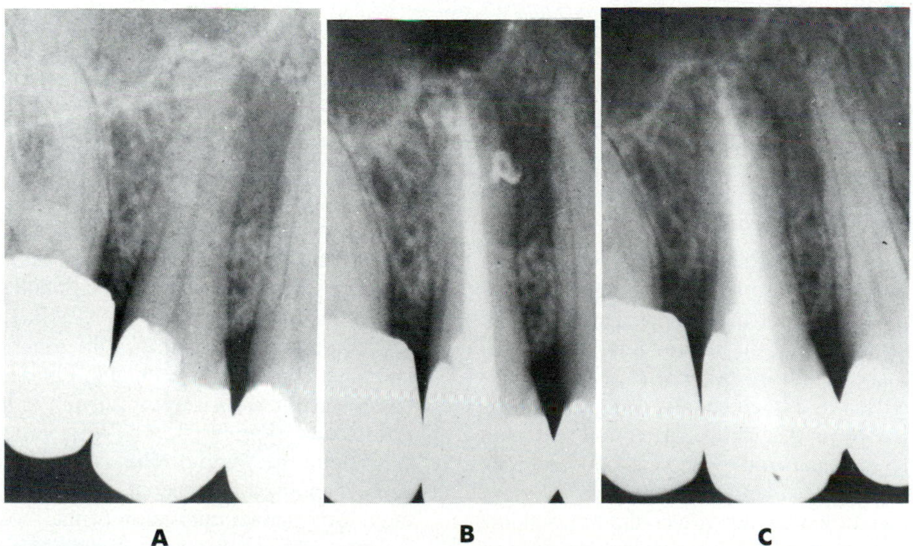

FIG. 9-35 Maxillary second premolar. **A,** Pretreatment. There is a possibility of lateral canals because of the unusual location of the radiolucency along the mesial aspect of the root. **B,** Canal filled by the lateral and vertical condensation method. Note the complex foramina and lateral canals. **C,** Two years later, complete osseous repair.

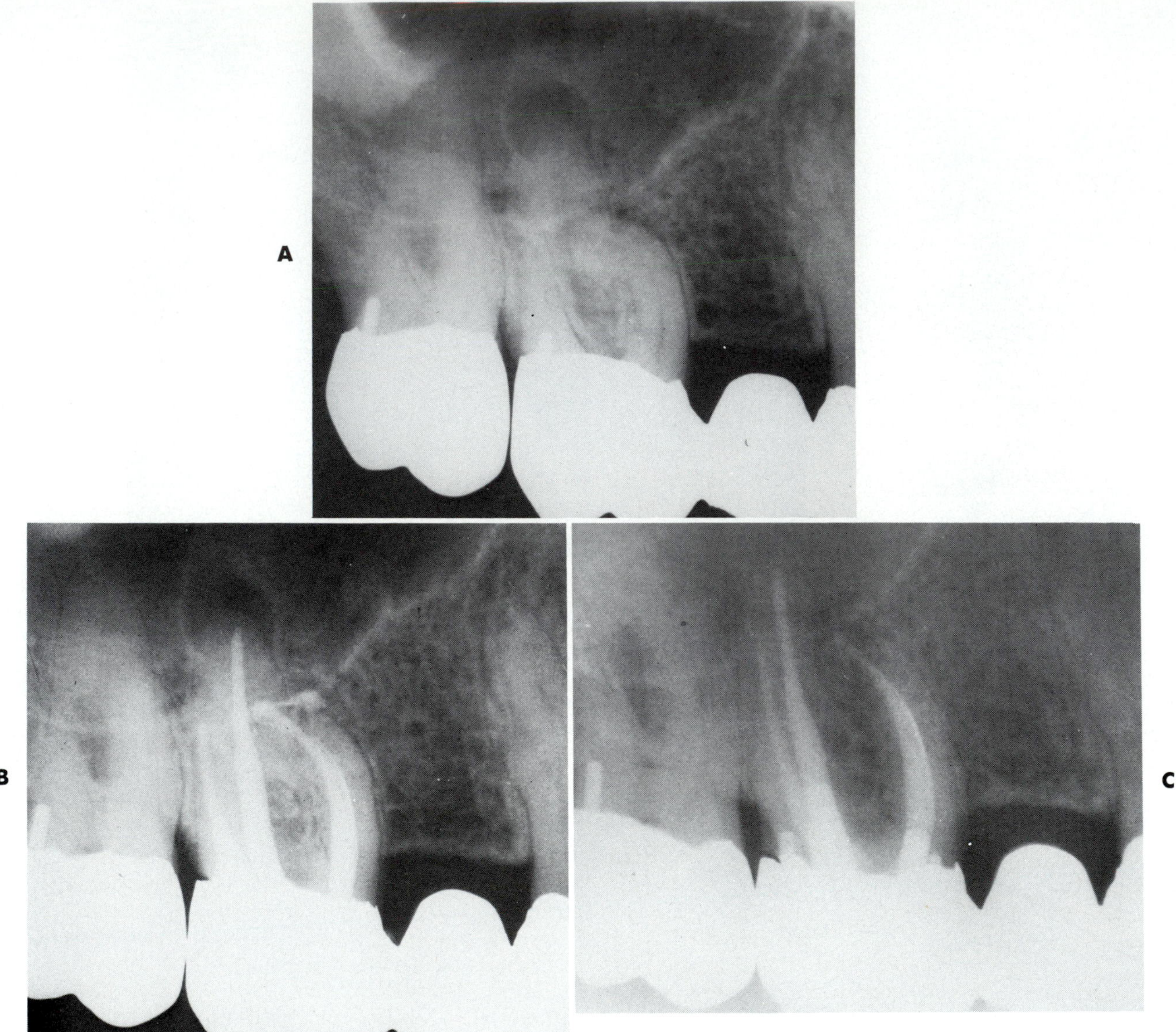

FIG. 9-36 Maxillary first molar. **A,** Bridge abutment with chronic apical periodontitis and a sinus tract. **B,** Canal filled with gutta-percha by lateral and vertical condensation. **C,** Eighteen months later, good healing.

Warm lateral condensation technique

Martin developed a cordless, rechargeable, battery-operated gutta-percha heat condenser for use in warm lateral condensation. The device, known as Endotec, is adapted with a small tip which is equal in size to a no. 30 file and a large tip equal to a size no. 45 file. The small tip, because of its flexibility, is capable of condensation in curved canals. The heat is thermostatically controlled by a mechanical activator button to soften the gutta-percha at a temperature between 600° and 650° F (315.5° C and 343.9° C). Although two studies[40,68] have shown that this temperature will not affect the surrounding periodontium, the effect of this high heat on the integrity of the gutta-percha must be taken into consideration. Gutta-percha is known to undergo partial decomposition at temperatures above 100° C.

The technique follows the lateral condensation procedure and can produce a three-dimensional filling superior to that obtained with the usual cold lateral condensation.[60a]

A significant advantage of the Endotec (Fig. 9-37) warm lateral condensation technique is its ability to soften and coalesce several gutta-percha points in the canal. In the traditional cold lateral condensation technique, the gutta-percha points are merely laminated together, leaving possible voids for potential leakage (Fig. 9-38, *A*). With Endotec warm lateral condensation, the gutta-percha is fused and compacted into a denser, more homogeneous mass (Fig. 9-38, *B*), creating a three-dimensional obturation of the root canal space. No special type of gutta-percha is required for use with the Endotec.

After the canal is coated with sealer and the master cone is placed to proper depth, the Martin heat condensor tip is introduced into the canal alongside the gutta-percha cone as with an ordinary spreader. A rubber stop marker can be used for

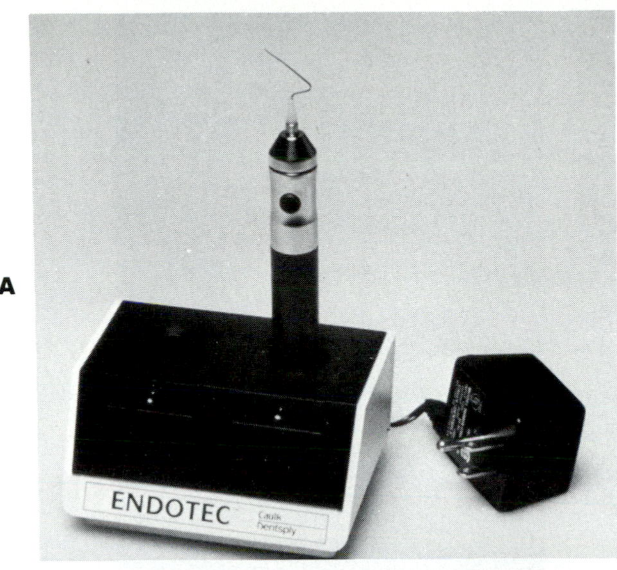

A

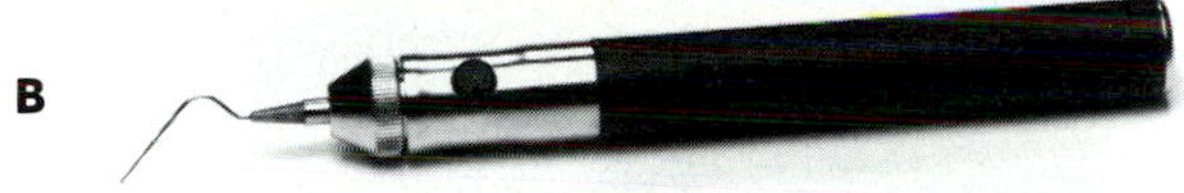

B

FIG. 9-37 Endotec warm lateral condensation. **A,** Endotec device in recharger. **B,** Endotec gutta-percha heat condenser showing mechanical activator button. (Courtesy Caulk/Dentsply, Milford, Del.)

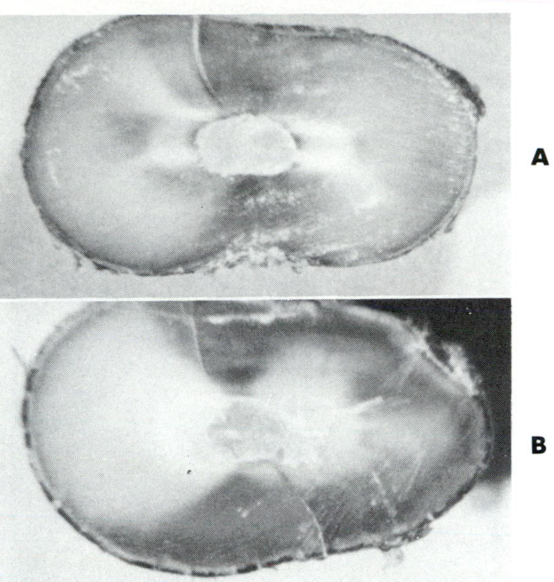

A

B

FIG. 9-38 Leakage study with methylene blue dye. **A,** Cold lateral condensation at 5 mm level shows dye penetration. **B,** Warm lateral condensation at 5 mm level shows no dye leakage. (Courtesy Dr. H. Martin.)

depth control to correlate with the canal length. The activator switch is then depressed, causing the tip of the instrument to become warm within 2 seconds. The heat condenser is gently forced apically and laterally into the canal with a rotary penetrating motion, causing the gutta-percha to spread laterally and apically for more complete obturation of the canal space. The heat condenser is then gently withdrawn, and an auxiliary cone is inserted in the space just created by the condenser tip. The same procedure is repeated—adding, spreading, and condensing several gutta-percha cones until the canal is compactly filled.

Since the gutta-percha mass has been softened by the heat condenser, little exertion is required to spread and condense the material apically and laterally. It has been shown in trial use that three or four more gutta-percha cones can be added when the heat condenser is used, as compared with the regular lateral condensation technique. If strong pressure is desired, the normal plugger or spreader may be used to compact the thermoplasticized gutta-percha. Leakage studies[69,70] with methylene blue dye (Fig. 9-38) showed that warm lateral condensation is superior to cold lateral condensation in preventing apical dye penetration. Another study,[73] using a leakage model in vitro, reported that the Endotec warm lateral condensation has the least leakage, compared with Ultrafil and lateral condensation. The forces required to condense adequately the thermosoftened gutta-percha are less stressful with the Endotec condenser than those used in cold lateral condensation, as demonstrated by photoelastic stress studies.[67] This would lessen the chance of vertical root fractures.

Thermopact

A new efficient heating device for use in either the lateral or vertical warm gutta-percha condensation technique was described by Sauveur.[96] The Thermopact (Degussa, France PB 125-223 Neuilly Sur Seine; Fig. 9-39) consists of a unit containing a transformer and an electronically controlled circuit for heat generation and control, and a handpiece adapted with different-sized spreaders and a heat carrier. The temperature can be selected, regulated, and maintained at any desired level from 40° C to 70° C.

When heated, gutta-percha cones can be transformed from beta phase (solid form) to alpha phase (plasticized form) at temperatures ranging from 42° C to 49° C. This difference in temperature is due to the difference in formulation by the various manufacturers of gutta-percha cones. When the temperature goes from 53° C to 59° C, the gutta-percha is transformed from alpha phase to the amorphic phase, with some changes in structural and physical properties.

Sauveur[96] observed that chemicals accord great importance on the effect of temperature on the structure of gutta-percha, whereas clinicians, when performing endodontic treatment, seem rather oblivious of the amount of heat to which the gutta-percha is subjected. When gutta-percha burns under high temperature, it looses its organic matrix and homogeneity. The remaining material consists of a white powder of zinc oxide, its principal component. He therefore suggested that when one is using the Thermopact device, the operating temperature should be set precisely and maintained constant. It should range within the limits of the gutta-percha going from beta (or solid) phase to alpha (or plasticized) phase, at approximately 42° C; or from the alpha plasticized phase to the amorphic phase, where partial decomposition begins to occur, approximately at 60° C. The Thermopact should therefore be ideally set and maintained at 42° C for warm lateral condensation, and at about 59° C for warm vertical compaction.

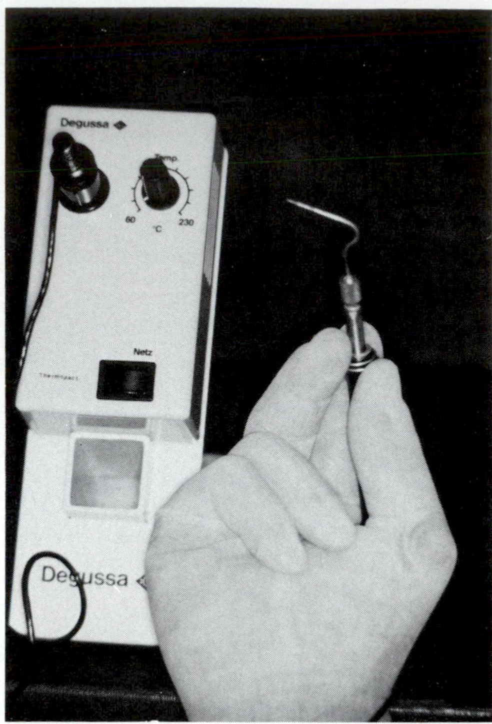

FIG. 9-39 The Thermopact device for use in warm lateral condensation or in warm vertical compaction. The temperature can be set electronically and maintained precisely at 42° C for warm lateral condensation, and at 59° C for vertical compaction to prevent overheating and possible decomposition of the gutta-percha. (Courtesy Dr. G. Sauveur, Paris, France.)

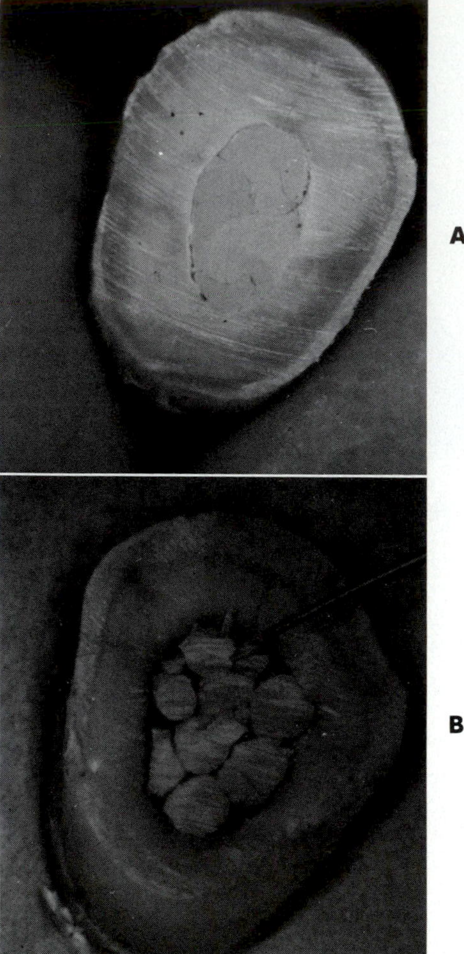

FIG. 9-40 Lateral condensation techniques. **A,** Warm lateral condensation with the Thermopact, no sealer used, showing compactness of gutta-percha mass. **B,** Cold lateral condensation, no sealer used, showing significant spaces between gutta-percha cones. (Courtesy Dr. G. Sauveur, Paris, France.)

With the Thermopact device set and maintained at 42° C, *warm lateral condensation* is carried out in a manner similar to the traditional cold lateral condensation method. The difference is that the warm spreaders soften and depress the gutta-percha laterally, allowing the instruments to gently and deeply penetrate to the desired apical level. Therefore more gutta-percha cones can be added successively in the space created by the warm spreader and coalesced into a denser mass. The technique produces a homogeneously compacted filling with accurate control of apical extrusion, maximal gutta-percha, and minimal sealer (Fig. 9-40).

Regular spreaders may be also heated and stocked in a glass bead container with temperature set to 60° C. When inserted into the root canal, the spreader would have a temperature of around 45° C. This temperature is sufficient to heat the gutta-percha from beta solid phase to alpha plasticized phase, allowing for a more effective lateral condensation. Dipping the heated spreader in silicone oil will prevent gutta-percha from sticking to it upon withdrawal.

When the *warm gutta-percha vertical compaction method* is used, the Thermopact device is adapted with a heat carrier. The temperature is set and maintained at 60° C. This temperature is sufficient to heat the gutta-percha from beta solid phase through alpha plasticized phase to the amorphic phase. The softened warm gutta-percha can be readily compacted apically into the irregularities of the root canal system.

Marciano and Michailesco,[64] in their differential scanning calorimetry study of gutta-percha, reported that heat carriers heated over a flame can reach an average temperature of 321.2° C. They can transmit a mean temperature of 140.7° C to the surface gutta-percha, giving rise to the partial decomposition of the gutta-percha which is known to occur with temperatures above 100° C. Since gutta-percha can be plasticized at temperatures ranging from 40° C to 60° C, the authors cited above suggested that new devices used to plasticize gutta-percha be designed with these data in consideration.

Warm lateral condensation can effectively provide a denser, more compact obturation with a maximum amount of gutta-percha and a minimum amount of sealer (Figs. 8-52, *A*, 9-38). The minimal condensing pressure used to obtain a compact and accurate filling is a decided advantage in the prevention of root fractures.

Sectional method

The sectional method varies slightly with different clinicians; but in essence, it consists of filling the canal with sections of gutta-percha 3 to 4 mm in length (Fig. 9-41).

A plugger is selected, and a suitable marker is engaged on the instrument for length control. The plugger is introduced into the canal so it will reach a point 3 or 4 mm from the apex.

A gutta-percha cone approximately the size of the canal is

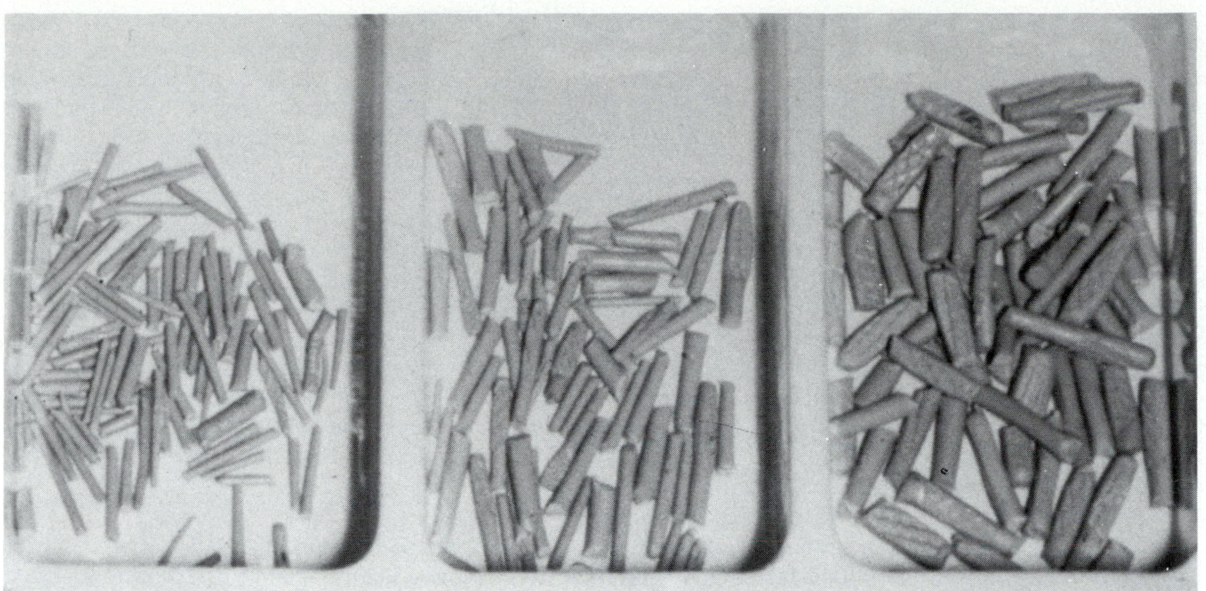

FIG. 9-41 Precut sections of gutta-percha, of different diameters, for use in the sectional method.

fitted a few millimeters short of the apex and cut in 3- to 4-mm sections.

After the end of the plugger is warmed over the Bunsen burner, the apical section of gutta-percha is tacked to it. The section of gutta-percha is dipped into eucalyptol and then carried to the apical foramen. Some clinicians coat the canal walls with a thin layer of sealer before inserting the gutta-percha. *Moving the plugger back and forth through a lateral arc will cause it to release from the section of gutta-percha.*

A radiograph is exposed to verify the position of the cone. If the cone is short, the next smaller plugger, with a rubber band marker for length control, may be used to pack the cone farther apically.

Additional sections of gutta-percha are inserted to fill the canal completely. If the need for a dowel is contemplated, the filling process may be stopped after the condensation of several sections of gutta-percha.

This technique is useful in filling tube-type canals or severely curved canals but requires very precise length control by the clinician. If too much pressure is used, the apical section of gutta-percha may be forced into the periapical space or vertical root fracture may result.

Three-dimensional obturation: the rationale and application of warm gutta-percha with vertical condensation

Clifford J. Ruddle

CURRENT OBTURATION TECHNIQUES

Dramatic improvements in endodontic therapy have occurred on multiple fronts. Perhaps the most intriguing advancement for many dentists is observing obturation potentials of various techniques. Justifiably, practitioners are constantly searching for obturation techniques that are safe, predictable, expeditious, easily reversible, *and* three dimensional (Fig. 9-43, Part 2).

Certain obturation techniques currently receiving significant marketing campaigns fail to address the importance of canal preparation and have evolved as "simplified" attempts to obturate underprepared and, hence, uncleaned—canals.[15] Some of these obturation techniques are potentially more three-dimensional than the older time-honored lateral condensation technique. On the other hand, many of these so-called three-dimensional obturation techniques have distinct clinical disadvantages such as lack of control, dimensional instability, inconsistency, lack of ready reversibility, and alteration of physical properties of gutta-percha resulting in greater leakage. Clinicians must be discouraged from selecting obturation techniques, designed around inadequate canal preparation, that create needless complications to nonexistent problems.

PHYSICAL PROPERTIES OF GUTTA-PERCHA

The well-understood physical and thermomolecular properties of gutta-percha are described in Chapter 13.* Gutta-percha is a long-chain hydrocarbon and is an isoprene unit of naturally obtained rubber. When heated, thermal conductivity through gutta-percha occurs over a limited range of 4 to 5 mm. Therefore, vertical condensation and effective adaptation of thermosoftened gutta-percha can only occur over a range of 4 to 5 mm. Gutta-percha need be heated only 3° C to 8° C above body temperature (to 40° C to 45° C) to become sufficiently moldable so that it can be easily compacted into the infinite geometric configurations of the root canal system. Repeated gutta-percha heatings slowly increases and progressively transfers heat through the length of the gutta-percha master cone, transforming it from a semirigid to a moldable state. Vertically condensing gutta-percha as it cools slightly from a maximum of 45° C to body temperature at 37° C produces an optimally adapted and dimensionally stable material. To consis-

*References 30, 31, 35, 65, 98.

tently meet these obturation objectives any syringeable gutta-percha technique must include intermittent vertical compactions of injected thermosoftened gutta-percha every 4 to 5 mm to insure canal adaptation *and* to discourage shrinkage and loss of volume.

ARMAMENTARIUM

Pluggers

Caulk Dental Company (Milford, Del.) manufactures a set of Schilder pluggers utilized to pack thermosoftened gutta-percha into the root canal system (Fig. 9-42). There are nine instruments in the set, and the series ranges from the smallest plugger size 8, and increases by half sizes, 8½, 9, 9½, . . ., to the largest plugger size 12. The size 8 plugger is 0.4 mm in diameter at its working end, 8½ (0.5 mm), . . ., and so on. The posterior set of pluggers as they are designed can easily be used in all teeth and give the clinician about 23 mm of working length. Additionally, the pluggers have reference lines at 5-mm intervals, enabling the clinician to know the depth of the plugger in the root canal system at all times. Rubber stops can be placed on the pluggers to further orientate the clinician as to the desired depth of placement and their safe use. Generally, three pluggers are used for any one root canal preparation, selecting pluggers whose diameter is just slightly less than that of the canal preparation at any given level. The largest-diameter plugger must work passively, unimpeded by dentinal walls over a range of a few millimeters in the coronal one third (Color Plate 1, *A*), a smaller-diameter plugger is chosen that can work passively but effectively in the middle third (Color Plate 1, *B*), and a smallest plugger is selected that can work easily to within 4 to 5 mm from the canal terminus (Color Plate 1, *C*). The pluggers selected must be prefit before packing so that the clinician knows with confidence that when a plugger meets resistance, it is on a cushion of thermosoftened gutta-percha and *not* on unyielding dentinal walls.

Heat Source

Analytic Technology (Redmond, Wash.) has developed several heating units designed to thermosoften gutta-percha (Fig. 9-43, Part 1, *A*). The author prefers the 5004 unit for a variety of reasons. This small and highly efficient unit can be set at the desired temperature and the clinician can activate the heat carrier by merely touching a designated area on the probe. Almost instantly the carrier becomes red-hot, transferring heat into the gutta-percha. If the 5004 Touch 'n Heat unit is used correctly, the temperature imparted into the gutta-percha cannot exceed 45° C, insuring a stable beta phase gutta-percha. Because of the thermomolecular properties of gutta-percha, heat is transferred about 4 to 5 mm apically along the master cone from the point of heat contact.[31,65] Thermosoftened gutta-percha has compaction potential; and vertical condensation is employed to achieve three-dimensional obturation (Fig. 9-43, Part 2, *B*).

Gutta-Percha Gun

As discussed shortly, following the down-packing and corking of the apical third, the most efficient way to back-pack the root canal system is to use the Obtura II gutta-percha gun made by Texceed (Costa Mesa, Calif.) (Fig. 9-53). This well-designed and well-engineered gun allows the clinician to select the appropriate gauge size and safely squeeze off uniformly heated aliquots of gutta-percha against the previously corked apex. These thermosoftened segments are readily compacted into the root canal system in an apical to coronal direction.

CONE FIT

After optimal canal preparation and appropriate drying techniques a nonstandardized cone of gutta-percha is selected of a size that closely resembles the dimension of the cleaned and shaped canal. The greater taper of these master cones, as compared to the standardized gutta-percha, ensures more effective

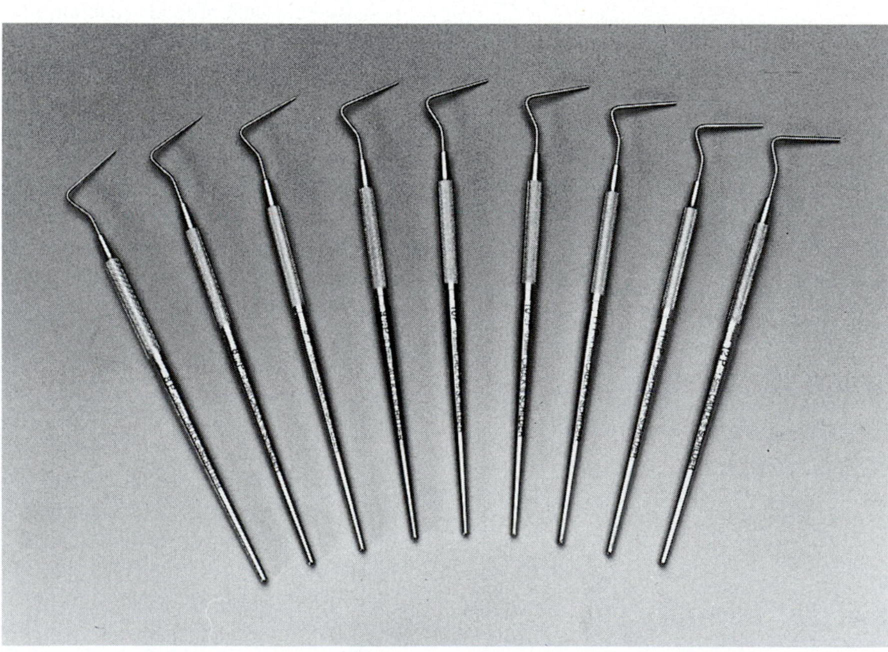

FIG. 9-42 Armamentarium for vertical condensation of warm gutta-percha. Assembled are a graded series of posterior root canal pluggers.

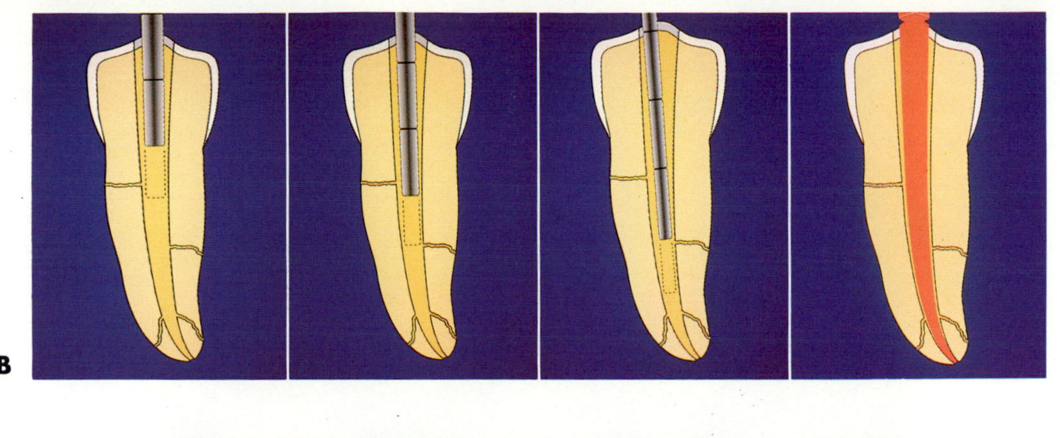

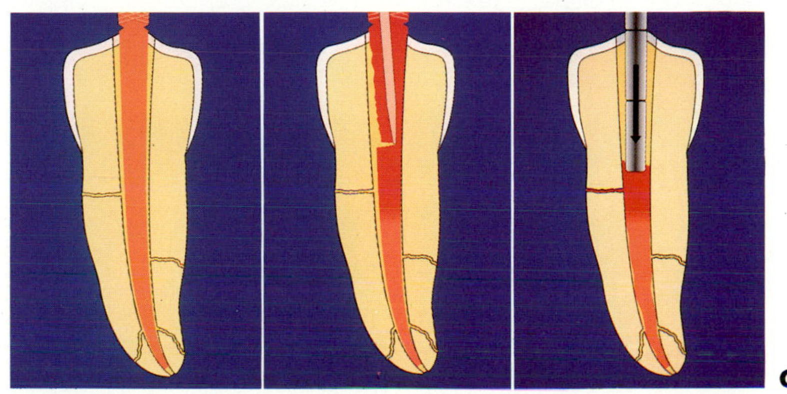

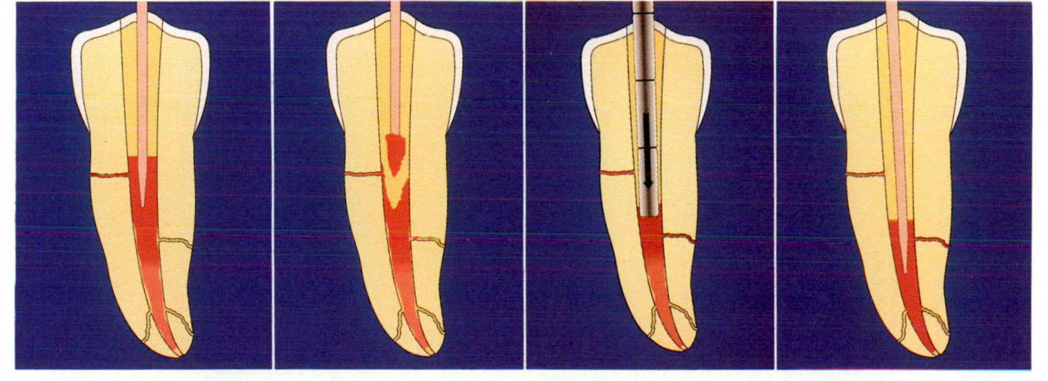

COLOR PLATE 1 A, A large size plugger is selected that will work passively and effectively over a range of a few millimeters in the coronal third. **B**, A smaller plugger is selected that will work passively and effectively over a range of few millimeters in the middle third. **C**, The smallest size plugger is selected that will work passively and effectively over a range of a few millimeters to within 4 to 5 mm of the canal terminus. **D**, A nonstandardized gutta-percha master cone is selected and adjusted so it is loose in the coronal and the middle third, fits to the canal terminus, and is snug in its apical extent. **E**, The master cone is trimmed back appropriately from the canal terminus or consistent most apical drying point. **F**, The heat carrier is activated and the useless portion of the master cone is seared off with the tip of the carrier at the level of the CEJ in single-rooted teeth. Note the limited transfer of heat through the gutta-percha. **G**, The large prefit plugger generates the first wave of condensation and compacts warm gutta-percha vertically and automatically laterally into the root canal system. **H**, The activated heat carrier becomes red-hot almost instantly and is allowed to plunge about 3 to 4 mm into the gutta-percha coronally. Note the progressive apical transfer of heat through the gutta-percha master cone. **I**, The heat carrier is deactivated and, after momentary hesitation, the cooling instrument is removed along with a bite of gutta-percha. **J**, A smaller prefit plugger captures the maximum cushion of rubber and carries a wave of warm gutta-percha into the narrowing cross-sectional diameters of the preparation. This second wave of condensation fills the system three dimensionally over a range of 4 to 5 mm. **K**, The heat carrier is activated, plunges another 3 to 4 mm into the gutta-percha, and carries a heat wave through the gutta-percha to its terminus.

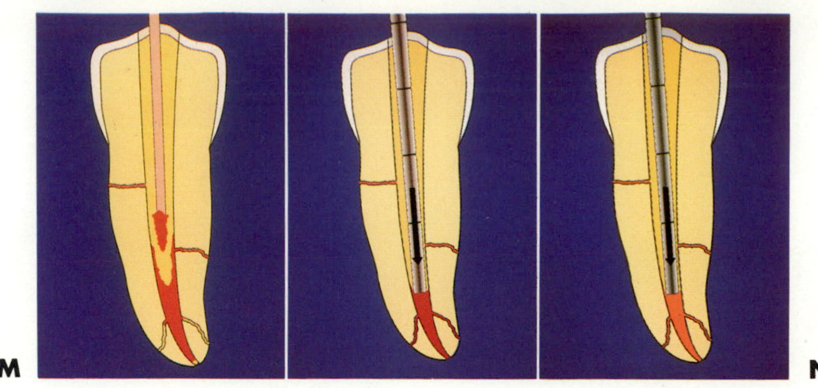

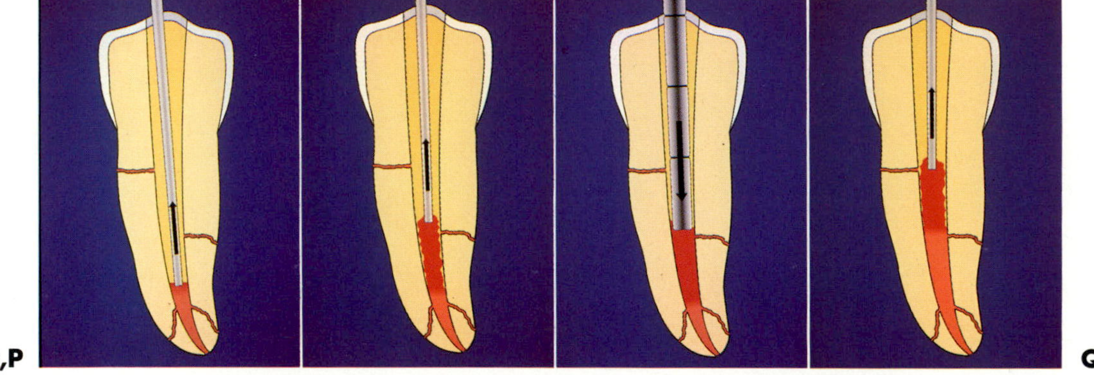

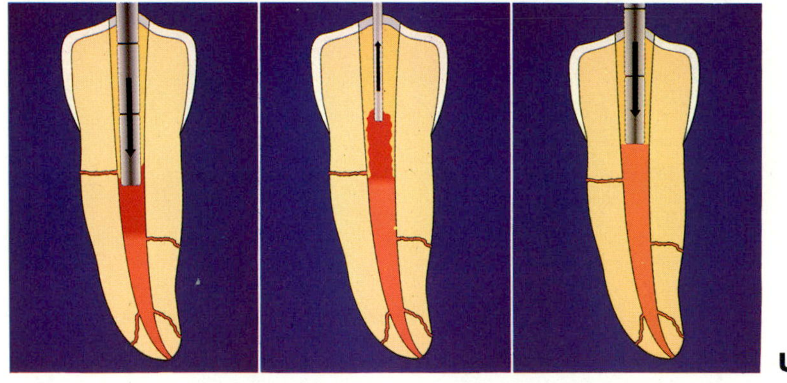

COLOR PLATE 1, cont'd. L, Removing another "bite" of gutta-percha allows for deeper plugger placement and action. **M**, The smallest prefit plugger effectively creates the final wave of condensation and delivers warm gutta-percha into multiple portals of exit, resulting in apical corkage. **N**, Continuous condensation as the gutta-percha cools to 37° C produces an optimally adapted and dimensionally stable material. **O**, Initially the hot needle of the Obtura II gutta-percha gun is placed against, and resoftens, the gutta-percha coronally. **P**, Holding the gutta-percha gun lightly and syringing easily allows the gun to back out of the canal while injecting a uniformly heated 4 to 5 mm segment of warm gutta-percha. **Q**, A prefit plugger three dimensionally packs thermosoftened gutta-percha, generating a reverse wave of condensation. Stepping the plugger circumferentially around the canal preparation while using short firm strokes eliminates space and ensures a dense solid core of gutta-percha. **R**, Injection of another uniformly heated aliquot of gutta-percha. Again, the needle is placed against the previously packed gutta-percha apically and, while injecting, the gun will back out of the canal. **S**, A larger prefit plugger generates another reverse wave of condensation three dimensionally, filling the canal with warm gutta-percha laterally and in depth over a range of 4 to 5 mm. **T**, Reheating the coronal aspect of the gutta-percha core and injecting the final aliquot of thermosoftened gutta-percha. **U**, The largest prefit plugger delivers the thermosoftened gutta-percha three dimensionally against the walls of the preparation, completing the back-packing phase.

obturation, as we will see subsequently. Generally, a "medium" nonstandardized master cone is selected and fitted so that the rate of taper of the master cone is less than but parallels the rate of taper of the prepared canal; the master cone can be inserted to full working length, not further, and upon removal exhibits apical tug-back (Color Plate 1, *D*). Master cones can be further customized by heat, glass slabs, or cold rolling with a spatula. A diagnostic film confirms the master cone's position and all the operative steps to date. Before packing, the master cone is cut back about 0.5 mm from the canal terminus or consistent drying point (Color Plate 1, *E*). In irregularly shaped orifices/canals a supplemental point typically of size fine-medium or medium should be placed lateral to the master cone to enhance compaction. It is simple to fit a master cone into a well-prepared canal and, when properly performed, this ensures that obturation is controlled, complete, and quick.

SEALER

Kerr pulp canal sealer (Romulus, Mich.) is the sealer of choice for this technique because of:

1. flow, lubrication, and viscosity;
2. biocompatability,
3. virtual nonresorbability,
4. quick setting time, and
5. prostaglandin inhibition. (Zinc oxide and eugenol combine to form zinc eugenate, a prostaglandin inhibitor. Prostaglandins are known pain mediators.)

Kerr pulp canal sealer completely sets and is essentially inert within 15 to 30 minutes, thus significantly reducing the inflammatory responses noted with sealers that take 24 to 36 hours to set fully. The amount of sealer used in the warm gutta-percha with vertical condensation technique is minimal in that only a thin film will occupy the dentin/gutta-percha interface. A thin sealer film has been shown to be significantly less pre-

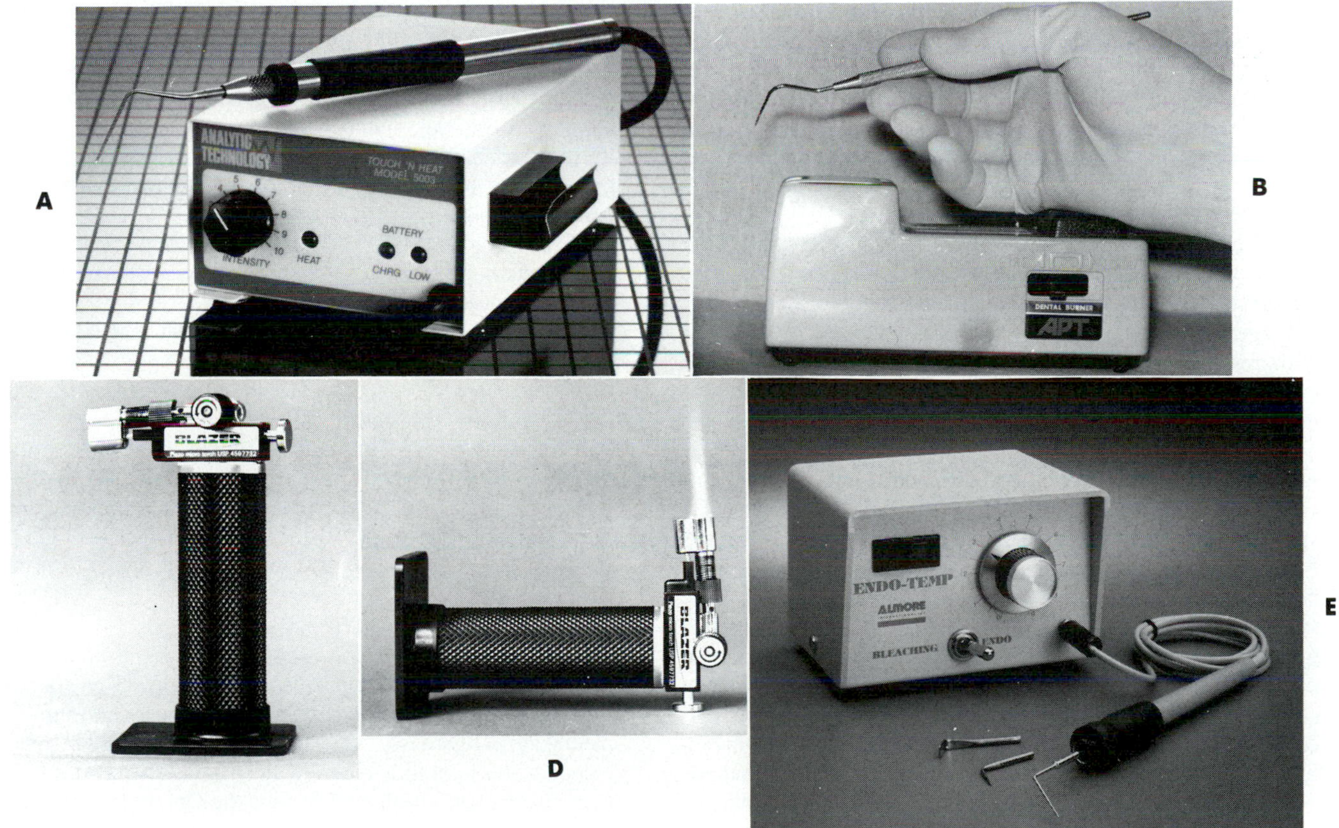

FIG. 9-43 (Part 1) Heating devices for warm gutta-percha compaction technique. **A,** Touch 'n Heat portable battery-powered (rechargeable) heating device, model no. 5004. Instrument tip will heat to glowing within seconds, ready for use in softened gutta-percha techniques. The device may also be used for hot pulp testing or bleaching by changing the tips and adjusting the heat level. (Courtesy Analytic Technology, Redmont, Wash.) **B,** Portable chairside butane gas burner APT. A convenient and effective heat source (Phoenix Dent Co., Ltd., Tokyo, Japan). **C,** Piezo-Micro refillable butane torch, an excellent open flame source with electronic ignition for trigger-quick flame, **D,** The Piezo-Micro torch is more stable when laid horizontally during use (Blazer Products, New York). **E,** Endo-Temp self-heating unit for use in warm gutta-percha techniques (Endo-mode) or for bleaching (bleaching mode) and preparation of post space. (Courtesy Almore International, Portland, Ore.)

disposed to washing out.[14] Most obturation techniques must rely on sealer pools to initially fill the space between the gutta-percha cones and the *gutta-percha–dentin* interface, but over time these lakes of cement more readily undergo dissolution and shrinkage.

SEALER AND MASTER CONE PLACEMENT

The amount of Kerr pulp canal sealer used is typically one small bead of cement carried into the carefully dried canal preparation with the last working file that can fit to the canal terminus. The file carrying the sealer is placed into the preparation to full length and gently worked in short up-and-down circumferential strokes, so that the cement is streaked along the canal walls. Additionally, the prefitted master cone is lightly buttered with cement in its apical one third and the cone is slowly and carefully teased to place to further distribute a uniform layer of cement along the length of the canal preparation and to prevent cement from being displaced periapically. The operator is now ready to pack.

VERTICAL CONDENSATION OF WARM GUTTA-PERCHA

The objective of this obturation technique is to continuously and progressively carry a wave of warm gutta-percha along the length of the master cone starting coronally and ending in apical corkage (Fig. 9-43, Part 2, *C*). The vertical condensation of warm gutta-percha is conducted in a heat-sustained compaction cycle and is performed in the following manner.

Down-Packing

Following sealer placement and master cone insertion, the heat carrier is activated and the useless portion of the cone is seared off and removed at the orifice level (Color Plate 1, *F*). The apical extent of the largest prefit plugger is lightly coated with any root canal sealer powder, to prevent adhesion to the tacky gutta-percha and is used to vertically pack the thermosoftened mass apically (Color Plate 1, *G*). To capture the maximum cushion of warm gutta-percha, the plugger is stepped circumferentially around the canal while plugging apically with firm, short strokes. This cycle is completed by a sustained firm apical press held for a few seconds. Tactilely, the clinician will feel the thermosoftened mass of gutta-percha begin to stiffen as it cools during vertical condensation. The apical and automatic lateral movement of thermosoftened gutta-percha readily and three-dimensionally adapts to the preparation over a range of 4 to 5 mm and is termed a *wave of condensation*. Compacting thermosoftened gutta-percha apically moves this mass into narrowing cross-sectional diameters of the preparation, creating a piston effect on the entrapped cement, producing significant sealer hydraulics. It should be noted that the master gutta-percha cone has not been heat-altered in the middle and apical one-third yet. This completes the first heating and compaction cycle.

Immediately the probe of the Touch 'n Heat unit is introduced into the orifice, is activated, and is allowed to plunge 3 to 4 mm into the coronal most extent of the gutta-percha (Color Plate 1, *H*). The heat-activating element is then released and the clinician pauses just momentarily, allowing the instrument tip to begin cooling, then removes the heat carrier along with an adherent bite of gutta-percha (Color Plate 1, *I*). Two important events have occurred. The first result of this action is the progressive apical transfer of heat along the master cone another 4 to 5 mm. The second result of removing a bite of gutta-percha is that a smaller prefit plugger can be placed progressively deeper into the root canal preparation where it can vertically pack warm gutta-percha. Again, gutta-percha will three-dimensionally fill the preparation laterally and in depth over a range of 4 to 5 mm, producing a second wave of condensation, piston effect, and resultant sealer hydraulics (Color Plate 1, *J*). The down-pack continues in a heat sustained compaction cycle.

Through heating, gutta-percha removal, and vertical condensation of warm gutta-percha, the cycle continues usually about 3 or 4 times, depending on root length, until the smallest prefit plugger approaches the apical one-third and can be placed within 4 to 5 mm of the canal terminus.

Following the final heating and gutta-percha removal cycle (Color Plate 1, *K* and *L*), the transfer of heat is progressive into the apical one-third of the gutta-percha master cone, reaching a maximum temperature of about 45° C. The smallest prefit plugger need not be placed closer than 4 to 5 mm of the canal terminus and can predictably deliver a thermosoftened wave of gutta-percha into the narrowing cross-sectioned diameters of the canal, resulting in apical corkage (Color Plate 1, *M*). The plugger action is firm, short, vertical strokes capturing the maximum cushion of rubber; a sustained vertical press on the plugger will produce the final wave of condensation. Stepping the plugger circumferentially along the canal perimeter while plugging apically during the gutta-percha cooling cycle will effectively offset any potential for shrinkage and allow for controlled predictable apical corkage[65] (Color Plate 1, *N*). It is important to note that it is impossible to overextend gutta-percha periapically if:

1. The clinician has a continuous tapering canal preparation whose diameter is narrowest apically.
2. The master cone is fitted correctly.
3. Analytic Technology's Touch 'n Heat unit is used correctly (gutta-percha temperature will not exceed 45° C).
4. The heated tip/pluggers are not placed closer than 4 to 5 mm from canal terminus.

A periapical working film taken during or at the conclusion of the down-pack frequently reveals filled lateral canals coronal to the apical mass of gutta-percha and packed multiple apical portals of exit (Fig. 9-43, Part 2, *D*). The material in the previously cleaned lateral canals is gutta-percha, sealer, or a combination of the two.

Back-Packing

The down-pack is completed, and if a dowel is desirable, then dowel restorative selection and placement can follow immediately. Otherwise, sealing the entire canal is recommended, so as not to leave radicular voids. The most effective and efficient back-pack technique is the Obtura II gutta-percha gun.

The smallest 23-gauge needle is attached to the Obtura II gutta-percha gun, and the hot, precurved needle is inserted into the canal until it comes into contact with previously packed gutta-percha apically. The hot tip of the precurved needle will resoften the most coronal aspect of the apical core of gutta-percha, ensuring cohesion and homogeneity during back-packing procedures (Color Plate 1, *O*). Holding the Obtura II gutta-percha gun lightly, the clinician firmly and slowly squeezes the trigger, injecting a controlled 4- to 5-mm segment of uniformly thermosoftened gutta-percha against the previously corked apical third (Color Plate 1, *P*). If this is properly performed, the clinician feels the Obtura II gutta-percha

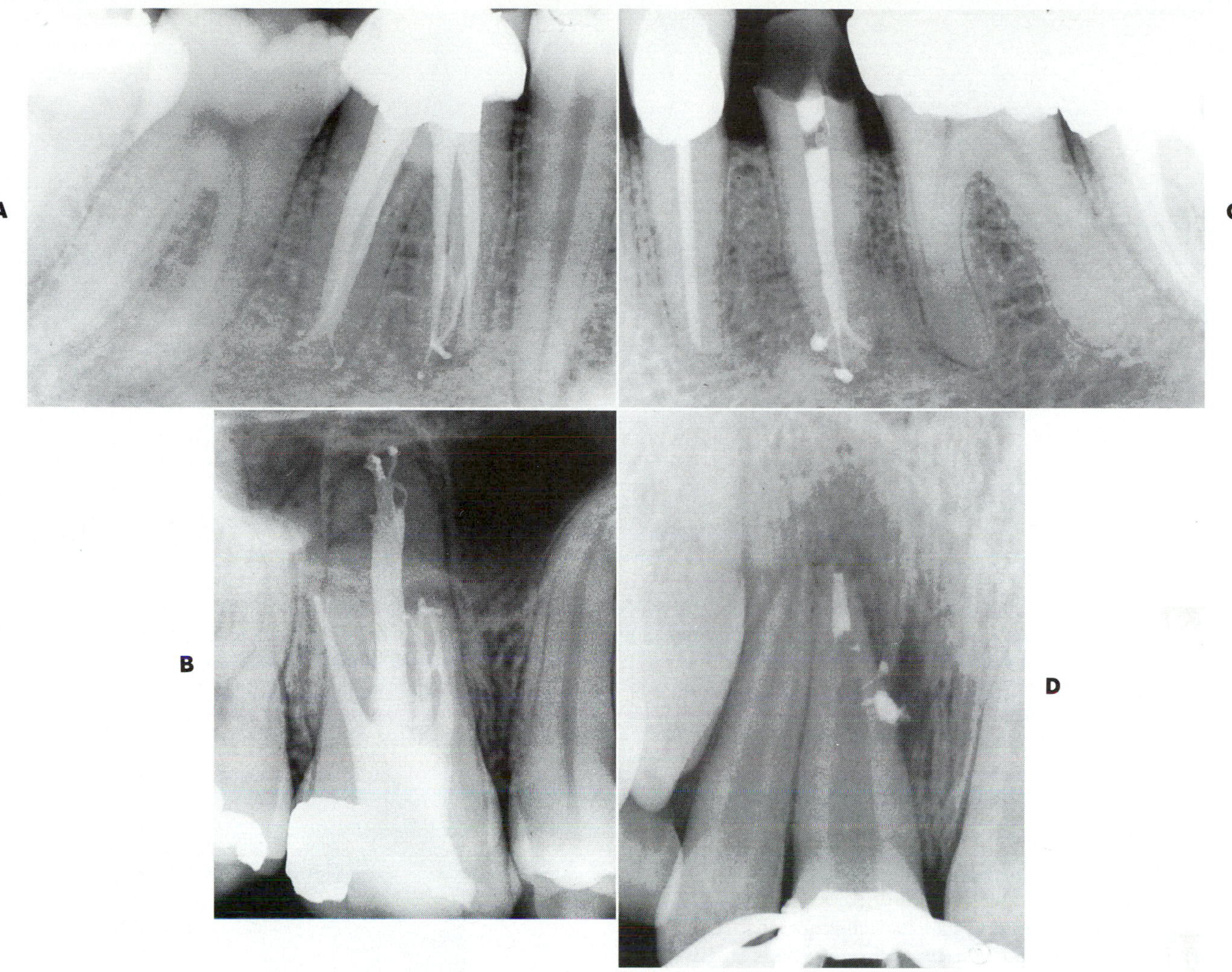

FIG. 9-43 (Part 2) A, Following three-dimensional obturation, note the anastomosing systems in the mesial root and the multiple apical portals of exit associated with each root. **B,** Following obturation of this complex canal system, note the MB root containing two anastomosing canal systems and the multiple portals of exit associated with all apices. **C,** Completed treatment of the primary system containing three apical portals of exit. **D,** Periapical working film of a maxillary central incisor taken at the conclusion of the ''downpack'' reveals three filled lateral canals coronal to the corked apical one-third.

gun back out of the canal easily and progressively when small aliquots of warm gutta-percha are injected. The smallest prefit plugger is used in short vertical strokes and is stepped circumferentially around the preparation, enabling the clinician to capture a maximum cushion of rubber, generating a reverse wave of condensation (Color Plate 1, *Q*). Through a series of gutta-percha injections and vertical condensations the canal is filled (Color Plate 1, *U*). The pulp chamber floor of multirooted teeth should be covered with a thin layer of sealer and gutta-percha syringed into the chamber floor. Using an appropriate plugger, the thermosoftened gutta-percha is plugged vertically, allowing for the obturation of furcal canals.

At this stage, a radiograph should be taken to confirm that the root canal system is densely obturated to the canal terminus. Frequently, a sealer puff will be noticed adjacent to the portals of exit, which ensures clinically that the root canal system has been eliminated in its entirety (Fig. 9-43, Part 2). Because of a well-fitted master cone, sealer puffs generally are larger laterally and smaller or nonexistent apically. Surplus sealer is thoroughly excavated from the pulp chamber with organic solvents to prevent residual sealer from infiltrating the dentinal tubules, where longitudinal crown darkening could result. The clinical crown can now be restored in the appropriate manner.

[The section contributed by Dr. Ruddle ends here.]

Gutta-Percha Altered by Solvents

Chloropercha is made by dissolving gutta-percha in chloroform. The chloropercha paste has been used by some clinicians as the sole canal-filling material. This technique is unsound because of the excessive shrinkage of the filling after evaporation of the chloroform; however, used as a sealer in conjunction with a well-fitted primary cone, chloropercha can fill accessory canals and the root canal space successfully. The technique is used by a few clinicians in perforation cases and in filling unusually curved canals that cannot be negotiated sufficiently (Fig. 9-44) or canals with ledge formation. In view of the FDA's lack of approval of chloroform, it would be prudent to substitute xylol, turpentine or eucalyptol. For purposes of this discussion, however, *chloroform* will be used.

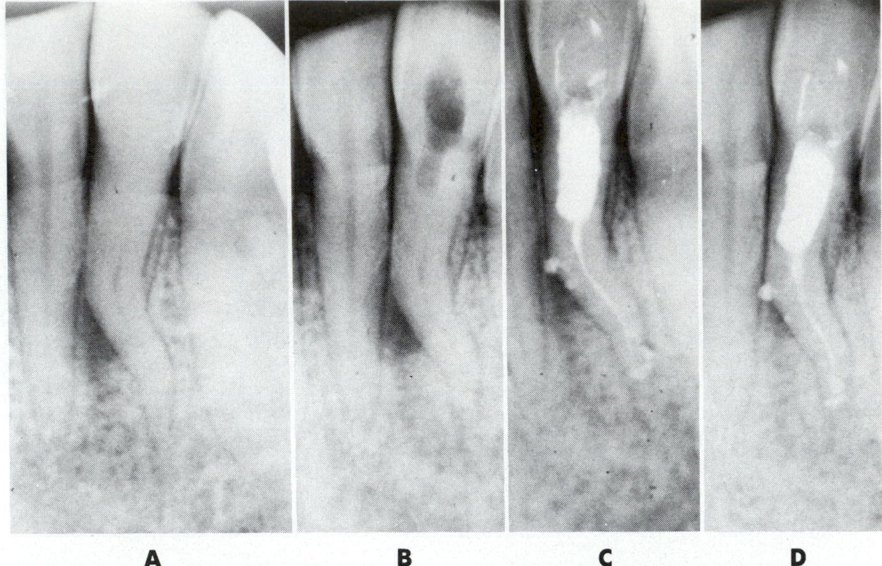

FIG. 9-44 Mandibular lateral incisor. **A,** Pretreatment. Note the calcification of the coronal half of the pulp cavity and the narrow bayonet canal. **B,** Checking the direction of the cut made by a no. 2 long-shanked round bur mounted on a miniature contraangle handpiece for better vision and access. **C,** The canal could not be negotiated but was filled in its entirety by a combination of chloropercha diffusion and forceful vertical condensation. Note the well-filled lateral canals and multiple foramina. **D,** Posttreatment. Within 5 months there was significant bone repair.

Modified chloropercha methods

There are two modifications of the chloropercha method: the Johnston-Callahan and the Nygaard-Østby.

Johnston[53] modified the Callahan[13] chloropercha technique to develop the *Johnston-Callahan diffusion technique*. By this method, the canal is repeatedly flooded with 95% alcohol and then dried with absorbent points. It is then flooded with Callahan's rosin-chloroform solution for 2 to 3 minutes. More chloroform is added if the paste becomes too thick by diffusion or evaporation. A suitable gutta-percha cone is inserted and compressed laterally and apically with a stirring motion of the plugger until the gutta-percha is entirely dissolved in the chloroform-rosin solution in the canal. Additional points are inserted, one at a time, and dissolved in the same way. A plugger is used to apply lateral and vertical pressure to force the chloropercha into the accessory canals and multiple foramina. Care must be exercised to prevent overfilling, because freshly prepared chloropercha is toxic before evaporation. As chloroform from the chloropercha evaporates, it causes a significant dimensional change of the filling, and possibly loss of the apical seal.[154] If sufficient time is allowed for the chloroform to become dissipated in the course of the filling operation and the gutta-percha is compressed to form a homogeneous mass, successful fillings can be obtained by this method (Fig. 9-45).

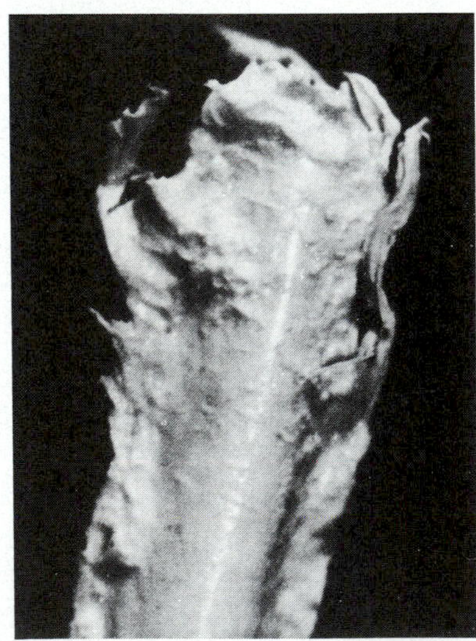

FIG. 9-45 Chloropercha filling. This filling is homogeneous with excellent replication of the apical portion and mold interface. (Original magnification ×25.) (Courtesy Drs. M. Wong, D.D. Peters, L. Lorton, and W. Bernier.)

Nygaard-Østby[83] modified the chloropercha method by adding a preparation made of finely ground gutta-percha, Canada balsam, colophonium, and zinc oxide powder mixed with chloroform in a Dappen dish or watch glass. After the canal walls are coated with Kloroperka, the primary cone, dipped in sealer, is forcefully inserted apically, pushing the partially dissolved tip of the cone to its apical seat. Additional cones dipped in sealer are packed into the canal to obtain a satisfactory filling (Fig. 9-46). Nygaard-Østby suggested additional lateral condensation; but, to avoid overfilling with the chloropercha technique, the use of a spreader is delayed until a subsequent appointment. At this sitting, chloroform is used to soften and remove the coronal chloropercha to a point slightly below the apical third of the canal. Spreading is done thoroughly in the

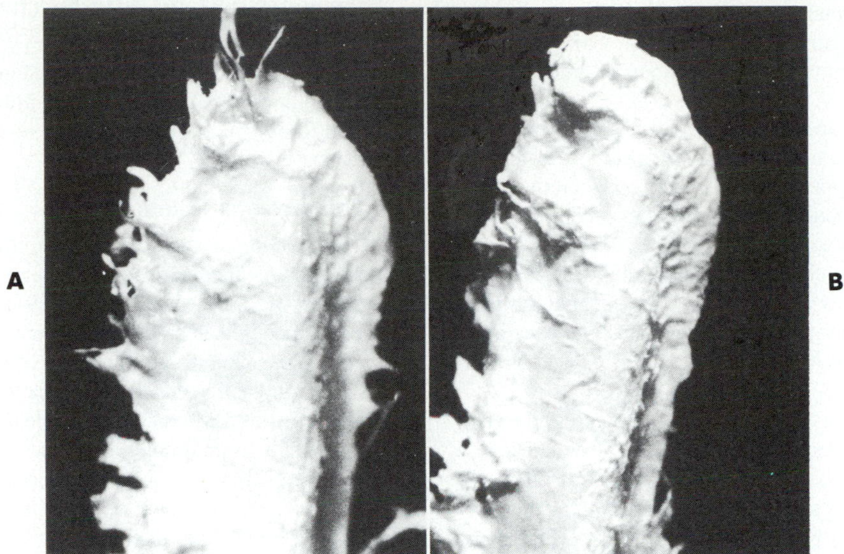

FIG. 9-46 Kloropercha filling. This filling is homogeneous with excellent replication of the apical portion and mold interface. **A,** Immediately after filling. **B,** Three weeks after filling. (Original magnification ×25.) (Courtesy Drs. M. Wong, D.D. Peters, L. Lorton, and W. Bernier.)

coronal two thirds of the canal. The undisturbed apical section acts as a plug to prevent overfilling.

Gutta-Percha–Eucapercha Method

Investigations by the FDA[27] have shown chloroform to be a potential carcinogen. The Council on Dental Therapeutics of the American Dental Association has decided to delete chloroform from *Accepted Dental Therapeutics*. This action may serve to eliminate the clinical use of chloroform in dentistry. Although I am not aware of any cases of malignancy traced to chloroform used in endodontic therapy, a few clinicians[72,79,84] have advocated the use of eucalyptol (also an organic solvent) in place of chloroform by revising the old gutta-percha–eucapercha technique.

Eucalyptol is derived from eucalyptus trees and is the major constituent of eucalyptus oil.[61] It has much less local tissue toxicity than does chloroform and is used in medicine as a decongestant and rubefacient. Although it takes much longer than chloroform to dissolve gutta-percha (minutes versus seconds), eucalyptol can be heated up to about 30° C (86° F) in a Dappen dish and will dissolve gutta-percha into eucapercha in about a minute. Eucalyptol is reported to have antibacterial and antiinflammatory properties.[79,80] Both properties are desirable characteristics of a root canal–filling ingredient.

Technique

The endodontic cavity preparation is done as usual to obtain a smooth tapered preparation. Since the gutta-percha–eucapercha can be diffused and made to flow into narrow and curved canals, the endodontic preparation does not have to be very extensive apically. Usually a no. 25 or 30 file at the apical foramen is adequate. The preparation should present a definite apical constriction, to prevent an undue amount of eucapercha from being forced beyond the confines of the root canal system.

The primary cone should be fitted very tightly, to about 1 or 1.5 mm short of the radiographic apex; it should possess a definite tug-back. The canal is irrigated and dried and is then rechecked with a small file set at full working length to ensure the patency of the canal all the way to the apical foramen.

The large well of the Dappen dish is filled about two-thirds full with eucalyptol. Segments of gutta-percha are placed in the eucalyptol. The Dappen dish is held with pliers over the flame of an alcohol lamp or Bunsen burner for 20 to 30 seconds. This warms the eucalyptol and increases its ability to dissolve gutta-percha. The Dappen dish is then placed over the work counter, and the contents are stirred with a plastic instrument until the gutta-percha segments are dissolved. The eucapercha mixture turns into a cloudy mass.

The prefitted primary cone is held with the cotton pliers at the full working length. The apical half of the cone is dipped into the warm eucapercha mixture and rotated for 30 to 45 seconds. The length of time depends on how short the cone was fitted; the shorter the fit at the apical foramen, the longer the gutta-percha cone must be rotated in the eucapercha mixture. A primary cone can be dipped in the warm eucapercha for about a minute without losing its basic shape. The eucapercha-coated cone is inserted into the canal until the beaks of the pliers coincide with the operating landmark on the incisal or occlusal surface.

A radiograph is exposed to determine the position of the cone in the canal. Vertical and lateral condensation is then done to complete the filling procedure. On occasion, a few drops of warm eucalyptol can be added to the pulp cavity to help soften the filling mass and move the gutta-percha–eucapercha apically. Prefitted and premeasured pluggers are used for vertical condensation. Additional accessory cones are added and fused to the gutta-percha–eucapercha mass to fill the canal system three-dimensionally.

To facilitate insertion of the accessory cones, it is best not to dip them in the eucapercha mixture. The correctness and compactness of the filling are again verified with a radiograph.

Gross overfilling can usually be effectively controlled if the canal was prepared with an apical constriction acting as a matrix against which the gutta-percha–eucapercha mass is condensed.

The gutta-percha–eucapercha technique, if carried out properly, can effectively fill lateral and accessory canals. However, the fine canals will not appear as radiopaque as when the gutta-percha is used in conjunction with a root canal cement sealer containing barium sulfate.

The mixture of eucapercha in the Dappen dish can be saved by covering the dish with a paper cup. The eucapercha mixture will last an entire day without much evaporation, as compared with the chloropercha which evaporates in a few minutes.

Using India ink in a dye-penetration study to assess the sealing quality in extracted teeth filled with lateral condensation method, chloroform-dipped, and eucalyptol-dipped techniques, investigators[119] found no significant statistical difference among the three test groups at the 0.05 level. The investigators concluded that eucalyptol may prove to be an adequate substitute for chloroform in softening gutta-percha, although they suggested that additional research on eugenol toxicity be carried out.

Others[39] have compared the apical seal produced by four obturation techniques. Sixty-four extracted human teeth were obturated by the lateral condensation method using unmodified gutta-percha, and gutta-percha dipped variously in eucalyptol, in chloroform, or in eucapercha paste. They found that "significantly more apical leakage occurred in the eucapercha group than in the other three groups." They also reported that modification of the gutta-percha master cone with solvent does not improve the apical seal in vitro." If modification is desired, dipping the master cone in either eucalyptol or chloroform produces an apical seal superior to that achieved with eucapercha."

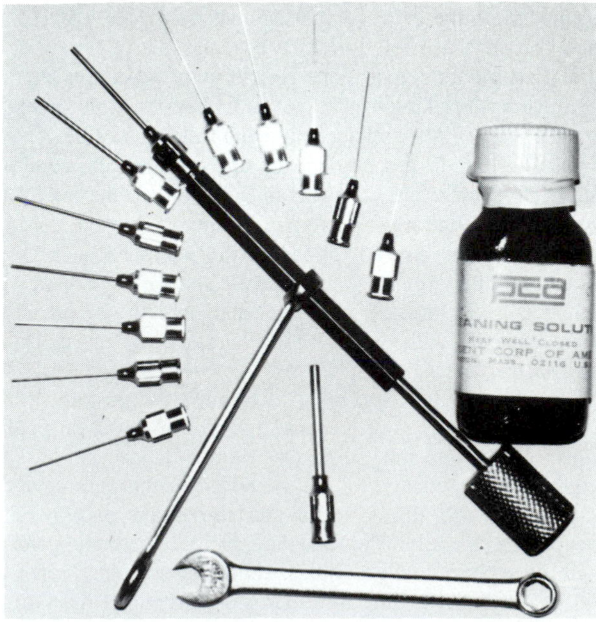

FIG. 9-47 Pressure syringe and accessories for expressing root canal cement. (Courtesy Pulpdent Corporation of America, Boston, Mass.)

Thermoplasticized Gutta-Percha Injection-Molded Method

Obturation of the root canal system, using a thermoplasticized gutta-percha delivered by a pressure syringe previously heated to 160° C, was introduced in 1977 by a group at Harvard/Forsyth.[121]

Experimental technique

The root canal systems of the extracted human teeth were thoroughly cleaned and shaped to receive gutta-percha. The endodontic pressure syringe (Fig. 9-47) was adapted with a threaded needle selected from sizes 18 to 22 gauge so it would negotiate the canal to within 4 mm of the root apex (Fig. 9-48). The thermoplasticized gutta-percha was injected into the root canal until the desired obturation level had been reached. Radiographic examination showed the injected gutta-percha to be of uniform density, with occasional small voids possibly caused by air entrapment when no sealer was used. Investigators[121] reported that when sealer was used, no voids along the root canal walls could be detected radiographically. The injection-molded gutta-percha seemed to be capable of filling multiple foramina and other apical ramifications (Fig. 9-49).

The time required to inject the gutta-percha into the prepared canal was reported to be less than 20 seconds. To prevent possible voids left by the needle, manual condensation with pluggers may be used because the gutta-percha remains plastic as long as 2 to 3 minutes after injection. Although the syringe and needle were heated to 160° C, the actual temperature of the extruded gutta-percha was cooler and well tolerated by human mucosa. No adverse effects were noticed in clinical tests. Dye penetration studies showed that the thermoplasticized gutta-percha injection-molded technique provided a seal comparable to the more conventional obturation methods.[121] The investigation cited above showed that effective root canal obturation could be achieved in vitro, so the technique was modified and improved for in vivo use.

The early endodontic pressure syringe delivery system was cumbersome. Furthermore, both patient and clinician had to be protected from a device using temperature in excess of 155° C. Subsequently, a more efficient, less cumbersome delivery system was developed and patented.[44]

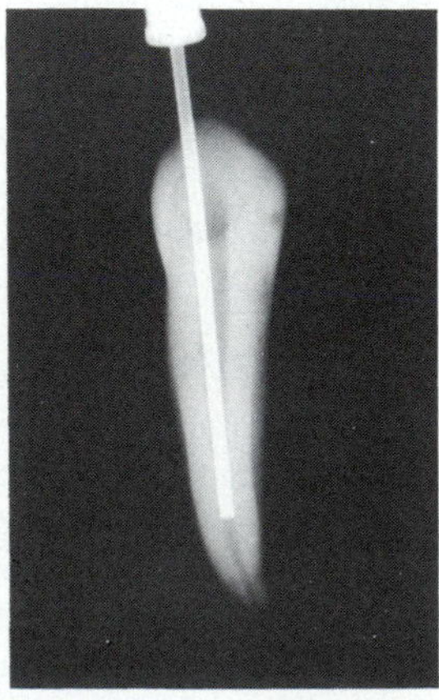

FIG. 9-48 Radiographic confirmation of the needle positioned within the apical third of the prepared root canal.

Obtura and PAC 160

The improved delivery system for the thermoplasticized gutta-percha injection-molding technique is manufactured commercially as the Obtura (Texceed Co., Costa Mesa, Calif.). It consists of an electrical control unit, a pistol-grip syringe, and specifically designed gutta-percha pellets for use with the Obtura system. The syringe is adapted with silver needles as applicator tip. Relatively flexible silver needles of different sizes (18, 20, 22, and 25 gauge) are used to introduce the plasticized gutta-percha into the prepared canal. By using a silver needle as the applicator tip, the plasticized gutta-percha can be injected through a needle as small as 25 gauge. The silver needle keeps the gutta-percha warm as it flows through the tip, which can be bent for easy canal access. Injection time averages less than 20 seconds. Upon completion of the injection, the gutta-percha remains sufficiently plastic for 2 to 3 minutes, which is adequate time for manual condensation. *To counterbalance the effect of shrinkage when the softened gutta-percha hardens, continuous plugger pressure must be maintained until it solidifies.*

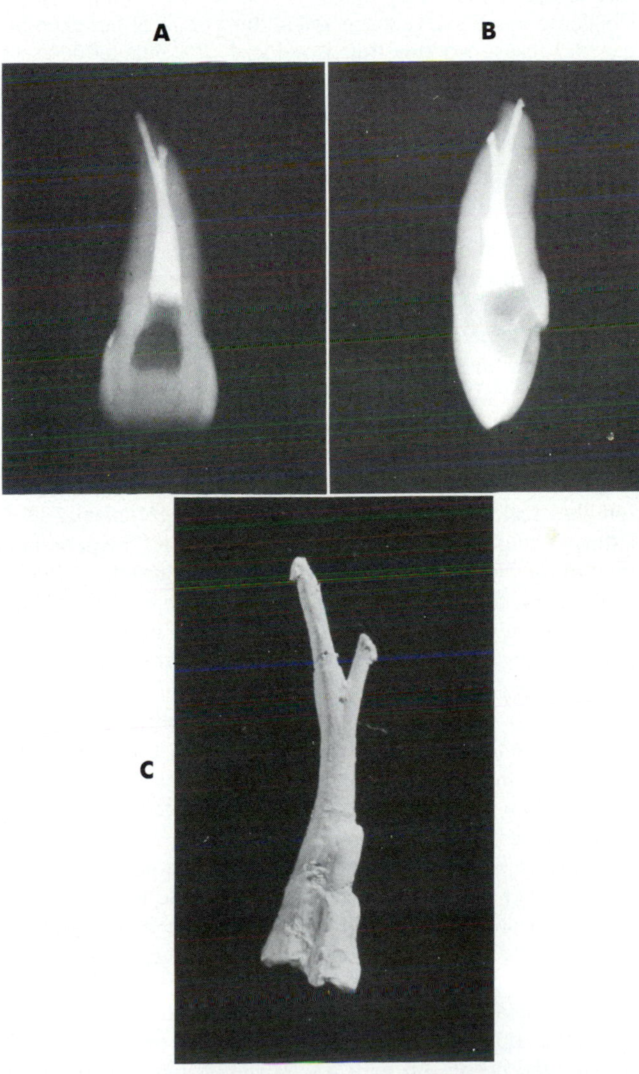

FIG. 9-49 A, Labial-lingual view of a root canal obturated with thermoplasticized gutta-percha. **B,** Mesial-distal view. **C,** Recovered root canal filling of injected thermoplasticized gutta-percha. Note the accessory canal and the irregular outline of the canal proper. (Courtesy Dr. F. Yee.)

Thermoplasticized gutta-percha injection technique

Cavity preparation. The success of any endodontic obturation method, particularly of the thermoplasticized gutta-percha injection technique, depends largely on an adequate canal preparation. An endodontic cavity preparation with a slight flare to accommodate the needle size and definite constriction or minimal opening at the apical terminus makes it easier to obtain a three-dimensionally well-condensed gutta-percha filling with minimal apical extrusion (Fig. 9-50).

Injection technique. *Ideally the selected needle should be able to reach within 3 to 5 mm from the apical terminus passively* (Fig. 9-50). As the *applicator tip is fragile,* caution should be used not to exert any force on the tip. The last instrument used to prepare the body of the canal, or a paper point, is employed to wipe the canal walls with a slow-setting zinc oxide–eugenol-base sealer or AH-26, which acts as a lubricant and sealant. More sealer is needed in a narrow or very curved canal to aid the flow of the gutta-percha. After the consistency of the gutta-percha is tested (Fig. 9-53, *D*), the needle is placed in the canal to full depth and the gutta-percha is now passively injected by squeezing the trigger mechanism. It is very important that the injection be done by applying pressure on the trigger mechanism and not by forcing the fragile applicator needle downward or inward. As the warmed gutta-percha flows and fills the canal space, the back-pressure gradually raises the needle out of the canal. The Obtura device does not melt the gutta-percha into a running liquid state. The gutta-percha flowing out of the applicator tip is semisolid. It has enough viscosity and adhesiveness to stay in maxillary canals. The temperature control unit can also be adjusted to control the viscosity of the softened gutta-percha.

Usually, the entire canal is filled at one time. When two

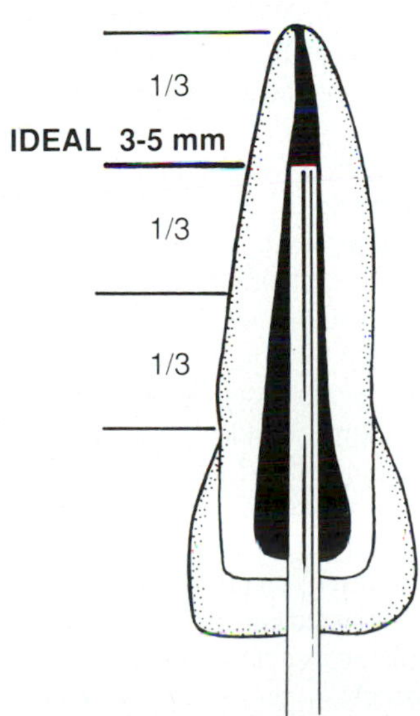

FIG. 9-50 Thermoplasticized gutta-percha injection-molding technique. The needle applicator tip ideally should be able to reach within 3 to 5 mm of apical terminus passively. (Redrawn from Obtura technique manual.)

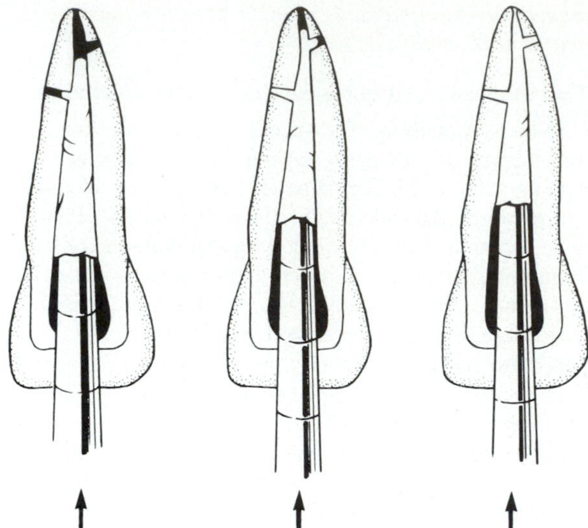

FIG. 9-51 When entire canal is filled at one time, compaction is done using progressively larger to smaller pluggers. Freshly injected gutta-percha is sticky; pluggers are dipped in isopropyl alcohol to prevent stickiness. (Redrawn from Obtura technique manual.)

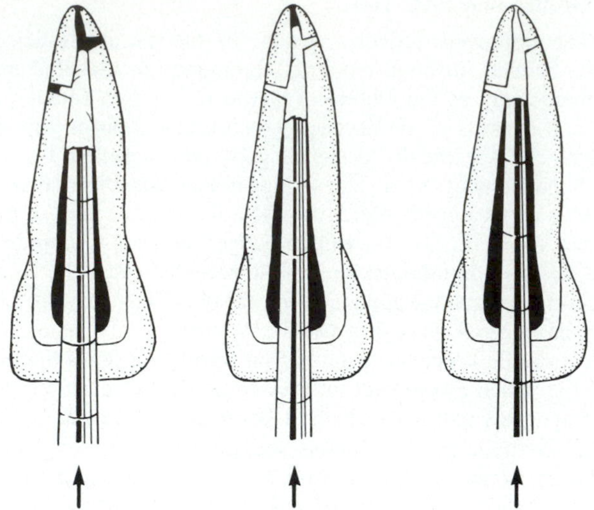

FIG. 9-52 When segmental filling technique is used, compaction is accomplished by starting with smaller pluggers first. Condense immediately when apical third of canal has been injected, because working time is reduced. The plugger does not have to be pushed all the way to the apex to ensure complete three-dimensional filling. (Redrawn from Obtura technique manual.)

canals join, they can be injected at the same time; the canal with easier access is injected first. The puttylike thermoplasticized gutta-percha is then gently compacted with pluggers that have been dipped into isopropyl alcohol, used as a separating medium. Freshly injected gutta-percha is sticky and may be pulled out without a separating medium. Condensation is done by using larger, then progressively smaller pluggers (Fig. 9-51).

When the gutta-percha feels rubbery and resistant, a rapidly developed radiograph will verify whether the apical terminus has been reached and sealed. If not, condensation is repeated with smaller pluggers until the apex has been sealed as shown by a radiograph. Working time varies from 3 to 5 minutes, depending on the canal size. The volume of gutta-percha in larger canals retains its warmth longer than that in smaller canals.

Some clinicians prefer the segmental or incremental filling technique. After the apical third of the canal has been injected, condensation is done with smaller pluggers. Once the apical seal is verified by a radiograph, the remainder of the canal is progressively and rapidly back-filled and condensed with larger pluggers (Fig. 9-52).

To compensate for shrinkage upon cooling, continuous manual condensation force should be used until the gutta-percha cools and solidifies. Vertical condensation with selected pluggers serves also to minimize or prevent small voids caused by possible air entrapment, thereby improving the density and compactness of the root canal filling.

The thermoplasticized injection-molded gutta-percha method appears promising as a new and rapid way to fill the root canal system of straight or gently curved roots.

Torabinejad and coworkers[110] used the scanning electron microscope to evaluate in vitro the thermoplasticized injection-molded gutta-percha fillings on the basis of their adaptation to the surrounding dentinal walls, the presence of voids, and the extent and thickness of the cement sealer. Their study indicated that the root canal system was obturated at least as well by the injection of thermoplasticized gutta-percha in conjunction with sealer as by other generally accepted methods of obturation.

Guttmann and colleagues[37] evaluated the response of the periodontium to the temperature generated by the Obtura thermoplasticized gutta-percha injection technique on dogs' teeth. No identifiable tissue changes were observed within three observation periods: immediate, 24 hours, and 72 hours. Therefore they feel that the technique appears to be technically safe, although long-term evaluation of the response of the periodontium to the elevated temperature change is warranted.

Although the reduction of chair time is an important benefit, the presently available needle sizes make it difficult to introduce them deeply enough apically in narrow canals. The flow of gutta-percha through the silver needle is affected by the thickness of the silver walls, which influences heat transmission, and the diameter of the lumen, which affects frictional resistance. Insufficiently heated gutta-percha will not flow properly into the prepared canal and may interfere with successful three-dimensional obturation.

As the injection of thermoplasticized gutta-percha was developed over time, serious efforts were made to improve its technology and delivery systems. Presently there are two popular systems: (1) *High temperature: Obtura II system* (Texceed Corp., Costa Mesa, Calif.). This system uses gutta-percha heated to 160° C and injected through a silver needle applicator tip. The thermoplasticized gutta-percha extrudes through the needle tip with a temperature range of 62° C to 65° C.[37] (2) *Low temperature: Ultrafil system* (Hygienic Corp., Akron, Ohio) heats the gutta-percha to 70° C for injection into the root canal space.

The Obtura II system is a second-generation device (Fig. 9-53). A much improved version of the previous Obtura in-

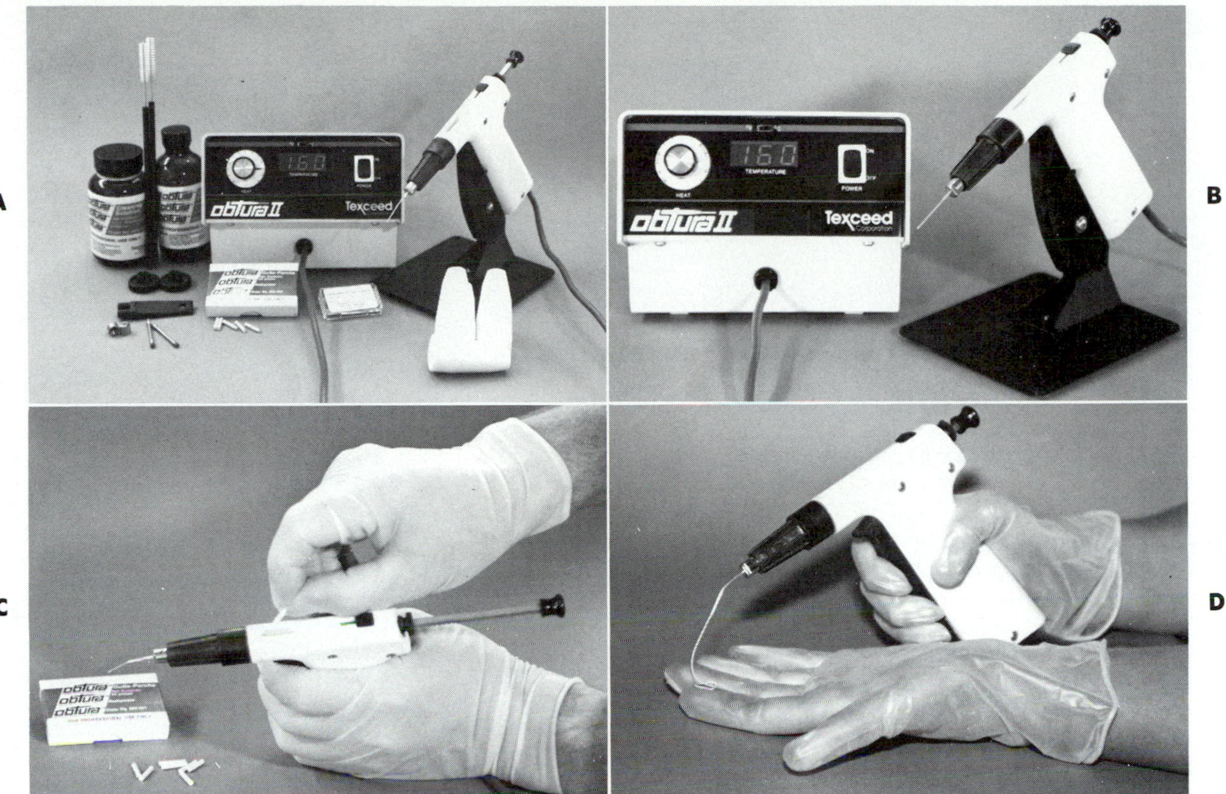

FIG. 9-53 The Obtura II, an improved delivery system for the thermoplasticized gutta-percha injection technique. **A,** The complete Obtura II heated gutta-percha system. **B,** Electrical control unit with pistol grip syringe handpiece. **C,** Loading gutta-percha into the barrel of the handpiece. **D,** At operating temperature, the gutta-percha is extruded from the needle. It is a viscous fluid and sticky at this temperature, has good consistency, and is not uncomfortable to the touch. (Courtesy Texceed Corp., Costa Mesa, Calif.)

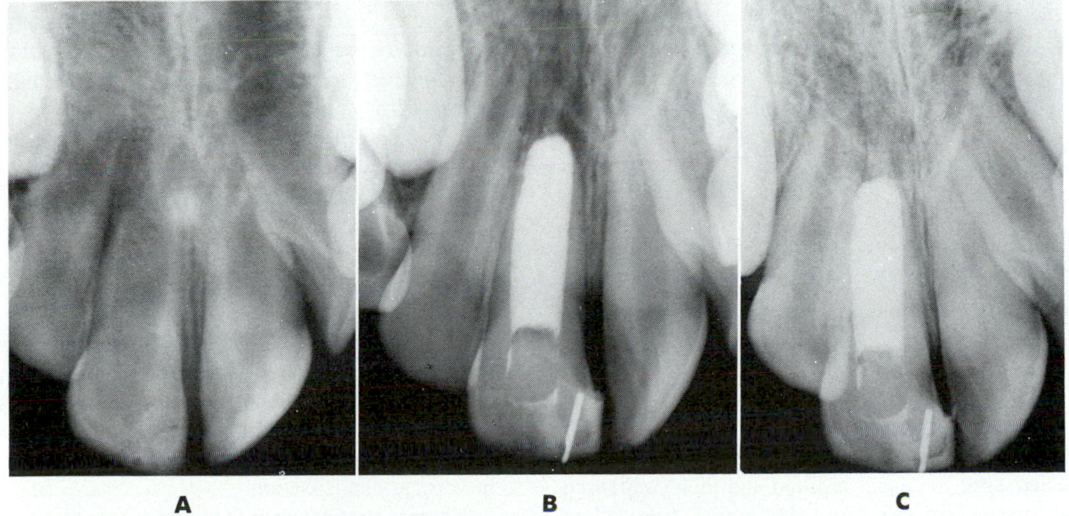

FIG. 9-54 A, Central incisor with incomplete apex formation and periapical tissue changes. Patient's family was traveling and therefore did not permit apexification procedure. **B,** Large root canal space with open apex obturated precisely without apical excess with thermoplasticized gutta-percha injection-molding technique as described under Figure 9-60. **C,** Two-year checkup radiograph obtained when patient's family was transferred back to the United States shows good healing. (Courtesy Dr. J. Marlin.)

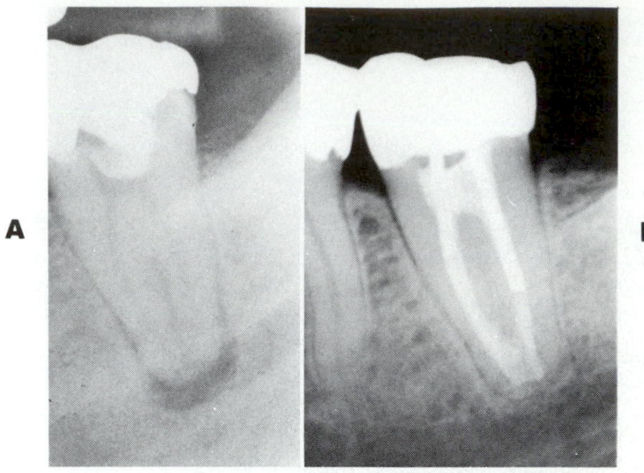

FIG. 9-55 A, Preoperative radiograph of mandibular molar with periapical lesion. **B,** Two-year recall checkup radiograph of root canal filling shows good healing. Canal system filled with injection-molded thermoplasticized gutta-percha showing "weblike" internal anatomy in apical third. (Courtesy Dr. J. Marlin.)

strument, it incorporates many improvements and refinements gained from modern technology. The pistol-grip syringe is made of stronger plastic material that is more resistant to higher temperature. Its highly polished chamber is precisely fitted with a newly designed and well-sealed round plunger. This improves the flow of the softened gutta-percha and is easier to clean after use. The control unit is equipped with a digital readout of temperature and fail-safe circuitry with precise temperature control. Better-designed and -fitted disposable silver needles enhance the injection of thermoplasticized gutta-percha and aid in infection control.

The thermoplasticized gutta-percha injection-molding technique seems to be capable of filling multiple foramina and other irregular configurations of the root canal system (Figs. 9-54 to 9-59). It must be emphasized, however, that canal preparation for all injection-filling techniques requires a slightly flaring body and *a definite constriction at the apex*. The apical constriction limits the flow of the softened gutta-percha within the confines of the canal space. This makes it easier to compact densely the filling materials into the irregularities, fins, grooves, and cul-de-sacs of the complex canal system without undue extrusion.

Injection-molding technique in canals with a large apical foramen

Canals with large apical openings may be fitted first with a tightly fitted master cone to within 1 mm of working length. After the root canal has been filled with the master cone and sealer, the bulk of the master cone is removed with a heated instrument to a point 6 to 8 mm from the apex to allow for the placement of the injection needle. The thermoplasticized gutta-percha is injected until the canal is filled and then condensed vertically with preselected pluggers. This two-step procedure of filling the canal with a master cone and sealer, followed by vertical condensation of the injectable gutta-percha into the canal space, is gaining more popularity with clinicians.[86] It combines the versatility and thoroughness of compaction of the softened gutta-percha into the root canal space with more efficient control of apical extrusion of the filling materials.

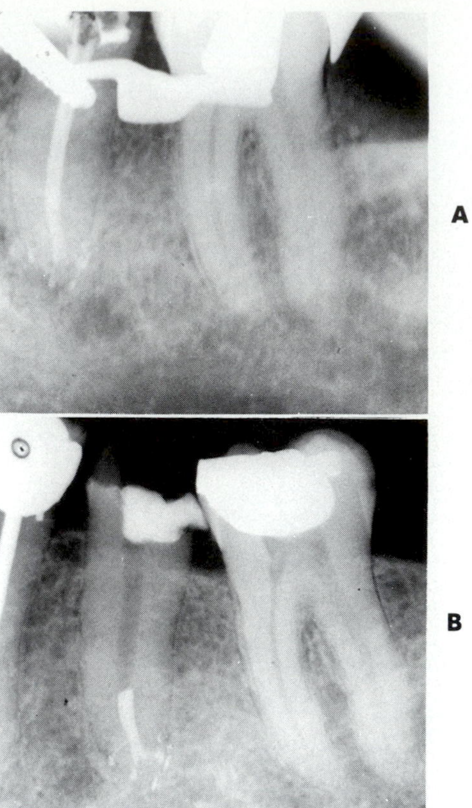

FIG. 9-56 A, Mandibular second bicuspid obturated with injection-molded thermoplasticized gutta-percha. Postfilling radiograph showing multiple accessory canals filled and thickened PDL. **B,** Six-month recall radiograph with space for post and core buildup shows complete periapical healing. (Courtesy Dr. J. Marlin.)

Another obturation method for a canal with a large apical opening is to place the largest needle applicator tip at the canal orifice entrance. The injection is done in a 360-degree circular manner, to deposit a plug of gutta-percha *only in the occlusal third of the canal space*. The plug of gutta-percha is then compacted circumferentially toward the apex, moving it by increments of 2 to 3 mm at a time, verified by radiographs, until the apex is reached (Fig. 9-60). Once the plug of gutta-percha has reached the apex, vertical pressure of the condenser is maintained without forward apical push until the gutta-percha solidifies. The remainder of the canal is then safely and quickly back-filled.

Vertical condensation of thermoplasticized gutta-percha is less forceful, compared with vertical compaction of the warm gutta-percha filling technique. It is particularly useful when obturating canals with a fragile, weak root or a root with a suspected vertical fracture, as less pressure and stress are involved in vertical condensation.

When a *vertical root fracture* is suspected, only the apical third of the root canal is filled with gutta-percha. It is advisable to fill the occlusal two thirds of the canal and the coronal access cavity with an adhesive composite glass isonomer, such as Ketac silver. The crown of the tooth is subsequently protected with a full crown. Stewart[107] reported several successfully managed cases of vertical crown and root fractures, which

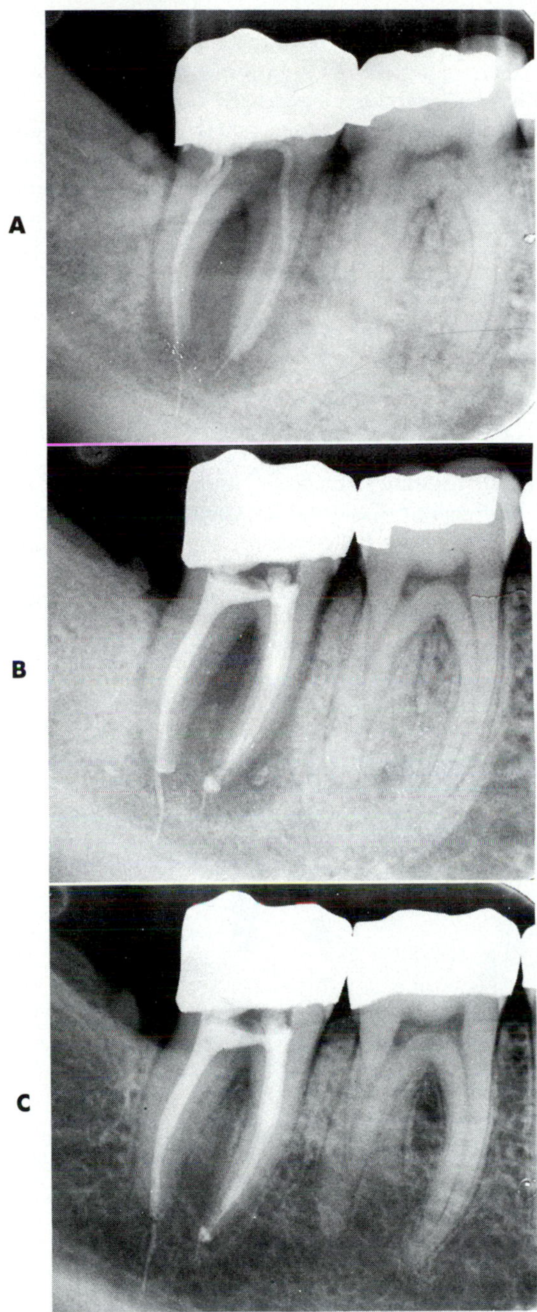

FIG. 9-57 A, The referring dentist felt the endodontic treatment failure was due to the distal root "overfill" and requested surgical removal of the overfill and curettage of the periradicular lesion of this mandibular second molar. **B,** Tooth retreated nonsurgically and canals reobturated with PAC-160 injection-molded thermoplasticized gutta-percha. **C,** Sixteen-month recall radiograph showed good continued healing of the supporting tissues. This case demonstrated two important points: (1) Canals must be totally obturated so as to heal predictably, and (2) the presence of biocompatible gutta-percha in the apical region of a properly treated root canal system seems to be inconsequential. (Courtesy Dr. G. John Schoeffel.)

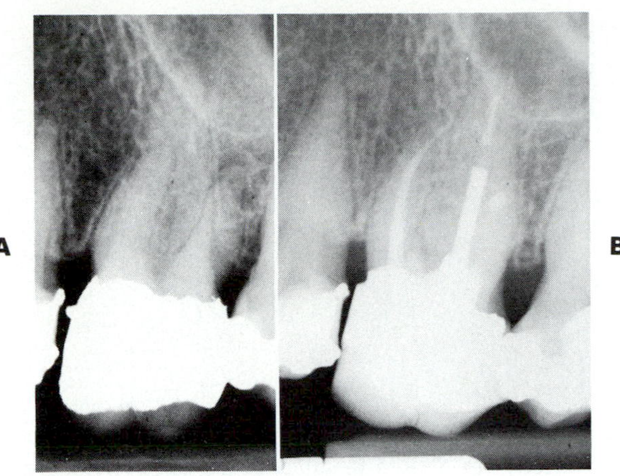

FIG. 9-58 Retrofilling with injection-molded thermoplasticized gutta-percha. **A,** Maxillary first molar with completely calcified disto-buccal canal and periapical tissue changes on the palatal and disto-buccal roots. **B,** Two-year recall radiograph. The mesio-buccal and palatal roots were obturated nonsurgically; the disto-buccal root had apicoectomy and retrofilling. All three roots were filled with injection-molded thermoplasticized gutta-percha. Good osseous repair is evident. (Courtesy Dr. J. Marlin.)

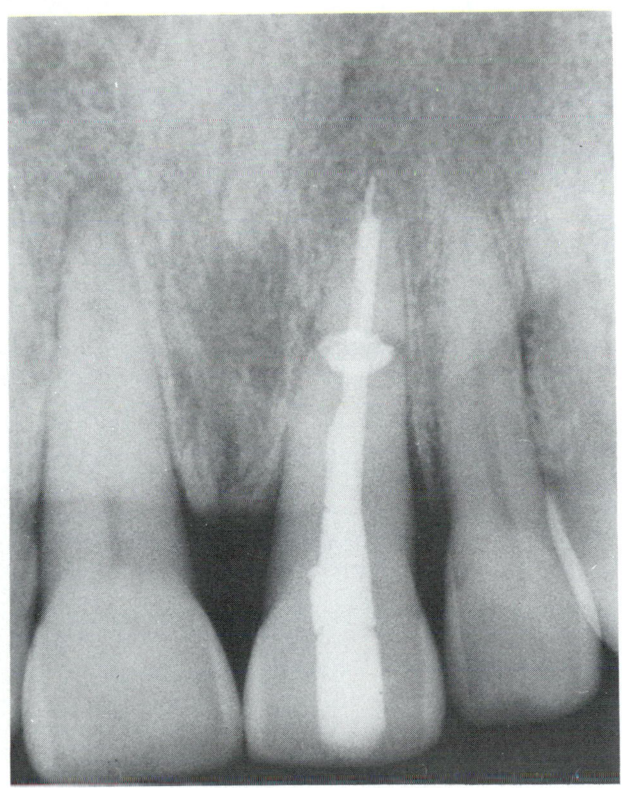

FIG. 9-59 Fractured central incisor. Both segments were successfully obturated with PAC-160 (Fig. 9-57) gutta-percha without excessive overfilling in the area of the fracture line. The apical 1.5 mm was instrumented to a size 45 file, and the remainder to a size 100 file, to accommodate the pressure dynamics necessary for thorough obturation in this unique situation. (Courtesy Dr. C.J. Schoeffel.)

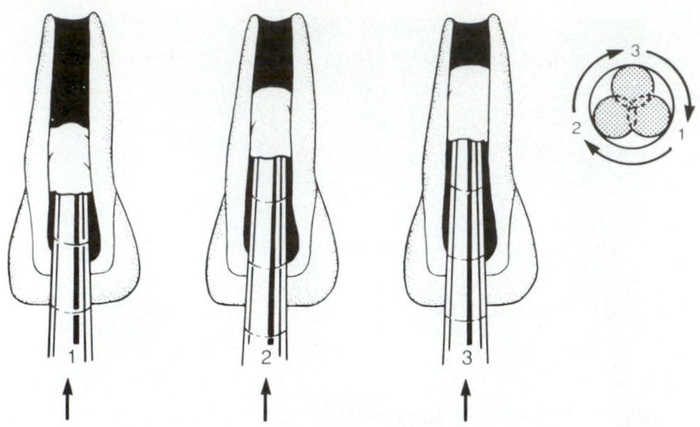

FIG. 9-60 Open apex compaction technique. The largest needle applicator tip is used to inject in a 360° circle a plug of gutta-percha only in the coronal third of the canal. With large condensing pluggers, the mass of gutta-percha is compacted circumferentially, moving it 2 to 3 mm at a time, guiding the progress with radiographs. Once the apex is reached, plugger pressure is maintained until the gutta-percha solidifies. (Redrawn from Obtura technique manual.)

in the past normally would have been condemned as hopeless problems. *Calcium hydroxide treatment is carried out first, until there is evidence of periadicular healing, before the canal is obturated with gutta-percha or filled with a reinforced Ketac silver bonding composite,* which also serves as post and core. A full veneer crown is used to protect the crown of the tooth (Figs. 9-61 and 9-62).

The thermoplasticized gutta-percha injection delivery method has been used in an expanded variety of cases. It has been used efficiently to obturate canals with internal resorption, to inject around broken instruments, or in surgical applications to repair radicular defects, perforations, and retrofillings. With experience and imagination, clinicians are finding new applications for the thermoplasticized gutta-percha injection-molding technique.

Variations in gutta-percha thermoplasticizing technology

Technologic variations in the art of thermoplasticizing gutta-percha to improve and facilitate its compaction into the canal space have been suggested by several clinicians.

Use of ultrasound. Moreno[77,78] from Mexico used an ultrasonic scaling unit (Cavitron) to supply heat for plasticizing gutta-percha to obtain better compaction. The no. 25 file at-

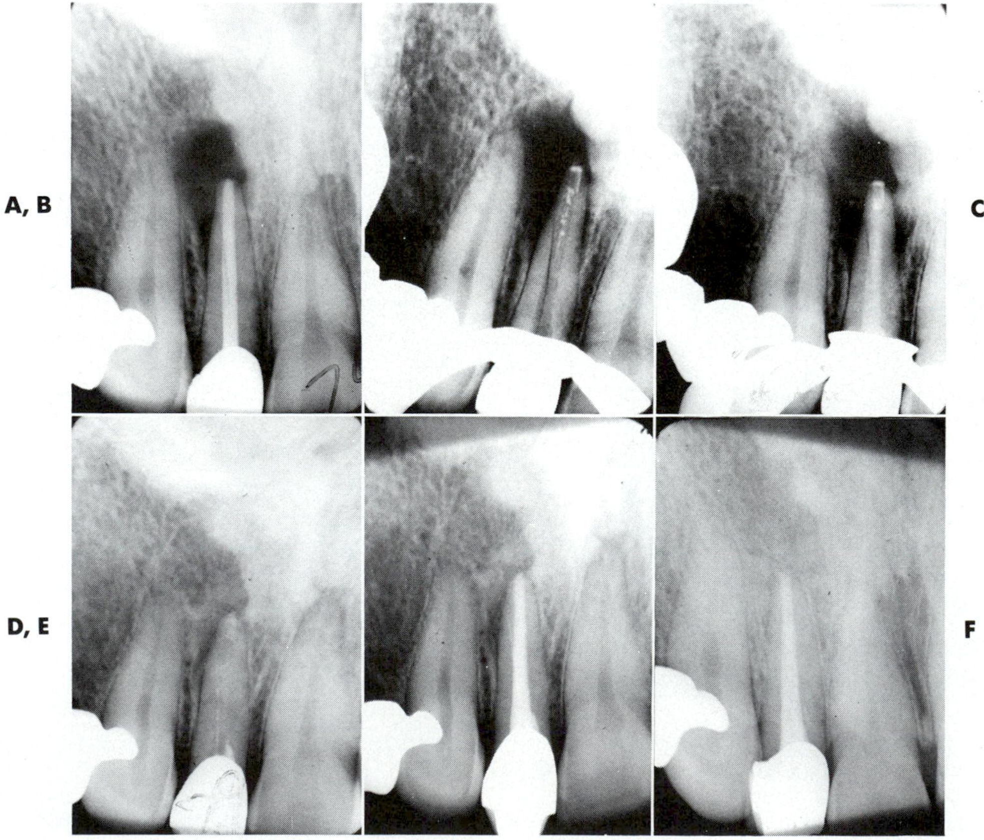

FIG. 9-61 A, The patient had a large periradicular lesion. A line seen in the gutta-percha caused suspicion of a vertical root fracture. **B,** Removal of the gutta-percha and exposure of the classic vertical fracture. **C,** Tooth being treated with $Ca(OH)_2$ and contrast medium. **D,** Healing of the supporting structures is obvious. **E,** The root canal has been sealed with gutta-percha. There is evidence of continued healing of the periradicular tissues. **F,** Ten years after treatment. Healing is complete and there is no longer evidence of the fracture. (From Stewart G: J Endod 14(1):50, 1988.)

tached to the PR 30 insert of the ultrasonic unit is placed alongside the primary gutta-percha point and sealer to a depth about 5 mm short of the working length. The ultrasonic unit with the rheostat set at 1 is activated for 3 to 4 seconds. The ultrasound thermal energy released by vibratory motion of the ultrasonically activated file plasticizes the gutta-percha. Upon removal of the file, the spreader is inserted immediately to create room for auxiliary cones. The softened primary cone allows a deeper penetration of the spreader, and a greater number of auxiliary cones can therefore be used to obtain better compaction.

In a leakage study using iodine-131 to compare this modified technique with regular lateral condensation, Moreno[78] reported that the mean leakage for regular lateral condensation was 2 mm (1 to 3 mm), versus a mean leakage of 0.6 mm for the modified technique.

Another clinician, Martin,[71] suggested softening the apical gutta-percha with the ultrasonic enlarging instrument that he helped develop (Dentsply Cavi-Endo device). The thermoplasticized gutta-percha allows deeper and more efficient penetration of spreaders and pluggers and a better lateral and vertical compaction of the gutta-percha mass.

Thermoplasticized low-temperature (70° C) gutta-percha injection-filling technique. As the injection technique of thermoplasticized gutta-percha to fill the root canal system gained popularity, clinicians developed ingenious injection systems. *It is entirely possible that in the not too distant future canal obturation will consist of injecting an ideal filling material in the canal space with a well-perfected injection device.*

In two studies[19,75] investigators developed and tested a new way to fill the root canal system; this method, which uses a low-temperature (70° C) plasticized gutta-percha, is called the Ultrafil System. The system consists of an injection syringe, gutta-percha cannulas with a needle attached, and a small portable 120-V heater with preset thermostatically controlled temperature (Fig. 9-63, *A*). The gutta-percha used contains the same ingredients as gutta-percha points; however, there appears to be a greater proportion of paraffin. A process developed by the Hygienic Corporation allows the gutta-percha to flow at 70° C. For convenience, the gutta-percha is packed into a prototype cartridge-needle combination or cannules (Fig. 9-63, *A*). Each disposable cannule contains enough gutta-percha to fill a multirooted tooth. When first introduced the cannules of gutta-percha of the Ultrafil System were available in only one viscosity. Presently, Ultrafil gutta-percha comes in three different viscosities for use in various clinical situations and techniques. The original *Regular Set* in white cannule and the *FirmSet* in blue cannule have the highest flow properties. They are used primarily for simple injection techniques where the gutta-percha will not be compacted manually. The FirmSet gutta-percha sets in 4 minutes, the Regular Set in 30 minutes. To counteract the concern about expansion and shrinkage of the injected gutta-percha, a third product, the *Endoset* gutta-percha, was introduced, which can be condensed

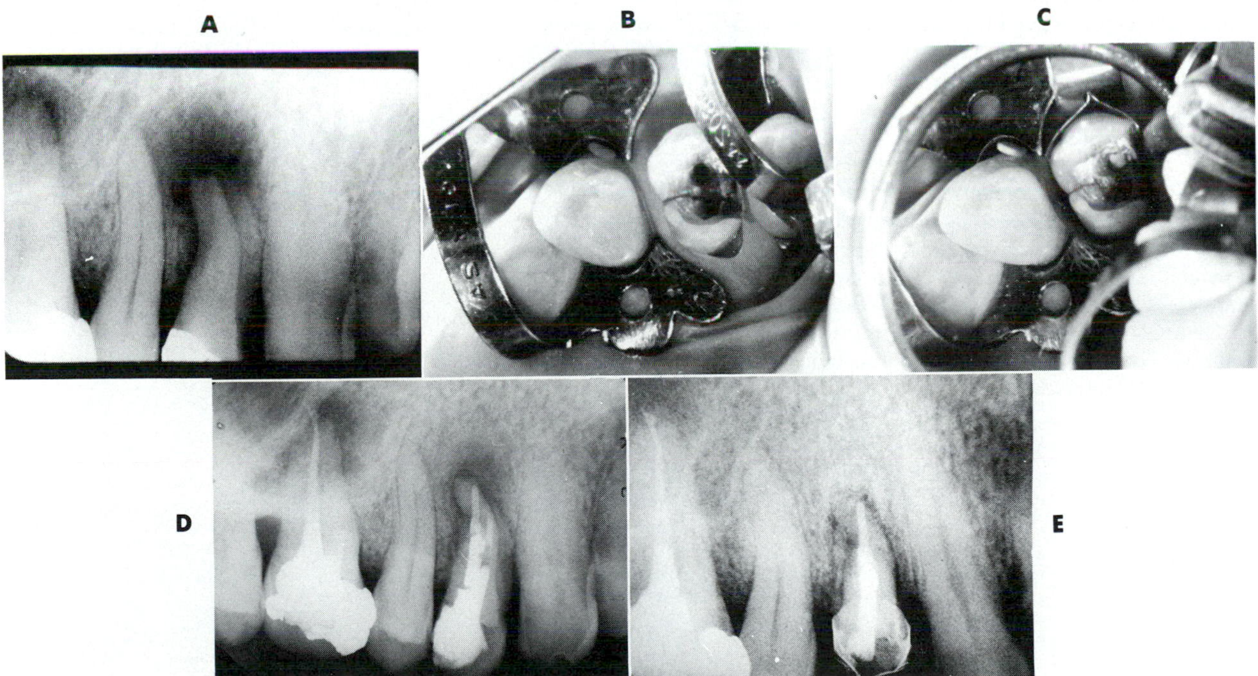

FIG. 9-62 A, Film shows a large periradicular defect as well as apical root resorption. **B,** The rubber dam in place supported by two premolar clamps. There is an obvious fracture running along the floor of the pulp chamber and involving the distomarginal wall. **C,** The crown of the tooth is being held together with a matrix band. There are gutta-percha plugs in the openings of the root canals to prevent the reinforced glass ionomer from entering the canals when the crown is restored. **D,** The root canals have been sealed with a modified glass ionomer. There is evidence of continued healing. **E,** Four months after root canal sealing, the crown preparation has been completed and continued healing of the periradicular tissues is evident. (From Stewart G: J Endod 14(1):50, 1988.)

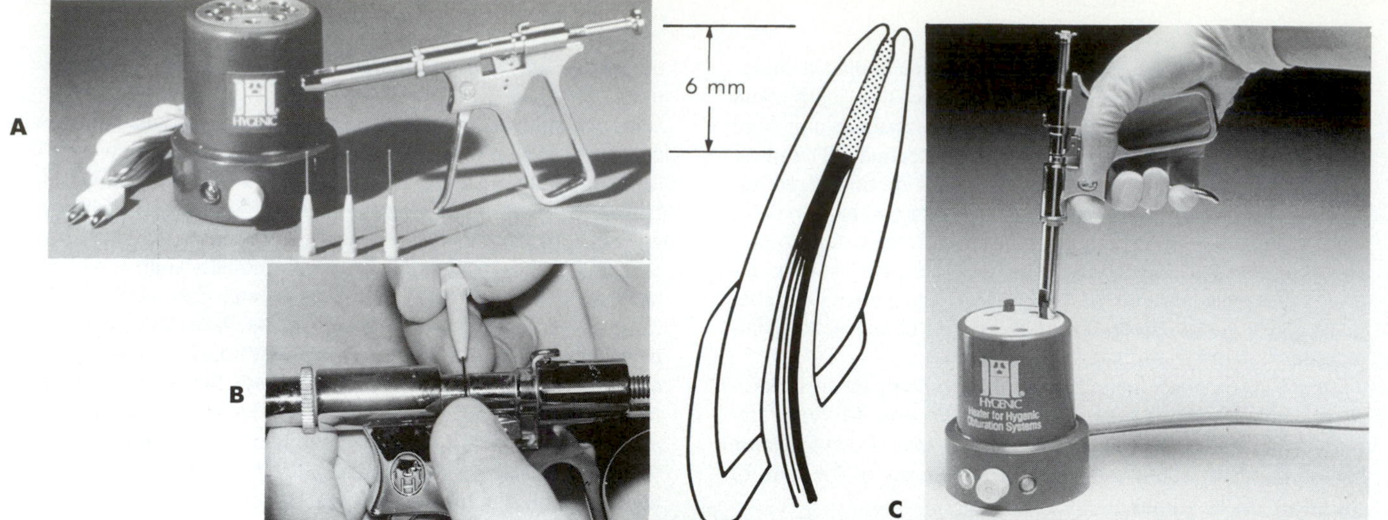

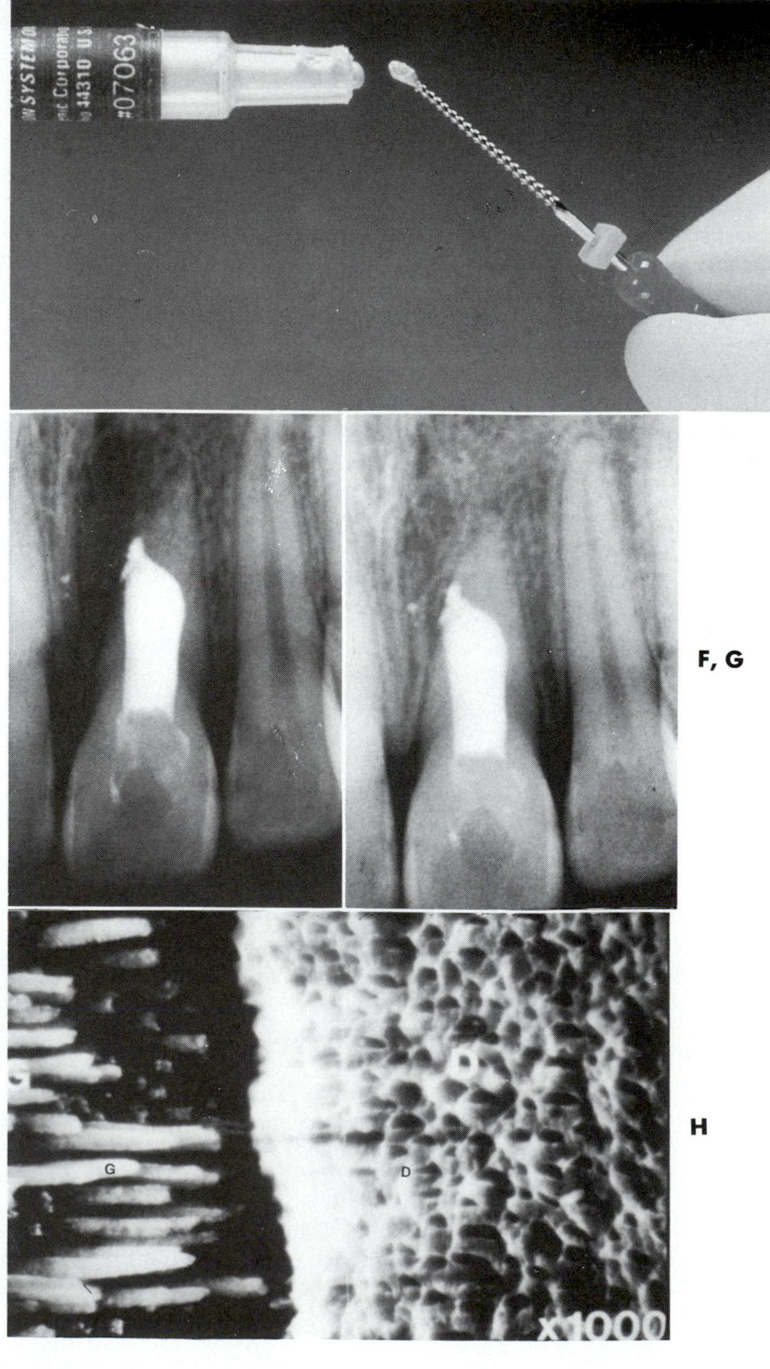

FIG. 9-63 A, Ultrafil low-temperature injection system. Portable heater, pressure syringe, cartridge-needles, gutta-percha cannulas. **B,** Cannula needle can be custom bent or precurved by drawing the needle over the syringe barrel while pressing the needle against the syringe. **C,** The cannula needle is inserted to within 6 mm of the apical terminus. Note the apical constriction of the prepared canal. Ultrafil gutta-percha injection technique. **D,** Syringe-cannula combination is replaced in heater between injection to keep gutta-percha in flowable state. **E,** Sterile K file inserted 2 to 3 mm in the SuccessFil syringe to pick up a small amount of gutta-percha for creating an apical plug. **F,** Internal resorption shown by postfilling radiograph. **G,** One-year recall radiograph shows good healing. **H,** Scanning electron micrograph shows projections of the low-temperature gutta-percha *(G)* filling penetrating into dentinal *(D)* tubules. (Original magnification, ×1000.) (**A, D, E,** Courtesy The Hygienic Co., Akron, Ohio; **C,** redrawn from The Hygienic Co. Technical Bulletin; **F-H,** Courtesy Dr. A.E. Michanowicz.)

immediately after injection. The Endoset gutta-percha, in green cannule, is slightly less fluid and more viscous. It is used primarily for all techniques that require condensing with either a plugger or a spreader. The final setting time of the Endoset gutta-percha is 2 minutes. As with all other gutta-percha obturation techniques the use of a sealer is mandatory[24] with the Ultrafil injection system.

To gain better canal access and visibility during injection, *the cannula needle is prefitted in the canal to a depth of about 6 mm from the apical terminus and custom bent or precurved accordingly prior to heating*. Curving is done by placing the cannula needle over the barrel of the syringe and drawing the needle over the syringe barrel with the thumb (Fig. 9-63, *B*). Bending the needle with a pair of pliers may crimp or damage it and prevent the free flowing of gutta-percha.

The cannulas are then placed in the portable heater with the temperature preset at 90° C (194° F) and heated for a minimum of 15 minutes before use. The Ultrafil cannulas should not remain in the heater longer than 4 hours; otherwise the properties of the gutta-percha are adversely affected. The cannulas can be reheated; however, when the cumulative time exceeds 4 hours, they should be discarded. When not in use, the cannulas are best kept under refrigeration. One cannule is ample to fill one tooth, although partially used cannulas can be reused.

The thermoplasticized gutta-percha will flow for approximately 1 minute after the cannula is removed from the heater and loaded onto the syringe. To ensure good results, the injection procedure must be smoothly and promptly executed. It takes usually 15 to 30 seconds to fill most canals without the need for manual condensation.

The trigger is squeezed slowly and released to extrude some gutta-percha through the needle before inserting it into the canal to within 6 to 8 mm from the apical terminus (Fig. 9-63, *C*). Since the gutta-percha cools faster in the needle than in the body of the cannula, constant flow must be maintained during injection. Care must be taken not to bind the needle tightly against the canal walls.

It is important to understand the concept of "passive injection," to prevent excessive internal pressure buildup within the cannule. The plasticized gutta-percha is not forced out of the cannula as in a hypodermic injection technique. It should be allowed to flow out of the needle at its own rate by means of a squeeze-release-pause-squeeze-release motion on the trigger. As the plasticized gutta-percha fills the canal, the back-pressure created by the free-flowing gutta-percha will gradually "lift" or "push" the needle out of the canal. Withdrawing the needle without feeling this back-pressure could result in voids or incomplete filling.

When obturating a multirooted tooth, after filling one canal the clinician must replace the syringe-cannula combination in the heater for at least 45 seconds before repeating the injection procedure in the next canal. This will assure sufficient flowability of the gutta-percha between each canal injection (Fig. 9-63, *I*).

The Ultrafil technique does not advocate manual compaction. If desired, pluggers should be dipped in isopropyl alcohol before use to prevent adhesion and dislodgment of the tacky gutta-percha. Hand condensation with pluggers is done with a *light tapping pressure* rather than a forceful vertical compaction.

A *sequential obturation technique* may be used, if desired. A set of three pluggers is prefitted at working length less 1 mm at midcanal and at the coronal third. After lightly coating the canal walls with sealer a small increment of SuccessFil gutta-percha is deposited and an apical plug is condensed (see Fig. 9-63, *E*). A small amount of Endoset gutta-percha is then injected and condensed with light tapping with a small plugger wet with alcohol as a separating medium. Meanwhile, after injecting, the syringe-cannula combination is always replaced on the heater for reheating to ensure sufficient flow of the gutta-percha for the next incremental injection. An additional amount of gutta-percha is injected and condensed lightly with a larger plugger. The process is continued until the canal is obturated. When obturating a multirooted tooth, placing paper points in canals not being filled helps maintain canal access.

The New Trifecta Technique and Trifecta Kit

To further improve the Ultrafil system's versatility and adaptability for varied obturation techniques, the Hygienic Corporation had added a New SuccessFil gutta-percha syringe containing 1 ml of high-viscosity gutta-percha and a set of SuccessFil titanium and plastic cores to the Ultrafil Kit and new names were coined: The New Trifecta Technique and Trifecta Kit.

The titanium and plastic cores are available in size 20 to 40 (titanium) and size 25 to 80 (plastic). The cores are prepared for use by carefully coating them with the high-viscosity gutta-percha from the SuccessFil syringe, which has been heated in the heater a minimum of 15 minutes. Precoated cores are stored in a cool area until needed. They are sterilized in 5.25% sodium hypochlorite and rinsed in alcohol before use.

Although the Trifecta Kit contains titanium and plastic cores to provide an obturation technique combining injectable Ultrafil gutta-percha with solid core delivery of SuccessFil gutta-percha to gain "complete apical control and exact placement of gutta-percha" for the prevention of overfills or short fills, the Hygienic Corporation pamphlet emphasizes the removal of the solid core: "The Trifecta Technique removes the core, leaving just gutta-percha and sealer in the canal as the root canal filling." However, in order to obtain a three dimensionally dense and well-compacted obturation it is most important to inject additional Ultrafil FirmSet or Endoset gutta-percha and to condense with a plugger or spreader to prevent voids created by the removal of the solid core.

Grassi et al[32] in their study of changes of physical properties of raw gutta-percha (unrefined, unfilled), of gutta-percha points, and of the two forms of Ultrafil gutta-percha (Regular Set [white], FirmSet [blue]) reported "melting temperatures of the Ultrafil materials are depressed by about 20° C from that of the raw gutta-percha and the gutta-percha point material." The Ultrafil gutta-percha samples melt at temperatures ranging from 38° C to 44° C, and the raw gutta-percha and gutta-percha points melt at a temperature ranging from 46° C to 59° C. "The Ultrafil blue and white material exhibit melting temperatures 14° C to 19° C lower than that of the point material." This lowering of the melting temperature is due to the amount of milling (mastication), which is the process of mixing raw gutta-percha with its other components. With an increase in mastication processing, there is a decrease in molecular weight and melting temperature. "When the Ultrafil material was compared with the gutta-percha points, the blue material had approximately the same amount of shrinkage (2.6%);

the white material shrank slightly less (2.2%). The raw gutta-percha, being 100% polymer, had the greatest amount of shrinkage (4.6%)."

The Ultrafil injection technique was tested with and without a root canal sealer and was found to create a good apical seal (Fig. 9-63, *D* and *E*). An in vitro study[75] utilizing methylene blue dye to investigate the sealing properties of the low-temperature (70° C) gutta-percha injection technique showed that the injected gutta-percha sealed as well as or slightly better than the lateral condensation technique using gutta-percha cones and Grossman's sealer. Another study,[19] utilizing radioactive isotopes to quantitatively determine leakage, had similar results. The low-temperature injection gutta-percha with Grossman's sealer had the least amount of leakage, followed by the lateral condensation with gutta-percha and Grossman's sealer. When used without sealer, the low-temperature injection gutta-percha showed slightly greater isotope leakage than the other two groups. Overall, the three groups showed a good apical seal with only minimal leakage.

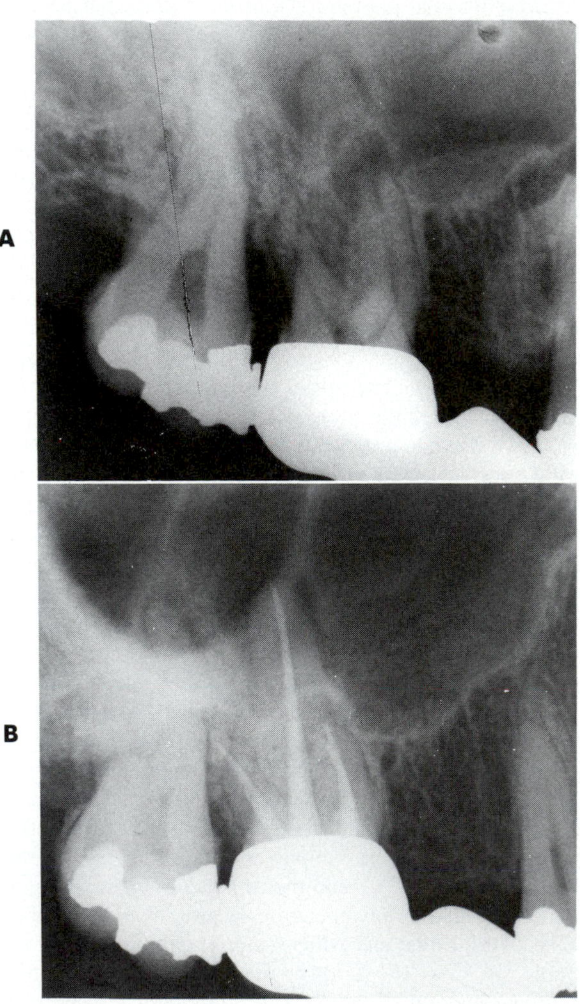

FIG. 9-64 A, Prefilling radiograph of tooth no. 3 with chronic apical periodontitis. An accessory canal is apparent at the apex of the mesiobuccal root. **B,** Postfilling radiograph showing the root filled with sealer and master cone, condensed and injected with Ultrafil FirmSet. The accessory canal appears to be filled. (Courtesy Dr. A. Michanowicz.)

Other investigators[24] reported that neither the lateral condensation nor the injected thermoplasticized gutta-percha technique provides an apical seal to ink penetration when used without a root canal sealer, even with the smear layer removed. An effective apical seal could be obtained with both techniques when they were used with a sealer. The presence or absence of the smear layer had no significant effect on the apical seal in vitro. It was recommended that the use of injected thermoplasticized gutta-percha be accompanied by the use of a sealer, whether or not the smear layer has been removed.

Like all injection techniques, the Ultrafil technique stresses the importance of maintaining the integrity of the apical foramen; therefore *a constriction or "stop" at the dentin-cementum junction must be maintained to restrict the flow of gutta-percha beyond the apex*. The canal is flared back from the apical foramen and should be prepared to receive a 22-gauge needle inserted approximately 6 mm from the working length, since the plasticized gutta-percha will flow 6 to 8 mm to reach the apex. This size can be obtained by enlarging the middle third of the canal with a No. 2 or 3 Gates-Glidden bur or a No. 70 file.

In case of an open apex, an apical "stop" or plug may be created by any of the following three methods:

1. "Dry-file the canal walls and pack the dentin chips at the apex, using a file or a finger plugger" (Hygienic Corporation UltraFil pamphlet). Dentin chips can be produced by a Hedström file or Gates-Glidden bur.
2. Fit a primary cone very snugly at the apex. After cementation, remove most of the cone with a hot endodontic excavator spoon or a hot plugger. The remaining apical section will act as a stop. The injected thermoplasticized gutta-percha will flow around the gutta-percha point but not beyond the apex (Figs. 9-64 and 9-65).
3. For most cases, the creation of an *apical plug* or stop is advisable. Select a K file one size smaller than the last apical file and set a stop marker at working length. Sterilize the file and insert about 2 to 3 mm of its tip in the

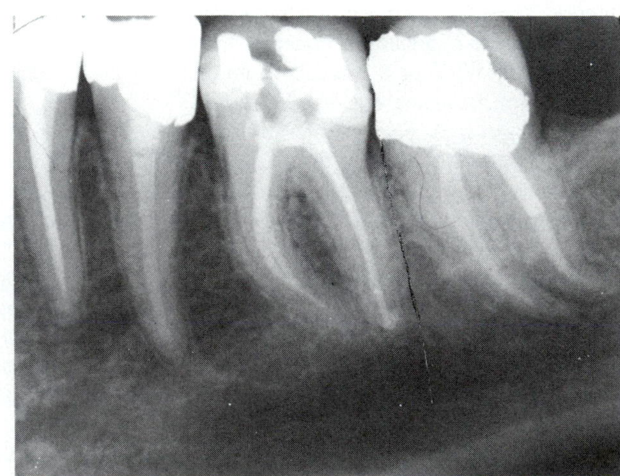

FIG. 9-65 Postfilling radiograph of tooth no. 19 obturated with a combination of sealer and master cone, condensed and injected with Ultrafil FirmSet. Teeth 18, 20, and 21 were filled with lateral condensation technique. The radiographic density appears similar. (Courtesy Dr. A. Michanowicz.)

preheated SuccessFil gutta-percha syringe, to pick up a small amount of the high-viscosity gutta-percha (Fig. 9-63, *E*). Without twisting the file, immediately insert it into the canal to the full working length. Immediately rotate the file counterclockwise to deposit the gutta-percha at the apex. The high-viscosity gutta-percha will remain at the apex as the file is quickly withdrawn. In curved canals a wiggling motion is used to remove the file. With a small plugger prefitted within 1 mm of the working length, condense the still soft gutta-percha to eliminate the void left by removal of the file. Alcohol is used as a separating medium (Hygienic Corporation pamphlet).

The Ultrafil system using low temperature (70° C) in conjunction with a sealer appears promising. The minimal amount of time required to fill the root canal system, and the fact that manual condensation is not needed, offer additional appeal. The Ultrafil Trifecta system has evolved into an obturation technique that offers more versatility and adaptability for varied obturation techniques and also greater control of overfills and short fills to three-dimensionally obturate the root canal system. Because it is relatively nontechnique sensitive and adheres to traditionally accepted standards, it has gained increased acceptance with clinicians.

Thermafil endodontic obturators

An innovative approach to obturating the root canal system with stainless steel files and thermally plasticized gutta-percha, in conjunction with a sealer, was reported by Johnson in 1978.[52] Mynol (Mynol Chemical Co., Broomall, Pa.) gutta-percha is used to coat the last file used to prepare the apex of the root canal system. The file is prenotched so that it will break at a predetermined point, depending on whether the need for a dowel is anticipated. A small amount of sealer is used to coat the canal walls. The gutta-percha–coated file is warmed in a flame until the gutta-percha glistens. The file with the thermally plasticized gutta-percha is inserted into the canal with a firm apical pressure to the working length. While pressure is maintained, the shank of the file is twisted off or broken off by bending it back and forth, and is removed. The gutta-percha is then condensed vertically around the file with a small lubricated plugger. Johnson obtained impressive results with this technique.

Since then, Johnson's technique has been refined, improved, systematized, and made commercially available as the *Thermafil Endodontic Obturators* (Tulsa Dental Products, Tulsa, Okla.). Originally the Thermafil Obturator device is a specifically designed flexible stainless steel, titanium, or plastic carrier coated with alpha phase gutta-percha and adapted with a sliding rubber stop for precise length measurement and control during canal insertion at obturation time.

Alpha phase gutta-percha has the same chemical formula as the commonly used gutta-percha points that are in the beta phase. The difference lies in the fact that the alpha phase gutta-percha has been annealed with a proprietary process to obtain a different crystalline structure and physical properties. When plasticized by heat, alpha phase gutta-percha has excellent flow characteristics. It becomes sticky and more adhesive and exhibits a wetting phenomenon, causing it to adhere to the helix-shaped core of the stainless steel carrier. This wetting phenomenon allows the gutta-percha to be transported into the canal toward the apex without being stripped from the helical flutes of the central carrier. When heated, beta phase gutta-percha, as used in conventional points, becomes deformable but has poor flow characteristics and less stickiness.

The Thermafil technique, when used properly, can provide a rapid three-dimensional obturation of the canal with precise apical control, because it eliminates the time consumed in the fitting, apical placement, and condensation of a master cone. *The carrier is not the primary cone for obturation. It acts as a carrier and condenser for the thermally plasticized alpha phase gutta-percha* and seems to be capable of forcing the softened gutta-percha to the apex and, laterally, to fill the irregularities of root canal walls and accessory canals (Fig. 9-66).

Thermafil obturators are sized from 20 to 140 and are color coded to correspond to endodontic instruments (Fig. 9-67). They can be used effectively in small and curved canals, owing to the flexibility of the carriers. In a severely curved canal the Thermafil metal carrier may be precurved with thumb and index finger before it is heated, to facilitate its placement. Thermafil plastic carriers are inherently flexible and need not be precurved.

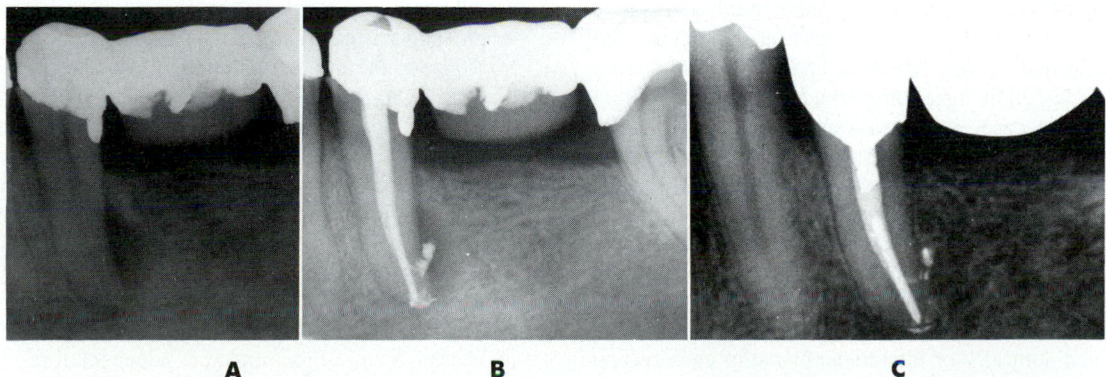

FIG. 9-66 Mandibular second premolar obturated with Thermafil technique. **A,** Pretreatment. The location of the periradicular lesion suggests the possibility of lateral canals along the distal aspect of the root. **B,** Postfilling radiograph showing lateral canals filled. **C,** Three years later; good osseous repair. (Courtesy Dr. B. Johnson.)

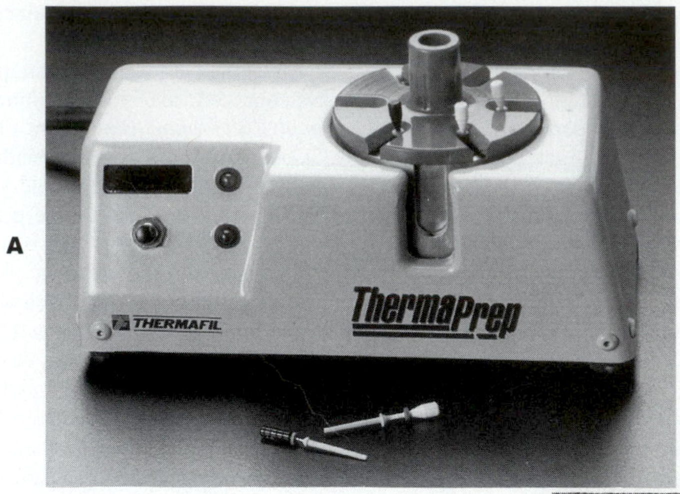

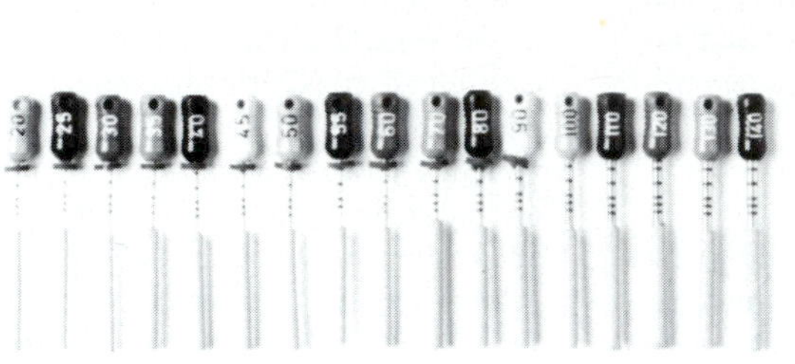

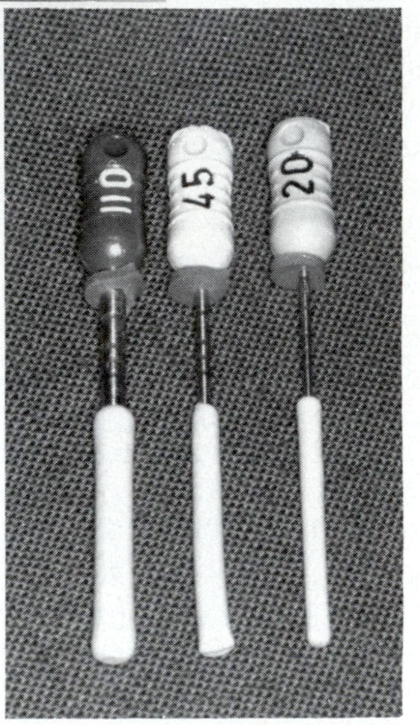

FIG. 9-67 A, Therma Prep oven provides a stable heat source with more control and uniformity for the heating of Thermafil obturators and plastic and metal carriers. **B,** Thermafil obturators (sizes 20 to 140) are color coded and sized to correspond to endodontic instruments. **C,** Close-up of sizes 20, 45, and 110. (Courtesy Thermafil, Tulsa Dental Products, Tulsa, Okla.)

Thermafil procedure. In the Thermafil obturation procedure, the canal preparation has less flare in its occlusal half compared with that in the vertical compaction or the thermoplasticized gutta-percha injection methods. As with all obturation methods, the canal preparation must be performed carefully and completely with good débridement and proper cleansing and shaping. Difficulties encountered in this technique are often due to inadequate canal preparation. The goal of canal preparation is to create a smoothly tapering funnel-shaped canal with its terminus at the apical constriction. The step-back technique from the apex or crown down are effective and popular canal preparation methods. Copious irrigation, particularly when activated sonically or ultrasonically, after each recapitulation enhances débridement and maintains canal patency. When the canal preparation is completed, the last file used in the apical terminus must fit easily without binding.

Final working length verification and selection of obturator. The length of the master apical file, or preferably an appropriate Size Verification Carrier, is verified by a radiograph. This ensures that the selected Thermafil obturator of the same size as the master apical file or the Size Verification Carrier will go to the full working length without being forced by rotation or twisting. The silicone stop marker is then adjusted to reflect this measurement on the shaft of the Thermafil obturator. The obturator is placed in a 5.25% sodium hypochlorite solution for 1 minute to disinfect the gutta-percha and then is washed in 70% alcohol solution.

The canal is thoroughly dried, then coated with a *very light coating of sealer* by means of a paper point or sonic applicator. Although the Thermafil corporation recommends the use of Therma Seal, a biocompatible noneugenol resin sealer with a good dentin adhesion and flow rate, others sealers such as AH-26, Sealapex (Kerr Dental Products Romulus, Mich.), Roth's, or Kerr pulp canal sealer may be used. Sealers that set too quickly when in contact with heat, such as Hygienic's CRCS or Kerr's Tubliseal, or sealers that exhibit extreme flow

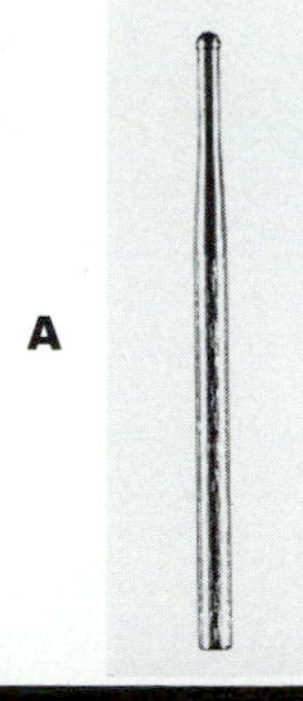

FIG. 9-68 A, Prepi bur. Smooth, round-headed bur for cutting the thermatic plastic obturator for post space preparation. Thermafil normal obturation procedure. **B,** The Thermafil obturator has been heated in the blue zone of an open flame until the gutta-percha develops a surface sheen and begins to expand slightly. Ready for insertion into canal. **C,** Thermafil device inserted into canal to previously marked working length. **D,** The shaft is severed 1 to 2 mm above canal orifice with a no. 37 inverted cone bur and removed. (Courtesy Dr. B. Johnson.)

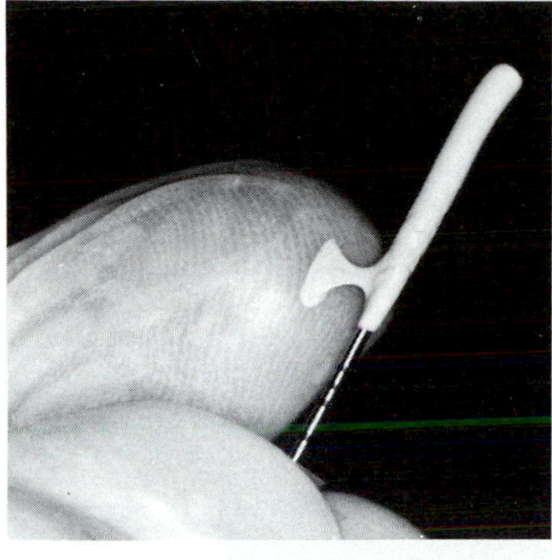

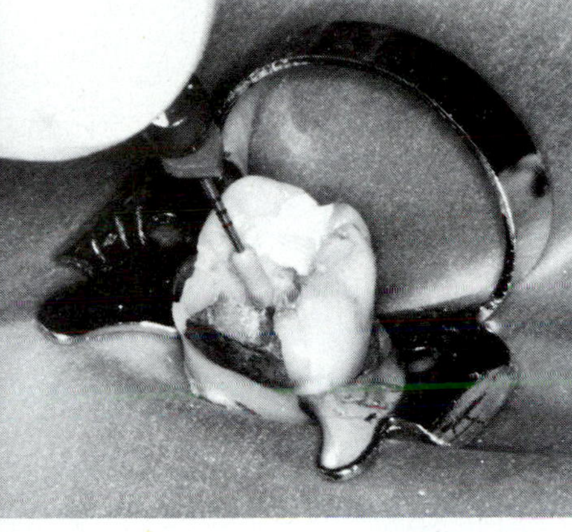

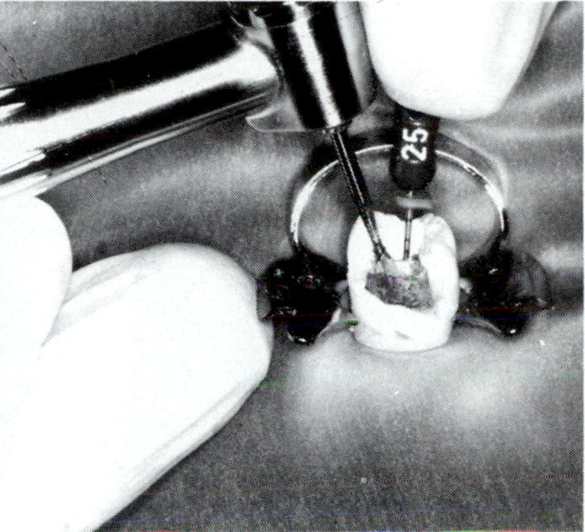

characteristics such as Wach's paste or Lee's Endofil are not recommended for the Thermafil technique.[85]

Heating of Thermafil obturators. Thermafil obturators may be heated over an open flame or in the Therma Prep oven. One study[16] reported different results with regard to apical leakage of roots filled with the Thermafil technique. Some of the problems may be due to insufficient heating or overheating of the gutta-percha before insertion. An oven is now available that offers a stable heat source with more control and uniformity for plasticizing the gutta-percha (Fig. 9-67). The oven is useful for heating plastic obturators which cannot be heated over an open flame.

When an open flame is used, a few passes of the Thermafil metal obturator in the cooler blue zone of the flame are sufficient to heat the alpha phase gutta-percha to proper consistency. Rotating the device between the fingers will ensure even heating. When the gutta-percha develops a surface sheen and begins to expand slightly, the device is inserted with firm apical pressure into the canal until it reaches the previously marked working length (Fig. 9-68, *B* and *C*).

When the Therma Prep oven is used it must be preheated at least 20 minutes before the obturators are heated. Smaller-sized obturators no. 20 to 35 require a minimum of 3 to 4 minutes' heating time and should not be heated more than 7 to 10 minutes. Plastic obturators no. 25 to 35 will suffer carrier deformation if heated longer than 10 minutes. Larger-sized obturators no. 40 to 140 take about 5 to 7 minutes to plasticize and should not be heated longer than 15 to 20 minutes. A timer must be used to ensure correct heating time. When obturating multirooted teeth it is more time efficient to obturate smaller canals first, as the larger obturators take more time to plasticize. An oven-plasticized obturator will exhibit a definite surface sheen, similar to that of an obturator heated over a flame. After removing the obturator from the oven the clinician has about 8 to 10 seconds' working time. Firm apical pressure is used to insert the Thermafil obturator to the previously marked working length. As the oven can heat three to six obturators at one time it is a good precaution to heat an extra obturator of each size. If an additional obturator is needed for any reason, the obturation procedure can proceed without loss of time or concern that the sealer might set while waiting for another obturator to be plasticized.

After radiographic verification the carrier shaft is severed to a point 1 to 2 mm above the canal orifice while applying firm finger pressure to the obturator handle (Fig. 9-68, *C*). The handle is removed and discarded. A small condenser lubricated with vaseline or lidocaine topical anesthetic is used to condense vertically the gutta-percha around the shaft. When filling a multirooted tooth, the same steps are repeated for the other canals after the removal of any excess of gutta-percha that may block their orifices.

When the use of a dowel or post is anticipated, the Thermafil device is notched with a fissure bur at a predetermined point to allow for adequate post space (Fig. 9-69, *A*). A properly notched carrier should have enough axial strength for insertion, yet be weak enough to fracture when twisted off after complete seating. The heated Thermafil device should be inserted to the full working length without rotation. Rotating the device during insertion may cause premature separation. The excess shaft is removed by maintaining firm apical pressure on the instrument while *twisting it counterclockwise*. The counterclockwise rotation pumps gutta-percha toward the apex and causes the instrument to snap off. Rotating an insufficiently notched carrier in a clockwise direction may screw it

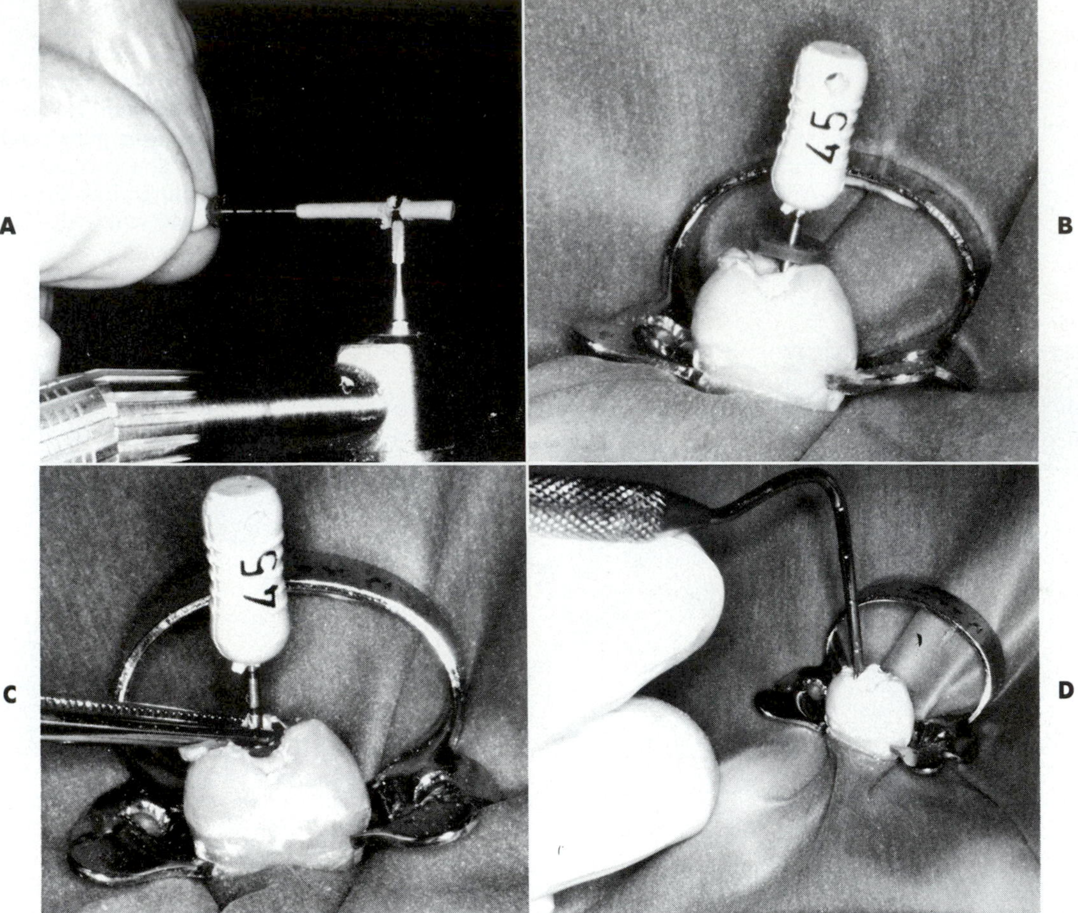

FIG. 9-69 Thermofil obturation when a post is planned for eventual placement. **A,** Nicking the carrier lightly with a no. 1558 fissure bur while rotating device until the tip is close to severing (approximately to a diameter of 13 to 18 thousandths of an inch). **B,** Device inserted into canal to previously determined working length after the gutta-percha has been heated as described. **C,** Cotton pliers pushing rubber stop against the orifice while handle is pulled out of canal. **D,** Plugger pushed on wet cotton pellet, compacting gutta-percha to fill any voids left by removal of shaft. (Courtesy Dr. B. Johnson.)

past the apex. It is therefore very important for the clinician to practice notching on several old files to gain the needed experience. After the removal of the occlusal portion of the handle and shaft, a small lubricated plugger is used to compact the gutta-percha over the severed top of the carrier. The canal is now ready for post preparation.

If a post is needed in a canal filled with a thermatic plastic obturator, a friction grip, long-shank bur with smooth noncutting round head called the *Prepi bur* is used (Fig. 9-68, *A*). The bur used in a high-speed handpiece with water spray generates frictional heat to melt away the plastic and remove the gutta-percha to the appropriate depth for subsequent post preparation. The bur's smooth noncutting head eliminates the risk of root perforation. It is available in assorted sizes to facilitate post space preparation in canals of different sizes.

If dowel construction is only planned for eventual placement, the canal may be filled with gutta-percha as follows: A pair of cotton pliers is used to slide the rubber stop marker against the canal orifice. While the rubber stop is pressed down with the cotton pliers, the severed handle is pulled out, leaving the gutta-percha behind in the canal space. The rubber stop marker is then removed, and a wet cotton pellet is placed over the canal orifice. Vertical condensation is carried out by pushing on the cotton pellet with a proper sized plugger to fill compactly any voids left by the removal of the shaft (Fig. 9-69, *B-D*).

The Thermafil obturation method, when properly used, can deliver the gutta-percha precisely where it is needed with good apical control. The technique can be used effectively in curved and narrow canals as well as in canals with large apical openings. Recent studies[16,36,85] have reported favorably on the sealing ability of the Thermafil obturators. The technique has gained increased popularity among practicing dentists in the United States and abroad.

CANAL OBTURATION WITH PASTES

Pastes may be either soft or semisolid. They are composed mostly of zinc oxide with various additives, to which glycerin or an essential oil (usually eugenol) is added. They can be freshly mixed before use (soft paste) or come premixed and ready for use (Cavit, a semisolid paste).

Pastes have been used as the sole canal-filling material.

Some paste formulas contain iodoform, which is radiopaque and absorbable. Maisto and Erausquin[62] suggested a slowly absorbable, antiseptic paste of iodoform and other additives and used it in conjunction with gutta-percha points. Overfilling can cause the patient to experience a great deal of discomfort until absorption takes place. To consistently obtain a dense nonporous filling using a creamy paste, in comparison with the more reliable use of a solid cone and sealer to obturate the canal space, is rather difficult. The hazard of relying on absorbable pastes as filling materials lies in the difficulty of eliminating entrapped air within the filling. If the entrapped air creates voids near the apical foramen, both leakage and percolation of exudate into the canal space may occur. Also, in the absence of positive pressure, pastes cannot effectively fill accessory canals.

One instance in which pastes, despite their low density and their tendency to be easily forced out beyond the apical foramen, may prove useful is in the filling of root canals of primary teeth. The paste will be absorbed along with the physiologic resorption of the roots. A thick paste made of zinc oxide and eugenol may be packed into the canals of primary molars by means of a Jiffy tube and pluggers. Radiographic verification is used to control the depth of the paste filling to confine it within the canal space.

Pressure Syringe Injection Technique

Krakow and Berk[58] popularized the pressure syringe developed by Greenberg[33] (Fig. 9-47). The pressure syringe provides an effective method of introducing the sealer into the canal. The root canal may be filled entirely with cement without a solid core of gutta-percha or silver cone.

A modified Wach's extrafine cement is mixed, loaded in the pressure syringe, and introduced with a fine needle to about 2 mm from the apical foramen. The position of the needle is determined by a marker and verified by a radiograph. The cement is extruded by giving the handle of the syringe a quarter turn. Additional cement is extruded from the syringe into the canal by stages until the canal is completely filled with cement.

The pressure syringe injection technique seems to be useful for filling fine, tortuous canals that cannot be negotiated with instruments, filling primary teeth, and filling some large canals. The control of excessive extrusions of cement into the periapical space can be a difficult task.

N-2 and Related Pastes

N-2 root canal-filling material, introduced by Sargenti,[76] may be called a paste. N-2 is advocated for use in "sterilizing" and filling the root canal, usually in one treatment. During the past 30 years, N-2 as a root canal-filling material and the N-2 method have been the objects of considerable controversial discussion. The material and technique employed appear to be a modification of the so-called mummification technique no longer popular in the United States but still practiced in some parts of Europe.

The composition and name of N-2 have been changed repeatedly during the last 25 years. Preparations of N-2 (R-C, RC-2B, RET-B, etc.) contain (along with zinc oxide and eugenol) paraformaldehyde (basis of many of the old mummification techniques), an organic mercury compound (phenylmercuric borate), lead oxide, and corticosteroids.

Scientific studies[12] have indicated the potential danger of the N-2 formulas to patients. The material has essentially been banned in a number of countries, in California, and in several branches of the U.S. Armed Forces. Therefore, no further discussion of the techniques or their use seems appropriate in this book.

Problems Inherent in Injection Technique

All pastes, cements, plastic and plasticized materials, or resins placed into the canal space by pumping, spiraling with a Lentulo, or injection with pressure syringes share some common difficulties or problems.

1. It is difficult to control *overextension,* with its attendant tissue inflammatory responses and discomfort. The literature is replete with case histories ranging from mild reactions to severe reactions with bone loss and paresthesia.[3,76,114] Although initial reports on silicone resins[59,106] appear favorable, practically all filling materials are toxic and cause inflammatory tissue responses, particularly materials containing formaldehyde and its derivatives.[17,81] Zinc oxide–eugenol, a long-time standard against which other sealers were measured, is quite toxic[4] when compared with N-2, Rickert's, and Cavit. As the cement sealers reach their final set, the initial inflammatory reaction usually subsides and healing takes place unless the material continues to break down, releasing toxic products of some of its components. In all pumping or injection filling methods the maintenance of an apical constriction is of paramount importance. Recent improvements in pressure syringe design provided some degree of control of overfillings.
2. It is difficult to control *underextension* with injection or pumping techniques. There is no assurance of sealing efficacy, since it is not easy to precisely and securely control or compact viscous or pasty materials. This may lead to incomplete obturation, with partially filled canal spaces. Underextension along with material resorption and solubility would lead to fluid percolation, with subsequent periapical inflammation. In a study using Adaptic, AH-26, Cavit, Durelon, and ZOE cement placed in canals by pressure syringe, Fogel reported that after 30 days all filling exhibited seepage, with AH-26 showing the least marginal leakage.[26]
3. It is difficult to prevent *voids* in the body of the filling. If a void is located opposite a patent accessory canal or the foramen, fluid percolation would occur and complete healing may be in jeopardy. Sealant materials containing relatively more radiopacifiers such as lead, silver, bismuth, iodine, or barium may give the impression of compactness despite the presence of minor voids in the body of the filling. Eucapercha or chloropercha pastes pumped into the canal space will shrink substantially as the solvent evaporates. Voids are likely to develop, and the seal may be affected.[123] The Ultrafil low-temperature (70° C) gutta-percha injection technique does not advocate hand compaction after injection. This poses a serious question of possible void development or poor density resulting from shrinkage of gutta-percha as it cools from 70° C to body temperature. Additionally, during the mixing of a paste or silicone resin, a too rapid stirring or whipping motion is to be avoided because it may incorporate air bubbles in the mixture.
4. It is difficult to effectively and securely fill the complex root canal system, including accessory canals, with pastes, cements, or plastic materials because of the *lack of positive pressure.*

On the basis of the attributes and shortcomings of cements, pastes, and plastic or plasticized materials used without a solid core, one cannot help but feel a strong reservation about their routine use.

Solid Core Material with a Cement Sealant

On the basis of published studies, the most reliable and predictable endodontic seal available at present is that of a solid core compacted into the canal space with a cement sealant. The core material should be able to be plasticized enough to allow for as minimal a reliance on the sealant as possible. The sealant acts as cement to fill discrepancies between the core material and canal walls, including patent accessory canals. Gutta-percha is the currently recommended core material. Popular sealant cements include Rickert's and Grossman formulas and the resin AH-26; a newly introduced silicone resin or rubber sealant has also gained increasing popularity.

The choice of obturation method or a combination of methods best suited to treat and fill three-dimensionally a specific root canal system is left substantially to the discretion of the individual clinician.

However, regardless of the obturation technique used, a well-cleansed and shaped canal with a tapered flare and a definite constriction or minimal opening at the dentin-cementum junction makes it easier to obtain a well-compacted three-dimensional filling of the root canal system.

Lee Endo Fill has not received the support of the profession; therefore the technique will not be described in detail in this edition. (Interested readers may refer to the fifth edition of this book for details of this technique.)

Filling with Dentin Chips and Apical Plug

In the perpetual search for biocompatible materials, and as a result of the desire to keep irritating products from apical contact, clinicians became increasingly interested in dentin chip filling. Dentinal plugs inadvertently formed, even while clinicians were trying to avoid forming them, seemed to create an effective apical barrier against which healing could occur. A deliberate dentin-chips filling technique was born. Essentially it consists of filling at least the apical 1 mm of the root apex with dentin chips to block the foramen. Other materials, usually gutta-percha with a sealer, are then compacted against this apical plug barrier, or "biologic seal."

Dentin chips are produced only after the canal has been properly debrided and shaped, sanitized, and dried. A Hedström file or a Gates-Glidden bur is used to produce dentin powder from the occlusal two thirds of the canal. A small plugger or the blunt end of a paper point may be utilized to push the dentin chips apically. Care must be taken to gather scattered chips raised by the file or bur around the pulp chamber floor and to pack them apically. A file 1 or 2 sizes larger than the master key file or a very small plugger or a paper point may be used for this purpose. With a no. 15 or 20 file the apical plug is tested for completeness of density. A dense plug of at least 1 mm in thickness should offer resistance to perforation by the file. The canal is then obturated with gutta-percha in conjunction with a sealer or with other plastic materials or silicone rubber.

This technique is popular mostly in Europe. One study[6] reported apical closure with "osteodentin" proportional to the thickness of the dentin plug, with some incomplete calcification across all the serial sections. Another study[112] found healing in monkey teeth into which apical plugs had been introduced. Still another study[89] found more rapid healing where dentin plugs had been created, even when the foramen was perforated. Investigators[21] found that dentin plugs were most effective in confining irrigating solutions and filling materials within the canal space.

However, other investigations reflect less favorably on the technique. Recently it was found[51] that leakage was greater in teeth with dentin plugs than in those without. Others[10,122] also found the apical plug to be of dubious value.

Infected dentin chips may be a serious deterrent to healing[48] and may actually irritate and hinder repair.[111]

Calcium Hydroxide Pastes as Sealers and Apical Plugs

The success of calcium hydroxide and calcium phosphate formulations in achieving apical closure in cases of open apices has stimulated the use of calcium compounds as sealers, paste fillings, or apical plugs.[49,55,59,79,85] One study[90] reported that calcium hydroxide plugs and dentin plugs resulted in significant calcification at the foramen. However, the calcification observed with the dentin plugs was more complete than that observed with calcium hydroxide plugs. Another investigation[46] found that calcium hydroxide plugs produce a periapical response that overall is indistinguishable from that produced by dentin plugs.

Calcium hydroxide or calcium compounds may be carried into the canal by means of a small amalgam carrier normally used in retrofilling. The Messing amalgam carrier, particularly the newly designed carrier with curved tips, may be suitable for this purpose. A small plugger or paper point is used to push and pack the material apically, forming an apical plug or barrier against which the core material, usually gutta-percha, and a sealant are condensed.

The search for the perfect filling material continues. Some clinicians have experimented with calcium compounds such as Proplast or used a cross-linked collagen-calcium phosphate gel to induce dentinogenesis and cementogenesis and apical closure. Others used silicone resin as a sole sealant and filling, delivered by a precision micrometer syringe, not to mention the use of ultrasonic devices to enhance sealer placement and canal obturation.[115]

The quest for a beyond-the-space-age endodontic filling material has many ardent followers. This would be a magical material that satisfies all of Grossman's requirements and other requirements as listed on page 223; a material fluid enough and viscous enough to flow into all the ramifications of the root canal system and form a mechanical and even chemical bond with the dentinal tubules; a perfectly biocompatible material capable of inducing dentinogenesis and cementogenesis and apical closure. When the ideal material and the perfect delivery system become a reality, the task of obturating the "pathways of the pulp" will be a joyful labor of love.

APICAL EXTENT OF ROOT CANAL FILLINGS

The question whether the canal should be filled flush with, short of, or beyond the radiographic apex merits clarification. The radiographic apex is where the root apex appears on the radiograph to join the periodontal ligament. The vast majority of endodontists prefer filling the canal to the dentin-cementum junction (essentially the apical foramen) so as not to impinge on the periapical tissues, permitting, hopefully, physiologic

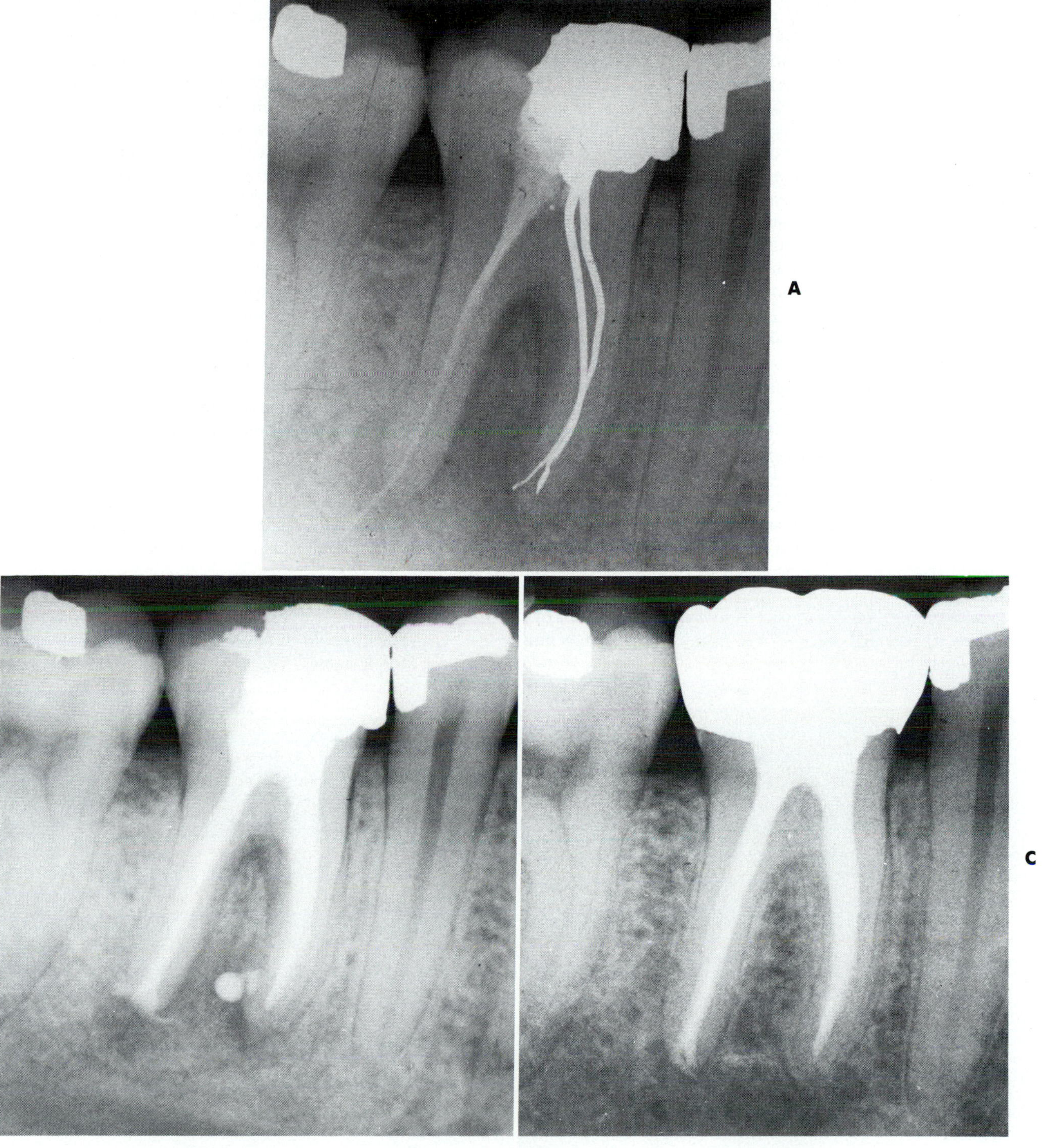

FIG. 9-70 Mandibular first molar filled with silver cones. **A,** Note the grossly overextended and underfilled distal canals and the loose cones in the mesial canals. **B,** After removal of the cones. Retreatment with gutta-percha cones as the filling material. Note the overfilling and the extruding cement. **C,** Eighteen months later, good osseous repair with complete absorption of sealer.

closure of the root canal by cementum. The vertical position of the dentin-cementum junction varies with each tooth. It may be located 0.5 to 2 or 3 mm from the radiographic apex. Filling the canal so it appears flush with the radiographic apex produces esthetically pleasing radiographs; however, in reality, the filling is probably slightly overextended beyond the apical foramen, especially in roots curved in a buccal-lingual direction. Because of the physics of dental radiography, the true extent of root curvature seldom appears on the radiograph (Chapter 4). The most desirable vertical extent of the root canal filling is a homogeneously dense filling extending 0.5 to 1 mm short of the radiographic apex. An overwhelming majority of successful cases have been obturated in this manner (Fig. 9-7). In cases of vital extirpation, fillings slightly underextended are much more comfortable to the patient than are fillings extended to the radiographic apex.

Contrary to the old suggestion of filling to the radiographic apex or slightly beyond in cases with an area of rarefaction, we have observed countless successful cases with periapical lesions filled nonsurgically to 0.5 to 2 mm short of the radiographic apex. Emphasis should be on how densely and how well the entire root canal space is obturated.

Schilder[97] emphasized the distinction between overfilling and underfilling and between overextension and underextension.

In *overfilling,* the canal space is entirely obturated, with a surplus of material extruding beyond the apical foramen (Fig. 9-70). In overfilling, the apical seal is obtained and success is the usual outcome of treatment (Figs. 9-4, 9-5, 9-35, and 9-36).

In *underfilling,* the canal space is incompletely filled, leaving voids as potential areas of recontamination and infection (Fig. 9-6, *A*).

Overextension and *underextension* refer merely to the vertical extent of the root canal filling, independent of its volume.[97] An overextended filling may actually be grossly underfilled; there may be large dead spaces or voids in the pulp canal, leading to fluid percolation and ultimate failure (Fig. 9-70, *A*).

A serious effort to compact the filling material vertically, therefore, should be made to obtain a dense, homogeneous-appearing filling in its entire mass. A filling may seem dense from the buccal-lingual view but may be grossly underfilled from the mesial-distal view (Fig. 9-71). Although the tight apical seal is of prime importance for the success of endodontic treatment, the sealing of patent accessory canals at locations other than the root apex is no less important in enhancing the chance of success toward that perfect 100%. An endodontic implant (not FDA approved) used to improve the crown/root ratio is an intentional overfilling with metal cones. Many failures observed in endodontic implants come from lack of an apical seal. Concern for an apical seal has led many clinicians to overfill the canal in an effort to obtain a tight seal or an apical "button" at the foramen (Fig. 9-72, *A*).

Sealers currently in use are more or less toxic when freshly mixed. Gross excess of filling materials beyond the apical foramen is an *unnecessary* invasion of the attachment apparatus, resulting in needless postfilling pain and discomfort. Fortunately, tissue tolerance to commonly used filling materials is high, the excess sealer usually is absorbed, and the prognosis is for ultimate success (Fig. 9-70, *B*).

PATIENT INSTRUCTION AFTER CANAL OBTURATION

The patient should be advised that the tooth may be slightly tender for a few days. The discomfort may be due to sensitiv-

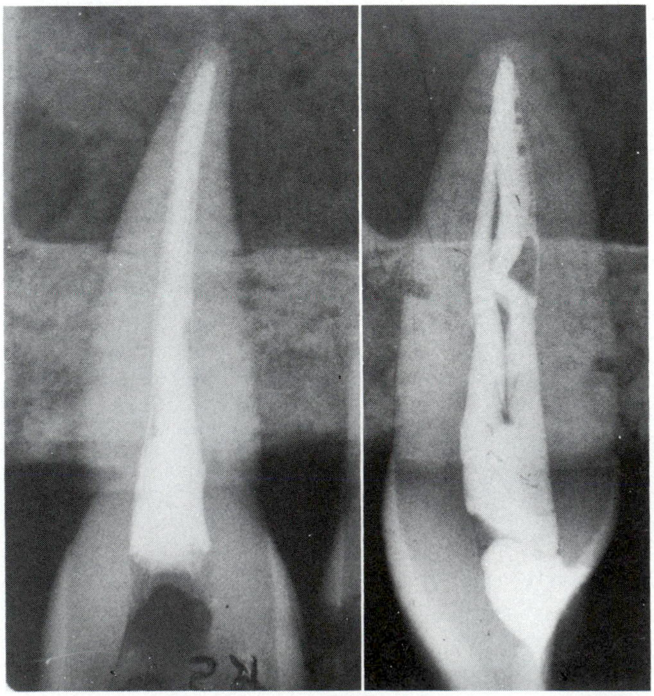

A B

FIG. 9-71 A, Labial-lingual view of a central incisor. The canal appears well-filled. **B,** Mesial-distal view. Note the gross underfilling and the large voids in the body of the filling.

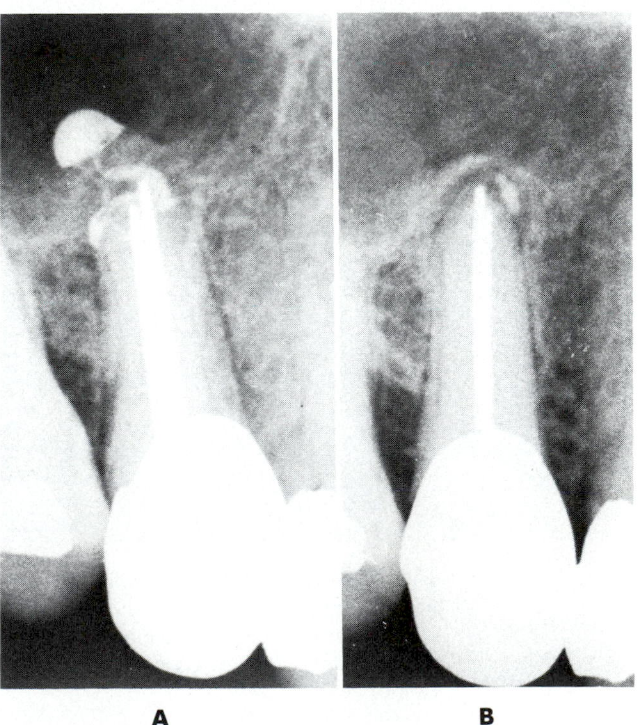

A B

FIG. 9-72 A, Maxillary premolar filled with silver cones. Note the massive excess of sealer extruded into the maxillary sinus. **B,** Nine months later, almost complete absorption of sealer.

ity to the possible excess of filling materials pushed beyond the apical foramen. Excess sealer is usually absorbed in a few months (Fig. 9-72, *B*). Pain from temporary apical inflammation may be relieved by nonsteroidal antiinflammatory drugs, analgesics, and frequent warm saline rinses (1 level teaspoon salt per 8-ounce glass of very warm water). The patient is advised to hold the warm water in the affected area for 10 seconds, empty the mouth, and repeat the procedure until the entire glass of warm salt water has been used. If swelling occurs, cold compresses or an ice bag should be applied on the face over the affected area: on 10 minutes, off 5 minutes, for several hours. This intraoral warming and extraoral chilling is usually effective in relieving postendodontic swelling and discomfort. Antiinflammatory drugs such as corticosteroids together with an antibiotic may be prescribed in severe cases. The patient should be advised not to chew unduly on the tooth until it is protected by a permanent restoration.

RECALL CHECKUP

A recall checkup for clinical evaluation of tissue repair and healing progress should be arranged before the patient is dismissed. If bone loss is extensive or the therapy was unusual or prolonged, the first recall checkup should be within 3 months; in most cases, patients are recalled in 6 months. A comparison of the new radiograph with the preceding one should show continued regeneration of bone. Complete bone regeneration and healing require a few months to more than one year. The periapical tissue of an endodontically treated tooth without an area of rarefaction should continue to appear normal at the recall checkup. The radiograph of a successful root canal filling should show the periodontal ligament with a uniform thickness and the lamina dura continuous along the lateral surfaces of the root and around the apex. A break in the continuity of the lamina dura around the apex should be questioned as evidence of possible pathologic disturbance. The root canal filling should appear homogeneously dense and filled to the dentin-cementum junction. The tooth should be entirely comfortable to the patient and be serviceable as a useful member of the masticating apparatus.

SUMMARY

The aim of canal obturation is to fill the entire volume of the root canal space, including patent accessory canals and multiple foramina, completely and densely with biologically inert and compatible filling materials. Regardless of the technique used, a serious effort should be made to obtain a hermetic apical seal and contain the filling material within the confines of the root canal. An endodontic cavity preparation with a slight flare and a definite constriction or minimal opening at the dentin-cementum junction makes it easier to obtain a three-dimensional, well-condensed gutta-percha filling with minimal apical excess. Needless invasion of the periapical space with gross excess of filling materials has no biologic justification and must be avoided.

REFERENCES

1. Alexander JB, and Gordon TM: A comparison of the apical seal produced by two calcium hydroxide sealers and a Grossman-type sealer when used with laterally condensed gutta-percha, Quint Int 16:615, 1985.
2. Allison D, Weber C, and Walton R: The influence of the method of canal preparation on the quality of apical and coronal obturation, J Endod 5:298, 1979.
3. Antrim DD: Evaluation of the cytotoxicity of root canal sealing agents on tissue culture cells in vitro: Grossman's sealer, N_2 (permanent), Rickert's sealer and Cavit, J Endod 2:111, 1978.
4. Barkhordar RA, and Nguyen NT: Paresthesia of the mental nerve after overextension with AH-26 and gutta-percha: report of case, J Am Dent Assoc 110:202, 1985.
5. Barry GN, and Fried IL: Sealing quality of two polycarboxylate cements used as root canal sealers, J Endod 1:107, 1975.
6. Baume L, Holz J, and Risk LB: Radicular pulpotomy for category III pulps, parts I to III, J Prosthet Dent 25:418, 1971.
7. Benner MD, et al: Evaluation of a new thermoplastic gutta-percha obturation technique using ^{45}Ca, J Endod 7:500, 1981.
8. Block RM, et al: Cell-mediated immune response to dog pulp tissue altered by Kerr (Rickert's) sealer via the root canal, J Endod 4:110, 1978.
9. Block RM, et al: Cell-mediated response to dog pulp tissue altered by N_2 paste within the root canal, Oral Surg 45:131, 1978.
10. Bowman GA: History of dentistry in Missouri, Fulton, Mo, 1983, Ovid Bell Press.
11. Brady JE, Himal VT, and Weir JC: Periapical response to an apical plug of dentin fillings intentionally placed over root canal overcementation, J Endod 11:323, 1985.
12. Brewer DL: Histology of apical tissue reaction to overfill (Sargenti formula vs gutta-percha-Grossman), J Calif Dent Assoc 3:58, 1975.
13. Callahan JR: Resin solution for the sealing of the dentinal tubuli and as an adjuvant in the filling of root canals, J Allied Dent Soc 9:53, 1914.
14. Casanova F: Understanding of some clinically significant physical properties of Kerr sealer through investigation. Thesis, Boston University, 1975.
15. Chohayeb A: Comparison of conventional root canal obturation techniques with Thermafil obturators, JOE 18:1992.
16. Clark CS, El Deeb ME: Apical sealing ability of metal versus plastic carrier thermafil obturators, J Endod 19:4, 1993.
17. Cohler CM, et al: Studies of Sargenti's technique of endodontic treatment: short term response in monkeys, J Endod 6:473, 1980.
18. Crane DL, et al: Biological and physical properties of an experimental root canal sealer without eugenol, J Endod 6:438, 1980.
19. Czonstkowsky M, Michanowicz AE, and Vasquez JA: Evaluation of an injection of thermoplasticized low-temperature gutta-percha using radioactive isotopes, J Endod 11:71, 1985.
20. Dow PR, and Ingle JI: Isotope determination of root canal failure, Oral Surg 8:1100, 1955.
21. El Deeb ME, Nguyen TTQ, and Jensen JR: The dentinal plug: its effects on confining substances to the canal and on the apical seal, J Endod 9:355, 1983.
22. Erausquin J, and Muruzabal M: Response to periapical tissues in the rat molar to root canal fillings with Diaket and AH-26, Oral Surg 21:786, 1966.
23. Erausquin J, and Muruzabal M: Tissue reactions to root canal cements in the rat molar, Oral Surg 26:360, Sept 1968.
24. Evans JT, and Simon JS: Evaluation of the apical seal produced by injected thermoplasticized gutta-percha in the absence of smear layer and root canal sealer, J Endod 12:101, 1986.
25. Feldman G, and Nyborg H: Tissue reaction to root canal filling material, Odontol Revy 15:33, 1964.
26. Fogel BA: A comparative study of five materials for use in filling root canal spaces, Oral Surg 43:284, 1977.
27. Food and Drug Administration: Memorandum to state drug officials, Washington, DC, 1974, US Government Printing Office.
28. Formaldehyde—an assessment of its health effect, National Academy of Sciences, March 1980.
29. Goldberg F, and Gurfinkel J: Analysis of the use of Dycal with gutta percha points as an endodontic filling technique, Oral Surg 47:78, 1979.
30. Goldman A, Schilder H, and Aldrich W: The thermomechanical properties of gutta percha, II. The history and molecular chemistry of gutta-percha, Oral Surg 37:954, 1974.
31. Goodman A, Schilder H, and Aldrich W: The thermomechanical

properties of gutta-percha. IV. A thermal profile of the warm gutta-percha packing procedure, Oral Surg 51:544, 1981.

32. Grassi MD, et al: Changes in the physical properties of the ultrafil low-temperature (70° C) thermoplasticized gutta-percha system. J Endod 11:517, 1989.
33. Greenberg M: Filling root canals in deciduous teeth by an injection technique, Dent Dig 67:574, 1961.
34. Grossman LI, Oliet S, and Del Rio C: Endodontics, ed 11, Philadelphia, 1988, Lea & Febiger.
35. Gurney BF, Best EJ, and Gervasio G: Physical measurements of gutta-percha, Oral Surg 32:260, 1971.
36. Gutmann JL, et al: Apical leakage of root treated teeth obturated with plastic Thermafil (AADR Abstracts, No. 52) J Dent Res 71:1992.
37. Gutmann JL, et al: Evaluation of heat transfer during root canal obturation with thermoplasticized gutta-percha. II. In vivo response to heat levels generated, J Endod 13:441, 1987.
38. Guttuso J: Histopathologic study of rat connective tissue response to endodontic materials, Oral Surg 16:7, 1963.
39. Haas SB, et al: A comparison of four root canal filling techniques, J Endod 15:596, 1989.
40. Hand R, Huget E, and Tsaknis P: Effects of a warm gutta-percha technique on the lateral periodontium, Oral Surg 42:395, 1976.
41. Harnden DG: Tests for carcnogenicity and mutagenicity, Int Endod J 14:35, 1981.
42. The hazards of formaldehyde, Alert Sheet, US Consumer Product Safety Commission (Bulletin), March 1980.
43. Hendry JA, et al: Comparison of calcium hydroxide and zinc oxide and eugenol pulpectomies in primary teeth of dogs, Oral Surg 54:445, 1982.
44. Herchowitz SB, Marlin J, and Stiglitz MR: US patent No. 831714.
45. Hoen MM, LaBounty GL, and Keller DL: Ultrasonic endodontic sealer placement, J Endod 14:169, 1988.
46. Holland GR: Periapical response to apical plugs of dentin and calcium hydroxide in ferret canines, J Endod 10:71, 1984.
47. Holland R, et al: Apical hard tissue deposition in adult teeth of monkeys with use of calcium hydroxide, Aust Dent J 25:189, 1980.
48. Holland R, et al: Tissue reaction following apical plugging of the root canal with infected dentin chips, Oral Surg 49:366, 1980.
49. Holland R, et al: Root canal treatment with calcium hydroxide. III. Effect of debris and pressure filling, Oral Surg 47:185, 1979.
50. Hovland EJ, and Dumsha TC: Leakage evaluation in vitro of the root canal sealer cement Sealapex, Int Endod J 18:179, 1985.
51. Jacobson EL, Bery PF, and BeGole EA: The effectiveness of apical dentin plugs in sealing endodontically treated teeth. J Endod 11:289, 1985.
52. Johnson WB: A new gutta-percha filling technique, J Endod 4:184, 1978.
53. Johnston HB: The principle of diffusion applied to the Callahan method of pulp canal filling, Dent Summ 43:743, 1927.
54. Jones G: The use of Silastic as an injectable root canal obturating material, J Endod 6:552, May 1980.
55. Kapsimalis P, and Evans R: Sealing properties of endodontic filling materials using radioactive isotopes, Oral Surg 22:386, 1966.
56. Keane K, and Harrington GW: The use of a chloroform-softened gutta-percha master cone and its effect on the apical seal, J Endod 10:57, 1984.
57. Kennedy WA, Walker WA, and Gough RW: Smear layer removed effects on apical leakage, J Endod 1:21, 1986.
58. Krakow AA, and Berk H: Efficient endodontic procedure with the use of a pressure syringe, Dent Clin North Am, p. 387, 1965.
59. Lee H, and Teigler D: Review of biological safety testing of Endo-Fill, research report RR-82-101, South El Monte, Calif, 1982, Lee Pharmaceuticals.
60. Leonardo MR, Leal JM, and Simoes Filho AP: Pulpectomy: immediate root canal filling with calcium hydroxide, Oral Surg 49:441, 1980.
60a. Liewehr F et al: Improved density of gutta-percha after warm lateral condensation, J Endo 19:489, 1993.
61. Lysenko LV: Antiphlogistic action of eucalyptus oil azulene, Farmakol Toksikol 30:341, 1967.
62. Maisto OA, and Erausquin J: Reacción de los tejidos periapicales del molar de la rata a las prastas de obturación reabsorbibles, Rev Assoc Odontol Argent 53:12, 1965.
63. Manhart JJ: The calcium hydroxide method of endodontic sealing, Oral Surg 54:219, 1982.
64. Marciano J, and Michailesco PM: Dental gutta-percha: chemical composition, x-ray identification, enthalpic studies, and clinical implications, J Endod 15:14, 89.
65. Marlin J, and Schilder H: Physical properties of gutta-percha when subjected to heat and vertical condensation, Oral Surg 361:872, 1973.
66. Martin H, and Cunningham W: Endosonic endodontics: the ultrasonic synergistic system, Int Dent J 198-203, 1984.
67. Martin H, and Fischer E: Photoelastic stress evaluation of Endotec vs lateral condensation, Oral Surg (accepted for publication).
68. Martin H, and Jeffries S: Endotec heat transfer: in vitro, Oral Surg (submitted for publication).
69. Martin H, and LaBounty G: Endotec (warm lateral) vs lateral condensation bacterial leakage, Oral Surg (submitted for publication).
70. Martin H, and LaBounty G: Endotec (warm lateral) vs lateral condensation leakage, Oral Surg 70:325, 1990.
71. Martin H: Personal communication, April 1985.
72. Maruzzela JC, and Sicurella NA: Antibacterial activity of essential oil vapors, J Am Pharm Assoc 49:692, 1960.
73. McComb D, and Smith DC: Comparison of the physical properties of polycarboxylate-based and conventional root canal sealers, J Endod 2:228, Aug 1976.
74. McElroy DL, and Wach EC: Endodontic treatment with a zinc oxide–Canada balsam filling material, J Am Dent Assoc 56:801, 1958.
75. Michanowicz AE, and Czonstkowsky M: Sealing properties of an injection-thermoplasticized low-temperature (70° C) gutta-percha: a preliminary study, J Endod 10:563, 1984.
76. Mohammad AR, et al: Cytotoxicity evaluation of root canal sealers by the tissue culture-agar overlay technique, Oral Surg 45:768, 1978.
77. Moreno A: Thermomechanical softened gutta-percha technique, J Mex Dent Assoc 33:13, 1976.
78. Moreno A: Thermomechanically softened gutta-percha root canal filling, J Endod 3:186, 1977.
79. Morse DR, and Wilcko JM: Gutta percha—eucapercha: a new look at an old technique, Gen Dent 26:58, 1978.
80. Morse DR, et al: A comparative tissue toxicity evaluation of the liquid components of gutta-percha root canal sealers, J Endod 7:545, 1981.
81. Newton CW, Patterson SS, and Kafrawy AH: Studies of Sargenti's technique of endodontic treatment: six-month and one-year responses, J Endod 6:509, 1980.
82. Nicholson RJ, et al: Tissue response to an acrylic reinforced gutta percha, J Calif Dent Assoc 7:55, 1979.
83. Nygaard-Østby B: Introduction to endodontics, Oslo, 1971, Scandinavian University Books.
84. Ochi S: Studies on the cellular response to various root canal filling materials, Bull Exp Biol 14:1, 1964.
85. Oguntebi BR, and Shen C: Effect of different sealers on thermoplasticized gutta-percha root canal obturations, J Endod 18:363, 1992.
86. Olson AK, Hartwell GR, and Weller NR: Evaluation of the controlled placement of injected thermoplasticized gutta-percha, J Endod 15:3, 1989.
87. Olsson B, Sliwkowski A, and Langeland K: Subcutaneous implantation for the biological evaluation of endodontic materials, J Endod 7:355, 1981.
88. O'Neil KJ, Pitts DS, and Harrington GW: Evaluation of the apical seal produced by the McSpadden Compactor and by lateral condensation with a chloroform-softened primary cone, J Endod 9:190, 1983.
89. Oswald RJ, and Friedman CE: Periapical response to dentin fillings, Oral Surg 49:344, 1980.

89a. Pitt Ford T, and Rowe A: A new root canal sealer based on calcium hydroxide, J Endod 15:286, July 1989.
90. Pitts DL, Jones JE, and Oswald RJ: A histological comparison of calcium hydroxide plugs and dentin plugs used for the control of gutta-percha root canal filling material, J Endod 10:283, 1984.
91. Rappaport HM, Lilly GE, and Kapsimalis P: Toxicity of endodontic filling materials, Oral Surg 18:785, 1964.
92. Rising DW, Goldman M, and Brayton SM: Histologic appraisal of three experimental root canal filling materials, J Endod 1:172, 1975.
93. Russin TP, et al: Apical seals obtained with laterally condensed, chloroform softened gutta percha and Grossman's sealer, J Endod 6:678, 1980.
94. Saito S: Characteristics of glass ionomer cements and clinical application, J Dent Med 10:1, 1979.
95. Sargenti A: Endodontic course for the general practitioner, ed 4, Brussels, 1965, European Endodontic Society.
96. Sauveur G: Amelioration des techniques d' obturation endodontiques a la gutta: Thermopack, Inf Dent 15:1327, 1986.
97. Schilder H: Filling root canals in three dimensions, Dent Clin North Am, p. 723, 1967.
98. Schilder H, Goodman A, and Aldrich W: The thermomechanical properties of gutta-percha, III. Determination of phase transition temperatures for gutta-percha, Oral Surg 38:109, 1974.
99. Seltzer S, et al: Tissue reactions to polycarboxylate cements, J Endod 2:208, 1976.
100. Seltzer S, Soltanoff W, and Smith J: Periapical tissue reactions to root canal instrumentation beyond the apex and root canal fillings short of and beyond the apex, Oral Surg 36:725, 1973.
101. Smith DC: Some observations on endodontic cements. Paper presented at the meeting of the Canadian and American Association of Endodontics, April 1972.
102. Solomon SM, and Oliet S: Rejuvenation of aged (brittle) endodontic gutta percha cones, J Endod 5:233, 1979.
103. Spangberg L: Biologic effect of root canal filling materials, Odontol Tdskr 77:502, 1969.
104. Spangberg L: Biological effects of root canal filling materials, Odontol Revy 20:133, 1969.
105. Spielman A, Gutman D, and Laufer D: Anesthesia following endodontic overfilling with AH26, Oral Surg 52:554, 1981.
106. Spradling PM, and Senia ES: The relative sealing ability of paste-type filling materials, J Endod 8:543, 1982.
107. Stewart GG: The detection and treatment of vertical root fractures, J Endod 14:47, 1988.
108. Tamse A, et al: Paresthesia following overextension of AH26: report of two cases and review of the literature, J Endod 8:88, 1982.
109. Torabinejad M, Kettering JD, and Bakland LK: Evaluation of systemic immunological reactions to AH-26 root canal sealer, J Endod 5:196, 1979.
110. Torabinejad M, et al: Scanning electron microscopic study of root canal obturation using thermoplasticized gutta-percha, J Endod 4:250, 1978.
111. Torneck CD, Smith JS, and Grindall P: Biologic effects of procedures on developing incisor teeth, II. Effect of pulp injury and oral contamination, Oral Surg 35:378, 1973.
112. Tronstad L: Tissue reactions following apical plugging of the root canal with dentin chips in monkey teeth subjected to pulpectomy, Oral Surg 45:297, Feb 1978.
113. von Fraunhofer JA, and Branstetter J: The physical properties of four endodontic sealer cements, J Endod 8:126, 1982.
114. Wennberg A: Biological evaluation of root canal sealers using in vitro and in vivo methods, J Endod 6:784, 1980.
115. West L, LaBounty G, and Keller D: Obturation quality utilizing ultrasonic cleaning and sealer placement followed by lateral condensation with gutta-percha, J Endod 15:507, 1989.
116. Wollard R, et al: Scanning and electron microscopic examination of root canal filling materials, J Endod 2:98, 1976.
117. Wong M, Peters DD, and Lorton L: Comparison of gutta-percha filling techndiques: compaction (mechanical), vertical (warm), and lateral condensation techniques, part 1, J Endod 7:151, 1981.
118. Wong M, et al: Comparison of gutta-percha filling techniques: three chloroform-gutta percha filling techniques, part 2, J Endod 8:4, 1982.
119. Yancich PO, Hartwell GR, and Portell FR: A comparison of apical seal: chloroform versus eucalyptol-dipped gutta-percha obturation, J Endod 15:16, 1989.
120. Yates J, and Hembree J: Microleakage of three root canal cements, J Endod 6:591, 1980.
121. Yee FS, et al: Three dimensional obturation of the root canal using injection-molded, thermoplasticized dental gutta-percha, J Endod 3:168, 1977.
122. Yee RDJ, Newton CW, and Patterson SS: The effects of canal preparation and leakages characteristic of the apical dentin plug, J Endod 10:308, 1984.
123. Zakariasen KL, and Stadem PS: Microleakage associated with modified eucapercha and chloropercha root-canal-filling techniques, Int Endod J 15:67, 1982.
124. Zmener O, and Dominguez FV: Tissue response to a glass ionomer used as an endodontic cement, Oral Surg 56:198, 1983.

Self-assessment questions

1. A well-fitted root canal
   a. prevents microbial leakage.
   b. exhibits radiopacity.
   c. extends beyond the apical constriction.
   d. needs no root canal cement.
2. Appropriate time for obturation is
   a. when the canal is free of hemorrhage.
   b. when the canal has ceased to exude tissue fluids.
   c. when the tooth is symptomatic.
   d. before post cementation.
3. Root-filling materials must be
   a. low cost.
   b. easily dissolved.
   c. rigid.
   d. biocompatible.
4. Root canal cements should
   a. be bactericidal.
   b. be bacteriostatic.
   c. set quickly.
   d. be radiolucent.
5. Tug-back is achieved and the canal is ready for filling
   a. when the gutta-percha has extended beyond the apex.
   b. when the gutta-percha is easily removed from the root canal.
   c. when the gutta-percha placed to apical constriction exhibits resistance on removal.
   d. after cementation.
6. Calcium hydroxide root canal sealers
   a. are the most biocompatible.
   b. are irritating to the periapical tissue.
   c. should be used exclusively.
   d. prevent postobturation pain.
7. The "string-out test" for root canal sealer is achieved when, using a spatula, the cement can be raised from the glass slab
   a. ½ inch.
   b. 2 inches.
   c. 1 inch.
   d. 3 inches.

Chapter 10

Records and Legal Responsibilities

Edwin J. Zinman

EXCELLENT ENDODONTIC THERAPY VIA EXCELLENT RECORDS

Importance

Endodontic therapy records serve as an important map, guiding the clinician along the correct road toward diagnosis and treatment. Documentation is essential to attaining endodontic excellence.

Content

Endodontic treatment records should include the following information:

1. Name of patient
2. Date of visit
3. Medical and dental history (periodically updated)
4. Chief complaints
5. Radiographs of diagnostic quality
6. Clinical examination findings
7. Differential and final diagnosis
8. Treatment plan
9. Prognosis
10. Referral, including patient refusals (if any)
11. Progress notes, including complications
12. Completion notes
13. Canceled or missed appointments and stated reasons
14. Emergency treatment
15. Patient concerns and dissatisfactions
16. Planned follow-ups
17. Drug and laboratory prescriptions
18. Patient noncompliance
19. Consent forms
20. Accounting
21. Recalls

Function

Dental records should document the following information:

1. Course of the patient's dental disease and treatment by recorded diagnosis, treatment, and prognosis.
2. Communication among the treating dentist and other health care providers, consultants, subsequent treating practitioners, and third-party carriers.
3. Official professional business record in dental-legal matters documenting a sound plan of dental management.
4. Necessity and reasonableness of care and treatment for evaluation by peer review and insurance carriers.
5. The standard of care was followed.

Patient Information Form

A patient information form provides data essential for identification and office communication. Name, address, business address, and telephone numbers are needed to contact the patient for scheduling purposes or to inquire about treatment sequelae. Similar information about the patient's spouse, relative, or a close friend who can be notified in an emergency is also required. In the event the patient is a minor, the responsible parent or guardian should provide the information. Often questions about dental insurance and financial responsibility are included to avoid any misunderstandings later and to fulfill federal requirements regarding truth in lending for installment payments of four or more, regardless of interest charges, or any late payment charges.[1,2] Patient information and history forms should be updated periodically, or as the need arises (Fig. 10-1).

[1]Morris WO: Dental litigation, ed 2, 1977, The Michie Co.
[2]Federal Truth in Lending Act, 15 USC §1601 et seq.

PATIENT INFORMATION

Name: __________ Social Security No. __________ Date: __________

Date of Birth: __________ If minor, Parents' Names: __________

Marital Status: Single Married Separated Widowed Divorced

Address: __________ Phone: __________ Fax: __________

City: __________ State: __________ Zip Code: __________

REFERRED BY: __________ Patient Driver's License #: __________

Occupation: __________ Employer: __________ How long? __________

Business Address: __________ Phone: __________

City: __________ State: __________ Zip Code: __________

Name of Spouse: __________

Occupation: __________ Employer: __________ How Long: __________

Business Address: __________ Phone: __________

City: __________ State: __________ Zip Code: __________

PERSON RESPONSIBLE FOR ACCOUNT: __________

Address (if different from patient): __________

City: __________ State: __________ Zip Code: __________ Phone: __________

Relationship to patient: __________

DENTAL INSURANCE CARRIER:

__________ Group # __________ Local # __________

Name of Insured Person __________ Social Security No. __________

Relationship to Patient: __________

SECOND DENTAL INSURANCE CARRIER (if dual coverage):

__________ Group # __________ Local # __________

Name of Insured Person __________ Social Security No. __________

Relationship to Patient: __________

Date: __________ Signature: __________

FIG. 10-1 Patient information form.

Health History

Past and present health status should be thoroughly reviewed by the dentist before proceeding, so that dental treatment can be safely initiated. Health questionnaires open avenues for discussion about problems of major organ systems, important biochemical mechanisms, such as blood coagulation, and any immunocompromise. As a result of this review, the dentist may suggest or insist that the patient be examined by a physician or tested by a laboratory under medical supervision to determine whether a suspected medical problem may require attention before endodontic therapy proceeds or whether treatment modifications should be made (e.g., because of drug sensitivity).[3,4]

Every health history form should request information about any current medical therapy and the name of the treating physician to be contacted in the event of emergency. Consultation with the patient's physician may be indispensable to the patient's welfare.

Medical histories must be updated periodically, at least annually. The patient should be asked to review the original history. If there are no changes, the patient should date and sign the original history form. Otherwise, the patient should identify each medical change and date and sign the form as a medical update. If the patient provides an entirely new, updated form (rather than changing data on the old form), earlier medical histories are always retained for future reference.

[3]Keeling D: Malpractice claim prevention, J Calif Dent Assoc 3(8):55, 1975
[4]Weichman J: Malpractice prevention and defense, J Calif Dent Assoc 3:58, 1975.

Dental History

The dental history should include past dental difficulties. A positive response should suggest further consultation with the patient and consideration for obtaining the prior treating dentist's written records and radiographs for elucidation.[5,6]

Diagnostic and Progress Records

Diagnostic and progress records often combine the "fill-in" and "check-off" types of forms. *Fill-in* or essay-type forms allow greater latitude of response to a question, resulting in a more detailed description. One drawback, however, is that it also is open to oversights unless a dentist is very conscientious in noting all clinical information.

An essay-type health history response, alone, is inefficient. A *check-off* format is efficient and more practical. Forms with questions that reveal pertinent data alert the clinician to medical or dental conditions that may warrant further consideration or consultation before proceeding. Moreover, such records document missing medical information the patient failed to provide. Therefore, at the end of the check-off portion of the medical history, there should be an essay question so that the patient can provide any other pertinent medical information.

Radiographs

Radiographs are essential for diagnosis and also as additional documentation of the pretreatment condition of the patient. A panographic radiograph is not diagnostically accurate for endodontics and therefore is used only as a screening device.[7] Diagnostic quality periapical radiographs are essential aids in diagnosis and midtreatment endodontic therapy, to verify the final result, and for follow-up comparisons at recall examinations.

Evaluation and Diagnosis

Diagnosis includes discussing history of the current problem, clinical examination, pulpal testing, and recorded radiographic results. If therapy is indicated, the reasons can be discussed with the patient in an organized way. When other factors affect the prognosis (e.g., strategic importance or restorability of the tooth), the clinician should consider further consultation before initiating any treatment.

Differential Diagnosis

Sound endodontics begins with a proper diagnosis. Otherwise, unnecessary or risky treatment follows. Generally, the following tests should be performed to arrive at a correct and accurate diagnosis:

1. Thermal testing
2. Electrical testing, if possible
3. Percussion
4. Palpation
5. Mobility
6. Periodontal evaluation

Negative, as well as positive, pulpal testing results should be recorded. In the mind of a jury, Peer Review committees, and insurance consultants, if test results were not recorded, the tests may be regarded as not ever having been done.

---

[5]Morris WO: Dental litigation, ed 2, 1977, The Michie Co.

[6]Terezhalmy G, and Bottomley W: General legal aspects of diagnostic dental radiography, Oral Surg 48:486, 1979.

[7]See Chapter 5.

Treatment Plan

Treatment records should contain a written plan that includes all aspects of the patient's oral health. Treatment plans should be coordinated, preferably in writing, with other jointly treating dentists. If another aspect of the patient's dental care not under your direct supervision is not proceeding properly, initiate contact with the other dentist and advise the patient of the problem. For instance, endodontic treatment will probably fail if underlying periodontal pathology is ignored and untreated. Therefore, treat the patient's whole mouth, not just the pulp remnants.

If the scope of the examination or treatment is intentionally limited, such as a screening examination or emergency endodontic therapy, the limited scope of the visit should be recorded. Otherwise, the chart appears as if the examination was superficial, or the treatment incomplete and substandard. If a suspicious apical lesion is to be reevaluated, record the future evaluation date. Otherwise, the chart appears as if the dentist ignored a potential pathological condition such as suspected fracture. General soft tissue examination with cancer check is a standard part of any complete dental examination.

Consent Form

Following endodontic diagnosis, the benefits, risks, treatment plan, and alternatives to endodontic treatment, including the patient's refusal of treatment, are presented to the patient or guardian to document acceptance or rejection of the consultation recommendations. The patient (or guardian) signs and dates the consent form, including any video informed consent. Later changes in the proposed treatment plan should also be discussed and initialed by the patient, to indicate continued acceptance and to acknowledge understanding of any new risks, alternatives, or referrals.

Treatment Record—Endodontic Chart

A suggested chart is presented herein to facilitate recording of information pertinent to the diagnosis, recommendations, and treatment of the endodontic patient (Fig. 10-2). Systematic acquisition and arrangement of data from the patient questionnaire, and also clinical and radiographic examinations, expedite accurate diagnosis and recording of endodontic treatment in detail with minimal clinician time. Chart format and use are described below.

General patient data

Patient name, address, phone number(s), and referring doctor are printed or typed in the corresponding space at the patient's initial office visit.

Appointment schedule and business record

This section is divided into two parts:

1. The first portion is completed by the treating dentist or staff after the diagnosis and treatment plan have been formulated and presented to the patient. Tooth number and quoted fee are posted. Treatment plan is recorded by simply circling the appropriate description. Under *Special Instructions,* specific treatment requests by the referring dentist are circled. Details of planned adjunctive procedures (e.g., hemisection, root resection) may be written in the adjacent space. Along with information from the patient data section, the dentist uses this for general reference during future treatment. The dental secretary also

LAST NAME	FIRST NAME	AGE

DENTAL HISTORY: **CHIEF COMPLAINT** **SYMPTOMATIC** **ASYMPTOMATIC**

SYMPTOMS Location	Chronology	Quality	Affected By	Prior Tx	Initial:
localized referred diffuse radiating	Inception Clinical Course: constant momentary intermittent lingering	sharp intensity dull + ++ +++ spontaneous pulsating provoked steady reproducible enlarging occasional	hot palpation cold manipulation biting head position chewing activity percussion time of day	Tx: restorative Yes No emergency Yes No RCT Yes No Sx Pre-Tx: Yes No Sx Post-Tx: Yes No	TOOTH R — L

MEDICAL HISTORY

Heart Condition angina coronary surgery pacemaker Rheumatic Fever / Murmur Hypertension / Circulatory Immunosuppression	Anemia / Bleeding Diabetes / Kidney Hepatitis / Liver Herpes Thyroid / Hormonal Asthma / Respiratory Ulcers / Digestive Migraine / Headaches	Epilepsy / Fainting Sinusitis / ENT Glaucoma / Visual Mental / Neural Tumor / Neoplasms Alcoholism / Addictions Infectious Diseases Venereal Disease	Allergies: penicillin / antibiotics aspirin / Tylenol codeine / narcotics local anesthetic N_2O/O_2 Other:	Major Medical Prob: Females: Pregnant _______month Recent Hosp. Operation: Current Medical TX: Medicaitons: Initial:

CLINICAL FINDINGS

EXAMINATION RADIOGRAPHIC: Tooth	RADIOGRAPHIC: Attachment Apparatus	CLINICAL: Tooth	CLINICAL: Soft Tissues
WNL caries restoration calcification resorption fracture perforation / deviation prior RCTx/RCF separated instrument canal obstruction post / build-up open apex	PDL normal PDL thickened alveolar bone, WNL diffuse lucency circumscribed lucency resorption apical lateral hypercementosis osteosclerosis perio:	WNL discoloration caries pulp exposure prior access attrition / abrasion fracture restoration amalgam composite glass ionomer inlay / onlay temporary crown abutment	WNL extra-oral swelling intra-oral swelling sinus tract lymphadenopathy TMJ perio: B / M — D / L

DIAGNOSTIC TESTS: Tooth #						
periodontal						
mobility						
percussion						
palpation						
cold						
hot						
EPT						
transillum-ination						
cavity						
bite / chewing						
date:						

DIAGNOSIS PULPAL	PERIAPICAL	ETIOLOGY		PROGNOSIS ENDODONTIC	PERIODONTAL	RESTORATIVE
WNL reversible pulpitis irreversible pulpitis necrosis prior RCTx/RCF	WNL acute apical periodontitis acute apical abscess chronic periapical inflammation phoenix abscess osteosclerosis	idiopathic caries restoration attrition / abrasion developmental	trauma periodontal orthodontic prior RCTx intentional	favorable questionable poor hopeless	favorable questionable poor hopeless	favorable questionable poor hopeless

Initial:

PT. CONSULT ___ Examination Findings ___ Treatment Plan ___ Periodontal Status ___ Restoration ___ Fracture ___ Discoloration ___ Surgery ___ Recall ___ Prognosis ___ Consent Form ___ Video consent Initial:

TREATMENT DATE mo	day	yr	CONS pt.	Dr.	PRE-TREATMENT local	R.D.	rel oc.	O.D.	CLEANING / SHAPING access	pulpec.	canal	test	final	G.G.B.	s. file	cotton	temp	OBTURATION G.P.	sealer	tech.	post	post space	B-U	temp	SURG I&D	REA	hemisection	exploratory	curettage	S. R.	Rx analgesic	Antibiotic	CaOH2	X-Ray	electrosurgery	bleach	retreatment	doctor initial	chairside init.

CANAL	REF	Elec.	X-Ray	Adj.	Final	Size	Rx	MEDICATION	DOSE DISP	INSTR.
B F									x	q h
L P									x	q h
MB									x	q h
ML									x	q h
DB									x	q h
DL									x	q h

FIG. 10-2 Endodontic treatment record.

uses the information when scheduling appointments and establishing financial arrangements.
2. The remaining second portion is completed by business personnel. Financial agreements, third-party coverage, account status, and appointment data, including the day, date, and scheduled procedure, are recorded.

Portions of the following diagnosis and treatment sections may be completed by either the dentist or the chairside assistant. The dentist should review and approve entries.

Dental history

Chief Complaint should note if the patient is symptomatic at the time of examination. Narrative facts regarding the presenting problem are then recorded. Additional details of the chief complaint obtained during successive questioning are recorded by circling the applicable descriptive adjective within each symptom parameter. The pain intensity index (0 to 10) or pain classification (mild +, moderate ++, severe +++) should be registered alongside the appropriate description. For accurate assessment of the effects of prior dental treatment pertaining to the examination site, a summary account of such procedures should be documented. All pretreatment signs and symptoms should be described.

Medical history

Reference information (e.g., personal physician's name, address, and phone, patient's age, date of last physical examination) are recorded. Obtain a detailed medical history by completing a survey of the common diseases and disorders significant to dentistry along with a comprehensive review of corresponding organ systems and physiologic conditions. Specific entities that have affected the patient are circled. Essential remarks regarding these entries (e.g., details of consultations with the patient's physician) should be documented in the space below. A review of the patient's medical status (including recent or current conditions, treatment, and medications) completes the health history. Medical histories should be updated at least annually and at reevaluation visits, particularly if evidence of failing endodontic procedures necessitates retreatment.

Examination

Following the dental and medical history, findings obtained from the various phases of the clinical and radiographic examinations are recorded. Lists in each category afford the clinician a systematic format for recording details pertinent to a proper diagnosis. Appropriate descriptions are circled, followed by the necessary notations in the accompanying spaces. Tabular arrangement allows easier recording and comparison of diagnostic test data acquired from one tooth on different dates or from different teeth on one day. As for entries in the dental history, a pain intensity index (0 to 10) or pain classification (mild +, moderate ++, severe +++) should be used whenever possible to document diagnostic test results.

Diagnosis

Careful analysis of accumulated examination data should result in the determination of an accurate pulpal and periapical diagnosis. Clinical conditions are circled, as are the probable etiologic factors for the presenting problem. Alternative modalities of therapy are considered and analyzed. The recommended treatment plan is circled, followed by a prognostic assessment of the intended therapeutic course.

Patient consultation

Patients should be advised of each diagnosis and should consent to the treatment plan before therapy is instituted. Consultation should include an explanation of reasonable alternative treatment approaches and rationales, as well as any preexisting conditions and consequences, including risks from nontreatment or delayed treatment that may affect the outcome of intended therapy. Such discussion is documented by simply completing and endorsing the checklist.

Treatment

All treatment rendered on a given date is documented by placing a check mark (√) within the designated procedural category. Only the most frequent retreatment procedures are included for tabulation. Descriptions of occasional procedures or explanatory treatment remarks should be entered in writing. A separate dated entry should be made for each patient visit, phone communication (e.g., consultations with the patient or other doctors), and correspondence (e.g., biopsy report, treatment letters).

Individual root canal lengths are recorded by (1) circling the corresponding anatomic designation and the method of length determination (e.g., radiograph or electronic measuring device), (2) writing the measurement (in millimeters), and (3) indicating the reference point.

For any medication prescribed, refilled, or dispensed the record should show the date and type of drug, including dosage, quantity, and instructions for use, in the treatment table under *Rx*. Periodic recall intervals, dates, and findings are entered in the spaces provided.

Abbreviations

Abbreviated records can be frustrating if the practitioner is unable to decipher his or her own handwritten entries. Use standard or easily understood abbreviations. Pencil entries are legally valid, but ink entries are less vulnerable to a plaintiff's claim of erasure or record alteration. However, even a short pencil is better than a long memory. Records remember but patients and dentists alike may forget.

A sample completed endodontic chart (Fig. 10-3) illustrates its proper utilization. An explanatory key listing the standard abbreviations used in the chart is provided in Figure 10-4.

Computerized Treatment Records

Increasingly, dentists are utilizing computerized record storage. To avoid a claim of record falsification, whatever computer system is utilized should be able to demonstrate that records indicating earlier treatment were not recently falsified. Technology, such as the WORM system, which will identify tampering of computer data, is not foolproof, since it cannot detect tampering where an entire disk of recent origin has been substituted for an earlier version. Practitioners periodically should print out a hard copy of data maintained in the computer and should hand-initial and date the hard copy as written verification of the computer records.

Record Size

Brief records risk incomplete documentation. There is no harm in writing too much but great danger in recording too little. Standard 8½ by 11 inch or larger clinical records possess the advantage of providing the treating dentist adequate space for clinical notes.

MIDDLE INITIAL

FIRST NAME

LAST NAME

LAST NAME	FIRST NAME	DR MR. MISS MRS.	ADDRESS	HOME PHONE S.F. BUSINESS PHONE T.L.

REF. DR.	REF. DR. ADDRESS	REF. DR. PHONE

TOOTH	FEE		TREATMENT PLAN	SURGERY	SPECIAL INSTRUCTIONS
R — L 30		(CONSULT) EET	(RCT) AE PE (ME)	$Ca(OH)_2$	POST SPACE (PREFORMED POST/B.U.) COMP (AMAL) TEMP. CR. Distal Canal

INSURANCE S D	AMT DUE	REC'D	DATE	DAY	TIME	PRO-CEDURE	X-RAY	REMARKS:
PRE-AUTH Y N								
% COVERED								
VERIFIED								
FORM SIGNED								
PT. INFORMED								
PT. PORTION								
INS SENT								

DATE MO	DAY	YR	REMARKS	SIGNATURE
2	14	94	Pt. urged to have a cast metal crown	
			made as soon as possible. Confirming	A.E./S.C.
			letter to referring doctor.	

FIG. 10-3 Treatment record section used to detail progress and events.

Continued.

LAST NAME	FIRST NAME	TOOTH	FEE	TREATMENT PLAN	SPECIAL INSTRUCTIONS
		R — L 30		(CONSULT) (RCT) SURGERY EET AE PE (ME) Ca(OH)$_2$	POST SPACE (PREFORMED POST / B-U) COMP (AMAL) TEMP. CR

DENTAL HISTORY — CHIEF COMPLAINT: (symptomatic) asymptomatic — Onlay placed 2 weeks ago. Diffuse pain began several days later. Pt. cannot localize the pain. Pain increases with heat / cold / chewing.

SYMPTOMS Location	Chronology	Quality	Affected By:	Prior Tx
Right side V1 – V3	Inception: 10 days	(sharp) dull	Intensity + (++) +++	(hot) + (cold) +++ palpation manipulation	Tx: restorative (Yes) No — onlay; emergency Yes (No); RCT Yes (No)
localized referred (diffuse) (radiating)	Clinical Course: (constant) momentary intermittent (lingering)	(pulsating) steady enlarging	spontaneous provoked (reproducible) occasional	biting (chewing) + percussion; head position activity time of day	Sx Pre-Tx: Yes (No); Sx Post-Tx: (Yes) No — Initial: A. E.

MEDICAL HISTORY — Physician Name: Dr. M. Welby — Address: 450 Sutter — Phone: 555-1212 — Last Physical: 2-11-93 — Pt. Age: 52

			Allergies:	
Heart Condition	Anemia / Bleeding	Epilepsy / Fainting	(penicillin) antibiotics	Major Medical Prob:
angina	Diabetes / Kidney	Sinusitis / ENT	aspirin / Tylenol	Females: Pregnant _____ mo.
coronary	Hepatitis / Liver	Glaucoma / Visual	codeine / narcotics	Recent Hosp./Operation:
surgery	Herpes	Mental / Neural	local anesthetic	Current Medical TX:
pacemaker	Thyroid / Hormonal	Tumor / Neoplasms	Latex	Medications:
Rheumatic Fever / Murmur	Asthma / Respiratory	Alcoholism / Addictions	N_2O / O_2	Medical Status:
Hypertension / Circulatory	(Ulcers) / Digestive	Infectious Diseases	Other:	
Immunocompromised	Migraine / Headaches	Venereal Disease		

Initial: A. E.

EXAMINATION

RADIOGRAPHIC Tooth	RADIOGRAPHIC Attachment Apparatus	CLINICAL Tooth	CLINICAL Soft Tissues
WNL	PDL normal	WNL	(WNL)
caries	(PDL thickened)	discoloration	extra-oral swelling
(restoration)	alveolar bone, WNL	caries	intra-oral swelling
(calcification) mesial	diffuse lucency	pulp exposure	sinus tract
resorption	circumscribed lucency	prior access	lymphadenopathy
fracture	resorption	attrition/abrasion	TMJ
perforation/deviation	apical	fracture	perio:
prior RC Tx / RCF	lateral	(restoration)	2 B
separated instrument	hypercementosis	amalgam	3 M — D 3
canal obstruction	osteosclerosis	composite	L 2
post / build-up	perio:	inlay (onlay)	
open apex		temporary	
		crown	
		abutment	

DIAGNOSTIC TESTS

Tooth No.	29	30	31
perio.	WNL	WNL	WNL
mobility	+1	WNL	WNL
percussion	WNL	+	WNL
palpation	WNL	WNL	WNL
cold	WNL	+++	WNL
hot	WNL	++	WNL
EPT			
transillum.			
cavity			
date:	2-14-94		

Recommend endo-tx #30

DIAGNOSIS

PULPAL	PERIAPICAL	ETIOLOGY		PROGNOSIS ENDODONTIC	PERIODONTAL	RESTORATIVE
WNL	(WNL)	idiopathic	trauma	(Favorable)	(Favorable)	(Favorable)
reversible pulpitis	acute apical periodontitis	caries	periodontal	questionable	questionable	questionable
(irreversible pulpitis)	acute apical abscess	(restoration)	orthodontic	poor	poor	poor
necrosis	chronic periapical inflammation	attrition / abrasion	prior RC Tx	hopeless	hopeless	hopeless
prior RC Tx / RCF	phoenix abscess	developmental	intentional RCT			
	osteosclerosis					

PT. CONSULT: ✓ Examination Findings; ✓ Treatment Plan; ✓ Periodontal Status; ✓ Restoration; ✓ Fracture; ___ Discoloration; ✓ Surgery; ✓ Recall; ✓ Prognosis; ✓ Consent Form; ___ Video consent; Initial: S. C.

mo	day	yr	pt.	Dr.	local	R.D.	reloc.	O.D.	access	pulpec.	canal	test	final	G.G.B.	s. file	cotton	temp	G.P.	sealer	tech.	post	B-U	temp	I&D	retro	S.R	analg	Ab	REMARKS
2	14	94	✓		✓	✓			✓	✓	✓	✓	✓	✓	✓	✓	✓										①		Lido-2% c̄
2	21	94			✓	✓									✓			✓	✓	L/c	D + amalgam core								epi· 1=100,000

(Column groups: TREATMENT DATE; CONS; PRE-TREATMENT; CLEANING / SHAPING; OBTURATION; SURG; Rx; REMARKS)

CANAL	REF	Elec.	X-Ray	Adj	Final	Size	Rx	MEDICATION	DOSE	DISP	INSTR.	RECALL	DATE	REMARKS
B F							①	Ibuprofen	600	x 20	1 q 4 h PRN	12 mos	2/29/94	WNL - crowned
L P										x	q h			
MB	MBC		✓	21.0	21.0	25				x	q h			
ML	MLC		✓	21.0	21.5	25				x	q h			
DB	BG		✓	21.5	22.5	30				x				
DL	BG		✓	20.5	21.0	35				x				

FIG. 10-3, cont'd. Treatment record section used to detail progress and events.

Ab	=	Antibiotic
ABS	=	Abscess
access	=	Access cavity
analg.	=	Analgesic
apico	=	Apicoectomy
B-U	=	Buildup of tooth
canal	=	Identify canal that has been cleaned and shaped
cotton	=	Placed in pulp chamber between treatments
ENDO	=	Endodontics
epin	=	Epinepherine
final	=	Final file
G.G.B.	=	Gates-Glidden bur
G.P.	=	Gutta-percha
I & D	=	Incision and drainage
L.A. or local	=	Local anesthetic
O.D.	=	Open and drain
perio	=	Periodontal
post	=	Preformed or custom post
pt	=	Patient
pulpec	=	Pulpectomy
R.D.	=	Rubber dam
Rel occ	=	Relieved occlusion
resorp.	=	Resorption
retro	=	Retrograde procedure
S/R	=	Suture removal
s.file	=	Serial filing
S/D	=	Single insurance or dual coverage
sealer	=	Type of sealer used
tech.	=	Technique for canal obturation
temp	=	Temporary restoration
test	=	Test file
WNL	=	Within normal limits
Y/N	=	Insurance preauthorized? Yes or No

FIG. 10-4 Standard abbreviation key.

Identity of Entry Author

It is inconsequential whether a dentist or an auxiliary records the clinical entries. What is important is that the correct clinical information is recorded. Each person who makes an entry should record the date and initial the entry. Otherwise, the author's identity may be forgotten should the individual who recorded the entry be needed in a legal proceeding. For instance, initializing the entry makes it easier to identify the particular dentist or auxiliary who, since recording, is now employed elsewhere.

Patient Record Request

Patient requests for records must be honored. It is unethical to refuse to transfer patient records, upon patient request, to another treating dentist.[8] Moreover, it is illegal in some states, subjecting the dentist to discipline and fines should the records not be provided to the patient upon written request, even if an outstanding balance is owed.[9]

Patient Education Pamphlets

Patient education pamphlets may be utilized in litigation as evidence that a patient who was properly informed and given endodontic alternatives, instead chose extraction. Such pamphlets include the ADA's "Your Teeth Can be Saved by Endodontic Root Canal Treatment" or the AAE's "Saving Teeth Through Endodontic Therapy." Indicate in the patient's chart that the patient was shown or given the pamphlet(s).

Recording Referrals

Every dentist, including an endodontic specialist, has a duty to refer under appropriate circumstances. No one is perfect, and consultations with additional experts or specialists may become necessary. Otherwise, a dentist appears to be the jack-of-all-trades but master of none.

All referrals should be recorded, lest they be forgotten. Consider a carbonless, two-part referral card. Provide the original to the patient to take to the referral dentist and place the copy in the chart.

Record Falsification

Records must be complete, accurate, legible, and dated. All diagnosis, treatments, and referrals should be recorded. Al-

[8] American Dental Association: Principles of ethics and code of professional conduct, Section 1B.
[9] See, e.g., California Health and Safety Code §1795.12(g).

though alterations are always proscribed, subsequent additions may be added to expand, correct, define, modify, or clarify so long as they are dated to indicate a belated entry, rather than one contemporaneous with treatment.

To correct an entry, line out but do not erase or obscure the erroneous entry. Place and date the correction on the next available line in the chart. Handwriting and ink experts utilize infra-red technology to prove falsified additions, deletions, or substituted records. If records are proven to be falsified, the dentist may be subject to punitive damages in civil litigation. In addition, the dentist may be subject to license revocation for intentional misconduct.[10] Professional liability insurance policies will likely not indemnify a dentist for the punitive damages portion of a verdict based upon fraud or deceit.

Altered records prove the dentist has not been honest. When patient records have been requested or subpoenaed, it is wise to refrain from examining them, to avoid anxiety and the temptation to clarify an entry. Alteration of records is a cause of large settlements. Dental records are business documents. Do not be cavalier about making belated changes. Insurance carriers may deny renewal of professional liability coverage if the dentist has fraudulently altered dental records.

Records are (1) subject to audits by insurance carriers for documentation that treatment was performed, (2) reviewed by peer review committees; and (3) subject to subpoena by state licensing boards or agencies for disciplinary proceedings. Accordingly, incomplete or missing records expose the dentist not only to civil liability for professional negligence but to criminal penalties for offenses such as insurance fraud.[11]

LEGAL RESPONSIBILITIES

Malpractice Prophylaxis

Good dentists keep good records. Therefore, remember the three *R*s of malpractice prophylaxis: *records, records,* and *records*. Records represent the single most critical evidence a dentist can present in court as confirmation of accurate diagnosis and proper treatment.

Prophylaxis is the cornerstone of good dental care because it provides a healthy dental foundation based on prevention. Likewise, endodontic treatment performed with the requisite standard of care not only saves endodontically treated teeth but also helps insulate the treating dentist from a lawsuit for professional negligence. Sound endodontic principles carefully applied protect both dentist and patient. Careful attention to the principles of due care reduces avoidable or unreasonable risks associated with endodontic therapy.

Standard of Care

Good endodontic practice, as defined by the courts, is the standard of reasonable care legally required to be performed by the treating dentist. The standard of care does not require dental perfection, ideal care, or, by analogy, an A+ grade, in endodontics. Instead, the legal standard is that *reasonable* degree of skill, knowledge, or care ordinarily possessed and exercised by dentists under similar circumstances in diagnosis and treatment.[12]

Although the standard of care is a flexible standard that accommodates individual variations in treatment, it is objectively tested based on what a reasonable dentist would do. Reasonable conduct, at a minimum, constitutes legally due care. Additional precautionary steps that rise above the minimum floor of reasonableness and approach the ceiling of ideal care are laudable but not legally mandated.

Dental Negligence Defined

Dental negligence is defined as a violation of the standard of care (i.e., an act or omission that a reasonably prudent dentist under similar circumstances would not have done).[13] Negligence is equated with carelessness or inattentiveness.[14] Malpractice is a lay term for such professional negligence. Simply stated, dental negligence occurs if a dentist either (1) fails to possess a reasonable degree of education and training in order to act prudently or (2) despite reasonable schooling and continuing education, acts (or fails to act) unreasonably or imprudently.

One simple test to determine if a particular treatment outcome results from negligence is to ask the following question: Was the treatment result reasonably avoidable? If the answer is Yes, it is probably malpractice. If the answer is No, it is probably an unfortunate misadventure that occurs despite the best of care by other reasonable dentists, but it is not malpractice.

Locality Rule

The locality rule, which provides for a different standard of care in different communities, is becoming outdated. Originating in the 19th century, the rule was designed to acknowledge differences in facilities, training, and equipment between rural and urban communities.[15]

The trend across the country is to move from a locally-based standard to a statewide standard, at least for generalists. For endodontists usually a national standard of care is applied, considering that the AAE Board is national in scope. Thus, no disparity generally exists between small town and urban endodontics standards, considering advances in communication, transportation, and education.

Peoria dentists should not be any more or less careful than Pittsburgh dentists. A dentist should provide proper endodontic care to a patient regardless of where the treatment is performed. Rather than focusing on different standards for different communities, other more important considerations include endodontic advances, availability of facilities, and whether the dentist is a specialist or general practitioner.

The locality rule has two major drawbacks. In some small areas dentists may not wish to testify as expert witnesses against other local dentists. Also, the rule allows a small group of dentists in an area to establish a local standard of care inferior to what the law requires.

Standards of Care: Generalist versus Endodontist

A general practitioner performing treatment ordinarily performed exclusively by specialists, such as complicated endodontic surgery, advanced periodontal surgery, or full bony im-

---

[10]Calif Bus Prof code §1680(s).
[11]Tulsa dentist found guilty of mail fraud, conspiracy, Tulsa World, Jan 12, 1993.
[12]Folk v Kick, 53 CA3d 176, 185; 126 CR 172 (1975); see also California Book of Approved Jury Instructions, Civil, 6.00 et seq.

[13]Mathis v Morrissey 11 Cal App 4th 332 (1992); Folk v Kilk, 53 Cal App 3d 176, 185 (1975); 126 Cal Rptr 172; Am Jur 2d, Physicians and surgeons and other healers, 138, 1972.
[14]*Webster's Dictionary*, 1987, p. 250.
[15]See 18 ALR 4th 603.

paction surgery, will be held to the specialist's standard of care. A generalist should refer to a specialist rather than perform procedures that are beyond the general practitioner's training or competency, to avoid the likely result that a subsequent treating specialist will regard the generalist's therapy as below the specialist's standard.

Approximately 80% of U.S. general practitioners provide some type of endodontic therapy, and by the year 2000, U.S. endodontic cases are expected to exceed 30 million annually. The expansion of this specialty into the realm of the generalist can be linked to (1) refinements in root canal preparation and filling techniques now taught in dental schools, (2) continuing education courses, and (3) significant improvements in the armamentarium of instruments, equipment, and materials available to dentists.

Higher Standard of Care for Endodontist—Extended Diagnostic and Treatment Responsibilities

Endodontists, as specialists, are generally held to a higher standard of skill, knowledge, and care than general practitioners.[16] However, endodontists should not forget their general dentist training. Even though a patient may be referred for a specific procedure or undertaking, the endodontist cannot overlook sound biologic principles inherent in the treatment of any patient, lest that dentist be found liable. A specialist may also be held liable for failing to conduct an independent examination and instead relying solely on the information referral card or observations of the referring dentist, should the diagnosis or therapeutic recommendations prove incorrect.[17]

Without performing an independent examination, the endodontist risks misdiagnosis, and resulting incorrect treatment. Prevention of misdiagnosis or incorrect treatment requires accurate medical/dental history and clinical examination not only of the specific tooth (or teeth) involved but also the general oral condition. Obvious problems, such as oral lesions, periodontitis, or gross decay, should be noted in the chart and the patient advised regarding a referral for further examination or testing or consultation with the referring dentist.

Radiographs from the referring dentist should be reviewed for completeness, clarity, and diagnostic accuracy. Usually the endodontist takes a new radiograph to verify current status prior to treatment.

Poor oral hygiene may be indicative of periodontal disease. In such cases endodontic treatment may be secondary to bringing the periodontal condition under control. Referral to a periodontist may be necessary before endodontic treatment or upon completion.

In summary, it is necessary for the endodontist to (1) be alert to any contributory medical or dental condition within the area of treatment, (2) undertake an independent examination of the treatment area without relying solely on the referring dentist, and (3) perform at least a cursory general dental examination of the patient's mouth.[18]

Ordinary Care Equals Prudent Care

"Ordinary" is commonly understood (outside its legal context) to mean "lacking in excellence" or "being of poor or mediocre quality." As expressed in the context of actions for negligence, however, "ordinary" care has assumed a technical-legal definition somewhat different from its common meaning. *Black's Law Dictionary,* 4th edition, describes ordinary care as "that degree which persons of ordinary care and prudence are accustomed to use or employ . . . that is, reasonable care."

In adopting this distinction, the courts have defined ordinary care as "that degree of care which people ordinarily prudent could be reasonably expected to exercise under circumstances of a given case."[19] It has been equated with the reasonable care and prudence exercised by ordinarily prudent persons under similar circumstances.[20] It is not extraordinary or ideal care.

Although the standard required of a professional cannot be that of the most highly skilled practitioner, neither can it be that of the average member of the profession, since those who have less than median skill may still be competent and qualify.[21] By such an illogical definition, half of all dentists in a community would automatically fall short of the mark and be negligent as a matter of law. "We are not permitted to aggregate into a common class the quacks, the young men who have not practiced, the old ones who have dropped out of practice, the good, and the very best, and then strike an average between them."[22] Rather, the reasonably prudent dentist is the standard and not the average or mediocre practitioner. Even if 90% of dentists perform a certain treatment unreasonably, no matter how great the number who do it wrong, that never makes it right.

Customary Practice versus Negligence

Customary practice may constitute evidence of the standard of care, but it is not the only determinant. Moreover, if the customary practice constitutes negligence, it is not reasonable dentistry merely because it is customary among a majority of dentists.[23]

Typical negligent custom examples include dentists and hygienists who customarily fail to probe[24] or take diagnostic quality radiographs,[25] do not refer for complicated procedures beyond the ken of their training,[26] disregard aseptic practices such as rubber gloves and face masks,[27] do not employ rubber dams for endodontics,[28] fail to install or periodically check valves in dental units to prevent water retraction suck-back

[16]Carmichael v Reitz 17 Cal App 3d 958 (1971); Cal BAJI, No 6.01.

[17]Howard WW, and Parks AL: The dentist and the law, p 156; St. Louis, 1973, Times Mirror/Mosby College Publishing, O'Brien v Stover (8th Cir) 443 F2d 1013 (1971); Sinz v Owens 33 Cal 2d 749, 205 P.2d 3, 8 ALR 2d 757 (1949).

[18]Fraijo v Hartland Hospital 99 Cal App 3d 331 (1979).

[19]California BAJI 3.16; Switzer v Atchison, Topeka & Santa Fe Railroad Co, 7 Cal App 2d 661, 666, (1935); 47 p 2d 353; see 57A Am Jur 2d (Rev ed), Negligence §144 et seq.

[20]Switzer v. Atchison, Topeka, & Santa Fe Railroad Co, 7 Cal App 2d 661, 666; 47 P 2d 353, (1935); Restatement 2d, Torts, §283, 289.

[21]Restatement 2d, Torts, §299A, Comment (e).

[22]61 Am Jur 2d, Physicians and surgeons and other healers, §110.

[23]Barton v Owen, 71 Cal App 3d 484, 492–493, 139 Cal Rptr 494(1979).

[24]American Academy of Periodontology, Periodontal Screening and Recording 1992.

[25]Rohlin M, et al: Observer performance in the assessment of periapical pathology: a comparison of panoramic with periapical radiography, Dentomaxillofac Radiogr 20; 127, 1991; Zeider S, Ruttimann U, and Webber R: Efficacy in the assesment of intraosseous lesions of the face and jaws in asymptomatic patients, Radiology 162:691, 1987.

[26]Seneris J. Hass 45 Cal 2d 811, 826, 291 P2d 915, 53 ALR 2d 124 (1955).

[27]Recommendations for preventing transmission of human immunodeficiency virus and hepatitis B virus to patients during exposure-prone invasive procedures, MMWR 40:1, 1991; Recommended infection practices in dentistry, MMWR 35:237, 1986.

[28]Simpson v Davis, 219 Kan 584, 549 P2d 950 (1976).

cross-contamination,[29] and routinely diagnose pulpal disease without pulpal testing.[30]

Merely because a majority of practitioners in a community practice a particular method does not establish the standard of care, if such customary practice is unreasonable or imprudent.[31] Ultimately, the courts determine what is or is not reasonable dental practice, considering the available dental knowledge and weighing the risks and benefits of a particular procedure.

The law does not require dental perfection.[32] Instead, the legal yardstick by which such conduct is measured is what a reasonably prudent practitioner would do under the same or similar circumstances regardless of how many or how few practitioners conform to such a standard.

In one case, the evidence was undisputed that virtually no ophthalmologist in the entire state routinely tested for glaucoma patients under the age of 40, since the incidence was only 1 in 25,000 patients. Nevertheless, the Supreme Court of Washington State held that the defendant ophthalmologist was negligent as a matter of law irrespective of customary practice.[33]

There is little excuse for failing to routinely chart periodontal pockets before rendering endodontic therapy, no matter how many other dentists in the community fail to do so. The benefit of recognition of periodontal disease by probing and of pulpal disease by testing substantially outweighs the virtually nonexistent risks of conducting these procedures. A lame legal defense likely to invoke a jury's wrath is to claim that a necessary diagnostic or prophylactic procedure is "too time consuming," when the dental and medical health of the patient are placed at risk for failure to adopt prudent practices.

Compliance with a safety statute does not conclusively establish due care, since regulations require only minimal care and not necessarily prudent care or what the law regards as due care.[34]

Negligence per se

A civil liability duty of care may be imposed by statutes and safety ordinances. For example, violation of a health safety statute may create a presumption of negligence on the part of the dentist.[35]

Although at trial plaintiff ordinarily has the burden of proving negligence, a rebuttable presumption of negligence is created if the following conditions are met:

1. Violation of a statute, ordinance, or regulation of a public entity occurs;
2. The violation caused injury;
3. Injury resulted from an occurrence that the statute, ordinance, or regulation was designed to prevent; *and*
4. Person suffering injury was one of the persons for whose protection the statute, ordinance, or regulation was adopted.[36]

If plaintiff establishes the presumption of negligence per se, the burden then shifts to the defendant to rebut plaintiff's case.

Foreseeability of Unreasonable Risk

Each endodontic procedure has some degree of inherent risk. The standard of care requires that the dentist avoid unreasonable risks that may harm the patient. Treatment is deemed negligent when some unreasonable risk of harm to the patient would have been foreseen by a reasonable dentist. Failure to follow the dictates of sound endodontic practice increases the risk of negligence-induced deleterious results. Accordingly, prophylactic endodontic negligence law is designed to prevent foreseeable risks of injury which are reasonably avoidable.

It is not necessary that the exact injuries that occur be foreseeable. Nor is it necessary to foresee the precise manner or circumstances under which the injuries are inflicted. It is enough that a reasonably prudent dentist would foresee that injuries of the same general type would be likely to occur in the absence of adequate safeguards.[37]

Informed Consent Principles

In general

The legal doctrine of informed consent requires that the patient be advised of reasonably foreseeable material risks of endodontic therapy, the nature of the treatment, reasonable alternatives, and the consequences of nontreatment.[38] This doctrine is based on the legal principle that individuals have the right to do with their own bodies as they see fit, including the right to lose teeth, regardless of recommended dental treatment. Thus, once the dentist has informed the patient of the diagnosis, recommended corrective treatment or alternative therapy, and the likely risks and prognosis of treatment compared with not proceeding with recommended therapy, an adult of sound mind is entitled to elect to do nothing about existing endodontic disease rather than elect corrective treatment.

To be effective, a patient's consent to treatment must be an informed consent. Accordingly, a dentist has a fiduciary duty to disclose all information *material to the patient's decision*.[39] The scope of a dentist's duty to disclose is measured by the amount of knowledge a patient needs to make an informed choice. Material information is that which the dentist knows or should know would be regarded as significant by a reasonable person in the patient's position when deciding to accept or reject a recommended endodontic procedure.

If a dentist fails to reasonably disclose, and a reasonable person in the patient's position would have declined the procedure had adequate disclosure been given, the dentist may be liable if an undisclosed risk manifests. Beyond the foregoing minimal disclosure, a dentist must also reveal such additional information as a skilled practitioner of good standing would

---

[29]Miller C: Cleaning, sterilization and infection, J Am Dent Assoc 48:54, 1993; Williams JF, Johnston AM, Johnson B et al: Microbial contamination of dental unit waterlines, J Am Dent Assoc 124:59, 1993.

[30]Chapter 1.

[31]Barton v Owen, 71 Cal App 3d 484, 492–493 (1977); 139 Cal Rptr 494.

[32]Gurdin v Dongieux, 468 So2d 1241 (1985).

[33]Helling v Carrey, 83 Wash2d 514 (1974); 519P.2d 981; but see, Meeks v Marx 15 Wash App 571, 556 P2d 1158 (1974).

[34]Texas & Pacific Railway Co v Behymer, 189 US 468, 470, 47 L Ed 905, 23 S Ct622 (1903).

[35]McGee v Cessna Aircraft Co, 139 Cal App 3d 179, 188 Cal Rptr 542 (1983).

[36]Cal Evid Code §669.

[37]Restatement 2d, Torts, §282 et seq.; Witkin BE Summary of California Law, §751 (1988).

[38]Scaria v St. Paul Fire & Marine Insurance Co, 68 Wis 201, 227 NW2d 647 (1975); Zinman E: Informed consent to periodontal surgery. Advise before you incise, J West Soc Periodontol 24:101, 1976.

[39]Cobbs v Grant, 8 Cal 2d 229, 104 Cal Rptr 505, 502 P2d 1 (1972); BAJI 6.11.

provide under similar circumstances. However, a minicourse in endodontics is not required.

Application of standard

Informed consent is a flexible standard that considers the reasonably foreseeable consequences depending on the clinical situation present both before and during treatment. For instance, a fractured endodontic instrument left in the canal presents a varied foreseeable likelihood of root canal failure or impaired success, depending on whether the fracture occurred in the coronal, middle, or apical third of the root canal. Therefore, the dentist must advise the patient of relative risks of future failure because of the retained instrument, and treatment alternatives available to correct the problem, so that the patient can make an intelligent choice among apicoectomy, referral to an endodontist for attempted retrieval, or watchful waiting with close observation at recall visits.

Adequate disclosure includes clinical judgment and experience, which assesses current research and applies it to the clinical needs of each patient. According to the laws of aeronautic engineering, the bumblebee should not fly. Beekeepers, entomologists, flowers, and stung persons know otherwise. So it is with competent clinicians who practice applied dental science in daily practice. Advances in theoretical methods of therapy are great if they "fly," but should be reconsidered if the clinician cannot get off the ground with recommended treatment. Today's advances may be tomorrow's retreat if materials, devices, or instruments lacking adequate long-term study of proven safety and efficacy are utilized. Therefore, the dentist should disclose personal clinical failures, if these results are at odds with published results of other clinicians, so the patient may make an intelligent choice of therapists.

Material disclosure concerns whether the patient was provided sufficient information for a reasonable patient to achieve a general understanding of the proposed treatment or procedure, including any dentally acceptable reasonable alternatives, predictable nonremote inherent risks of serious injury, and likely consequences should the patient refuse proposed therapy. Informed consent applies only to inherent risks of nonnegligent treatment since a patient's "consent" to negligent treatment is voidable as contrary to public policy.[40] For instance, a patient who refuses necessary diagnostic radiographs should be refused treatment. Even a superb dentist is not Superman with x-ray vision.

Advice regarding different schools of thought

After advising proper treatment, if other reasonable dentists would disagree or if there are other respectable schools of thought on the correct treatment may be material information that should be disclosed to the patient in the course of obtaining consent. For example, assume for purposes of illustration that there are two schools of thought concerning the optimal treatment for retrofilling and apicoectomy. One school posits that a retrograde with IRM is the appropriate procedure, while the minority review asserts that retrograde with super EBA is the preferred treatment. Assume further than an explanation of these two different methods of treatment constitutes material information for the purposes of informed consent. The mere fact that there is a disagreement within the relevant endodontic community does not establish that the selection of one procedure as opposed to the other constitutes negligent endodontic therapy. Since competent endodontists regularly use both procedures, a patient would face an insuperable task in proving dental negligence (i.e., that the endodontist failed "to have the knowledge and skill ordinarily possessed, and to use the care and skill ordinarily used, by reputable specialists practicing in the same field and in the same or a similar locality and under similar circumstances").

On the other hand, the specialist would have a duty under these hypothetical circumstances to disclose the two recognized schools of treatment so that the patient could be sufficiently informed to make the final, personal decision. An endodontist, being the expert, appreciates the risks inherent in the procedure prescribed, the risks of a decision not to undergo the treatment, and the probability of a successful outcome of the treatment. Once this information has been disclosed, that aspect of the endodontist's expert function has been performed. The weighing of these risks against the individual subjective fears and hopes of the patient is not an expert skill. Such evaluation and decision is a nondental judgment reserved for the patient alone.[41] In this hypothetical situation, failure to disclose such material information would deprive the patient of the opportunity to weigh the risks; consequently the dentist would have failed in the duty of disclosure.

Avoiding patient claims

If a dentist fails to obtain adequate informed consent, a plaintiff can recover damages even in the absence of any negligent treatment. Therefore, discussions of treatment risks with the patient must be documented. Informed consent forms are very helpful, although not legally mandated since a jury may believe that the patient was informed orally. Equally, if not more, important than consent forms, is a notation in the chart that informed consent risks and alternatives were discussed by the dentist and understood and accepted by the patient. Patients may mentally block out frightening information. Trauma and a potent anesthetic can create retrograde amnesia. Therefore, document in your chart risks, benefits, and alternatives provided to the patient.

Follow only the patient-authorized and consented-to treatment plan. If an emergency precludes advising treatment risks to the patient, lack of informed consent is defensible as implied consent, since no reasonable person would refuse necessary nonelective emergency treatment.

Record any recommended but refused treatment, and the patient's refusal reason. Such an example follows:

> *Patient refused endodontic referral for consultation with Dr. Jones since husband was laid off work last month and cannot afford, but understands detrimental risks of delay.*

Patients may initial the refusal on the chart to be extra cautious, but it is not mandatory.

Reasonable familiarity with a new product or technique is required before it is used. In addition, a patient is entitled to know the dentist's personal experience with a particular mo-

[40]Tunkl v Regents of University of California, 60 Cal2d 92, 32 Cal Rptr 33, 383 P2d 441 (1963).

[41]Cobbs v Grant, 8 Cal3d 229, 243, 104 Cal Rptr 505, 502 P2d 1 (1973).

ENDODONTIC INFORMED CONSENT

I understand the goal of Endodontic Root Canal treatment is to retain a tooth that may otherwise require extraction. Although Endodontic Root Canal treatment usually has a high degree of clinical success, it is a dental-biological procedure, whose results cannot be guaranteed. Occasionally, Endodontic Root Canal treatment may fail, with resulting tooth loss. A permanent (outside) restoration, such as crown or onlay, will be placed afterwards by my restorative dentist. I agree to notify my restorative dentist immediately following completion of the root canal treatment so that a restoration may be placed over my root canal-filled tooth. Following completion of endodontic root canal treatment, fracture and loss of my root canal-filled tooth due to brittleness may be more likely to occur unless my root canal-filled tooth is restored within a month following completion of endodontics.

Payment

I also acknowledge full responsibility for the payment of such services for my root canal treatment and agree to pay for them, in full, AT or BEFORE COMPLETION, unless other specific arrangements are made with the secretary. One (1) percent interest per month or 12 percent per annum is billed on account balances over 31 days past due.

Insurance Assignment

I authorize my insurance carrier to pay any dental benefits of my plan directly to this dental office. I also authorize release of any information necessary to process my dental insurance claim.

Signed: Patient or Parent ____________________

Date: ______________

Witness: ______________

FIG. 10-5 Informed consent form documents the patient's understanding of the proposed endodontic root canal treatment.

dality because the patient has a right to chose between reasonable alternatives, one of which is to seek care from a dentist who has more experience with a particular modality or product. A dentist who fails to obtain informed consent is liable for injury caused by a product or instrument, just as if the dentist's treatment was negligently performed. In other words, the fact that the dentist followed precisely the manufacturer's instructions is no defense if the dentist did not provide adequate information concerning a product or instrument risk to permit the patient to intelligently weigh the information and give informed consent.

Endodontic Informed Consent (Figs. 10-5 and 10-6)

Using statistics presented in national literature regarding success rates for endodontic procedures is insufficient disclosure to fulfill the legal requirements of informed consent if the practitioner's own statistical experience varies significantly from national statistics.[42]

Among specialists, the reported incidence of treatment complications in endodontics is, fortunately, relatively low. Based on a Southwest Endodontic Society retrospective study, a reasonable endodontist or a practitioner with similar abilities should disclose the following facts to patients:[43]

1. Endodontic therapy cannot be guaranteed.
2. Although endodontic therapy is usually successful, a small percentage of teeth are lost despite competent endodontic care, owing to complications or treatment failure.
3. Overfilling or underfilling of root canals occurs in 2% to 4% of cases, which may contribute to treatment failure.
4. Slight-to-moderate transient postoperative pain may occur; severe postoperative pain occurs in very few cases.
5. Irreparable damage to the existing crown or restoration secondary to endodontic treatment is uncommon.

Video Informed Consent

Animated video informed consent shown to the patient is a dynamic method of providing informed consent. Since the video informed consent is considered part of the dentist's records, in the event the patient disputes having ever been ad-

[42]Hales v Pittman, 118 Ariz305 (1978); 576 P2d 493, 499-500; Shelter v Rochelle, 2 Ariz App at 370, 409 P2d at 86 (1965).

[43]Selbst: Understanding informed consent and its relationship to the incidence of adverse treatment events in conventional endodontic therapy, J Endod 16:387, 1990.

PHOTOGRAPHIC CONSENT

I, ____________________, consent to photographic color slides of my teeth or face to be taken by Dr. ________________ or his staff for reproduction and viewing by other dentists for scientific or educational purposes inscientific publications or at dental meetings.

Date: ____________________

____
Signature of patient or legal guardian

Witness: ____________________

FIG. 10-6 Photography consent form.

vised of (1) the nature of endodontic disease, (2) the availability of endodontic specialists, or (3) the relative indications for nonsurgical versus surgical endodontic care, the videotape can be played back to the jury as proof that the patient was informed. It is doubtful a jury would believe a forgetful patient who admits having previously viewed the videotape, since the videotape refreshes the stream of memories that have otherwise faded away into the unconscious.

A patient who can view the videotape is more likely to understand the informed consent disclosure. If a picture is worth a thousand words, a moving picture is worth a thousand pictures. After viewing the videotape and discussing its contents with the dentist, the patient should sign a video consent form, verifying that the video was viewed and all of the patient's questions were answered.

Ethics

Endodontics is one of the seven dental specialties recognized by the ADA. Although any licensed dentist may legally practice endodontics, it is unethical to announce that one specializes in endodontics absent specialty training or being "grandfathered" into endodontic practice. It is ethically unpermissible for a general practitioner to characterize his or her practice as "limited to endodontics."[44] A general practitioner who desires to emphasize or limit his or her practice to endodontics is ethically permitted only to advertise as follows: *General Practitioner—Endodontics.*

Referrals to Other Dentists

Every dental practitioner, including specialists, will at some time need to refer a patient to a specialist for treatment in order to comply with the standard of care required of a reasonable and prudent dentist.[45]

Generally, if the referral takes place within the same dental practice, the legal doctrine of *respondeat superior* ("let the master answer") may be applicable. Under this rule, a dentist is liable for the dental negligence of a person acting as his agent, employee, or partner.[46] This is determined by whether the referring practitioner controls the means of providing diagnosis and treatment.[47]

If the referral is made, even within the same physical environment, to an "independent contractor" endodontist who does not diagnose or treat under the direction or supervision of the referring dentist, and that referring dentist has no right of control as to the mode of performing the treatment, then the principle of agency and responsibility for the acts of another does not apply.[48]

To ensure that the referred dentist is not considered the agent of the referring dentist within the same facility, fees for the referral dentist should not be set by the referring dentist. Nor should the fees be divided equally or shared based on some other arrangement. Also, the referral dentist should bill separately and exercise independent diagnostic and therapeutic judgment. Advise the patient that the referral dentist is independent of the referring dentist.

Surgical versus Nonsurgical Endodontics

Litigation to determine whether nonsurgical or surgical endodontics was the proper treatment choice will not be decided by any one clinician, the ADA, AAE, or the ablest of judges. Rather, after considering all of the evidence, including experts,

[44]American Dental Association: Principles of ethics and code of professional conduct, §§ 5-C and 5-D: California Dental Association, Principle of Ethics, §§8 and 9.

[45]Simone v Sabo, 37 Cal2d 253, 231 P2d 19 (1951)

[46]Restatement 2d, Agency, §§228-237.

[47]Restatement 2d, Agency §§228-237.

[48]Mission Insurance Co v Worker's Comp Appeals Board, 123 Cal App 3d 211 (1981).

a jury—not of a dentist's peers but of a patient's peers—will decide. Depending on the individual case, the jury may decide that either a combination of nonsurgical and surgical endodontic therapy, rather than one method exclusively, should have been attempted. The jury may also decide that the patient should have been advised of the availability of such alternative therapy.

Product Liability

Today's dentist, exploring ways to improve the quality and success of endodontic therapy, is constantly presented with new dental products and techniques.

For prescribing and using drugs or other agents, the ADA's *Principles of Ethics,* Section 10, provides this guideline:

> The dentist has an obligation not to prescribe, dispense, or promote the use of drugs or other agents whose complete formulas are not available to the dental profession. He also has the obligation not to prescribe or dispense, except for limited investigative purposes, any therapeutic agent, the value of which is not supported by scientific evidence. The dentist has the further obligation of not holding out as exclusive any agent, method, or technique.

Broken Instruments

Save broken or defective instruments such as a needle whose broken portion becomes lodged in a patient. The instrument manufacturer may be liable because the product was defective rather than the dentist being liable for dental negligence.[49]

Equipment and Supplies

Keep equipment in good repair and check the condition frequently. Carefully note the manufacturer's instructions and all warnings on both medications and appliances, and inform your staff. Infection control in operating dental equipment is mandatory, such as updating and maintaining dental units with check valves to prevent water retraction or suck-back. Inspect check valves monthly and change clogged valves.[50] Water retraction testers, at no charge to the dentist, are available from some manufacturers.[51] Alternatively, disassemble the handpiece and run water through the line for a few seconds, then stop. If a bubble of water is visible at the end of the water hose holes, the check valve is operating properly. If the bubble of water is not visible, water may be sucked back owing to an absent or clogged check valve. An absent or clogged check valve is a source of cross-contamination.

Drugs

Exercise extreme caution when administering or prescribing dangerous drugs. Write cautionary directions on prescriptions for sedative or narcotic drugs which the pharmacist should place on the prescription container as a patient reminder. For example, for the appropriate drugs, prepare a prescription rubber stamp or obtain pre-printed prescriptions, which state:

> Do not drive or operate dangerous machinery after taking medication since drowsiness is likely to occur. Alcohol, sedative, or tranquilizing drugs will cause drowsiness if taken in combination with this prescribed drug.

The ADA and AMA both provide prescription drug warning pads. Document in the chart the drug information forms provided with the prescription.

Dentist's Liability for Staff's Acts or Omissions

A dentist is liable for the acts or omissions of the dentist's staff under the doctrine of *respondeat superior* ("let the master answer"). This is termed *vicarious liability,* which means that the dentist is responsible not because he or she did anything wrong personally, but because the dentist assumes legal responsibility for his or her employees and agents while they are acting in the course and scope of their employment.

The dentist should instruct the staff in advising patients regarding posttreatment complaints. For example, if the staff ignores signs of infection, such as difficulty swallowing or breathing or elevated temperature, and dismisses the patient's complaints as normal postoperative swelling, the dentist may be held liable for injury to the patient, such as cellulitis, Ludwig's angina, brain abscess, or other complications.

Be cautious when delegating responsibilities. Give clear instructions to ensure that your staff properly represents you and your practice methods. Do not let auxiliaries practice beyond their competency level or license. For example, the dentist should check an assistant-placed restoration prior to patient dismissal. Staff members should not make final diagnoses or handle patient complaints without the dentist's involvement. Instruct staff to ask appropriate questions and to relay the patient's answers to the dentist, so that the dentist can determine what should be done.

Abandonment

Once endodontic treatment is initiated, the dentist is legally obligated to complete the treatment regardless of the patient's payment of any outstanding balance. This requirement is posited on the legal premise that any person who attempts to rescue another from harm must reasonably complete the rescue with beneficial intervention unless another rescuer (dentist) is willing to assume the undertaking.[52] Another view is that, should a patient be placed in a position of danger, unless further treatment is performed, the dentist must institute reasonable therapeutic measures to ensure that adverse consequences do not result.[53]

A dentist performing endodontic therapy should have reasonable means of communicating with patients after regular office hours to avoid a claim for abandonment. A recorded message is inadequate if the dentist fails to check for recorded messages frequently. Therefore, answering services and/or computer-directed beepers are required by the standard of care.

If the dentist providing endodontic therapy is away from the office for an extended period, a substitute on-call dentist should be available for any endodontic emergency and to answer patients' emergency calls. The endodontic treating dentist should arrange in advance for emergency service with a covering dentist rather than simply leaving a name on the answering machine or with the answering service, without first determining the availability of the covering dentist. Otherwise, the covering dentist may be away and unavailable for emergency care.

[49] Restatement 2d, Torts, §402A.

[50] Miller C: Cleaning, sterilization and disinfection: basics of microbial killing for infection control, J Am Dent Assoc 124:48, 1993.

[51] A-Dec, for instance.

[52] Lee v Deubre, Tex Civ App 362 SW 2d 900 (1962); Clark v Hoek, 219 Cal Rptr 845 (1985)

[53] McNamara v Emmons, 36 Cal App 2d 199 (1939); 97 P2d 503; Small v Wegner, Mo 267 SW 2d 26, 50 ALR 2d 170 (1954).

To avoid an abandonment claim, several prophylactic measures apply:

1. No legal duty requires a dentist to accept all patients for treatment. A dentist may legally refuse to treat a new patient, despite severe pain or infection, except for racial or handicapped reasons.[54] If treatment is limited to emergency measures only, be certain that the patient is advised that only temporary emergency endodontic therapy is being provided and not complete treatment. Record on the patient's chart, for instance:

   > Emergency treatment only. Endodontic treatment of tooth number ____ to be completed with another dentist.

   Also, the patient should acknowledge that treatment is limited to the existing emergency by endorsing an informed consent to emergency endodontics:

   > I agree to emergency endodontic treatment of my tooth and have been advised that (1) emergency treatment is for temporary relief of pain and (2) further root canal treatment is necessary to avoid further complications, including, but not limited to, pain, infection, fracture, abscess, or loss of tooth.

2. No legal duty requires a dentist to continue former patients on recalls or emergency care once treatment is complete. Thus, completion of endodontic treatment for tooth no. 19 at a prior visit does not legally obligate the dentist to initiate endodontic therapy for tooth no. 3, whose endodontic disease began after the last treatment of tooth no. 19.
3. Any patient may be discharged from a practice for any arbitrary reason, except racial or handicap discrimination, so long as all initiated treatment is completed. Accordingly, a former patient who evokes memories of a "frictional" relationship, who is financially irresponsible, or who arrives at the office after an absence of several years with an acute apical abscess in a site where previous care was not rendered, may legally be refused treatment.
4. It is not considered abandonment if a patient is given reasonable notice to seek endodontic treatment with another dentist and is willing to seek endodontic services elsewhere.[55] Thus if rapport with the patient dissolves, do not hesitate to suggest that each of you would be better served if any remaining endodontic treatment were performed elsewhere by a different dentist.

   Should you wish to discontinue treatment, you may do so, provided it is not done at a time when the patient's dental health will be jeopardized. To avoid a claim of abandonment, do as follows:

   1. Notify the patient of the plan to discontinue treatment after a certain date.
   2. Allow enough time for the patient to obtain substitute service, usually 30 days.
   3. Offer to make emergency service available until a new dentist is obtained.
   4. Make records, radiographs, and other information about the patient available to the new dentist.
   5. Do not discontinue treatment if it would jeopardize the patient's health.
   6. Allow the patient to select a new practitioner or suggest referral by the local dental society if a referral service exists.
   7. Document in your records, and send a certified letter to the patient, verifying all of the above.

Expert Testimony

The standard of care that a dentist must possess and exercise is peculiarly within the knowledge of dental experts. However, there are occasional exceptions where the conduct involved is within the common knowledge of laypersons, in which case expert testimony is not required. In determining whether expert testimony is required to establish negligence, one California court commented: "The correct rule on the necessity of expert testimony has been summarized by Bob Dylan: 'You don't need a weatherman to know which way the wind blows.' "[56] Operating on the contralateral side owing to mismounted radiographs or marking the wrong tooth on an endodontic referral card are examples of negligent conduct within the common knowledge of laypersons.

MALPRACTICE INCIDENTS

Screw Posts

Screw posts represent a restorative anachronism. The risk of root fracture is too great compared to the benefit, particularly when reasonable and superior passive alternatives exist (see Chapter 22). Even if the screw post is contemplated to be placed passively, the temptation to turn the screw is too great, considering human nature. Screw posts are not currently a reasonable and prudent treatment choice.

Paresthesia

Endodontic surgery in the vicinity of the mental foramen carries with it the risk of injury to the mental nerve. Consequently, advise the patient in lay terms, before any surgery is performed, that there is a risk of temporary or permanent anesthesia or paresthesia. Have the patient execute a written informed consent form confirming that you advised him or her of this risk.

Failure of Treatment

A dentist should not guarantee success of treatment. It is foolish to assure the patient that you will save a tooth or achieve a perfect result.[57] Endodontic failures may occur despite the best endodontic care.[58]

To avoid claims based on failed endodontics, the patient should be advised in advance of treatment of the inherent but relatively small risk of failure. It may be adequate to advise the patient of the high statistical probability of success in endodontics so long as the clinical condition of the tooth and the

---

[54]McNamara v Emmons, 36 Cal App 2d 199 (1939); 97 P2d 503; Small v Wegner, Mo 267 SW 2d 26, 50 ALR 2d 1970 (1954); The Americans with Disabilities Act, Publ No. 101-336; Americans with Disabilities Act Title III Regulations, 28 CFR Part 36, Nondiscrimination on the basis of disability by public accommodations and in commercial facilities, U.S. Department of Justice, Office of the Attorney General; and Americans with Disabilities Act Title I Regulations, 29 CFR Part 1630, Equal employment opportunity for individuals with disabilities, U.S. Equal Employment Opportunity Commission.

[55]Murray v US, Va Civ App, 329 F2d 270 (1964).

[56]Jorgensen v Beach 'N' Bay Realty, Inc, 125 Cal App 3d 155, 177 Cal Rptr 882 (1981) quoting "Subterranean Homesick Blues" from *Bringing It All Back Home,* accord, Easton v Strassburger, 152 Cal App 3d 90, 199 Cal Rptr 383, 46 ALR4th 521 (1984).

[57]Christ v Lipsitz, 160 Cal Rptr 498; 99 Cal App 3d 894 (1980).

[58]Ingle J, and Beveridge E: Endodontics, ed 2, Philadelphia, 1976, Lea & Febiger, pp 34, 597; Maloccurrence does not per se equal malpractice; Gurdin v Dongieux, 468 So2d 1241 (1985).

clinician's past success rate warrant such representation.[59] Factors to be considered in avoiding representing the national success rate of endodontics vis-à-vis a particular dentist in a given clinical situation are (1) a tooth whose periodontal status is questionable, and (2) a clinician who is known to have an unusually high rate of endodontic failures.

An endodontic treating dentist is also liable for failure to disclose evident pathology in the quadrant being treated. The patient should be advised of any periodontal disease that adversely affects the prognosis of abutment teeth for partial dentures or bridges. A dentist should also advise of cysts, fractures, or lesions of suspected neoplasms. Also be careful not to ignore any evident pathology which, if untreated, may adversely affect the dental or medical health of the patient. A dentist who fails to plan treatment properly plans for treatment to fail.

The doctrine of informed consent protects both the dentist and the patient so there will be no surprises or patient disappointment if an adverse result occurs. Should a nonnegligent failure or poor result occur, the availability of a signed informed consent form may serve as a reminder to the patient that the risk of complications was discussed in advance of treatment and that, unfortunately, the patient's endodontic treatment came out on the wrong end of the statistical curve.

Slips of the Drill

A slip of the drill, like a slip of the tongue, may be unintentional, but it nevertheless causes harm. When a cut tongue or lip occurs, it is usually the result of operator error. To paraphrase Alexander Pope, to err is human, but to forebear divine. To increase the likelihood that a patient will forebear from filing suit because of a cut lip or tongue, the clinician should follow these steps:

1. Inform the patient that you indeed regret the injury to the patient. This is not a legal admission of guilt, but rather an admission that you are a compassionate human being.
2. Repair the injured tissue yourself or refer the patient to an oral or plastic surgeon, depending on the extent of the injury and whether a plastic revision due to scarring is likely.
3. Advise the patient that you will pay the bill for the referred treatment of the oral or plastic surgeon. Indeed, have the oral or plastic surgeon send the bill directly to you for payment. Send the oral or plastic surgeon's bill to your professional liability carrier. Most carriers will pay the claim under the medical payments provisions of the general liability policy for an "accident" rather than as a malpractice incident compensable under the professional liability policy. Call the patient periodically to check on healing and recovery.

Electrosurgery

Electrosurgery can cause problems if mishandled. Damage to the oral cavity caused by poor use of electrosurgical devices consists primarily of gingival and osseous necrosis and sloughing distal to the surgical field, and pulpal necrosis of affected teeth.

All equipment should be properly maintained and certified to meet American National Standard/American Dental Association Specification No. 44 on Electrical Safety Standards. Check current equipment to see that units meet ANSI standards and that electrical cords and other components are in good repair. Electrical receptacles should meet the requirements of the National Electrical Code for circuit grounding and ground fault protection. During use, the dispersive electrode plate should be well away from metal parts of the dental chair and the patient's clothing. Skin contact can cause burns. Use of plastic mirrors, saliva ejectors, and evacuator tips is strongly recommended.

Reasonable versus Unreasonable Errors of Judgment

Although a dentist is legally responsible for unreasonable errors in judgment, mistakes occasionally do happen despite adherence to the standards of reasonable care. Maloccurrence does not alone prove malpractice unless the maloccurrence is caused by a malpractice error.[60]

For example, accessory or fourth canals on molar teeth are frequently difficult to locate and tax the best of operators. Failure to locate an accessory or fourth canal does not conclusively constitute an unreasonable error of judgment. Rather, this may represent a reasonable error of judgment in the performance of endodontics. Nevertheless, if the additional canal was readily apparent radiographically, the existence of a fourth canal should have been considered and treatment should have extended to it.

Treatment of the Incorrect Tooth

A reasonable, nonnegligent mistake of judgment may occur owing to difficulty in localizing the source of endodontic pain. Vital pulps may on occasion be sacrificed in an attempt to diagnose the source of pain. Nevertheless, it is unreasonable, and therefore inexcusable, to treat the wrong tooth because it is recorded incorrectly on the referral slip or because the radiographs are mounted incorrectly or reversed.

If the wrong tooth is treated because of an unreasonable mistake of judgment the dentist should be sympathetic, waive payment for all endodontic treatment, and offer to pay the fee for crowning the unnecessarily treated tooth.

Swallowing of an Endodontic Instrument

Use of a rubber dam in endodontics is mandatory.[61] Even if the endodontically treated tooth is broken-down and cannot be clamped, a rubber dam, regardless of required modification, should be used in all instances (see Chapter 4). Not only is microbial contamination thereby reduced, but also the risk of a patient's aspirating or swallowing an endodontic instrument (Fig. 10-7).

If a patient swallows a file, it is likely due to the dentist's failure to observe the standard of care. If such an incident does occur, the dentist should (1) advise the patient that you regret what occurred, (2) refer the patient for immediate medical care, including radiography, to determine if it is lodged in the bronchus or stomach so that appropriate measures are taken to remove it, and (3) offer to pay for the patient's out-of-pocket medical expenses.

---

[59]Hales v Pittman, 118 Ariz305, 576 P 22 493 (1978).

[60]Gurdin v Dongieux, 468 So 2d 1241 (1985); Tropani v Holzer, 158 Cal App 2d 1, 321 P2d 803.

[61]Simpson v Davis, 219 Kan584; 549 P2d 950 (1976).

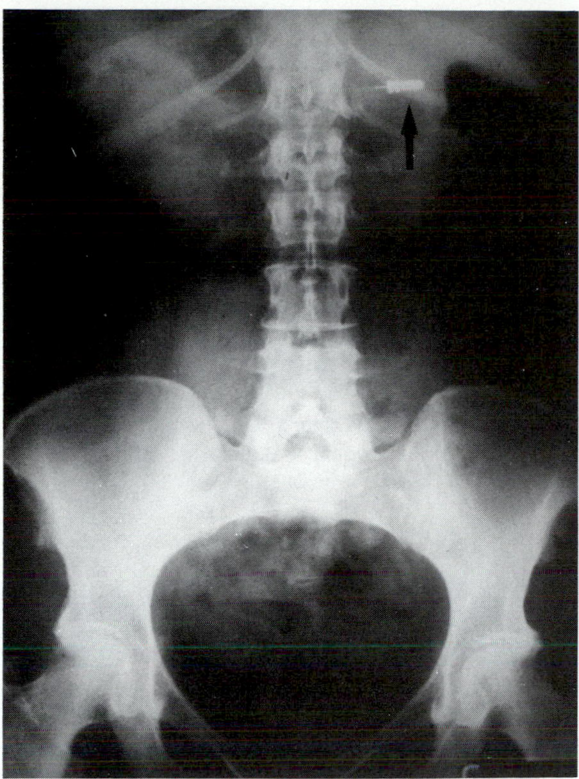

FIG. 10-7 Swallowed endodontic instrument demonstrates the wisdom of using a rubber dam.

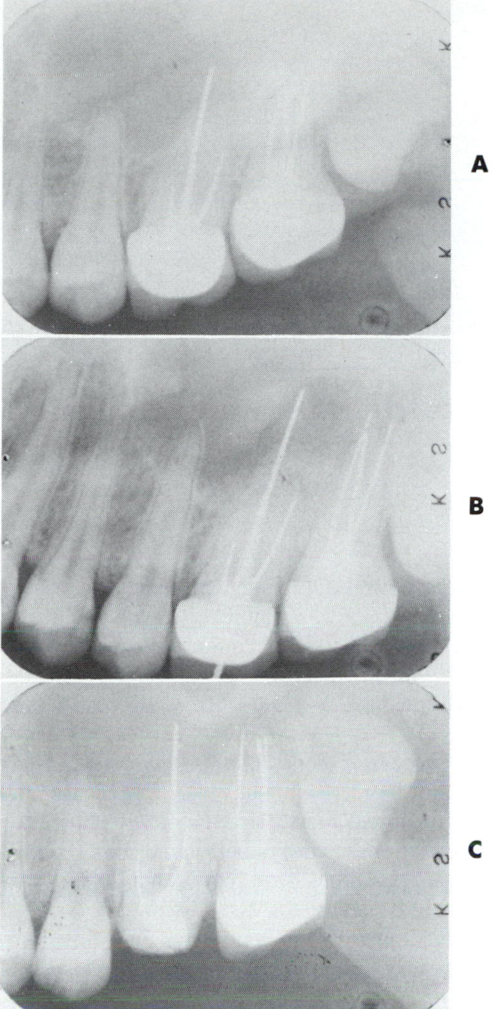

FIG. 10-8 Gross overfill into sinus with a silver point, which ultimately caused sinusitis and loss of tooth no. 14 as a result of endodontic failure.

Overfill of a Canal

A very slight overfill of a canal can occur without violating the standard of care (Chapter 9). Gross overfills usually indicate faulty technique. Nevertheless, so long as the overfill is not in contact with vital structures, such as the mandibular nerve or sinuses, permanent harm is unlikely.

If, however, severe postoperative pain is foreseeable as a result of the overfilling, the patient should be advised of the likelihood of postoperative discomfort because of contact of the sealant material with the surrounding tissue. Similarly, if the overfill is slight or increased postoperative pain is unlikely, the patient need not be advised, lest it cause unnecessary alarm. However, a note should be made on the patient's chart of the overextension—and of the reason for not informing the patient. Fortunately, slight to moderate overfillings with inert conventional endodontic sealers like gutta-percha with Grossman's paste usually repair themselves and produce no irreversible changes.

Current Usage of Silver Points

Use of silver points in lieu of gutta-percha or other conventional endodontic filling materials represents a departure from today's standard of care. Figure 10-8 represents gross overfilling with a silver point that ultimately caused the loss of tooth no. 14 as a result of endodontic failure.

Use of N-2 (Sargenti Paste)

Dental literature reports that permanent paresthesias are associated with gross overfilling with paraformaldehyde sealant (N-2) but are not reported with conventional sealants (Fig. 10-9). Current use of paraformaldehyde-containing endodontic sealants is not merely the result of a philosophical difference between two respectable schools of thought. Rather, the distinction is between the reasonable and prudent school of thought that advocates conservative conventional endodontics, and the imprudent, radical school of paraformaldehyde providers who risk permanent, deleterious injury with N-2 overfills. Stated otherwise, no matter how many N-2 practitioners do it, their sheer number does not make it right.

A dentist may be liable for fraudulent concealment or intentional misrepresentation, or as a coconspirator, if obvious dental disease due to the negligence of another dentist is detected and the patient is falsely advised that none exists. For instance, if a gross overfill of a paraformaldehyde sealant is evident radiographically and the patient reports that another dentist caused the overfill, which resulted in paresthesia, a subsequent treating dentist may be liable who defends such gross negligence by advising the patient that the paresthesia will probably disappear shortly and that using N-2 merely reflects a philosophical difference rather than substandard practice.

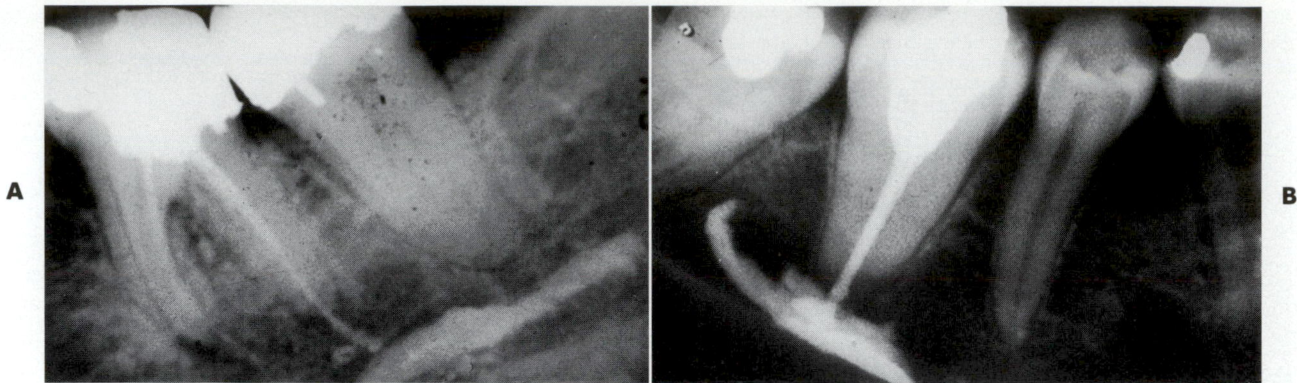

FIG. 10-9 A and **B,** Overextensions of Sargenti paste filling the inferior alveolar canal. Both cases could have been avoided if the practitioners had selected a conventional sealing material and used a technique that emphasizes length control.

The federal Food, Drug, and Cosmetic Act, enacted in 1938 and amended in 1962, prohibits interstate shipment of an unapproved drug or individual components utilized to compound the drug.[62] On February 12, 1993, the FDA dental advisory panel confirmed that N-2's safety and effectiveness remain unproven. N-2 may not be shipped interstate nor may it be distributed intrastate if any of the N-2 ingredients were acquired interstate. Mail order shipments of N-2 from out-of-state pharmacies in quantities greater than for single-patient use are considered a bulk sales order rather than a prescription, thus violating FDA regulations.[63] A San Francisco jury awarded punitive damages against the N-2-distributing New York pharmacy for knowingly shipping N-2 in violation of FDA regulations and with deliberate disregard for patient safety.[64]

PROPHYLACTIC ENDODONTIC PRACTICE

Periodontal Examination

Competent endodontic treatment begins with adequate diagnostic procedures, as discussed in Chapters 1 and 2. An adequate periodontal evaluation must accompany each endodontic diagnosis, which requires a diagnostic radiograph, clinical visualization, evaluation of the periodontal tissues, and probing for periodontal pockets with a calibrated periodontal probe, particularly in furcation areas.[65]

Although endodontic treatment may be successful, tooth loss may nevertheless result from progress of any residual untreated periodontitis. Consequently, a periodontal evaluation and prognosis are mandatory, so that the patient and dentist can make an informed and intelligent choice about whether to proceed with endodontics, a combination of periodontal and endodontic treatment (Chapter 17), or extraction.

Each tooth undergoing endodontic therapy, as well as adjacent teeth, should be probed with a calibrated periodontal instrument to obtain six measurements per tooth. Pockets of 4 mm or greater should be recorded on the patient's chart. If no pockets exist, then WNL (within normal limits), or a similar abbreviation, should be noted. Mobility should also be charted and designated class I, II, or III. Gingival recession, furcations and mucogingival deficiencies should be recorded.

A dentist who treats with endodontic success but ignores loss of periodontal attachment may misdiagnose or fail to appreciate the risk of failure because of poor periodontal prognosis. The endodontic treating dentist should not assume that a periodontal evaluation has been performed by another dentist, even the referring dentist. Instead, an independent periodontal evaluation should be done.

If clinically significant periodontal disease is present, the endodontic treating dentist should consult with the restorative dentist to determine whether the periodontal disease will be properly treated or referred in conjunction with endodontic treatment. A patient should be advised of any compromise of the endodontically treated tooth's periodontal status, in order to comply with required informed consent disclosure.

Preoperative and Postoperative Radiographs

1. A current preoperational diagnostic periapical radiograph is mandatory.
2. Working films are necessary to verify canal length (if an electronic canal-measuring devise is not used) and the apical extent of the gutta-percha fill.
3. Posttreatment radiographs are essential for determining the adequacy of the endodontic seal, as discussed in Chapter 8.

Patient Rapport

Good patient relations are 15% dependent upon your competency to cure and 85% upon demonstrating to the patient that you care enough to always give your professional best.

Rapport between dentist and patient reduces the likelihood the patient will sue. Develop rapport by demonstrating genuine interest in the patient and making the patient feel like the most valued one in the practice.

Patients feel important if they are seated in the operatory within a reasonable time after arriving. The longer a patient is kept waiting, the more frustration and animosity will build up. If the patient cannot be seen within a reasonable time, a staff

---

[62]USCA §§301 et seq.

[63]Cedars N Towers Pharm, Inc v U.S.A., Fla Fed Dist Ct No 77-4965 (Aug. 18, 1978).

[64]Irsheid v Elbee Chemists and Available Products, Inc, San Francisco Super Ct, Docket No 908373 (1992).

[65]McFall W, et al: Presence of periodontal data in patient records of general practices: patient records, J Periodontol 59:445, 1988.

member should communicate the reason, and, if appropriate, offer to reschedule the appointment. Staff or doctor should telephone the patient at the end of the day following any difficult procedure or surgery as a patient reminder to follow post-operative instructions and to check on the patient's status. Any patient complaints and symptoms should be recorded, as well as noncompliance with instructions, as evidence of the patient's contributory negligence.

Rapport Building Blocks

Sir William Osler advised, "Listen to the patient. He's trying to tell you what's wrong with him." The best communicators listen more than they speak. When they do speak, it is mostly to clarify what the patient has said. Difficult doctor-patient relationships create poor communications. Improved understanding of the patient's complaints fosters better rapport, aids treatment, and reduces the likelihood of litigation.

In handling the patient's complaints ask, "What do *you* think is causing the problem?" Otherwise, you may solve the patient's dental problem but not the patient's perceived problem. Failing to clarify the patient's expectations about diagnoses and recommended treatment leaves the patient with unresolved worries and concern. For instance, a patient may fear that a retained endodontic file is carcinogenic unless this fear is allayed with a careful explanation.

Do not rush the visit. Full attention to the patient's complaints, good eye contact, and respectful addressing of the patient gains rapport, improves communication, and prevents lawsuit. Care more, not less, lest you be judged careless.

Avoid questions that require a yes or no answer. Instead, ask what are the patient's problems. Rephrase the patient's complaints to prevent miscommunication. Then ask if you have summarized the patient's complaints accurately. Summarizing clarifies understanding by repeating important points. Inquire if there are any remaining questions. Nonverbal communication can be a powerful tool. For instance, shake hands initially and/or comfort with an outstretched hand if pain is provoked.

Emotions are the dominant force behind most malpractice claims. Patients who feel misled, betrayed, or abandoned become angry and seek vindication of their rights more than financial compensation. Thus, maintain a tactful and courteous approach and be attentive to patients' needs and complaints. Always make sure that your communications with the patient are clear, even to the point of being repetitious, by asking if the patient has any questions. Never abandon a patient in the middle of a course of treatment and always be available to provide follow-up care. Avoid telephone diagnosis. If you do so, follow-up with a chart note.

Good telephone communication is a matter of asking the right questions, such as asking a post-operative patient if there is difficulty breathing or swallowing, as well as the degree and location of swelling. In cases of suspected infection, remain at a telephone where you can be reached until the patient or family member calls you back with a temperature reading to verify the patient is afebrile.

Do not make off-the-cuff diagnoses. One dentist dismissed a patient's party guest's endodontic problem as sensitivity due to gum recession and recommended a desensitizing toothpaste. A lawsuit resulted from inadequate follow-up despite mere cocktail chatter.

Keep conversations professional. Making light of a minor occurrence, like the dropping of an instrument, with a quip about your "one-drink-too-many" at lunch, may seem funny at the time you said it but may not sound so funny if the patient soberly reiterates your quip to the jury.

Do not let a patient's flattery of your abilities undermine your best professional judgment. Heroic measures usually result in treatment failures, a dissatisfied patient, and, ultimately, a law suit for uninformed consent despite the patient's virtually hopeless prognosis.

A patient dissatisfied with prior treatment, such as a patient with a bag full of dentures or bridges made by other competent dentists, should signal a waving red flag to stop, rather than proceeding with treatment. Young practitioners are more apt to walk into unreasonable treatment traps where more experienced practitioners fear to tread.

A compassionate and concerned dentist who is able to demonstrate that the patient is cared about, as well as cared for, avoids many malpractice actions. Thus when an iatrogenic mishap occurs, it behooves the clinician to be frank and forthright with the patient. Moreover, concealment of negligence may extend the statute of limitations, since most states with discovery statutes construe discovery as the date upon which the patient discovered the negligent cause of the injury and not the date of the injury itself.[66] Furthermore, belated discovery of injury from another dentist evokes a feeling of betrayal in the patient and destroys any rapport that would otherwise dissuade the patient from instituting litigation.

Fees

Clarify fees and payment procedures before initiating treatment. If the dental treatment becomes more extensive than originally planned, discuss the increased charges and reasons with the patient before continuing treatment. Resist charging for untoward complications such as extended postoperative visits or retrieving broken instruments.

An overzealous receptionist who places payment pressure on a dissatisfied patient, or the dentist who sues to collect a fee from an already displeased patient, may invite a countersuit for malpractice. Refunding fees or paying for the treatment fee of the subsequent treating dentist under the general liability rather than professional liability portion of your insurance policy is usually much less expensive than a week in court and a jury award for a patient's pain and suffering. If you do sue for your fee, do so only if your treatment is beyond reproach and your records substantiate proper diagnosis, treatment, and informed consent options.

Post Perforations

Post selection is important for avoiding perforations. Although perforations may occur without violating the standard of care, certain results circumstantially imply that the standard of care was not met. Generally, posts should not exceed one third of the mesial-distal width of a tooth and should follow the canal anatomy. Excessively large posts violate these guidelines and unreasonably increase the risk of perforation or tooth fracture.

---

[66]Dolan v Borelli, 13 Cal App 4th 816 (1993); Franklin v Albert, 411 NE2d 458 (Mass. 1980). Note, 38 Mont L Rev 399, 1977; Annot, 80 ALR 2d 368, §7b, 1961.

Advances in Endodontics

Technological advances are touted as ideal endodontics. However, the standard of care is a minimal standard of reasonably acceptable practice rather than the ideal. Thus, the reasonable and prudent practitioner is not required to know and use all of the latest technological advances in endodontics. On the other hand, the reasonable and prudent practitioner must keep current with available advances.

Microsurgical endodontics is an example of so-called cutting-edge endodontics. Nonetheless, the great expense of this technique, and the fact that most endodontics can be accomplished successfully without superpower optics, does not mean that standard of care requires microsurgical endodontics. Use of magnifying loupes or similar devices is adequate in most instances.

If studies demonstrate significantly superior results for some alternative to surgical endodontics, the informed consent standard of care may one day require that the patient be advised of the alternative technique, even if it is more expensive. That day has not yet come nor is it inevitable. There may be more than one path to success. So long as the dentist utilizes reasonably acceptable techniques, and informs the patient of reasonable alternatives, the standard of care is met. Moreover, today's surgical advance may be tomorrow's retreat. Breast and TMJ implants are two examples of inadequately tested technology that proved disastrous.[67]

Other Dentist's Substandard Treatment

Do not be overly protective of blatant examples of another dentist's substandard dental treatment. Upon discovery of a gross violation of the minimum standard of dental care, a dentist has an ethical responsibility to report the matter to one's local dental society peer review and/or the dental licensing board or agency.[68] If you do not, and the patient later discovers poor treatment, then you could be sued as a co-conspirator to fraudulent concealment of another practitioner's neglect.

Corroborate your suspicion of prior care deficiencies by obtaining the patient's written authorization for transfer of a copy of the prior dentist's records including radiographs. If still in doubt after obtaining and reviewing the records, consider speaking with the prior dentist to learn what occurred previously.

Peer Review

If, despite good rapport, candid disclosure, and an offer to pay corrective medical or surgical bills the patient is still unsatisfied, the clinician should consider referring the patient to Peer Review. Peer Review committees award damages only for out-of-pocket losses, not for pain and suffering or lost wages. Consequently, even if the committee's decision is adverse to the dentist, the damage award will probably be less than a jury's verdict. If Peer Review finds for the dentist, the patient may be discouraged from proceeding further with litigation. Peer Review proceedings, including the committee's decision, are not admissible at trial for either side.[69]

[67]Federal Register 58:43442-43445, Aug. 16, 1993; Randall T: Antibodies to silicone detected in patients with severe inflammatory reactions, J Am Med Assoc 268:14, 1992.

[68]ADA principles of ethics and code of professional conduct, 1-G Justifiable Criticism, J Am Dent Assoc 123:102, 1992.

[69]Cal Evid Code §1157.

Insurance carriers will usually honor and pay a Peer Review committee award, since a fair adjudication of the merits has been determined. The award is usually less than a jury would award, and defense costs and attorney's fees are saved.

Human Immunodeficiency Virus (HIV) and Endodontics

A dentist may not ethically refuse to treat an HIV-seropositive patient solely because of the diagnosis.[70] Although in the 1980s no federal law had clearly extended the protection of the handicapped laws to AIDS patients, federal congressional action in 1990 extended this protection to the dental office setting with the passage of the Americans with Disabilities Act.[71] Many states already offer additional protection under state law.[72]

Confidentiality for patients disclosing their HIV status is important, since an inadvertent disclosure to an insurance carrier or to other third parties, without any need to know, may result in cancellation of the patient's health, disability, or life insurance, resulting in a claim against the dentist whose office disclosed such information without authorization. Therefore, employees should sign the confidentiality agreement contained in Fig. 10-10. In signing, the staff may be alerted to appreciate the seriousness and importance of maintaining the confidentiality of patient health histories, since the medical history may document AIDS, venereal disease, or another socially stigmatizing diseases.

Should a patient request the dentist not to inform the staff of the patient's HIV status, the dentist should refuse to treat, since this information is essential to staff members. For example, an accidental needlestick with HIV-infected blood, which carries a risk of approximately one chance in 250 of seroconversion, may occur. Current medical protocol includes prophylactic administration of AZT either to prevent or to slow the manifestation of AIDS for deep-penetrating, accidental needlestick exposure.

Although a treating dentist risks devastating a dental practice by informing patients that the dentist has contracted AIDS, the legal risk of not informing the patient is also great indeed. The health care provider may be required to advise patients of positive HIV test results under the doctrine of informed consent (advising of a known risk of harm, i.e., accidental exposure).[73] Even if the patient never contracts AIDS, the patient may nonetheless bring an action for intentional concealment as a variant of informed consent and seek to recover emotional distress and punitive damages. Conversely, patients may be legally liable for lying on their health history regarding their HIV status.[74]

Infective Endocarditis

If warranted by the patient's medical history, consult with the patient's physician to determine the necessity of antibiotic prophylaxis against infective endocarditis in accordance with

[70]Davis M: Dentistry and AIDS: an ethical opinion, J Am Dent Assoc (suppl 9-5), 1989.

[71]Americans with Disabilities Act, Pub L 101-336.

[72]Decision and order of the New York City Commission on Human Rights, Whitmore v The Northern Dispensary, 17 Aug, 1988; California court upholds ban on AIDS discrimination, ADA News 5 Feb 1990.

[73]Doe v U.S. Attorney General, ND Calif. Dec. 28, 1992. No. c-88-3820

[74]Boulais v Lustig, Los Angeles Super Ct BC038105 [$102,500 jury verdict to an ungloved surgical technician].

DENTAL AUXILIARY CONFIDENTIALITY AGREEMENT

I, ______________________, have been informed by
(Dental Assistant)
______________________, DDS, that all dental, medical,and
(Dentist Name)
financial information concerning patients is confidential.

As a condition of employment, I agree to maintain the confidentiality of all oral and written information, including treatment charts, and to not disclose such information to any unauthorized outside persons, including any family members, except upon request and authorization by the patient, the patient's agent, or supervising dentist.

I understand and agree that breach of this employment agreement shall constitute good cause for my discharge from employment. I acknowledge that I may by personally liable for any violation of a patient's privacy or civil rights committed by me without consent of the patient, or the patient's agent, or approval by above-named dentist.

Date: ______________ ______________________________
Signature of Dental Assistant

Witness: ______________

FIG. 10-10 Dental auxiliary confidentiality agreement.

current American Heart Association Guidelines. If the physician does not appear knowledgeable about those guidelines, provide a copy of the guidelines to the physician. If the physician advises that deviation from AHA guidelines is appropriate, ask the physician why. Record your discussions with the physician in the patient's chart.

Communications with the physician should be specific, since the physician may not appreciate dental treatment. The following format might be used:

Dear Doctor:

Your patient requires dental treatment that will result in transient bacteremia. Does the patient have a heart valve defect that increases the risk of infective endocarditis? If so, please advise of the diagnosed defect and recommended prophylactic antibiotic and dosage.

Please also advise if your recommendation is in accordance with the enclosed American Heart Association current guidelines concerning bacterial endocarditis relating to dental treatment.

Thank you for your anticipated cooperation.

Enclosure: 1991 American Heart Association Guidelines.

Patient with joint prostheses require premedication only at the orthopedist's discretion. There are no ADA, AHA, or American Academy of Orthopedic Surgeons mandatory requirements.

CONCLUSION

If the dentist performs endodontics within the standard of care, as described in this chapter, there should be little concern that a lawsuit for professional negligence will be successful. Suggested "prophylactic" measures in this chapter will reduce the chances of litigation by reducing avoidable risks associated with endodontic care.

Both the patient and dentist benefit from risk reduction. It is far better for the dentist to take the extra minute to *do it right,* rather than to subject a patient to a lifetime of misery for an expedient but risky wrong.

Self-assessment questions

1. Which of the following statements is true?
   a. Alteration of records is forbidden.
   b. Alteration of records is permitted if dated.
   c. Additions to records are forbidden.
   d. Additions to records are permitted if dated.
2. Standard of care, as defined by courts,
   a. requires absolute perfection.
   b. describes what a reasonably careful and prudent clinician would do under similar circumstances.
   c. does not allow for individual variations of treatment.
   d. is equivalent to customary practice.
3. The doctrine of informed consent does *not*
   a. require that a patient be advised of reasonably foreseeable risks of treatment.
   b. require that the patient be advised of reasonable alternatives.
   c. require that the patient forfeit his right to do as he sees fit with his own body.
   d. require that the patient be advised of the consequences of non-treatment.
4. To make sure a dentist to whom one refers a patient is not considered to be an agent of the referring dentist, the referring dentist should
   a. verbally inform the patient of that fact.
   b. inform the patient in writing.
   c. enter a disclaimer in the patient's record.
   d. inform the patient that the referral is a suggestion only.
5. A dentist may legally
   a. refuse to treat a new patient despite severe pain and infection.
   b. be bound to see former patients on recall after treatment is completed.
   c. discharge a patient from his practice at any time.
   d. refuse to treat a patient who has an outstanding balance on his account.
6. If a patient who is HIV seropositive requests that the dentist not inform the staff of his condition, the dentist should
   a. refuse to treat the patient.
   b. tell the staff in private, then treat the patient using extra precautions.
   c. not tell the staff, but treat the patient with great caution.
   d. not tell the staff and require the patient to sign a private guarantee that the patient will be liable if someone contracts the virus.
7. If a patient swallows a file and the dentist had not placed a rubber dam, the dentist should
   a. offer to pay for any medical expenses incurred as a result.
   b. not offer to pay for medical expenses, which is an admission of guilt.
   c. not mention who should pay medical expenses and try to infer that the patient is to blame (e.g., sudden movement, difficult case).
   d. apologize for the mishap, and suggest that the patient have medical evaluation only if a problem develops as a result.
8. An endodontist may be held liable who
   a. informs the patient that her general practitioner is performing substandard care (the general practitioner may hold the endodontist liable).
   b. fails to disclose to the patient and/or referring dentist evident pathosis other than the tooth they are treating.
   c. fails to locate a very small canal that is not evident radiographically.
   d. mistakenly initiates treatment on the wrong tooth in a difficult diagnosis situation.
9. Of the following, the dentist's *best* approach to avoiding legal action by patients is to
   a. tell all patients that he/she (the dentist) does not carry malpractice insurance.
   b. attend Continuing Education courses frequently to remain informed of current techniques.
   c. refer all major patient complaints to peer review.
   d. demonstrate genuine interest in the welfare of each patient.

PART TWO

THE SCIENCE OF ENDODONTICS

Chapter 11

Pulp Development, Structure and Function

Henry O. Trowbridge
Syngcuk Kim

By definition, the pulp is a soft tissue of mesenchymal origin residing within the pulp chamber and root canals of teeth. At its periphery is a layer of highly specialized cells, the odontoblasts. The close relationship between the odontoblasts and dentin is one of several reasons why the dentin and pulp should be considered as a functional entity, sometimes referred to as the *pulp-dentin complex*. Certain peculiarities are imposed on the pulp by the rigid mineralized dentin in which it is enclosed. Thus, it is situated within a low-compliance environment that limits its ability to increase in volume during episodes of vasodilatation and increased vascular permeability. In this situation, careful regulation of blood flow is critically important.

The dental pulp is in many ways similar to other connective tissues of the body, but its special characteristics deserve serious consideration. Even the mature pulp bears a strong resemblance to embryonic connective tissue; and yet at its periphery is a layer of highly sophisticated cells, the odontoblasts. The pulp chamber is filled with nerves, vascular tissue, fibers, ground substance, interstitial fluid, odontoblasts, fibroblasts, and other minor cellular components. Since each of these constituents is relatively incompressible, the total volume of blood within the pulp chamber cannot be increased, although reciprocal volume changes can occur between arterioles and venules.

No true arteries or veins enter or leave the pulp, so the circulatory system of the pulp is actually a microcirculatory system whose largest vascular components are arterioles and venules. Unlike most tissues, the pulp lacks a true collateral system and is dependent upon the relatively few arterioles entering through the root foramina and the occasional arteriole through a lateral canal. Since with age there is a gradual reduction in the luminal diameters of these foramina, the vascular system of the pulp decreases progressively.

The pulp is also a rather unique sensory organ. Being encased in a protective layer of dentin, which in turn is covered with enamel, it might be expected to be quite unresponsive to stimulation; yet, despite the low thermal conductivity of dentin, the pulp is undeniably sensitive to thermal stimuli such as ice cream and hot drinks. Later in this chapter we will consider the unusual mechanism that allows the dentin-pulp complex to function as such an exquisitely responsive sensory system.

Following tooth development the pulp retains its ability to form dentin throughout life. This enables the vital pulp to partially compensate for the loss of enamel or dentin caused by mechanical trauma or disease. How well it serves this function depends on many factors, but the potential for regeneration and repair is as much a reality in the pulp as in other connective tissues of the body.

It is the purpose of this chapter to try to bring together what is known about the development, structure, and function of the dentin-pulp complex in the hope that this knowledge will provide a firm biologic basis for clinical decision making.

DEVELOPMENT

Embryologic studies have shown that the pulp is derived from the cephalic neural crest. Neural crest cells arise from the ectoderm along the lateral margins of the neural plate and migrate extensively. Those that travel down the sides of the head into the maxilla and mandible contribute to the formation of the tooth germs. The dental papilla, from which the

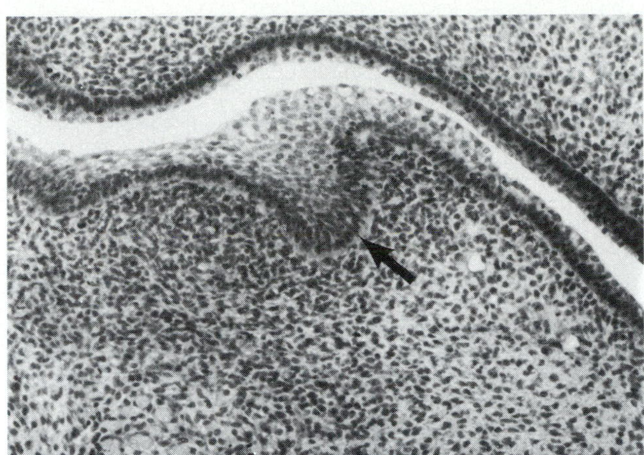

FIG. 11-1 Dental lamina *(arrow)* arising from the oral ectoderm.

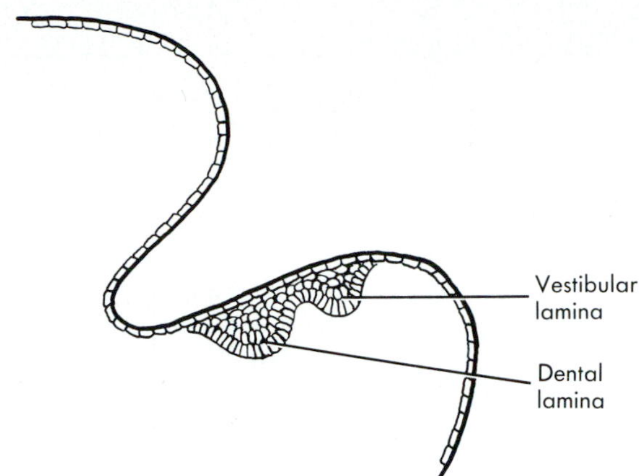

FIG. 11-2 Diagram showing formation of the vestibular and dental lamina from oral ectoderm.

mature pulp arises, develops as ectomesenchymal cells proliferate and condense adjacent to the dental lamina at the sites where teeth will develop (Fig. 11-1). It is important that we remember the migratory potential of ectomesenchymal cells, for later in this chapter we will consider the ability of pulp cells to move into areas of injury and replace destroyed odontoblasts.

During the sixth week of embryonic life, tooth formation begins as a localized proliferation of ectoderm associated with the maxillary and mandibular processes. This proliferative activity results in the formation of two horseshoe-shaped structures, one on each process, that are termed the primary dental laminae. Each primary dental lamina splits into a vestibular and a dental lamina (Fig. 11-2).

Numerous studies have indicated that the embryonic development of any tissue is promoted by interaction with an adjacent tissue.[70,144] The complex epithelial-mesenchymal coactions occurring during tooth development have been studied extensively (for reviews, see Ruch,[145] Slavkin,[152] and Thesleff[160]). Cell-to-cell and cell-to–extracellular matrix (ECM) interactions direct the differentiation of ameloblasts and odontoblasts by causing these cells to change gene expression.

The timing and position of epithelia and mesenchyme are thought to reside in the sequential expression of cell transmembrane linkage molecules such as integrin, cell surface adhesion molecules (CAMs), and substrate adhesion molecules (SAMs, for discussion, see Edelman[34]). CAMs mediate morphogenesis through controlled cell proliferation, specific cell-cell adhesion, and migration. Cells contain membrane proteins called integrins, which are specific receptors for CAMs. Laminin is the CAM of basement membranes. It contains binding domains for heparan sulfate, type IV collagen, and cells. SAMs carry out cell-matrix interactions. The best-studied SAMs of the ECM are the fibronectins, a family of glycoproteins that bind to fibrin, collagen, heparan sulfate, and cell surfaces.

Growth Factors

Growth factors are polypeptides produced by cells that initiate proliferation, migration, and differentiation of a variety of cells. It can be assumed that growth factors are involved in signaling in epithelial-mesenchymal interactions that regulate tooth morphogenesis and cell differentiation. Epidermal growth factor has been shown to play a role in tooth development by stimulating proliferation of cells in the enamel organ and preodontoblasts.[168] It has been hypothesized that transforming growth factor-β_1 (TGF-β_1) may regulate changes in the composition and structure of ECM.[160] A fibroblast growth factor may also be involved in the determination and differentiation of odontoblasts.

From the onset of tooth formation, a dental basement membrane (DBM) exists between the inner dental epithelium and the dental mesenchyme. The DBM consists of a thin basal lamina, which is formed by the epithelial cells, and a layer of ECM derived from the dental mesenchyme. The basal lamina is composed of an elastic network composed of type IV collagen, which has binding sites for other basement membrane constituents such as laminin, fibronectin, and heparan sulfate proteoglycans. Laminin binds to type IV collagen and also to receptors on the surface of preameloblasts and ameloblasts. The DBM also contains mesenchyme-derived type I and type III collagen, hyaluronate, heparan sulfate, and chondroitin 4 and 6 sulfates. Odontoblast cell surface proteoglycans function as receptors for matrix molecules. Signals from components of the matrix influence the migration and differentiation of odontoblasts. The composition of the DBM changes during tooth development, and these alterations appear to modulate the successive steps in odontogenesis. With the differentiation of odontoblasts, type III collagen disappears from the predentin matrix, and fibronectin, which surrounds preodontoblasts, is restricted to the apical pole of mature odontoblasts.[106]

The initial stage of development of the dental papilla is characterized by proliferative activity beneath the dental lamina at sites corresponding to the positions of the prospective primary teeth. Even before the dental lamina begins to form the enamel organ, a capillary vascular network develops within the ectomesenchyme, presumably to support the increased metabolic activity of the presumptive tooth buds.[57] This primordial vascularization is thought to play a key role in induction of odontogenesis.

Although formation of the tooth is a continuous process, as a matter of convenience the process has been divided into three

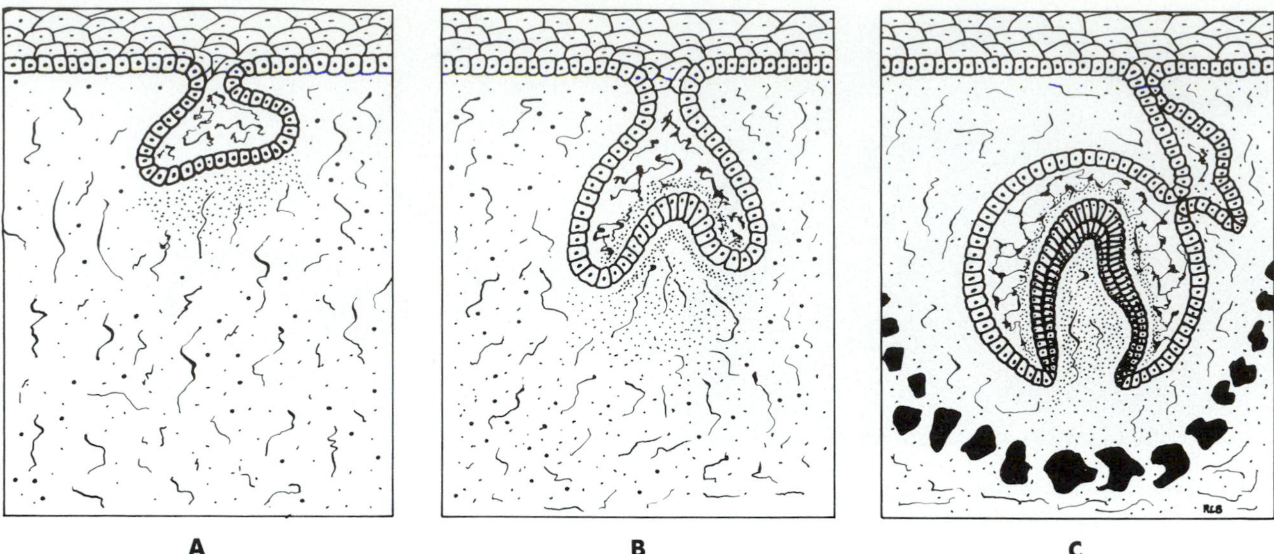

FIG. 11-3 Diagrammatic representation of **A,** the bud, **B,** the cap, and **C,** the bell stages of tooth development.

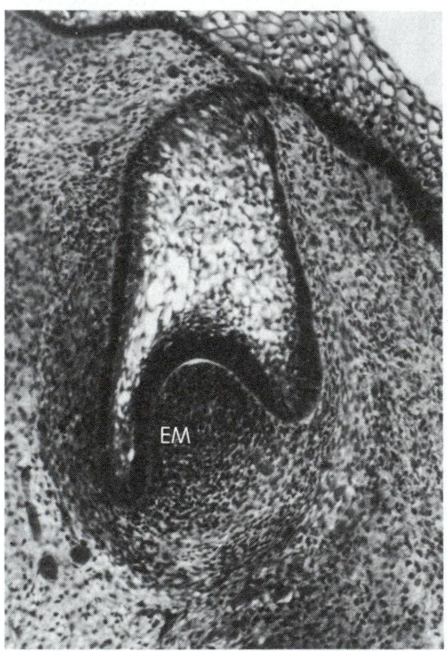

FIG. 11-4 Cap stage of tooth development. The condensed ectomesenchyme *(EM)* that will form the dental papilla lies subjacent to the concave aspect of the enamel organ.

stages: bud, cap, and bell (Fig. 11-3). The *bud* is the initial stage of tooth development, wherein the epithelial cells of the dental lamina proliferate and produce a budlike projection into the adjacent ectomesenchyme. The *cap* stage is reached when the cells of the dental lamina have proliferated to form a concavity that produces a caplike appearance (Fig. 11-4). The outer cells of the "cap" are cuboidal and constitute the outer enamel epithelium. The cells on the inner or concave aspect of the cap are somewhat elongated and represent the inner enamel epithelium. Between the outer and inner epithelia is a network of cells termed the stellate reticulum because of the branched reticular arrangement of the cellular elements. The rim of the enamel organ (i.e., where the outer and inner enamel epithelia are joined) is termed the cervical loop. As the cells forming the loop continue to proliferate, there is further invagination of the enamel organ into the mesenchyme. The organ assumes a bell shape, and tooth development enters the *bell* stage (Fig. 11-5). During the bell stage the ectomesenchyme of the dental papilla becomes partially enclosed by the invaginating epithelium. Also during this stage the blood vessels become established in the dental papilla.

The condensed ectomesenchyme surrounding the enamel organ and dental papilla complex forms the dental sac and ultimately develops into the periodontal ligament (Fig. 11-5). As the tooth bud continues to grow, it carries a portion of the dental lamina with it. This extension is referred to as the lateral lamina. During the bell stage the lateral lamina degenerates and is invaded and replaced by mesenchymal tissue. In this way the epithelial connection between the enamel organ and the oral epithelium is severed. The free end of the dental lamina associated with each of the primary teeth continues to grow and form the successional lamina (Fig. 11-5). It is from this structure that the tooth germ of the succedaneous tooth arises. As the maxillary and mandibular processes increase in length, the permanent first molar arises from posterior extensions of the dental lamina. After birth the second and third molar primordia appear as the dental laminae proliferate into the underlying mesenchyme.

Differentiation of epithelial and mesenchymal cells into ameloblasts and odontoblasts, respectively, occurs during the bell stage of tooth development. This differentiation is always more advanced in the apex of the "bell" (the region where the cusp tip will develop) than in the area of the cervical loop. From the loop upward toward the apex the cells appear progressively more differentiated. The preameloblasts differentiate at a faster rate than the corresponding odontoblasts so that at any given level mature ameloblasts appear before the odon-

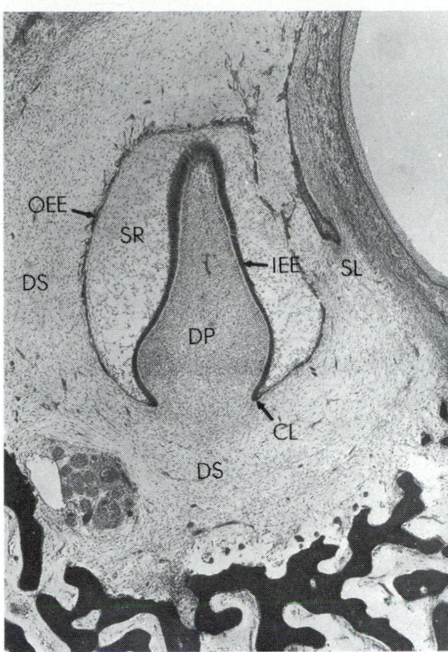

FIG. 11-5 Bell stage of tooth development showing the outer enamel epithelium *(OEE),* stellate reticulum *(SR),* inner enamel epithelium *(IEE),* dental papilla *(DP),* cervical loop *(CL),* successional lamina *(SL),* and dental sac *(DS).*

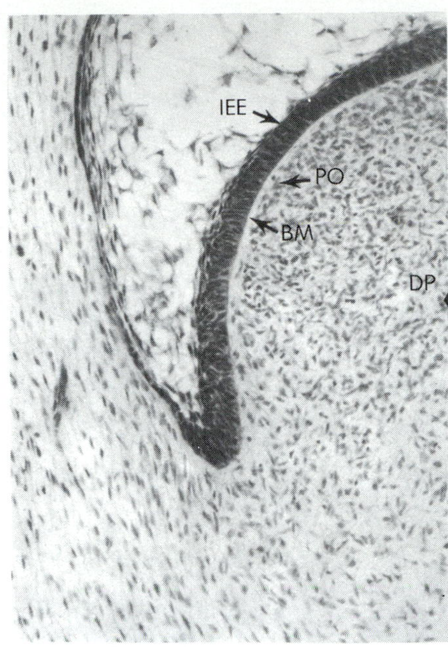

FIG. 11-6 Bell stage shows preodontoblasts *(PO)* aligned along the basement membrane *(BM),* separating the inner enamel epithelium *(IEE)* from the dental papilla *(DP).*

toblasts have fully matured. In spite of this difference in rate of maturation, dentin matrix is formed before enamel matrix.

During the bell stage of development there is still mitotic activity among the relatively immature cells of the inner enamel epithelium in the region of the cervical loop. As they commence to mature into ameloblasts, mitotic activity ceases and the cells elongate and display the characteristics of active protein synthesis (i.e., an abundance of rough endoplasmic reticulum [RER], a well-developed Golgi complex, and numerous mitochondria).

As the ameloblasts undergo differentiation, changes are taking place across the basement membrane in the adjacent dental papilla. Thanks to some excellent studies,[144,156] a comprehensive picture of dentin development has emerged. Prior to differentiation of odontoblasts, the dental papilla consists of sparsely distributed polymorphic mesenchymal cells with wide intercellular spaces (Fig. 11-6). With the onset of differentiation a single layer of cells, the presumptive odontoblasts (preodontoblasts), align themselves along the basement membrane separating the inner enamel epithelium from the dental papilla (Fig. 11-6). These cells stop dividing and elongate into short columnar cells with basally situated nuclei (Fig. 11-7). Several cytoplasmic projections from each of these cells extend toward the basal lamina. At this stage the preodontoblasts are still relatively undifferentiated.

As the odontoblasts continue to differentiate, they become progressively more elongated and take on the ultrastructural characteristics of protein-secreting cells. Cytoplasmic processes from these cells extend through the dental basement membrane toward the basal lamina, and more and more collagen fibrils appear within the ECM. Large fan-shaped bundles 1000 to 2000 Å in diameter (sometimes referred to as *von Korff fibers*) become oriented more or less at right angles to the basal lamina. Smaller collagen fibers approximately 500 Å in diameter also accumulate; these lie more parallel to the basal lamina. A study on collagen gene expression during mouse molar tooth development found type I but no type III collagen mRNA in odontoblasts.[4] Both type I and type III collagen mRNA was detected in most of the various mesenchymal cells of the dental papilla. Others have reported that the dentin of bovine and human teeth contains only type I collagen.[109,113] This indicates that all collagen fibers in dentin originate from odontoblasts.

Dentinogenesis first occurs in the developing tooth at sites where the cusp tips or incisal edge will be formed. It is in this region that odontoblasts reach full maturity and become tall columnar cells, at times attaining a height of 50 μm or more (Fig. 11-7). The width of these cells remains fairly constant at approximately 7 μm. Production of the first dentin matrix involves the formation, organization, and maturation of collagen fibrils and proteoglycans. As more collagen fibrils accumulate subjacent to the basal lamina, the lamina becomes discontinuous and eventually disappears. This occurs as the collagen fibers become organized and extend into the interspaces of the ameloblast processes. Concurrently the odontoblasts extend several small processes toward the ameloblasts. Some of these become interposed between the processes of ameloblasts, resulting in the formation of enamel spindles (dentinal tubules that extend into the enamel). Membrane-bound vesicles bud off from the odontoblast processes and become interspersed among the collagen fibers of the dentin matrix. These vesicles subsequently play an important role in the initiation of mineralization (this subject will be discussed later). With the onset of dentinogenesis the dental papilla becomes the dental pulp.

As predentin matrix is formed, the odontoblasts commence to move away toward the central pulp, depositing matrix at a

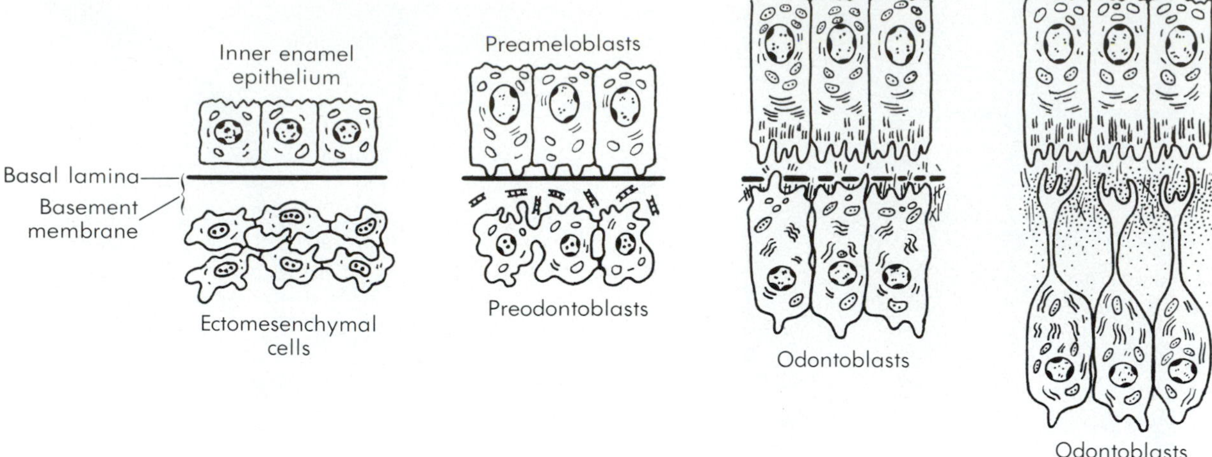

FIG. 11-7 Diagrammatic representation of the stages of odontoblast differentiation.

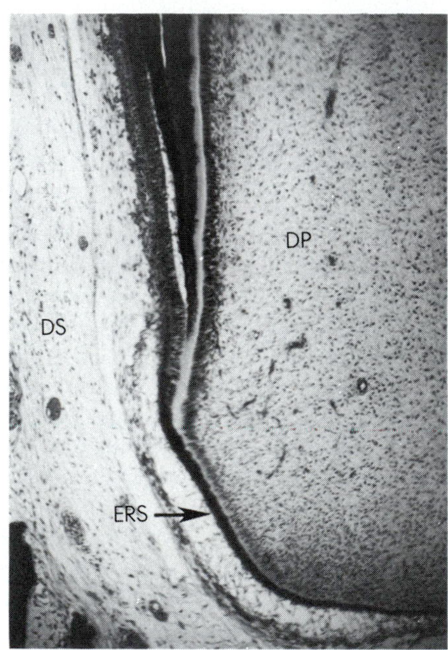

FIG. 11-8 Root development showing dental pulp *(DP)*, dental sac *(DS)*, and epithelial root sheath *(ERS)*.

rate of approximately 4 to 8 μm per day in their wake. Within this matrix a process from each odontoblast becomes accentuated and remains to form the primary odontoblast process. It is around these processes that the dentinal tubules are formed.

Root

Root development commences after the completion of enamel formation. The cells of the inner and outer enamel epithelia, which comprise the cervical loop, begin to proliferate and form a structure known as Hertwig's epithelial root sheath (Fig. 11-8). This sheath determines the size and shape of the root or roots of the tooth. As in the formation of the crown, the cells of the inner enamel epithelium appear to influence the adjacent mesenchymal cells to differentiate into preodontoblasts and odontoblasts. As soon as the first layer of dentin matrix mineralizes, gaps appear in the root sheath, allowing mesenchymal cells from the dental sac to move into contact with the newly formed dentin. These cells then differentiate into cementoblasts and deposit cementum matrix on the root dentin.

Epithelial Rests of Malassez

The epithelial root sheath does not entirely disappear with the onset of dentinogenesis. Some cells persist within the periodontal ligament and are known as epithelial rests of Malassez. Although the number of these rests gradually decreases with age, it has been shown that at least some of them retain the ability to undergo cell division[177] (Fig. 11-9). [1] *If in later life a chronic inflammatory lesion develops within the periapical tissues as a result of pulp disease, proliferation of the epithelial rests may produce a periapical (radicular) cyst.*

Accessory Canals

Occasionally during formation of the root sheath a break develops in the continuity of the sheath, producing a small gap. When this occurs, dentinogenesis does not take place opposite the defect. The result is a small "accessory" canal between the dental sac and the pulp. An accessory canal can become established anywhere along the root, thus creating a periodontal-endodontic pathway of communication and a possible portal of entry into the pulp if the periodontal tissues lose their integrity. *In periodontal disease the development of a periodontal pocket may expose an accessory canal and thus allow microorganisms or their metabolic products to gain access to the pulp.*

DENTIN

Fully mature dentin is composed of approximately 65% inorganic material by weight, nearly all in the form of hydroxyapatite crystals. Collagen accounts for about 20% of dentin. Citrate, chondroitin sulfate, noncollagenous protein, lactate, and lipid account for approximately 2%. The remaining 13% consists of water. By volume, inorganic matter makes up 45% of dentin; organic molecules 33%; and water 22%. A charac-

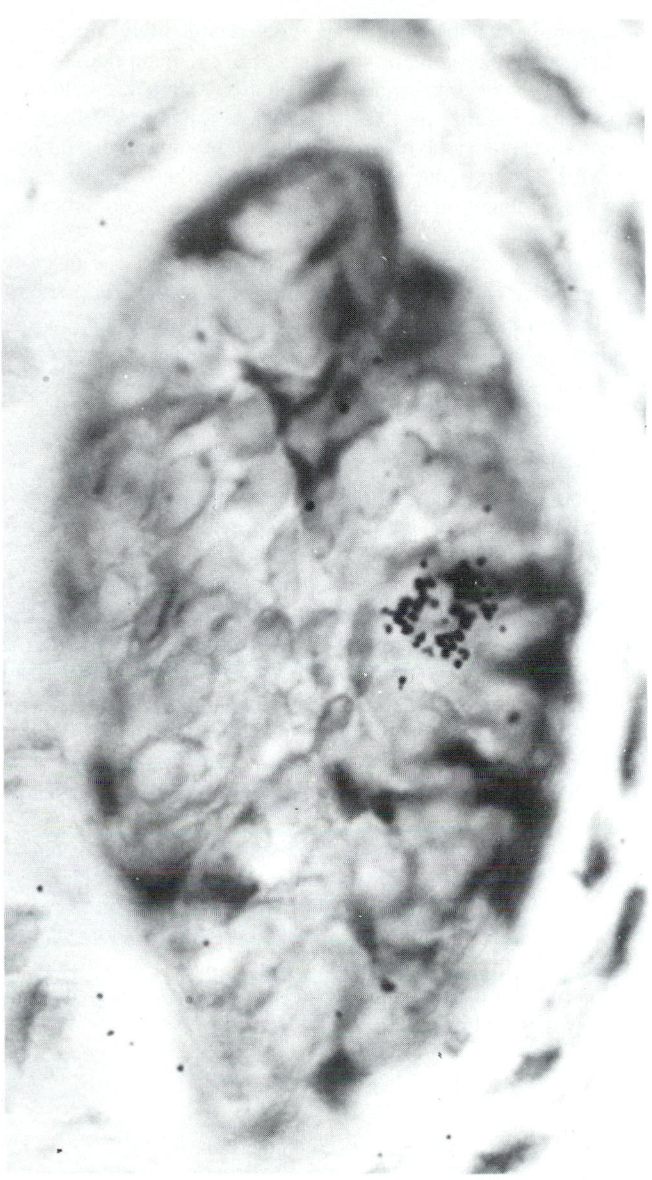

FIG. 11-9 Radioautograph of an epithelial rest cell showing ^{3}H-thymidine labeling of the nucleus. The cell is preparing to divide. (From Trowbridge HO, and Shibata F: Periodontics 5:109, 1967.)

teristic of human dentin is the presence of tubules that occupy from 20% to 30% of the volume of intact dentin. These tubules house the major cell processes of odontoblasts. The elasticity of dentin provides flexibility for the overlying brittle enamel.

Dentin and enamel are closely bound together at the dentin-enamel junction (DEJ), and dentin joins cementum at the dentin-cementum junction (DCJ). Electron microscopy has revealed that the hydroxyapatite crystals of dentin and enamel are intermixed in the area formerly occupied by the basal lamina of the inner enamel epithelium.[83] Since the basal lamina is dissolved prior to the onset of dentinogenesis, no organic membrane separates the crystals of enamel from those of dentin. It is well known clinically that the DEJ is an area of considerable sensitivity. The reason for this is not clear, but it is thought that the branching of the dentinal tubules in the region of the DEJ plays a role.

Types

Developmental dentin is that which forms during tooth development. That formed physiologically after the root is fully developed is referred to as *secondary dentin*. Developmental dentin is classified as *orthodentin,* the tubular form of dentin found in the teeth of all dentate mammals. Mantle dentin is the first formed dentin and is situated immediately subjacent to the enamel or cementum. It is typified by its content of the thick fan-shaped collagen fibers deposited immediately subjacent to the basal lamina during the initial stages of dentinogenesis. Spaces between the fibers are occupied by smaller collagen fibrils lying more or less parallel with the DEJ or DCJ. The width of mantle dentin in human teeth has been estimated at 80 to 100 μm.[11,121]

Circumpulpal dentin is formed after the layer of mantle dentin has been deposited, and it constitutes the major part of developmental dentin. The organic matrix is composed mainly of collagen fibrils, approximately 500 Å in diameter, that are oriented at right angles to the long axis of the dentinal tubules. These fibrils are closely packed together and form an interwoven network.

Predentin is the unmineralized organic matrix of dentin situated between the layer of odontoblasts and the mineralized dentin. Its macromolecular constituents include type I and type II trimer collagens, several proteoglycans (dermatan sulfate, heparan sulfate, hyaluronate, keratan sulfate, chondroitin-4-sulfate, chondroitin-6-sulfate), glycoproteins, glycosaminoglycans (GAGs), gamma-carboxyglutamate-containing proteins (GLA-proteins) and dentin phosphoprotein, a tissue-specific molecule which is unique to the odontoblast cell lineage.[29,152] Chondroitin-4-sulfate and chondroitin-6-sulfate accumulate near the calcification front.

Mineralization

Mineralization of dentin matrix commences within the initial increment of mantle dentin. Calcium phosphate crystals begin to accumulate in matrix vesicles within the predentin.[20] Presumably these vesicles bud off from the cytoplasmic processes of odontoblasts. Although matrix vesicles are distributed throughout the predentin, they are most numerous near the basal lamina. The apatite crystals grow rapidly within the vesicles, and in time the vesicles rupture. The crystals thus released mix with crystals from adjoining vesicles to form advancing crystal fronts that merge to form small globules. As the globules expand, they fuse with adjacent globules until the matrix is completely mineralized.

Apparently matrix vesicles are involved only in mineralization of the initial layer of dentin. As the process of mineralization progresses, the advancing front projects along the collagen fibrils of the predentin matrix. Hydroxyapatite crystals appear on the surface and within the fibrils and continue to grow as mineralization progresses, resulting in an increased mineral content of the dentin.

Dentinal Tubules

Tubules form around the odontoblast processes and thus traverse the entire width of the dentin from the DEJ or DCJ to the pulp. They are slightly tapered, with the wider portion situated toward the pulp. This tapering is the result of the progressive formation of peritubular dentin, which leads to a continuous decrease in the diameter of the tubules toward the enamel.

In coronal dentin the tubules have a gentle S shape as they extend from the DEJ to the pulp. The S-shaped curvature is presumably a result of the crowding of odontoblasts as they migrate toward the center of the pulp. As they approach the pulp, the tubules converge because the surface of the pulp chamber has a much smaller area than the surface of dentin along the DEJ.

The number and diameter of the tubules at various distances from the pulp have been determined (Table 11-1).[56] Investigators[1] found the number and diameter of dentinal tubules to be similar in rats, cats, dogs, monkeys, and humans, indicating that mammalian orthodentin has evolved amazingly constantly.

Lateral tubules containing branches of the main odontoblastic processes have been demonstrated by other researchers,[91] who suggested that they form pathways for the movement of materials between the main processes and the more distant matrix. It is also possible that the direction of the branches influence the orientation of the collagen fibrils in the intertubular dentin.

Near the DEJ the dentinal tubules ramify into one or more terminal branches (Fig. 11-10). This is due to the fact that during the initial stage of dentinogenesis the differentiating odontoblasts extended several cytoplasmic processes toward the DEJ but, as the odontoblasts withdrew, their processes converged into one major process (Fig. 11-7).

TABLE 11-1. Mean number and diameter per square millimeter of dentinal tubules at various distances from the pulp in human teeth

Distance from pulp (mm)	Number of tubules ($1000/mm^2$)		Tubule diameter (μm)	
	Mean	Range	Mean	Range
Pulpal wall	45	30-52	2.5	2.0-3.2
0.1-0.5	43	22-59	1.9	1.0-2.3
0.6-1.0	38	16-47	1.6	1.0-1.6
1.1-1.5	35	21-47	1.2	0.9-1.5
1.6-2.0	30	12-47	1.1	0.8-1.6
2.1-2.5	23	11-36	0.9	0.6-1.3
2.6-3.0	20	7-40	0.8	0.5-1.4
3.1-3.5	19	10-25	0.8	0.5-1.2

From Garberoglio R and Brännström M: Arch Oral Biol 21:355, 1976.

Peritubular Dentin

Dentin lining the tubules is termed *peritubular dentin,* whereas that between the tubules is known as *intertubular dentin* (Fig. 11-11). Presumably precursors of the dentin matrix that is deposited around each odontoblast process are synthesized by the odontoblast, transported in secretory vesicles out into the process, and released by reverse pinocytosis. With the formation of peritubular dentin there is a corresponding reduction in the diameter of the process.

Peritubular dentin represents a specialized form of orthodentin not common to all mammals. Because of its lower content of collagen, peritubular dentin is more quickly dissolved in acid than is intertubular dentin.

It has also been shown that peritubular dentin is more highly mineralized and therefore harder than intertubular dentin.[49,53,105,112,183,205] Because of its hardness, peritubular dentin may provide added structural support for the intertubular dentin. The matrix of peritubular dentin also differs from that of intertubular dentin in having relatively fewer collagen fibrils and a higher proportion of sulfated proteoglycans.

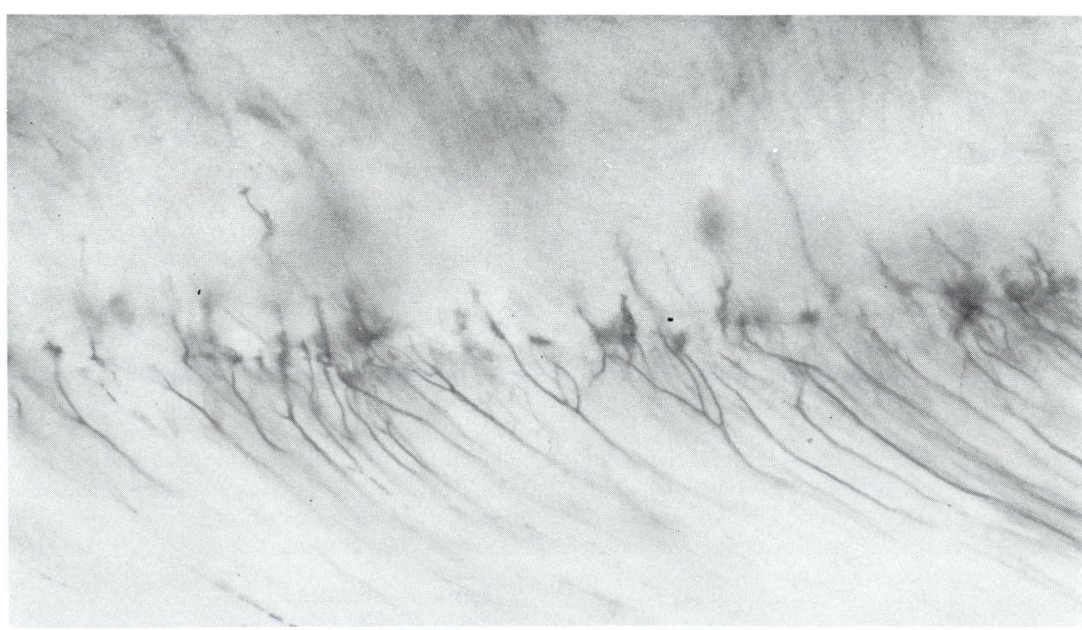

FIG. 11-10 Ground section of a tooth demonstrating branching of the dentinal tubules near the DEJ. This branching may account for the increased clinical sensitivity at the DEJ.

Intertubular Dentin

Intertubular dentin is located between the rings of peritubular dentin and constitutes the bulk of circumpulpal dentin (Fig. 11-11). Its organic matrix consists mainly of collagen fibrils having diameters of 500 to 1000 Å. These fibrils are oriented approximately at right angles to the dentinal tubules.

Dentinal Sclerosis

Partial or complete obturation of dentinal tubules may occur as a result of aging or develop in response to stimuli such as attrition of the tooth surface or dental caries.[153] When tubules become filled with mineral deposits, the dentin becomes sclerotic. Dentinal sclerosis is easily recognized in histologic ground sections because of its translucency, which is due to the homogeneity of the dentin since both matrix and tubules are mineralized. Studies using dyes, solvents, and radioactive ions[14,15,42,45,119,128] have shown that sclerosis results in decreased permeability of dentin. Thus dentinal sclerosis, by limiting the diffusion of noxious substances through the dentin, helps to shield the pulp from irritation.

One form of dentinal sclerosis is thought to represent an acceleration of peritubular dentin formation. This form appears to be a physiologic process, and in the apical third of the root it develops as a function of age.[153] Dentinal tubules can also become blocked by the precipitation of hydroxyapatite and whitlockite crystals within the tubules.[159] This type occurs in the translucent zone of carious dentin as well as in attrited dentin and has been termed "pathological sclerosis."[183]

Interglobular Dentin

The term *interglobular dentin* refers to organic matrix that remains unmineralized because the mineralizing globules fail to coalesce. This occurs most often in the circumpulpal dentin just below the mantle dentin where the pattern of mineralization is more likely to be globular than appositional. In certain dental anomalies (e.g., vitamin D–resistant rickets and hypophosphatasia) large areas of interglobular dentin are a characteristic feature (Fig. 11-12).

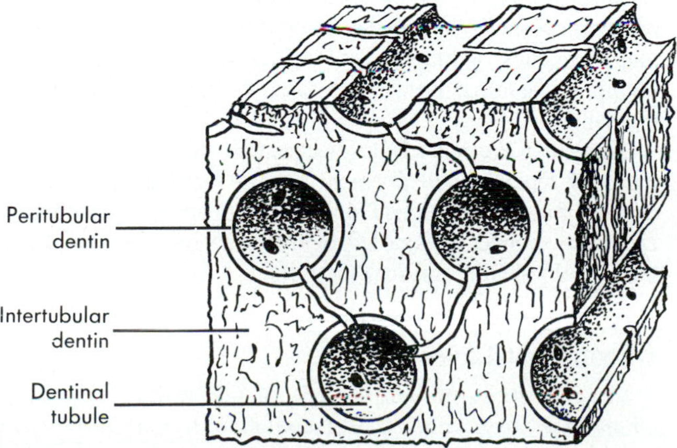

FIG. 11-11 Diagram illustrating peritubular and intertubular dentin. (From Trowbridge HO: Dentistry 82 2(4):22-29, 1982.)

Dentinal Fluid

Free fluid occupies about 22% of the total volume of dentin. This fluid is an ultrafiltrate of blood in the pulp capillaries and its composition resembles plasma in many respects. The fluid flows outward between the odontoblasts into the dentinal tubules and eventually escapes through small pores in the enamel. It has been shown that the tissue pressure of the pulp is approximately 6 mm Hg.[71] Consequently, there is a pressure gradient between the pulp and the oral cavity that accounts for the outward flow of fluid. Exposure of the tubules by tooth fracture or during cavity preparation often results in the movement of fluid to the exposed dentin surface in the form of tiny droplets. This outward movement of fluid can be accelerated by dehydrating the surface of the dentin with compressed air, dry heat, or the application of absorbent paper. The rapid flow of fluid through the tubules is thought to be a cause of dentin sensitivity. (See pp. 318-319.)

Bacterial products or other contaminants may be introduced into the dentinal fluid as a result of dental caries, restorative procedures, or growth of bacteria beneath restorations.[22,23,171] Dentinal fluid may thus serve as a sump from which injurious agents can percolate into the pulp, producing an inflammatory response.[13]

Dentin Permeability

The permeability of dentin has been well characterized (for reviews, see Pashley[137,138]). Dentinal tubules are the major channels for fluid diffusion across dentin. Since fluid permeation is proportional to tubule diameter and number, dentin permeability increases as the tubules converge on the pulp (Fig. 11-13). The total tubular surface near the DEJ is approximately 1% of the total surface area of dentin,[137] whereas close to the pulp chamber the total tubular surface may be nearly 45%. Thus from a clinical standpoint it should be recognized that dentin beneath a deep cavity preparation is much more permeable than dentin underlying a shallow cavity. For the same reason peripheral dentin is stronger than dentin near the pulp.

One study[48] found that the permeability of radicular dentin is much lower than that of coronal dentin. This was attributed to a decrease in the density of the dentinal tubules from approximately 42,000 per square millimeter in cervical dentin to about 8000 tubules per square millimeter in radicular dentin. These investigators found that fluid movement through outer radicular dentin was only approximately 2% that of coronal dentin. The low permeability of outer radicular dentin should make it relatively impermeable to toxic substances such as bacterial products emanating from plaque.

Factors modifying dentin permeability include the presence of odontoblast processes in the tubules, the presence of collagen fibers in the tubules, and the sheathlike lamina limitans that lines the tubules. Thus the functional or physiological diameter of the tubules is only about 5% to 10% of the anatomic diameter (i.e., the diameter seen in microscopic sections).[117]

In dental caries an inflammatory reaction develops in the pulp long before the pulp actually becomes infected.[27,143,171] This indicates that bacterial products reach the pulp in advance of the bacteria themselves. Dentinal sclerosis beneath a carious lesion reduces this permeation by obstructing the tubules, thus decreasing the concentration of irritants that are introduced into the pulp.

The cutting of dentin during cavity preparation produces mi-

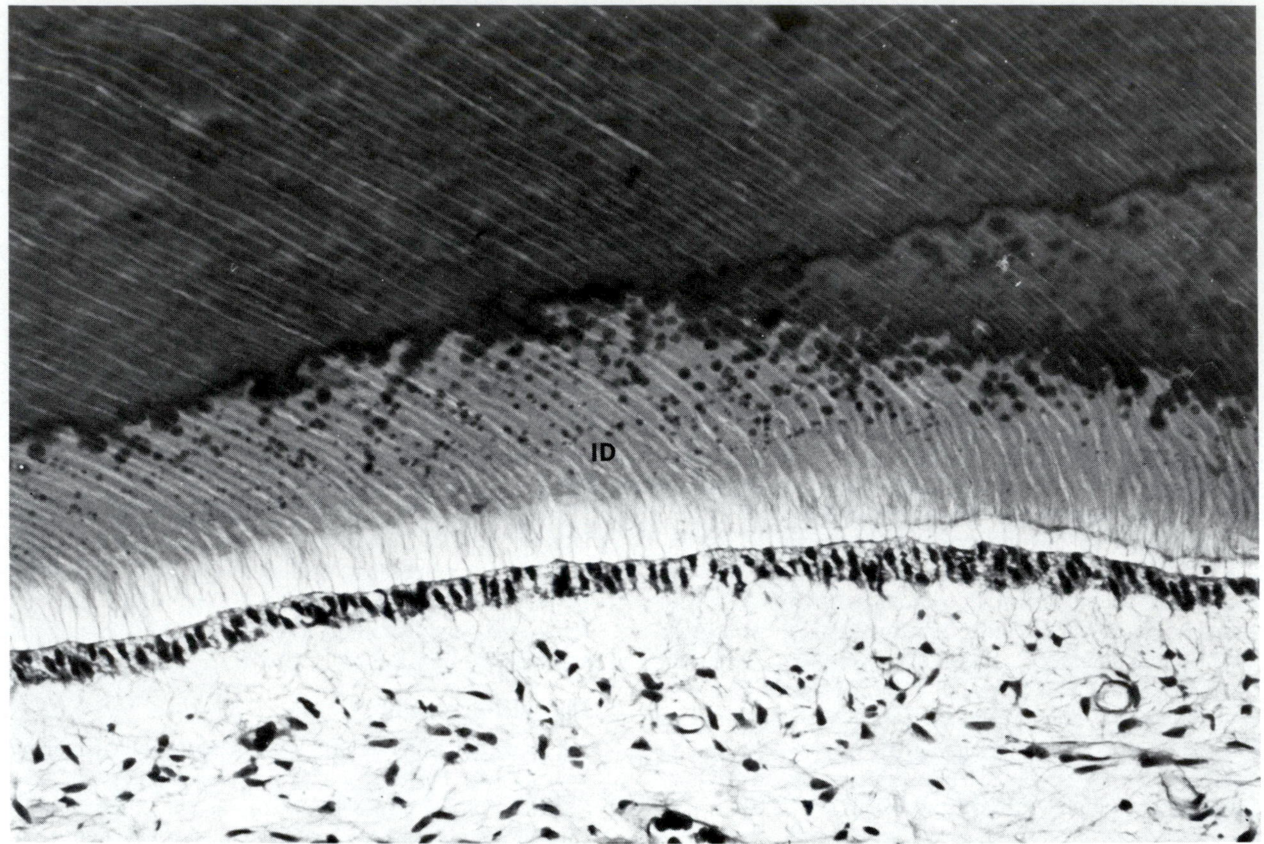

FIG. 11-12 Section showing interglobular dentin *(ID)* in a deciduous incisor from a 3-year-old boy with childhood hypophosphatasia.

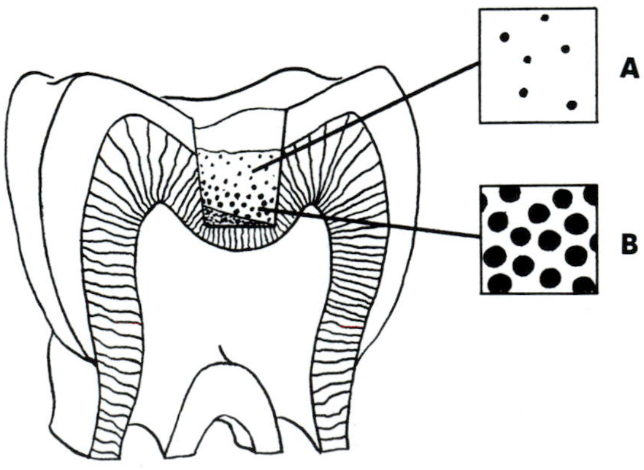

FIG. 11-13 Diagram illustrating the difference in size and number of tubules in the dentinal floor between a shallow, *A*, and a deep, *B*, cavity preparation. (From Trowbridge HO: Dentistry 82 2(4):22-29, 1982.)

crocrystalline grinding debris that coats the dentin and clogs the orifices of the dentinal tubules. This layer of debris is termed the smear layer. Because of the small size of the particles, the smear layer is capable of preventing bacteria from penetrating dentin.[118] Removal of the grinding debris by acid etching greatly increases the permeability of the dentin by decreasing the surface resistance and widening the orifices of the tubules. Consequently, the incidence of pulpal inflammation may be increased significantly if cavities are treated with an acid cleanser, unless a cavity liner or base is used.

In vital teeth bacteria do not readily pass through exposed dentinal tubules into the pulp. Constrictions and irregularities within the dentinal tubules are capable of arresting 99.8% of the bacteria that enter the dentin surface.[118,135] In teeth from which the pulps have been removed, bacteria pass into the pulp in a relatively short time.[31] Presumably this is due to the resistance offered by the presence of dentinal fluid and odontoblast processes in the tubules of vital teeth. It is also possible that antibodies or other antimicrobial agents may be present within the dentinal fluid in response to bacterial infection of the dentin.

Since they are not motile, bacteria advance through the tubules by repeated cell division.[118] If a force such as the hydraulic pressure generated during mastication or impression taking is applied to exposed dentin, bacteria may be driven through the dentin and into the pulp.

MORPHOLOGIC ZONES OF THE PULP

Odontoblast Layer

The outermost stratum of cells of the healthy pulp is the odontoblast layer (Figs. 11-14 and 11-15). This layer is located immediately subjacent to the predentin. Since the odontoblast processes are embedded within the dentinal tubules, the odontoblast layer is composed principally of the cell bodies of odontoblasts. Additionally, capillaries and nerve fibers may be found among the odontoblasts.

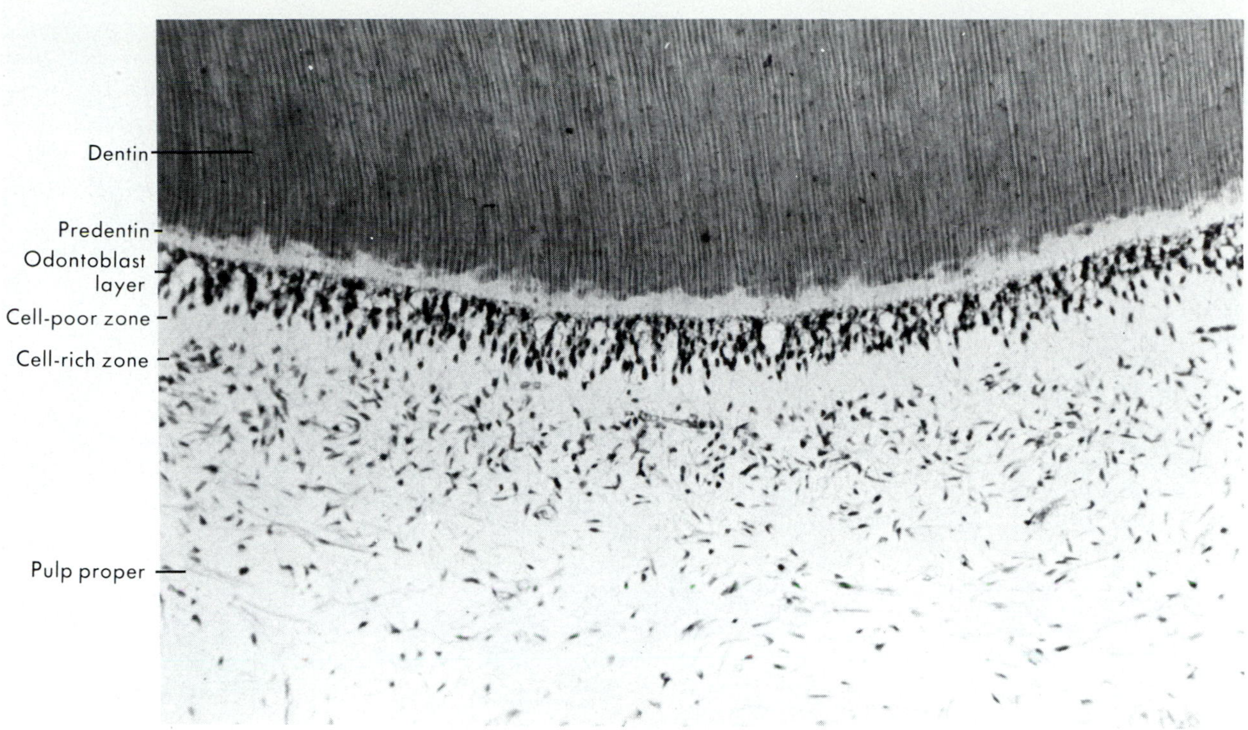

FIG. 11-14 Morphologic zones of the mature pulp.

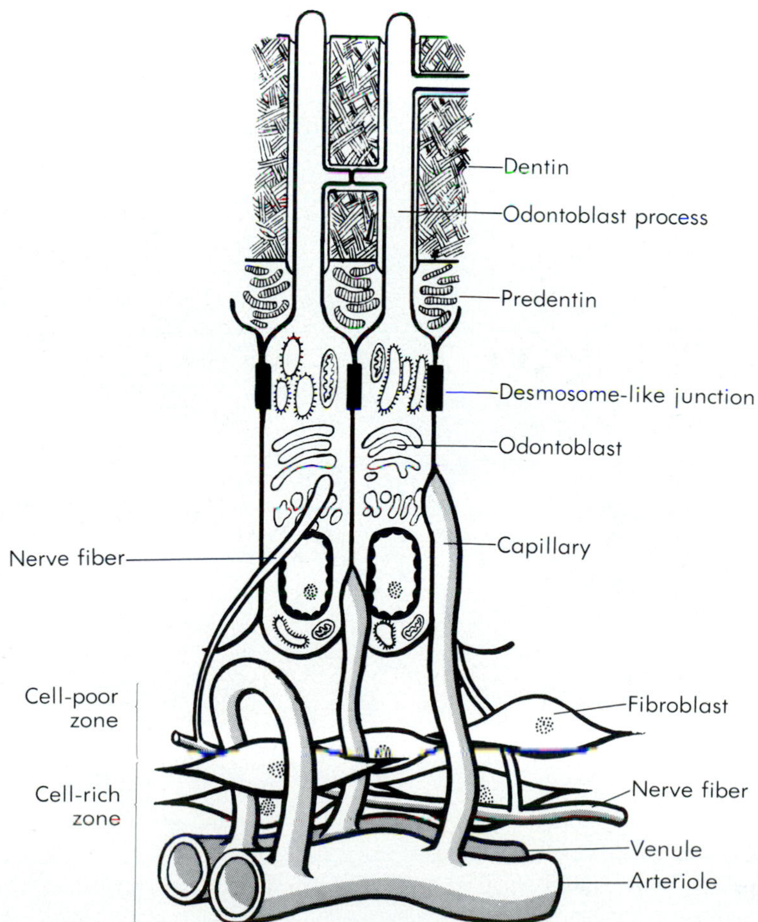

FIG. 11-15 Diagrammatic representation of the odontoblast layer and subodontoblastic region of the pulp.

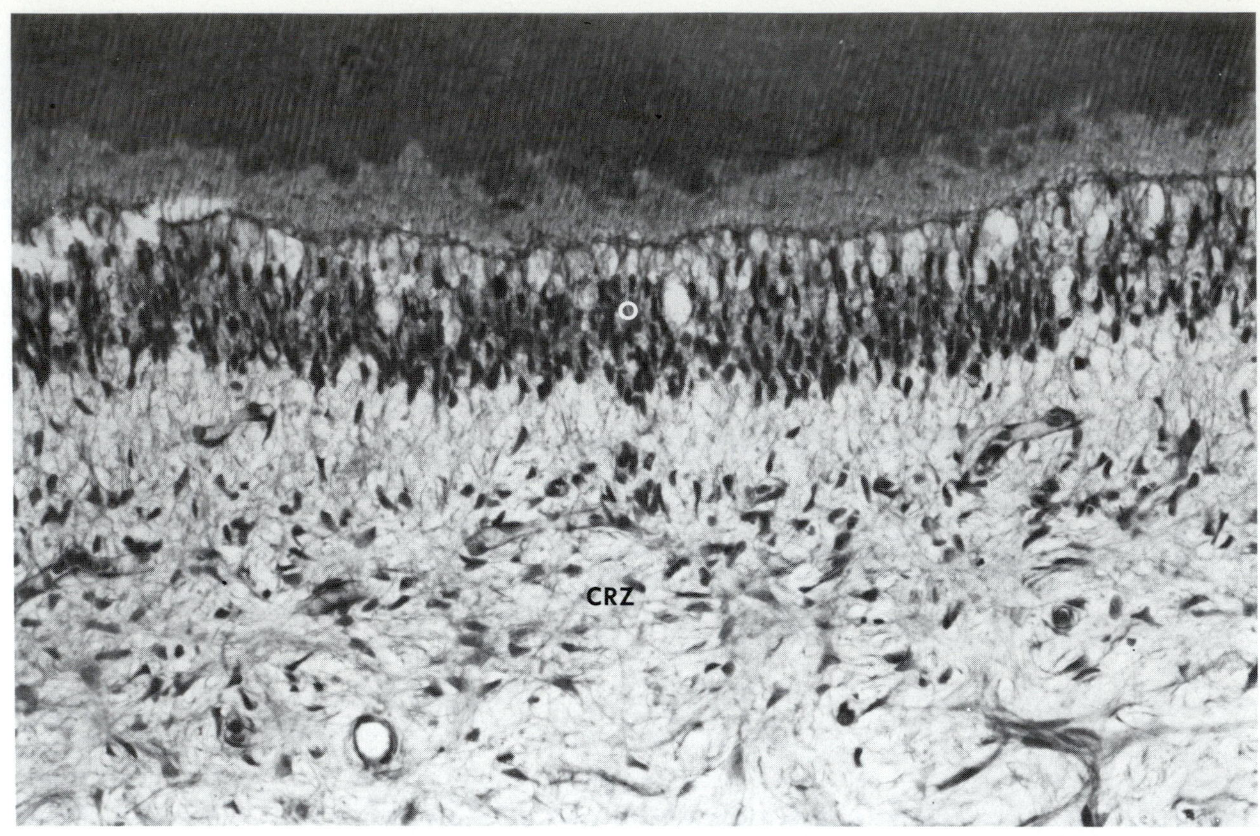

FIG. 11-16 Tall columnar odontoblasts *(O)* of the coronal pulp. Note the presence of the cell-rich zone *(CRZ)*.

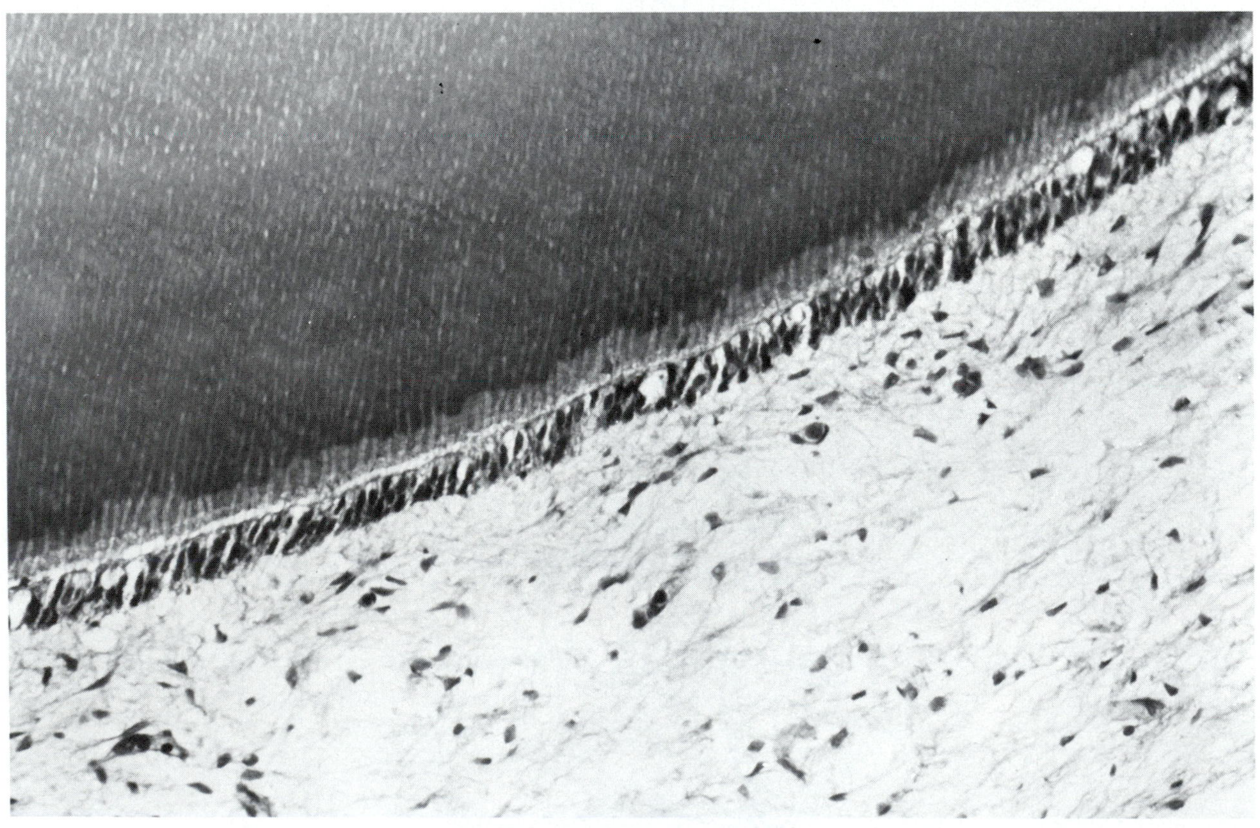

FIG. 11-17 Low columnar odontoblasts of the radicular pulp. The cell-rich zone is inconspicuous.

In the coronal portion of a young pulp the odontoblasts assume a tall columnar form. The tight packing together of these tall slender cells produces the appearance of a palisade. The odontoblasts vary in height; consequently, their nuclei are not all at the same level and are aligned in a staggered array. This often produces the appearance of a layer three to five cells in thickness. Between odontoblasts there are small intercellular spaces approximately 300 to 400 Å in width.

The odontoblast layer in the coronal pulp contains more cells per unit area than in the radicular pulp. Whereas the odontoblasts of the mature coronal pulp are usually columnar (Fig. 11-16), those in the midportion of the radicular pulp are more cuboidal (Fig. 11-17). Near the apical foramen the odontoblasts appear as a flattened cell layer. Since there are fewer dentinal tubules per unit area in the root than in the crown of the tooth, the odontoblast cell bodies are less crowded and are able to spread out laterally. The cell body of most of the odontoblasts borders on the predentin; the odontoblast process, however, passes on through the predentin into the dentin.

Between adjacent odontoblasts there are three types of specialized cell-to-cell junctions.[76,78,99] Spot desmosomes (macula adherens) located in the apical part of odontoblast cell bodies mechanically join odontoblasts together. Numerous gap junctions (nexuses) provide low-resistance pathways through which electrical excitation can pass between odontoblasts (Fig. 11-18). These junctions are most numerous during the formation of primary dentin. Gap junctions and desmosomes have also been observed joining odontoblasts to the processes of fibroblasts in the subodontoblastic area. Tight junctions (zonula occludens) are found mainly in the apical part of odontoblasts in young teeth. These structures consist of linear ridges and grooves which close off the intercellular space. It appears that tight junctions determine the permeability of the odontoblast layer by restricting the passage of molecules, ions, and fluid

A

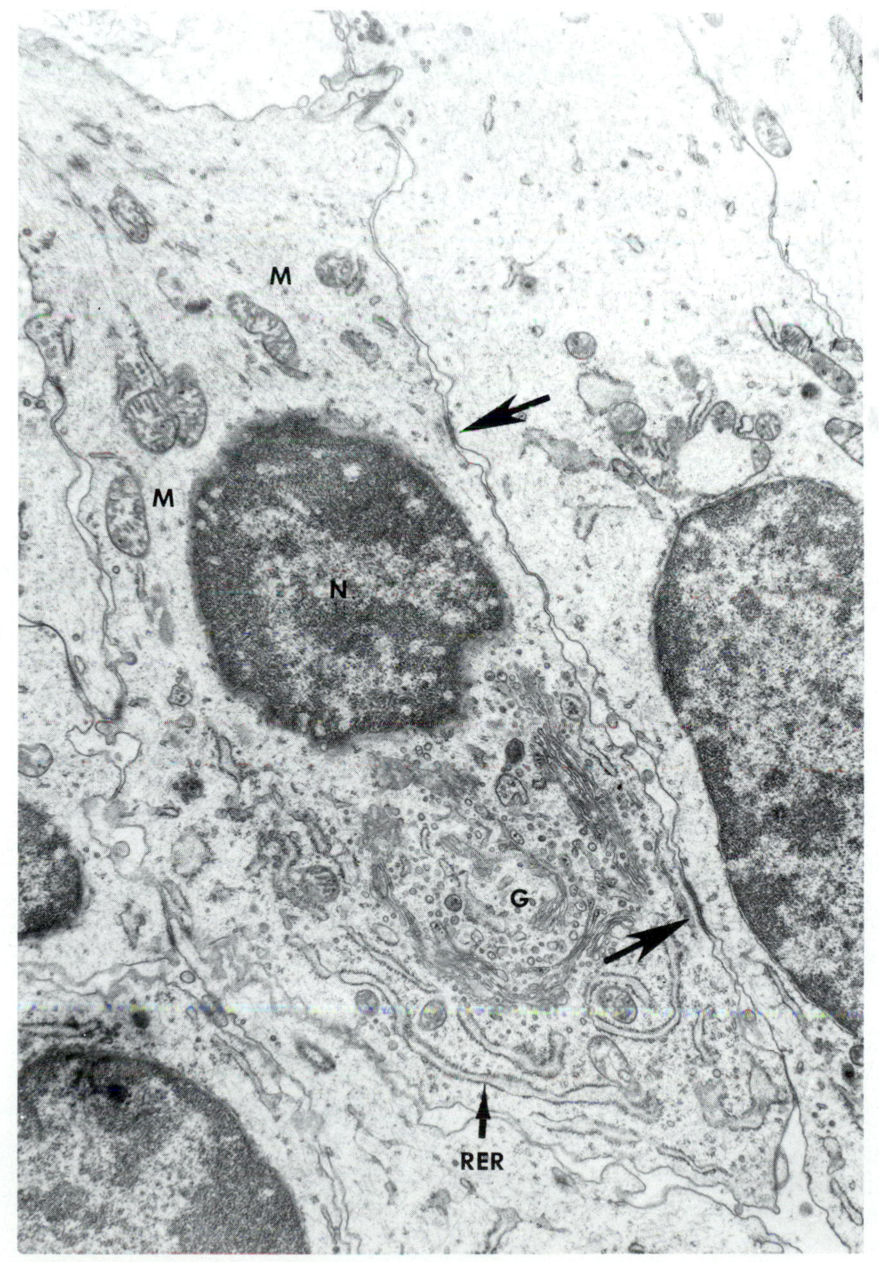

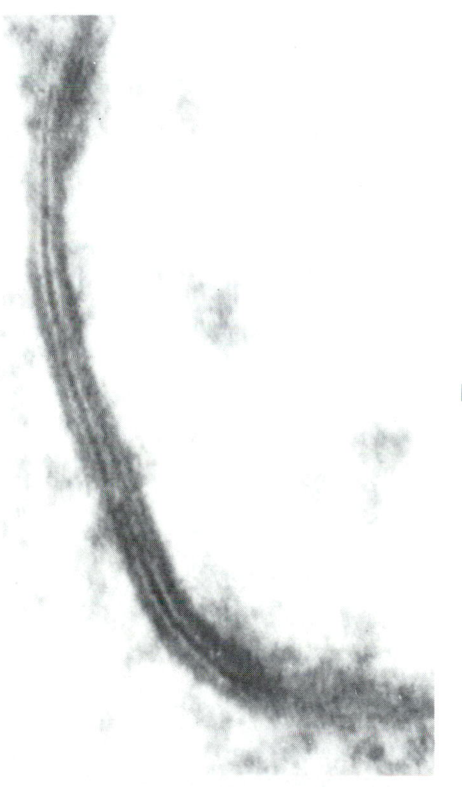

B

FIG. 11-18 A, Electron micrograph of a mouse molar odontoblast demonstrating gap junctions *(arrows),* nucleus *(N),* mitochondria *(M),* Golgi complex *(G),* and rough endoplasmic reticulum *(RER).* **B,** High magnification of a section fixed and stained with lanthanum nitrate to demonstrate a typical gap junction. (Courtesy Dr. Charles F. Cox, School of Dentistry, University of Michigan.)

between the extracellular compartments of the pulp and predentin.[178]

In addition to odontoblasts, class II antigen–expressing dendritic cells have been observed in the odontoblast layer. These cells are discussed below.

Cell-Poor Zone

Immediately subjacent to the odontoblast layer in the coronal pulp there is often a narrow zone approximately 40 μm in width that is relatively free of cells (Figs. 11-14 and 11-15). It is traversed by blood capillaries, unmyelinated nerve fibers, and the slender cytoplasmic processes of fibroblasts. The presence or absence of the cell-poor zone depends upon the functional status of the pulp. It may not be apparent in young pulps rapidly forming dentin or in older pulps where reparative dentin is being produced.

Cell-Rich Zone

Usually conspicuous in the subodontoblastic area is a stratum containing a relatively high proportion of fibroblasts compared with the more central region of the pulp (Fig. 11-14). It is much more prominent in the coronal pulp than in the radicular pulp. Besides fibroblasts, the cell-rich zone may include a variable number of macrophages and lymphocytes.

On the basis of evidence obtained in rat molar teeth, it has been suggested[58] that the cell-rich zone forms as a result of peripheral migration of cells populating the central regions of the pulp, commencing at about the time of tooth eruption. Although cell division within the cell-rich zone is a rare occurrence in normal pulps, death of odontoblasts causes a great increase in the rate of mitosis.[59] Since irreversibly injured odontoblasts are replaced by cells that migrate from the cell-rich zone into the odontoblast layer,[47] this mitotic activity is probably the first step in the regeneration of the odontoblast layer.

Pulp Proper

The pulp proper is the central mass of the pulp (Fig. 11-14). It contains the larger blood vessels and nerves. The connective tissue cells in this zone are fibroblasts, or pulpal cells.

CELLS OF THE PULP

Odontoblast

Because it is responsible for dentinogenesis both during tooth development and in the mature tooth, the odontoblast is the most characteristic cell of the dentin-pulp complex. During dentinogenesis the odontoblasts form the dentinal tubules, and their presence within the tubules makes dentin a living tissue.

Dentinogenesis, osteogenesis, and cementogenesis are in many respects quite similar. Therefore it is not surprising that odontoblasts, osteoblasts, and cementoblasts have many similar characteristics. Each of these cells produces a matrix composed of collagen fibers and proteoglycans that is capable of undergoing mineralization. The ultrastructural characteristics of odontoblasts, osteoblasts, and cementoblasts are likewise similar in that each exhibits a highly ordered RER, a prominent Golgi complex, secretory granules, and numerous mitochondria. In addition, these cells are rich in RNA and their nuclei contain one or more prominent nucleoli. These are the general characteristics of protein-secreting cells.

Perhaps the most significant differences between odontoblasts, osteoblasts, and cementoblasts are their morphologic characteristics and the anatomic relationships between the cells and the structures they produce. Whereas osteoblasts and cementoblasts are polygonal to cuboidal in form, the fully developed odontoblast of the coronal pulp is a tall columnar cell. In bone and cementum the osteoblasts and cementoblasts become entrapped in the matrix as osteocytes or cementocytes respectively. The odontoblasts, on the other hand, leave behind cellular processes to form the dentinal tubules. Lateral branches between the major odontoblast processes interconnect the processes through canals just as osteocytes and cementocytes are linked together through the canaliculae in bone and cementum. This provides for intercellular communication as well as circulation of fluid and metabolites through the mineralized matrix.

The ultrastructural features of the odontoblast have been the subject of numerous investigations.[55,88,158] The cell body of the active odontoblast has a large nucleus that may contain up to four nucleoli (Figs. 11-18 and 11-19). The nucleus is situated at the basal end of the cell and is contained within a nuclear envelope. A well-developed Golgi complex, centrally located in the supranuclear cytoplasm, consists of an assembly of smooth-walled vesicles and cisternae. Numerous mitochondria are evenly distributed throughout the cell body. RER is particularly prominent, consisting of closely stacked cisternae forming parallel arrays that are dispersed diffusely within the cytoplasm. Numerous ribosomes closely associated with the membranes of the cisternae mark the sites of protein synthesis. Within the lumen of the cisternae, filamentous material

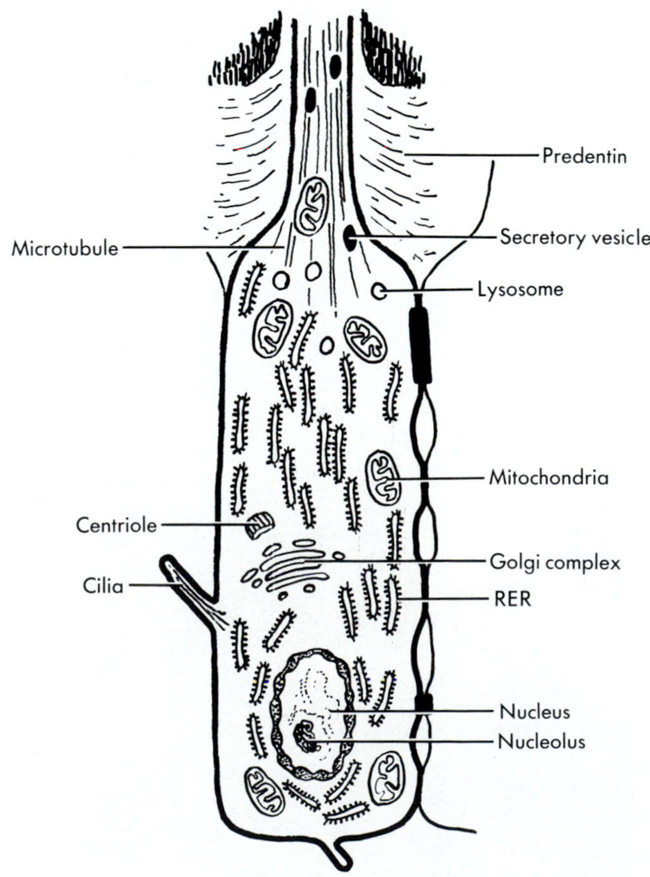

FIG. 11-19 Diagram of a fully differentiated odontoblast.

probably representing newly synthesized protein can be observed.

Apparently the odontoblast synthesizes only type I collagen and an unusual type I trimer having three alpha chains. In addition to proteoglycans and collagen, the odontoblast secretes phosphophoryn, a phosphoprotein involved in extracellular mineralization. This substance is unique to dentin and is not found in any other mesenchymal cell lines.[29,182]

Acid phosphatase activity occurs in the Golgi complex and in lysosomes located in the cell body close to the predentin.[90] Some activity extends into the basal portion of the odontoblast process. It has been suggested that lysosomal enzymes such as acid phosphatase may be involved in digesting material that has been resorbed from the predentin matrix, possibly proteoglycans associated with mineralization.[38,90] The odontoblast also secretes alkaline phosphatase, an enzyme that is closely linked to mineralization but whose precise role is yet to be illuminated.

In contrast to the active odontoblast, the resting or inactive odontoblast has a decreased number of organelles and may become progressively shorter. These changes can begin with the completion of root development.

Odontoblast Process

Cytoplasmic microtubules extend from the cell body into the odontoblast process. These straight structures follow a course that is parallel with the long axis of the cell and impart the impression of rigidity. Although their precise role is unknown, theories as to their functional significance suggest that they may be involved in cytoplasmic extension, transport of materials, or simply the provision of a structural framework.

Microtubules and microfilaments are the principal ultrastructural components of the odontoblast process and its lateral branches.[80] These structures have a preferential arrangement parallel with the long axis of the process. The plasma membrane of the odontoblast process closely approximates the wall of the dentinal tubule. Localized constrictions in the process occasionally produce relatively large spaces between the tubule wall and the process.[50,161] Such spaces may contain collagen fibrils and fine granular material which presumably represents ground substance. The peritubular dentin matrix lining the tubule is circumscribed by an electron-dense limiting membrane.[161] A space separates the limiting membrane from the plasma membrane of the odontoblast process. This space is usually narrow except in areas where, as mentioned previously, the process is constricted.

The extent to which the odontoblast process extends outward in the dentin has been a matter of considerable controversy. It has long been thought that the process is present throughout the full thickness of dentin.[8,140,165] However, many ultrastructural studies using scanning and transmission electron microscopy have described the process as being limited to the inner third of the dentin.[25,77,161] On the other hand, studies employing scanning electron microscopy have described the process in peripheral dentin, often extending to the DEJ.[60,92,187] One investigator[161-163] has shown that the lumen of the dentinal tubule is surrounded by an electron-dense structure, the lamina limitans, which is indistinguishable from the odontoblast process, and he has suggested that this is what others have described as being the odontoblast process. Using antibodies directed against microtubules, investigators have demonstrated immunoreactivity throughout the dentinal tubule, suggesting that the process extends throughout the entire thickness of dentin.[150-151] Obviously this problem warrants further study. Since high-speed drilling can disrupt odontoblasts, it would be of considerable clinical importance to establish conclusively the extent of the odontoblast processes in human teeth. With this knowledge the clinician would be in a better position to estimate the impact of restorative procedures on the underlying odontoblast layer.

The odontoblast is considered to be a fixed postmitotic cell in that once it has fully differentiated it apparently cannot undergo further cell division. If this is indeed the case, the life-span of the odontoblast coincides with the life-span of the viable pulp.

Relationship of Structure to Function

Isotope studies have shed a great deal of light on the functional significance of the cytoplasmic organelles of the active odontoblast.[52,185] In experimental animals the intraperitoneal injection of collagen precursors such as ^{3}H-proline is followed by autoradiographic labeling of the odontoblasts and predentin matrix (Fig. 11-20). Rapid incorporation of the isotope in the RER soon leads to labeling of the Golgi complex in the area where the procollagen is packed and concentrated into secretory vesicles. Labeled vesicles can then be followed along their migration pathway until they reach the base of the odontoblast process. Here they fuse with the cell membrane and release their tropocollagen molecules into the predentin matrix by the process of reverse pinocytosis. It is now known that collagen fibrils precipitate from a solution of tropocollagen and that the aggregation of fibrils occurs on the outer surface of the odontoblast plasma membrane. Fibrils are released into the predentin and increase in thickness as they approach the calcification front. Whereas fibrils at the base of the odontoblast process are approximately 150 Å in diameter, fibrils in the region of the calcification front have attained a diameter of about 500 Å.

Similar tracer studies[184] have elucidated the pathway of synthesis, transport, and secretion of the predentin proteoglycans. The protein moiety of these molecules is synthesized by the RER of the odontoblast whereas sulfation and addition of the GAG moieties to the protein molecules takes place in the Golgi complex. Secretory vesicles then transport the proteoglycans to the base of the odontoblast process, where they are secreted into the predentin matrix. Proteoglycans, principally chondroitin sulfate, accumulate near the calcification front. The role of the proteoglycans is speculative, but mounting evidence suggests that they act as inhibitors of calcification by binding calcium. It appears that just before calcification the proteoglycans are removed, probably by lysosomal enzymes secreted by the odontoblasts.[38]

Fibroblast (Pulp Cell)

Fibroblasts of the pulp appear to be tissue-specific cells capable of giving rise to cells that are committed to differentiation as odontoblasts, given the proper signal. These cells produce the collagen fibers of the pulp, and since they degrade collagen, they are also responsible for collagen turnover.

Although distributed throughout the pulp, fibroblasts are particularly abundant in the cell-rich zone. The early-differentiating fibroblasts are polygonal and appear to be widely separated and evenly distributed within the ground substance.[7] Cell-to-cell contacts are established between the mul-

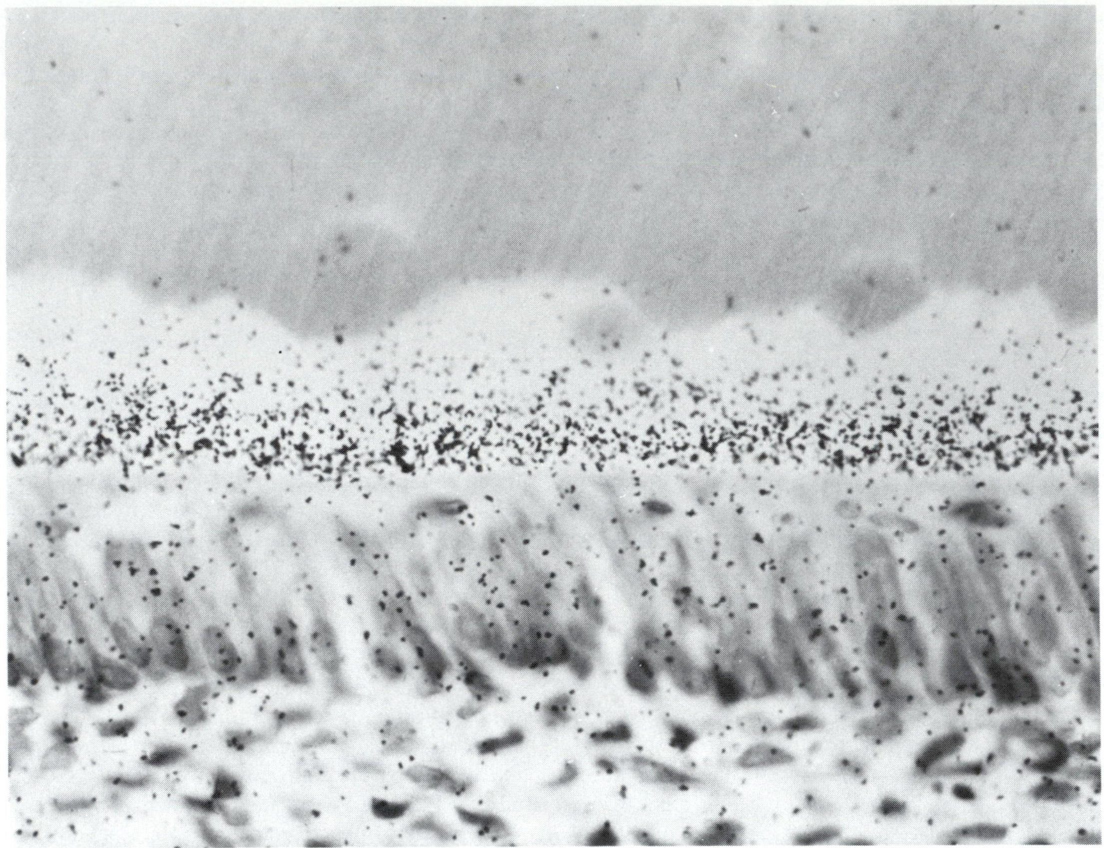

FIG. 11-20 Radioautograph demonstrating odontoblasts and predentin in a developing rat molar 1 hour after intraperitoneal injection of ^{3}H-proline.

tiple processes that extend out from each of the cells. Many of these contacts take the form of gap junctions, which provide for electronic coupling of one cell to another. Ultrastructurally the organelles of the immature fibroblasts are generally in a rudimentary stage of development, with an inconspicuous Golgi complex, numerous free ribosomes, and sparse RER. As they mature, the cells become stellate in form and the Golgi complex enlarges, the RER proliferates, secretory vesicles appear, and the fibroblasts take on the characteristic appearance of protein-secreting cells. Along the outer surface of the cell body, collagen fibrils commence to appear. With an increase in the number of blood vessels, nerves, and fibers there is a relative decrease in the number of fibroblasts in the pulp.[7]

A colleague once remarked that the fibroblasts of the pulp are very much like Peter Pan in that they never grow up. There may be an element of truth in this statement, for these cells do seem to remain in a relatively undifferentiated modality as compared to fibroblasts of most other connective tissues.[65] This perception has been fortified by the observation of large numbers of reticulin fibers in the pulp.[140] Reticulin fibers, once believed to be precollagenous in nature and therefore the product of immature cells, have an affinity for silver stains and are similar to the argyrophilic fibers of the pulp. However, in a careful review of the subject, Baume[11] concluded that because of distinct histochemical differences, reticulin fibers, such as those of gingiva and lymphoid organs, are not present in the pulp. He suggested that these pulpal fibers be termed *argyrophilic collagen fibers*. The fibers apparently acquire a GAG sheath, and it is this sheath that is impregnated by silver stains. In the young pulp the nonargyrophilic collagen fibers are sparse, but they progressively increase in number as the pulp ages.

Many experimental models have been developed to study wound healing in the pulp, particularly dentinal bridge formation following pulp exposure or pulpotomy. One study[47] demonstrated that mitotic activity preceding the differentiation of replacement odontoblasts appears to occur primarily among fibroblasts. Thus, it appears that pulpal fibroblasts can be regarded as odontoprogenitor cells.

Macrophage

Tissue macrophages, or histiocytes, are monocytes that have left the bloodstream, entered the tissues, and differentiated into macrophages. These cells are quite active in endocytosis and phagocytosis. In addition, a proportion of macrophages participate in immune responses as accessory cells by processing and presenting antigen to lymphocytes (for review see Trowbridge[174]). The processed antigen is bound to class II (Ia) histocompatibility antigens on the macrophage where it can interact with specific receptors present on immunocompetent T cells. Such interaction is obligatory for induction of cell-mediated immunity. Macrophages also produce a large variety of soluble factors including interleukin-1 and other cytokines.

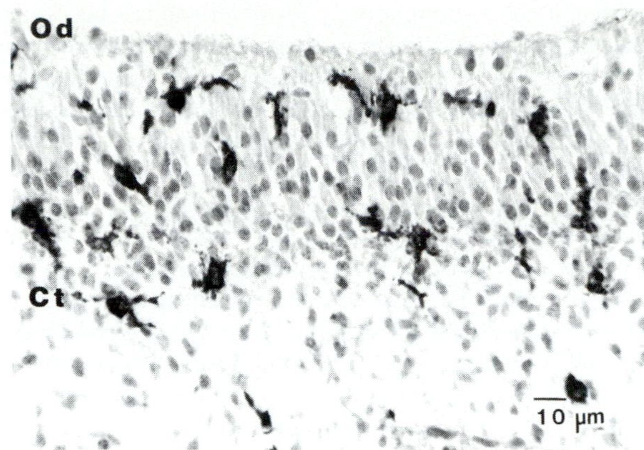

FIG. 11-21 Class II antigen-expressing dendritic cells in the odontoblast layer *(Od)* and subodontoblastic connective tissue *(Ct)* in normal rat incisor pulp, as demonstrated by immunocytochemistry. (From Jontell M, et al: J Dent Res 67:1263, 1988.)

Dendritic Cell

Dendritic cells, like macrophages, are accessory cells of the immune system. Similar cells are found in the epidermis and mucous membranes, where they are called *Langerhans' cells*. Dendritic cells are primarily found in lymphoid tissues, but they are also widely distributed in connective tissues, including the pulp (Fig. 11-21).[89,132] These cells are termed *antigen-presenting cells* and are characterized by dendritic cytoplasmic processes and the presence of cell surface class II antigens. Like macrophages, they phagocytose and process antigens but are otherwise only weakly phagocytic. Together with macrophages and lymphocytes, dendritic cells are believed to participate in immunosurveillance in the pulp.

Lymphocytes

Hahn and colleagues[62] reported finding T lymphocytes and B lymphocytes in normal pulps from human teeth. T8 (suppressor) lymphocytes were the predominant T-lymphocyte subset present in these pulps. Lymphocytes have also been observed in the pulps of impacted teeth.[102] The presence of macrophages, dendritic cells, and lymphocytes indicates that the pulp is well-equipped with cells required for the initiation of immune responses.

Mesenchymal Cell

Some authors hold the view that primordial mesenchymal cells persist in adult tissues as "undifferentiated" mesenchymal cells. However, during wound healing well-differentiated fibroblasts undergo rapid serial division to give rise to new fibroblasts. Consequently, there is no need to postulate that in the pulp new mesenchymal cells arise from cells other than pulpal fibroblasts.

Mast Cell

Mast cells are widely distributed in connective tissues, where they occur in small groups in relation to blood vessels. One investigator[39] reported the presence of mast cells in inflamed as well as uninflamed human pulps. This cell has been the subject of considerable attention because of its dramatic role in inflammatory reactions. The granules of mast cells contain heparin, an anticoagulant, as well as histamine, an inflammatory mediator.

METABOLISM

The metabolic activity of the pulp has been studied by measuring the rate of oxygen consumption and the production of carbon dioxide or lactic acid by pulp tissue in vitro.[43,44,146] More recent investigations[64] have employed the radiospirometry method.

Because of the relatively sparse cellular composition of the pulp, the rate of oxygen consumption is low in comparison to that of most other tissues. During active dentinogenesis, metabolic activity is much higher than following the completion of crown development.[44,146] As would be anticipated, the greatest metabolic activity is found in the region of the odontoblast layer.[43]

In addition to the usual glycolytic pathway, the bovine pulp has the ability to produce energy through a phosphogluconate (pentose phosphate) shunt type of carbohydrate metabolism,[46] suggesting that the pulp may be able to function under varying degrees of ischemia. This could explain how the pulp manages to withstand periods of vasoconstriction resulting from the use of infiltration anesthesia employing epinephrine-containing local anesthetic agents.[94]

Several commonly used dental materials (e.g., eugenol, zinc oxide-eugenol, calcium hydroxide, silver amalgam) have been shown to inhibit oxygen consumption by pulp tissue, indicating that these agents may be capable of depressing the metabolic activity of pulpal cells.[45,87] One study[64] found that application of orthodontic force to human premolars for 3 days resulted in a 27% reduction in respiratory activity in the pulp.

GROUND SUBSTANCE

Ground substance comprises the matrix in which connective tissue cells and fibers are embedded. Whereas the fibers and cells of the pulp have recognizable shapes, the ground substance is described as being amorphous. The cells that produce connective tissue fibers also synthesize the major constituents of ground substance.

Ground substance can be thought of as a sol (fluid colloidal system) or a gel that cannot be easily squeezed out of the connective tissue. In this respect it differs from tissue fluid that can be removed largely by drainage alone. Early in embryonic development the ground substance is quite fluid, whereas in mature connective tissue it tends to be viscous or gel-like. This may help to limit the spread of bacteria.

The principal molecular components of interstitial ground substance are proteoglycans and glycoproteins. Proteoglycans consist of polysaccharide chains (GAGs) linked covalently to a protein molecule. In the pulp the principal proteoglycans include hyaluronic acid,* dermatan sulfate, heparan sulfate, and chondroitin sulfate.[114] The ability of connective tissue to retain water is ascribed to the GAGs. The proteoglycan content of pulp tissue decreases approximately 50% with tooth eruption.[109] During active dentinogenesis, chondroitin sulfate is the principal proteoglycan, particularly in the odontoblast-predentin layer, where it is somehow involved with mineralization, but with tooth eruption hyaluronic acid and dermatan sulfate increase and chondroitin sulfate decreases greatly.

Ground substance glycoproteins help form extracellular

*Since there is still some doubt as to whether hyaluronic acid is linked to protein, it should probably be referred to as a GAG rather than a proteoglycan.

fibrils or basement membranes, or serve as adhesive molecules that bond to cell surfaces and other matrix molecules. In this way they participate in the formation of connective tissue matrices. Fibronectin is a major surface glycoprotein that, together with collagen, forms an integrated fibrillary network that influences adhesion, motility, growth, and differentiation of cells. Laminin, an important component of basement membranes, binds to type IV collagen and cell-surface receptors. Tenascin is another substrate adhesion glycoprotein.

The consistency of a connective tissue such as the pulp is largely determined by the proteoglycan components of the ground substance. The long GAG chains of the proteoglycan molecules form relatively rigid coils constituting a network that holds water, thus forming a characteristic gel. Hyaluronic acid in particular has a strong affinity for water and is a major component of ground substance in tissues with a large fluid content, such as Wharton's jelly. The water content of the pulp is very high (approximately 90%), and thus the ground substance forms a cushion capable of protecting cells and vascular components of the tooth.

Ground substance also acts as a molecular sieve in that it excludes large proteins and urea. Cell metabolites, nutrients, and wastes pass through the ground substance between cells and blood vessels. In some ways ground substance can be likened to an ion-exchange resin since the polyanionic charges of the GAGs bind cations. Additionally, osmotic pressures can be altered by excluding osmotically active molecules. Thus the proteoglycans can regulate the dispersion of interstitial matrix

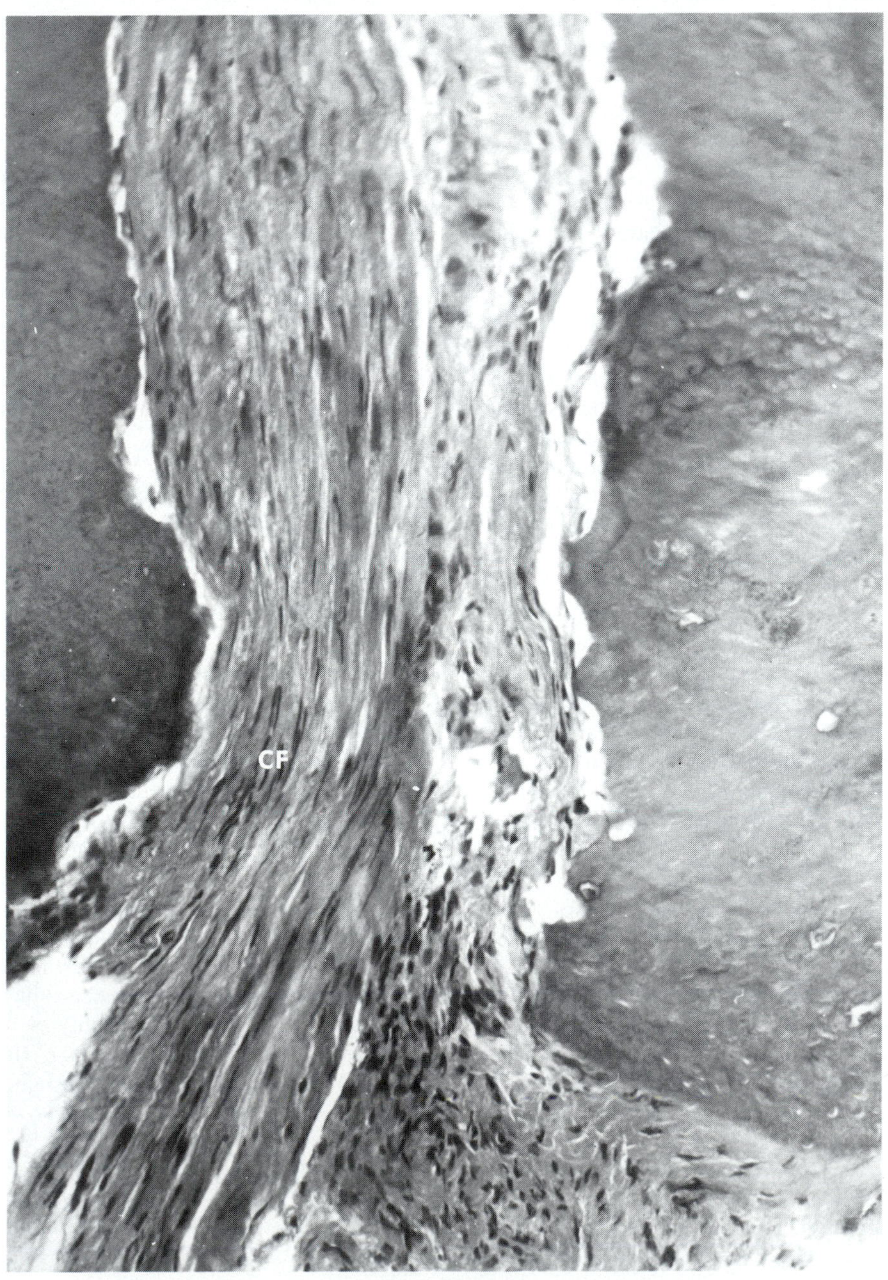

FIG. 11-22 Dense bundles of collagen fibers *(CF)* in the apical pulp.

solutes, colloids, and water and in large measure determine the physical characteristics of the pulp.

Degradation of ground substance can occur in certain inflammatory lesions in which there is a high concentration of lysosomal enzymes. Proteolytic enzymes, hyaluronidases, and chondroitin sulfatases of lysosomal as well as bacterial origin are examples of the hydrolytic enzymes that can attack components of the ground substance. The pathways of inflammation and infection are strongly influenced by the state of polymerization of the ground substance components.

FIBERS OF THE PULP

Two types of structural proteins are found in the pulp: collagen and elastin. However, elastin fibers are confined to the walls of arterioles and, unlike collagen, are not a part of the intercellular matrix.

A single collagen molecule, referred to as tropocollagen, consists of three polypeptide chains, designated as either α-1 or α-2 depending upon their amino acid composition and sequence. The different combinations and linkages of chains making up the tropocollagen molecule has allowed collagen to be classified into a number of types. Type I is found in skin, tendon, bone, dentin, and pulp. Type II occurs in cartilage. Type III is found in most unmineralized connective tissues. It is a fetal form found in the dental papilla as well as the mature pulp. In the bovine pulp it comprises 45% of the total pulp collagen during all stages of development.[104] Type IV collagen is found only in basement membranes.

In collagen synthesis the protein portion of the molecule is formed by the polyribosomes of the RER of connective tissue cells. The proline and lysine residues of the polypeptide chains are hydroxylated in the cisternae of the RER, and the chains are assembled into a triple helix configuration in the smooth endoplasmic reticulum. The product of this assembly is termed procollagen, and it has a terminal unit of amino acids known as the telopeptide of the procollagen molecule. When these molecules reach the Golgi complex, they are glycosylated and packaged in secretory vesicles. The vesicles are transported to the plasma membrane and secreted via exocytosis into the extracellular milieu, thus releasing the procollagen. Here the terminal telopeptide is cleaved by a hydrolytic enzyme and the tropocollagen molecules begin aggregating to form collagen fibrils. It is believed that aggregation of tropocollagen is somehow mediated by the GAGs. The conversion of soluble collagen into insoluble fibers occurs as a result of cross-linking of tropocollagen molecules.

The small collagen fibers of the pulp stain black with silver impregnation stains and are thus referred to as *argyrophilic fibers*. Collagen fibers in the young pulp are characteristically small and irregularly oriented.[67] The presence of collagen fibers passing from the dentin matrix between odontoblasts into the dental pulp has been reported in fully erupted teeth.[19] These fibers are often referred to as *von Korff fibers*. Larger collagen fiber bundles, more often seen in older pulps, are not argyrophilic but can be demonstrated with special histochemical methods such as Gomori's trichrome stain or Mallory's analine blue. The highest concentration of these larger fiber bundles is usually found in the radicular pulp near the apex (Fig. 11-22). Thus, Torneck[170] advises that, during pulpectomy, if the pulp is engaged with a barbed broach in the region of the apex this generally affords the best opportunity to remove it intact.

INNERVATION

The pulp is a sensory organ capable of transmitting information from its sensory receptors to the central nervous system. Regardless of the nature of the sensory stimulus (i.e., thermal change, mechanical deformation, injury to the tissues), all afferent impulses from the pulp result in the sensation of pain. The innervation of the pulp includes both *afferent* neurons, which conduct sensory impulses, and *autonomic* fibers, which provide neurogenic modulation of the microcirculation and perhaps regulate dentinogenesis, too.

In addition to sensory nerves, sympathetic fibers from the superior cervical ganglion appear with blood vessels at the time the vascular system is established in the dental papilla. In the adult tooth sympathetic fibers form plexuses, usually around pulpal arterioles.[5] Stimulation of these fibers results in constriction of the arterioles and a decrease in blood flow. Sympathetic fibers have also been found lying independent of blood vessels in close association with the region of the odontoblasts. Both adrenergic and cholinergic fibers have been found in close relation to odontoblasts.[10,81] It is thought that autonomic nerve fibers may somehow be involved in the regulation of dentin formation.

Nerve fibers are classified according to their function, diameter, and conduction velocity, as shown in Table 11-2. Most of the nerves of the pulp fall into two main categories, A-δ and C fibers. The principal characteristics of these fibers are summarized in Table 11-3.

TABLE 11-2. Classification of nerve fibers

Type of fiber	Function	Diameter (μm)	Conduction velocity (m/sec)
A-α	Motor, proprioception	12-20	70-120
A-β	Pressure, touch	5-12	30-70
A-γ	Motor, to muscle spindles	3-6	15-30
A-δ	Pain, temperature, touch	1-5	6-30
B	Preganglionic autonomic	<3	3-15
C dorsal root	Pain	0.4-1.0	0.5-2
sympathetic	Postganglionic sympathetic	0.3-1.3	0.7-2.3

TABLE 11-3. Characteristics of sensory fibers

Fiber	Myelination	Location of terminals	Pain characteristics	Stimulation threshold
A-δ	Yes	Principally in region of pulp-dentin junction	Sharp, pricking	Relatively low
C	No	Probably distributed throughout pulp	Burning, aching, less bearable than A-δ fiber sensations	Relatively high, usually associated with tissue injury

During the bell stage of tooth development, "pioneer" nerve fibers enter the dental papilla following the path of blood vessels.[40] While only unmyelinated fibers are observed in the dental papilla, a proportion of these fibers are probably A fibers that have not yet become myelinated. Myelinated fibers are the last major structures to appear in the developing human dental pulp.[7] The number of nerve fibers gradually increases and some branching occurs as the fibers near the dentin, but during the bell stage very few fibers enter the predentin.

The sensory nerves of the pulp arise from the trigeminal nerve and pass into the radicular pulp in bundles via the foramen in close association with arterioles and venules (Fig. 11-23). Each of the nerves entering the pulp is invested within a Schwann cell, and the A fibers acquire their myelin sheath from these cells. With the completion of root development the myelinated fibers appear grouped in bundles in the central region of the pulp (Fig. 11-24). Most of the unmyelinated C fibers entering the pulp are located within these fiber bundles; the remainder are situated toward the periphery of the pulp.[142]

Investigators[84] found that in the human premolar the number of unmyelinated axons entering the tooth at the apex reached a maximum number shortly after tooth eruption. At this stage they observed an average of 1800 unmyelinated axons and upwards of 400 myelinated axons, although in some teeth fewer than 100 myelinated axons were present. The number of A fibers gradually increased to upwards of 700 five years after eruption. *The relatively late appearance of A fibers in the pulp helps to explain why the electric pulp test tends to be unreliable in young teeth.*[53,54]

A quantitative study of nerve axons 1 to 2 mm above the root apex of fully developed human canine and incisor teeth has been conducted.[85] It reported a mean of 361 and 359 myelinated axons in canines and incisors respectively. The number of unmyelinated axons was much greater, with means of 2240 for canines and 1591 for incisors. Thus, approximately 80% of the nerves were unmyelinated fibers. However, some myelinated fibers may lose their sheaths before entering the apex or, in young teeth, they may not yet have acquired a sheath. Consequently, it is difficult to accurately assess the true proportion of myelinated and unmyelinated fibers entering the pulp.

The nerve bundles pass upward through the radicular pulp together with blood vessels. Once they reach the coronal pulp, they fan out beneath the cell-rich zone, branch into smaller bundles and finally ramify into a plexus of single nerve axons known as the plexus of Raschkow (Fig. 11-25). Full development of this plexus does not occur until the final stages of root formation.[41] It has been estimated that each fiber entering the pulp sends at least eight branches to the plexus of Raschkow. There is prolific branching of the fibers in the plexus, producing a tremendous overlap of receptor fields.[68] It is in the plexus that the A fibers emerge from their myelin sheaths and, while

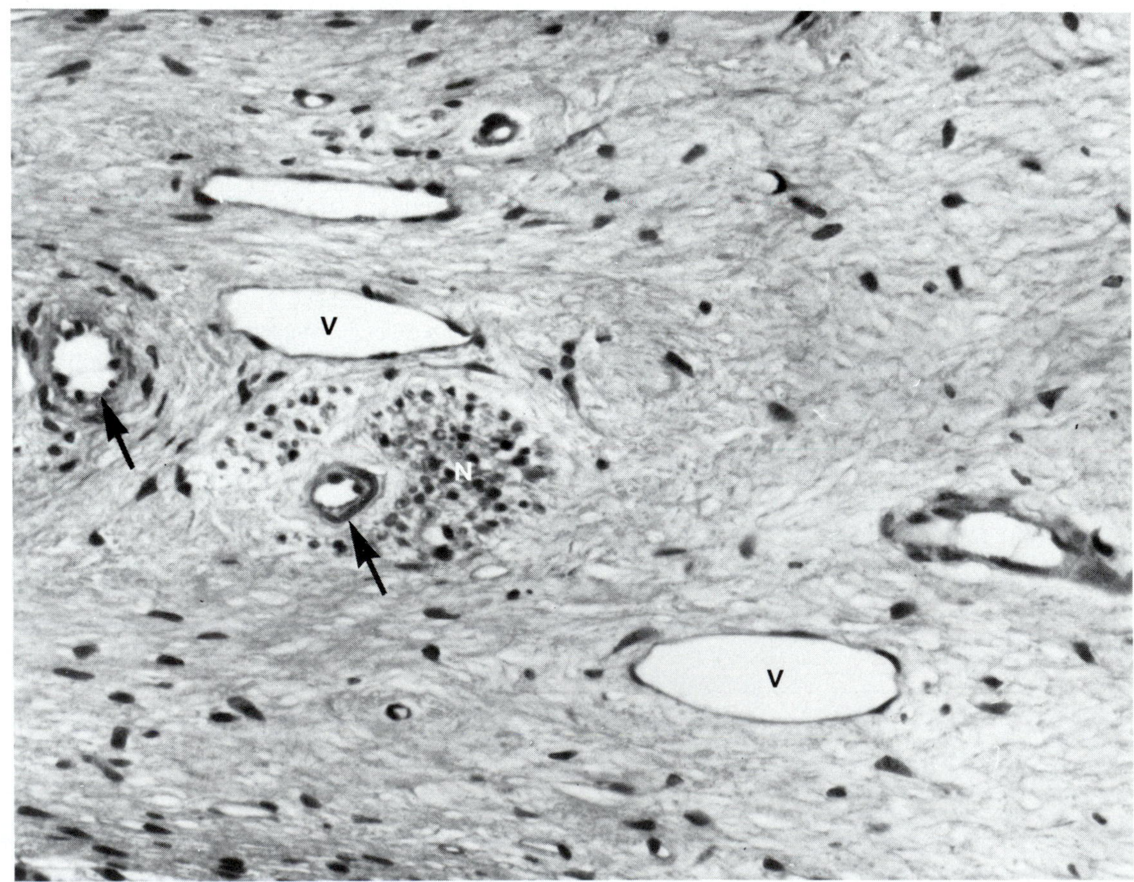

FIG. 11-23 Cross section of the apical pulp of a young human premolar demonstrating the nerve fiber bundle *(N)*, arterioles *(arrows)*, and venules *(V)*.

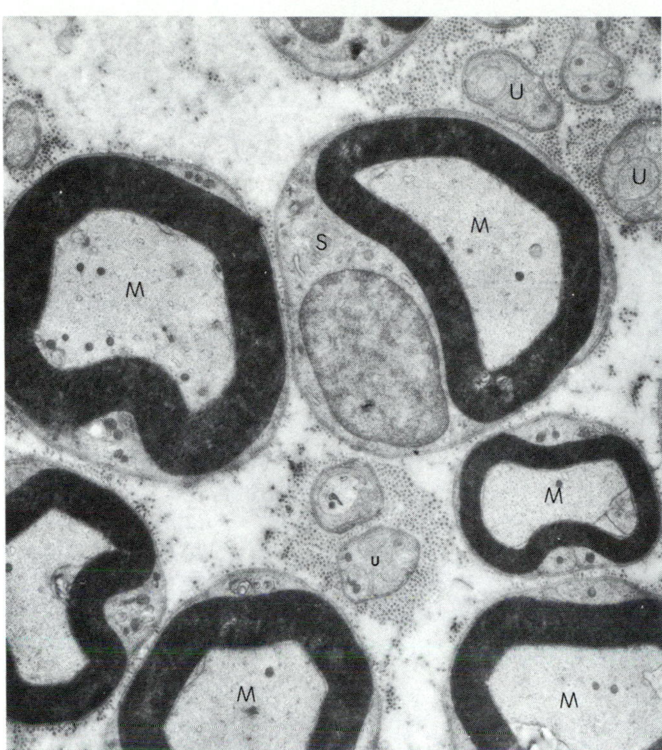

FIG. 11-24 Electron micrograph of the apical pulp of a young canine tooth showing in cross section myelinated nerve axons *(M)* within Schwann cells *(S)*. Smaller, unmyelinated axons *(U)* are enclosed singly and in groups by Schwann cells. (Courtesy Dr. David C. Johnsen, School of Dentistry, Case Western Reserve University.)

still within Schwann cells, branch repeatedly to form the subodontoblastic plexus (Fig. 11-26). Finally, terminal axons exit from their Schwann cell investiture and pass between the odontoblasts as free nerve endings (Figs. 11-27 and 11-28).

One investigator[61] studied the distribution and organization of nerve fibers in the dentin-pulp border zone of human teeth. On the basis of their location and pattern of branching, he described several types of nerve endings (Fig. 11-29). He found simple fibers that run from the subodontoblastic nerve plexus towards the odontoblast layer but do not reach the predentin. These fibers terminate in extracellular spaces in the cell-rich zone, the cell-poor zone, or the odontoblast layer. Other fibers extend into the predentin and run straight or spiral through a dentinal tubule in close association with an odontoblast process. Most of these intratubular fibers extend into the dentinal tubules for only a few microns, but a few may penetrate as far as 100 or so microns. He also observed complex fibers that reach the predentin and branch extensively (Fig. 11-30). The area covered by a single such terminal complex often reached thousands of square microns.

The anatomic relationships between the odontoblasts, their processes, and the intratubular nerve endings has been studied by several investigators.[6,76] It appears that these fibers lie in a groove or gutter along the surface of the odontoblast process.[77] Toward their terminal ends the nerve fibers twist around the process like a corkscrew. The cell membranes of the odontoblast process and the nerve fiber are closely approximated and run closely parallel for the length of their proximity.

Intratubular nerve endings are most numerous in the area of the pulp horns where as many as one in four tubules contain fibers.[79,107] The number of intratubular fibers decreases in other parts of the dentin, and in root dentin only about one

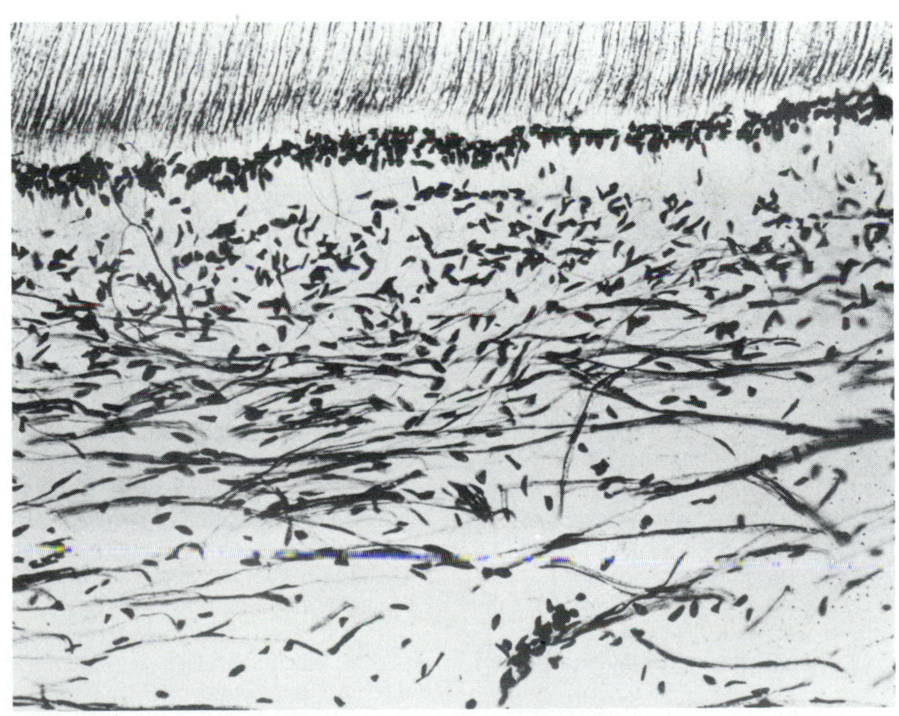

FIG. 11-25 Parietal layer of nerves (plexus of Raschkow) below the cell-rich zone. (From Avery JK: J Endod 7:205, 1981.)

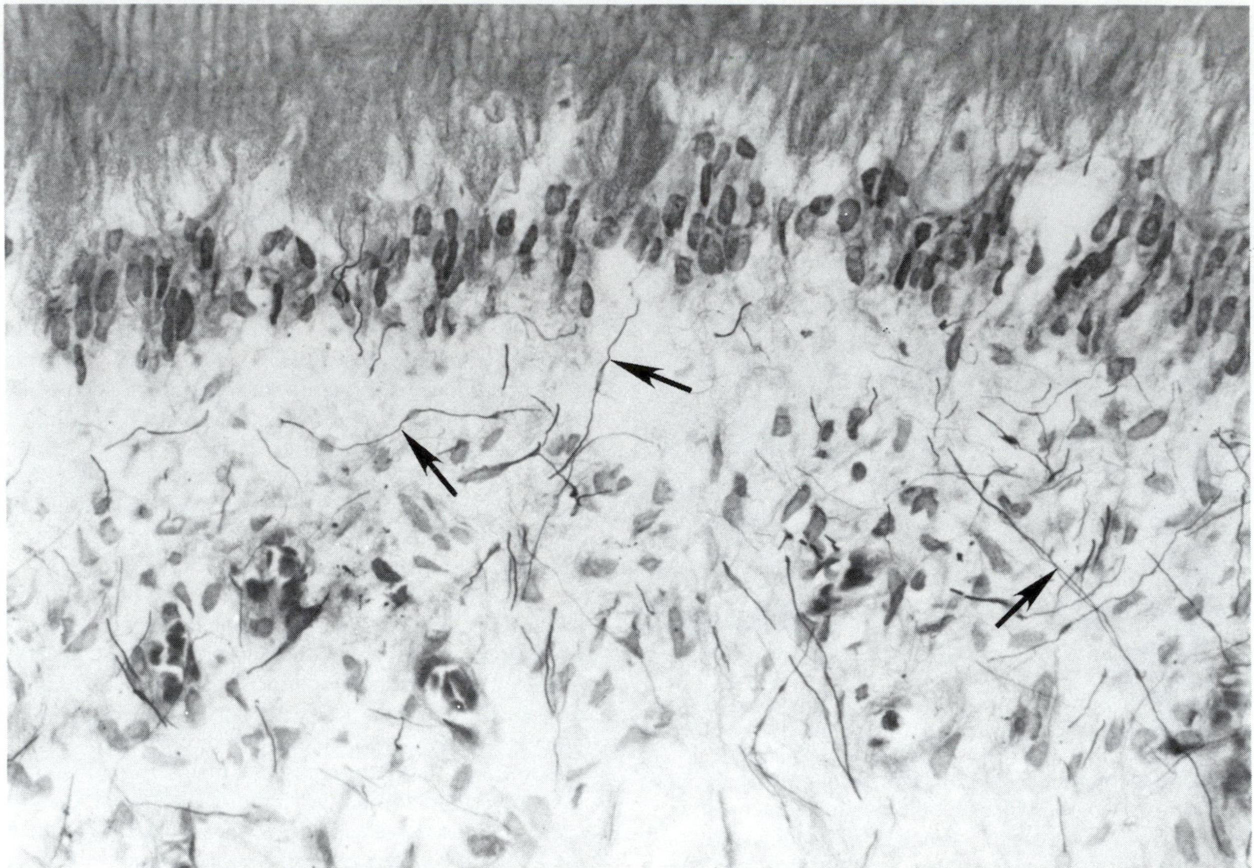

FIG. 11-26 Nerve fibers *(arrows)* in the subodontoblastic area as demonstrated by the Pearson silver impregnation method.

tubule in ten contains a fiber.[107] The functional significance of the intratubular fibers is by no means established, and there is still some question as to whether they are autonomic or sensory fibers. It has even been suggested that they may be passively trapped in the tubules during the final stage of dentin formation.[32]

Although it may be tempting to speculate that the odontoblasts and their associated nerve axons are functionally interrelated and that together they play a role in dentin sensitivity, evidence for this is lacking. If the odontoblast were acting as a receptor cell,* it would synapse with the adjacent nerve fiber. However, Byers[30] was unable to find synaptic junctions that could functionally couple odontoblasts and nerve fibers together. With regard to the membrane properties of odontoblasts, it has been reported that the membrane potential of the odontoblast is low (around −30 mV) and that the cell does not respond to electrical stimulation.[101,186] Thus, it would appear that the odontoblast does not possess the properties of an excitable cell. Furthermore, the sensitivity of dentin is not diminished following disruption of the odontoblast layer.[24,108]

The extent to which dentin is innervated has been the subject of numerous investigations. With the possible exception of the intratubular fibers discussed above, dentin is totally devoid of sensory nerve fibers. This offers an explanation as to why pain-producing agents such as acetylcholine and potassium chloride do not elicit pain when applied to exposed dentin.[2] Similarly, application of topical anesthetic solutions to dentin does not decrease its sensitivity.

In addition to sensory nerves, sympathetic fibers from the superior cervical ganglion appear with blood vessels at the time the vascular system is established in the dental papilla. In the adult tooth sympathetic fibers form plexuses, usually around pulpal arterioles.[5] When stimulated, these fibers cause constriction of the arterioles, resulting in a decrease in blood flow. Sympathetic fibers have also been found lying independent of blood vessels in the region of the odontoblasts. It is thought that these nerve endings may be involved in the regulation of dentin formation. One study reported finding both adrenergic and cholinergic nerve endings among the odontoblasts.[10]

Another study showed that a reduction in pulpal blood flow induced by stimulation of sympathetic fibers leading to the pulp results in depressed excitability of pulpal A fibers.[36] The excitability of C fibers is less affected than that of A fibers by a reduction in blood flow.[169]

Pulpal nerve fibers contain neuropeptides such as neuropeptide Y, calcitonin gene–related peptide (CGRP), vasoactive intestinal polypeptide (VIP), tyrosine hydroxylase, and substance P.[111,136,182] Release of these peptides can be triggered by such things as tissue injury, complement activation, antigen-antibody reactions, or antidromic stimulation of the in-

*A receptor cell is a nonnerve cell capable of exciting adjacent afferent nerve fibers. Synaptic junctions connect receptor cells to afferent nerves.

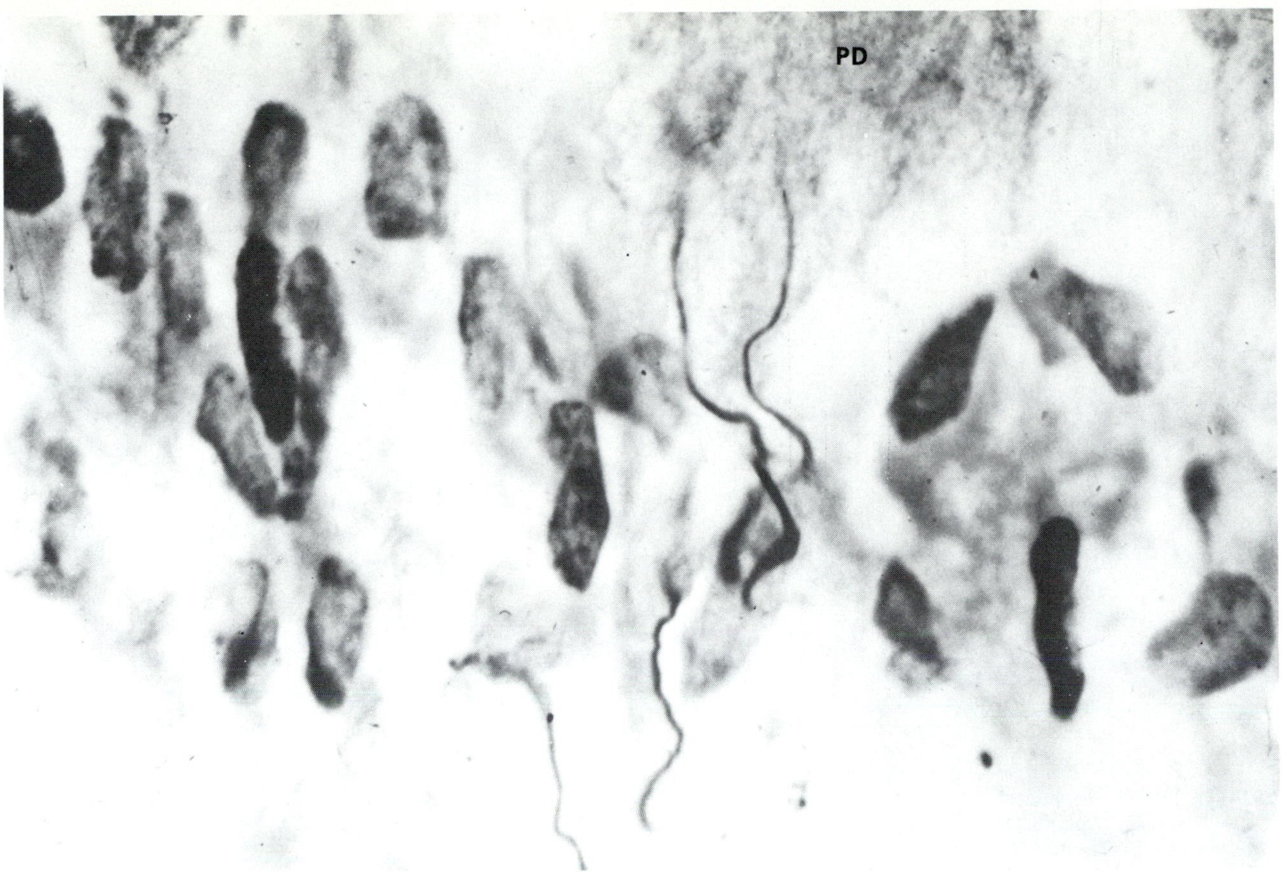

FIG. 11-27 Nerve fibers passing between odontoblasts to the predentin *(PD)*.

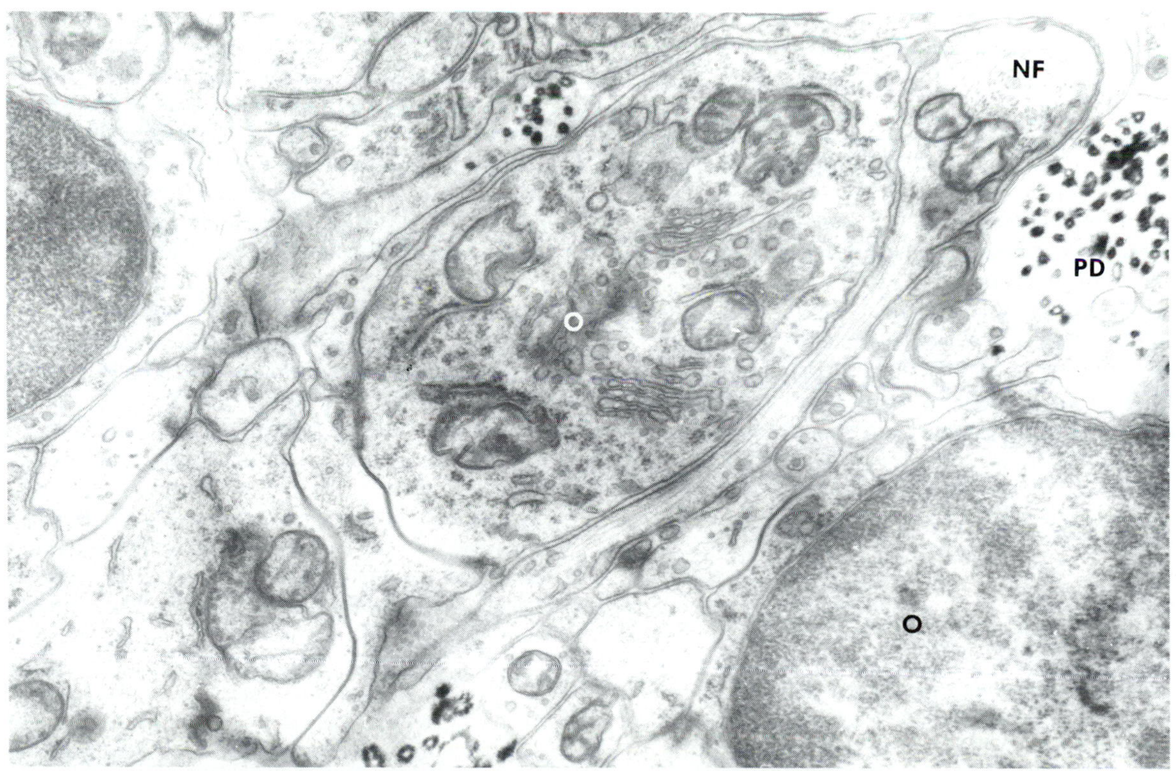

FIG. 11-28 Unmyelinated nerve fiber *(NF)* without a Schwann cell covering located between adjacent odontoblasts *(O)* overlying pulp horn of a mouse molar tooth. Predentin *(PD)* can be seen at upper right. Within the nerve there are longitudinally oriented fine neurofilaments, microvesicles, and mitochondria. (From Corpron RE and Avery JK: Anat Rec 175:585, 1973.)

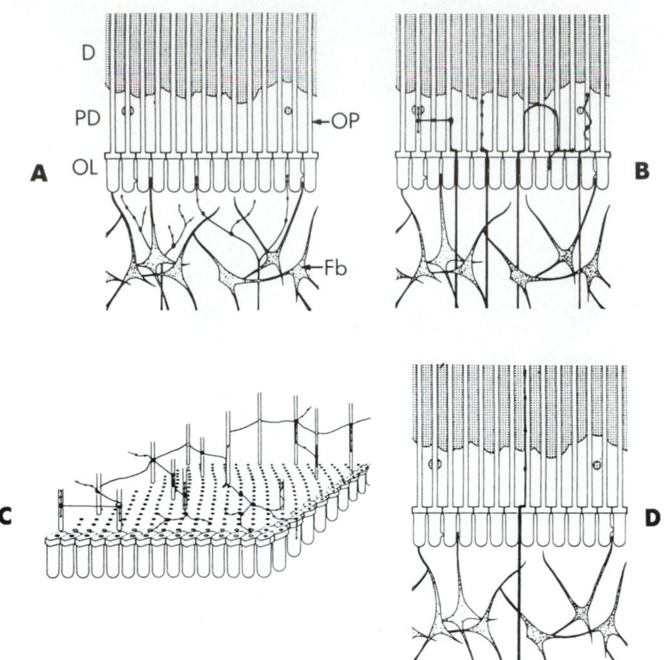

FIG. 11-29 Schematic drawing showing four types of nerve fibers in the pulpodentinal border zone. **A,** Fibers running from the subodontoblastic plexus to the odontoblast layer but not the predentin. *D,* Dentin; *PD,* predentin; *OP,* odontoblast process; *OL,* odontoblast layer; *Fb,* fibroblast. **B,** Fibers extending into dentinal tubules in the predentin. **C,** Complex fibers that branch extensively in the predentin. **D,** Intratubular fibers extending into the dentin. (Courtesy T. Gunji, Niigata University, Japan.)

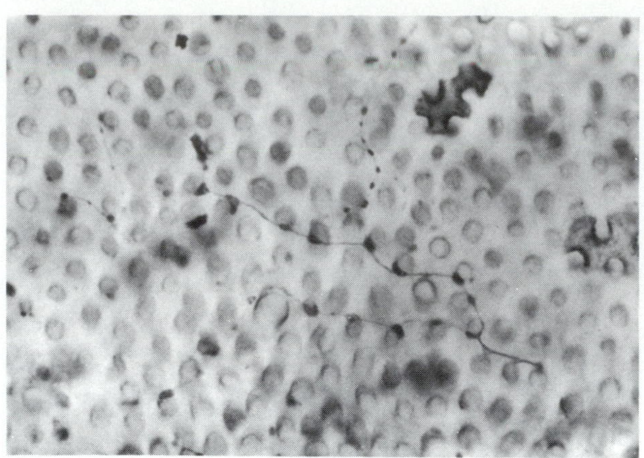

FIG. 11-30 Histologic section showing a terminal branch of a complex predentinal nerve fiber. (Courtesy T. Gunji, Niigata University, Japan.)

ferior alveolar nerve. Once released, vasoactive peptides produce vascular changes that are similar to those evoked by histamine and bradykinin.

The electric pulp tester delivers a current sufficient to overcome the resistance of enamel and dentin and stimulate the A-δ fibers at the pulp-dentin border zone. C fibers of the pulp do not respond to the conventional pulp tester because significantly more current is needed to stimulate them.[129] Bender[12] and others found that in anterior teeth the optimum placement site of the electrode is the incisal tooth edge, as the response threshold is lowest at the incisal edge and increases as the electrode is moved toward the cervical region of the tooth.

Of considerable clinical interest is the evidence that nerve fibers of the pulp are relatively resistant to necrosis.[37,123] This is apparently due to the fact that nerve bundles in general are more resistant to autolysis. Even in degenerating pulps, the nerve fibers could still respond to stimulation.[37] It may be that C fibers remain excitable even after blood flow has been compromised in the diseased pulp, for C fibers are better able to maintain their functional integrity in the presence of hypoxia.[169] This may help to explain why instrumentation of the root canals of apparently nonvital teeth sometimes elicits pain.

SENSITIVITY OF DENTIN

The mechanisms underlying dentin sensitivity have been the subject of keen interest in recent years. How are stimuli relayed from the peripheral dentin to the sensory receptors located in the region of the pulp-dentin border zone? Converging evidence indicates that *movement of fluid in the dentinal tubules is the basic event in the arousal of pain* (see review by Trowbridge[172]). It now appears that pain-producing stimuli such as heat, cold, air blasts, and probing with the tip of an explorer have in common the ability to displace fluid in the tubules.[21,26,176] Brännström and his group in Stockholm[21,22,28] are responsible for advancing the hydrodynamic theory of dentin sensitivity. This theory helps to explain how fluid movement in the dentinal tubules is translated into electrical signals by sensory receptors located in the pulp.

In experiments on humans, brief application of heat or cold to the outer surface of premolar teeth evoked a painful response before the heat or cold could have produced temperature changes capable of activating sensory receptors in the underlying pulp.[176] The evoked pain was of very short duration, 1 or 2 seconds. The thermal diffusivity of dentin is relatively low; yet the response of the tooth to thermal stimulation is rapid, often less than a second. How best can this be explained? Evidence suggests that thermal stimulation of the tooth results in a rapid movement of fluid in the dentinal tubules that results in the deformation of the sensory nerve terminals in the underlying pulp. Heat would expand the fluid within the tubules, causing it to flow towards the pulp, whereas cold would cause the fluid to contract, producing an outward flow. Presumably the rapid movement of fluid across the cell membrane of the sensory receptor activates the receptor. All nerve cells have membrane channels through which charged ions pass, and this current flow, if great enough, can stimulate the cell and cause it to transmit impulses to the brain. Some channels are activated by voltage, some by chemicals and some by mechanical pressure. In the case of pulpal nerve fibers that are activated by hydrodynamic forces, pressure would increase the flow of sodium and potassium ions through pressure-activated channels, thus initiating generator potentials.

The dentinal tubule is a capillary tube having an exceedingly small diameter.* Therefore, the effects of capillarity are significant, as the narrower the bore of a capillary tube, the

*To appreciate fully the dimensions of dentin tubules, understand that the diameter of the tubules is much smaller than that of red blood cells.

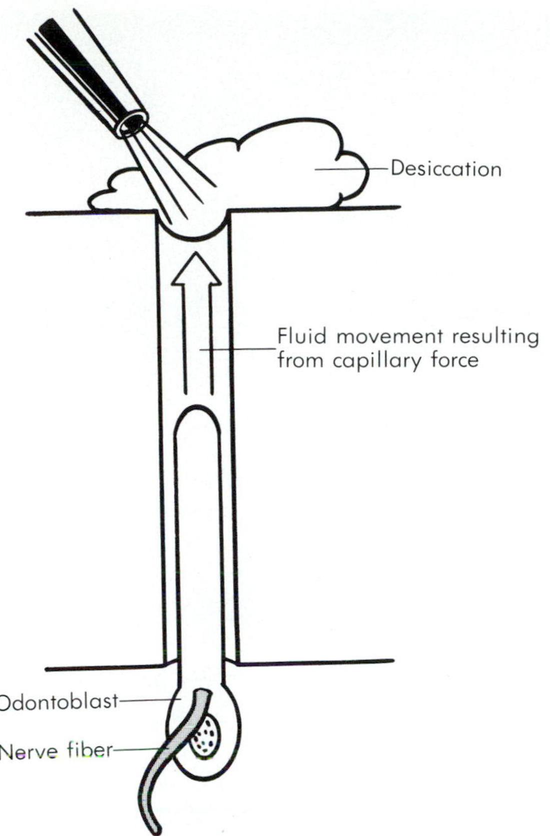

FIG. 11-31 Diagram illustrating movement of fluid in the dentinal tubules resulting from dehydrating effect of a blast of air from an air syringe.

greater the effect of capillarity. Thus, if fluid is removed from the outer end of exposed dentinal tubules by dehydrating the dentinal surface with an airblast or absorbent paper, capillary forces will produce a rapid outward movement of fluid in the tubule (Fig. 11-31). According to Brännström[22] desiccation of dentin can theoretically cause dentinal fluid to flow outward at a rate of 2 to 3 mm per second. In addition to air blasts, dehydrating solutions containing hyperosmotic concentrations of sucrose or calcium chloride can produce pain if applied to exposed dentin.[3,110]

Investigators have shown that it is the A fibers rather than the C fibers that are activated by stimuli such as heat, cold, and air blasts applied to exposed dentin.[125,126] However, if heat is applied long enough to increase the temperature of the pulp-dentin border several degrees Celsius the C fibers may respond, particularly if the heat produces injury. It seems that the A fibers are only activated by a very rapid displacement of the tubular contents.[127] Slow heating of the tooth produced no response until the temperature reached 43.8° C, at which time C fibers were activated, presumably because of heat-induced injury to the pulp.

It has also been shown that pain-producing stimuli are more readily transmitted from the dentin surface when the exposed tubule apertures are wide and the fluid within the tubules is free to flow outward.[86] For example, other researchers found that acid treatment of exposed dentin to remove grinding debris opens the tubule orifices and makes the dentin more responsive to stimuli such as air blasts and probing.[75]

Perhaps the most difficult phenomenon to explain is pain associated with light probing of dentin. Even light pressure of an explorer tip can produce strong forces.* Presumably these forces mechanically compress the openings of the tubules and cause sufficient displacement of fluid to excite the sensory receptors in the underlying pulp. Considering the density of the tubules in which hydrodynamic forces would be generated by probing, thousands of nerve endings would be simultaneously stimulated, thus producing a cumulative effect.

Another example of the effect of strong hydraulic forces that are created within the dentinal tubules is the phenomenon of odontoblast displacement. In this reaction the cell bodies of odontoblasts are displaced upward into the dentinal tubules, presumably by a rapid movement of fluid in the tubules produced when exposed dentin is desiccated, as with the use of an air syringe or cavity-drying agents (Fig. 11-32). Such displacement results in loss of the odontoblasts since cells thus affected soon undergo autolysis and disappear from the tubules. (Displaced odontoblasts may eventually be replaced by cells that migrate from the cell-rich zone of the pulp, as discussed below.)

The hydrodynamic theory can also be applied to an understanding of the mechanism responsible for hypersensitive dentin. Hypersensitive dentin is associated with the exposure of dentin normally covered by cementum. The thin layer of cementum is frequently lost as gingival recession exposes cementum to the oral environment and cementum is subsequently worn away by brushing, flossing, or the use of toothpicks. Once exposed, the dentin may respond to the same stimuli that any exposed dentin surface responds to—mechanical pressure, dehydrating agents, etc. Although the dentin may at first be very sensitive, within a few weeks the sensitivity usually subsides. This densitization is thought to occur as a result of gradual occlusion of the tubules by mineral deposits, thus reducing the hydrodynamic forces. Additionally, the deposition of reparative dentin over the pulpal ends of the exposed tubules probably also reduces sensitivity.[173]

Currently, the treatment of hypersensitive teeth is directed toward reducing the functional diameter of the dentinal tubules so as to limit fluid movement. In order to accomplish this objective, there are several possible treatment modalities (for discussion, see Trowbridge[175]): (1) formation of a smear layer on the sensitive dentin by burnishing the exposed root surface; (2) application of agents such as oxalate compounds that form insoluble precipitates within the tubules; (3) impregnation of the tubules with plastic resins; (4) application of dentin bonding agents to seal off the tubules.

Painful Pulpitis

From the foregoing it is apparent that pain associated with the stimulation of the A-δ fibers does not necessarily signify that the pulp is inflamed or that tissue injury has occurred. The A-δ fibers have a relatively low threshold of excitability, and painful pulpitis is more likely to be associated with nociceptive C fiber† activity. The clinician should carefully examine

*A force of 10 g (0.022 lb) applied to an explorer having a tip 0.002 inch in diameter would produce a pressure of 7000 psi on the dentin.

†A nociceptive fiber is a pain-conducting fiber that responds to stimuli capable of injuring tissue.

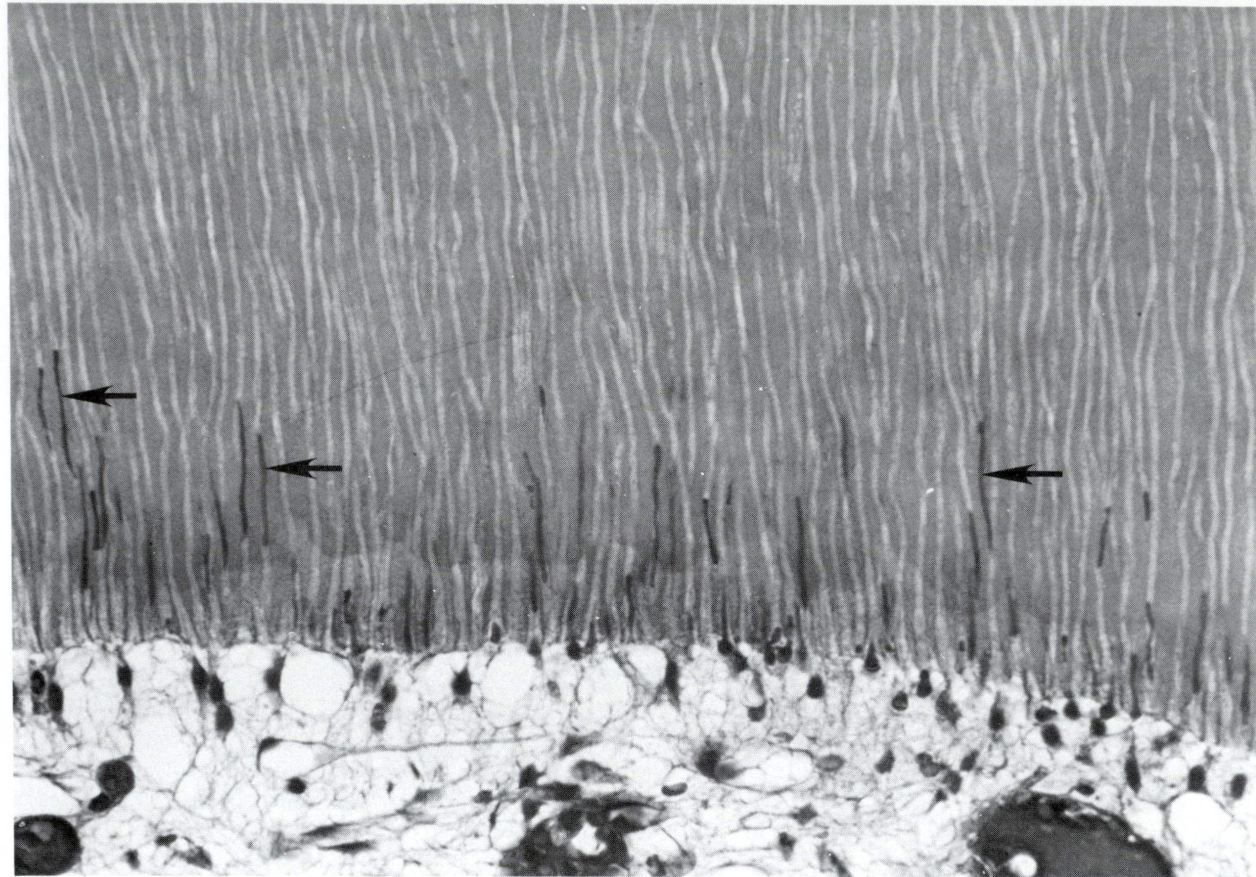

FIG. 11-32 Nuclei of odontoblasts *(arrows)* displaced up into the dentinal tubules.

symptomatic teeth to rule out the possibility of hypersensitive dentin, cracked fillings, or dentinal fractures, each of which may initiate hydrodynamic forces, before establishing a diagnosis of pulpitis.

Pulpitis, or inflammation of the pulp, may be either painless or painful, but pain seems to be the exception rather than the rule. It is recognized that the stimulation threshold of nerve fibers that mediate pain is lowered by sustained inflammation. In this case the inflamed pulp may become hypersensitive to all stimuli. Clinically it has been observed that the sensitivity of dentin is increased when the underlying pulp becomes acutely inflamed, and the tooth may be more difficult to anesthetize. Although a precise explanation for this hyperalgesia* is lacking, apparently the localized elevations in tissue pressure that accompany acute inflammation play an important role.[155,179]

Clinically, we know that when a pulp chamber of a painful tooth with an abscessed pulp is opened, drainage soon produces a reduction in the level of pain. This suggests that pressure may contribute to hyperalgesia. In addition, algogenic (i.e., pain-producing) agents are known to alter the sensitivity threshold of sensory fibers. Endogenous chemical mediators of inflammation such as bradykinin, 5-hydroxytryptamine (5-HT), and prostaglandins are either directly or indirectly algogenic and thus may be capable of exciting sensory nerves of the pulp. Investigators[130,133] found that 5-HT is able to sensitize intradental fibers to hydrodynamic stimuli such as cold, air blasts, and osmotic stimulation, thus suggesting that inflammatory mediators may increase the sensitivity of dentin. Unmyelinated fibers are activated by bradykinin and histamine.[128] These agents produced a dull, aching pain when placed in deep cavities in human teeth.[134]

Recently, leukotriene B_4 was shown to have a long-lasting sensitizing effect on intradental nerves, suggesting that it may potentiate nociceptor activity during pulpal inflammation.[112]

Pain associated with an inflamed or degenerating pulp may be either provoked or spontaneous. The hyperalgesic pulp may respond to stimuli that usually do not evoke pain, or the pain may be exaggerated and persist longer. On the other hand, the tooth may commence to hurt spontaneously in the absence of any external stimulus. There is not a satisfactory explanation as to why a pulp that has been inflamed but asymptomatic for weeks or months suddenly begins to ache at 3:00 o'clock in the morning. Such unprovoked pain usually manifests itself as a dull, aching, poorly localized sensation qualitatively different from the brief, sharp, well-localized sensation associated with hydrodynamic fluid movement within the dentinal tubules.

One researcher[124] has done much to elucidate the role of hydrostatic pressure changes in the activation of pulpal nerve fibers. In his experiment involving dogs and cats both positive and negative pressure changes were introduced into the pulp by means of a cannula inserted in the dentin. Using single-

**Hyperalgesia,* lowering of the pain threshold.

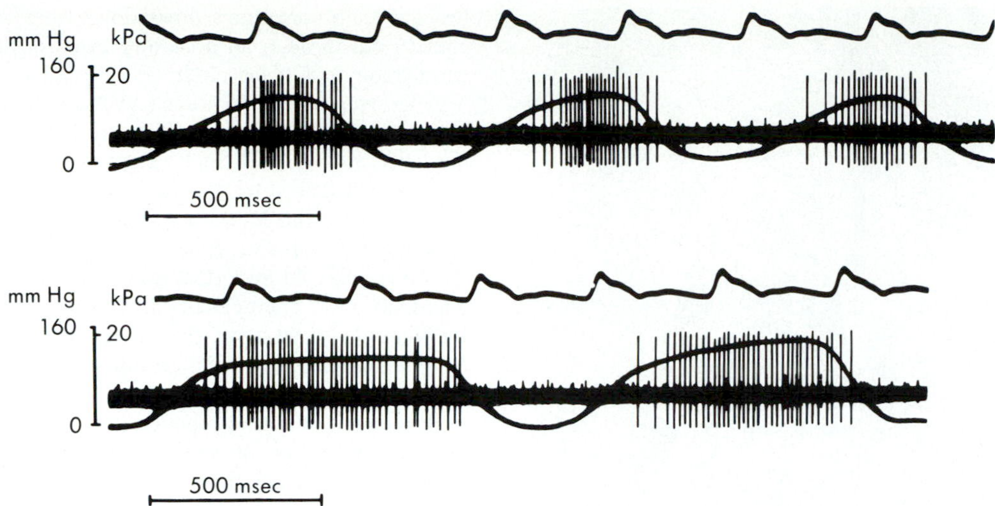

FIG. 11-33 Response of a single dog pulp nerve fiber to repeated hydrostatic pressure stimulation pulses. The lower solid wavy line of each recording indicates the stimulation pressure applied to the pulp. The upper line *(kPa)* is the femoral artery blood pressure curve recorded to indicate the relative changes in the pulse pressure and the heart cycle. (From Närhi M: Proc Finn Dent Soc 74[suppl 5]:1, 1978.)

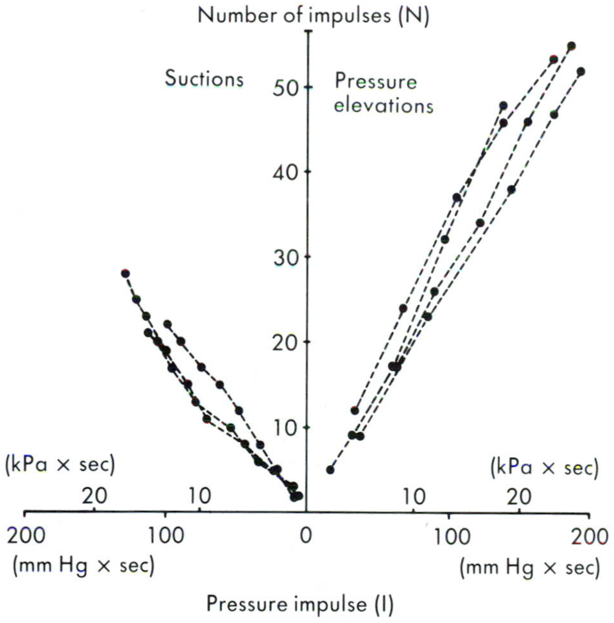

FIG. 11-34 Relationship between the number of nerve impulses *(N)* and the pressure impulse *(I)* of a small group of pulpal cat nerve fibers with three suction stimuli and four pressure elevations. The pressure impulse is labeled as both mm Hg × sec and kPa × sec. (From Närhi M: Proc Finn Dent Soc 74[suppl 5]:1, 1978.)

fiber recording techniques, he found a positive correlation between the degree of pressure change and the number of nerve impulses leaving the pulp. He theorized that the pressure changes produced local deformities in the pulp tissue, resulting in a stretching of the sensory nerve fibers (Figs. 11-33 to 11-35).

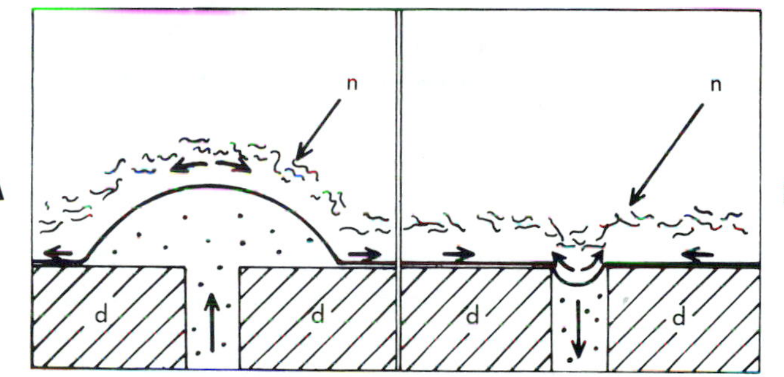

FIG. 11-35 Theoretical effect of hydrostatic pressure changes on the area of stimulation in the pulp. *d,* Dentin; *n,* nerve endings. **A,** Positive pressure. **B,** Suction. (From Närhi M: Proc Finn Dent Soc 74[suppl 5]:1, 1978.)

VASCULAR SUPPLY

Hemodynamics

Blood from the dental artery enters the tooth via arterioles having diameters of 100 μm or less. These vessels pass through the apical foramen or foramina in company with nerve bundles (Fig. 11-23). Smaller vessels may enter the pulp via lateral or accessory canals. The arterioles course up through the central portion of the radicular pulp and give off branches that spread laterally toward the odontoblast layer, beneath which they ramify to form a capillary plexus (Fig. 11-36). As the arterioles pass into the coronal pulp, they fan out toward the dentin, diminish in size, and give rise to a capillary network in the subodontoblastic region (Figs. 11-37 and 11-38). This network provides the odontoblasts with a rich source of metabolites.

Capillary blood flow in the coronal portion of the pulp is

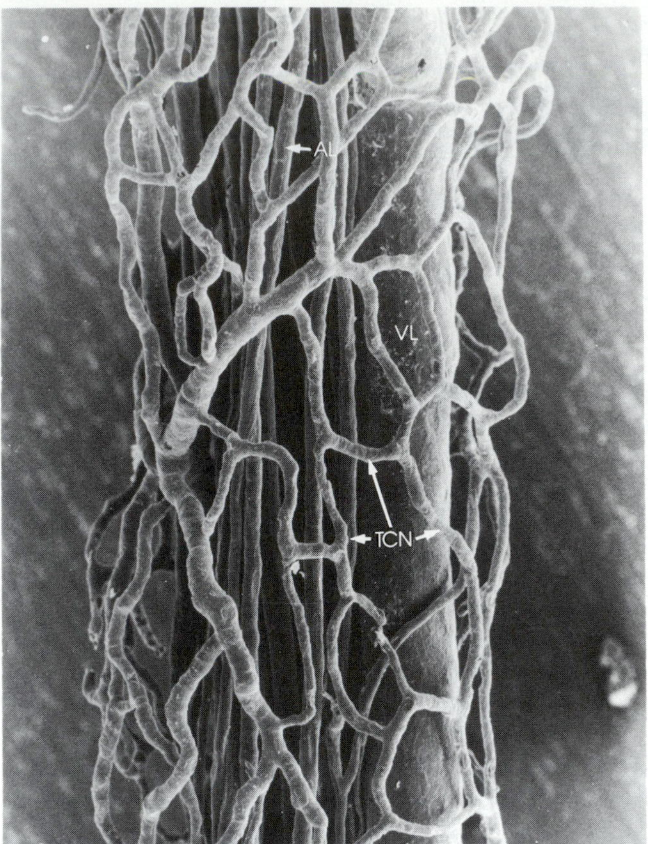

FIG. 11-36 High-power scanning electron micrograph of vascular network in the radicular pulp of a dog molar showing the configuration of the subodontoblastic terminal capillary network *(TCN)*. Venules *(VL)* and arterioles *(AL)* are indicated. (Courtesy Dr. Y. Kishi, Kanagawa Dental College, Kanagawa, Japan.)

nearly twice that in the root portion.[97,139] Moreover, blood flow in the region of the pulp horns is greater than in other areas of the pulp.[116]

The subodontoblastic capillaries are surrounded by a basement membrane, and occasionally fenestrations (pores) are observed in their walls.[141] These fenestrations are thought to provide rapid transport of fluid and metabolites from the capillaries to the adjacent odontoblasts. In addition, one study[66] observed numerous pinocytic vesicles in the capillaries of the hamster pulp and suggested that these structures might also be important in the transcapillary transport of metabolites. In young teeth, capillaries commonly extend into the odontoblast layer, thus assuring an adequate supply of nutrients for the metabolically active odontoblasts.

Blood passes from the capillary plexus first into postcapillary venules and then into progressively larger venules (Fig. 11-37). Venules in the pulp have unusually thin walls, which may facilitate the movement of fluid in or out of the vessel. The muscular coat of these venules is thin and discontinuous. The collecting venules become progressively larger as they course to the central region of the pulp. The largest venules have a diameter that may reach a maximum of 200 μm; thus they are considerably larger than the arterioles of the pulp. According to one study,[100] the principal venous drainage in multirooted teeth sometimes flows down only one root canal or courses out through an accessory canal in the bifurcation or trifurcation area of the tooth.

Arteriovenous anastomoses (AVAs) may be present in both the coronal and radicular portions of the pulp, particularly in the latter.[100,107,157,176] Such vessels provide a direct communication between arterioles and venules, thus bypassing the capillary bed. The AVAs are relatively small venules, having a diameter of approximately 10 μm.[97] It is hypothesized that the AVAs play an important role in the regulation of the pulp circulation.[93,97] Theoretically they could provide a mechanism for shunting blood away from areas of injury where damage to the microcirculation may result in thrombosis and hemorrhage.

Recently it has been reported that the fraction of blood in the coronal pulp of cat canines is 14.4%.[181] The average capillary density was found to be 1404 per square millimeter, which is higher than in most other tissues of the body.

Among the oral tissues, the pulp has the highest volume of blood flow, but it is substantially lower than blood flow in the major visceral organs (Fig. 11-39). This reflects the fact that the respiratory rate of pulp cells is relatively low.[43]

Regional blood flow distribution in the pulps of dogs has been studied.[93] As would be anticipated, pulpal blood flow was greater in the peripheral layer of the pulp (i.e., the subodontoblastic capillary plexus) than in the central area.

It appears that blood flow in the pulp is largely under the control of the adrenergic sympathetic system.[97] The walls of arterioles and venules are associated with smooth muscle that is innervated by unmyelinated sympathetic fibers. When stimulated, these fibers transmit impulses that cause the muscle fibers to contract, thus decreasing the diameter of the vessel (vasoconstriction). It has been shown experimentally that electrical stimulation of sympathetic fibers leading to the pulp results in a decrease in pulpal blood flow.[35,93,167] Activation of α-adrenergic receptors by the administration of epinephrine-containing local anesthetic solutions may result in a marked decrease in pulpal blood flow.[94] Functional evidence for cholinergic parasympathetic regulation of pulpal blood flow is lacking. However, the presence of cholinergic nerve endings among odontoblasts in mouse and monkey pulps has been reported along with the suggestion that these fibers may influence dentinogenesis.[9]

One investigation measured tissue and intravascular pressures in the pulps of cats.[167] The tissue pressure was estimated to be approximately 6 mm Hg. Pressure in the arterioles, capillaries, and venules was 43, 35, and 19 mm Hg, respectively (Fig. 11-40).

Blood circulation in an inflamed pulp involves very complex pathophysiologic reactions that have not been fully elucidated, in spite of numerous studies (for reviews see Heyeraas[73] and Kim and others[96]). A unique feature of the pulp is that it is rigidly encased within dentin. This places it in a low-compliance environment, much like the brain and bone marrow. Thus, pulp tissue has limited ability to expand, so vasodilatation and increased vascular permeability evoked during an inflammatory reaction result in an increase in pulpal hydrostatic pressure.[179] Presumably, any sudden rise in intrapulpal pressure would be distributed equally within the area of pressure increase, including the blood vessels. Theoretically, if tissue pressure increases to the point that it equals the intravascular pressure, the thin-walled venules would be

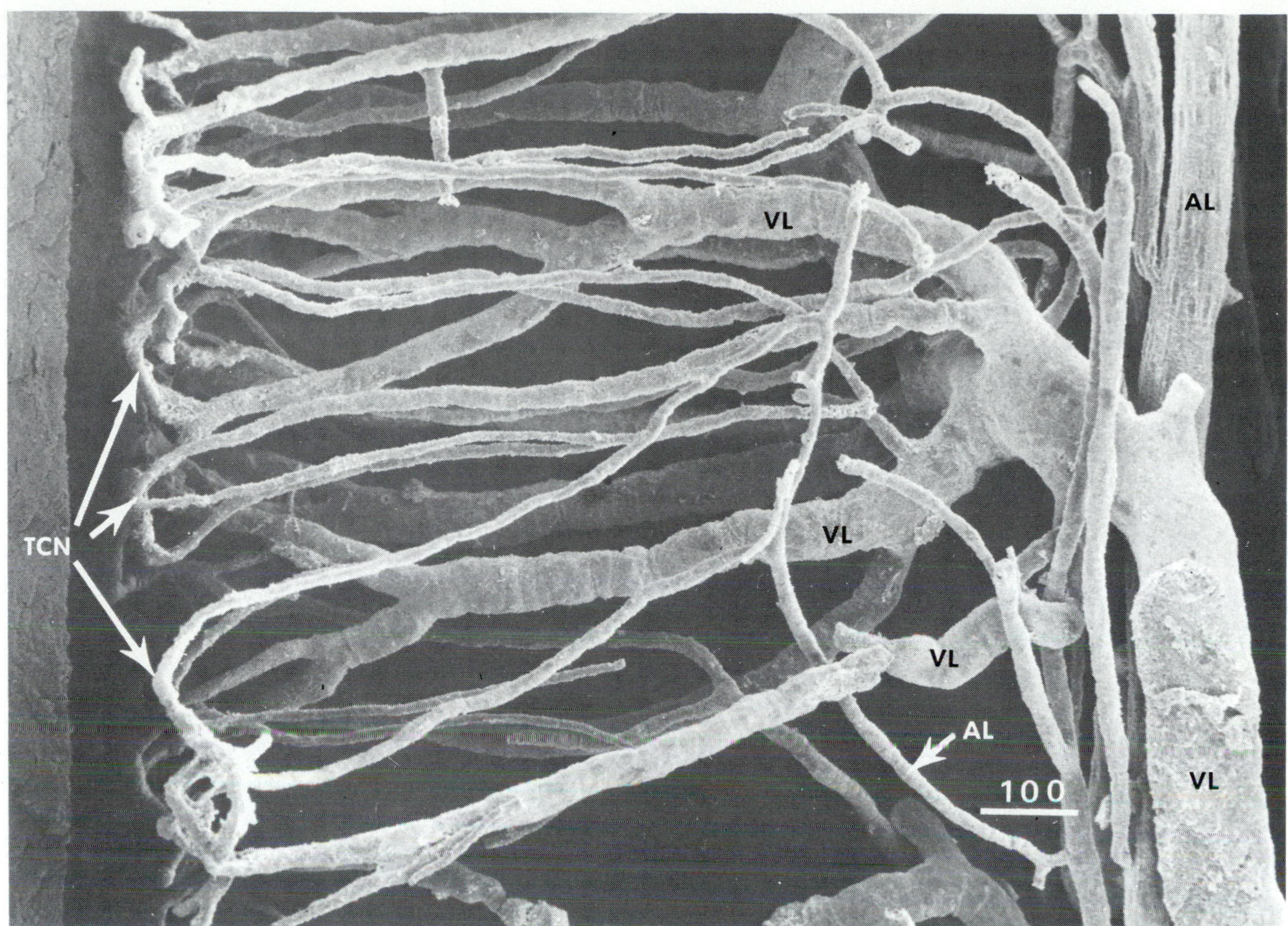

FIG. 11-37 Subodontoblastic terminal capillary network *(TCN)*, arterioles *(AL)*, and venules *(VL)* of young canine pulp. Dentin would be to the far left and the central pulp to the right. The bar is 100 μm. (From Takahashi K, et al: J Endod 8:131, 1982.)

compressed, thereby increasing vascular resistance and reducing pulpal blood flow.[95] This could explain why injection of vasodilators such as bradykinin into an artery leading to the pulp results in a reduction rather than an increase in pulpal blood flow.[98,166] However, it is possible that an increase in intrapulpal tissue pressure would promote absorption of tissue fluid back into the blood and lymphatic vessels, thus reducing the pressure. In this case blood flow could increase, in spite of a marked elevation in tissue pressure.[72] Obviously, a combined multidisciplinary approach is needed in order to better understand the intricate circulatory changes occurring during the development of pulpal inflammation.

Lymphatics

The existence of lymphatics in the pulp has been a matter of debate, since it is not easy to distinguish between venules and lymphatics by ordinary light microscopic techniques. Recently, however, studies utilizing light- and electron-microscopy have described lymphatic capillaries in human and in feline dental pulps (Fig. 11-41).[18,115]

REPAIR

The inherent healing potential of the dental pulp is well recognized. As in all other connective tissues, repair of tissue injury commences with débridement by macrophages followed by proliferation of fibroblasts, capillary buds, and the formation of collagen. Local circulation is of critical importance in wound healing and repair. An adequate supply of blood is essential to transport inflammatory elements into the area of pulpal injury and to provide the young fibroblasts with nutrients from which to synthesize collagen. Unlike most tissues, the pulp has essentially no collateral circulation; and for this reason it is theoretically more vulnerable than most other tissues. Thus, in the case of severe injury, healing would be impaired in teeth with a limited blood supply. It is well recognized that the highly cellular pulp of a young tooth, with a wide open apical foramen and rich blood supply, has a much better healing potential than does an older tooth, with a narrow foramen and a restricted blood supply.

Dentin that is produced in response to the injury of primary odontoblasts has been known by several different names:

Irregular secondary dentin
Irritation dentin
Tertiary dentin
Reparative dentin

The term most commonly applied to irregularly formed dentin is *reparative* dentin, presumably because it so frequently forms in response to injury and appears to be a component of the reparative process. It must be recognized, however, that this type of dentin has also been observed in the pulps of normal unerupted teeth without any obvious injury.[102,131]

It will be recalled that secondary dentin is deposited circumpulpally at a very slow rate throughout the life of the vital tooth. In contrast, the formation of reparative dentin occurs at the pulpal surface of primary or secondary dentin at sites corresponding to areas of irritation. For example, when a carious lesion has invaded dentin, the pulp usually responds by depositing a layer of reparative dentin over the dentinal tubules of the primary or secondary dentin which communicate with the carious lesion (Fig. 11-42). Similarly, when occlusal wear removes the overlying enamel and exposes the dentin to the oral environment, reparative dentin is deposited over the exposed tubules. In general, the amount of reparative dentin formed in response to caries or attrition of the tooth surface is proportional to the amount of primary dentin that is destroyed. Thus the formation of reparative dentin allows the pulp to retreat behind a barrier of mineralized tissue.

Compared to primary dentin, reparative dentin is less tubu-

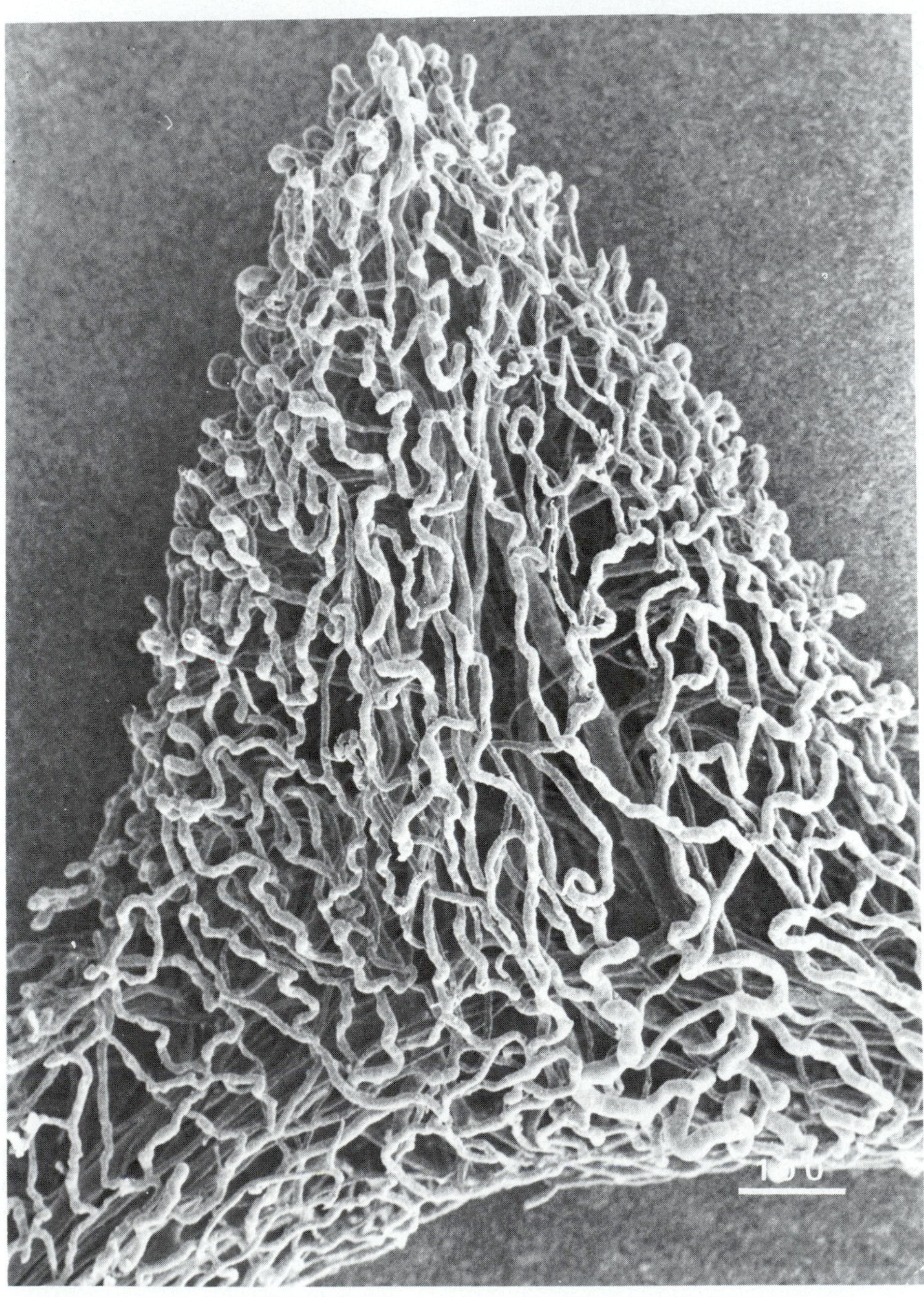

FIG. 11-38 Scanning electron micrograph of the terminal capillary network in the pulp horn of a dog molar. (Courtesy Professor K. Takahashi, Kanagawa Dental College, Kanagawa, Japan.)

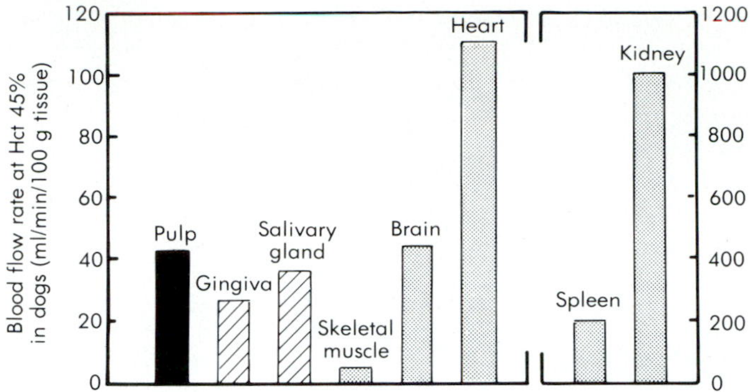

FIG. 11-39 Blood flow per 100 g tissue weight for various organs and tissues at 45% hematocrit *(Hct)* in dogs. (From Kim S: J Endod 11:465, 1985.)

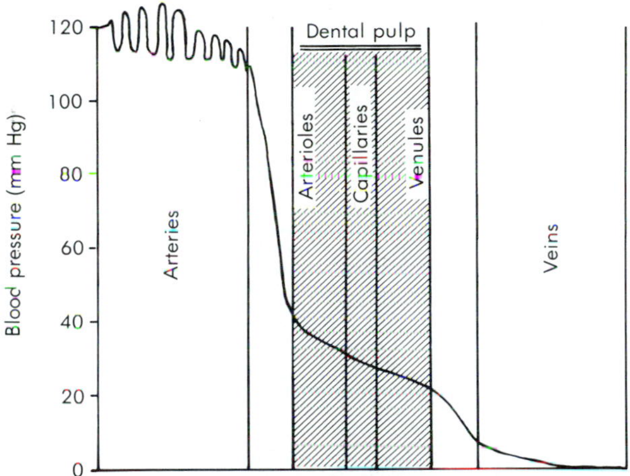

FIG. 11-40 Blood pressure fall along extrapulpal and intrapulpal blood vessels. (Modified from Heyeraas KJ: J Dent Res 64(special issue):585, 1985.)

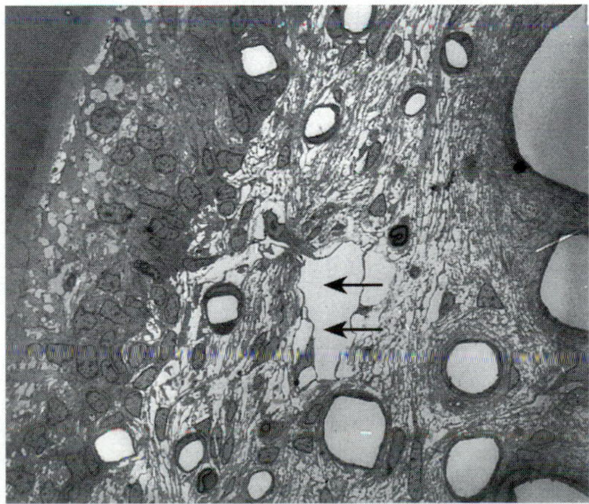

FIG. 11-41 Electron micrograph showing lymphatic vessel *(arrows)* in a feline dental pulp. (From Bishop MA, and Malhotra M: Am J Anat 187:247, 1990.)

lar and the tubules tend to be more irregular with larger lumina. In some cases no tubules are formed. The cells that form reparative dentin are not as columnar as the primary odontoblasts of the coronal pulp and are often cuboidal (Fig. 11-43). The quality of reparative dentin (i.e., the extent to which it resembles primary dentin) is quite variable. If irritation to the pulp is relatively mild, as in the case of a superficial carious lesion, the reparative dentin formed may resemble primary dentin in terms of tubularity and degree of mineralization. On the other hand, reparative dentin deposited in response to a deep carious lesion may be relatively atubular and poorly mineralized with many areas of interglobular dentin. The degree of irregularity of reparative dentin is probably determined by factors such as the amount of inflammation present, the extent of cellular injury, and the state of differentiation of the replacement odontoblasts.

The poorest quality of reparative dentin is usually observed in association with marked pulpal inflammation. In fact, the dentin may be so poorly organized that areas of soft tissue are entrapped within the dentinal matrix. In histologic sections these areas of soft tissue entrapment impart a Swiss cheese appearance to the dentin (Fig. 11-44). As the entrapped soft tissue degenerates, products of tissue degeneration further contribute to the inflammatory stimuli assailing the pulp.

It has been reported[33] that trauma caused by cavity preparation which is too mild to result in the loss of primary odontoblasts does not lead to reparative dentin formation, even if the cavity preparation is relatively deep. This evidence would suggest that reparative dentin is formed principally by replacement cells.[120] For many years it has been recognized that destruction of primary odontoblasts is soon followed by increased mitotic activity within fibroblasts of the subjacent cell-rich zone. It has been shown that the progeny of these dividing cells

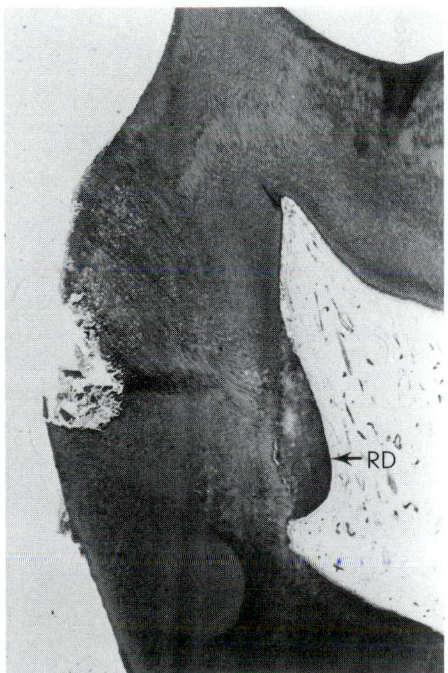

FIG. 11-42 Reparative dentin *(RD)* deposited in response to a carious lesion in the dentin. (From Trowbridge HO: J Endod 7:52, 1981.)

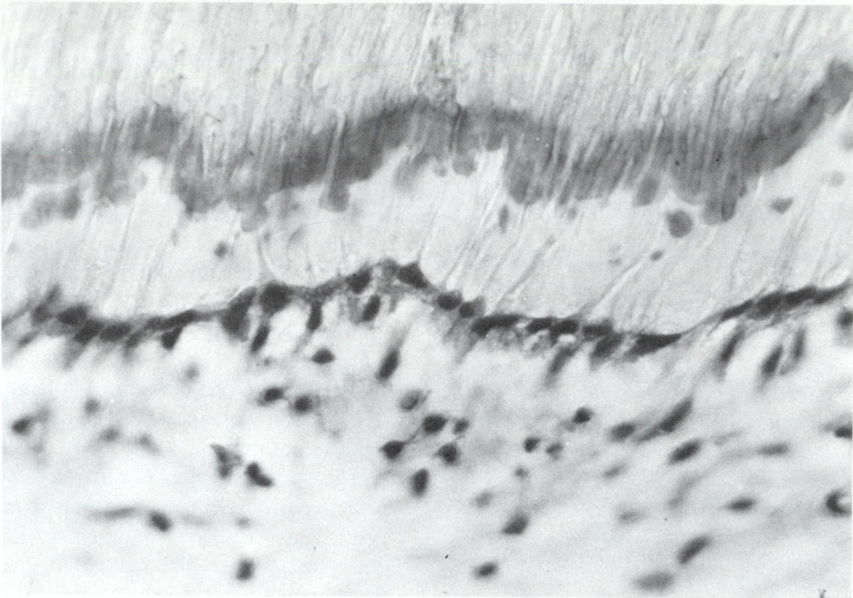

FIG. 11-43 Layer of cells forming reparative dentin. Note the decreased tubularity of reparative dentin as compared to the developmental dentin above.

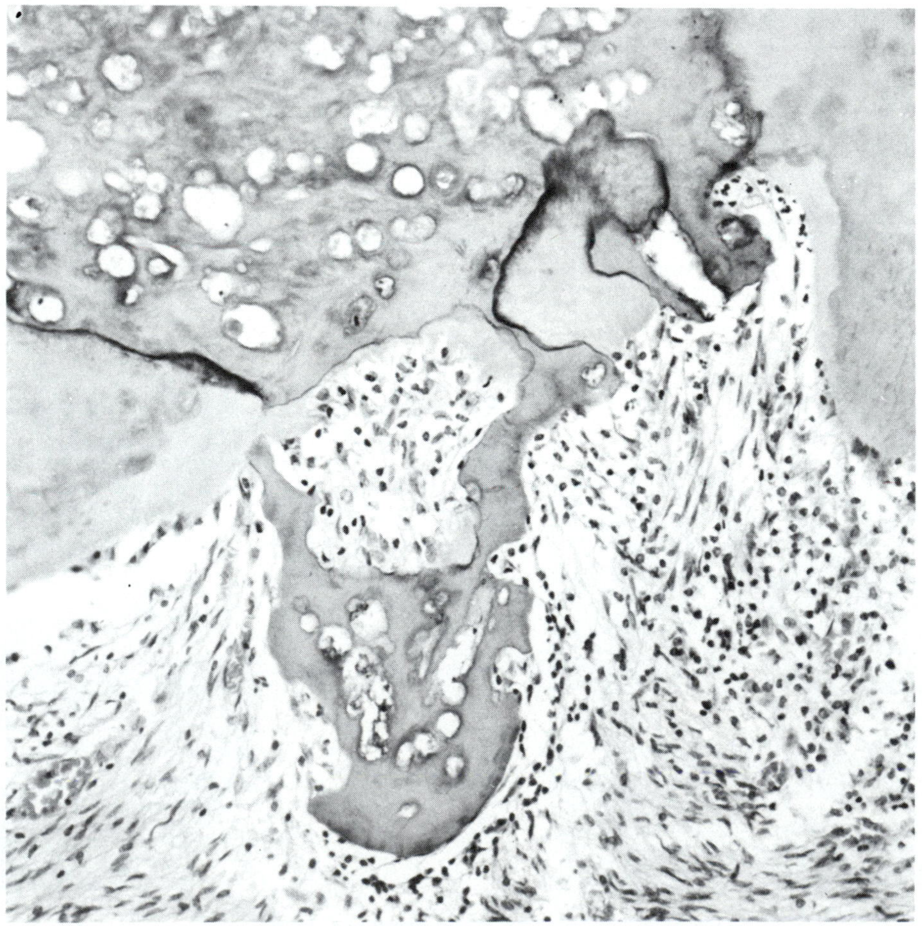

FIG. 11-44 Swiss cheese type of reparative dentin. Note the numerous areas of soft tissue inclusion and infiltration of inflammatory cells in the pulp.

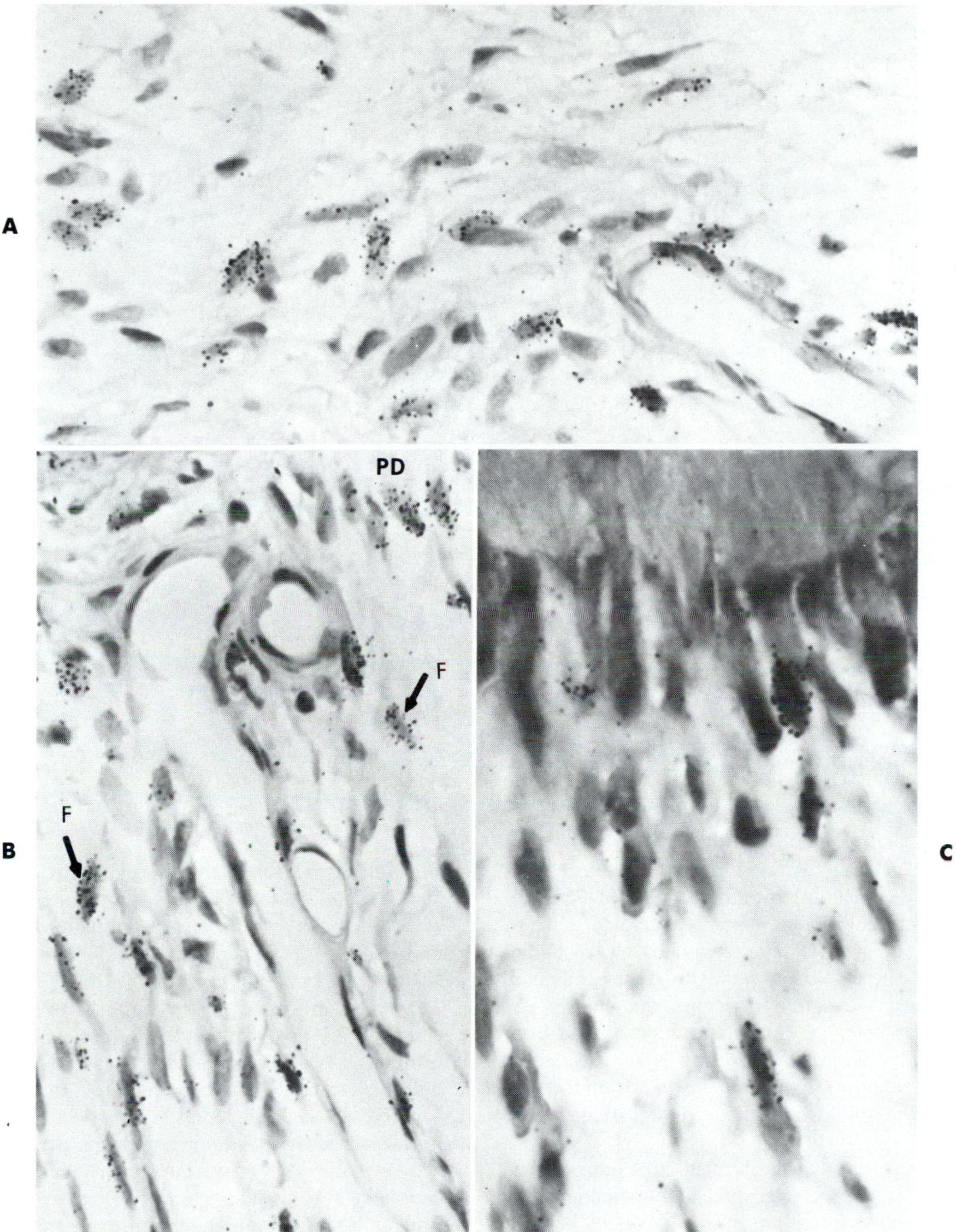

FIG. 11-45 Autoradiographs from dog molars illustrating uptake of ^{3}H-thymidine by pulp cells preparing to undergo cell division following pulpotomy and pulp capping with calcium hydroxide. **A,** Two days after pulp capping. Fibroblasts, endothelial cells, and pericytes beneath the exposure site are labeled. **B,** By the fourth day preodontoblasts adjacent to the predentin *(PD)* as well as fibroblasts *(F)* are labeled, which suggests that differentiation of preodontoblasts occurred within 2 days. **C,** Six days after pulp capping, new odontoblasts are labeled and tubular dentin is being formed. (Tritiated thymidine was injected 2 days after the pulp capping procedure in **B** and **C.**) (From Yamamura T, et al: Bull Tokyo Dent Coll 21:181, 1980.)

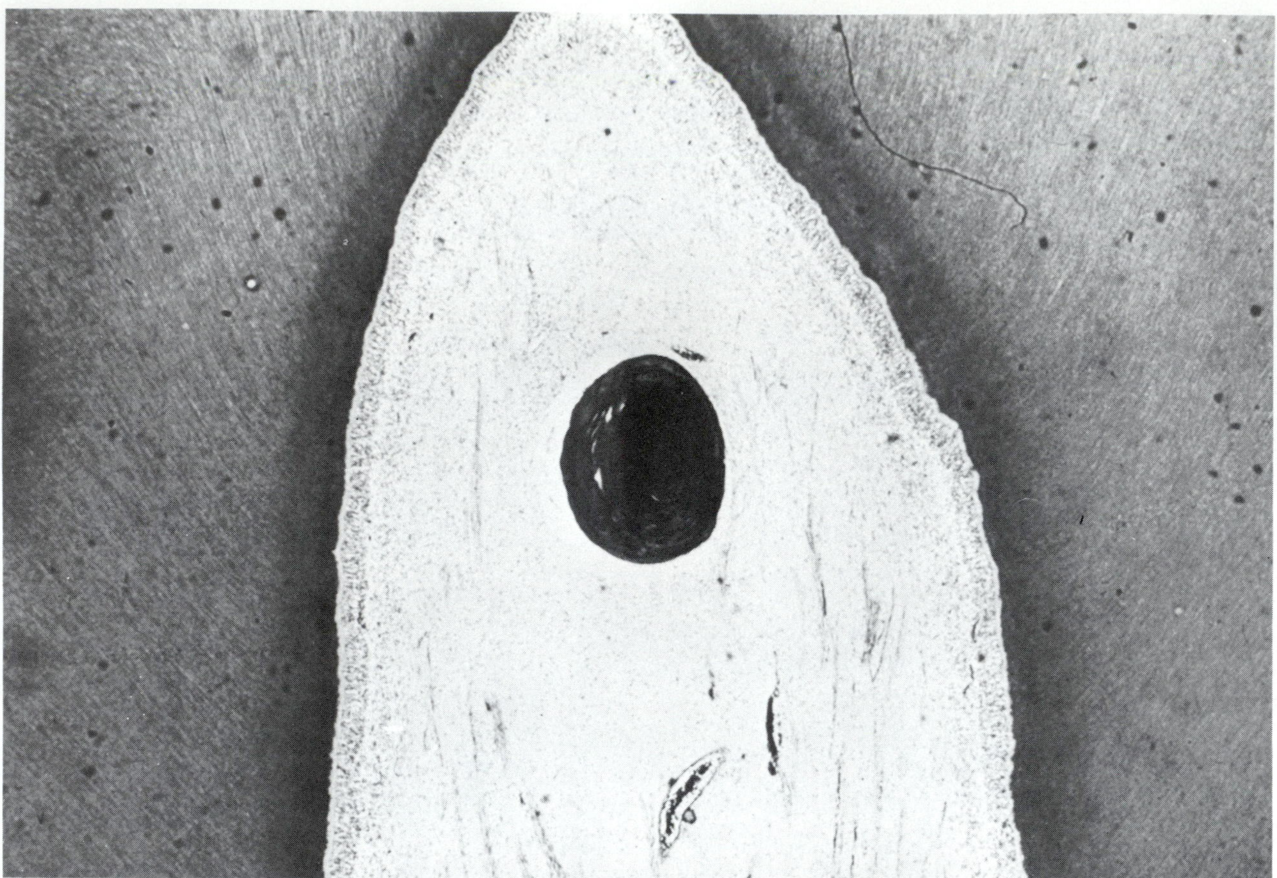

FIG. 11-46 Pulp stone with a smooth surface and concentric laminations in the pulp of a newly erupted premolar extracted in the course of orthodontic treatment.

differentiate into functioning odontoblasts.[47] Other investigators[188,189] have studied dentin bridge formation in the teeth of dogs and found that pulpal fibroblasts appeared to undergo dedifferentiation and revert to undifferentiated mesenchymal cells (Fig. 11-45). These cells divided and the new cells then redifferentiated in a new direction to become odontoblasts. Recalling the migratory potential of ectomesenchymal cells from which the pulpal fibroblasts are derived, it is not difficult to envision the differentiating odontoblasts moving from the subodontoblastic zone into the area of injury to constitute a new odontoblast layer.

Baume[11] has suggested that the formation of atubular "fibrodentine" results in the secondary induction of odontoblast differentiation, provided a capillary plexus develops beneath the fibrodentin. This is consistent with the observation made by other researchers[189] that the newly formed dentin bridge is composed first of a thin layer of atubular dentin upon which a relatively thick layer of tubular dentin is deposited. The fibrodentin* was lined by cells resembling mesenchymal cells, whereas the tubular dentin was associated with cells closely resembling odontoblasts.

Still other researchers[154] studied reparative dentin formed in response to relatively traumatic experimental class V cavity preparations in human teeth. They found that seldom was reparative dentin formed until about the 30th postoperative day, although in one case dentin formation was observed on day 19. The rate of formation was 3.5 μm per day for the first 3 weeks after the onset of dentin formation. Then it decreased markedly. By postoperative day 132, dentin formation had nearly ceased. Assuming that most of the odontoblasts were destroyed during cavity preparation, as was likely in this experiment, it is probable that the lag phase between cavity preparation and the onset of reparative dentin formation represented the time required for the proliferation and differentiation of new replacement odontoblasts.

Does reparative dentin protect the pulp or is it simply a form of scar tissue? To serve a protective function, it would have to provide a relatively impermeable barrier that would exclude irritants from the pulp and compensate for the loss of developmental dentin. The junction between developmental and reparative dentin has been studied.[148] This study found, in addition to a dramatic reduction in the number of tubules, that the walls of the tubules along the junction were thickened and often occluded with material similar to peritubular matrix. Furthermore, others[119] have reported that the junction is less permeable to dyes than is normal developmental dentin. These observations would indicate that the junctional zone between developmental and reparative dentin is an area of relatively low permeability.

One group studied the effect of gold foil placement on human pulps[164] and found that this was better tolerated in teeth in which reparative dentin had previously been deposited beneath the cavity than in teeth that were lacking such a deposit.

*Actually, the term *osteodentin* was used rather than fibrodentin.

It would thus appear that reparative dentin can protect the pulp, but it must be emphasized that this is not always the case. It is well known that reparative dentin can be deposited in a pulp that is irreversibly inflamed and that its presence does not necessarily signify a favorable prognosis (Fig. 11-44). The quality of the dentin formed, and hence its ability to protect the pulp, to a large extent reflects the environment of the cells producing the matrix.

Periodontally diseased teeth have smaller root canal diameters than do teeth that are periodontally healthy.[103] The root canals of such teeth are narrowed by the deposition of large quantities of reparative dentin along the dentinal walls.[149] The decrease in root canal diameter with increasing age, in the absence of periodontal disease, is more likely to be the result of secondary dentin formation.

In one study, it was shown in a rat model that scaling and root planning frequently result in reparative dentin formation along the pulpal wall opposite the instrumented root surface.[69]

Fibrosis

Not uncommonly the cellular elements of the pulp are largely replaced by fibrous connective tissue. It appears that in some cases the pulp responds to noxious stimuli by accumulating large fiber bundles of collagen rather than by elaborating reparative dentin. However, fibrosis and reparative dentin formation often go hand in hand, indicating that both are expressions of a reparative potential.

PULPAL CALCIFICATIONS

Calcification of pulp tissue is a very common occurrence. Although estimates of the incidence of this phenomenon vary widely, it as safe to say that one or more pulp calcifications are present in at least 50% of all teeth. In the coronal pulp calcification usually takes the form of discrete pulp stones (Fig. 11-46), whereas in the radicular pulp it tends to be diffuse (Fig. 11-47). Some authors believe that pulp calcification is a pathologic process related to various forms of injury,[63,147] whereas others regard it as a natural phenomenon.[74,82]

Pulp stones range in size from small, microscopic particles to accretions that occupy almost the entire pulp chamber (Fig. 11-48). Histologically, two types of stones are recognized: (1) those that are round or ovoid with smooth surfaces and concentric laminations (Fig. 11-46) and (2) those that assume no particular shape, lack laminations, and have rough surfaces (Fig. 11-49). Both types have an organic matrix composed principally of collagen fibrils in which hydroxyapatite crystals are embedded. The laminated stones appear to grow by the addition of collagen fibrils to their surface, whereas the unlaminated stones develop via the mineralization of preformed collagen fiber bundles. In the latter type the mineralization front seems to extend out along the coarse fibers, making the surface of the stones appear fuzzy (Fig. 11-50). Often these coarse fiber bundles appear to have undergone hyalinization, thus resembling old scar tissue.

Pulp stones that form around epithelial cells (remnants of Hertwig's epithelial root sheath) are termed denticles. Presumably the epithelial remnants induce adjacent mesenchymal cells to differentiate into odontoblasts. Characteristically these pulp stones are found near the root apex and contain dentinal tubules.

Quite frequently, small mineralizations are observed in association with the walls of arterioles, even in normal pulps of young teeth (Fig. 11-51). Such deposits usually project out-

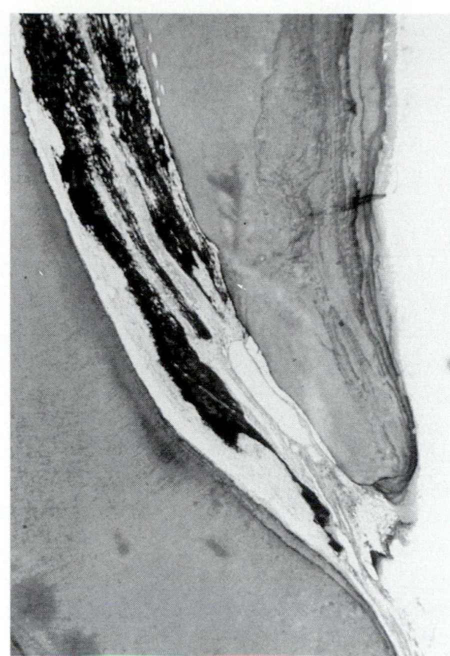

FIG. 11-47 Diffuse calcification near the apical foramen.

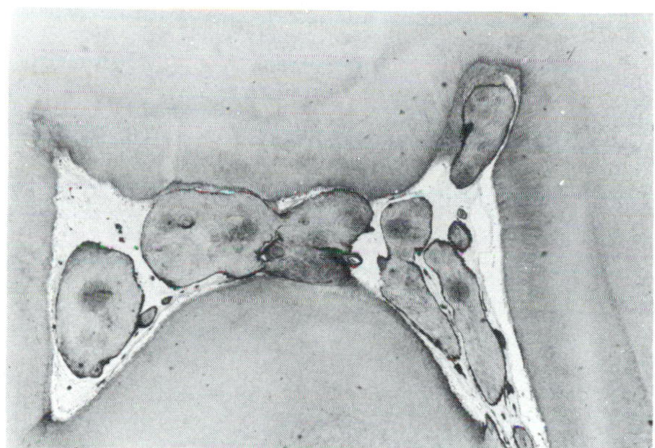

FIG. 11-48 Pulp stones occupying much of the pulp chamber.

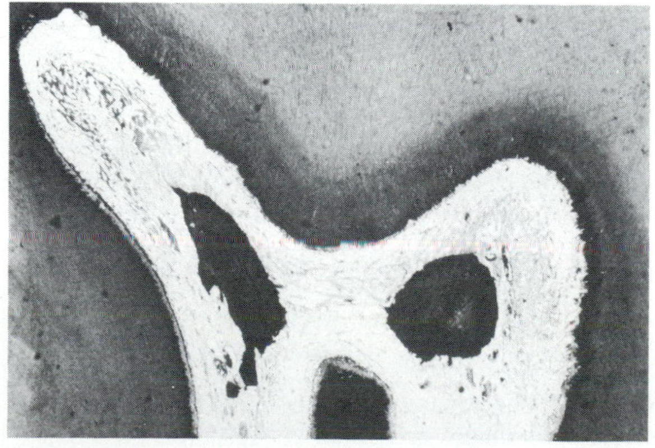

FIG. 11-49 Rough surface form of pulp stones. Note the hyalinized appearance of collagen fibers in the pulp.

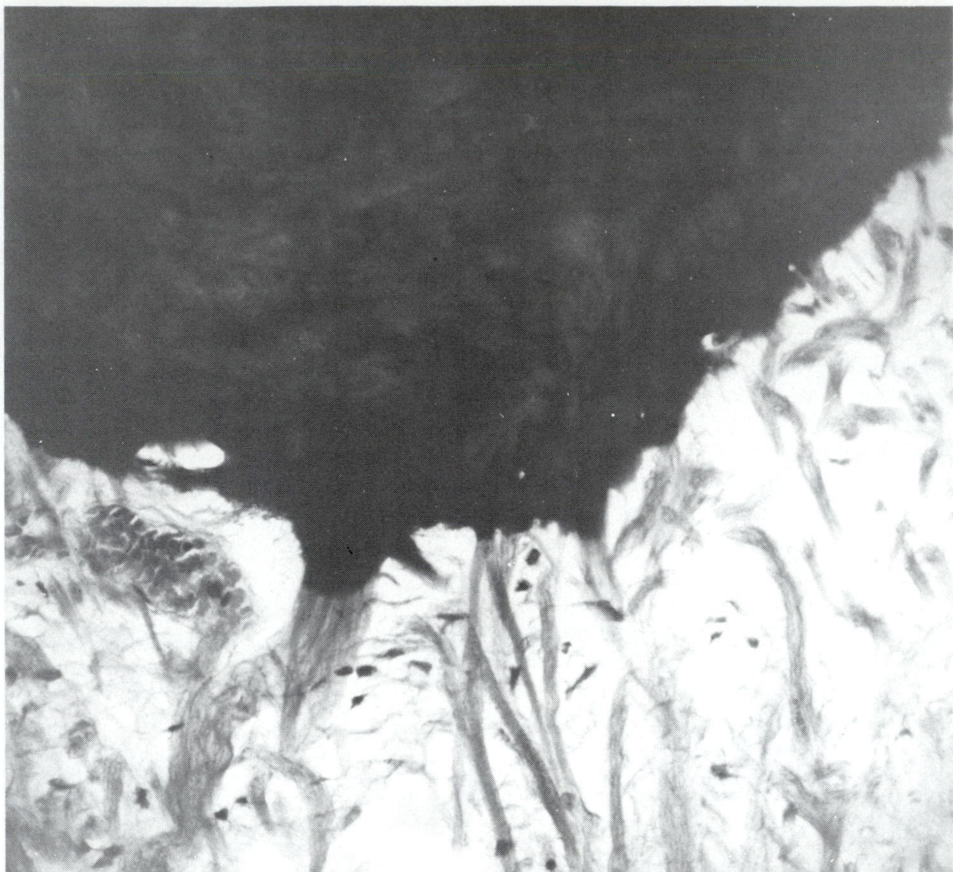

FIG. 11-50 High-power view of a pulp stone from Fig. 11-49 showing the relationship of mineralization fronts to collagen fibers.

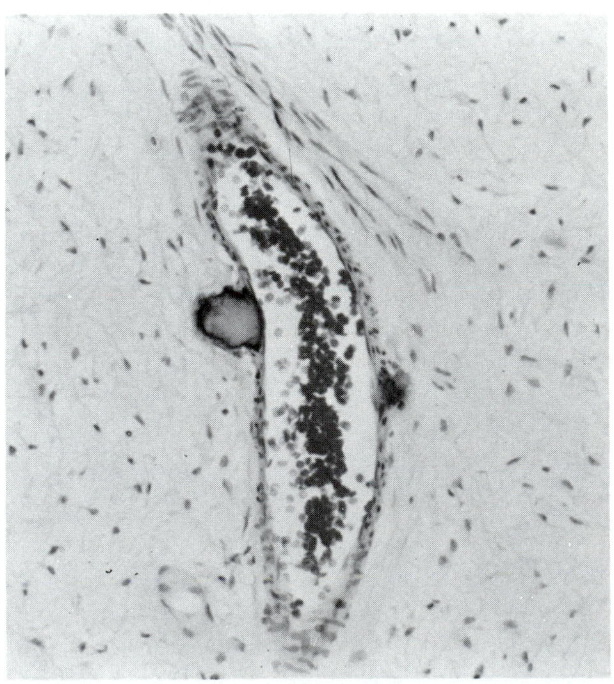

FIG. 11-51 Mineralized mass projecting from the wall of an arteriole in an otherwise normal young pulp.

ward from the vessel wall and do not encroach on the lumen.

The cause of pulpal calcification is largely unknown. Calcification may occur around a nidus of degenerating cells, blood thrombi, or collagen fibers. Many authors believe this represents a form of dystrophic calcification. In this type calcium is deposited in tissues where degenerative changes are occurring. When cells degenerate, calcium phosphate crystals may be deposited within the cell, initially within the mitochondria, because of the increased membrane permeability to calcium that results from a failure to maintain active transport systems within the cell membranes. Thus degenerating cells serving as a nidus may initiate calcification of a tissue. In the absence of obvious tissue degeneration the cause of pulpal calcification is enigmatic. It is often difficult to assign the term *dystrophic calcification* to pulp stones, since they so often occur in apparently healthy pulps. For example, pulpal calcifications have been reported in teeth that have not erupted,[102] suggesting that functional stress need not be present for calcification to occur. Calcification in the mature pulp is often assumed to be related to the aging process. However, in a study involving 52 impacted canines from patients between 11 and 76 years of age Nitzan and co-workers[131] found that concentric denticles demonstrated a constant incidence for all age groups, indicating no relation to aging. Diffuse calcifications, on the other hand, increased in incidence to age 25 years and thereafter remained constant in successive age groups.

Although soft tissue collagen does not usually calcify, it is not at all uncommon to find calcification occurring in old hy-

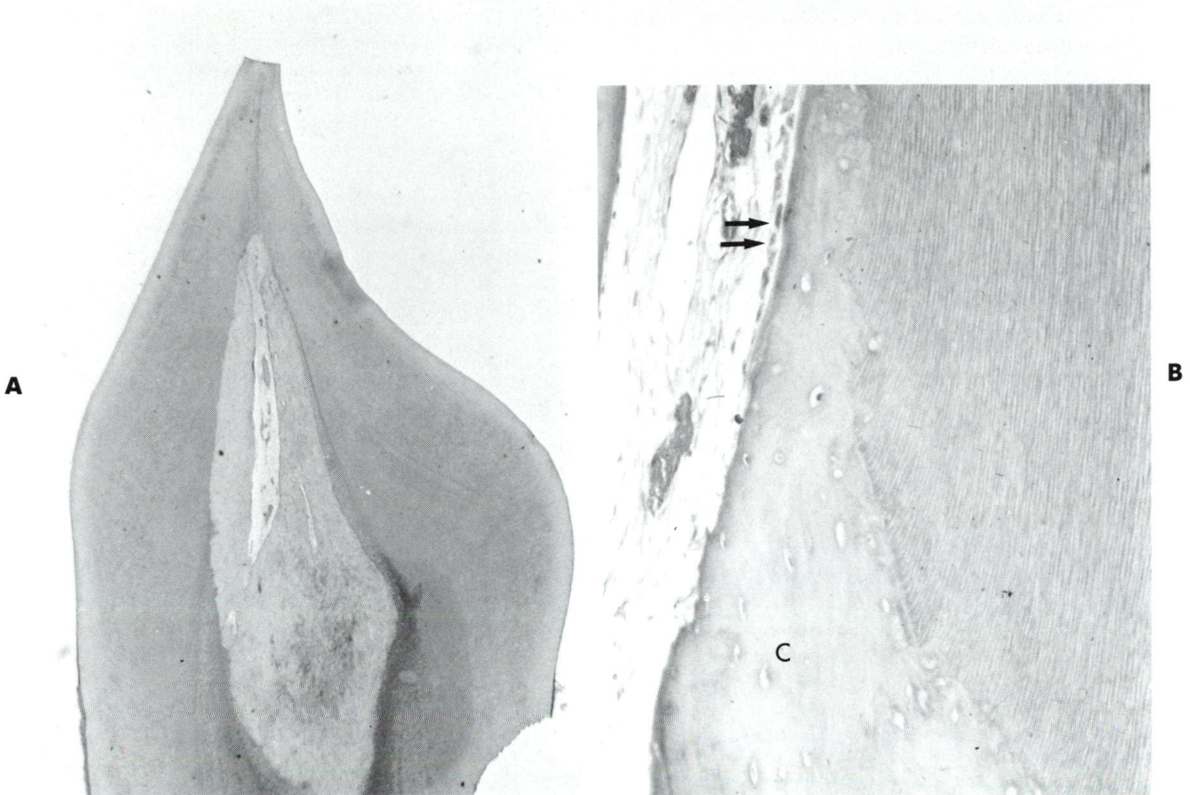

FIG. 11-52 A, Calcific metamorphosis of pulp tissue following luxation of tooth as a result of trauma. Note presence of soft tissue inclusion. **B,** High-power view showing cementoblasts *(arrows)* lining cementum *(C),* which has been deposited on the dentin walls.

alinized scar tissue in the skin. This may be due to the increase in the extent of cross linking between collagen molecules, since increased cross linkage is thought to enhance the tendency for collagen fibers to calcify. There may thus be a relationship between pathologic alterations in collagen molecules within the pulp and pulpal calcification.

Diffuse calcification is most often found in the perivascular adventitia and vascular walls within the radicular pulp. This form of pulpal calcification increases with age and seems to accompany the decrease in vascularity and innervation that are thought to represent age changes in the pulp.

Calcification replaces the cellular components of the pulp and may possibly embarrass the blood supply, although concrete evidence for this is lacking. Pain has frequently been attributed to the presence of pulp stones; but because calcification so often occurs in pathologically involved pulps, it is difficult to establish a cause-and-effect relationship, particularly since pulp stones are so frequently observed in teeth lacking a history of pain. (Perhaps their greatest endodontic significance is that they may hinder root canal instrumentation.) Investigators[16] have described the effect of calcification on aging pulp.

Calcific Metamorphosis

Luxation of teeth as a result of trauma may result in calcific metamorphosis, a condition that can in a matter of months or years lead to partial or complete radiographic obliteration of the pulp chamber. The cause of radiographic obliteration is excessive deposition of mineralized tissue resembling cementum or, occasionally, bone on the dentin walls (Fig. 11-52). Histologic examination invariably reveals the presence of some soft tissue, and cells resembling cementoblasts can be observed lining the mineralized tissue.

Clinically, the crowns of teeth affected by calcific metamorphosis may show a yellowish hue as compared with adjacent normal teeth. This condition usually occurs in teeth with incomplete root formation. Trauma results in disruption of blood vessels entering the tooth, thus producing pulpal infarction. The wide periapical foramen allows connective tissue from the periodontal ligament to proliferate and replace the infarcted tissue, bringing with it cementoprogenitor and osteoprogenitor cells capable of differentiating into either cementoblasts or osteoblasts, or both.

AGE CHANGES

Continued formation of secondary dentin throughout life gradually reduces the size of the pulp chamber and root canals.[122] In addition, certain regressive changes in the pulp appear to be related to the aging process. There is a gradual decrease in the cellularity as well as a concomitant increase in the number and thickness of collagen fibers, particularly in the radicular pulp.[17,122] The odontoblasts decrease in size and number and may disappear altogether in certain areas of the pulp, particularly on the pulpal floor over the bifurcation or trifurcation areas of multirooted teeth.

Decrease in size of the pulp is thought to be related to a reduction in the number of nerves and blood vessels.[15,16] Fibrosis appears to occur in relation to the pathways of degenerated vessels or nerves, and the thick collagen fibers may serve as foci for pulpal calcification.

There is also evidence that aging results in an increase in the resistance of pulp tissue to the action of proteolytic enzymes[190] as well as hyaluronidase and sialidase,[17] suggesting an alteration of both collagen and proteoglycans in the pulps of older teeth.

The main changes in dentin associated with aging are the increase in peritubular dentin, dentinal sclerosis, and the number of dead tracts.* Dentinal sclerosis produces a gradual decrease in dentinal permeability as the dentinal tubules become progressively reduced in diameter.

REFERENCES

1. Ahlberg K, Brännström M, and Edwall L: The diameter and number of dentinal tubules in rat, cat, dog and monkey. A comparative scanning electronic microscopic study, Acta Odontol Scand 33:243, 1975.
2. Anderson DJ, Curwen MP, and Howard LV: The sensitivity of human dentin, J Dent Res 37:669, 1958.
3. Anderson DJ, Matthews B, and Goretta C: Fluid flow through human dentine, Arch Oral Biol 12:209, 1967.
4. Andujar MB, et al: Differential expression of type I and type III collagen genes during tooth development, Development 111:691, 1991.
5. Anneroth G, and Nordenberg KA: Adrenergic vasoconstrictor innervation in the human dental pulp, Acta Odontol Scand 26:89, 1968.
6. Arwill T: Studies on the ultrastructure of dental tissues. II. The predentin-pulpal border zone, Odontol Rev 18:191, 1967.
7. Avery JK: Structural elements of the young normal human pulp, Oral Surg 32:113, 1971.
8. Avery JK: Dentin. In Bhaskar SN, ed: Orban's oral histology and embryology, ed 9, St. Louis, 1980, Times Mirror/Mosby College Publishing.
9. Avery JK: Repair potential of the pulp, J Endod 7:205, 1981.
10. Avery JK, Cox CF, and Chiego DJ Jr: Presence and location of adrenergic nerve endings in the dental pulps of mouse molars, Anat Rec 198:59, 1980.
11. Baume LJ: The biology of pulp and dentine. In Myers HM, ed: Monographs in oral science, vol 8, Basel, 1980, S Karger AG.
12. Bender IB, et al: The optimum placement-site of the electrode in electric pulp testing of the 12 anterior teeth, J Am Dent Assoc 118:305, 1989.
13. Bergenholtz G: Effect of bacterial products on inflammatory reactions in the dental pulp, Scand J Dent Res 85:122, 1977.
14. Berggren H: The reaction of the translucent zone of dentine to dyes and radioisotopes, Acta Odontol Scand 23:197, 1965.
15. Bernick S: Effect of aging on the nerve supply to human teeth, J Dent Res 46:694, 1967.
16. Bernick S, and Nedelman C: Effect of aging on the human pulp, J Endod 1:88, 1975.
17. Bhussry BR: Modification of the dental pulp organ during development and aging. In Finn SB, ed: Biology of the dental pulp organ: a symposium, Birmingham, 1968, University of Alabama Press.
18. Bishop MA, and Malhotra M: An investigation of lymphatic vessels in the feline dental pulp. Am J Anat 187:247, 1990.
19. Bishop MA, Malhotra M, and Yoshida S: Interodontoblastic collagen (von Korff fibers) and circumpulpal dentin formation: an ultrathin serial section study in the cat. Am J Anat 191:67, 1991.
20. Bonucci E: Matrix vesicles and their role in calcification. In Linde A, ed: Dentin and dentinogenesis, vol I, Boca Raton, Fla, 1984, CRC Press, pp 135-154.

*The term *dead tract* refers to a group of dentinal tubules in which odontoblast processes are absent. Dead tracts are easily recognized in ground sections as the empty tubules refract transmitted light and the tract appears black in contrast to the light color of normal dentin.

21. Brännström M: The transmission and control of dentinal pain. In Grossman LJ, ed: Mechanisms and control of pain, New York, 1979, Masson Publishing USA.
22. Brännström M: Dentin and pulp in restorative dentistry, Nacka, Sweden, 1981, Dental Therapeutics AB.
23. Brännström M: Communication between the oral cavity and the dental pulp associated with restorative treatment, Oper Dent 9:57, 1984.
24. Brännström M, and Åström A: A study of the mechanism of pain elicited from the dentin. J Dent Res 43:619, 1964.
25. Brännström M, and Garberoglio R: The dentinal tubules and the odontoblast processes, Acta Odontol Scand 30:291, 1972.
26. Brännström M, and Johnston G: Movements of the dentine and pulp liquids on application of thermal stimuli. An in vitro study, Acta Odontol Scand 28:59, 1970.
27. Brännström M, and Lind PO: Pulpal response to early dental caries, J Dent Res 44:1045, 1965.
28. Brännström M, Lindén L-A, and Åström A: The hydrodynamics of the dental tubule and of pulp fluid. A discussion of its significance in relation to dentinal sensitivity, Caries Res 1:310, 1967.
29. Butler WT, et al: Recent investigations on dentin specific proteins. Proc Finn Dent Soc 88 (Suppl 1):369, 1992.
30. Byers MR: Large and small trigeminal nerve endings and their association with odontoblasts in rat molar dentin and pulp. In Bonica JJ, Liebeskind JC, and Able-Fessard DG, eds: Advances in pain research and therapy, vol 3, New York, 1979, Raven Press.
31. Chirnside IM: Bacterial invasion of nonvital dentin, J Dent Res 40:134, 1961.
32. Corpron RE, and Avery JK: The ultrastructure of intradental nerves in developing mouse molars, Anat Rec 175:585, 1973.
33. Diamond RD, Stanley HR, and Swerdlow H: Reparative dentin formation resulting from cavity preparation, J Prosthet Dent 16:1127, 1966.
34. Edelman GM: Cell adhesion and the molecular processes of morphogenesis, Ann Rev Biochem 54:135, 1985.
35. Edwall L, and Kindlová M: The effect of sympathetic nerve stimulation on the rate of disappearance of tracers from various oral tissues, Acta Odontol Scand 29:387, 1971.
36. Edwall L, and Scott D Jr: Influence of changes in microcirculation on the excitability of the sensory unit in the tooth of the cat, Acta Physiol Scand 82:555, 1971.
37. England MC, Pellis EG, and Michanowicz AE: Histopathologic study of the effect of pulpal disease upon nerve fibers of the human dental pulp, Oral Surg 38:783, 1974.
38. Engström C, Linde A, and Persliden B: Acid hydrolases in the odontoblast-predentin region of dentiogenically active teeth, Scand J Dent Res 84:76, 1976.
39. Farnoush A: Mast cells in human dental pulp, J Endod 10:250, 1984.
40. Fearnhead RW: The neurohistology of human dentine, Proc Roy Soc Med 54:877, 1961.
41. Fearnhead RW: Innervation of dental tissues. In Miles AEW, ed: Structure and chemical organization of teeth, vol 1, New York, 1967, Academic Press, Inc.
42. Fish EW: Experimental investigation of the enamel, dentine, and dental pulp, London, 1932, John Bale Sons & Danielson, Ltd.
43. Fisher AK: Respiratory variations within the normal dental pulp, J Dent Res 46:424, 1967.
44. Fisher AK, et al: The influence of the stage of tooth development on the oxygen quotient of normal bovine dental pulp, J Dent Res 38:208, 1959.
45. Fisher AK, et al: Effects of dental drugs and materials on the rate of oxygen consumption in bovine dental pulp, J Dent Res 36:447, 1957.
46. Fisher AK, and Walters VE: Anaerobic glycolysis in bovine dental pulp, J Dent Res 47:717, 1968.
47. Fitzgerald M, Chiego DJ, and Heys DR: Autoradiographic analysis of odontoblast replacement following pulp exposure in primate teeth, Arch Oral Biol 35:707, 1990.
48. Fogel HM, Marshall FJ, and Pashley DH: Effects of distance of the pulp and thickness on the hydraulic conductance of human radicular dentin, J Dent Res 67:1381, 1988.

49. Frank RM: Etude au microscope électronique de l'odontoblaste et du canalicule dentinaire humain, Arch Oral Biol 11:179, 1966.
50. Frank RM: Ultrastructure of human dentine. In Fleisch H, Blackwood HJJ, and Owen M, eds: Third European symposium on calcified tissues, New York, 1966, Springer-Verlag New York, Inc.
51. Frank RM: Ultrastructural relationship between the odontoblast, its process and the nerve fibre. In Symons NBB, ed: Dentine and pulp, Dundee, 1968, University of Dundee.
52. Frank RM: Etude autoradiographique de la dentinogenèse en microscopie électronique à l'aide de la proline tritiée chez le chat, Arch Oral Biol 15:583, 1970.
53. Fulling H-J, and Andreasen JO: Influence of maturation status and tooth type of permanent teeth upon electrometric and thermal pulp testing, Scand J Dent Res 84:286, 1976.
54. Fuss Z, et al: Assessment of reliability of electrical and thermal pulp testing agents, J Endod 12:301, 1986.
55. Garant PR, and Cho M-I: Ultrastructure of the odontoblast. In Butler WT, ed: The chemistry and biology of mineralized tissues, Birmingham, Ala, 1985, Ebsco Media.
56. Garberoglio R, and Brännström M: Scanning electron microscopical investigation of human dentinal tubules, Arch Oral Biol 21:355, 1976.
57. Gaunt WA: The vascular supply to the dental lamina during early development, Acta Anat 37:232, 1959.
58. Gotjamanos T: Cellular organization in the subodontoblastic zone of the dental pulp. II. Period and mode of development of the cell-rich layer in rat molar pulps, Arch Oral Biol 14:1011, 1969.
59. Gotjamanos T: Mitotic activity in the subodontoblastic cell-rich layer of adult rat molar pulps, Arch Oral Biol 15:905, 1970.
60. Grossman ES, and Austin JC: Scanning electron microscope observations on the tubule content of freeze-fractured peripheral vervet monkey dentine (Ceropithecus pygerythrus), Arch Oral Biol 28:279, 1983.
61. Gunji T: Morphological research on the sensitivity of dentin, Arch Histol Jpn 45:45, 1982.
62. Hahn C-L, Falkler WA Jr, and Siegel MA: A study of T cells and B cells in pulpal pathosis, J Endod 15:20, 1989.
63. Hall DC: Pulpal calcifications—a pathological process? In Symons NBB, ed: Dentine and pulp, Dundee, 1968, University of Dundee.
64. Hamersky PA, Weimer AD, and Taintor JF: The effect of orthodontic force application on the pulpal tissue respiration rate in the human premolar, Am J Orthod 77:368, 1980.
65. Han SS: The fine structure of cells and intercellular substances of the dental pulp. In Finn SB, ed: Biology of the dental pulp organ, Birmingham, 1968, University of Alabama Press.
66. Han SS, and Avery JK: The ultrastructure of capillaries and arterioles of the hamster dental pulp, Anat Rec 145:549, 1963.
67. Harris R: Histogenesis of fibroblasts in the human dental pulp, Arch Oral Biol 12:459, 1967.
68. Harris R, and Griffin CJ: Fine structure of nerve endings in the human dental pulp, Arch Oral Biol 13:773, 1968.
69. Hattler AB, and Listgarten MA: Pulpal response to root planning in a rat model, J Endod 10:471, 1984.
70. Hay ED, and Meier S: Tissue interaction in development. In Shaw JH, et al, eds: Textbook of oral biology, Philadelphia, 1978, WB Saunders Co.
71. Heyeraas KJ: Pulpal, microvascular, and tissue pressure, J Dent Res 64 (special issue):585, 1985.
72. Heyeraas KJ: Interstitial fluid pressure and transmicrovascular fluid flow. In Inoki R, Kudo T, and Olgart LM, eds: Dynamic aspects of dental pulp, London, 1990, Chapman and Hall, pp 189-198.
73. Heyerass KJ, and Kvinnsland I: Tissue pressure and blood flow in pulpal inflammation. Proc Finn Dent Soc 88 (suppl 1):393, 1992.
74. Hill TJ: Pathology of the dental pulp, J Am Dent Assoc 21:820, 1934.
75. Hirvonen T, and Närhi M: The excitability of dog pulp nerves in relation to the condition of dentine surface, J Endod 10:294, 1984.
76. Holland GR: Membrane junctions on cat odontoblasts, Arch Oral Biol 20:551, 1975.
77. Holland GR: The extent of the odontoblast process in the cat, J Anat 121:133, 1976.
78. Holland GR: Lanthanum hydroxide labelling of gap junctions in the odontoblast layer, Anat Rec 186:121, 1976.
79. Holland GR: The incidence of dentinal tubules containing more than one process in the cuspal dentin of cat canine teeth, Anat Rec 200:437, 1981.
80. Holland GR: The odontoblast process: form and function, J Dent Res 64 (special issue):499, 1985.
81. Inoue H, Kurosaka Y, and Abe K: Autonomic nerve endings in the odontoblast/predentin border and predentin of the canine teeth of dogs, J Endod 18:149, 1992.
82. James VE, Schour I, and Spence JM: Biology of the pulp and its defense, J Am Dent Assoc 59:903, 1959.
83. Johansen E: Ultrastructure of dentine. In Miles AEW, ed: Structural and chemical organization of the teeth, vol 2, New York, 1967, Academic Press, Inc.
84. Johnsen DC, Harshbarger J, and Rymer HD: Quantitative assessment of neural development in human premolars, Anat Rec 205:421, 1983.
85. Johnsen D, and Johns S: Quantitation of nerve fibers in the primary and permanent canine and incisor teeth in man, Arch Oral Biol 23:825, 1978.
86. Johnson G, and Brännström M: The sensitivity of dentin. Changes in relation to conditions at exposed tubule apertures, Acta Odontol Scand 32:29, 1974.
87. Jones PA, Taintor JF, and Adams AB: Comparative dental material cytotoxicity measured by depression of rat incisor pulp respiration, J Endod 5:48, 1979.
88. Jones SJ, Boyde A: Ultrastructure of dentin and dentinogenesis. In Linde A, ed: Dentin and dentinogenesis, vol I, Boca Raton, Fla, 1984, CRC Press, pp 81-134.
89. Jontell M, and Bergenholtz G: Accessory cells in the immune defense of the dental pulp. Proc Finn Dent Soc 88(suppl 1):345, 1992.
90. Katchburian E, and Holt SJ: Ultrastructural studies on lysosomes and acid phosphatase in odontoblasts. In Symons NBB, ed: Dentine and pulp, Dundee, 1968, University of Dundee.
91. Kaye H, and Herold RC: Structure of human dentine. I. Phase contrast, polarization, interference, and bright field microscopic observations on the lateral branch system, Arch Oral Biol 11:355, 1966.
92. Kelley KW, Bergenholtz G, and Cox CF: The extent of the odontoblast process in rhesus monkeys *(Macaca mulatta)* as observed by scanning electron microscopy, Arch Oral Biol 26:893, 1981.
93. Kim S: Regulation of blood flow of the dental pulp: macrocirculation and microcirculation studies, doctoral thesis, New York, 1981, Columbia University.
94. Kim S, et al: Effects of local anesthetics on pulpal blood flow in dogs, J Dent Res 63:650, 1984.
95. Kim S: Neurovascular interactions in the dental pulp in health and inflammation. J Endod 14:48, 1990.
96. Kim S, et al: Effects of selected inflammatory mediators on blood flow and vascular permeability in the dental pulp, Proc Finn Dent Soc 88 (suppl 1):387, 1992.
97. Kim S, Schuessler G, and Chien S: Measurement of blood flow in the dental pulp of dogs with the ^{133}xenon washout method, Arch Oral Biol 28:501, 1983.
98. Kim S, et al: Effects of bradykinin on pulpal blood flow in dogs, J Dent Res 61:293, 1982.
99. Köling A: Structural relationships in the human odontoblast layer, as demonstrated by freeze-fracture electron microscopy, J Endod 14:239, 1988.
100. Kramer IRH: The distribution of blood vessels in the human dental pulp. In Finn SB, ed: Biology of the dental pulp organ, Birmingham, 1968, University of Alabama Press.
101. Kroeger DC, Gonzales F, and Krivoy W: Transmembrane potentials of cultured mouse dental pulp cells. Proc Soc Exptl Med 108:134, 1961.
102. Langeland K, and Langeland LK: Histologic study of 155 impacted teeth, Odontol Tidskr 73:527, 1965.

103. Lantelme RL, Handleman SL, and Herbison RJ: Dentin formation in periodontally diseased teeth, J Dent Res 55:48, 1976.
104. Lechner JH, and Kalnitsky G: The presence of large amounts of type III collagen in bovine dental pulp and its significance with regard to the mechanism of dentinogenesis, Arch Oral Biol 26:625, 1981.
105. Lefèvre R, Frank RM, and Voegel JC: The study of human dentine with secondary ion microscopy and electron diffraction, Calcif Tiss Res 19:251, 1976.
106. Lesot H, Osman M, and Ruch JV: Immunofluorescent localization of collagens, fibronectin and laminin during terminal differentiation of odontoblasts, Dev Biol 82:371, 1981.
107. Lilja J: Innervation of different parts of the predentin and dentin in young human premolars, Acta Odontol Scand 37:339, 1979.
108. Lilja J, Noredenvall K-J, and Brännström M: Dentin sensitivity, odontoblasts and nerves under desiccated or infected experimental cavities, Swed Dent J 6:93, 1982.
109. Linde A: The extracellular matrix of the dental pulp and dentin, J Dent Res 64 (special issue):523, 1985.
110. Lindén LA, and Brännström M: Fluid movements in dentine and pulp, Odontol Rev 18:227, 1967.
111. Luthman J, Luthman D and Hökfelt T: Occurrence and distribution of different neurochemical markers in the human dental pulp. Arch Oral Biol 37:193-208, 1992.
112. Madison S, et al: Effect of leukotriene B4 on intradental nerves, J Dent Res 68(special issue)243:494, 1989.
113. Magloire H, et al: Distribution of type III collagen in the pulp parenchyma of the human developing tooth. Light and electron microscope immunotyping, Histochemistry 74:319, 1982.
114. Mangkornkarn C, and Steiner JC: In vivo and in vitro glycosaminoglycans from human dental pulp, J Endod 18:327, 1992.
115. Marchetti C, and Piacentini C: Examin au microscope photonique et au microscope électronique des capillaires lymphatiques de la pulpe dentaire humaine, Bulletin du Groupement International Pour la Récherche Scientifique en Stomatologie et Odontologie 33:19, 1990.
116. Meyer MW, and Path MG: Blood flow in the dental pulp of dogs determined by hydrogen polarography and radioactive microsphere methods, Arch Oral Biol 24:601, 1979.
117. Michelich V, Pashley DH, and Whitford GM: Dentin permeability: a comparison of functional versus anatomical tubular radii, J Dent Res 57:1019, 1978.
118. Michelich VJ, Schuster GS, and Pashley DH: Bacterial penetration of human dentin in vivo, J Dent Res 59:1398, 1980.
119. Miller WA, and Massler M: Permeability and staining of active and arrested lesions in dentine, Br Dent J 112:187, 1962.
120. Mjör IA: Dentin-predentin complex and its permeability: pathology and treatment overview, J Dent Res 64(special issue):621, 1985.
121. Mjör IA, and Pindborg JJ: Histology of the human tooth, Copenhagen, 1973, Einar Munksgaard.
122. Morse DR: Age-related changes of the dental pulp complex and their relationship to systemic aging, Oral Surg 72:721, 1991.
123. Mullaney TP, Howell RM, and Petrich JD: Resistance of nerve fibers to pulpal necrosis, Oral Surg 30:690, 1970.
124. Nähri M: Activation of dental pulp nerves of the cat and the dog with hydrostatic pressure, Proc Finn Dent Soc 74(suppl 5):1, 1978.
125. Närhi MVO, Hirvonen TJ, and Hakumäki MOK: Activation of intradental nerves in the dog to some stimuli applied to the dentine, Arch Oral Biol 27:1053, 1982.
126. Närhi M, et al: Role of intradental A- and C-type nerve fibers in dental pain mechanisms. Proc Finn Dent Soc 88 (suppl 1):507, 1992.
127. Närhi M, et al: Activation of heat-sensitive nerve fibers in the dental pulp of the cat, Pain 14:317, 1982.
128. Närhi M, et al: Functional differences in intradental A- and C-nerve units in the cat, Pain Suppl 2:S242 (abstract), 1984.
129. Närhi M, et al: Electrical stimulation of teeth with a pulp tester in the cat, Scand J Dent Res 87:32, 1979.
130. Ngassapa D, Närhi M, and Hirvonen T: The effect of serotonin (5-HT) and calcitonin gene-related peptide (CGRP) on the function of intradental nerves in the dog, Proc Finn Dent Soc 88 (suppl 1):143, 1992.
131. Nitzan DW, et al: The effect of aging on tooth morphology: a study on impacted teeth, Oral Surg 61:54, 1986.
132. Okiji T, et al: An immunohistochemical study of the distribution of immunocompetent cells, especially macrophages and Ia antigen-presenting cells of heterogeneous populations, in normal rat molar pulp. J Dent Res 71:1196, 1992.
133. Olgart L: Influence of pharmacologic agents on blood flow and sensory nerves in the pulp. In Grossman LI, ed: The mechanism and control of pain, New York, 1979, Masson Publishing USA, Inc.
134. Olgart L: Pain research using feline teeth, J Endod 12:458, 1986.
135. Olgart L, Brännström M, and Johnson G: Invasion of bacteria into dentinal tubules. Experiments in vivo and in vitro, Acta Odontol Scand 32:61, 1974.
136. Olgart L, et al: Release of substance P-like immunoreactivity from the dental pulp, Acta Physiol Scand 101:510, 1977.
137. Pashley DH: Dentin conditions and disease. In Lazzari G, ed: CRC handbook of experimental dentistry, Boca Raton, Fla, 1893, CRC Press.
138. Pashley DH: Dentin permeability: theory and practice. In Spangberg L, ed: Experimental endodontics, Boca Raton, Fla, 1989, CRC Press.
139. Path MG, and Meyer MW: Heterogeneity of blood flow in the canine tooth of the dog, Arch Oral Biol 25:83, 1980.
140. Provenza DV: Oral histology. Inheritance and development, Philadelphia, 1964, JB Lippincott Co.
141. Rapp R, et al: Ultrastructure of fenestrated capillaries in human dental pulps, Arch Oral Biol 22:317, 1977.
142. Reader A, and Foreman DW: An ultrastructural qualitative investigation of human intradental innervation, J Endod 7:161, 1981.
143. Reeves R, and Stanley HR: The relationship of bacterial penetration and pulpal pathosis in carious teeth, Oral Surg 22:59, 1966.
144. Ruch JV: Odontoblast differentiation and the formation of the odontoblast layer, J Dent Res 64(spec iss):489, 1985.
145. Ruch JV: Epithelial-mesenchymal interactions in formation of mineralized tissues. In Butler WT, ed: The chemistry and biology of mineralized tissues, Birmingham, Ala, 1985, Ebsco Media.
146. Sasaki S: Studies on the respiration of the dog tooth germ, J Biochem 46:269, 1959.
147. Sayegh FS, and Reed AJ: Calcification in the dental pulp, Oral Surg 25:873, 1968.
148. Scott JN, and Weber DF: Microscopy of the junctional region between human coronal primary and secondary dentin, J Morphol 154:133, 1977.
149. Seltzer S, Bender IB, and Ziontz M: The interrelationship of pulp and periodontal disease, Oral Surg 16:1474, 1963.
150. Sigal MJ, et al: The odontoblast process extends to the dentinoenamel junction: an immunocytochemical study of rat dentine, J Histochem Cytochem 32:872, 1984.
151. Sigal MJ, et al: A combined scanning electron microscopy and immunofluorescence study demonstrating that the odontoblast process extends to the dentinoenamel junction in human teeth, Anat Rec 210:453, 1984.
152. Slavkin HC: Molecular biology of dental development: a review. In Davidovitch Z, ed: The biological mechanisms of tooth eruption and root resorption, Birmingham, Ala, 1988, Ebsco Media.
153. Stanley HR, et al: The detection and prevalence of reactive and physiologic sclerotic dentin, reparative dentin and dead tracts beneath various types of dental lesions according to tooth surface and age, J Oral Pathol 12:257, 1983.
154. Stanley HR, White CL, and McCray L: The rate of tertiary (reparative) dentin formation in the human tooth, Oral Surg 21:180, 1966.
155. Stenvik A, Iverson J, and Mjör IA: Tissue pressure and histology of normal and inflamed tooth pulps in Macaque monkeys, Arch Oral Biol 17:1501, 1972.
156. Symons NBB: The microanatomy and histochemistry of dentinogenesis. In Miles AEW, ed: Structural and chemical organization of the teeth, vol 1, New York, 1967, Academic Press, Inc.

157. Takahashi K, Kishi Y, and Kim S: A scanning electron microscope study of the blood vessels of dog pulp using corrosion resin casts, J Endod 8:131, 1982.
158. Takuma S, and Nagai N: Ultrastructure of rat odontoblasts in various stages of their development and maturation, Arch Oral Biol 16:993, 1971.
159. Takuma S, et al: Electron microscopy of carious lesions in human dentin, Bull Tokyo Dent Coll 8:143, 1967.
160. Thesleff I, and Vaahtokari A: The role of growth factors in determination and differentiation of the odontoblast cell lineage. Proc Finn Dent Soc 88 (suppl 1):357, 1992.
161. Thomas HF: The extent of the odontoblast process in human dentin, J Dent Res 58(D):2207, 1979.
162. Thomas HF: The lamina limitans of human dentinal tubules, J Dent Res 63:1064, 1984.
163. Thomas HF, and Payne RC: The ultrastructure of dentinal tubules from erupted human premolar teeth, J Dent Res 62:532, 1983.
164. Thomas JJ, Stanley HR, and Gilmore HW: Effects of gold foil condensation on human dental pulp, J Am Dent Assoc 78:788, 1969.
165. Tomes J: On the presence of the fibrils of soft tissue in the dentinal tubules, Philos Trans 146:515, 1856.
166. Tönder KJH: Effect of vasodilating drugs on external carotid and pulpal blood flow in dogs: "stealing" of dental perfusion pressure, Acta Physiol Scand 97:75, 1976.
167. Tönder KJH, and Naess G: Nervous control of blood flow in the dental pulp in dogs, Acta Physiol Scand 104:13, 1978.
168. Topham RT, et al: Effects of epidermal growth factor on tooth differentiation and eruption. In Davidovitch Z, ed: The biological mechanisms of tooth eruption and root resorption, Birmingham, Ala, 1988, Ebsco Media.
169. Torebjörk HE, and Hanin RG: Perceptual changes accompanying controlled preferential blocking of A and C fiber responses in intact human skin nerves, Exp Brain Res 16:321, 1973.
170. Torneck CD: Dentin-pulp complex. In Ten Cate AR: Oral histology: development, structure, and function, ed 2, St. Louis, 1985, Times Mirror/Mosby College Publishing.
171. Trowbridge HO: Pathogenesis of pulpitis resulting from dental caries, J Endod 7:52, 1981.
172. Trowbridge HO: Intradental sensory units: physiological and clinical aspects, J Endod 11:489, 1985.
173. Trowbridge HO: Mechanisms of pain induction in hypersensitive teeth. In Rowe NH, ed: Hypersensitive dentin: origin and management, Ann Arbor, 1985, University of Michigan.
174. Trowbridge HO: Immunological aspects of chronic inflammation, J Endod 16:54, 1990.
175. Trowbridge HO: Review of current approaches to in-office management of tooth hypersensitivity, Dent Clin North Am 34:561, 1990.
176. Trowbridge HO, et al: Sensory response to thermal stimulation in human teeth, J Endod 6:405, 1980.
177. Trowbridge HO, and Shibata F: Mitotic activity in epithelial rests of Malassez, Periodontics 5:109, 1967.
178. Turner DF: Immediate physiological response of odontoblasts. Proc Finn Dent Soc 88 (suppl 1):55, 1992.
179. Van Hassel HJ: Physiology of the human dental pulp, Oral Surg 32:126, 1971.
180. Veis A, Tsay TG, and Kanwar Y: The preparation of antibodies to dentin phosphophoryns. In Ruch JV, and Belcourt AB, eds: Tooth morphogenesis and differentiation, vol 125, Paris, 1984, Inserm Symposia Series.
181. Vongsavan N, and Matthews B: The vascularity of dental pulp in cats, J Dent Res 71:1913, 1992.
182. Wakisaka S: Neuropeptides in the dental pulp: their distribution, origins and correlation, J Endod 16:67, 1990.
183. Weber DF: Human dentine sclerosis: a microradiographic study, Arch Oral Biol 19:163, 1974.
184. Weinstock A, Weinstock M, and Leblond CP: Autoradiographic detection of 3H-fucose incorporation into glycoprotein by odotonblasts and its deposition at the site of the calcification front in dentin, Calif Tiss Res 8:181, 1972.
185. Weinstock M, and Leblond CP: Synthesis, migration and release of precursor collagen by odontoblasts as visualized by radioautography after 3H-proline administration, J Cell Biol 60:92, 1974.
186. Winter HF, Bishop JG, and Dorman HL: Transmembrane potentials of odontoblasts, J Dent Res 42:594, 1963.
187. Yamada T, et al: The extent of the odontoblast process in normal and carious human dentin, J Dent Res 62:798, 1983.
188. Yamamura T: Differentiation of pulpal cells and inductive influences of various matrices with reference to pulpal wound healing, J Dent Res 64(special issue):530, 1985.
189. Yamamura T, et al: Differentiation and induction of undifferentiated mesenchymal cells in tooth and periodontal tissue during wound healing and regeneration, Bull Tokyo Dent Coll 21:181, 1980.
190. Zerlotti E: Histochemical study of the connective tissue of the dental pulp, Arch Oral Biol 9:149, 1964.

Self-assessment questions

1. Blood vessels become established in the dental papilla
   a. before the formation of the cervical loop.
   b. during the bud stage of tooth formation.
   c. during the bell stage of tooth formation.
   d. during the cap stage of tooth formation.
2. Root development begins
   a. before enamel formation.
   b. concurrently with enamel formation.
   c. after completion of enamel formation.
   d. before Hertwig's epithelial root sheath formation.
3. The cell-rich zone
   a. is more prominent in the radicular pulp than in the coronal pulp.
   b. exhibits increased mitotic activity following death of odontoblasts.
   c. is the result of the central migration of cells from the periphery following completion of dentin formation.
   d. contains mainly macrophages and endothelial cells and few fibroblasts.
4. Although similar in function, the odontoblast differs from the osteoblast and cementoblast in
   a. morphologic characteristics.
   b. ultrastructure.
   c. matrix production.
   d. being a protein-secreting cell.
5. The extent to which the odontoblast process extends outward in dentin
   a. has been shown conclusively in recent years.
   b. varies with the age of the tooth.
   c. depends on continued mitotic activity of the odontoblast.
   d. is unrelated to the effects on the pulp of restorative procedures.
6. Fibroblasts
   a. are the least numerous cells of the pulp.
   b. are capable of giving rise to cells that may differentiate into macrophages.
   c. increase in numbers as blood vessels and nerves decrease with age.
   d. undergo active differentiation in the pulp, as do fibroblasts of other connective tissues.

7. The pathways of pulpal inflammation and infection are strongly influenced by
   a. the two structural proteins in the pulp: collagen and elastin.
   b. dental materials that depress pulpal metabolic activity.
   c. the state of polymerization of the ground substance components in the pulp.
   d. osmotic pressures as regulated by proteoglycans.
8. Water content of the pulp is approximately
   a. 30%.
   b. 50%.
   c. 70%.
   d. 90%.
9. Regardless of the nature of the sensory stimulus, all afferent impulses from the pulp result in the sensation of
   a. proprioception.
   b. pain.
   c. heat.
   d. touch.
10. The nerve fibers of the pulp are
    a. mainly myelinated fibers at the time of tooth eruption.
    b. easily damaged by inflammation.
    c. only sensory.
    d. unevenly distributed throughout the pulp.
11. Fluid movement in dentinal tubules is known as the
    a. hydrodynamic theory.
    b. osmotic pressure.
    c. mechanical deformation theory.
    d. hydraulic theory.
12. Painful pulpitis associated with an inflamed or degenerating pulp
    a. is caused by a decrease in intrapulpal pressure.
    b. results from a reduction of nerve cell permeability.
    c. is associated with stimulation of A fibers.
    d. is most likely due to nociceptive C-fiber activity.
13. Volume of blood flow in the pulp
    a. is least in the regions of the pulp horns.
    b. is greater in the root portion than in the crown portion.
    c. is greater than the blood flow in most visceral organs.
    d. is largely under the control of the adrenergic sympathetic system.
14. A healthy dental pulp responds to an injury by
    a. developing an effective collateral circulation to transport inflammatory elements to the area.
    b. decreasing in blood flow throughout the pulp.
    c. initiating an inflammatory response, usually followed by partial or complete necrosis.
    d. forming reparative dentin at the pulpal surface corresponding to areas of irritation.
15. Pulpal calcifications
    a. may compromise the pulpal blood supply.
    b. are of no significance in root canal therapy.
    c. have an organic matrix of collagen in all sizes.
    d. occur only after eruption.
16. Calcific metamorphosis
    a. is caused by increased activity of odontoblasts.
    b. may lead to complete obliteration of the pulp space.
    c. usually occurs in association with a constricted apical foramen.
    d. histologically resembles acellular cementum.
17. Growth factors are likely to be involved in tooth formation. What is at least one probable function of these factors?
    a. Signaling epithelial-mesenchymal interactions.
    b. One of the eruptive forces located in the apical region.
    c. Disruption of Hertwig's epithelial root sheath.
    d. Collagen maturation in the dental papilla.
18. The cell type to which the dendritic cell is most similar is:
    a. fibroblast.
    b. t-lymphocyte.
    c. mesenchymal cell.
    d. macrophage.
19. Lymphatics in the dental pulp
    a. have not been demonstrated.
    b. would not be necessary because of the extensive vascular network.
    c. cannot be demonstrated morphologically because they are identical to venules.
    d. participate in the removal of tissue fluids.
20. What would be the closest estimate of the number of tubules exposed with a full crown preparation of average depth that would have a surface area of 100 mm^2?
    a. 5000
    b. 50,000
    c. 500,000
    d. 5,000,000
21. When the pulp is injured it responds with inflammation. Why does it not have good capability for recovery if badly damaged?
    1. It has no collateral blood supply.
    2. It lacks lymph drainage.
    3. Pulp C.T. cells are incapable of mitosis.
    4. It is encased in a noncompliant environment.
       a. 1 & 2
       b. 1 & 3
       c. 1 & 4
       d. 2 & 3

Chapter 12

Periapical Pathology

James H. S. Simon

The inflammatory response associated with periapical pathology has been traditionally taught similar to an inflammatory response anywhere in the body. For example, when a splinter (irritant or antigen) is stuck into the skin, there is an immediate acute inflammatory response. If the splinter is not removed, chronic inflammatory cells infiltrate the site and fibroblasts isolate and wall off the reaction with a fibrous capsule. However, if the irritant is removed, then healing either by repair or regeneration occurs. This has been assumed to occur also with a periapical lesion. Once bacteria and their products reach the apical area they encounter polymorphonuclear neutrophils (PMNs) and macrophages. If this process is allowed to continue, chronic inflammatory cells, lymphocytes, plasma cells, and fibroblasts wall off the irritating agents. If the irritant is removed (i.e., if the canal is cleaned, shaped, and filled), then healing should occur similar to healing after the splinter is removed.

Historically, when x-rays first began to reveal dark areas at the apices of teeth, wholesale extraction of these "bags of infection" was recommended. This was the beginning of the focal infection era. In an early attempt to disprove the focal infection theory, Fish[15] implanted viable bacteria in the jaws of guinea pigs. He took a culture of *Staphylococcus aureus* on cotton wool and placed it in a hole drilled into the mandible. The guinea pigs were killed 4 to 40 days later. Histologic results showed that the infection remained localized regardless of the virulence of the organism or its invasive capacity. The bacteria were confined by polymorphonuclear leukocytes to the *zone of infection*. The next area, the *zone of contamination,* contained chronic round cells but no bacteria. Surrounding this zone was the *zone of irritation* with histiocytes as the predominant cell in addition to osteoclasts. Finally there was the *zone of stimulation* with mostly fibroblasts, capillary buds, and osteoblasts. This confirmed his view that, despite the abnormal x-ray appearance of the periapical lesion and the heavy round cell infiltration, bacteria could not be demonstrated histologically beyond the *zone of infection*. This experiment has been used to describe periapical lesions of teeth. The lucency is caused by the body's response to bacteria and their products located within the canal. It was felt that bacteria only got past the apical foramen in an acute alveolar abscess, where the body is temporarily overwhelmed by the bacteria. Recently Fish's study was duplicated with a strain of *S. aureus*. Osteomyelitis occurring up to 21 days after inoculation was shown histologically. Viable bacteria were found well beyond what Fish would have considered to be the *zone of infection*.

Until the mid-1970s it was believed that endodontic disease was caused mostly by aerobic *Staphylococci* and *Streptococci*. However, with the advent of practical methods for anaerobic culturing, it became apparent that endodontic disease begins as polymicrobial infections dominated by anaerobic species.[43] Kantz and Henry[24] introduced a new technique for anaerobic culturing that allowed for the identification of anaerobes in the pulpal and periapical tissues. Also, Sundquist[50] was the first to correlate symptoms (pain and suppuration) with the specific bacteria, black-pigmented *Bacteroides* organisms. Nair[38] believes that periapical lesions are infected only when they are acute and causing symptoms. This body of research clearly implicates bacteria in the disease process.

ARE PERIAPICAL LESIONS INFECTED?

This has been a controversial question over the years. Except with acute alveolar abscess, *histologic* studies in general have not been able to demonstrate viable bacteria in periapical

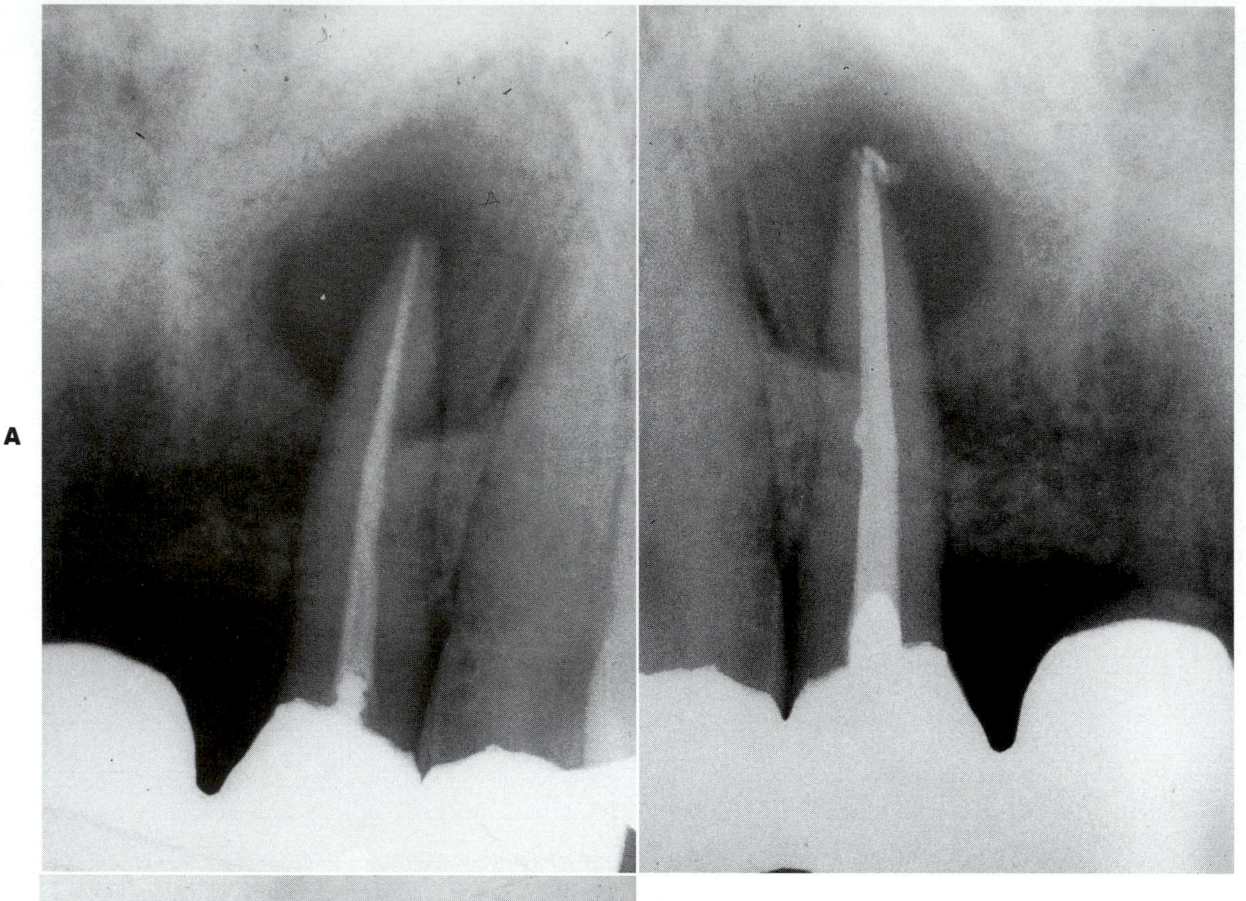

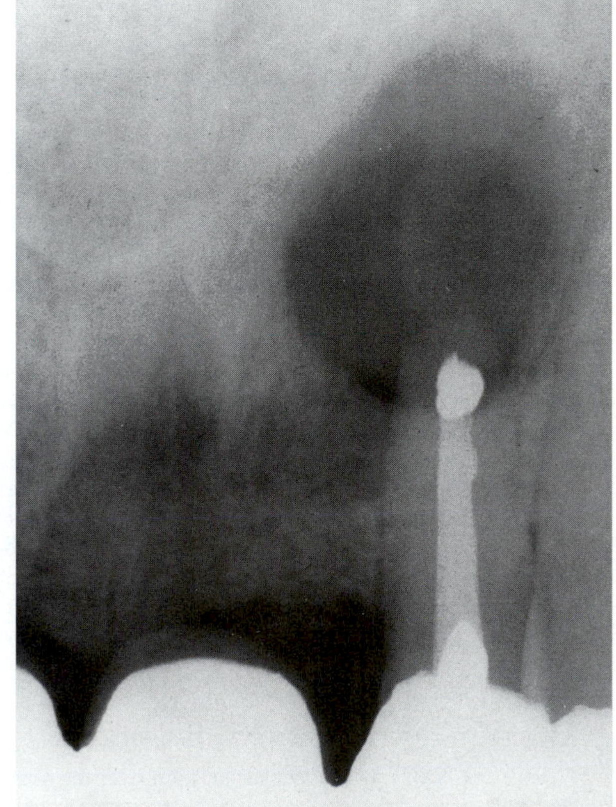

FIG. 12-1 A, Preoperative film of previously treated lateral incisor. A large periapical lucency is present. **B,** Nonsurgical retreatment of failing endodontic therapy. **C,** One year later the periapical lesion has still not responded to treatment. Surgical removal of the lesion and a retrofil amalgam has been placed. **D,** Histologic section of lesion showing PMNs and macrophages. (H&E stain.) **E,** Another section of the lesion showing "sulfur granules" or the presence of actinomycosis. **F,** One year recall showing healing by the formation of an apical scar.

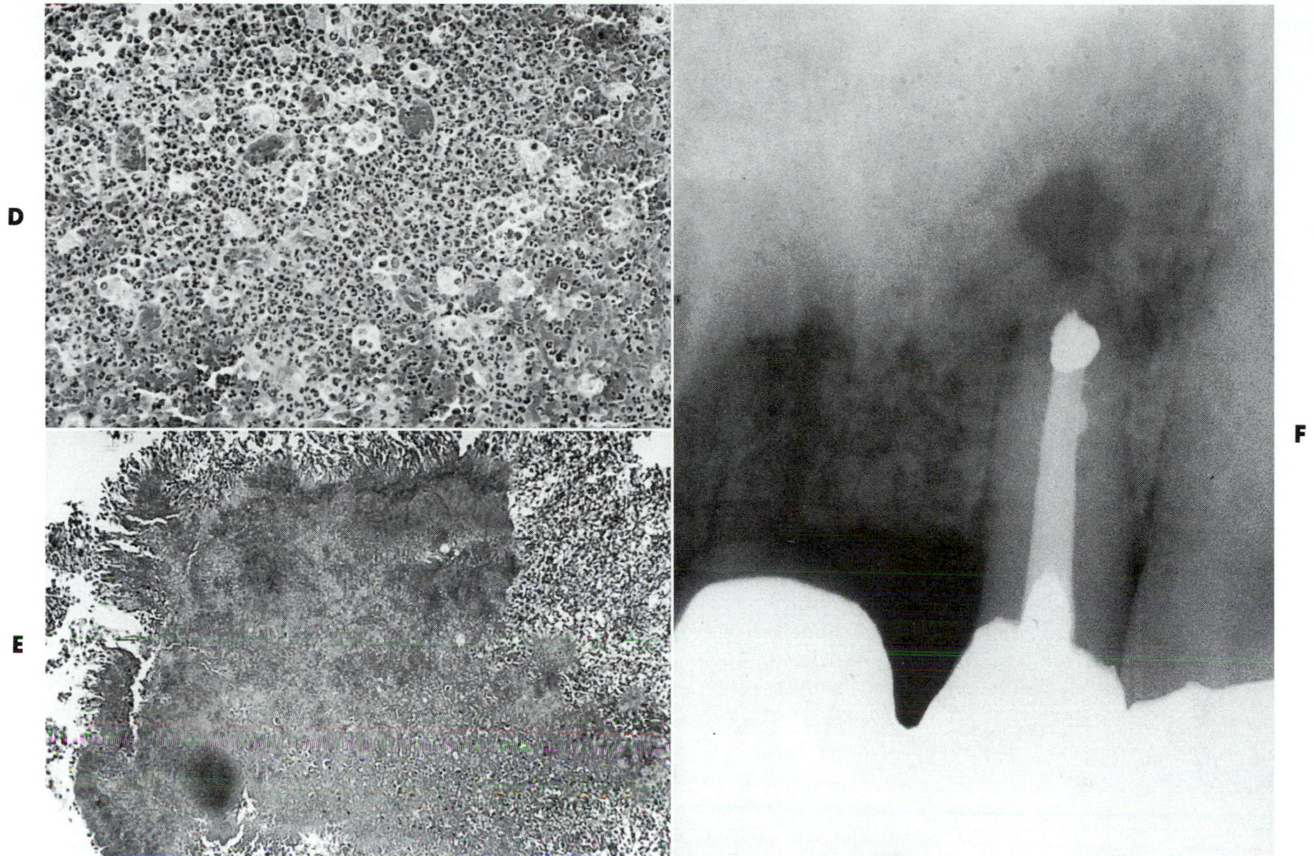

FIG. 12-1, cont'd For legend see opposite page.

lesions.[30,41,63] These findings persist to the present time.[62] However, a body of evidence is now forming that indicates many of these lesions may indeed be infected before and after endodontic treatment. In a recent study, Iwu[20] showed that 88% or 14 of 16 periapical granulomas were positive for bacteria when they were homogenized and *cultured*. In 1992 Wayman[54] studied 58 cases of periapical lesions. He cut these lesions in half and examined one half histologically and cultured the other half. In only 8 of 58 cases could he demonstrate bacteria *histologically*. However, when the other half of the lesion was *cultured* 51 of 58 cases were positive. He found 133 isolates, of which 87 were strict anaerobes, 37 were facultative anaerobes, and only 9 were aerobes. The bacteria[3] were found not only in periapical abscesses but also in granulomas and cysts.

With the demonstration of bacteria in periapical lesions it is not surprising to find reports of failure of nonsurgical endodontic therapy owing to the persistence of bacteria.* Sjogren, Burnett, Tronstad and Haponen all demonstrated live bacteria past the apices of endodontically treated teeth. Haponen[18] found, in 16 cases verified immunocytochemically, 13 had *Actinomycosis israelii,* 10 had *Actinomycosis propionica,* 6 had *Actinomycosis naeslundii,* and 9 had multiple bacteria. Therefore it is apparent that the pathogens (i.e., bacteria) can get past the apex of a tooth and may *survive* in the periapical tissues in spite of good nonsurgical endodontic therapy (Fig. 12-1).

At one time, the prevailing thought was that it was better to have these irritants outside the tooth, where the blood supply is richer and the body's own defense mechanism can neutralize the antigenic material. With the persistence of a periapical lesion after conventional endodontic therapy, it becomes apparent that the body's own defense mechanism may not always be capable of healing these lesions. Since the cause is now outside the canal, nonsurgical endodontic treatment may not be sufficient to effect healing.[10] Viable bacteria, endotoxin,[13,65] and foreign bodies,[26] once past the foramen, may require surgery to remove them. With current testing procedures it is now possible to demonstrate viable bacteria in the periapex. With improved techniques it is entirely possible that in the next decade we may find virus and virus particles in the periapex as pathogens.

The response to periapical disease is complex. Our tendency has been to oversimplify the process because of our incomplete understanding of the processes involved.

PERIAPICAL DISEASE

Endodontic pathology is a bacterial disease.[16,63] The periapex of the tooth becomes involved when bacteria invade the pulp, rendering it partially to totally necrotic. This was shown graphically in a classic study by Kakehashi, Stanley, and Fitzgerald[23] on gnotobiotic (germ-free) rats. They exposed the

*References 1, 2, 18, 48, 59, 60.

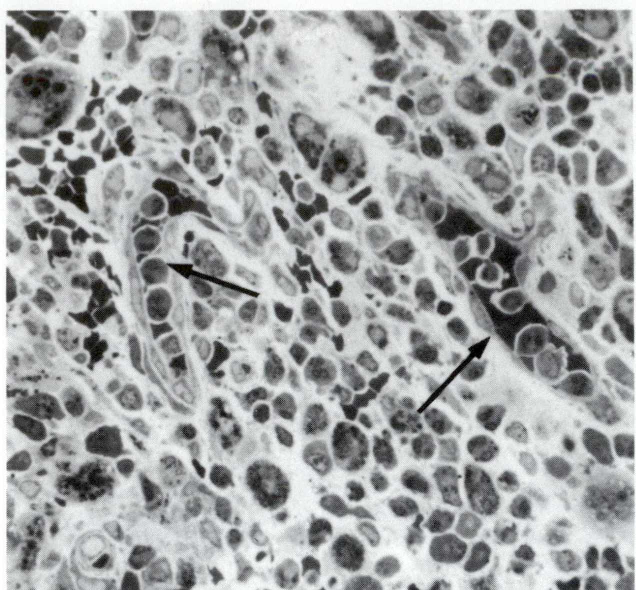

FIG. 12-2 Photomicrograph of an area of inflammation with two capillaries showing white and red cells flowing through the vessels *(arrows)*. (Original magnification, ×400.)

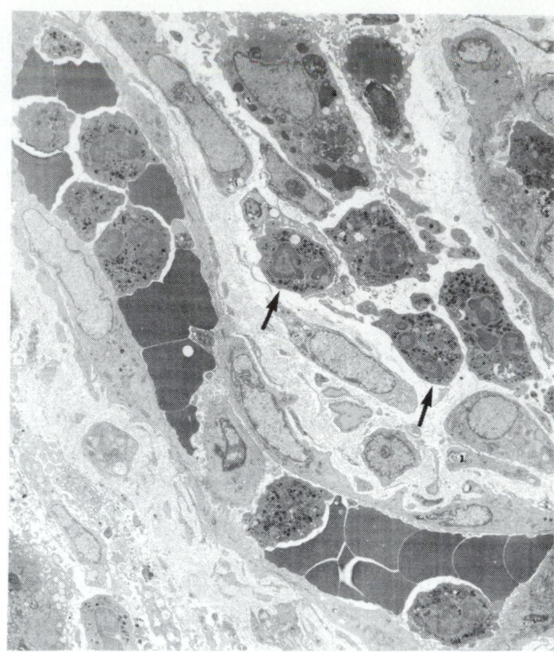

FIG. 12-3 Electron micrograph of a capillary with polymorphonuclear leukocytes and erythrocytes inside. Note PMNs in the extravascular tissue *(arrows)*. (Original magnification, ×3450.)

pulps of normal rats and left them open to the oral environment. Necrosis of the pulp ensued, followed by periapical inflammation and lesion formation. When the same procedure was performed on germ-free rats, the pulps not only remained vital and relatively uninflamed but the bur holes were repaired with dentin by the 36th day. The study demonstrated that without bacteria and their products, periapical lesions of endodontic origin *do not* occur. Confirmation came from a study by Moeller and colleagues[34] (1981) on nine monkeys. It was shown that noninfected necrotic pulp tissue did not induce periapical lesions or inflammatory reactions. However, if the pulp tissue subsequently was infected, periapical lesions and inflammation in the apical tissues ensued. Additionally, Korzen[27] demonstrated that it is a mixed infection and not a monoinfection that results in the more florid disease process. Thus, it is well established that periapical disease is the result of bacteria, their products, and the host response to them.

HOST RESPONSE

Inflammation

The basic disease process in both pulp and periapical disease is infection. The host responds to the infection with inflammation. Many definitions of inflammation exist, but none is precise. Menkin defined inflammation as the complex vascular, lymphatic, and local tissue reaction of a higher organism to an irritant.[33] Because inflammation is the host's response to an infection, the terms inflammation and infection are not interchangeable. The host can have an inflammatory response without the presence of infection (e.g., sunburn).

Vascular Changes

The initial vascular change in inflammation is a transient contraction of the microcirculation followed almost immediately by dilatation (Figs. 12-2 and 12-3). As the vessels dilate blood flow slows. The red blood cells move to the middle of the vessel (rouleaux formation) and the white blood cells move to the periphery and stick to the endothelial wall (margination, Fig. 12-4). The vasculature in the postcapillary venules becomes leaky owing to contraction of endothelial cells under the influence of histamine, which allows plasma to escape into the tissue spaces. Because of this leakage,[14,45,61] edema results, causing increased tissue pressure.

The immediate transient vascular response is most likely mediated by histamine, whereas the delayed vascular response is mediated by other vasoactive amines such as bradykinin. In addition, other plasma proteins such as fibrinogen pass into the tissues and contribute to the inflammatory response. Fibrinogen is converted to fibrin when it contacts the tissue collagen and form a meshwork to isolate the reaction (Fig. 12-5). The white blood cells that now line the endothelial wall of the vessels squeeze through the endothelial gaps and into the tissue by an ameboid movement called *diapedesis*.

Acute Inflammation

In acute inflammation the PMNs are the first cells to emigrate to the site of infection (Fig. 12-6), drawn there by chemotactic agents that are expressed either by the bacteria itself or by other mediators of inflammation. The monocytes are next attracted to the site. When these cells enter the tissues they are called *tissue macrophages* or *histiocytes* (Fig. 12-7). Neutrophils survive for hours, whereas macrophages last for days to months. Neutrophils are characterized by their lobulated nucleus, whereas macrophages have a single large nucleus. Both have extensive cytoplasmic granules containing lysosomal enzymes.

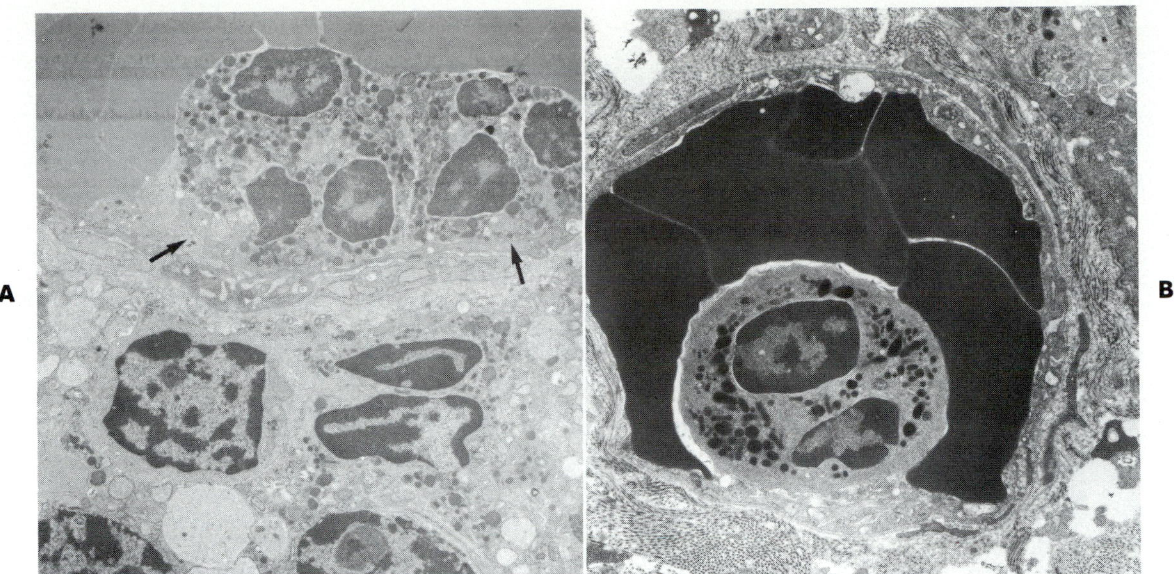

FIG. 12-4 A, Electron micrograph of a portion of a large vessel showing margination of two leukocytes *(arrows)*. (Original magnification, ×11,000). **B,** Smaller vessel with PMNS about to squeeze through the wall.

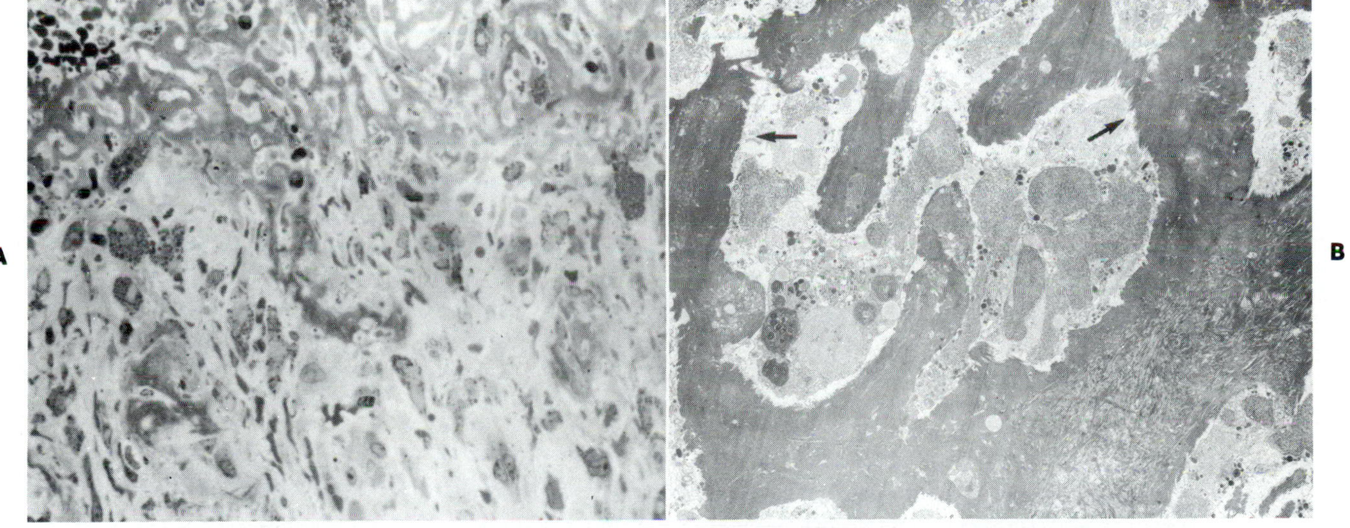

FIG. 12-5 A, One-micrometer section showing fibrin in the tissues walling off the resection. **B,** Ultrastructural picture of fibrin in the tissue *(arrows)*.

Phagocytosis

In the inflammatory process both PMNs and macrophages function as phagocytes (Fig. 12-8). The process of phagocytosis involves three stages:

1. Attachment of the phagocytic cell to the target cell or antigen. This is facilitated by opsonization by IgG, IgM, or C3b (from the complement system).
2. Ingestion of the cell or antigen. A cellular membrane extension envelops the opsonized antigenic material to form a phagosome. The phagosome fuses with cytoplasmic lysosomes that release their digestive enzymes in a process called *degranulation*.
3. Breakdown or degradation of the bacteria or antigen by:
   a. Lysosomal hydrolytic enzymes
   b. An acid pH in the vacuole
   c. Cationic proteins
   d. Lactoferrin
   e. Superoxide anion
   f. Hydrogen peroxide
   g. Peroxide-halide-myeloperoxidase

Thus, the process of phagocytosis includes attaching, ingesting, and then destroying the bacteria.

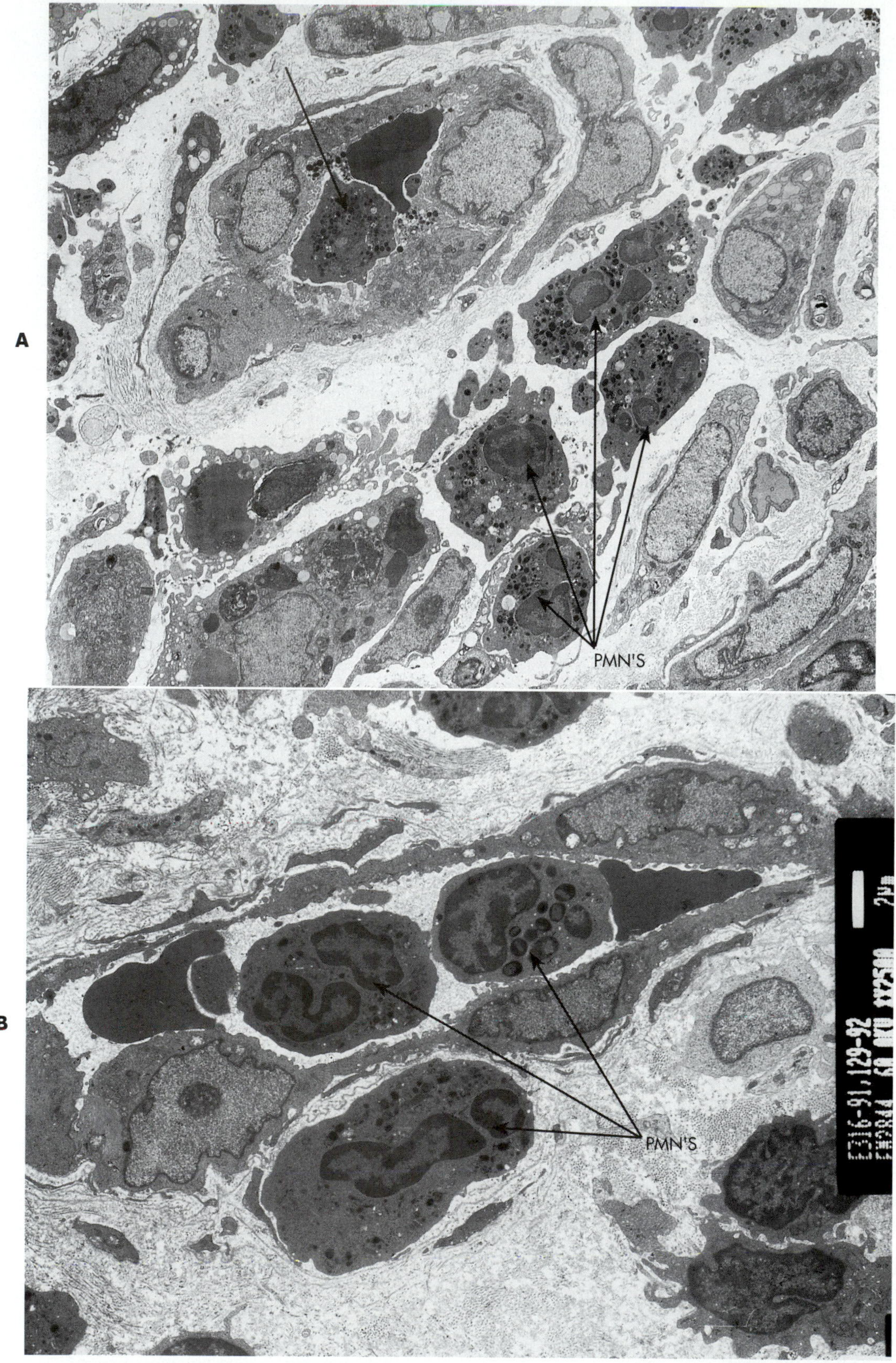

FIG. 12-6 A, Electron micrograph of a capillary containing an RBC and a PMN with numerous PMNs in the surrounding tissue. This is the beginning of acute inflammation. **B,** Longitudinal cut of a capillary with PMNs *(arrows)* in the lumen and a PMN in the tissue.

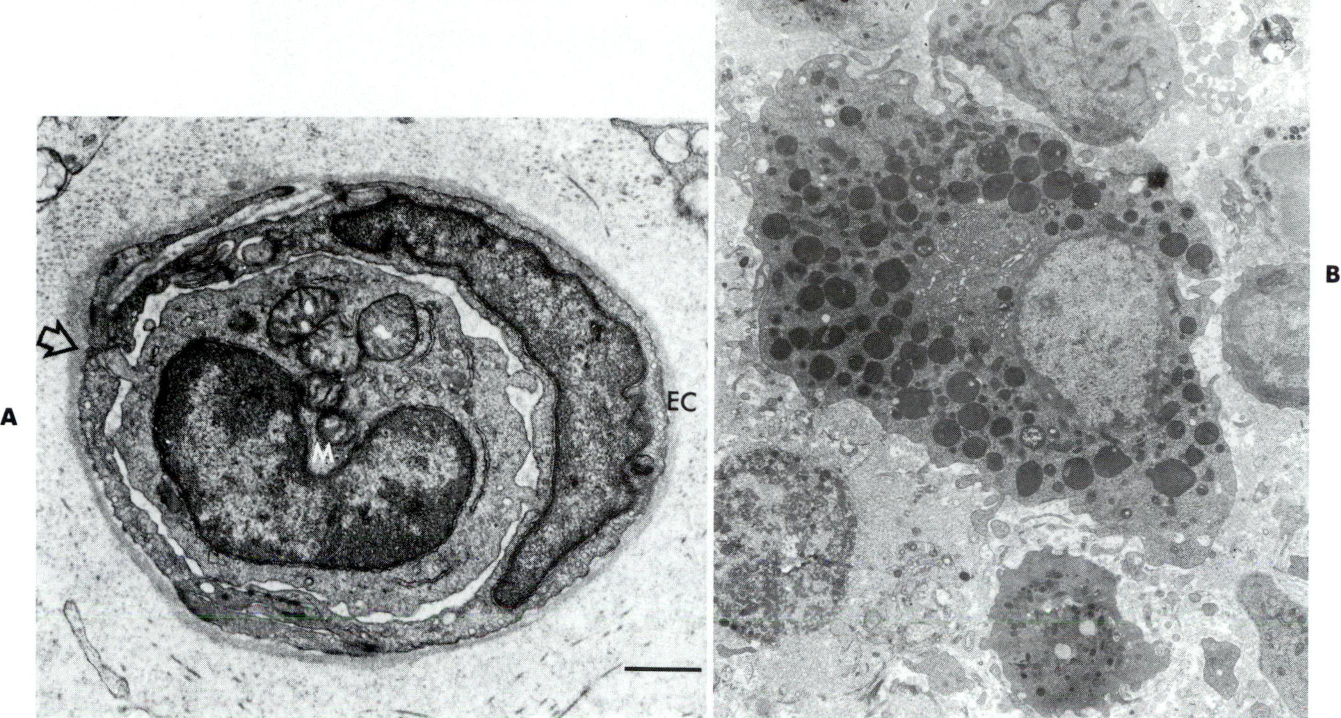

FIG. 12-7 A, Monocyte *(M)* in a capillary with three pseudopods extended. (Original magnification, ×12,900.) One pseudopod *(upper left)* is beginning to squeeze through the intercellular gap *(arrow)*. Note the prominent endothelial cells *(EC)*. **B,** Electron micrograph of a macrophage, now out in the tissue.

Mediators

Mediators are chemical substances that control the inflammatory response. Mediators may be exogenous (as from bacterial products) or endogenous. Endogenous mediators are classified as either plasma or tissue mediators. Mediators released from plasma include:

1. Bradykinin from the kinin system
2. Complement from the complement system
3. Factors from the clotting system

Mediators released from tissue include:

1. Vasoactive amines (released from mast cells and basophils). These are released in response to:
   a. Physical injury (i.e., trauma)
   b. Chemicals (i.e., neutrophilic lysosomal cationic protein)
   c. IgE-sensitized cells
   d. Exposure to complement C3a and C5a (anaphylatoxin)
2. Acidic lipids (i.e., SRS-A and prostaglandins, which are metabolites of arachidonic acid)[31,53]
3. Lysosomal components
   a. Cationic proteins
   b. Acid proteases
   c. Neutral proteases
4. Lymphocyte products (i.e., lymphokines from T cells)

Microscopically, the picture includes PMNs, macrophages, and the tissue response as a result of these chemical mediators. On the clinical level we can now account for the five cardinal signs of inflammation (Figs. 12-9 and 12-10):

1. Redness (increased dilatation of the vessels)
2. Swelling (escape of vascular fluid into the tissues causing edema)
3. Pain (release of pain mediators such as bradykinin and tissue pressure due to hyperemia and edema)
4. Heat (increased blood supply to the injured tissues)
5. Loss of function (due to pain and swelling)

ACUTE INFLAMMATION

The diagnosis of acute inflammation is both a histologic and a clinical one. Histologically, polymorphonuclear leukocytes and macrophages constitute the predominant acute inflammatory cells, but clinically the presence of pain usually denotes an acute condition. The other cardinal signs of acute inflammation may also be present: swelling, heat, redness, and loss of function.

Acute Apical Periodontitis

Acute apical inflammation is a very painful response that occurs before alveolar bone is resorbed. Apically, the vascular response to the antigens within the pulp produces edema. The edema and PMNs rapidly fill the periodontal ligament between the tooth and bone. Because the fluid is not compressible, any external pressure on the tooth forces the fluid against already sensitized nerve endings, resulting in exquisite pain. The tooth remains painful until the bone begins to be resorbed and space is created to accommodate the edema fluid. The patient may also complain of the tooth's feeling elevated in the socket, but no lesion is demonstrable on radiography.

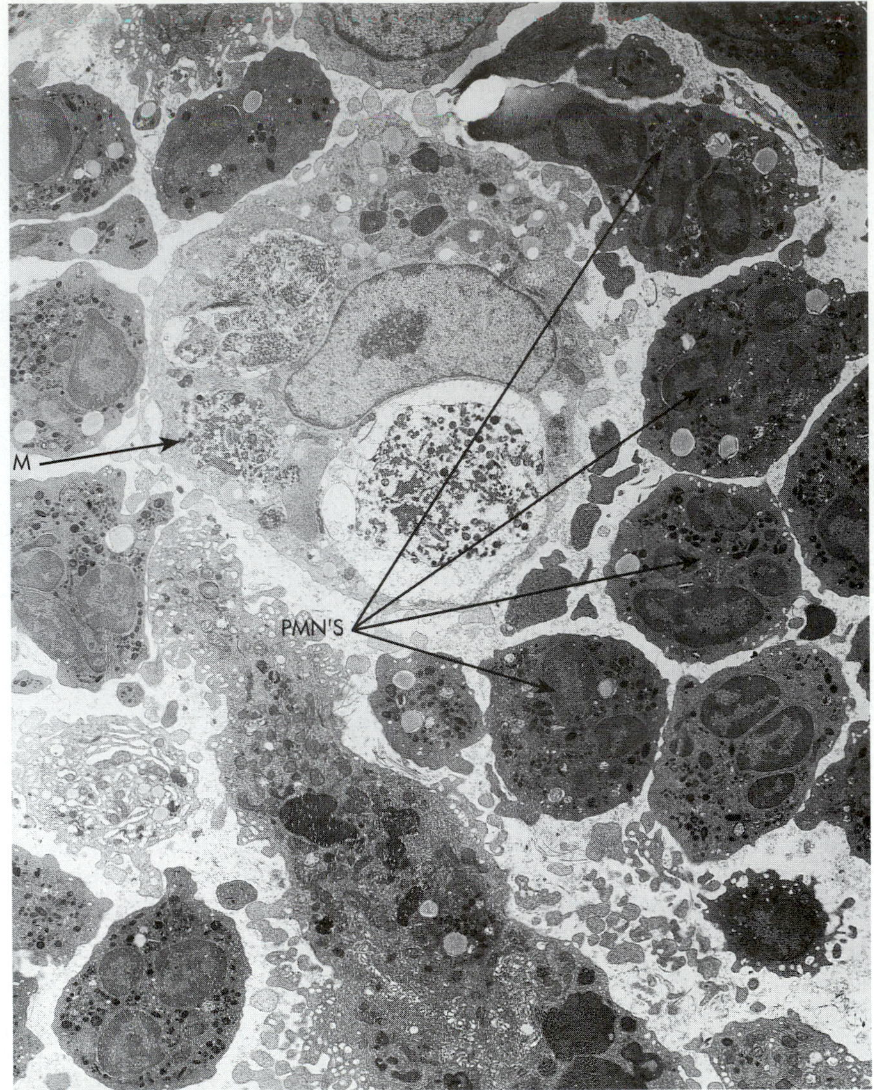

FIG. 12-8 Electron micrograph of a large macrophage *(M)* with a full phagosome in the cytoplasm. The cell is surrounded by PMNs *(arrows)*.

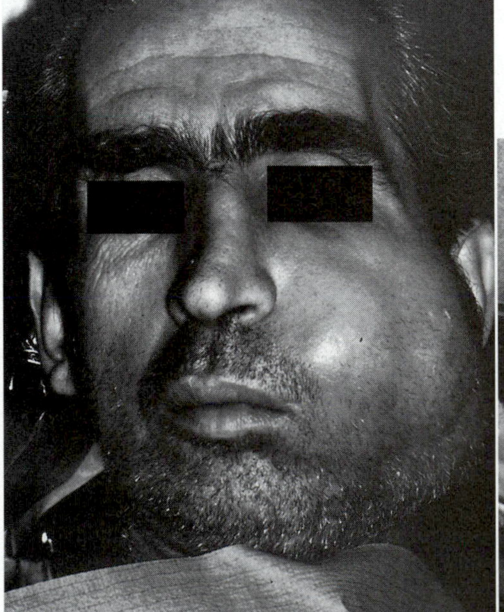

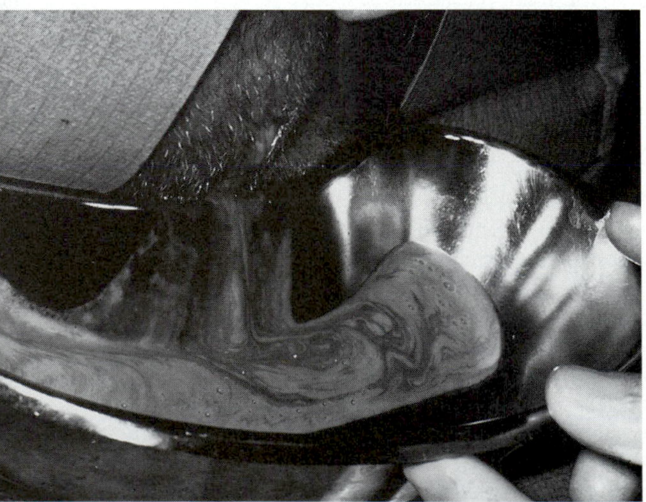

FIG. 12-9 A, Clinical photograph of an acute apical abscess. **B,** Pus and blood drain externally into a basin from the incised abscess.

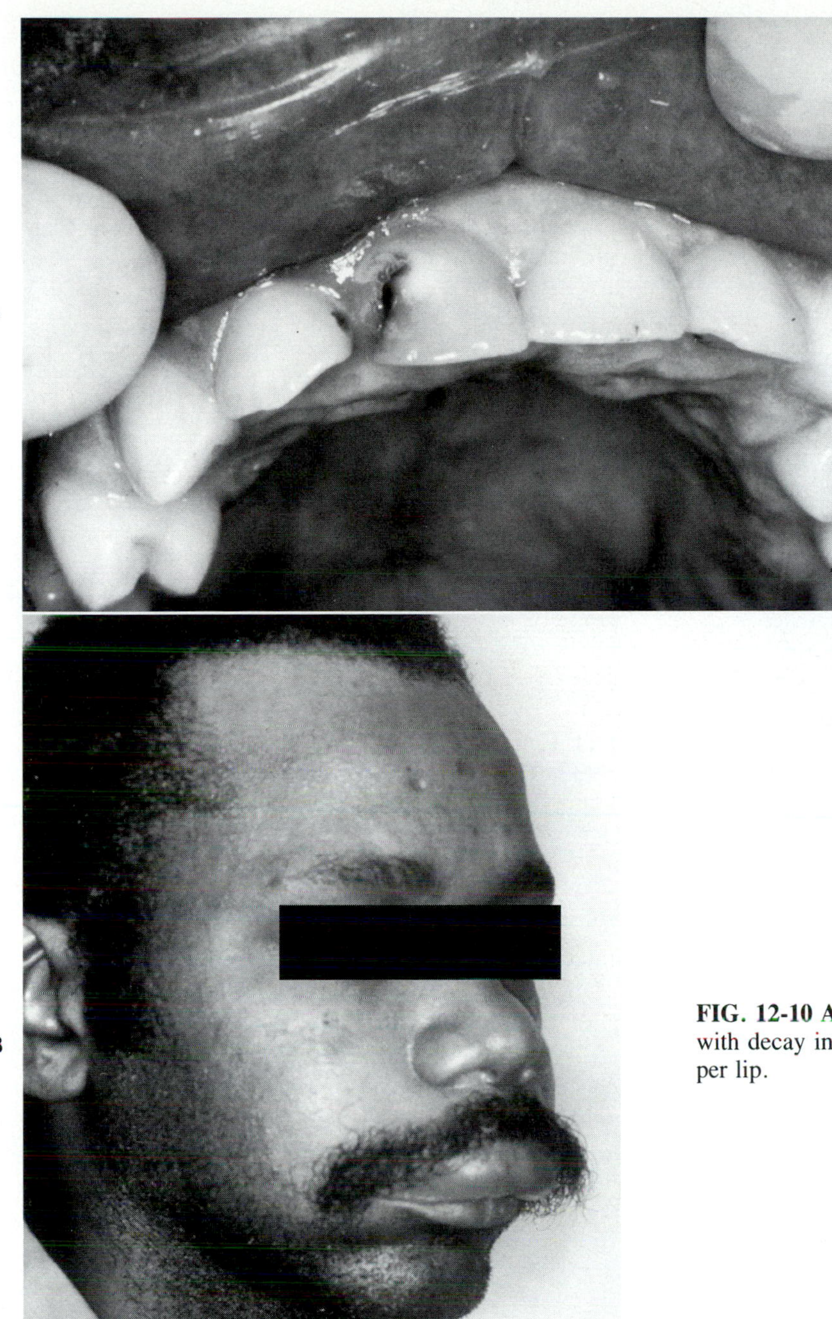

FIG. 12-10 **A,** Clinical photograph of upper right lateral incisors with decay into the pulp. **B,** Acute abscess with cellulitis of upper lip.

Acute apical abscess

An acute apical abscess may result when large numbers of bacteria get past the apex and elicit a severe inflammatory response. This response is acute, the predominant cell being the polymorphonuclear leukocyte. With the release of PMN lysosomal enzymes into the tissue space and the concomitant tissue degradation, an abscess forms (Figs. 12-9 and 12-10). An abscess is defined as a localized collection of pus which, microscopically, is composed of dead cells, debris, PMNs, and macrophages. Clinically, varying degrees of swelling occur, with pain. The patient complains of a feeling that the tooth is elevated out of the socket. Elevated temperature and malaise may follow. The body responds to this insult by trying to isolate the abscess and/or establish drainage either intraorally or extraorally. If drainage is not effective, the abscess may spread into fascial planes or spaces of the head and neck.

Phoenix Abscess

If a periapical radiolucency is present and an acute inflammatory response is superimposed on this preexisting chronic lesion it is termed a *phoenix abscess* (i.e., an acute exacerbation of an existing chronic inflammation; Fig. 12-11).

Healing

Healing can occur by either regeneration or repair. This distinction is important when considering what type of tissue forms after the antigenic agents are gone. If the tissue returns to its original state, it is called *regeneration*. If the original tissue is replaced with dense fibrous connective tissue, it is called *repair*.

Several cell types are involved in healing. Macrophages clean up the debris, fibroblasts repair the damage, and differentiated or undifferentiated cells regenerate the damaged tissues. Because of the increased oxygen demands during healing, proliferation of capillary buds also occurs.

A

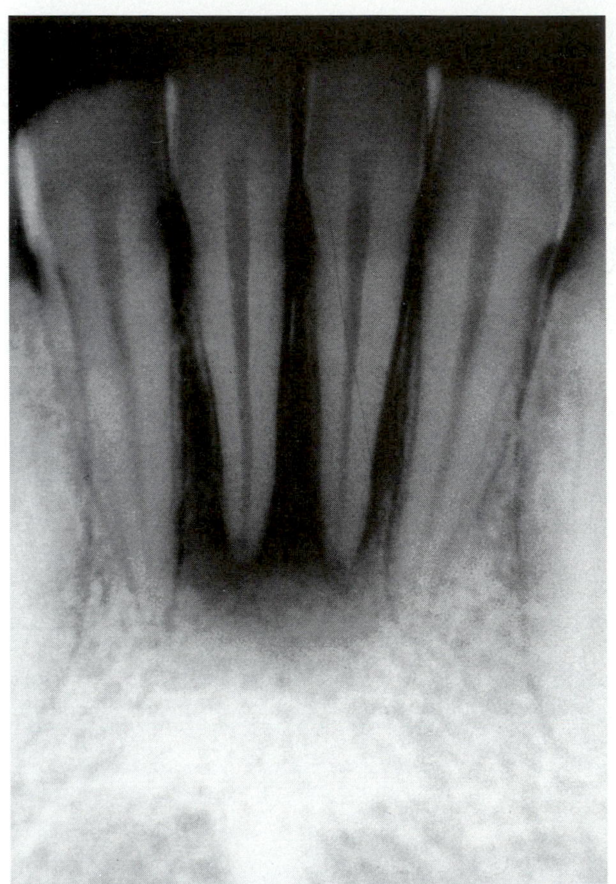

B

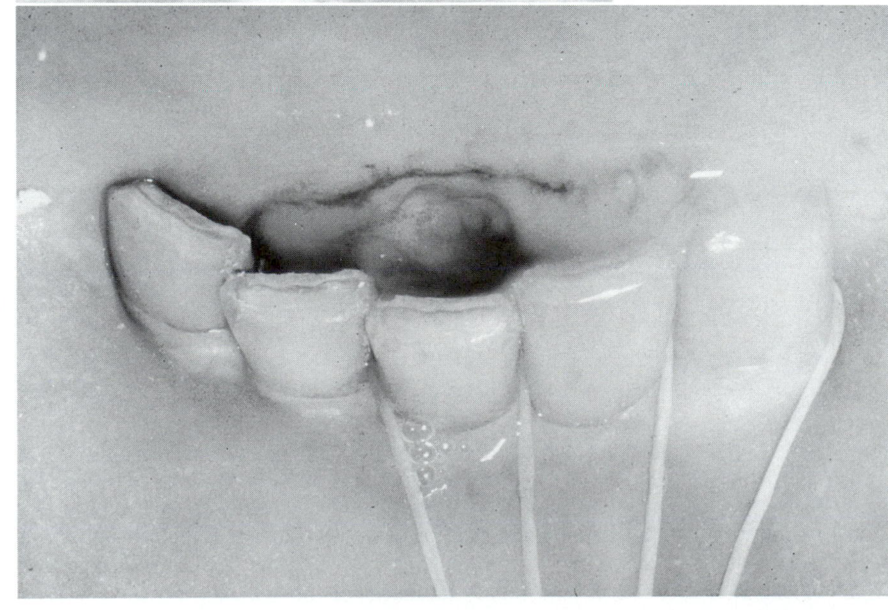

FIG. 12-11 A, Radiograph of lower anterior teeth with periapical lucency. **B,** Upon opening the central incisors, copious amounts of pus drained through the canals. The diagnosis is phoenix abscess.

Acute Osteomyelitis

Acute osteomyelitis can arise directly from an endodontic infection. Live bacteria are past the apex and now are multiplying in the marrow spaces and soft tissue of the bone. Osteomyelitis may be a serious progression of periapical infection that results in diffuse spread through the medullary spaces, ultimately leading to necrosis of bone. Acute osteomyelitis may be localized or spread throughout large areas of bone.[44] The patient usually has severe pain, an elevated temperature, and palpable lymph nodes. Although the teeth are loose and sore in the early stages, there may be no swelling, and radiographic changes are difficult to detect (Fig. 12-12). Microscopically the medullary spaces are filled predominately with neutrophils. There may or may not be pus formation. Other microscopic findings include bone resorption due to vigorous activity of the osteoclasts and the lack of osteoblasts.

If untreated, the acute form may progress to chronic disease. Clinically, chronic suppurative osteomyelitis is the same as acute except the symptoms are milder and radiographically diffuse bone resorption is evident. Osteomyelitis is a very serious extension of periapical disease and must be treated promptly and agressively (Fig. 12-13). This can be a disease of endodontic origin; however, the etiologic agent (bacteria) is now beyond the confines of the pulp and in the surrounding tissues. Endodontic therapy or extraction may not be an effective treatment option. More extensive surgical, hyperbaric oxygen, and antibiotic therapy may be required.

Chronic Inflammation

If the acute process does not heal but persists, the response becomes chronic. This is a change in both time and cell composition. The acute inflammatory process is an *exudative* re-

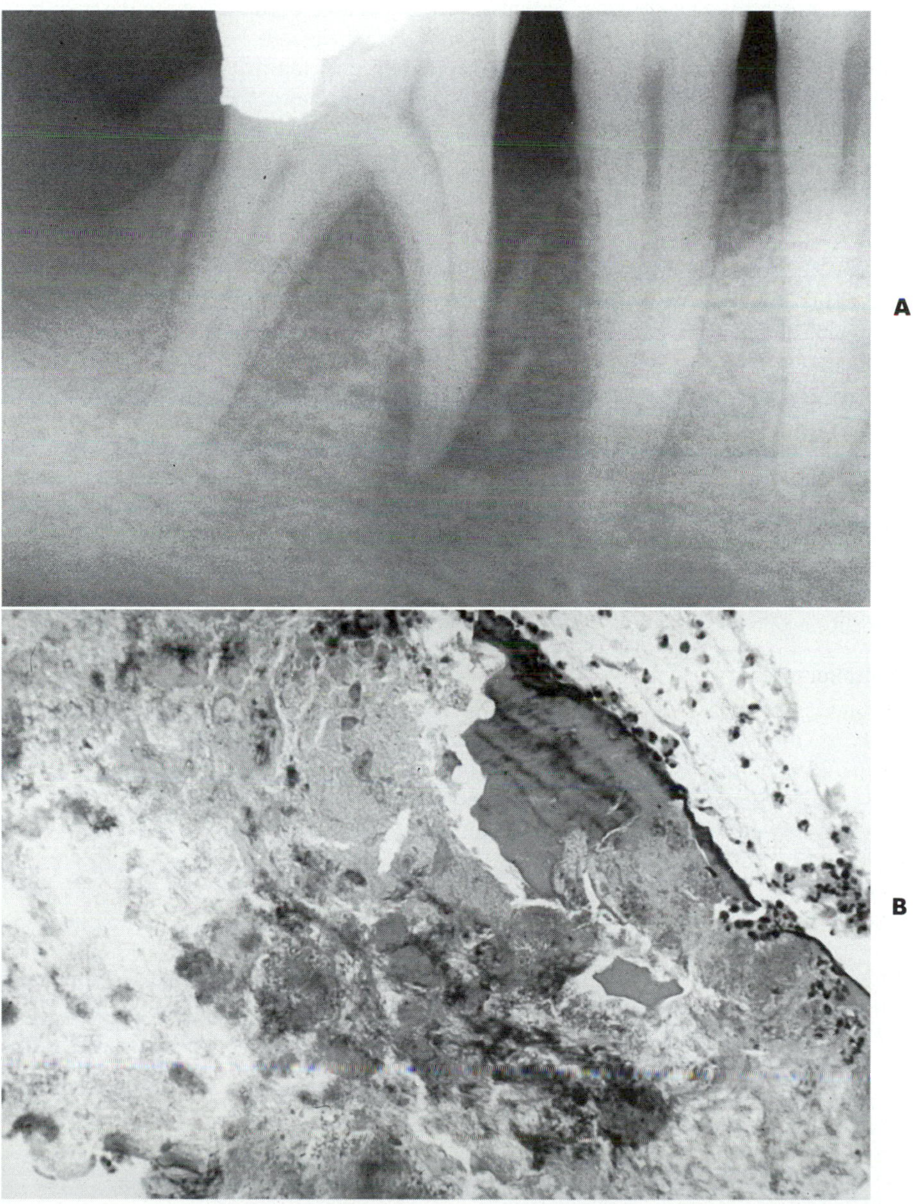

FIG. 12-12 A, Lower first molar area with a diffuse radiolucency. The molar was necrotic and did not respond to pulp testing procedures. **B,** Biopsy of the area reveals dead, avascular bone, debris, and bacteria. The diagnosis was acute osteomyelitis.

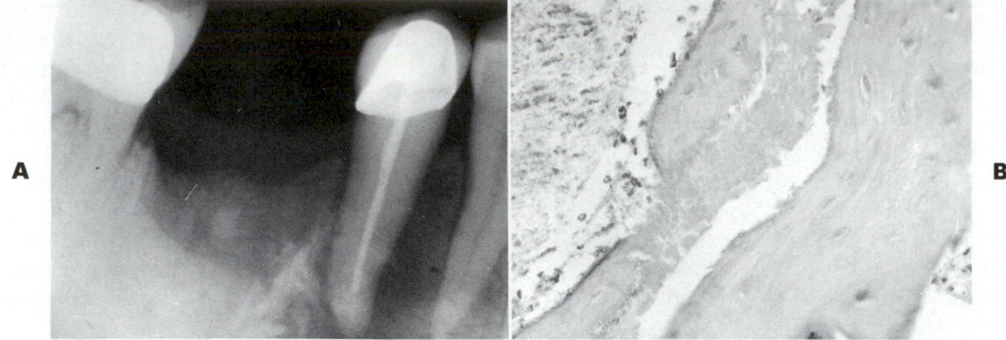

FIG. 12-13 A, Radiograph of chronic osteomyelitis showing extensive bone destruction in the mandible. **B,** Histologic section of necrotic bone with bacterial colonies.

sponse, whereas the chronic process is a *proliferative* response. Microscopically, proliferation of fibroblasts, vascular elements, and the infiltration of macrophages and lymphocytes are characteristic. In addition to the chronic inflammatory response, macrophages and lymphocytes elicit an immune response. The purpose of the immune system is to neutralize, inactivate, or destroy a stimulus (antigen or bacteria). This is accomplished by

1. Direct neutralization by antibody binding to the stimulus and/or destruction of the stimulus by sensitized lymphocytes.
2. Activation of biochemical and cellular mediator systems that can destroy the antigen.

People are either immunocompetent or immunodeficient. Immunocompetence is the ability to generate an immune response that can overcome many diseases and infections. Immunodeficient people cannot make this response and are thus afflicted with many inflammatory and infectious diseases. The host's ability to respond to an antigen has a genetic predisposition. This used to be referred to as *host resistance*. Diseases, immunosuppresive medications, and other insults can also alter the host's ability to mount an immune response.

Development of lymphocytes

Cell development begins shortly after conception in the yolk sac. The red blood cells (erythrocytes), granulocytes, macrophages, and lymphocytes differentiate from the hemopoietic stem cells. As fetal development progresses, these cells move to the spleen and liver and then on to the bone marrow. The immature lymphocytes go in two different directions[57]:

1. One group of stem cells migrates to the thymus gland, where they mature and become T cells (thymus-dependent lymphocytes). The T cells are concerned with cell-mediated immunity and control of the immune response. Following immunogen stimulation, these T cells become lymphoblasts and then multiply by clonal expansion. They do not have rough endoplasmic reticulum (RER) or make antibodies as plasma cells. However, the mediators they release (lymphokines) assist B cell expansion and differentiation into the antibody-producing plasma cell.
2. Another group of lymphocytes remain in the bone marrow and mature to form the B cells (bone marrow derived or bursa equivalent lymphocytes). The B cells give rise to antibody-forming plasma cells.

Both groups migrate to the peripheral lymphatic tissues: the lymph, blood, lymph nodes, spleen, Peyer's patches, appendix, and tonsils. While both T and B cells look identical microscopically, they can be differentiated. B cells can be identified by detecting the immunoglobulin and complement receptors on the cell membrane by using immunofluorescence techniques. T cells have the ability to form rosette clusters when exposed to sheep red blood cells.

Recognition

Each T cell and B cell has specific recognition sites on its membrane surfaces that chemically recognize and react with specific antigens.[12] Only a few cells of the total number have a specific site for a specific antigen. Thus, after the cell is stimulated, it rapidly reproduces by clonal expansion to produce enough cells for the specific antigen. Accessory cells, such as macrophages, process the antigen and present it to the T helper/inducer cell, which in turn triggers the differentiation of the B cells into blast cells. These cells mature into plasma cells (Fig. 12-14) that ultimately lead to antibody production. The life span of a plasma cell is approximately 12 hours.

Antigens (immunogens). Immunogens are any biologic or chemical macromolecule that can react with an antibody or cell product of the immune response. Antigens are usually:

1. Nonself, or foreign
2. Macromolecules
3. Usually proteins but can be carbohydrates, glycoproteins, or nucleic acids.

Lipids are not usually antigenic.

Each lymphocyte responds to a specific antigen, so two different antigens will not bind on its cell surface. The antigenic determinant is the area where the antibody actually recognizes the antigen.

Antibodies. Antibodies are immunoglobulins (proteins) that are synthesized by plasma cells. The plasma cell can secrete five classes of immunoglobulin molecules: IgG, IgA, IgM, IgE, and IgD (Fig. 12-15).[25,28,35,39,42] Each type is produced by a specific lymphocyte that can produce only that one type.

The function of the immunoglobulins may be summarized as follows:

IgG activates complement in the tissues and circulation. It has the highest serum concentration. IgG passes the placental barrier and is responsible for a newborn's initial immunity.[3,4,17]

IgM, the most efficient activator of complement, is mostly

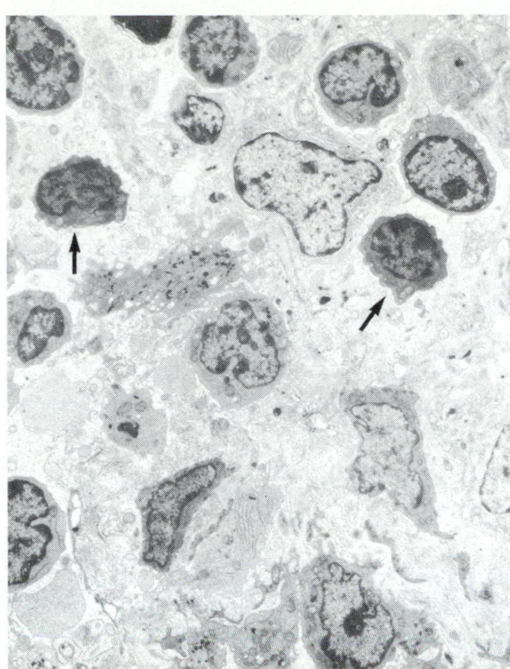

FIG. 12-14 Electron micrograph of numerous lymphocytes *(arrows)* in the lymphoblast stage transforming into plasma cells. Note the presence of a macrophage. (Original magnification, ×5,240.)

in circulation because it is a very large molecule. It is responsible for the initial immune response.

IgE binds to cell membranes of mast cells and basophils. After reacting with an immunogen, IgE will cause degranulation of these sensitized mast cells and basophils, resulting in the release of vasoactive factors that ultimately cause edema and swelling.[40,58]

IgA binds along epithelial surfaces in body secretions and blocks antigen entry across mucous membranes. It may also activate the alternative pathway of complement. Its highest concentration is in saliva.

IgD functions as a surface molecule (receptor) on cell membranes of maturing B lymphocytes.

For further information refer to Chapter 12.

Complement. Complement has 11 components (C1-C9, C1 has three parts) involving 23 to 26 proteins as split products. It is produced by the liver and macrophages and is found in circulation as an inactive form. Therefore, to exert its effect it must be activated.

There are two pathways for activation of the complement cascade[22]:

1. The *classical pathway* is triggered by an antigen/antibody reaction in the order C1–C4–C2–C3–C5–C6–C7–C8–C9. It can be activated by antigen complexes with IgG and IgM.
2. The *properdin* or the *alternative pathway* is triggered by cell surfaces and plant and bacterial carbohydrates but not by antigen/antibody reactions. This system is activated by properdin components that require the presence of C3b. The cascade does not require C1, C4, or C2. Therefore the path activates C3 and the cascade continues via the normal route: C3–C5–C6–C7–C8–C9. It can be activated by a variety of substances, including IgA, lysosomal enzymes, and gram-negative bacterial cell wall (endotoxin).

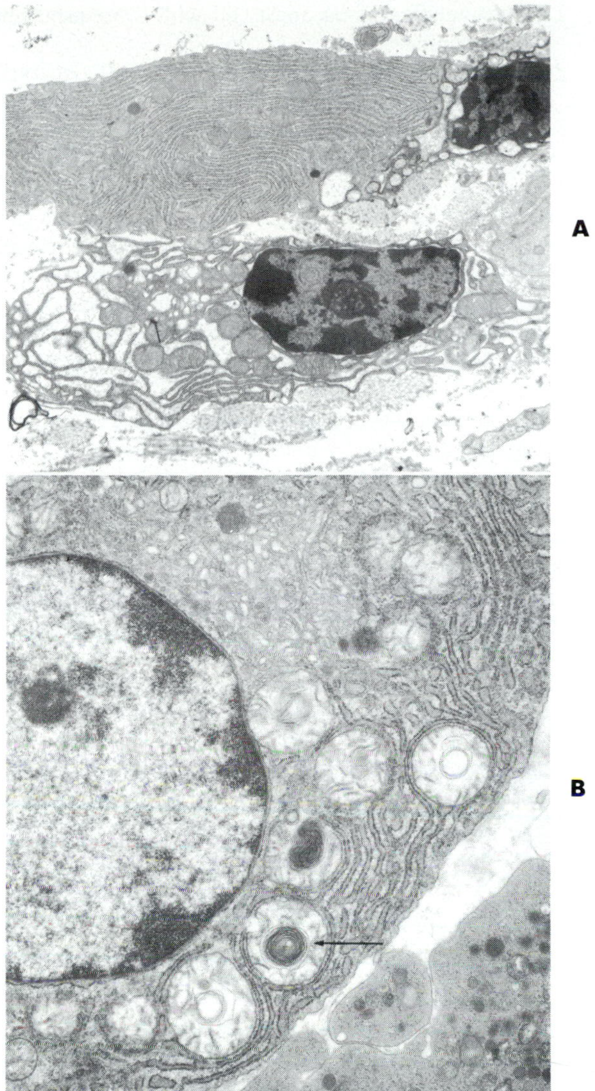

FIG. 12-15 A, Electron micrograph of two plasma cells, one with normal RER and the other with very dilated RER. This dilatation is thought to indicate immunoglobulin production and synthesis. (Original magnification, ×3,450.) **B,** High-power electron micrograph of part of a plasma cell showing the RER with ribosomes on the surface and myelin figures in the Golgi apparatus *(arrow)*. (Original magnification, ×23,700.)

In the complement systems C1 is the recognition unit, C2 to C4 is the activation unit, and C5 to C9 is the membrane attack unit. C1 binds with the antigen-antibody complex and triggers the entire sequence. C2 and C2a activate the kinin system that causes endothelial cells to contract, and therefore increase vascular permeability. C3a and C5a are anaphylatoxins; that is, they interact with mast cells and basophils that result in:

1. Degranulation of the mast cell with subsequent release of histamine
2. Production of arachidonic acid metabolites (leukotrienes and prostaglandins)
3. Release of enzymes to form bradykinin.

All of these increase vascular permeability. C3b binds to the cell membrane of the offending bacteria and acts as an opsonizing agent to assist in phagocytosis. C5a and C567 are chemotactic for PMNs, which release enzymes that destroy bacteria (and host tissues). C8 and C9 are responsible for cell lysis.

Complement can affect an antigen in three ways:

1. *Cytotoxicity*—Complement fragments C8 and C9, when bound to the antibodies that have opsonized the bacteria, will lysis the cell.
2. *Opsonization*—C3b allows binding of macrophages to the antigen.
3. *Chemotaxis for PMNs*—C5 and C567 draw PMNs into the affected area.

Immunopathologies. The immunopathologies are hypersensitivity reactions of the immune system that produce injury to the host.[54,55] These can be considered in two broad groups: antibody-mediated (types I, II, and III) and T cell mediated (type IV).[49]

1. *Antibody Mediated Hypersensitivities*—These reactions are mediated by antibodies that have sensitized basophils and/or mast cells.

   Type I: The primary exposure of the host to an antigen sensitizes the mast cells and/or basophils. The antibody IgE will prime the mast cells/basophils for the next exposure to the antigen. When that occurs, massive degranulation of these sensitized cells will result in the release of histamine and the production of arachidonic acid metabolites with their resulting biologic effects.

   Type II: IgG or IgM reacts with cell surface antigens and exerts a cytotoxic effect either by activating complement, which ultimately results in cell lysis, or phagocytosis by macrophages, PMNs, or K cells in a process known as *antibody-dependent cell-mediated cytotoxicity* (ADCC).

   Type III: Also mediated by IgG and IgM, it involves the fixation of complement. Free antigen (not cell or tissue bound) forms immune complexes with the antibodies.[37,56] This elicits the complement cascade. Complement components C5a and C567 are chemotactic for PMNs and macrophages. These subsequently phagocytose the immune complexes and release their lysosomal enzymes, which ultimately leads to tissue destruction of the host. Arthus' reaction is a type III hypersensitivity reaction.

2. *Type IV*—These T cell–mediated reactions develop slowly and reach their peak between 24 and 72 hours. Typically what happens is a sensitized individual encounters an antigen again. The accessory cell presents the antigen to the sensitized T cell, and T cells undergo blast transformation. The T cell expresses lymphokines and the macrophage releases lysosomal enzymes that damage the host tissues.

Evidence indicates that all of these inflammatory and immune processes may take place in the dental pulp and periapical tissues. Therefore, in the following descriptions, all these reactions may be occurring. This results in a microscopic picture that we label *chronic inflammation*.

Periapical Extension of Pulpal Inflammation

Periapical inflammation may begin before the pulp is totally necrotic. Bacterial products, mediators of inflammation, and deteriorating pulp tissue leak past the apex and evoke a chronic inflammatory response from the vessels in the periodontal ligament. This explains why it is possible to have a periapical radiolucency while some vital tissue remains in the apical canal (Fig. 12-16). The periapical inflammatory response is an extension of the pulpal inflammatory response.

Chronic Apical Periodontitis (Granuloma)

Chronic apical inflammation is a relatively low-grade, longstanding response to canal bacteria and irritants. Clinically, this lesion is usually asymptomatic and is revealed by an apical radiolucency. Microscopically the lesion is characterized by a predominance of lymphocytes, plasma cells, and macrophages surrounded by a relatively uninflamed fibrous capsule made up of collagen, fibroblasts, and capillary buds (Fig. 12-17). In the inflammatory area large, amorphous circles with very pale staining may be seen. These are Russell bodies and

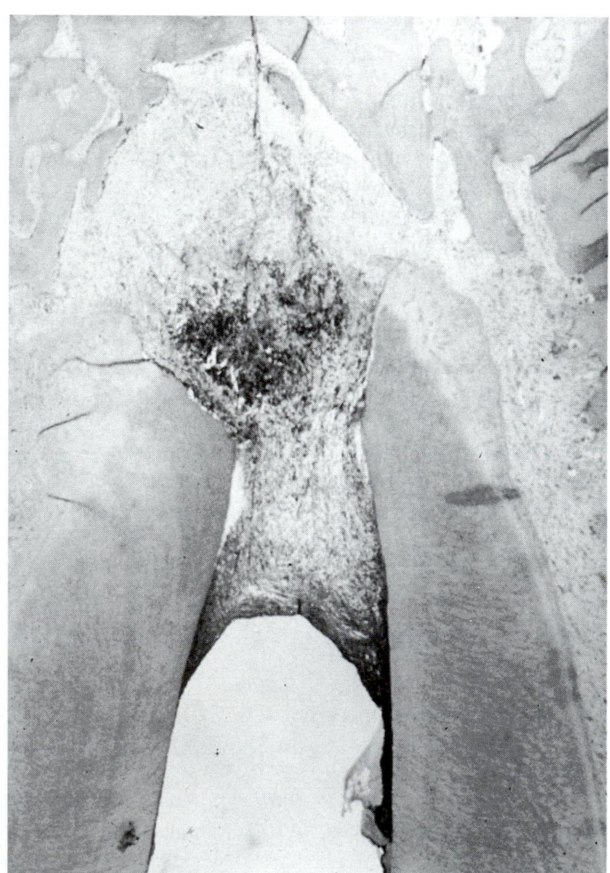

FIG. 12-16 Histologic section showing vital pulp tissue remaining in the canal with inflammation at the foramen and periapical bone resorption. (Courtesy Dr. Jacob Vaulderhaug.)

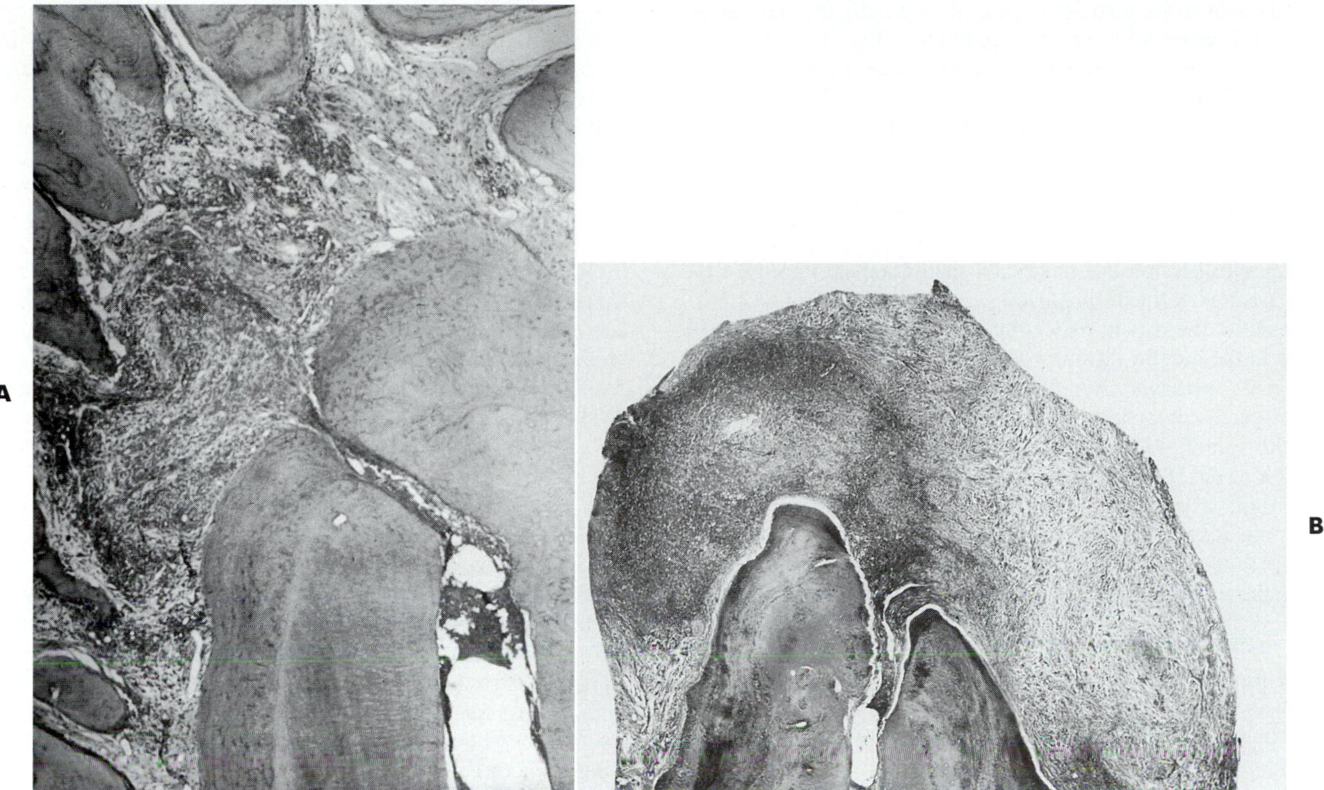

FIG. 12-17 A, Histologic section of necrotic canal with beginning periapical (granuloma) lesion formation. (Courtesy Dr. Jacob Vaulderhaug.) **B,** Histologic section of necrotic canal with chronic (granuloma) inflammatory lesion.

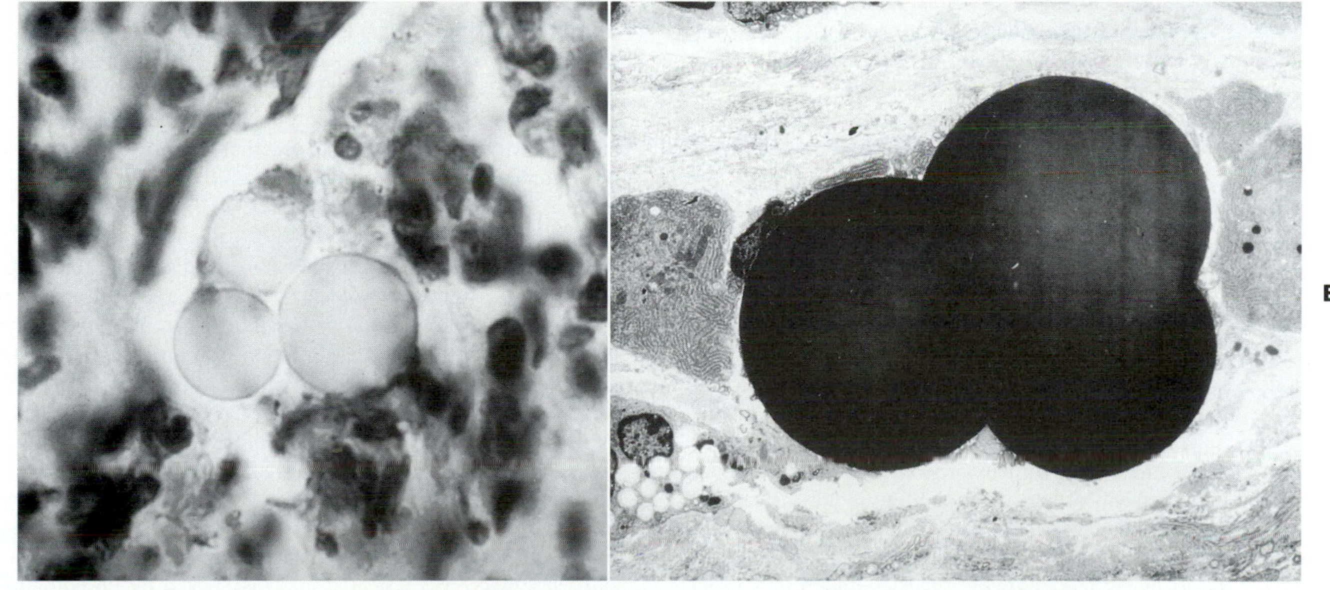

FIG. 12-18 A, Histologic section of granuloma shows three circular amorphous Russell bodies. (H&E stain; original magnification, ×400.) **B,** Electron micrograph of three Russell bodies that have coalesced. Note RER of associated plasma cell.

are thought to be associated with plasma cells that no longer have the capability to produce antibodies (Fig. 12-18). Cords or strands of proliferating epithelium may or may not be present. This lesion is usually not purely chronic in nature, since some PMNs may be seen scattered throughout the lesion.

Suppurative Apical Periodontitis (Granuloma with Fistulation)

An apical lesion that has established drainage through a sinus tract is termed *suppurative inflammation* (Fig. 12-19). Clinically, the patient may complain of a "gum boil" or a bad taste in the mouth. Pus may be expressed through the opening by gentle pressure. A radiograph should be exposed with a gutta-percha probe inserted into the tract to determine the cause of the lesion. Microscopically the tract may be filled with PMNs or pus. Chronic inflammatory cells may line the periphery, and, in later stages, epithelium may be present (Fig. 12-20). Studies estimate that epithelium lines the tract 10% to 30% of the time. Valderhaug has stated that the longer the tract persists the more likely it is to have an epithelial lining.

Foreign body reaction

A foreign body response may occur to many types of substances. The reaction can be acute and/or chronic. What usually distinguishes these lesions microscopically is the presence of multinucleate giant cells surrounding a foreign material (Fig. 12-21). If the material is soluble in the solutions used to prepare the histologic section the giant cells will appear to be surrounding a space. Usually the giant cells are surrounded by a chronic inflammatory infiltrate. The giant cells are thought to be formed by the fusion of several macrophages, creating a multinuclear cell (Fig. 12-22). These lesions may or may not be symptomatic. The cause is now beyond the apex, so surgery may be necessary to remove the foreign material and effect healing.

Osteosclerosis or condensing osteitis

The inflammatory response depends on the quality, duration, and virulence of the irritant. A very low-grade, subclinical response may lead to an increase in the bone density rather than resorption and lucency. This lesion may be clinically asymptomatic and radiographically can demonstrate increased trabeculation and opacity (Fig. 12-23). Microscopically, dense bone with growth lines is prevalent with a mild chronic inflammatory infiltrate in the marrow spaces. Not much is known about this lesion, but if it is associated with a necrotic or diseased pulp endodontic therapy may lead to healing.

Role of epithelium

One of the normal components of the lateral and apical periodontal ligament is the epithelial rests of Malassez. The term *rests* is misleading in that it evokes a vision of discrete islands of epithelial cells. It has been shown that these rests are actually a fishnet-like, three-dimensional network of epithelial cells. In many periapical lesions epithelium is not present and is presumed to have been destroyed.[46] If the rests remain, they may respond to the stimulus by proliferating in an attempt to wall off the irritants. The epithelium is surrounded by chronic inflammation, and this lesion is termed an epitheliated granuloma (a granuloma containing epithelium; Fig. 12-24, *A*). The epithelium continues to proliferate in an attempt to wall off the source of irritation (i.e., bacteria and products from the apical foramen). The term *bay cyst* has been coined for the microscopic representation of this situation (Fig. 12-24, *B*).[47] This is a chronic inflammatory lesion that has epithelium lining the lumen, but the lumen has a direct communication with the root canal system. It is not a true cyst, because a true cyst is a three-dimensional, epithelium-lined cavity with no communication between the lumen and the canal system (Fig. 12-24, *C*).

When periapical lesions are studied in relation to the root canal, completely epithelial lined cavities are found.[47] These are termed *true cysts*. There has been some confusion in the diagnosis when lesions are studied only on curetted biopsy material. Since the tooth is not attached to the lesion, orientation to the apex is lost. Therefore, the criterion used for diagnosis of a cyst is "a strip of epithelium that appears to be lining a cavity." It is apparent that curetting both a bay cyst and a true cyst could give the same microscopic diagnosis: a bay cyst could be sectioned in such a way that it could resemble or give the appearance of a true cyst.

The distinction between a bay and a true cyst is important from the standpoint of healing.[11] Endodontists state that they heal some cysts with nonsurgical root canal treatment, whereas surgeons state that cysts have to be surgically excised.[6,7,36] It may be that true cysts have to be surgically removed, but bay cysts that communicate with the root canal may heal with nonsurgical root canal therapy. Since root canal therapy can directly affect the lumen of the bay cyst, the environmental change may bring about resolution of the lesion. The true cyst is independent of the root canal system, so conventional therapy may have no effect on it. This would explain the discrepancy between the endodontic and surgical opinions on the treatment of cysts. The formation of a cyst and its progression from a bay cyst to a true cyst occurs over time. Vaulderhaug showed in monkeys that no cysts were formed until at least 6 months after the canal contents became necrotic. Thus, the longer a lesion has been present the greater is its chance of becoming a true cyst. The prevalence of true cysts is probably less than 10%.[47]

Another microscopic finding in epithelium is the occurrence of Rushton bodies. These have been described as hyaline (glasslike) bodies that occur only within the epithelium (Fig. 12-25). Formerly they were thought to be packed red blood cells. However, studies now show that they are not composed of erythrocytes but are probably an epithelial secretion.

Healing

Healing of periapical disease may lead to scar formation. This occurs when the tissue that was originally present is replaced with dense fibrous connective tissue after the irritant has been destroyed.[41] Scar formation may also occur after surgical intervention takes place, where both the buccal and the lingual cortical plates have been lost (Fig. 12-1). This shows as a radiolucency but does not require treatment. For all intents and purposes this lesion has healed. Microscopically there is an abundance of dense collagen bundles with some fibroblasts. In the earlier stages of healing, macrophages, fibroblasts, and capillary buds may be present (Fig. 12-26).

In summary, periapical disease is caused by combinations of bacteria, usually anaerobic, bacterial products, and the host's response to them (inflammation). The different periapical diagnoses only reflect different stages in the inflammatory

Text continued on p. 361.

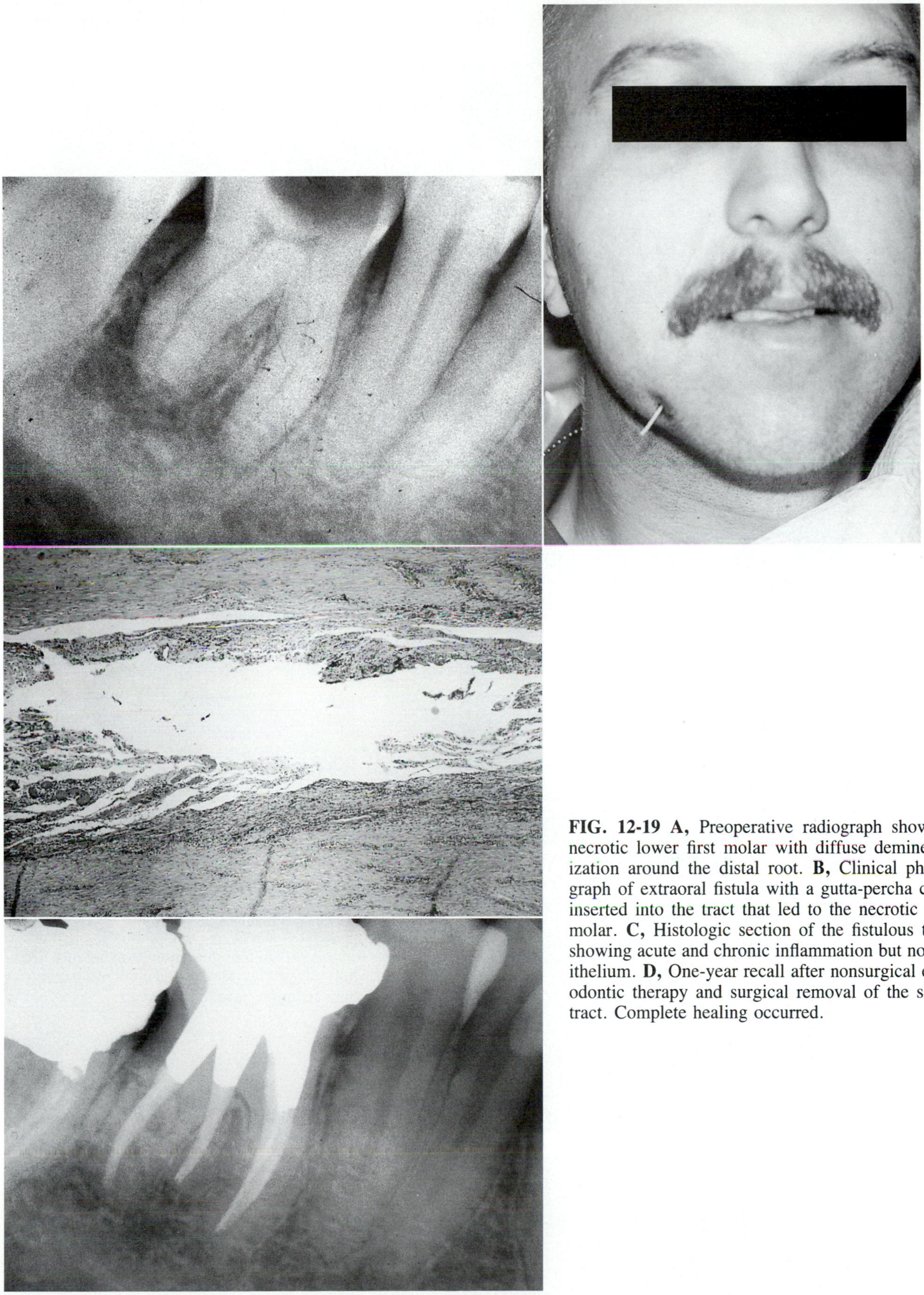

A

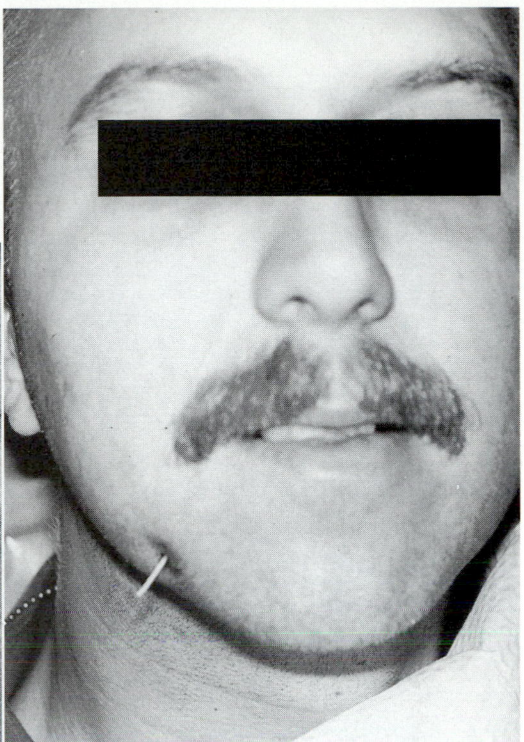

B

C

D

FIG. 12-19 A, Preoperative radiograph showing necrotic lower first molar with diffuse demineralization around the distal root. **B,** Clinical photograph of extraoral fistula with a gutta-percha cone inserted into the tract that led to the necrotic first molar. **C,** Histologic section of the fistulous tract showing acute and chronic inflammation but no epithelium. **D,** One-year recall after nonsurgical endodontic therapy and surgical removal of the sinus tract. Complete healing occurred.

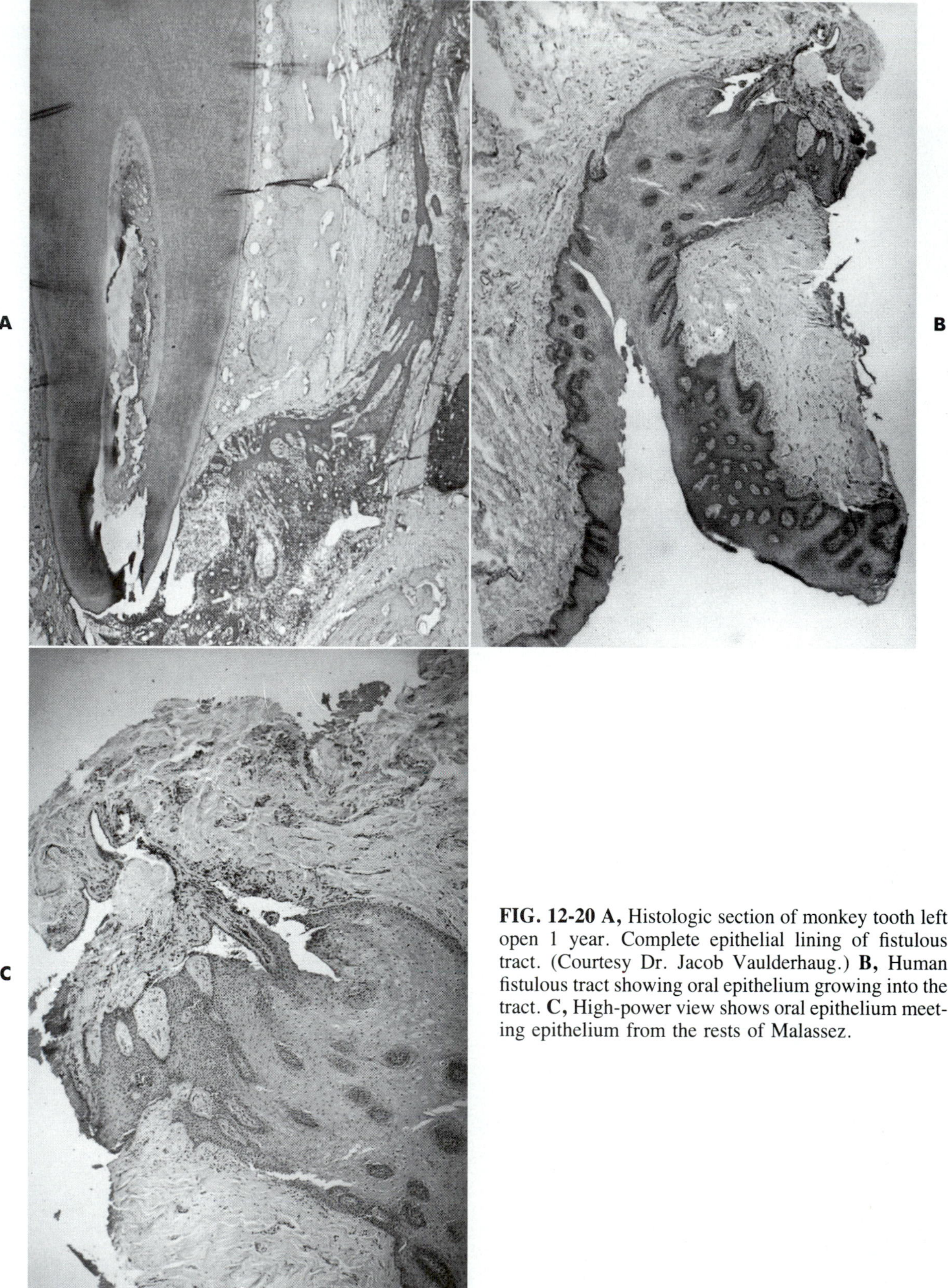

FIG. 12-20 A, Histologic section of monkey tooth left open 1 year. Complete epithelial lining of fistulous tract. (Courtesy Dr. Jacob Vaulderhaug.) **B,** Human fistulous tract showing oral epithelium growing into the tract. **C,** High-power view shows oral epithelium meeting epithelium from the rests of Malassez.

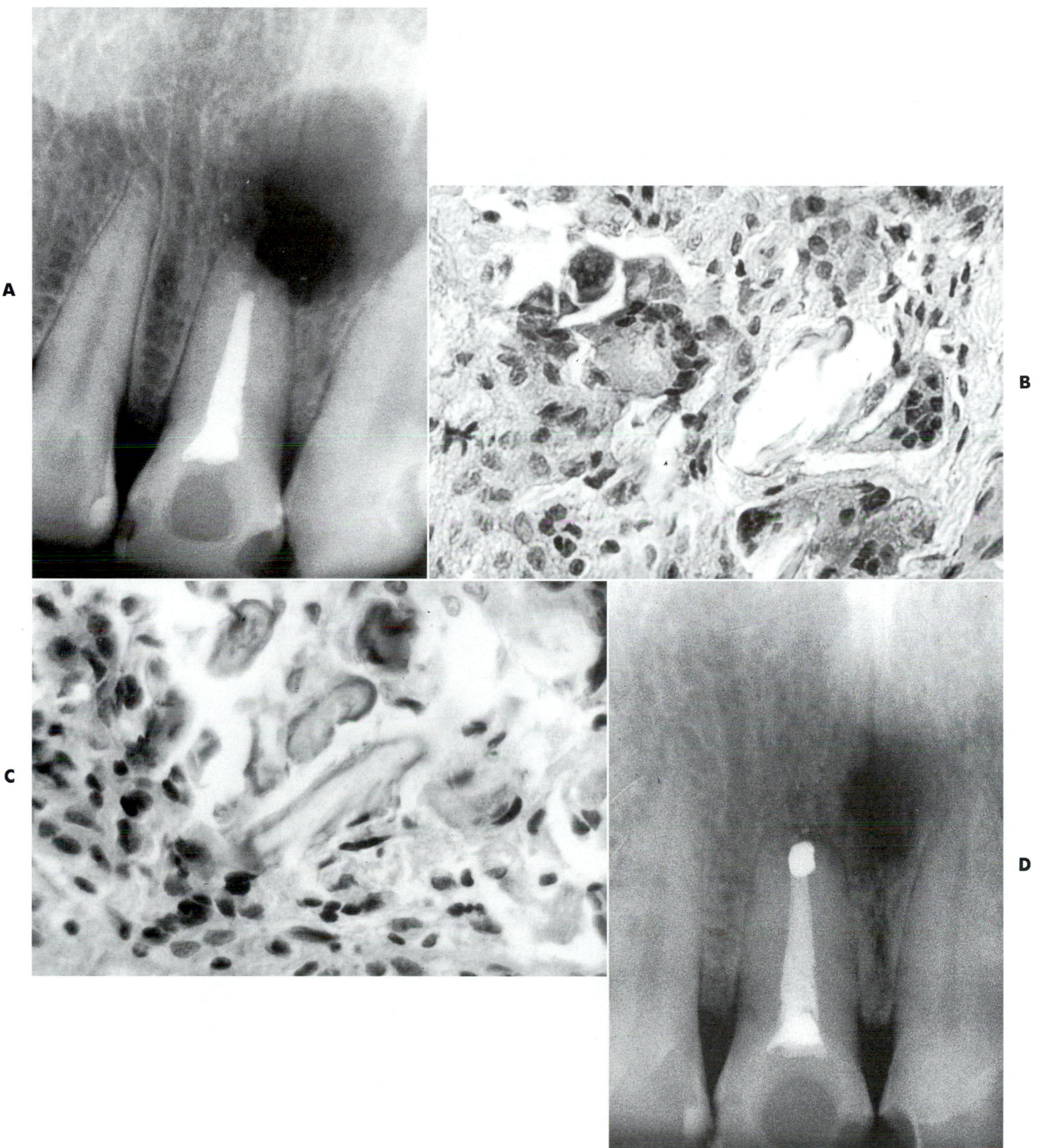

FIG. 12-21 A, A central incisor with large periapical lesion. Endodontic treatment was performed 27 years ago. **B,** Histologic section of lesion showing giant cells and foreign bodies. **C,** High-power view of foreign body particles. **D,** After surgical removal healing occurs 1 year later.

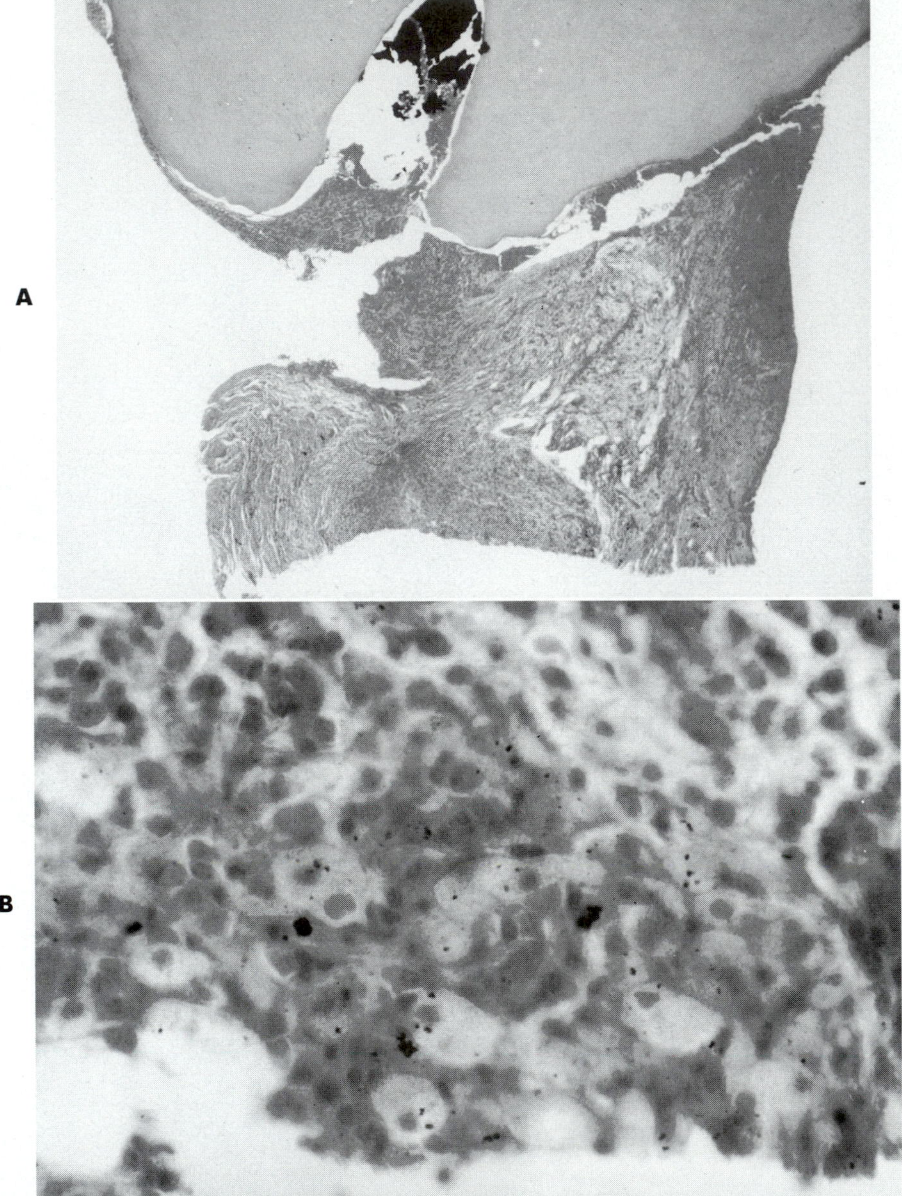

FIG. 12-22 A, Histologic section of necrotic lower bicuspid with attached periapical lesion. Note black foreign material in the canal. **B,** High-power view of central part of the lesion showing black foreign body particles and large macrophages.

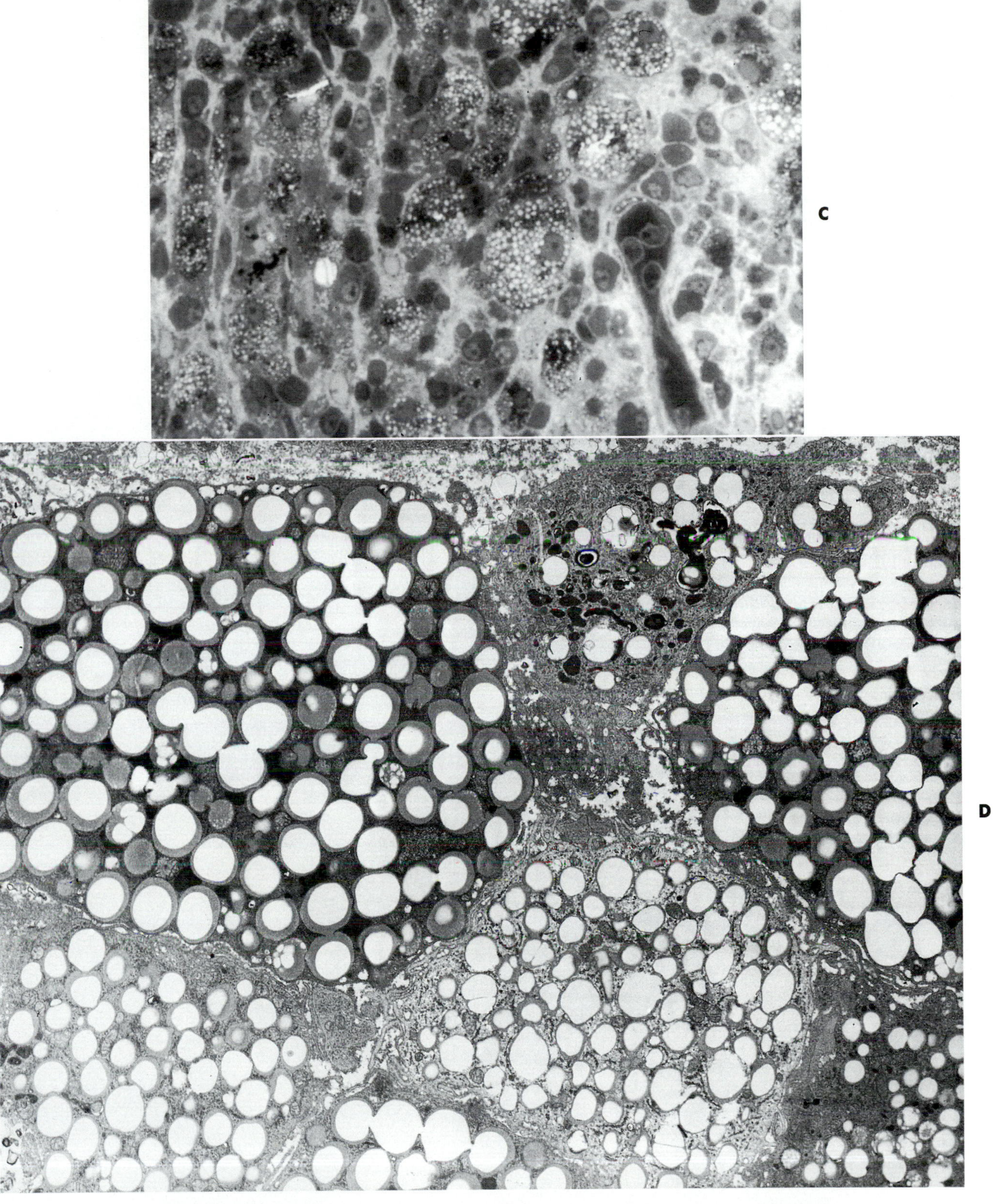

FIG. 12-22, cont'd C, One micron sections stained with methylene blue. Note large particles filling the cytoplasm of the macrophages. **D,** Transmission electron micrograph showing the entire cytoplasm of the macrophages full of foreign material. No cellular organelles are visible.

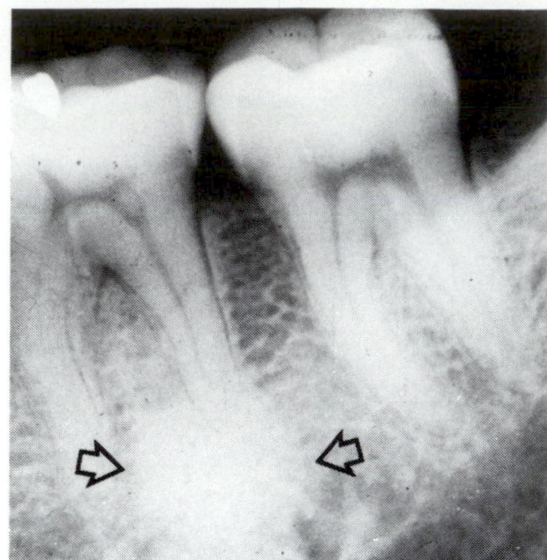

FIG. 12-23 Increased radiopacity *(arrows)* and trabeculation around the distal root of the mandibular first molar.

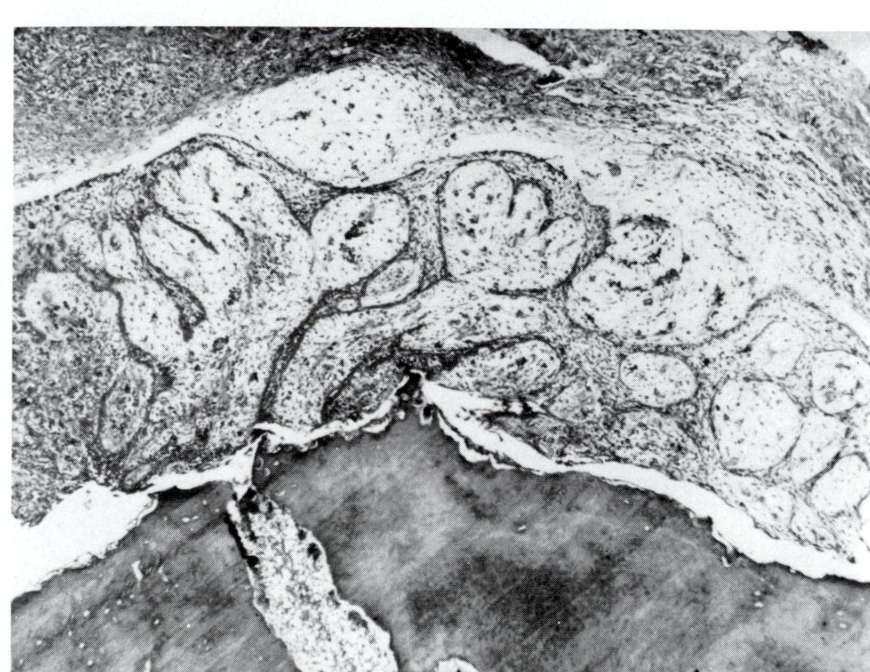

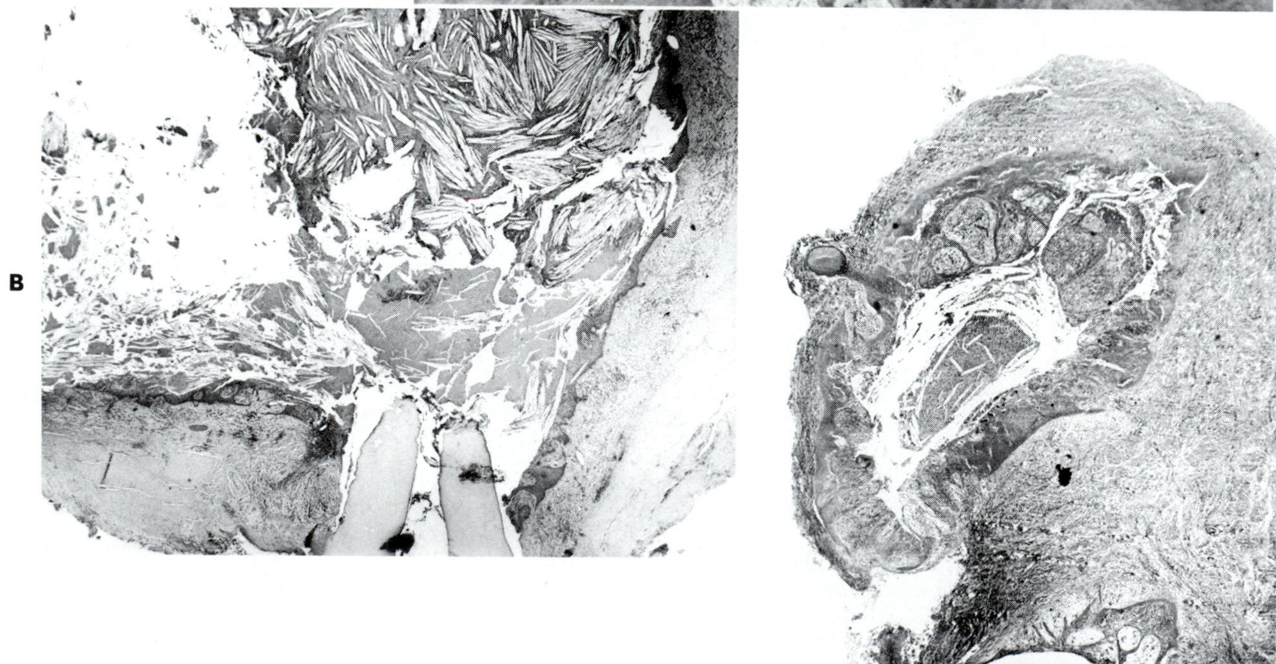

FIG. 12-24 A, Chronic apical periodontitis with proliferating cords of epithelium. **B,** Low-power photomicrograph of a bay cyst or apical periodontal pocket. The root canal opens directly into the lumen of this epithelium-lined lesion. **C,** Low-power photomicrograph of a true cyst. This is a cavity completely lined with epithelium that does not communicate with the root canal system.

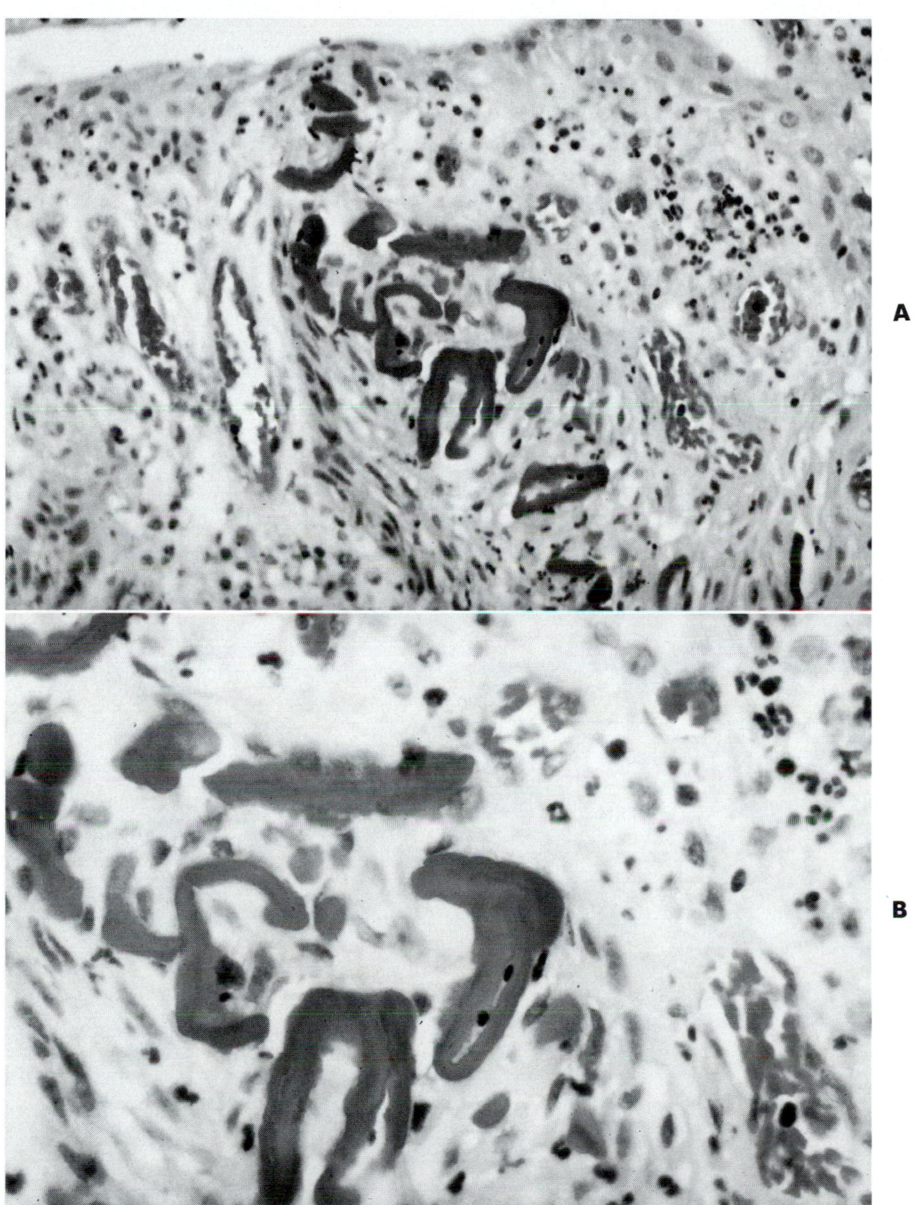

FIG. 12-25 A, Low-power photomicrograph of epithelium containing Rushton bodies. **B,** High-power view of "hyaline bodies."

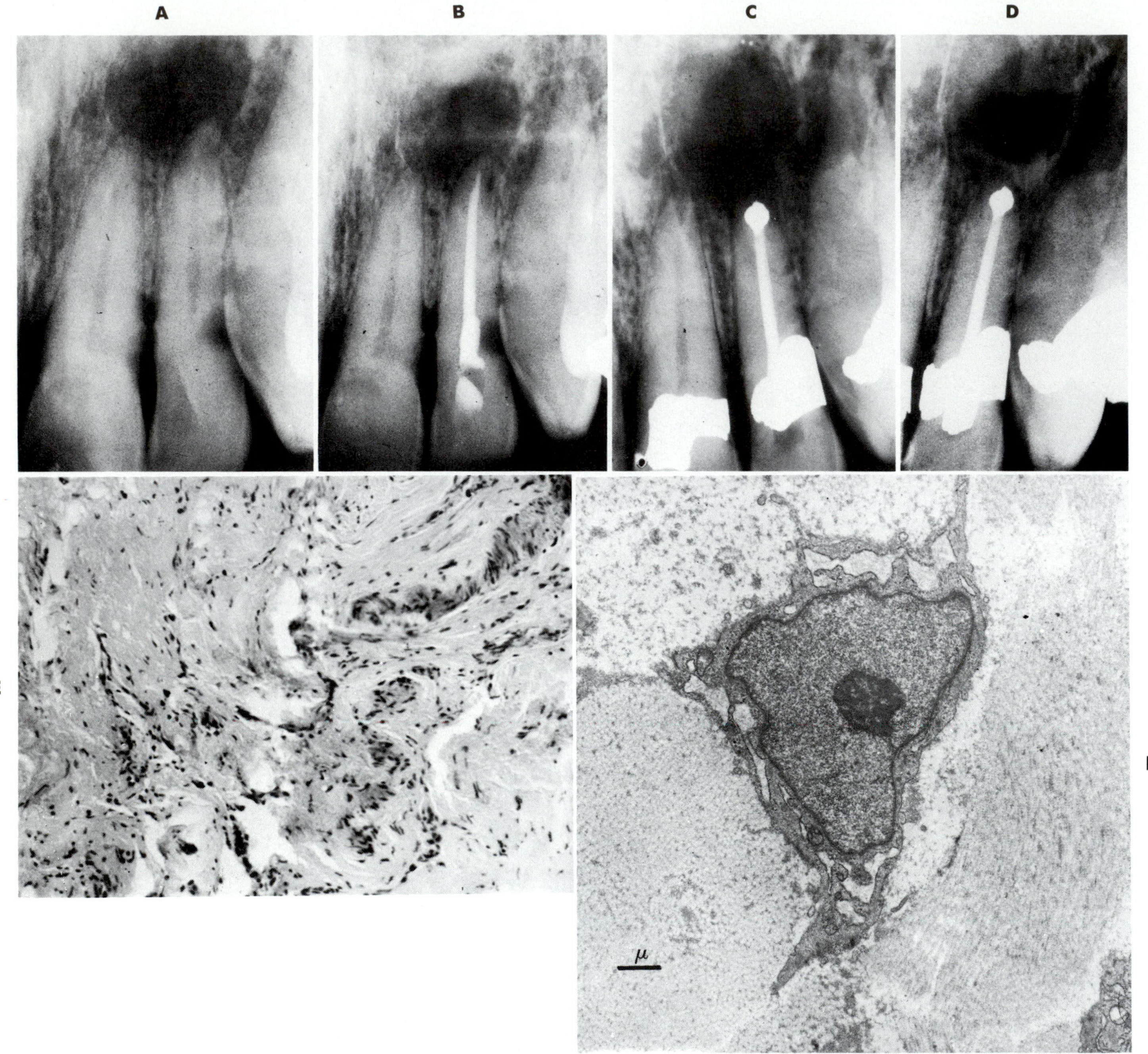

FIG. 12-26 A, Preoperative. **B,** Postoperative. **C,** Six months later. **D,** At 6-year recall. Note the apparent periapical healing. **E,** Biopsy of the lesion revealed dense connective tissue with scattered inflammatory cells. Diagnosis was an apical scar. (Original magnification, ×2200.) **F,** Fibroblast surrounded by dense collagen fibers. (Original magnification ×12,400.)

response. These lesions are not static but are capable of changing. They are static only under the microscope.

ACKNOWLEDGMENTS

A special thanks to David Mayeda, D.D.S., and Stephen Davis, D.D.S., for their contribution in the preparation of this manuscript; Sant Seckhon, Ph.D., and Nora L. Tong, M.A., of the Veterans Affairs Medical Center, Long Beach, California, for the transmission electron microscopic work displayed in this chapter.

REFERENCES

1. Barnett F, et al: Demonstration of *Bacteroides intermedius* in periapical tissue using indirect immunofluorescence microscopy, Endod Dent Traumatol 6:153, 1990.
2. Barnett F, et al: Ciprofloxacin treatment of periapical *Pseudomonas aeruginosa* infection, Endod Dent Traumatol 4:132, 1988.
3. Baumgartner JC, and Falkler WA Jr: Bacteria in the apical 5 mm of infected root canals, J Endod 17:380,1991.
4. Baumgartner JC, and Falkler WA Jr: Detection of immunoglobulins from explant cultures of periapical lesions, J Endod 17:105, 1991.
5. Baumgartner JC, and Falkler WA: Reactivity of IgG from explant cultures of periapical lesions with implicated microorganisms, J Endod 17:207, 1991.
6. Bhaskar SN: Periapical lesions—types, incidence, and clinical features, Oral Surg 21:657, 1966.
7. Bhaskar SN: Nonsurgical resolution of radicular cysts, Oral Surg 38:458, 1972.
8. Block RM, et al: A histopathologic, histobacteriologic, and radiographic study of periapical endodontic surgical specimens, Oral Surg 42:656, 1976.
9. Brynolf I: A histologic and roentgenologic study of the periapical region of human upper incisors, Odont Rev 18(suppl 2):1, 1976.
10. Bystrom A, et al: Healing of periapical lesions of pulpless teeth after endodontic treatment with controlled asepsis. Endod Dent Traumatol 3:58, 1987.
11. Cohen M: Pathways of inflammatory cellular exudate through radicular cyst epithelium: SEM study, J Oral Pathol 8:369, 1979.
12. Cymerman JJ, et al: Human T lymphocyte subpopulations in chronic periapical lesions, J Endod 10:9, 1984.
13. Dwyer TG, and Torabinejad M: Radiographic and histologic evaluation of the effect of endotoxin on the periapical tissues of the cat, J Endod 7:31, 1981.
14. Eisen HN: Immunology, ed 2, New York, 1980, Harper & Row.
15. Fish EW: Bone infection, J Am Dent Assoc 26:691, 1939.
16. Fouad A, et al: Induced periapical lesions in ferret canines: histologic and radiographic evaluation, Endod Dent Traumatol 8:56, 1992.
17. Greening AB, et al: Apical lesions contain elevated immunoglobulin G levels, J Endod 6:867, 1980.
18. Happonen RP: Periapical actinomycosis: a follow-up study of 16 surgically treated cases, Endod Dent Traumatol 2:205, 1986.
19. Hedman WJ: An investigation into residual periapical infection after pulp canal therapy, Oral Surg 4:1173, 1951.
20. Iwu C, et al: The microbiology of periapical granulomas, Oral Surg 69:502, 1990.
21. Reference deleted in proof.
22. Johannessen AC, et al: Deposits of immunoglobulins and complement factor C3 in human dental periapical inflammatory lesions, Scand J Dent Res 91:191, 1983.
23. Kakehashi S, Stanley HR, and Fitzgerald RJ: The effects of surgical exposure of dental pulps in germ-free and conventional laboratory rats, Oral Surg 20:340, 1965.
24. Kantz and Henry 1974.
25. Kettering JD, and Torabinejad M: Concentrations of immune complexes, IgG, IgM, IgE and C3 in patients with acute apical abscesses, J Endod 10:417, 1984.
26. Koppang HS, et al: Cellulose fibers from endodontic paper points as an etiologic factor in post-endodontic periapical granulomas and cysts, J Endod 15:369, 1989.
27. Korzen BH, Krakow AA, and Green DB: Pulpal and periapical tissue responses in conventional and noninfected gnotobiotic rats, Oral Surg 37:782, 1974.
28. Kuntz DD, et al: Localization of immunoglobulins and the third component of complement in dental periapical lesions, J Endod 3:68, 1977.
29. Lalonde ER, and Luebke RG: The frequency and distribution of periapical cysts and granulomas, Oral Surg 25:861, 1968.
30. Langeland K, Block RM, and Grossman LI: A histopathologic and histobacteriologic study of 35 periapical endodontic surgical specimens, J Endod 3:8, 1977.
31. McNicholas S, et al: The concentrations of prostaglandin E_2 in human periradicular lesions, J Endod 17:97, 1991.
32. Malmstrom M: Immunoglobulin classes of IgG, IgM, IgA and complement components C3 in dental periapical lesions of patients with rheumatoid disease, Scand J Rheumatol 4:57, 1975.
33. Menkin V: Dynamics of inflammation, New York, 1940, Macmillan Publishing Co, Inc.
34. Moller AJR, et al: Influence on periapical tissues of indigenous oral bacteria and necrotic pulp tissue in monkeys, Scand J Dent Res 890:475, 1981.
35. Morse DR, Lasater DR, and White D: Presence of immunoglobulin producing cells in periapical lesions, J Endod 1:338, 1975.
36. Mortensen H, Winther JE, and Birn H: Periapical granulomas and cysts: an investigation of 1600 cases, Scand J Dent Res 78:141, 1971.
37. Morton TH, Clagett JA, and Yavorsky JD: Role of immune complexes in human periapical periodontitis, J Endod 3:261, 1977.
38. Nair R: Light and electron microscopic studies of root canal flora and periapical lesions, J Endod 13:29, 1987.
39. Reference deleted in proof.
40. Nevins AJ, et al: Sensitization via IgE-mediated mechanism in patients with chronic periapical lesions, J Endod 11:228, 1985.
41. Patterson SS, Shafer WG, and Healey HJ: Periapical lesions associated with endodontically treated teeth, J Am Dent Assoc 68:191, 1964.
42. Piatelli A, et al: Immune cells in periapical granuloma; morphological and immunohistochemical characterization, J Endod 17:26, 1991.
43. Ranta K, Haapasalo M, and Ranta H: Monoinfection of root canals with *Pseudomonas aeruginosa,* Endod Dent Traumatol 4:269, 1988.
44. Roane JB, and Marshall FJ: Osteomyelitis: a complication of pulpless teeth, Oral Surg 34:257, 1972.
45. Roitt I, Brostoff J, and Male D: Immunology, London, 1985, Gower Medical Publishing.
46. Seltzer S, Soltanoff W, and Bender IB: Epithelial proliferation in periapical lesions, Oral Surg 27:111, 1969.
47. Simon JHS: Incidence of periapical cysts in relation to the root canal, J Endod 6:845, 1980.
48. Sjogren U, et al: Survival of *Arachnia propionica* in periapical tissue, Int Endod J 21:277, 1988.
49. Stabholz A, and McArthur WP: Cellular immune response of patients with periapical pathosis to necrotic dental pulp antigens determined by release of LIF, J Endod 4:282, 1978.
50. Sundquist G, Johansson E, and Sjogren U: Prevalence of black-pigmented *Bacteroides* species in root canal infections, J Endod 15:13, 1989.
51. Ten Cate AR: The epithelial cell rests of Malassez and the genesis of the dental cyst, Oral Surg 34:957, 1972.
52. Toller P: Origin and growth of cysts of the jaws, Ann R Coll Surg Engl 40:306, 1967.
53. Torabinejad M, et al: Concentrations of leukotriene B4 in symptomatic and asymptomatic periapical lesions, Endodont 18:205, 1992.
54. Torabinejad M, and Bakland LK: Immunopathogenesis of chronic periapical lesions, Oral Surg 46:685, 1978.
55. Torabinejad M, and Bakland LK: Prostaglandins: their possible role in the pathogenesis of pulpal and periapical disease, Part I, J Endod 6:733-769, 1980.
56. Torabinejad M, and Kettering JD: Detection of immune complexes in human dental periapical lesions by anticomplement immunofluorescence technique, Oral Surg 48:256, 1979.

57. Torabinejad M, and Kettering JD: Identification and relative concentration of B and T lymphocytes in human chronic periapical lesions, J Endod 11:122, 1985.
58. Torabinejad M, Kettering JD, and Bakland LK: Localization of IgE immunoglobulin in human dental periapical lesions by the peroxidase-antiperoxidase method, Arch Oral Biol 26:677, 1981.
59. Tronstad L, et al: Periapical bacterial plaque in teeth refractory to endodontic treatment, Endod Dent Traumatol 6:73, 1990.
60. Tronstad L, et al: Extraradicular endodontic infections, Endod Dent Traumatol 3:86, 1987.
61. Trowbridge H, and Emling RC: Inflammation, a review of the process, ed 3 Chicago, 1989, Quintessence Publishing Co., Inc.
62. Walton RE, and Ardjmand K: Histological evaluation of the presence of bacteria in induced periapical lesions in monkeys, J Endod 18:216, 1992.
63. Walton RE, and Garnick JJ: The histology of periapical inflammatory lesions in permanent molars in monkeys, J Endod 12:49, 1986.
64. Wayman B, et al: A bacteriological and histological evaluation of 58 periapical lesions, J Endod 18:152, 1992.
65. Wesselink PR, Thoden van Velzen SK, and Makkes PC: Release of endotoxin in an experimental model simulation the dental root canal, Oral Surg 45:789, 1978.

Self-assessment questions

1. In acute inflammation, the first cells to pass through the blood vessel walls into the tissue are
   a. eosinophils.
   b. lymphocytes.
   c. monocytes.
   d. polymorphonuclear neutrophils (PMNs).
2. Following monocyte white cell migration from the vessel to the tissue, the monocyte becomes a
   a. neutrophil.
   b. basophil.
   c. macrophage.
   d. histiocyte.
3. In the inflammatory process, which of the following cell types function as phagocytes?
   a. Macrophages and lymphocytes.
   b. Lymphocytes and neutrophils.
   c. Plasma cells and basophils.
   d. Neutrophils and macrophages.
4. Which of the following results may be expected following surgery when both the buccal and lingual cortical plates have been lost?
   a. Ankylosis.
   b. Scar tissue formation.
   c. Osteosclerosis.
   d. Normal bone regeneration.
5. A foreign body reaction is characterized by the presence of
   a. neutrophils.
   b. plasma cells.
   c. giant cells.
   d. fibroblasts.
6. Acute osteomyelitis is typically characterized by
   a. a draining sinus tract.
   b. a large diffuse radiolucency.
   c. necrotic bone.
   d. cellulitis.
7. T lymphocytes arise as immature cells in the
   a. bone marrow.
   b. thymus.
   c. lymph nodes.
   d. inflammatory lesion.
8. Which of the following would predominate in the zone of irritation?
   a. Bacteria.
   b. Chronic inflammatory cells.
   c. Capillary buds.
   d. Necrotic elements.
9. The periapical lesion that would most likely contain bacteria within the lesion is
   a. apical abscess.
   b. apical cyst.
   c. periapical granuloma.
   d. condensing osteitis.
10. Leukocytes move through the endothelium and into tissue by a process known as
    a. diapedesis.
    b. emigration.
    c. transudation.
    d. margination.
11. Opsonization facilitates
    a. mitosis of fibroblasts.
    b. chemotaxis of neutrophils.
    c. vasodilatation.
    d. phagocytosis.
12. A chemical mediator of inflammation that is responsible for early vascular response to injury is
    a. C_3a.
    b. C_5a.
    c. histamine.
    d. bradykinin.
13. The factor that is responsible for stimulating nerve endings to cause the pain associated with acute apical periodontitis is
    a. fluid pressure.
    b. histamine.
    c. complement.
    d. neutrophilic enzymes.
14. A sinus tract associated with a suppurative apical periodontitis usually
    a. is lined with epithelium.
    b. should be cauterized or removed surgically.
    c. will not heal unless the microorganisms are curetted from the apical area.
    d. requires no special treatment other than root canal treatment of the offending tooth.
15. What is the usual histologic picture of the pulp in a tooth with a chronic apical periodontitis (dental granuloma)?
    a. Pulpal abscess in the coronal pulp with chronic inflammation in the radicular pulp.
    b. Necrotic pulp.
    c. The majority of the pulp exhibits chronic inflammation.
    d. Chronic inflammation in the coronal pulp and the radicular pulp appears normal.
16. Chronic apical periodontitis (granuloma) presents a histologic picture that is most consistent with
    a. infection.
    b. early cyst formation.
    c. healing.
    d. immune response.

Chapter 13

Microbiology and Immunology

James D. Kettering
Mahmoud Torabinejad

Most pulpal and periradicular diseases are induced as a result of direct or indirect involvement of oral bacteria. This was demonstrated nearly a century ago[83] and has been confirmed with more advanced bacteriologic and immunologic tests. Based on present knowledge, it appears that most changes in pulpal and periradicular tissues are of bacterial origin and have to be dealt with as infectious processes. Because bacteria play a major role in the pathogenesis of pulpal and periradicular lesions, a fundamental knowledge of endodontic microbiology is needed to understand (1) the role of bacteria in these diseases, (2) pathways of pulpal and periradicular infections, (3) the pulpal and periradicular responses to bacterial infection, and (4) the methods used to eradicate and control root canal infections during root canal therapy. Tronstad[139] has summarized recent developments in endodontic research, relating how these principles apply to the management of patients with endodontic problems.

THE ROLE OF BACTERIA IN PULPAL AND PERIRADICULAR DISEASES

The dental pulp has been described as a unique organ with limited capacity to heal after it is subjected to repeated insults.[107] The intact hard tissues of the tooth normally protect the pulp by acting as physical barriers to noxious irritants. These tissues can also be viewed as structures that, while protecting, can physically restrict pulpal inflammation during tissue injuries. Any pulpal injury can result in inflammation and its consequences, such as increased vascular permeability, vasodilatation, pain, hard tissue resorption, and, sometimes, pulpal necrosis. Although irritants can be physical, thermal, or chemical, microbes are considered to be the major cause of pulpal and periradicular pathosis.

Miller,[83] in 1890, demonstrated the presence of bacteria in necrotic human pulp tissue. Since then a number of studies have implicated bacteria as prerequisite for pulpal and periradicular diseases.[18,39,81] Most studies investigated the flora of infected root canals and have reported the presence of numerous species of bacteria. The predominant species frequently found in infected root canals were streptococci and micrococci, and a small percentage of anaerobic bacteria.[155] Depending on the culture media and techniques of bacterial identification, types and number of isolated organisms varied significantly. Early investigations found a small incidence of anaerobic bacteria, whereas recent studies have reported a prevalence as great as 90% for these bacteria in the infected root canals.[15,57,123]

To determine the importance of bacteria, Kakehashi and associates exposed the dental pulps of conventional and germ-free (gnotobiotic) rats to their own flora, which resulted in the development of pulpal and periradicular lesions in conventional rats, but failed to create lesions in germ-free rats.[56]

An investigation[64] studied the effects of normal oral flora and monoinfection *(Streptococcus mutans)* on the pulp and periradicular tissues of conventional and gnotobiotic rats. Its results showed that the severity of pulpal and periradicular inflammation were directly related to the quantity of microorganisms in the root canals and to how long these tissues were exposed to the microorganisms. Furthermore, it showed that the degree of inflammation was less severe with monoinfection than with mixed infection. Up to the early 1970s most microbiological studies on root canal flora reported primarily the presence of facultative bacteria in this system.[87] However, technological advances in the isolation of anaerobes, and increased awareness by the medical and dental professions of the role of anaerobes in various diseases, caused significant changes in medical and dental bacteriology. Based on the results of more recent studies, it appears that root canal infections are multibacterial and that anaerobic organisms, namely *Bacteroides* species, play a significant role in clinical signs and symptoms of pulpal and periapical disease.[118,123] *Bacteroides* species have recently undergone classification changes. New genus names, *Porphyromonas* and *Prevotella,* have been assigned to many of the *Bacteroides* organisms routinely mentioned in endodontic research and clinical reports. Since both genus names are still encountered, we list both for clarity.

Other investigators, in a series of experiments, examined the importance of bacteria in the development of periradicular lesions, composition of root canal, flora, and the influence of a combination of oral bacteria on periradicular tissues of monkeys. In one study[85] these researchers severed the pulps of teeth in monkeys. The amputated pulps were either immediately sealed aseptically or left open to be contaminated with indigenous oral flora for one week and then sealed. After 6 to 7 months, clinical, radiographic, and histologic examinations of the teeth that were sealed aseptically showed no pathologic changes in the periradicular tissues. In contrast, teeth with infected root canals had inflammatory reactions in their tissues. In another experiment,[36] the investigators mechanically devitalized the pulps of monkeys, left them exposed to oral flora for a week, and then sealed them for 3, 6, and 35 months. Bacteriologic examinations of infected root canals at the end of these observation periods showed that 85% to 98% of the isolated bacteria were anaerobic. The most frequently found anaerobic species were *Bacteroides* and gram-positive anaerobic rods. A small percentage of facultative anaerobic bacteria were also isolated from the infected root canals.

Like most bacteria, anaerobes require specific environmental conditions for growth. Several investigators have shown that anaerobic bacteria such as *Bacteroides* are usually isolated from mixed infections and acquire some of their nutritional needs from their accompanying infective organisms,[86,114,122] One study[42] reported that hemin and vitamin K were essential elements for the growth of certain strains of *Prevotella (Bacteroides) melaninogenica.*

Later, Socransky and Gibbons[114] showed in an animal study that these substances could be provided to *Prevotella (Bacteroides) melaninogenica* by gram-positive bacteria in mixed infections. Recent studies[75,77] suggest that presence of hemin or succinates significantly increases the virulence of *Porphyromonas (Bacteroides) gingivalis.*

Fabricius and co-workers[35] inoculated 75 root canals of monkeys with 11 bacterial species separately, or in combinations, and sealed the access cavities for a period of 6 months. Their bacteriologic and histologic examinations showed that mixed infections have a greater capacity to cause apical lesions than monoinfections. Furthermore, they reported that the *Bacteroides* strain did not survive in the root canals when inoculated as pure cultures. Enterococci survived as pure cultures, and facultative streptococci induced small periradicular lesions. Sundqvist[123] demonstrated a high correlation between presence of *Prevotella (Bacteroides) melaninogenica* and clinical and radiographic signs and symptoms of periradicular pathosis. Griffee and associates[44] also found a similar correlation between the presence of this organism and pain, sinus tract formation, and foul odor. Other researchers[159] found that *Peptococcus magnus* and *Bacteroides* species were commonly associated with symptomatic cases, whereas oral streptococci and enteric bacteria were isolated from asymptomatic cases. Recently, Haapsalo[48] reported on the bacteriology of 62 infected human root canals, giving special attention to the *Bacteroides* species. His results confirm the findings of previous investigations: almost all root canal infections are mixed, and acute symptoms are usually related to the presence of specific anaerobes, such as *Porphyromonas (Bacteroides) gingivalis, Porphyromonas (Bacteroides) endodontalis,* and *Prevotella (Bacteroides) buccae.*

Brook and colleagues[14] confirmed the polymicrobial nature of bacteria isolated from aspirates of periradicular abscesses in 39 patients, with anaerobic isolates being present in more than 70% of the bacteria recovered. Wasfy and co-workers[149] obtained similar results in the microbiologic evaluation of periradicular infections in 85 adult Egyptians, when they found that anaerobic bacteria were the predominant flora in specimen cultures. Anaerobes comprised 73% (190/259) of cultivable bacteria.

PATHWAYS OF PULPAL AND PERIAPICAL INFECTIONS

Under normal circumstances, pulp tissue and its surrounding dentin are protected by the enamel and cementum. Natural absence, caries, or iatrogenic removal of enamel or cementum exposes the dentin (and, eventually, the pulp tissue) to the injurious effects of mechanical, chemical, and microbial irritants. The major pathways of pulpal contamination are exposed dentinal tubules, direct pulp exposure, lateral and apical foramen, and blood-borne bacteria.

Dentinal Tubules

Following loss of enamel and/or cementum, the dentinal tubules become exposed to the bacteria in the oral cavity. The dentinal tubules extend from the pulp to the dentinoenamel and cementodentinal junction. The diameters of these tubules are approximately 2.5 μm near the pulp and about 1 μm at the dentinoenamel and cementodentinal junction.[41] Although an actual quantitation of the dentinal tubules has not been performed, their numbers are large: approximately 15,000 dentinal tubules in a square millimeter of dentin near the cementodentinal junction.[50] Because of the size and numbers of tubules in the dentin, microorganisms can enter, multiply, and invade numerous exposed tubules.

A number of investigators have demonstrated bacteria within the exposed dentinal tubules of vital and pulpless teeth.[26,91,106] Experiments in vivo and in vitro show that dentinal tubules of viable dentin are not easily invaded by oral microorganisms.[91] Slow invasion of viable dentin by bacteria might be due to the presence of natural resistance factors in the dentin and the pulp tissue.

Hoshino and associates[53] used anaerobic procedures to demonstrate the early bacterial invasion of unexposed dental pulps, which were covered by clinically sound dentin beneath the carious lesions. Six of nine teeth had bacterial invasion, the predominant organisms being obligate anaerobes. They concluded that the organisms isolated in this study had passed through some individual dentinal tubules on the way to invasion of the dental pulp.

One investigator[26] who demonstrated bacteria in the dentinal tubules of pulpless teeth attributed their presence to the invasion of these tubules after pulpal necrosis. Presence of bacteria, their by-products, and other irritants in the dentinal tubules usually results in inflammatory responses in pulpal tissue. Pulpal inflammation can also occur when dentinal tubules transport irritants from incipient caries to the pulp or when the tubules contain and permit passage of microorganisms present beneath the restorative dental materials or next to periodontal pockets.[1,10,79] Leakage studies[10,100] indicate that bacterial penetration around dental materials may contribute more to pathogenic changes in pulpal tissue than do the chemicals present in these materials. Another study[1] examined the presence of bacteria in the dentin of periodontally involved teeth and compared it with that of teeth with a healthy periodontium. They found more microorganisms in the dentin and pulpal tissue of the periodontally involved teeth than in those of normal teeth. Removal of cementum during periodontal therapy can expose numerous dentinal tubules to oral flora, which can allow penetration of microorganisms into the pulp tissue. Production of a smear layer during root manipulation and calcium and phosphate ions in saliva can delay invasion of the dentinal tubules by oral microorganisms.

Infection by this means is generally thought to occur as an advancing bacterial front, and it is, therefore, slow. Most authors believe that acid-producing bacteria (with gram-positive organisms predominating) invade the tubules and demineralize the walls. Proteolytic species follow, acting on the organic matrix, which is denuded in the enlarged dentinal tubules. The acids and other metabolites and toxic products diffuse faster than the bacteria, so that the odontoblasts are affected, possibly leading to their breakdown. If the advancing bacteria are eliminated, healing may occur. Dental caries is the most common cause of pulp injury and many pulp reactions may be longstanding infections from dentinal tubules, originating from the cavity bottom and walls as a result of leaky filling materials. If untreated, bacteria finally reach pulp tissue and the inflammation ensues. Bacterial numbers increase, PMN's infiltrate, and abscesses form, leading to the death of the pulp tissue. This route of infection appears to be selective for only a few bacterial strains, mostly facultatively anaerobic bacteria found in the oral flora.

Pulp Exposure

In addition to contaminated dentinal tubules, direct pulpal exposure as a result of traumatic injuries or tooth decay can obviously cause contamination of pulpal tissue.

As a consequence of pulpal exposure to oral flora, the pulp and its surrounding dentin can harbor bacteria and their byproducts. Depending on the virulence of the bacteria, host resistance, amount of circulation, and degree of drainage, pulp tissue may stay inflamed for an extended time or it may rather rapidly become necrotic. After pulpal necrosis, the entire root canal system becomes infected with various species of bacteria, which can diffuse from this system into the periodontal ligament through the apical foramen or lateral canals. Bacteria within the root canal system usually result in development of periradicular and, sometimes, lateral lesions.

If the pulp is exposed, as with caries for example, the pulp is exposed to the entire oral flora. Alpha-hemolytic streptococci, enterococci, and lactobacilli are most often found; other facultatively anaerobic organisms are present in smaller numbers. As the depth of the necrotic pulp increases, more species of obligately anaerobic bacteria become established. These include anaerobic gram-positive cocci and gram-negative rods and are favored by the low oxygen tension found in the necrotic parts of the pulp. The mixed complex of mainly anaerobic flora present can influence the symptoms that endodontic patients may experience.

Periodontal Ligament

Although a clear cause-and-effect relationship exists between root canal infection and periradicular or lateral lesions, penetration of bacteria in the opposite direction (toward the pulp) during periodontal disease is a subject of controversy and current investigation. Theoretically, patent lateral canals and apical foramina adjacent to periodontal pockets should provide access for oral microorganisms to the root canal system. When the pulp is infected through the apical foramen, it appears that an impaired state of the pulp is always a prerequisite for infection. Only a few species of facultatively anaerobic streptococci appear to be involved. Grossman[47] applied *Serratia marcescens* over the labial gingiva of dogs' and monkeys' teeth and traumatized them with a metal weight. After recovering the same organism from pulpal tissue, he concluded that the periodontal ligament provided pathways for passage of these organisms into the pulpal tissue.

Anachoresis

Another possible source of pulpal contamination and infection is anachoresis. This phenomenon is defined as a positive attraction of blood-borne microorganisms to inflamed or necrotic tissue during bacteremia. Csernyei,[28] for the first time in 1939, demonstrated the anachoretic effect of periapical inflammation in dogs. After an application of croton oil to the pulp tissues of rats' teeth and injection of microorganism into the bloodstream, Robinson and Boling[11,102] localized the same organisms in the damaged tissues. Later, other investigators confirmed their results histopathologically.[17,113] It has been long reported that dental extractions, and even toothbrushing, can produce bacteremia.[19,105] During bacteremia, circulating microorganisms can be attracted to and can be localized in inflamed or necrotic pulps. Despite its occurrence in experimental animals, the contribution of anachoresis as a major source of pulpal infection in humans has not been fully elucidated.

Regardless of their pathways, after entering the pulp tissue the bacteria colonize, multiply, and contaminate the entire root canal system, and, possibly, the periradicular tissues. Depending on the level of oxygen tension and the presence or absence of essential nutrients in the root canal system, specific groups of bacteria survive and establish the flora of infected root canals.

FLORA OF ROOT CANAL AND PERIRADICULAR LESIONS

Most root canal infections appear to be multibacterial. At the present time a number of investigators have been or are attempting to define the role of specific microorganisms or groups of bacteria in the pathogenesis of pulpal and periradicular lesions.

Darkfield microscopy[127] represents a limited method for identifying these organisms. Yet the technique has demonstrated that cocci, rods, filaments, spirochetes, and motile organisms are present and have all been identified in infected root canals. Trope and colleagues[140] suggested that a darkfield microscopic spirochete count of lesion exudates may be useful to differentiate between an endodontic lesion or a periodontal lesion. This could be significant since successful treatment results would depend on an accurate diagnosis. More sophisticated studies are required to conclusively identify individual or groups of bacteria as causative agents. At the same time it has been suggested that some pulpless teeth appear to be sterile, including those that show radiographic evidence of periradicular pathosis. This has been used to question the exact role of microorganisms in pathologic changes in the pulp and periradicular diseases. In view of the recent reports, however, the basis of such uncertainty lies in the limited technology and interpretation of experiments in these studies.

Early studies[27,155] generally reported a predominance of facultative organisms over obligately anaerobic species. *Streptococcus* (alpha and gamma) species, gram-negative cocci, and lactobacilli were most often recovered, with a variety of anaerobes (varying in their resistance to atmospheric oxygen) usually found in numbers that constituted less than 50% of the total isolates reported. Through the use of improved techniques, a large variety of bacteria (genera and species) have been isolated from root canals and periradicular lesions. A number of studies[57,90,154] have given information that allows us to recognize a few generalities. Organisms most often found appear to be normal or usual flora of the oral cavity; only rarely is a bacterium recovered that can be shown to originate from other parts of the body. The composition of the microbiota from different infected root canals shows much variability.[90,154] The variations that are reported relate to the distribution of anaerobes versus facultative organisms and the different bacterial forms and species. In those cases where quantitation was attempted, the total count of bacteria varied from tooth to tooth.[90,154]

In general, a mixed flora of bacteria can be isolated in the various studies. This mixture usually comprises five to eight species. Studies[48,93,123] have suggested that several *Bacteroides* species are more likely to be involved, rather than just one species. Such reports must be viewed in comparison with the more than 300 bacterial species that are known to reside in the oral cavity. Obviously, the organisms that do eventually become involved in root canal infections have to survive a harsh selection process. Although finding several different species at once is common, it is usual for one or two to dominate the mixture. Table 13-1 shows a range of bacteria that have been isolated from earlier modern studies, circa 1980 to 1982.

A number of organisms have been identified at the species level; however, it is not uncommon to find results reporting different members of specific genera. Although the explanations for this limited identification are probably varied, a prime reason may be the limited capabilities of such identification processes that were available in the respective research laboratories or even clinical laboratories. Nevertheless, the combined data clearly demonstrate the variations in types and numbers of microorganisms that were isolated and identified in this period.

As more studies are published we can better appreciate the multibacterial etiology of endodontic infections. Debelian and associates[29] recovered *Propionibacterium acnes* from root canals and blood samples taken during and after patient treatment. *Actinomyces israelii* was isolated from an unusual case of a persistent infection related to a root-filled tooth.[38] *Streptococcus mutans* (NCTC 10832) was reported to be noncarcinogenic in monoinfected gnotobiotic rats by Watts and Paterson,[150] but the same organism was associated with extensive periradicular inflammation 28 days after the creation of untreated pulpal exposures.

TABLE 13-1. Typical bacteriologic report of organisms identified (circa 1980 to 1982)

Organism	Relative no.
Aerobic	
Streptococcus salivarius	3
α-Hemolytic streptococci	2
γ-Hemolytic streptococci	1
Anaerobic	
Gram-positive cocci	
Peptococcus intermedius	2
Peptococcus constellatus	3
Peptococcus species	3
Peptostreptococcus micros	4
Microaerophilic streptococci	5
Gram-negative cocci	
Veillonella parvula	44
Gram-positive bacilli	
Actinomyces species	3
Eubacterium species	1
Lactobacillus species	3
Gram-negative bacilli	
Fusobacterium nucleatum	3
Fusobacterium species	2
Bacteroides melaninogenicus species	4
Bacteroides melaninogenicus asacccharolyticus	2
Bacteroides melaninogenicus intermedius	1
Bacteroides melaninogenicus melaninogenicus	2
Bacteroides oralis	3
Bacteroides corrodens	3
Bacteroides ochraceus	1
Bacteroides bivius	1
Bacteroides species	3

(Modified from Brook I, Grimm S, and Kielich RB: Bacteriology of acute periapical abscesses in children, J Endod 7:380, 1981.)

More recent studies[69,154] have taken advantage of improved procedures and sampling methods to accurately sample anaerobic niches and maintain microorganisms' viability. Improved identification procedures, often with mechanized systems using a computer-based microorganism library, now enable investigators routinely to identify organisms to the species level. Table 13-2 contains a typical list of bacteria that have been reported in these later studies; Table 13-3 presents a current report on bacterial species recovered from periradicular lesions with possible oral cavity communication (C) and with no obvious communication (N).[152]

The black-pigmented *Bacteroides* species have gained special prominence in the search for pathogens of endodontic infections.[93,121,138] This genus, a rather heterogeneous group of microorganisms, is now divided into eight separate species, including *B. asaccharolyticus, B. corporis, B. denticola, B. endodontalis,*[143-145] *B. gingivalis, B. intermedius, B. melaninogenicus,* and *B. loeschei*. These organisms are able to produce abscesses that are severe and spread rapidly. *B. intermedius* and *B. endodontalis* appear to produce localized abscesses.[13,93] Current classification names for these organisms include *Porphyromonas (gingivalis* and *endodontalis)* and *Prevotella (melaninogenica* and *intermedia)*.

Little or no information is available on the virulence of the

TABLE 13-2. Identity of bacterial strains isolated from 50 acute peripheral abscesses

Facultative anaerobes	No. of isolates
Streptococcus milleri	25
Streptococcus mitior	3
Streptococcus mitis	3
Streptococcus mutans	1
Lactobacillus fermentum	2
Lactobacillus salivarius	1
Actinomyces odontolyticus	1
Actinomyces naeslundii	1
Actinomyces meyeri	1
Arachnia propionica	1
Haemophilus parainfluenzae	2
Capnocytophaga ochracea	1
Eikenella corrodens	1
Total	43
Strict anaerobes	**No. of isolates**
Peptostreptococcus species	14
Peptococcus species	32
Streptococcus intermedius	3
Streptococcus constellatus	1
Propionibacterium acnes	1
Eubacterium lentum	1
Veillonella parvula	3
Bacteroides oralis	20
Bacteroides gingivalis	14
Bacteroides melaninogenicus	12
Bacteroides intermedius	5
Bacteroides ruminicola	6
Bacteroides distasonis	1
Bacteroides ureolyticus	1
Bacteroides capillosus	1
Bacteroides uniformis	1
Fusobacterium nucleatum	6
Fusobacterium mortiferum	1
Total	123

(From Lewis MAO, McFarlane TW, and McGowan DA: Quantitative bacteriology of acute dentoalveolar abscesses, J Med Microbiol 21:101, 1986.)

other black-pigmented *Bacteroides* species. Haapasalo[48] has summarized the frequency of isolation of these species in human dental root canal infections.

In contrast to the presence of numerous studies on root canal flora, information on the microbiota of periapical tissues subsequent to root canal infection is both limited and controversial. Quoting Kronfield,[65] Grossman[46] states that although a tooth with a granuloma may have an infected root canal, it usually has sterile periradicular tissue: *"A granuloma is not an area in which bacteria live, but in which they are destroyed."* The relative sterility of periradicular lesions of pulpal origin has been claimed by some investigators.[67,109,115] However, others have supported the concept that bacteria are present in periradicular lesions and that their presence initiates and perpetuates such lesions.[138]

The location of and certain combinations of organisms are starting to be recognized as significant. Baumgartner and Falkler[6] examined the apical 5 mm of root canals from 10 freshly extracted teeth. Of the 50 bacterial isolates, 34 (68%) were

TABLE 13-3. Bacterial species recovered from periradicular lesions with possible oral cavity communication (C) and with no obvious communication (N)

	Facultative anaerobes		Anaerobes		Aerobes	
Species	**C**	**N**	**C**	**N**	**C**	**N**
Gram-positive cocci						
Streptococcus salivarius			1			
S. mitis			1			
S. mutans			1			
S. constellatus			1			
S. M G intermedius			1			
S. intermedius	3			3		
S. anginosus constellatus			1	1		
S. milleri			1			
S. sanguis II			2	1		
Group F β-streptococcus					1	
Staphylococcus hominis					1	
S. auricularis				1		
S. epidermidis			5	7		
S. aureus			1			
S. capitis			1	2		
S. warneri			1			
Peptostreptococcus micros	10	4				
P. anaerobius	1					
P. magnus	1					
Gamella morbillorum			1	1		
Gram-negative cocci						
Viellonella parvula	1	3				
Moraxella osloensis					1	
Gram-positive rods						
Eubacterium lentum	3					
Actinomyces odontolyticus	2	1				
A. meyeri		1				
A. israelii	2					
Propionibacterium acnes	4	4				
Corynebacterium species					4	1
C. pyogenes					1	
Lactobacillus acidophilus	1					
L. casei		1				
Bacillus pumilus				1		
Bacillus species				1		
Bifidobacterium		1				
Gram-negative rods						
Fusobacterium nucleatum	8	5				
Fusobacterium necrophorum	2					
Fusobacterium varium	1					
Fusobacterium species		1				
Bacteroides intermedius	6					
Bacteroides gracilis	4	3				
Bacteroides melaninogenicus	2	1				
Bacteroides buccae	4					
Bacteroides oris	1					
Bacteroides distasonis		1				
Bacteroides porphomonas gingivalis		1				
Bacteroides fragilis		1				
Bacteroides loeschei		1				
CDC group M-S		1				
Pseudomonas aeruginosa					1	1
Total	56	30	18	18	9	2

(Modified from Wayman BE, et al: A bacteriological and histological evaluation of 58 periapical lesions, J Endod 18:152, 1992.)

strict anaerobes, demonstrating the predominance of such organisms in this site. Walton and Ardjmand[148] found bacterial masses at the apical foramen of induced periradicular lesions in monkeys and concluded that such masses could contaminate periradicular tissues during surgery or extraction and could give a false positive result upon microbiologic sampling. Watts and Paterson[151] found bacteria in only a minority of sections of root canals and periradicular tissues of albino rats, with and without traumatic pulpal exposures. More research needs to be conducted to clearly delineate this situation.

Studies recognizing synergy or a positive correlation between species are also available. Simonson and co-workers[110] reported a highly significant synergistic relationship between *Treponema denticola* and *P. (B.) gingivalis,* while Sundqvist[119] found strong positive correlations between *Fusobacterium nucleatum* and *Peptostreptococcus micros* and *Porphyromonas endodontalis, Selenomonas sputigena,* and *Wolinella recta*. Such results are consistent with the concept of a special and selective environment in the root canal that is due, in part, to the cooperative as well as antagonistic nature of the relationships between bacteria in the root canal. A greater response of the dental pulp to combinations of *Lactobacillus plantarium* and *S. mutans* (NTCC 10919) has also been reported.[95]

Microorganisms and/or their products have been shown to be directly responsible for tissue damage or immunological responses. Extracts of *P. (B.) gingivalis* were found to be toxic to cultivated human pulpal cells and L929 cells.[97] Extensive bone loss was associated with a periradicular infection with this organism,[112] and complement activation by lipopolysaccharides purified from gram-negative bacteria isolated from infected root canals.[52] Sundqvist[120] has reviewed the selective pressures in the bacterial interrelations and the nutritional supply from the root canal. He accurately notes that endodontic treatment, apart from directly eliminating bacteria, can disrupt the delicate ecology and deprive persisting bacteria of their nutritional source.

RESPONSES OF PULPAL AND PERIRADICULAR TISSUES TO BACTERIAL INFECTION

Except for their unique anatomic locations, dental pulp and periradicular tissues react to bacterial infections as do other connective tissues elsewhere in the body. The extent of damage as a result of bacterial penetration into these tissues, as in other tissues, depends on the virulence factors of participating bacteria and the resistance factor of the host tissues. The degree of pulpal and periradicular response to bacterial irritants varies from slight tissue inflammation to complete pulpal necrosis or acute periradicular osteomyelitis with systemic signs and symptoms of severe infection.

Dental caries contain numerous species of bacteria, such as *S. mutans,* lactobacilli, and *Actinomyces* organisms.[76] The population of microorganisms decreases to few or none in the deepest layers of the carious dentin.[156] Direct exposure of pulpal tissue to microorganisms is not a prerequisite for pulpal response and inflammation.[5,12]

As a result of the presence of microorganisms in the dentin, a variety of immunocompetent cells can be recruited to the dental pulp. It is initially infiltrated by chronic inflammatory cells, such as macrophages, lymphocytes, and plasma cells. The concentration of these cells increases as the decay progresses toward the pulp. Polymorphonuclear leukocytes are the predominant cells at the site of pulp exposure.[59,157]

Pulp studies in human and rat teeth have shown the presence of immunocompetent cells and cells that recognize foreign antigens.[54,55] As a result of the interaction of microorganisms and their by-products, various mediators of inflammation, such as neuropeptides, vasoactive amines, kinins, complement components, arachidonic acid metabolites, and cytokines are released.[137]

Neuropeptides are proteins generated from somatosensory and autonomic nerve fibers following injury. They include substrate P, calcitonin gene–related peptides, and neurokinins originating from the sensory nerve fibers, as well as dopamine β-hydrolase and neuropeptide Y originating from sympathetic nerve fibers. These substances, which participate in the process of inflammation and pain transmission, were recently demonstrated in intrapupal nerve fibers using immunohistochemistry.[20,146]

The importance of vasoactive amines, such as histamine, in the pathophysiology of pulpal inflammation has been demonstrated by the presence of histamine-like substances in the walls of blood vessels in experimentally induced pulpitis[129] and by a fourfold increase in the levels of pulpal histamine after application of heat.[30] High concentrations of kinins have been found in symptomatic human periapical abscesses.[134] Kinins are considered the main mediators of the pain associated with inflammatory responses. The complement system, when activated, causes enhanced phagocytosis, increased vascular permeability, and lysis of cellular antigens. The presence in inflamed pulp of the C3 complement fragment suggests that this system participates in the pathogenesis of pulpitis.[98]

Arachidonic acid is released from the phospholipids of cell membranes as a result of cell damage. When metabolized through the cyclooxygenase or lipoxygenase pathway, various prostaglandins, thromboxanes, and leukotrienes are produced. These metabolites have been identified in experimentally induced pulpitis, and their concentrations have been significantly reduced by the use of nonsteroidal antiinflammatory medications.[68]

Specific immune reactions can also initiate and perpetuate pulpal diseases. Various classes of immunoglobulins have been found in inflamed human dental pulp and in periradicular lesions.[7,61,98] An interaction between these immunoglobulins and antigens, such as bacteria or their by-products present in dental caries, can trigger antibody-mediated responses.[49,126] Bergenholtz and associates have induced Arthus'-type reactions in the pulp tissue of sensitized monkeys.[9] Bridging of IgE molecules on mast cells in the dental pulp by antigens can initiate type I (anaphylactic) reactions in this tissue.

Although lymphocyte subtypes present in inflamed pulpal tissues have not yet been identified, it is likely that some of these cells are T lymphocytes that participate in the cell-mediated immunological response as well. The degree of pulpal inflammation is dependent on the outcome of the interaction of microorganisms, their by-products, and the resistance factors present in pulpal tissue. Based on present evidence, it appears that *Bacteroides* species play an important role in pathogenesis and in clinical signs and symptoms of pulpal and periradicular diseases. Proteinases released from these microorganisms can degrade several important defensive proteins, such as immunoglobulins and complement components.[25,89,121]

Mild infections usually do not result in significant changes in the pulp. However, moderate-to-severe insults can cause a significant release of inflammatory mediators, which results in increased vascular permeability, vascular stasis, and migration of leukocytes to this tissue. The disturbed blood flow, combined with lysosomal enzymes released from disintegrated leukocytes, can cause small abscesses and necrotic foci in the pulp. Uncontrolled pulpal infection and/or aberrant inflammatory reactions can result in total pulp necrosis and colonization of bacteria in the root canal system.[128] Egress of these organisms or their by-products from the root canal system into the periradicular tissues is the main cause for the development of apical lesions.

Numerous studies have shown that the root canal system can act as a pathway for host sensitization.[4,58,92] As in human pulpal lesions, pathologic changes associated with human periradicular lesions are also mediated by nonspecific inflammatory reactions and/or specific immune responses (Fig. 13-1).[131]

Mast cells are normally found in connective tissues and have been found in human periradicular lesions.[96] Degranulation of these mast cells is usually stimulated by antigens bridging IgE molecules on the mast cells, with the subsequent release of vasoactive amines such as histamine. Mast cells discharging vasoactive amines into the periradicular tissues can, in turn, initiate an inflammatory response or aggravate an existing inflammatory process.[131]

Several investigators have found C3 complement components in human periradicular lesions.[66,74,98] The inciting activators of the classical and alternate pathways of the complement system include: IgM and IgG, bacteria and their by-products, lysosomal enzymes from PMNs, and clotting factors. Most of these activators have been found in pathologically involved periradicular lesions. Activation of the complement system in periradicular tissues can contribute to bone resorption either by destruction of the bone or by inhibition of new bone formation.[131]

Data from several studies indicate that immune responses contribute to the formation and perpetuation of human periradicular lesions. Altered host tissue, bacteria, and their toxins and by-products present in pathologically involved root canals have the antigenic potential to initiate such responses.[40,117]

The presence of potential allergens, IgE molecules, and mast cells in human periradicular tissues indicates that all the components of an IgE-mediated reaction are present in apical lesions and that type I immune reactions can occur in these tissues. The presence of various classes of immunoglobulins[61] and immunocompetent cells, and the detection of immune complexes and C3 fragments in human apical lesions, indicate that type II and type III immune reactions can also occur in periradicular tissues.[131]

In addition to B cells and their by-products immunoglobulins, cell-mediated reactions also participate in pathogenic changes in periradicular tissues. Natural killer cells as well as other T cells have been found in chronic human apical lesions.[63,132]

By using an indirect immunoperoxidase technique, we examined the presence and relative concentration of B and T lymphocytes and their subpopulations in human apical lesions.[132] Our findings showed that there were numerous B cells, suppressor T cells, and helper T cells in these lesions and that the T cells outnumbered the B cells significantly ($P = 0.0001$). These findings have been confirmed by other investigators who have shown that T cells are more numerous than B cells.[72,125]

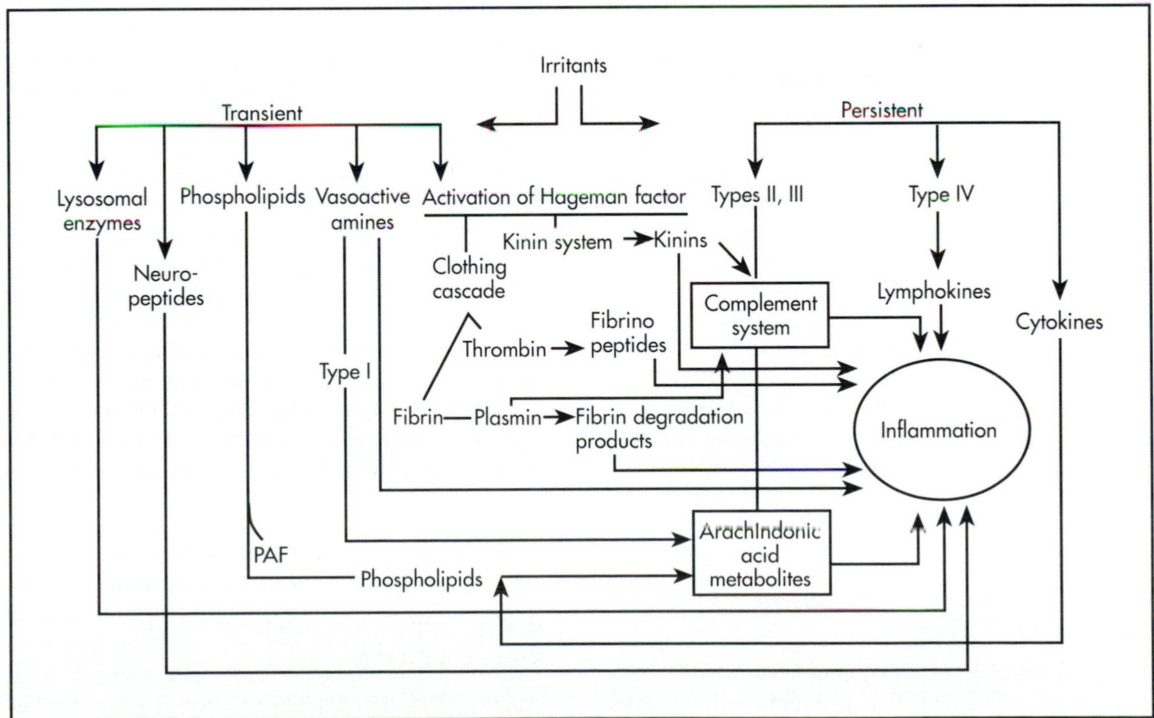

FIG. 13-1 Pathways of inflammation and bone resorption by nonspecific inflammatory mediators and specific immune reactions.

Subpopulations of T lymphocytes have been examined in humans and experimental animals.[2,116] Stashenko and Yu[116] enumerated helper and suppressor T cells in developing rat periradicular lesions. Their findings indicate that helper T cells are predominant during the active phase of lesion development, whereas suppressor T cells are associated with chronic lesions. The presence of different types of lymphocytes in human apical lesions suggests that various types of immune reactions participate in the pathogenesis of these lesions.[131] Based on present knowledge, it appears that nonspecific inflammatory and specific immune reactions contribute significantly to the protection—and under certain circumstances to the destruction—of pulpal and periradicular tissues.

In addition to well-defined mediators of inflammation such as neuropeptides, fibrinolytic peptides, kinins, lysosomal enzymes, complement components, and arachidonic acid metabolites,[78,130] a number of less well-characterized substances are released by a variety of cells. These soluble substances, which are capable of activating other cells, are referred to collectively as *cytokines*. When released from lymphocytes they are called *lymphokines,* and when released by monocytes they are referred to as *monokines*. Interleukins are substances that mediate communication between leukocytes. This heterogeneous group of proteins have several common features. Cytokines are glycoproteins secreted as a result of cellular stimulation and have low molecular weights. They are not stored within cells, are produced locally, have very short half-lives, and are extremely potent. They interact with cell surface receptors, which leads to a change in the patterns of cellular RNA and protein synthesis and cell behavior.

The major cytokines include interleukins, interferons, tumor necrosis factor, and colony-stimulating factors. Most interleukins cause T- and/or B-cell proliferation and can stimulate differentiation and proliferation of other inflammatory cells. Among interleukins, IL-1 and IL-6 are proinflammatory and chemotactic for inflammatory cells. Bone resorptive activity of IL-1 is probably due to its effect on osteoclast differentiation from hematopoietic progenitor cells and formation of osteoclast-like giant cells in cultured bone marrow.[71] Tumor necrosis factor (TNF) consists of two proteins (TNF-α and TNF-β) with similar biologic functions. TNF-α is produced mainly by macrophages, whereas TNF-β (lymphotoxin) is the product of activated lymphocytes. Both TNF molecules are potent stimulators of bone resorption and inhibit collagen formation.[71]

TNF has been found in periradicular tissue exudates of teeth with apical periodontitis.[104] IL-1 has also been found in human dental pulps of symptomatic carious teeth and third molars with pericoronitis,[32] in human chronic apical lesions,[3] and symptomatic apical lesions.[70] Studies in a rat model system have shown that higher levels of bone resorptive activity are present during the active phase of periradicular lesion expansion than in the chronic phase, and this activity may be due mainly to the presence of molecules in the cytokine molecular weight range of IL-1 and TNF.[117]

METHODS OF CONTROL AND ERADICATION OF ROOT CANAL INFECTIONS

Because bacteria initiate and perpetuate most pulpal and periradicular diseases, disinfection of pathologically involved root canal systems is considered paramount in endodontic therapy. The steps involved in the disinfection of root canals are isolation of the involved teeth, sanitation of the field of operation, and use of sterile instruments, as well as the removal of bacteria, their by-products, and debris. Special precautions taken to prevent recontamination of the cleaned root canal include obturation of the root canal in three dimensions and placement of leak-resistant permanent restorations. Lack of asepsis during root canal therapy, or its poor application, can result in complications for the patient, clinician, and/or dental auxiliaries.[21]

The presence of bacteria in the root canal system should be dealt with as an infectious process. Like other infectious sites in the body, root canal infections must be débrided mechanically, and under special circumstances supportive measures such as systemic antibiotics should be considered. Unlike causative agents of infections elsewhere in the body, those of root canal infections are within hard tissues and cannot easily be reached by defensive cells of the body. Because of its anatomic location and its complexity, disinfection of the root canal system is performed mainly by mechanical means and is aided by chemical substances.

ISOLATION AND SANITATION OF THE FIELD OF OPERATION

Use of physical barriers such as gloves and the rubber dam during root canal therapy reduces the incidence of reinfection and lessens the chance of cross-contamination. Human saliva contains numerous species of bacteria. Like other body fluids, saliva, gingival fluid, and, more importantly, blood should be considered infective and sources for the transmission of pathogenic bacteria and viruses. As described in Chapter 5, protective barrier techniques such as safety glasses, masks, plastic face shields, and gloves *must* be used to reduce the chance of cross-contamination. Regarding the use of gloves in dental practice, the Department of Health and Human Services has made the following recommendations: "Gloves must always be worn when touching blood, saliva, or mucous membranes. . . . When all work is completed on one patient, the hands must be washed and regloved before performing procedures on another patient. Repeated use of a single pair of gloves is not recommended, since such use is likely to produce defects in the glove material which will diminish its value as an effective barrier."[141] Despite these recommendations, some dental professionals still use no gloves at all or use rewashed gloves. An investigation has shown that rewashed gloves remain contaminated even after several washings.[158]

In addition to advocating the use of protective barriers, the Department of Health and Human Services has made strict recommendations regarding sterilization and disinfection of handpieces and other dental materials and equipment and has specifically recommended the use of rubber dam and high-speed vacuums to minimize generation of droplets and spatter.[141,142] An investigation tested the permeability of three weights of dental rubber dam materials to Phi-X-174 virus particles and *Escherichia coli* bacteria.[16] Results showed that in the absence of manufacturer's defects, rubber dams are capable of providing adequate physical barriers during dental procedures.

IRRIGANTS AND INTRACANAL MEDICATIONS

Because of the complexity of root canals, cleaning and shaping them with presently available instruments is almost impossible. To aid disinfection, irrigants, and sometimes intracanal medications, are used during root canal therapy. An ideal intracanal irrigant is a lubricant that can dissolve organic debris, has low toxicity and low surface tension, and is an effective disinfectant or sterilizer. A number of solutions, from distilled water to caustic acids, have been suggested as intracanal irrigants.

Despite its drawbacks, such as tissue toxicity and its inability to penetrate into the irregularities of the root canal system,[94,108] sodium hypochlorite is the most commonly used intracanal irrigant during root canal therapy. Studies have shown that the use of sodium hypochlorite reduces the bacterial population significantly.[23,43] This property of sodium hypochlorite is partly due to its antibacterial effect and to its flushing action as an intracanal irrigant.[101,108] In addition, the combination of ultrasound-energized intracanal instruments and constant irrigation has been advocated to enhance cleaning and disinfection of the root canal system.[24,45,111]

Studies have shown that some bacteria survive after "complete cleaning and shaping" and therefore can grow in the empty root canal when no intracanal medicament is used between appointments.[8,22,23] Because of our inability to completely eradicate microorganisms during cleaning and shaping, and the inability of present temporary filling materials to provide a bacteria-proof seal between appointments, the use of intracanal medications has been advocated to further reduce the number of microorganisms after cleaning and shaping and before obturation of the root canal system. Many chemicals—phenolics, aldehydes, antibiotics, steroids, and, recently, calcium hydroxide—have been used to disinfect the root canal, reduce pain, or render inert the canal contents.[99] Because of the anatomic configurations of the root canal system and the inherent properties of these medications, such as their toxicity and allergenicity, their routine use and their value as adjuncts to cleaning and shaping have been questioned.[147] Many studies have shown the bacteriocidal effect of calcium hydroxide against several species of bacteria.[48,51,103] Recent studies have also demonstrated the ability of calcium hydroxide to dissolve organic tissues and debris.[51,82] *Based on present knowledge of the properties of calcium hydroxide, as an intracanal medication it is preferable to other medications.* Calcium hydroxide paste can be placed into the cleaned root canal by injection or by intracanal instruments and can be flushed out by irrigating the root canal with sodium hypochlorite, alcohol, or sterile water.

CULTURING AND IDENTIFICATION TECHNIQUES

The aim of endodontic treatment is to eliminate the bacteria from the root canals of involved teeth and then to allow for resolution and repair of any damaged periradicular tissues. At one time various methods were used to check the sterility produced by routine endodontic treatment regimens. Currently, this routine culturing is not generally performed, because today's standard techniques have been shown to be effective in eliminating the majority of microorganisms. This has reduced the need to spend a great deal of time and money, which such techniques would require.

There are still several situations wherein bacterial sampling of root canals might be beneficial. Occasionally, conventional root canal therapy does not eliminate symptoms of endodontic infection. If unusual pathogens are present, culturing along with antibiotic-sensitivity testing may be the only way to determine accurately their presence and to select the most appropriate antibiotic.

A number of patients today may require more precise bacteriologic monitoring. These include patients who are (1) undergoing immunosuppressive therapy, (2) at high risk for endocarditis, or (3) have heart valve prostheses and may require a sampling at an early appointment to determine whether an antimicrobial susceptibility test may be needed. The wide range of microorganisms that may be encountered in infected root canals may not necessarily be treatable empirically.

Finally, a sterility check test culture may be taken as a teaching device. Such a sample placed in a medium that supports growth of a wide range of microorganisms simply requires a *growth–no growth* analysis to see if the operator has maintained aseptic technique in the field of operation. The actual process of sampling for microbial culture needs to be well understood if the results are to be interpreted with confidence.

Taking the Culture

The collecting of root canal samples requires the use of techniques that allows both facultative and anaerobic bacteria to grow. The clinician must keep in mind that contamination with normal oral flora as a result of contact with saliva or careless handling will cause false culturing results.

Good aseptic technique in the collection process is an absolute requirement. Next in importance is getting the sample to a microbiologic laboratory where it may be processed with as little delay as possible. A carrier medium should be used that maintains viability of all the organisms in the sample. The actual sampling technique is not difficult to master. It is important to remember that the initial preparation of the site will, in large part, determine the success or failure of a good culture sample.

It is best if the teeth to be sampled are first isolated and the crown and rubber dam disinfected.[84] Dressing should be removed and discarded. Care should also be taken to remove any excess disinfectant that might contaminate the bacteriologic sample. Antibacterial chemicals should not be placed into the root canal before sampling. Once the root canal is exposed, a sterile absorbent point is inserted into the canal to remove any trace of medication that might be present. This is then discarded. A fresh sterile absorbent point is inserted into the root canal and allowed to remain in place to absorb as much exudate (if any) as possible. If the canal is dry, it can be moistened with transport medium added to the canal, using a coarse sterile paper point. This point is removed using sterilized cotton pliers and placed as quickly as possible in a medium or transport solution. Speed of handling and careful choice of medium increase the chances of isolating the more fastidious microorganisms.

To sample an orofacial lesion or a submucosal abscess, the surface area must be disinfected. This sample can be collected by penetrating the lesion with a sterile needle and drawing the fluid into a sterile syringe. Air can be expelled from the syringe after withdrawal, and the needle can be plugged by sticking it into a rubber stopper. This procedure can be used to maintain an anaerobic atmosphere for sample transport, or the material can be transferred to a transport medium, as described above.

Once the sample is collected, it is important to get it to the microbiology laboratory as quickly as possible to ensure successful culturing results. Most dentists are not directly associated with a laboratory that is capable of isolating and identifying microorganisms from these samples. If such a laboratory is available, proper media and incubation procedures should be used to get both facultative and anaerobic organisms to grow.

Attempts to identify and quantify the different bacteria isolated will increase the amount of work required. If a hospital clinical laboratory or commercial laboratory is to be used, it is important to communicate the dentist's specific needs to the personnel involved in sample analysis. Such laboratories often report normal oral flora only in general terms. Once the laboratory realizes that a specific identification is needed, specific flora can be identified and reported.

If antimicrobial testing is needed, it should be done only on pure cultures, not mixtures of microorganisms. Final results are usually available in 4 to 7 days. One advantage of using a clinical or commercial laboratory is that many now use sophisticated, expensive automatic identification systems that rely on computer-based data systems that identify bacterial isolates. Such identities and antibiotic susceptibility tests done with these machines can often produce results in less than 24 hours.

The techniques used to study and identify bacteria are essentially familiar and common ones. Gram stain examination of an original sample shows the presence or absence of microbes (and identifies gram-positive and gram-negative species) and cells (epithelial, erythrocytes, PMNs). This technique is limited in the information it can express, however. No specific identification of genus or species is possible, and live organisms are not distinguished from dead microbes. It gives only an overview of the bacteria involved and the host's response to the infection.

The media that are routinely used in most diagnostic laboratories easily support the growth of the oral bacteria usually identified as causing endodontic infections. Blood agar enriched to support *Brucella* species' growth can serve as an excellent medium for both facultative and fastidious anaerobic microorganisms. Broth media (fluid thioglycolate or chopped meat broth) likewise allow the growth of both. Media that accommodate specific needs for organisms such as yeast, molds, or *Mycobacterium* species can be obtained readily and used, as determined by the microbiologist. Specific identification of a wide range of oral microorganisms can be readily achieved. Rare or unusual species may require media or techniques that are available only in the research laboratory setting.

In determining a final bacterial identification, immunologic techniques combined with standard identification procedures can increase accuracy and decrease the time factor.[33,34,133] Fluorescent antibody techniques use a chemical (fluorescent isothiocyanate, FITC) that can be attached to antibodies (polyclonal or monoclonal). A specific antibody-antigen (bacterial) complex will be easily seen when viewed with a fluorescence microscope. Such techniques have recently been used by several investigators.[60,93]

The enzyme-linked immunosorbent assay (ELISA) uses different labels that can be attached to antibodies instead of FITC. Such labels include horseradish peroxidase or alkaline phosphatase. ELISA tests can be used to identify antigens (bacteria) or to measure antibodies to known antigens. These are well-established procedures and have been used to study the involvement of specific bacteria in the development of pulpal and apical lesions.[37,62]

In radioimmunoassays (RIA) radioactive markers are attached to antibodies and are used in a manner similar to that described for ELISAs. Basically, RIA is still an experimental process in dental research, which may eventually be able to increase sensitivity in a variety of test systems. A disadvantage is the operator's having to work with radioactive materials, which require special handling, storage, and disposal.

When endodontic treatments are performed in two or three appointments, temporary restorations are used to seal the access cavity preparations between appointments. The most commonly used temporary restorations in root canal therapy are zinc oxide–eugenol (e.g., IRM), and Cavit.[153] A recent study[31] has shown that IRM was less leakproof than Cavit ($P < 0.05$) and TERM ($P < 0.05$); thermocoupling introduced on the fourth day of the experiment increased percolation of IRM, decreased tightness of Cavit, while TERM remained leakproof.

Obturation of the root canal system in three dimensions, and consequently elimination of spaces for bacterial growth, is the final step in eradicating infected root canals. Proper condensation of gutta-percha in conjunction with a root canal sealer usually provides an adequate seal after cleaning of the root canals. To avoid recontamination of the root canals and to ensure long-term success, the access cavity to the obturated root canal must be sealed with permanent filling materials.

Studies in vitro and in vivo have shown a high incidence of dye penetration into unprotected root-filled canals.[73,124] After cleaning and shaping and then obturation of 45 root canals, we purposely put the coronal portion of their filling materials in contact with *Staphylococcus epidermidis* or *Proteus vulgaris*.[136] The number of days required for these bacteria to penetrate the entire root canals was measured. Results revealed that more than 50% of the root canals were completely contaminated after 19 days of exposure to *S. epidermidis* and about 50% were also totally contaminated when their coronal surfaces were exposed to *P. vulgaris* for 42 days. The results of this investigation show the importance of a strong coronal seal after completion of root canal therapy.

SYSTEMIC USE OF MEDICATIONS DURING ROOT CANAL THERAPY

Analgesics and antibiotics are the major classes of medications used during the course of root canal treatment. Nonsteroidals are indicated only if an analgesic/anti-inflammatory effect is desired. Narcotics are useful only for the patient who clearly needs an analgesic with a sedative effect. Clinical studies have shown that the use of analgesics significantly reduces the incidence of interappointment emergencies.[80,136] Localized swellings usually do not require antibiotics; surgical drainage (I&D) and thorough canal débridement are much more effective.

Morse and co-workers,[88] in a study of patients with necrotic pulps and asymptomatic apical lesions, found a significant decrease in the incidence of flare-ups.

Until recently, antibiotics were indicated only if there was clinical evidence that a diffuse, rapidly spreading cellulitis had spread into fascial spaces. Because of the nature of root canal flora, however, no single antibiotic is always effective against all root canal infections. Penicillin remains the antibiotic of choice because it is effective against most bacteria found in infected root canals. In case of allergy, erythromycin is the drug of second choice. Because cleomycin produces a high concentration of this substance in the bone and is effective against anaerobic bacteria, it could be used as an alternative medication for patients who are allergic or nonresponsive to penicillin or erythromycin. Long-term use (more than 7 to 10 days) of cleomycin during root canal treatment is contraindicated. Judicious removal of irritants from the root canal system is the best and the most effective way to eradicate root canal infection.

REFERENCES

1. Adriaens PA, De Boever JA, and Loesche WJ: Bacterial invasion in root cementum and radicular dentin of periodontal diseases teeth in humans—a reservoir of periodontopathic bacteria, J Periodont 59:222, 1988.
2. Barkhordar RA, and Desouza YG: Human T-lymphocyte subpopulations in periapical lesions, Oral Surg 65:763, 1988.
3. Barkhordar RA, Hussain MZ, and Hayashi C: Detection of the IL-1β in human periapical lesions, Oral Surg 73:334, 1992.
4. Barnes GW, and Langeland K: Antibody formation in primates following introduction of antigens into the root canal, J Dent Res 45:1111, 1966.
5. Baume LJ: Dental pulp conditions in relation to carious lesions, Int Dent J 20:308, 1970.
6. Baumgartner JC, and Falkler WA: Bacteria in the apical 5 mm of infected root canals, J Endodont 17:380, 1991.
7. Baumgartner JC, and Falkler WA: Detection of immunoglobulins from explant cultures of periapical lesions, J Endodont 17:105, 1991.
8. Bence R, et al: A microbiologic evaluation of endodontic instrumentation in pulpless teeth, Oral Surg 35:676, 1973.
9. Bergenholtz Z, Ahlstedt S, and Lindhe J: Experimental pulpitis in immunized monkeys, Scand J Dent Res 85:396, 1977.
10. Bergenholtz G, et al: Bacterial leakage around dental restorations: its effect on the dental pulp, Oral Surg 11:439, 1982.
11. Boling LR, and Robinson HBG: Anachoretic effect in pulpitis, Arch Pathol 33:477, 1942.
12. Brannström M, and Lind PO: Pulpal response to early dental caries, J Dent Res 44:1045, 1965.
13. Brook I, Grimm S, and Kielich RB: Bacteriology of acute periapical abscesses in children, J Endod 7:380, 1981.
14. Brook I, Frazier EH, and Gher ME: Aerobic and anaerobic microbiology of periapical abscesses, Oral Microbiol Immunol 6:123, 1991.
15. Brown LR, and Rudolph CE: Isolation and identification of microorganisms from unexposed canals of pulp-involved teeth, Oral Surg 19:1094, 1957.
16. Buoncristiani J, Burch P, and Torabinejad M: Permeability of common dental barriers to small virus particles. Student Table Clinic, 1988, Loma Linda University.
17. Burke GW, and Knighton HT: The localization of microorganisms in inflamed dental pulps of rats following bacteremia, J Dent Res 39:205, 1960.
18. Burket LW: Recent studies relating to periapical infection, including data obtained from human necropsy studies. J Am Dent Assoc 25:260, 1938.
19. Burket LW, and Burn CG: Bacteremias following dental extraction. Demonstration of source of bacteria by means of a non-pathogen *(Serratia marcesens)*. J Dent Res 16:521, 1937.
20. Byers MR, et al: Effects of injury and inflammation on pulpal and periapical nerves, J Endod 16:78, 1990.
21. Bystrom A, and Sundqvist G: Bacteriologic evaluation of the efficacy of mechanical root canal instrumentation in endodontic therapy, Scand J Dent Res 89:321, 1981.
22. Bystrom A, Claesson R, and Sundqvist G: The antibacterial effect of camphorated paramonochlorophenol, camphorated phenol and calcium hydroxide in the treatment of infected root canals, Endod Dent Traumatol 1:170, 1985.
23. Bystrom A, and Sundqvist G: The antibacterial action of sodium hypochlorite and EDTA in 60 cases of endodontic therapy, Int Endod J 18:35, 1985.
24. Cameron JA: The use of ultrasonics in the removal of smear layer: a scanning electron microscope study, J Endod 9:289, 1983.
25. Carlsson J, et al: Degradation of the human proteinase inhibitors alpha$_1$-antitrypsin and alpha$_2$-macroglobulin by *Bacteroides gingivalis,* Infect Immun 43:644, 1984.
26. Chirnside I: Bacterial invasion of non-vital dentin, J Dent Res 40:134, 1961.
27. Crawford JJ, and Shankle RJ: Application of newer methods to study the importance of root canal and oral microbia in endodontics, Oral Surg 14:1109, 1961.
28. Csernyei AJ: Anachoretic effect of chronic periapical inflammation, J Dent Res 18:527, 1939.
29. Debelian GJ, Olsen I, and Tronstad L: Profiling of *Propionibacterium acnes* recovered from root canal and blood during and after endodontic treatment. Endod Dent Traumatol 8:248, 1992.
30. Del Balco AM, Nishimura RS, and Setterstrom JA: The effects of thermal and electrical injury on pulpal histamine levels, Oral Surg 41:110, 1976.
31. Deveaux E, et al: Bacterial leakage of Cavit, IRM and TERM, Oral Surg 74:634, 1992.
32. Desouza R, et al: Detection and characterization of IL-1 in human dental pulps, Arch Oral Biol 34:307, 1989.
33. Ebersole JL, et al: An ELISA for measuring serum antibodies to *Actinobacillus actinomycetemcomitans,* J Periodont Res 15:621, 1980.
34. Ebersole JL, et al: Serological identification of oral *Bacteroides* spp. by enzyme-linked immunosorbent assay, J Clin Microbiol 19(5):639, 1984.
35. Fabricius L, et al: Influence of combinations of oral bacteria on periapical tissues of monkeys, Scand J Dent Res 90:200, 1982.
36. Fabricius L, et al: Predominant indigenous oral bacteria isolated from infected root canals after varied times of closure, Scand J Dent Res 90:134, 1982.
37. Falkler WA, et al: Reaction of pulpal immunoglobulins to oral microorganisms by an enzyme-linked immunosorbent assay, J Endod 13:260, 1987.
38. Figures KH, and Douglas CWI: *Actinomyces* associated with a root-treated tooth: report of a case, Int Endod J 24:326, 1991.
39. Fish EW: Bone infection, J Am Dent Assoc 26:691, 1939.
40. Flood PM, et al: Immunological signals which control T cell responses, J Endod 18:435, 1992.
41. Garberoglio R, Brannström M: Scanning electron microscopic investigation of human dentinal tubules, Arch Oral Biol 21:355, 1976.
42. Gibbons RJ, and MacDonald JB: Hemin and vitamin K compounds as required factors for the cultivation of certain strains of *Bacteroides melaninogenicus,* J Bacteriol 80:164, 1980.
43. Grahnen H, and Krasse B: The effect of instrumentation and flushing of non-vital teeth in endodontic therapy, Odontol Rev 14:167, 1963.
44. Griffee MB, et al: The relationship of *Bacteroides melaninogenicus* to symptoms associated with pulpal necrosis, Oral Pathol 50:457, 1980.
45. Griffiths MB, and Stock CJ: The efficiency of irrigants in removing root canal debris when used with an ultrasonic preparation technique, Int Endod J 19:277, 1986.
46. Grossman LI: Bacteriologic status of periapical tissue in 150 cases of infected pulpless teeth, J Dent Res 38:101, 1959.
47. Grossman LI: Origin of microorganisms in traumatized pulpless sound teeth, J Dent Res 46:551, 1967.
48. Haapasalo M: *Bacteroides* spp in dental root canal infections, Endod Dent Traumatol 5:1, 1989.
49. Hahn CL, and Falkler WA: Antibodies in normal and diseased pulps reactive with microorganisms isolated from deep caries. J Endod 18:28, 1991.
50. Harrington GW: The perio-endo question: differential diagnosis, Dent Clin North Am 87:673, 1979.
51. Hasselgren G, Olsson B, and Cvek M: Effects of calcium hydroxide and sodium hypochlorite on the dissolution of necrotic porcine muscle tissue, J Endod 14:125, 1988.

52. Horiba N, et al: Complement activation by lipopolysaccharides purified from gram-negative bacteria isolated from infected root canals, Oral Surg 74:648, 1992.
53. Hoshino E, et al: Bacterial invasion of non-exposed dental pulp, Int Endod J 25:2, 1992.
54. Jontell M, et al: Dendritic cells and macrophages expressing class II antigens in the normal cat incisor pulp, J Dent Res 67:1263, 1988.
55. Jontell M, Gunraj MN, and Bergenholtz G: Immunocompetent cells in the normal dental pulp, J Dent Res 66:1149, 1987.
56. Kakehashi S, Stanley HR, and Fitzgerald RJ: The effects of surgical exposures of dental pulps in germ-free and conventional laboratory rats, Oral Surg 20:340, 1965.
57. Kantz WE, and Henry CA: Isolation and classification of anaerobic bacteria from intact pulp chamber of non-vital teeth in man, Arch Oral Biol 19:91, 1974.
58. Kennedy DR, Hamilton TR, and Syverton JT: Effects on monkeys of introduction of hemolytic streptococci into root canals, J Dent Res 36:496, 1957.
59. Kerosup E, et al: Ingestion of *Bacteroides buccae, Bacteroides oris, Porphyromonas gingivalis* and *Fusobacterium nucleatum* by human polymorphonuclear leukocytes in vitro, Oral Microbiol Immunol 5:202, 1990.
60. Kettering J, Payne W, and Prabhu S: Antibody levels against eleven oral microorganisms in an endodontic population, J Dent Res 67:202, 1988.
61. Kettering JD, Torabinejad M, and Jones SL: Specificity of antibodies present in human periapical lesions, J Endod 17:213, 1991.
62. Kettering JD, Torabinejad M, and Jones S: Identification of bacteria involved in pathogenesis of human periapical lesions by the ELISA technique, J Endod 14:198, 1988.
63. Kettering JD, and Torabinejad M: Presence of natural killer cells in human chronic periapical lesions. Int Endod J Vol. 26, 1993.
64. Korzen B, Krakow A, and Green D: Pulpal and periapical tissue responses in conventional and monoinfected gnotobiotic rats, Oral Surg 37:783, 1974.
65. Kronfeld R: Histopathology of the teeth and their surrounding structures, ed 2, Philadelphia, 1939, Lea & Febiger, p 209.
66. Kuntz DD, et al: Localization of immunoglobulins and the third component of complement in dental periapical lesions, J Endod 3:68, 1977.
67. Langeland K, Block RM, and Grossman LI: A histobacteriologic study of 35 periapical endodontic surgical specimens, J Endod 3:8, 1977.
68. Lessard GM, Torabinejad M, and Swope D: Arachidonic acid metabolism in canine tooth pulps and the effects of non-steroidal anti-inflammatory drugs, J Endod 12:146, 1986.
69. Lewis MAO, McFarlane TW, and McGowan DA: Quantitative bacteriology of acute dento-alveolar abscesses, J Med Microbiol 21:101, 1986.
70. Lim G, and Torabinejad M: Concentration of interleukin-1-β in symptomatic and asymptomatic human periradicular lesions, J Endod Abstract #10, 1992.
71. Lorenzo JA: Cytokines of bone metabolism: resorption and formation. In Kimbail ES (ed): Cytokines and inflammation, Boca Raton, Fla., 1991, CRC Press, pp 145-167.
72. Lukic A, et al: Quantitative analysis of the immunocompetent cells in periapical granuloma: correlation with the histological characteristics of the lesions. J Endod 16:119, 1990.
73. Madison S, Swanson KL, and Chiles SA: An evaluation of coronal microleakage in endodontically treated teeth. Part II. Sealer types, J Endod 13:109, 1987.
74. Malmstrom M: Immunoglobulin classes IgG, IgM, IgA and complement components C in dental periapical lesions of patients with rheumatoid disease, Scand J Rheumatol 4:57, 1975.
75. Mayrand D, and McBride BC: Ecological relationship of bacteria involved in a simple, mixed anaerobic infection, Infect Immun 27:44, 1980.
76. McKay GS: The histology and microbiology of acute occlusal dentin lesions in human permanent premolar teeth, Arch Oral Biol 21:51, 1976.
77. McKee AS, et al: Effect of hemin on the physiology and virulence of *Bacteroides gingivalis,* Infect Immun 52:349, 1986.
78. McNicholas S, et al: The concentration of prostaglandin E_2 in human peri-radicular lesions, J Endod 17:91, 1991.
79. Mejare B, Mejare I, and Edwardsson S: Acid etching and composite restorations. A culturing and histologic study on bacterial penetration, Endod Dent Traumatol 3:1, 1987.
80. Melton D, Baker K, and Walton R: Prophylactic administration of a nonsteroidal drug; effect on post-treatment endodontic pain, J Dent Res Abstract #556, 1986.
81. Melville TH, and Birch RH: Root canal and periapical floras of the infected teeth, Oral Surg 23:93, 1967.
82. Metzler RS, and Montgomery S: The effectiveness of ultrasonics and calcium hydroxide for débridement of human mandibular molars, J Endod 15:373, 1989.
83. Miller WD: Microorganisms of the human mouth, Philadelphia, 1890, S.S. White Dental Co., p 96.
84. Moller AJR: Microbiologic examination of root canals and periapical tissues of human teeth, Odont Tidskr 74:63, 1966.
85. Moller AJR: Influence on periapical tissues of indigenous oral bacteria and necrotic pulp tissue in monkeys, Scand J Dent Res 89:475, 1981.
86. Moorer WR, van Velzen SKT, and Wesselink PR: Abscesses formation induced in rabbits with bacteria-filled subcutaneous implants that simulate the infected dental root canal, Oral Surg 59:642, 1985.
87. Morse DR: Endodontic microbiology in the 1970s, Int Endod J 14:69, 1981.
88. Morse DR, et al: Infectious flare-ups and serious sequelae following endodontic treatment: a prospective randomized trial on efficacy of antibiotic prophylaxis in cases of asymptomatic pulpo-periapical lesions, Oral Surg 64:96, 1987.
89. Nilsson T, Carlsson J, and Sundqvist G: Inactivation of key factors of the plasma proteinase cascade systems by *Bacteroides gingivalis,* Infect Immun 50:467, 1985.
90. Oguntebi B, et al: Predominant microflora associated with human dental periapical abscesses, J Clin Microbiol 15:964, 1982.
91. Olgart L, Brannström M, and Johnson G: Invasion of bacteria into dentinal tubules. Experiments in vivo and in vitro, Acta Odontol Scand 32:61, 1974.
92. Page DO, Trump GN, and Schaeffer LD: Pulpal studies. I. Passage of ^{3}H tetracycline into circulatory system through rat molar pulps, Oral Surg 35:555, 1973.
93. Pantera EA, Zambon JJ, and Shih-Levine M: Indirect immunofluorescence for detection of *Bacteroides* species in human dental pulp, J Endod 14:218, 1988.
94. Pashley E, et al: Cytotoxic effects of NaOCl on vital tissue, J Endod 11:525, 1985.
95. Paterson RC, and Watts A: Pulp responses to two strains of bacteria isolated from human carious dentine (*L. plantarum* —NCTC 1406) and *Streptococcus mutans* (NCTC 10919) Int Endod J 25:134, 1992.
96. Perrini N, and Fonzi L: Mast cells in human periapical lesions: ultrastructural aspects and their possible physiopathological implications, J Endod 11:197, 1985.
97. Pissiotis E, and Spangberg LSW: Toxicity of sonicated extracts of *Bacteroides gingivalis* on human pulpal cells and L929 cells in vitro, J Endod 17:553, 1991.
98. Pulver WH, Taubman MA, and Smith DJ: Immune components in human dental periapical lesions, Arch Oral Biol 23:435, 1978.
99. Pumarola J, et al: Antimicrobial activity of seven root canal sealers, Oral Surg 74:216, 1992.
100. Qvist V: Marginal adaptation of composite restorations performed in vivo with different acid-etch restorative procedures, Scand J Dent Res 93:68, 1985.
101. Ram Z: Effectiveness of root canal irrigation, Oral Surg 44:306, 1977.

102. Robinson HBG, and Boling, LR: The anachoretic effect in pulpitis. I. Bacteriologic studies, J Am Dent Assoc 28:268, 1941.
103. Safavi K, et al: Comparison of antimicrobial effects of calcium hydroxide and iodine-potassium iodide, J Endod 11:454, 1985.
104. Safavi K, and Rossomando L: TNF identified in periapical tissue exudates of teeth with apical periodontitis, J Endod 17:12, 1991.
105. Sconyers JR, Crawford JJ, and Moriarty JD: Relationship of bacteremia to toothbrushing in patients with periodontitis, J Am Dent Assoc 87:616, 1973.
106. Seltzer S, and Bender IB: Pulp irritants: microbial. In: The dental pulp: biologic considerations in dental procedures, ed 3, Philadelphia, 1984, JB Lippincott Co, p. 176.
107. Seltzer S, and Bender IB: Pulp irritants: microbial. In: The dental pulp: biologic considerations in dental procedures, ed 3, Philadelphia, 1984, JB Lippincott, p. 187.
108. Senia ES, Marshall FJ, and Rosen S: The solvent action of sodium hypochlorite on pulp tissue of extracted teeth, Oral Surg 31:96, 1971.
109. Shindell E: A study of some periapical roentgenolucencies and their significance, Oral Surg 14:1057, 1961.
110. Simonson LG, et al: Bacterial synergy of *Treponema denticola* and *Porphyromonas gingivalis* in a multinational population, Oral Microbiol Immunol 7:111, 1992.
111. Sjogren U, and Sundqvist G: Bacteriologic evaluation of ultrasonic root canal instrumentation, Oral Surg 63:366, 1987.
112. Sjogren U, et al: Extensive bone loss associated with periapical infection with *Bacteroides gingivalis:* a case report, Int Endod J 23:254, 1990.
113. Smith LS, and Tappe G: Experimental pulpitis in rats, J Dent Res 41:17, 1962.
114. Socransky SS, and Gibbons RJ: Required role of *Bacteroides melaninogenicus* in mixed anaerobic infections, J Infect Dis 115:247, 1965.
115. Spangberg L, Engstrom B, and Langeland K: Biologic effects of dental materials. 3. Toxicity and antimicrobial effect of endodontic antiseptics in vitro, Oral Surg 36:856, 1973.
116. Stashenko P, and Yu SM: T helper and T suppressor cell reversal during the development of induced rat periapical lesions, J Dent Res 68:830, 1989.
117. Stashenko P, Yu SM, and Wang CY: Kinetics of immune cell and bone resorptive responses to endodontic infections, J Endod 18:422, 1992.
118. Sundqvist G: Bacteriological studies of necrotic dental pulps. Umea University odontological dissertation No. 7, Umea, Sweden, 1976, University of Umea.
119. Sundquvist G: Associations between microbial species in dental root canal infections, Oral Microbiol Immunol 7:257, 1992.
120. Sundqvist G: Ecology of the root canal flora, J Endod 18:427, 1992.
121. Sundqvist G, Johansson E, and Sjogren U: Prevalence of black-pigmented *Bacteroides* species in root canal infections, J Endod 15:13, 1989.
122. Sundqvist G, et al: Capacity of anaerobic bacteria from necrotic dental pulps to induce purulent infections, Infect Immun 25:685, 1979.
123. Sundqvist G, et al: Degradation of human immunoglobulins G and M and complement factors C3 and C5 by black-pigmented *Bacteroides,* J Med Microbiol 19:85, 1985.
124. Swanson KS, and Madison S: An evaluation of coronal microleakage in endodontically treated teeth, Part I. time periods, J Endod 13:56, 1987.
125. Tani N, et al: Comparative histological identification and relative distribution of immunocompetent cells in sections of frozen or formalin-fixed tissue from human periapical inflammatory lesions, Endod Dent Traumatol 8:163, 1992.
126. Tani N, et al: Immunobiological activities of bacteria isolated from the root canals of postendodontic teeth with persistent periapical lesions, J Endod 18:58, 1992.
127. Thilo B, et al: Dark-field observation of the bacterial distribution in root canals following pulp necrosis, J Endod 12:202, 1986.
128. Torabinejad M: Mediators of pulpal and periapical pathosis, Calif Dent Assoc J 14:21, 1966.
129. Torabinejad M, and Bakland LK: Prostaglandins: their possible role in pathogenesis of pulpal and periapical diseases. part II, J Endod 6:769, 1980.
130. Torabinejad M, Cotti E, and Jung T: The concentration of leukotriene B4 in symptomatic and asymptomatic lesions, J Endod 18:5, 1992.
131. Torabinejad M, Eby WC, and Naidorf LJ: Inflammatory and immunological aspects of the pathogenesis of human periapical lesions, J Endod 11:479, 1985.
132. Torabinejad M, and Kettering JD: Identification and relative concentration of B and T lymphocytes in human chronic periapical lesions, J Endod 11:122, 1985.
133. Torabinejad M, and Kettering JD: Immunological techniques in endodontal research. In Spanberg LS (ed): Experimental Endodontics, 1990, CRC Press, Boca Raton, Fla., pp. 155-172.
134. Torabinejad M, Midrou T, and Bakland L: Detection of kinins in human periapical lesions, J Dent Res 68, Abstract #156, 1989.
135. Torabinejad M, Ung B, and Kettering JD: In vitro bacterial penetration of coronally unsealed endodontically treated teeth, J Endod 16:566, 1990.
136. Torabinejad M, Kettering JD, McGraw JC, et al: Factors associated with endodontic interappointment emergencies of teeth with necrotic pulps, J Endod 14:261, 1988.
137. Torabinejad M, and Walton RE: Managing endodontic emergencies, JADA 122:99, 1991.
138. Tronstad L, et al: Anaerobic bacteria in periapical lesions of human teeth, J Endod 12:131, 1986.
139. Tronstad L: Recent development in endodontic research, Scand J Dent Res 100:52, 1992.
140. Trope M, Rosenberg E, and Tronstad L: Darkfield microscopic spirochete endodontic and periodontal abscesses, J Endod 18:82, 1992.
141. U.S. Department of Health and Human Services: Recommended infection-control practices for dentistry. MMWR 35:1, 1986.
142. U.S. Department of Health and Human Services: Recommendations for prevention of HIV transmission in health care settings. MMWR 36:75, 1987.
143. van Steenbergen TJM, et al: *Bacteroides endodontalis* sp. nov., and asaccharolytic black-pigmented *Bacteroides* species from infected dental root canals, Int J System Bacteriol 34:118, 1984.
144. van Winkelhoff AJ, Carlee AW, de Graaff J: *Bacteroides endodontalis* and other black-pigmented *Bacteroides* species in odontogenic abscesses, Infect Immun 49:494, 1985.
145. van Winkelhoff AJ, van Steenbergen JM, and de Graaf J: *Porphyromonas (Bacteroides) endodontalis:* its role in endodontal infections, J Endod 18:431, 1992.
146. Wakisaka S: Neuropeptides in the dental pulp: distribution, origin, and correlation, J Endod 16:67, 1990.
147. Walton RE: Intracanal medicaments, Dent Clin North Am 28:783, 1984.
148. Walton RE, and Ardjmand K: Histological evaluation of the presence of bacteria in induced periapical lesions in monkeys, J Endod 18:216, 1992.
149. Wasfy MO, et al: Microbiological evaluation of periapical infections in Egypt, Oral Microbiol Immunol 7:100, 1992.
150. Watts A, and Paterson RC: Pulp response to, and cariogenicity of, a further strain of *Streptococcus mutans* (NTCC 10832), Int Endod J 25:142, 1992.
151. Watts A, and Paterson RC: Detection of bacteria in histological sections of the dental pulp, Int Endod J 23:1, 1990.
152. Wayman BE, et al: A bacteriological and histological evaluation of 58 periapical lesions, J Endod 18:152, 1992.
153. Webber R, et al: Sealing quality of a temporary filling material, Oral Surg 46:423, 1978.
154. Williams BL, McCann GF, and Schoenknecht FD: Bacteriology of dental abscesses of endodontic origin, J. Clin Micro 18:770, 1983.

155. Winkler KC, and Van Amerongen J: Bacteriologic results from 4,000 root canal cultures, Oral Surg 12:857, 1959.
156. Wirthlin MR: Acid-reacting stains, softening and bacterial invasion in human carious dentin, J Dent Res 49:42, 1970.
157. Wu MK, Henry CA, and Gutman JL: Bacteriological effects of human neutrophils and sera on selected endodontic pathogenic bacteria in an anaerobic environment, Int Endod J 23:189, 1990.
158. Yetter CG, Torabinejad M, and Torabinejad A: An investigation on the safety of rewashed gloves, J Dent Hyg 63:358, 1989.
159. Yoshida M, et al: Correlation between clinical symptoms and microorganisms isolated from root canals of teeth with periapical pathosis, J Endod 13:24, 1987.

Self-assessment questions

1. Most root canal infections involve
   a. a single obligate anaerobic species.
   b. multiple anaerobic species only.
   c. mixed aerobic and anaerobic microorganisms.
   d. multiple aerobic species only.
2. Studies have demonstrated a correlation between clinical and radiographic signs and symptoms of periapical pathosis and the presence of
   a. *Streptococcus mutans.*
   b. *Prevotella melaninogenicus.*
   c. *Staphylococcus aureus.*
   d. no specific microorganism(s).
3. Which mediators of inflammation are considered also to be the main mediators of pain in inflammatory responses?
   a. Vasoactive amines.
   b. Kinins.
   c. Complement.
   d. Arachidonic acid.
4. The presence of which component of complement in the inflamed periapex suggests that the complement system participates in the pathogenesis?
   a. C1.
   b. C3.
   c. C7.
   d. C9.
5. Degranulation and release of histamine is usually stimulated by bridging which of the following on the mast cells?
   a. IgA.
   b. IgE.
   c. IgG.
   d. IgM.
6. Identification of lymphocytes in human periapical lesions has shown
   a. an absence of B lymphocytes.
   b. an absence of T lymphocytes.
   c. that T cells outnumber B cells.
   d. that B cells outnumber T cells.
7. In periapical lesions, suppressor T cells are associated with
   a. acute (developing) lesions.
   b. chronic lesions.
   c. healing lesions.
   d. foreign-body lesions.
8. Routine culturing of the root canal system is generally not practiced in today's treatment regimens because
   a. it is time consuming.
   b. important anaerobes cannot be recovered.
   c. standard RCT techniques effectively eliminate the majority of microorganisms.
   d. microorganisms play a minor role in endodontic pathosis.
9. When antibiotic therapy is indicated before, during, or after root canal treatment the drug of choice is
   a. clindamycin.
   b. erythromycin.
   c. penicillin.
   d. metronidazole.
10. Long-term administration of clindamycin is contraindicated because of the risk of developing
    a. severe gastrointestinal conditions.
    b. urticaria.
    c. photosensitivity.
    d. hypersensitivity.
11. Which one of the following is *least* likely to initiate an immune response?
    a. Necrotic tissue.
    b. Endotoxins.
    c. Autologous collagen.
    d. Viable bacteria.
12. What immunoglobulin predominates in a secondary humoral response?
    a. IgA.
    b. IgG.
    c. IgM.
    d. IgE.
13. Elevated levels of IgE have been identified in a periapical granuloma after canal instrumentation. This may represent which type of hypersensitivity reaction?
    a. Type I (immediate hypersensitivity).
    b. Type II (immediate cytotoxic hypersensitivity).
    c. Type III (immune complex hypersensitivity).
    d. Type IV (delayed hypersensitivity).
14. The cytokine, interleukin-1 (IL-1), has been identified in the inflamed pulp and inflamed periapical lesion. One important function is to
    a. result in bone resorption.
    b. neutralize bacterial endotoxins.
    c. inhibit inflammation.
    d. promote phagocytosis by macrophages.
15. The intracanal medication that has the best potential for effectiveness as an antimicrobial agent sealed in the canal is
    a. formocresol.
    b. 5.25% sodium hypochlorite.
    c. steroids.
    d. calcium hydroxide.
16. Coronal exposure of gutta-percha/sealer obturation to bacteria has shown that, throughout the canal, the bacteria
    a. penetrate very quickly (1 to 3 days) throughout obturation defects.
    b. penetrate very slowly (requires several months).
    c. do not penetrate.
    d. penetrate fairly quickly (1 week to 1 month).
17. Regarding the presence of bacteria, most studies show that the majority of periapical granulomas are
    a. supportive of numbers of anaerobes primarily.
    b. supportive of numbers of anaerobes *only,* primarily.
    c. supportive of numbers of variable, mixed flora.
    d. bacteria free.

Chapter 14

Instruments, Materials, and Devices

Leo J. Miserendino

The technical demands and level of precision required for successful performance of endodontic procedures have traditionally been achieved by careful manipulation of hand instruments within the root canal space and by strict adherence to the biologic and surgical principles, essential for disinfection and healing. The highly successful and predictable outcome of endodontic treatment afforded by adherence to traditional methods and principles has perhaps contributed to the tendency among most to view with skepticism or reject radical changes in methodology. On the other hand, the recent resurgence in popularity of mechanized or automated systems for preparation and sealing of the root canal may be interpreted to be the profession's preference for improving the speed or efficiency of treatment, with somewhat less emphasis on the precision or accuracy of endodontic procedures.

Although the armamentarium of endodontics has grown in complexity over the past 30 or more years, the basic instruments and materials most popular today differ very little from those commonly used at the turn of the century. Nevertheless, scientific and technologic advances have significantly increased the ability of the modern practitioner to provide a higher level of care than was achievable in the past. The development of improved materials and techniques have allowed treatment of clinical situations that previously would have been deemed hopeless.

As increasing numbers of patients have become aware of the advantages of endodontic treatment and the many benefits derived through preservation of the natural dentition, the demand for endodontic services has increased dramatically over the past two decades.[31] Concurrently, increasing numbers of clinicians have sought to develop the skills and techniques necessary to provide this valuable service to their patients, through formalized advanced and continuing education programs.

Though the literature appears to reflect disparate opinions on the safety and efficacy of specific products, and is dominated by preferences of individuals, the consensus on the basic aims and objectives of endodontic treatment essentially remains. The ultimate goal of endodontic instrumentation techniques and procedures continues to center on the established biologic and surgical principles of asepsis, débridement, and providing an environment that is conducive for healing and repair.

The purpose of this chapter is to provide clinicians and students with information on the biologic, physical, and mechanical properties of instruments, materials, and devices which either have been used or are currently available for use in endodontic treatment. Then they may have a basis for selecting instruments and materials appropriate for the variety of clinical problems they encounter.

REGULATIONS AND SAFETY STANDARDS

The instruments, materials, and equipment used in the practice of endodontics, by definition, fall within the jurisdiction of the Bureau of Medical Devices of the Food and Drug Administration of the Federal Government. Since 1966 the Council on Dental Materials, Instruments, and Equipment (CDMIE) of the American Dental Association (ADA) has assumed responsibility for evaluating and formulating standards for dental products by serving as secretariat for the American National Standards Institute (ANSI).

The primary function of the Council is to provide protection for dentists and their patients by determining the safety and effectiveness of dental products. The Council performs its duties principally through development of product specifications, and through its product certification and acceptance programs.

Formulation of product specifications is performed through the joint efforts of ANSI Committee MD-156 (medical devices) and CDMIE of the ADA. In addition to establishing minimum standards for the safety and efficacy of products, these specifications list the criteria for determining product quality by means of specific performance tests of physical, chemical, and biologic properties. Products that fulfill the requirements of the specification are eligible for Certification or Acceptance status by the CDMIE of the ADA.

Owing to our litigious society and increasing awareness of malpractice, practitioners are strongly advised, whenever possible, to select products that are recognized to be safe and effective for their intended application. Use of unapproved or otherwise experimental materials or products is solely the responsibility (and risk) of the dentist.

Many of the products described in this chapter have been found to be acceptable or approved for use in endodontics, but the fact that a product is described here should not be interpreted as an endorsement of its acceptability or appropriateness for use in endodontic practice. For a complete listing of products that have been certified or accepted by the CDMIE the reader is referred to *The Dentist's Desk Reference: Materials, Instruments and Equipment,* available through the ADA.

Guidelines for the safe use of dental instruments and material handling in the clinical practice of dentistry have been established by the Occupational Safety and Health Administration (OSHA) of the US Department of Labor. The purpose of these guidelines is to ensure a safe working environment for dental health care workers through the identification and proper handling of hazardous and infectious materials in the workplace. It is the responsibility of employers of dental health care workers to provide adequate training and a safe workplace for their employees through a formal hazards communication and training program.

Many materials used in endodontics and dentistry have the potential to be harmful if handled improperly. Similarly, any dental instrument may serve as a vector of infectious diseases once contaminated through use on patients. Information related to the potential risks and proper handling of dental materials is readily available from manufacturers and suppliers as material safety data sheets. Information related to the control and handling of infectious materials and instruments is also available through the ADA and other sources. Compliance with the guidelines established by OSHA and federal and state Environmental Protection Agencies is mandatory and enforceable under state and federal laws.

CLASSIFICATION OF INSTRUMENTS AND MATERIALS

The instruments, materials, and devices used in endodontics have been grouped according to use, by the International Standards Organization (ISO) and the Federation Dentaire Internationale (FDI) through a joint working group on dental instruments and materials. The development of worldwide standards for endodontic instruments and materials is guided by (Technical Committee) TC-106 JWG-1 (Joint Working Group) of FDI/ISO and its task groups on terminology, dimensions, physical properties, measuring systems, and quality controls.

Working independently, both FDI/ISO and ANSI groups continue to make progress in the development of international and national standards for endodontic instruments and materials. Considerable effort has been made to achieve harmony between international and national standards. While much of the work goes unfinished, there has been a tendency toward worldwide uniformity of endodontic instruments and materials through development of new standards and revision of existing ones.

TABLE 14-1. Classification of endodontic instruments and materials

ANSI	General description	ISO/FDI
28	Root canal files (K-type)	3630/1
58	Hedström files (H-type)	3630/1
63	Barbed broaches and rasps	3630/1
	Root canal enlargers	3630/2
71	Condensers, pluggers, spreaders	3630/3
73	Absorbent points	7551
78	Obturating points	6877
57	Root canal sealers	6876

A classification of instruments and materials commonly used in endodontic practice and their corresponding American (ANSI) and international (FDI/ISO) standards is given in Table 14-1. In addition to those listed are numerous unclassified or adjunctive items that deserve our attention and are presented in this chapter.

The chapter has been organized to include a discussion of the pertinent biologic and physical properties of instruments and materials available in the United States and elsewhere. General groupings of products have been made, according to their intended application in endodontics, and they are presented in sequence as they are used in clinical practice. In addition to diagnostic products, instruments and mechanical systems for root canal preparation and enlargement, materials and delivery systems for sealing (obturation) of the root canal space, auxiliary materials, devices and suggestions for future product development have been presented. It is hoped that the organization of information contained in this chapter will simplify reference for future needs.

MATERIALS, INSTRUMENTS, AND DEVICES FOR ENDODONTIC DIAGNOSIS

One of the most critical aspects of endodontic treatment is the formation of an accurate diagnosis. In addition to basic examination instruments such as the mouth mirror, explorer, and periodontal probe a number of specialized materials and devices are necessary for evaluating the pulpal and periapical status of teeth. A complete discussion of diagnostic procedures appears in Chapter 1.

Clinical assessment of pulp vitality is based on the patient's response to thermal, mechanical, or electrical stimuli applied to the surfaces of teeth.

Heat Testing

The best technique is to isolate the tooth with a rubber dam and bathe it with hot water as described in Chapter 1.

Cold Tests

The most common methods for cold testing teeth include application of ice, carbon dioxide "snow," or liquid refrigerants. A number of commercial products are available that can

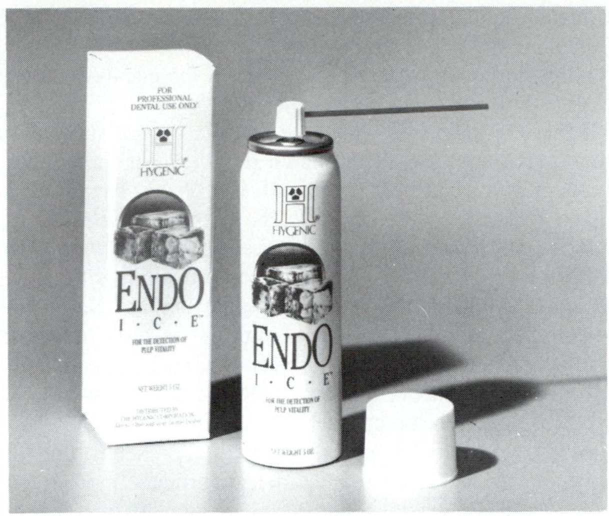

FIG. 14-1 Endo ice refrigerant (Hygenic) for thermal pulp testing.

be sprayed onto cotton pellets and applied to the teeth. Variations in temperature achieved may determine one's selection of a particular product. Carbon dioxide snow (−108° F) may be too cold for this purpose. Common ice (32° F), ethyl chloride (53° F), or Endo Ice (dichlorodifluoromethane, −21° F) may be a better alternative. Also, ethyl chloride is highly flammable, whereas Endo Ice (Fig. 14-1) is noncombustible.

Electric Pulp Tests

A variety of devices are available for testing pulp vitality based upon application of a direct current electrical stimulus of varying frequency. Most are battery-operated devices that afford some way of adjusting the level or rate of the applied stimulus. All require grounding to the patient for completion of the circuit and incorporate a stylus for application to the tooth. Some models (Fig. 14-2) display a digital readout of the response level; others possess adjustment dials and buttons for activation of the current. Those which gradually increase the intensity of the stimulus are preferred since they are less shocking to the patient.

A potentially more reliable method of assessing pulp vitality has been reported that involves the use of laser Doppler flowmetrics for measuring pulpal blood flow.[75,165] Therefore, the results obtained with electric pulp testing devices at present should be correlated with radiographic, thermal, and other clinical findings when formulating a pulpal diagnosis.

INSTRUMENTS FOR ROOT CANAL PREPARATION

Classification

According to the classification scheme established by ISO, endodontic instruments may be grouped as either hand-operated instruments (group I) or as engine-driven instruments (groups II and III). Included in group I instruments are barbed broaches, H-type (Hedström) files, K-type files, reamers, and R-type (rasp) files (Fig. 14-3). The intended use for this group of instruments can be limited solely to gross removal of pulp tissue and remnants (broaches) or to a combination of canal débridement and shaping (files, reamers, and rasps). Table

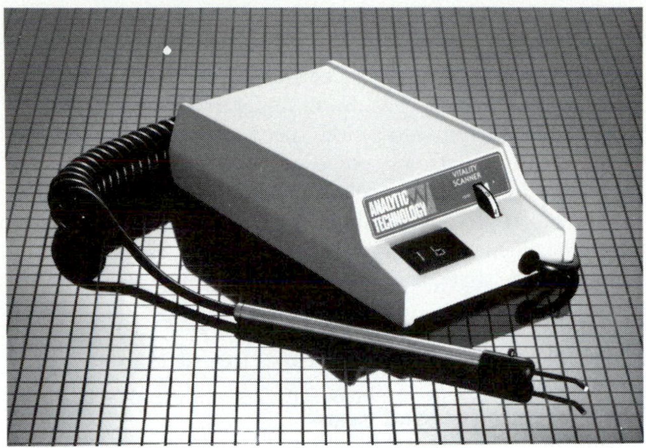

FIG. 14-2 Battery-operated electric pulp tester (Analytic Technology).

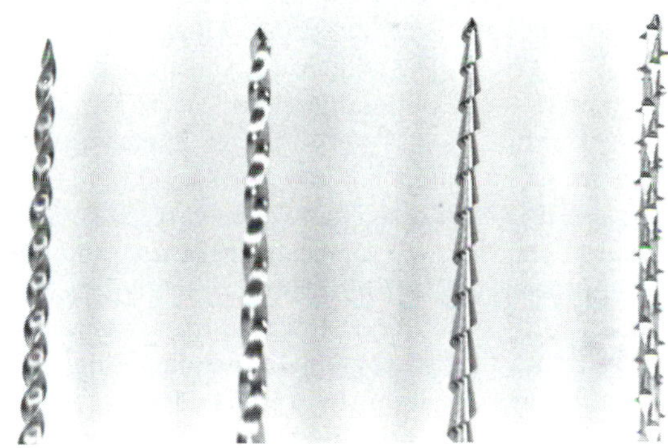

FIG. 14-3 Hand-operated instruments for canal preparation. *Left to right,* K-file, reamer, Hedström file, rasp.

TABLE 14-2. Size and color coding of endodontic instruments

	Diameter of instrument			
Size	D_0 (mm)	D_{16} (mm)	Color	Abbreviation
10	0.10	0.42	Purple	Pur
15	0.15	0.47	White	Wh
20	0.20	0.52	Yellow	Yel
25	0.25	0.57	Red	Red
30	0.30	0.62	Blue	Blu
35	0.35	0.67	Green	Grn
40	0.40	0.72	Black	Blk
45	0.45	0.77	White	Wh
50	0.50	0.82	Yellow	Yel
55	0.55	0.87	Red	Red
60	0.60	0.92	Blue	Blu
70	0.70	1.02	Green	Grn
80	0.80	1.12	Black	Blk
90	0.90	1.22	White	Wh
100	1.00	1.32	Yellow	Yel
110	1.10	1.42	Red	Red
120	1.20	1.52	Blue	Blu
130	1.30	1.62	Green	Grn
140	1.40	1.72	Black	Blk
150	1.50	1.82	White	Wh

14-2 lists information related to color coding and sizes of group I endodontic instruments.

Group II instruments may be described as group I instruments whose handle has been replaced with a latch-type adapter for insertion into a slow-speed contraangle handpiece. Group II instruments are composed of two parts, an operative cutting head and a latch-type attachment. Group III instruments are similar to group II instruments in that they have a latch-type attachment, but are fabricated from a single piece of metal—latch, shaft, and cutting head are composed all of one piece.

Physical and Mechanical Properties of Hand Instruments

Barbed broaches and rasps

The uniqueness of the design (Fig. 14-4) and method of fabrication of barbed broaches and rasps separates them from other intracanal hand instruments. They also differ from H-type and K-type instruments because of taper and length of the working portion of the shaft (10 mm).

The dimenional and physical performance requirements for these instruments are listed in specifications No. 63 (ANSI) and 3630-1 (ISO/FDI). The major difference between broaches and rasps lies in the depth and angle of cut in the wire shaft (core), which results in barbs of different heights and shapes. According to specification no. 63, barb height for broaches should be half the core diameter, whereas rasps should have barbs equal to one third the diameter of the tip. Additionally, the taper of broaches (0.007 mm/mm) is slightly less than half that of rasps (0.015 mm/mm). Because of this greater depth of cut in broaches than in rasps the remaining core thickness is much reduced, resulting in a more fragile instrument throughout its entire length. This major flaw in the design of the broach can easily lead to instrument fracture if it is not used cautiously.

Barbed broaches are used primarily for the removal of intact pulp tissue. The instrument is introduced slowly into the root canal until gentle contact with the canal walls is made. It is rotated 360 degrees either clockwise or counterclockwise, to entangle the pulpal tissue in the protruding barbs. It is then withdrawn directly from the root canal. If the maneuver is successful, the entire pulp comes out.

If the vital pulp is so inflamed that the gel-sol state of the ground substance has been altered by edema or the collagen fibrous network has been destroyed, it probably cannot be removed intact by a barbed broach. The instrument will only lacerate the already hemorrhagic tissues. Unless a necrotic pulp maintains a high degree of cellular or fibrous integrity, it will not lend itself to removal by the barbed broach. Because of these biologic realities and the design of the broach, this instrument has minimal use in clinical practice. Occasionally it will effectively retrieve a paper point or cotton dressing inadvertently lodged in the canal.

Rasps, being similar in design to barbed broaches, but having shallower and more rounded barbs, produce more rough-walled canal preparations than other instruments for canal enlargement and shaping. For this reason they have been superceded by H-type files, but they continue to be somewhat popular outside the United States.

K-Type Files and Reamers

Endodontic files and reamers are by far the most common intracanal instruments used today. The K-type file was first introduced at the turn of the century (1901) and receives the name *K-type* from the holder of its original patent, the Kerr Manufacturing Company.

More is known about K-type files and reamers than about other types of instruments in endodontics, not only because of their widespread acceptance but also because of the impetus given to instrument investigation by the development of national and international standards. K-type root canal instruments are, size for size, stiffer and stronger than comparable types of instruments (Fig. 14-5). This is mostly because of their mode of manufacture, wherein the grain structure of the fabricating wire is preserved and the entire bulk of metal in the working portion of the instrument makes up the blade with

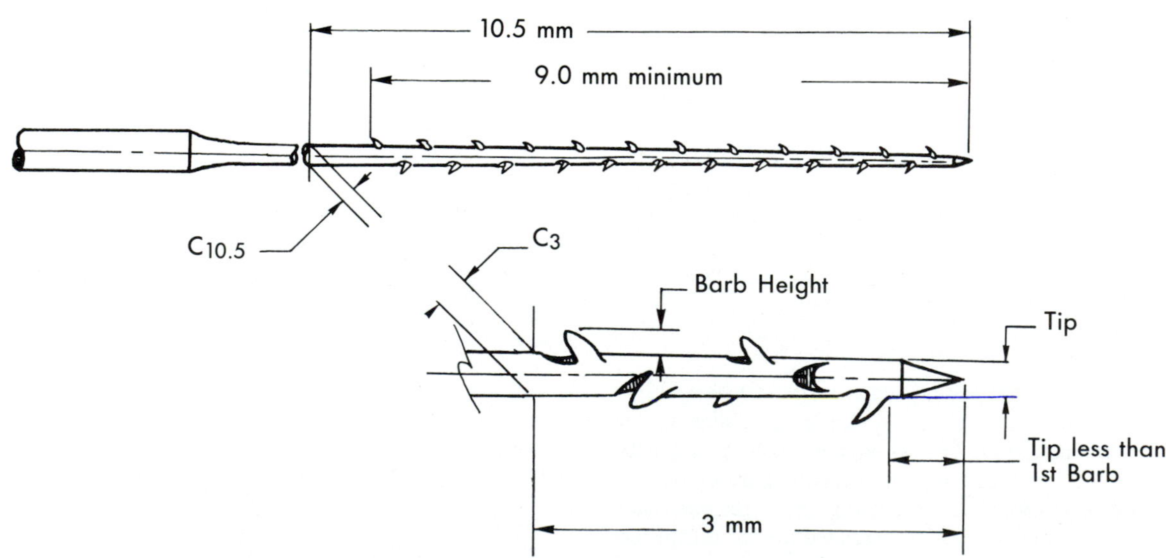

FIG. 14-4 Dimensional formula for barbed broaches and rasps according to ANSI specification no. 63.

its cutting edges. The ductility of the instrument, whether of carbon steel or stainless steel, varies according to the work hardening induced during drawing and fabrication.

Work hardening is a function of size, shape, and tightness of twist. For a given amount of twist, the larger instrument of the same shape will be more work hardened because of greater strains at its outer surfaces and edges. Similarly, a square-shafted (in cross section) instrument with greater bulk at the outer extremities will have more work hardening than a triangular-shafted instrument. The tighter the twist, the more work hardening is induced. A reamer has about half the twists of a file of the same size, and as a consequence has about half the work hardening. A No. 60 file is about three times larger than a No. 20 file, has approximately three fourths the number of twists, and is subjected to about two-and-one-half times more work hardening. Stainless steel is more ductile than carbon steel, but this means little as far as reamers are concerned; for clinical purposes stainless steel is more significant in files.

The cross-sectional shape of the shaft of the instrument can be important in clinical practice. The triangular shaft requires a one-third (120 degrees) rotation of the instrument to complete a cutting circle of the root canal wall, whereas the square shaft requires but a quarter turn to accomplish the same end (Fig. 14-6). An instrument having a triangular shaft gives a

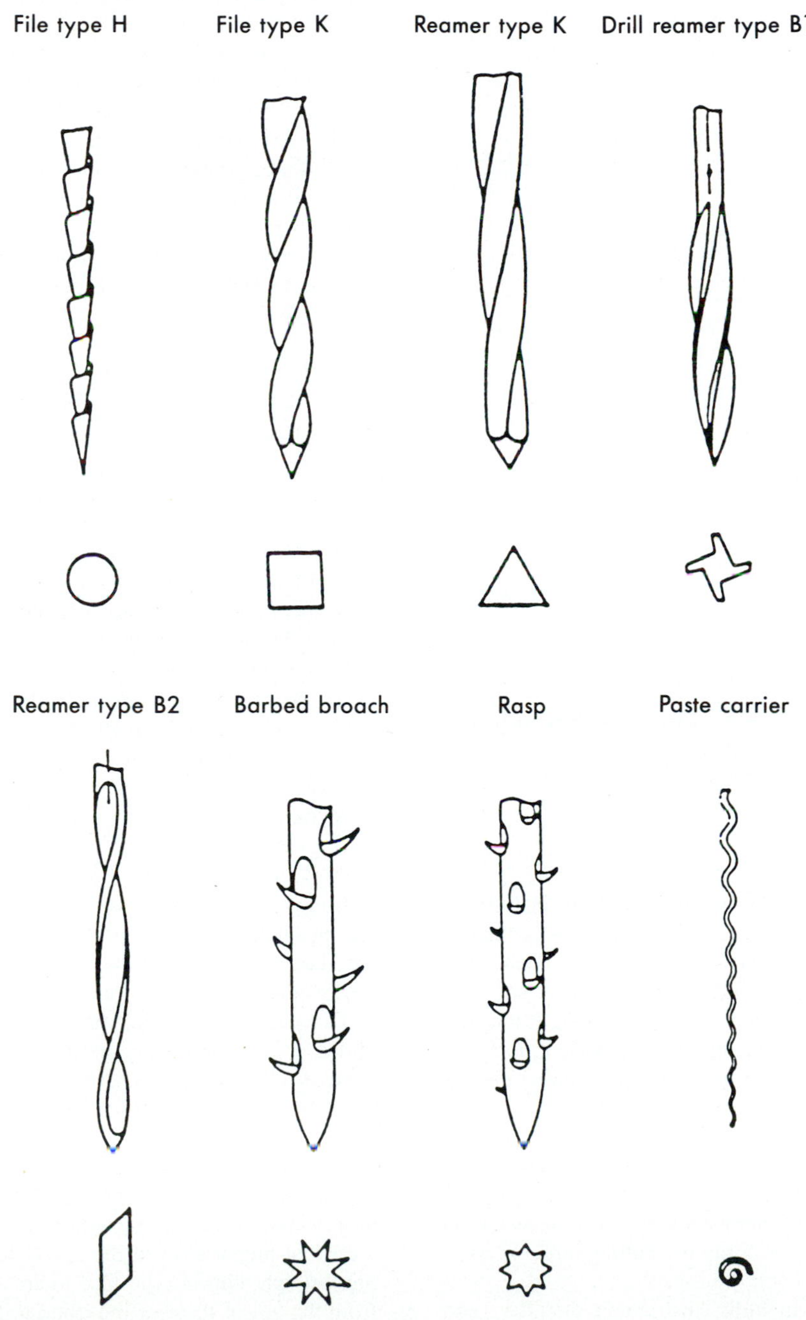

FIG. 14-5 Identification symbols and illustration of hand-operated and engine-driven intracanal instruments in accordance with ISO/FDI designations.

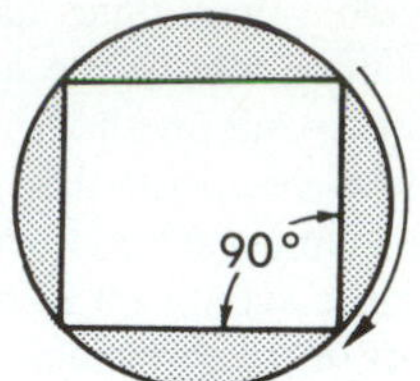

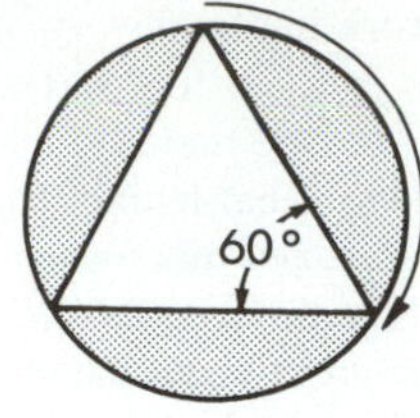

FIG. 14-6 Dynamics of cutting dentin by reaming action with square and triangular cross-sectional instruments. Stress concentration at the edge of the cutting blade creates cracks in the dentinal surface which propagate until chips are formed and separated from the canal surface.

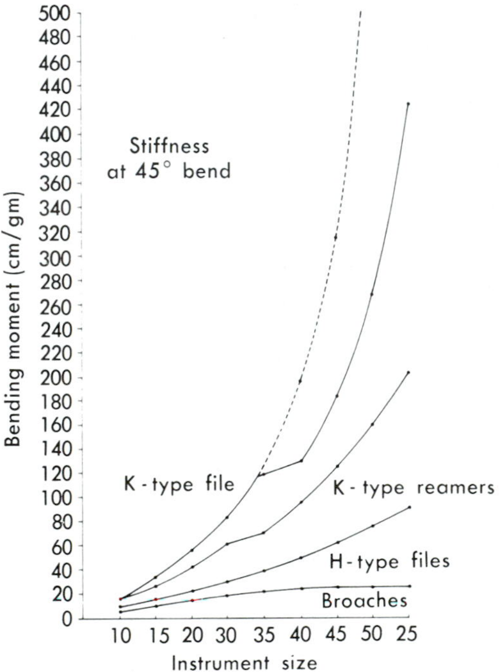

FIG. 14-7 Flexibility of endodontic instruments. The displacement of the curves for K-type files to the right reflects the change in shape from four-sided (square cross section) to three-sided (triangular cross section) instruments.

deeper cut with thicker cutting chips than does an instrument having a square shaft because of the triangular shaft's smaller contact angle with the root canal wall.[139] An instrument having a diamond-shaped or rhomboid shaft combines two acute edge angles and two obtuse edge angles, thus increasing the cutting efficiency of a four-sided instrument. When the blade engages the root canal wall in either instance, a large amount of compression and distortion occurs in the dentin, resulting in cracks that grow as tangents to the orbit of movement of the instrument's edge. When the cracks extend to certain distances, a chip from the surface 0.005 to 0.01 mm deep and 1 to 4 mm long breaks away. Whether a K-type file or reamer is being used, the net result is the same if a cutting circle is completed.[60]

Because of differences in bulk, instrument ductility, and contact angle with the root canal wall between the square-shafted file and the triangular-shafted file, the difference in clinical feel of the instruments and their consequences can be significant. Note that the curve for K-type files in Figure 14-7 changes abruptly between no. 30 and no. 35, as does the curve for K-type reamers between no. 25 and no. 30. This is because of a shift that some manufacturers make from square shafts in smaller instruments to triangular shafts in larger instruments. If the K-type files continued to be made with square shafts, the curve for stiffness would go on as indicated by the dotted line. If this change of instrument shaft shape is not perceived, and compensated for, the clinician is likely to experience an increase in instrument breakage by assuming a naturally increasing progression of applied forces during instrumentation.[89]

A root canal preparation that is round in cross section can be made only by rotary action of a K-type file.[159] In relatively straight root canals this can be accomplished 80% of the time at the apical 1-mm level. In severely curved canals it can be accomplished approximately 33% of the time at the same level.[133] Neither K-type files nor K-type reamers will produce any significant deviation from circular canal preparations when used with a reaming action; however, files used with filing action will produce significant deviations from circular preparations. Aside from being slightly more flexible and less susceptible to fracture, K-type reamers offer no advantage over K-type files.

H-type (Hedström) Files

The H-type file, more commonly known as the Hedström file, is frequently used in endodontic practice for flaring the canal from the apical region to the occlusal or incisal orifice. The design of the H-type file is such that the bulk of metal in the working blade supporting the cutting surfaces does not extend to the edges of the instrument but is a central core of metal (Fig. 14-8). This relationship between the overall size of the instrument and its inherent strength and flexibility can be deceptive, because the instrument is only as strong or as flexible as the central core of metal from which the cutting edges protrude. When placed in contact with a root canal wall, the cutting edges contact the wall at angles approaching 90 degrees and when the instrument is withdrawn exert an effective honing action.

A comparison of the common H-type instrument with a near 90-degree helical angle to a square-shafted K-type instrument is shown in Figure 14-9, which illustrates the extremes of the instrument types. What should be firmly kept in mind is that the designation H-type or K-type is a generic classification based on manufacturing process and does not apply to any single design or line of instruments.

To use root canal files for maximal effectiveness, Shoji[139,140] recommends the K-type file for preparation of the circular apical retention form and the H-type file for cleaning and shaping the coronal half of the root canal system. The sequence as adopted by many similarly inclined clinicians would be to clean and shape the canal by means of serial filing and recapitulation using K-type files with rotary twists of a quarter turn or more followed by withdrawal strokes, thereby creating a conical preparation to the apical foramen, and then following through with H-type files to create a flare for accessibility from the apical third of the canal to the occlusal or incisal orifice.

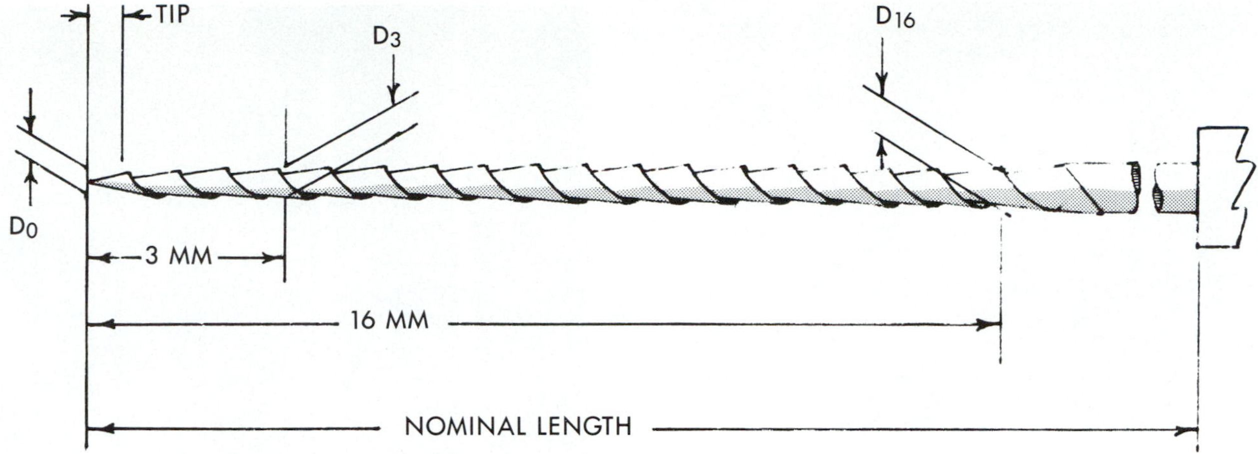

FIG. 14-8 Dimensional formula for H-type (Hedström) instruments according to ANSI specification no. 58.

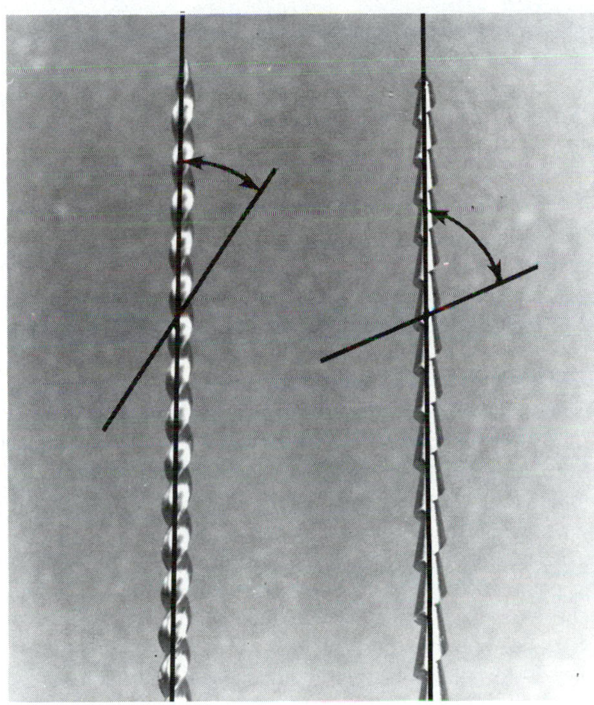

FIG. 14-9 Helical angle of K- and H-type instruments. Greater cutting efficiency is achieved in filing motion as the helical angle approaches 90 degrees to the dentin surface.

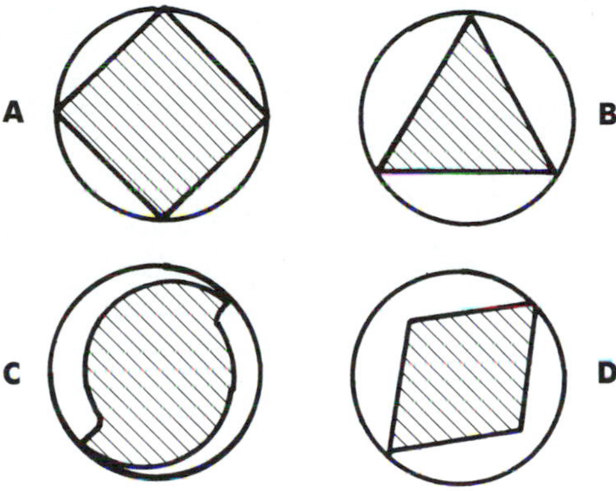

FIG. 14-10 Cross-sectional design of instruments. **A,** Square. **B,** Triangular. **C,** S-shaped. **D,** Rhomboid. Differences in bulk for these variations in cross-sectional design affect the flexibility and other physical properties.

Hybrid Instrument Designs

Modifications or departures from K-type, H-type, or R-type files have been made, that apparently are intended to alleviate some of the clinical difficulties encountered in instrumentation procedures; such as ledging or perforation of the root canal wall, or to aid in the penetration and enlargement of severely curved or constricted canals. Generally these modifications have consisted of (1) changes in the cross-sectional design (Fig. 14-10), (2) changes in the depth or angle of the cutting edges of the flutes, or (3) changes in the design of the tip of the instruments.

Minute variations in design have been reported to have a significant effect on an instrument's physical and mechanical properties, such as cutting efficiency,[7,111] torsional strength, and flexibility[40,76] as measured in laboratory comparisons. Others have presented clinical evidence in support of their theories that specific design modifications related to instruments govern their clinical performance and an operator's ability to successfully achieve the objectives of endodontic procedures.[125]

The K-Flex file (Fig. 14-11) introduced in 1981 appears to be the first serious effort to improve the K-file without mimicking the H-type's geometry or characteristics. For this reason it may be viewed as the forerunner of so-called hybrid instrument designs. The term *hybrid*, as it pertains to endodontic instruments, may be applied to those designs that attempt to integrate the strength and versatility of K-type files with the aggressive cutting properties of H-type instruments.[106]

Modifications of the cross-sectional design of K-type files from square to triangular or rhomboid (diamond-shaped) have resulted in significantly greater flexibility, especially in instruments of larger diameter.[40,76] The alternating flute depth re-

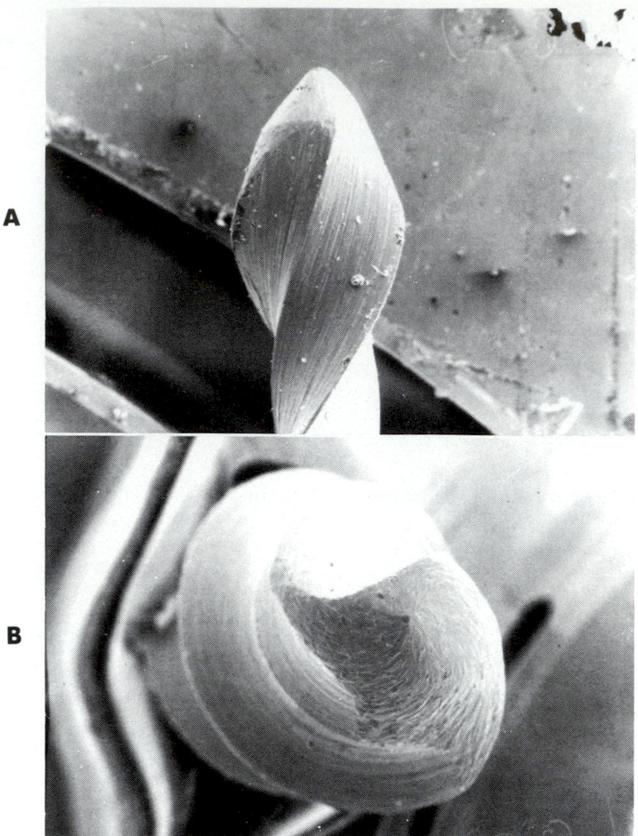

FIG. 14-11 A, Side view of K-Flex file. (Original magnification, ×50.) **B,** Top view of K-Flex file (original magnification, ×100) showing rhomboid cross section.

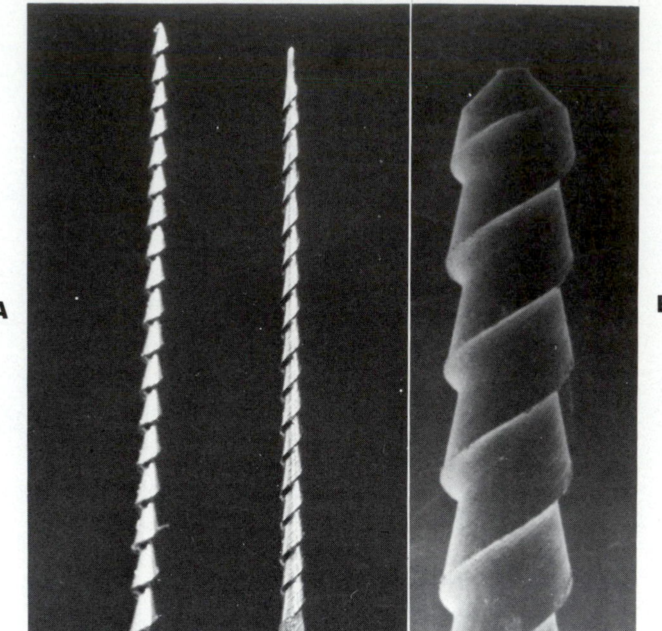

FIG. 14-12 A, H-type root canal files. Hedström *(left),* Unifile *(right).* **B,** S file. (Original magnification, ×50.)

sulting from the rhombic cross-sectional design may also be responsible for the apparent increase in debris removal from constricted canals, facilitated by a decrease in instrument bulk along the shaft.[101,111] Similarly, a 37.5% decrease in cross-sectional surface area is produced by a change from square to triangular design for the same-size instrument.[111,124]

Other cross-sectional variations of K-type and H-type geometry have been produced by milling or grinding, rather than by twisting the wire shaft. Two examples of such instruments are the Unifile and the S file (Fig. 14-12). These instruments possess an S-shaped cross section (Fig. 14-12, *B*) and flutes with geometric shapes not achievable by twisting, as with the K-type instruments. These varieties of instruments, by definition, belong to the H-type classification. For both of these instruments depth control is facilitated by a millimeter scale etched into the shaft between the cutting region and the handle. The S file displays a double helix ground into the shaft and an S-shaped cross section. Like the Unifile, the flutes are less deep than those of Hedström files, leaving greater bulk in the shaft. It differs from the Unifile since the angle of the flutes remains uniform through the length of the instrument and the depth of the flutes increases from the tip to the handle. Like the Hedström file, with its positive rake angle, cutting is most efficient in the withdrawal stroke; however, this design allows for cutting by reaming as well. According to its manufacturer, the potential for both apical preparation by reaming and coronal flaring by filing allows it to be used as a universal instrument for root canal preparation. Laboratory comparisons of the cutting efficiency of the S file and of other instrument designs tend to substantiate these claims.[106]

Variations in the Design of the Tip

Most recently, attention has shifted to the design of the tip of endodontic instruments. Specifications No. 28 and 58 state that the design of the tip of K-type and H-type instruments is optional. Early investigators of the effect of instrumentation procedures on the shape of the prepared root canal observed that the removal of cutting edges from the tip of the instrument could reduce the occurrence of ledging and perforation of curved roots.[102,163,164] More recent investigations further support the opinion that the tips of endodontic instruments (Fig. 14-13) possess potentially active cutting surfaces.[101,102,120,125]

The Flex-R file, developed by the Union Broach company, is one example of an instrument with a noncutting tip design (Fig. 14-14). The tip of this file has been modified to have a compound angle of 70 and 35 degrees without any active cutting edges (Fig. 14-15). The purpose of such a design is to guide the tip through curvatures and to reduce the risk of ledging and perforation. According to Roane,[125] its designer, the tendency for transportation during instrumentation of curved canals is inherent in the design of K-type files. Transportation or ledging commonly occurs at the outer curvature of the apical canal wall as a result of unbalanced forces and the presence of cutting edges on the tips of these (K-type) instruments. It is reasonable to assume that the energy stored by bending an instrument shaft creates a restoring force proportional to the inherent flexibility of the metal and the degree of curvature or bending. It is also plausible that when the sum of these forces is concentrated at the tip of the instrument, cutting of the outer

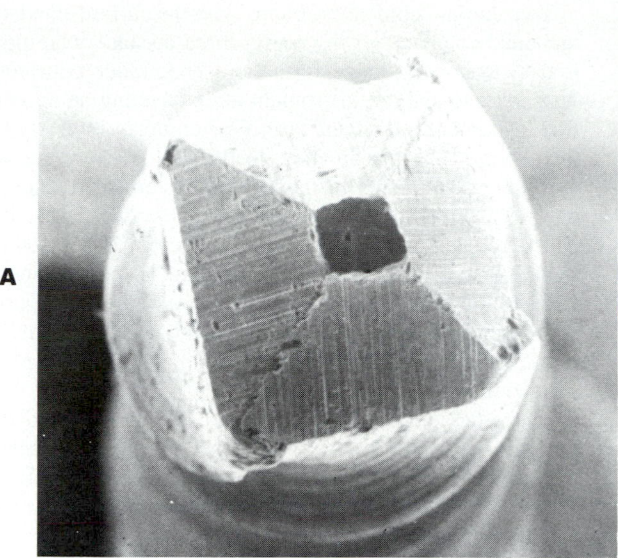

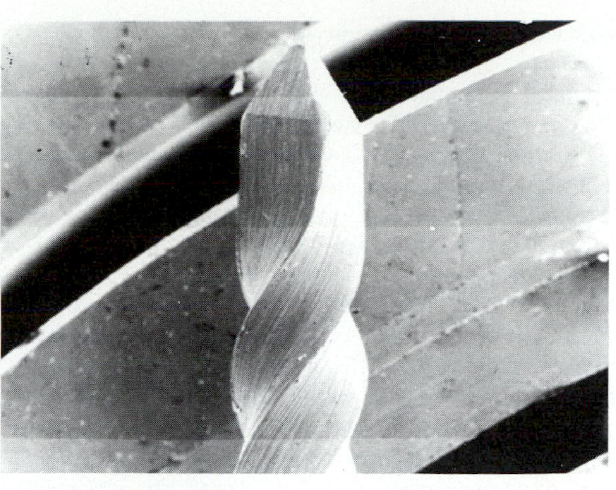

FIG. 14-13 A, Top view of Kerr K file. (Original magnification, ×100.) **B,** Side view of Kerr K file. (Original magnification, ×50.)

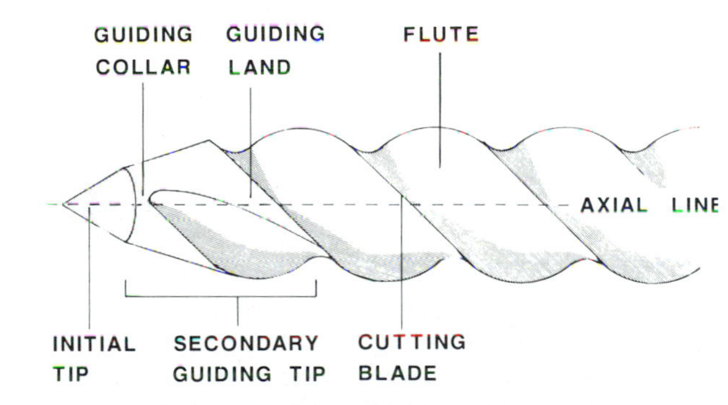

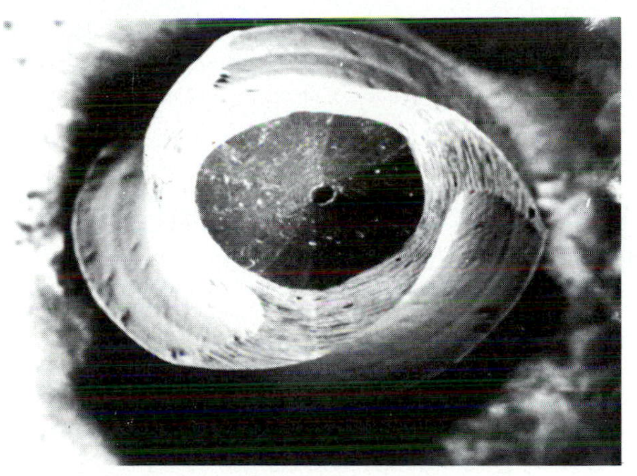

FIG. 14-14 A, Design features of Union Broach Flex-R file. Initial tip angle (70 degrees). Guiding collar angle (35 degrees). **B,** Top view of Flex-R file showing noncutting tip design. (Original magnification, ×100.)

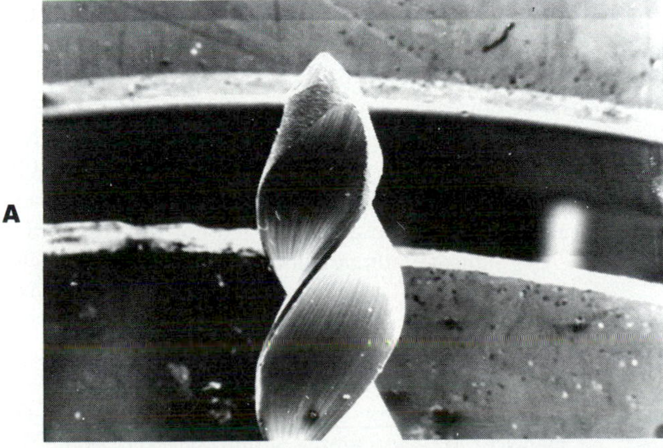

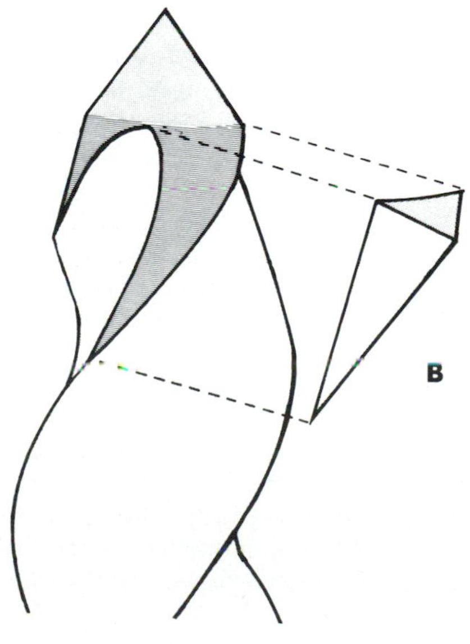

FIG. 14-15 A, Side view of Flex-R file showing the compound tip angle. (Original magnification, ×50.) **B,** Illustration of method of fabrication of guiding collar by removal of a section of the tip *(right)*.

dentin wall will occur more readily if cutting edges are prominent at the tip.

According to the manufacturer (Union Broach Corp., Long Island, N.Y.), the Flex-R file also differs from conventional designs in that the fluted edges are milled rather than twisted. This process allows control of instrument flexibility and cutting efficiency and influences torsional strength. By precise milling, the manufacturer is able to vary the angle of the cutting edge, which determines not only sharpness but also the cross-sectional area. The variation in cross-sectional area for different sizes of instruments can provide increased stiffness and torsional strength in smaller sizes or provide increased flexibility in larger sizes with minimal reduction in torsional strength.

A recent addition to the endodontic armamentarium is an unclassified hand instrument, called the Pathfinder, designed specifically to negotiate highly calcified and constricted root canals. This instrument, developed by the Kerr Manufacturing Company, is similar in appearance to the K-type file but possesses a narrower taper to uniformly distribute the axial stress along the instrument shaft, thus reducing the tendency to bend at the tip. These instruments come in presterilized single-unit packages and are available in 19-, 21-, and 25-mm lengths and two sizes, K1 and K2. The carbon steel shaft is reported to provide greater sharpness and strength for penetrating calcified root canals.

A new concept in instrument design

Herbert Schilder

"Standardized" measurements for manufacturing and designating files and reamers for enlarging root canals have been described in this chapter. Endodontic instruments for cleaning and shaping root canal systems have been newly introduced with a significant alteration to the current ISO formulation. In the current system the dimensional increase from one instrument to the next in a series of instruments when measured at D_0 is 0.02, 0.05, or 1.0 mm. That is, from the no. 06 instrument to the no. 10 instrument, each instrument in a series increases by 0.02 mm, from the no. 10 instrument to the no. 60 instrument each one in the series increases by 0.05 mm, and after instrument no. 60 each one increases by 0.10 mm at D_0 up to instrument no. 130.

The new instruments are based on a *constant percent* change of dimension at point D_0 rather than the *variable linear dimensional* changes incorporated in the current ISO standard.

Once a percent has been chosen to define the increase in size of endodontic files and reamers, or for that matter any instrument for shaping canals, the increase in dimension at the instrument defining point, D_0, is always parabolic (Fig. 14-16). Two outcomes of great clinical value are mathematically wedded to such a progression of instrument sizes.

First, fewer instruments are necessary to go from the narrowest to the widest instrument size than in the current endodontic armamentarium. Second, the instruments are automatically better spaced within the useful range, with more instruments at the beginning of the series and fewer at the end. For example, when a constant percent change of 29.17% is selected (K = 29.17%), eight instruments replace the eleven instruments currently provided between ISO series no. 10 and ISO series no. 60.

Two chronic clinical problems with the current standard had remained unaddressed for nearly three decades. One problem is that, to prevent ledge formation, endodontic educators advise never to skip an instrument after selecting an appropriate first instrument in a given case. Few clinicians actually follow this advice. The reason they do this is that there are simply too many instruments in the present system. For example, if one were to include all the instruments between nos. 06 and 140, there are 21 instruments in the current ISO system. The same full span of D_0 incremental increase is accomplished with 13 instruments in the new system! No one, of course, uses the entire range of instruments between 06 and 140 in any given case. Nevertheless, between 10 and 60 alone, there are 11 instruments in the present system!

The other unaddressed problem is the frequent difficulty found in negotiating narrow and curved canals, especially in their apical thirds. This often occurs because, in spite of the excellent matching capabilities of manufacturers, it is frequently difficult to find a no. 15 instrument constructed to ISO standards that easily follows a no. 10 instrument into narrow or curved canals. This difficulty represents a serious flaw in the current standard. The percent difference between a no. 10 instrument and a no. 15 instrument is an astounding 50%. On the other hand, the percent difference between a no. 60 and a no. 55 instrument is a mere 9%. No wonder that so many canals are blocked and clinicians frustrated in attempting to shape the apical thirds of canals, and that so many instruments are, quite often haphazardly, "skipped" in the final stages of canal preparation.

A comparison of percent incremental changes at D_0 in the current ISO series is revealing (Fig. 14-17). Where clinicians yearn for finer gradations, the largest percent changes currently exist! Where larger incremental changes are easily tolerated clinically, the smallest percent changes occur. Linearly defined instrument increments that may have appeared logical mechanically are not necessarily logical clinically. Note especially the illogical decrease in percent change between the 11 instruments counting from nos. 10 to 60 in the present system.

Currently, a series of instruments is available, constructed with a 29.17% constant increase between every successive instrument in the series. When K = 29.17%, 13 instruments in the new series replace 20 instruments between nos. 06 and 130 in the old ISO system and exclude two superfluous ISO instruments (ISO 140 and ISO 150) (please refer back to Fig. 14-16). Note that the new series is numbered 00, 0, and then 1 to 11. Easy points of reference for clinicians are that the new no. 1 corresponds precisely with the ISO no. 10 in the older system. The new no. 8 corresponds precisely with the old no. 60. The new system spans the gap between no. 10 and no. 60 in the old system with only 8 instruments instead of the 11 currently provided under the present ISO standard.

As indicated above, once a constant percentage increment is provided, the actual measurement changes at D_0 always increase parabolically. That automatically provides more instruments distributed in the smaller range of the series and fewer in the less-sensitive larger end of the series.

Figure 14-17 invites comparison of the actual D_0 measurements of the instruments within the ISO range 10 to 60 with the new instruments spanning the same range. It should be recalled immediately that the difference between the first two instruments in the new series is 29% rather than the current 50% difference between ISO 10 and ISO 15.

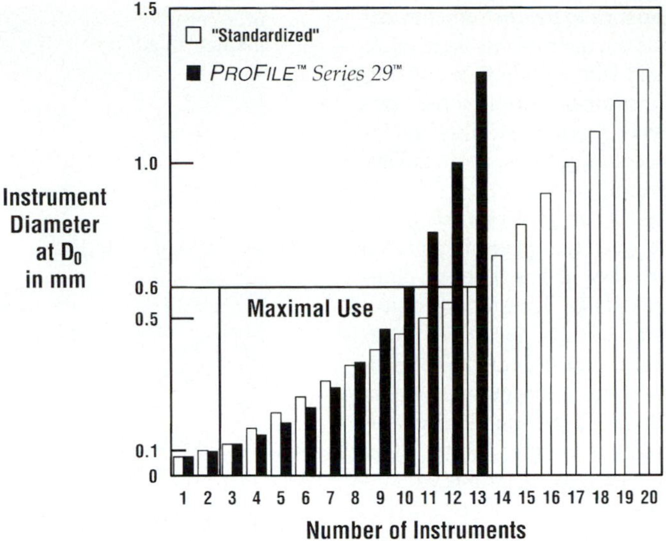

FIG. 14-16 In the new series 13 instruments replace 20 instruments in spanning the range of D_0 sizes from 0.06 to 1.3 mm. Note that in the new instrument series the increases are always decidedly more gradual at the beginning of the series. In the range of maximal use (the range in which most endodontic instruments are purchased) 8 instruments in the new series replace 11 instruments in the current ISO series. Most importantly, starting with an instrument of D_0 diameter of 0.1 mm (ISO 10 or new instrument series no. 1) each successive instrument in the new series is narrower at D_0 in the ISO series until the sixth instrument occurs at which time new instrument series no. 6 slightly exceeds ISO instrument no. 35.

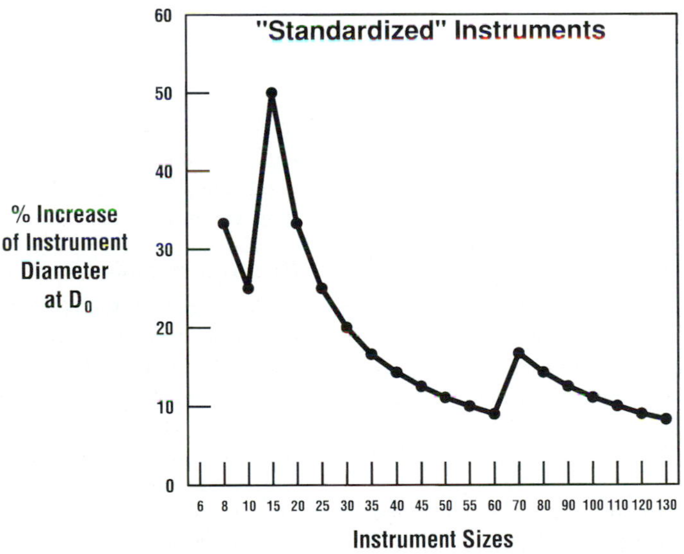

FIG. 14-17 Graphic representation of the chaotic percent incremental changes at D_0 with instruments manufactured in accordance with the current ISO specifications.

The difference between the second and third instruments in the new series is again 29% instead of the 33⅓% difference between ISO 15 and ISO 20. The parabolic nature of increase for the new instruments provides that the first five instruments used in succession in the new series are all narrower in diameter at D_0 than the first five instruments used in the current ISO system. In this example, not until the sixth successive instrument does the diameter at D_0 of the new series of instruments equal (in fact, slightly exceed) the diameter of the sixth successive ISO instrument (ISO 35). Two additional instruments take the operator to D_0 = 0.60 mm in the new system instead of the five instruments in the current ISO series.

Instruments constructed in accordance with these principles with the cooperation of several large manufacturers were tested by panels of endodontists and general dentists. The responses were uniformly favorable concerning the products of all three manufacturers. Indeed, the new sizing was so helpful in shaping around curves and in narrow canals that the various panel members often attributed characteristics to the instruments that they did not actually possess. Since the instruments were made with steel of the same flexibility and with cutting flutes of similar design as the equivalent ISO instruments of the same manufacturers, the common perception of greater flexibility and increased sharpness could be attributed only to the more advantageous sizing of the new instruments.

In summary, ISO $K = 0.02$, 0.05, or 0.10 mm for increment at D_0 was a great advance over the chaos it replaced nearly three decades ago. Nevertheless, it has inherent clinical flaws. One is that major increments at D_0 occur where minor ones are needed, and that subsequently negligible increments are provided where larger ones are indicated. The second is that too many successive instruments encourage random skipping of instruments and potential ledge formation. Instrument series based on K = a constant percentage, on the other hand, always span the same range with fewer instruments, better spaced within the useful range.

The principle is applicable to all endodontic-enlarging instruments, not simply reamers and files, and to engine-driven as well as to hand-manipulated instruments. With more universal use it is hoped that the ISO standard will be amended so that D_0 may be identified in terms of K = a constant percent. No change in the current ISO specified taper of 0.02 mm/mm between D_0 and D_{16} is currently recommended.

Instruments constructed according to this system are currently marketed by Tulsa Dental Products for hand use in stainless steel and nickel/titanium for K-type reamers and files, and for Hedström files, under the name Profile-Series 29. Appropriately sized gutta-percha cones matching the new instrument sizes will be generally available.

[Dr. Schilder's contribution ends here.]

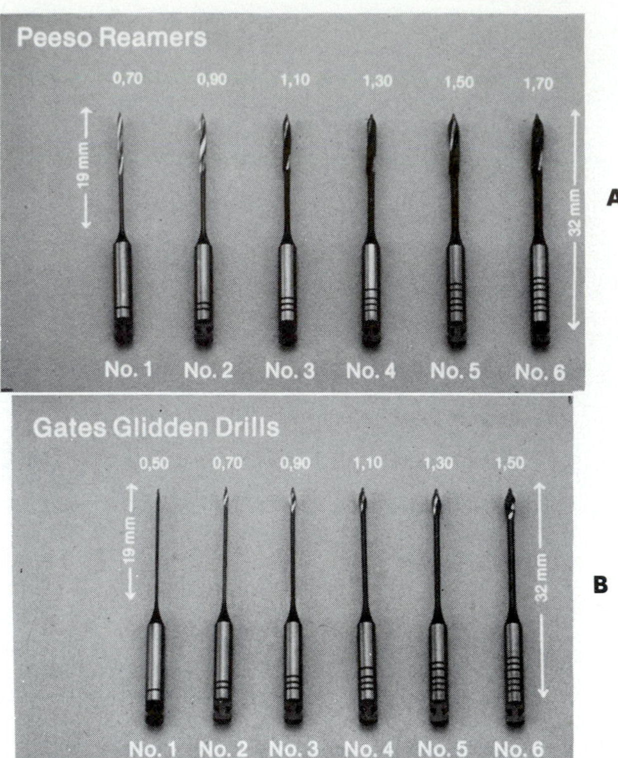

FIG. 14-18 A, Sizing and dimensions of Peeso-type engine reamers (Union Broach). **B,** Sizing and dimensions of Gates-Glidden engine reamers (Union Broach).

Power-Driven Instruments

As stated earlier, the resurgence in popularity of mechanized systems for preparing and enlarging the root canal is an indication of a desire for greater speed and efficiency of treatment.

A number of mechanized systems for enlargement of the root canal have been devised. Generally they can be divided into three groups: (1) latch-type rotary instruments for use in conventional handpieces; (2) endodontic files, reamers, and broaches for use in specialized reciprocal or oscillating handpieces; and (3) instruments used in specialized vibratory endodontic devices.

Rotary Instruments

Two types of instruments have been designed for use in slow-speed dental handpieces according to the ISO-FDI classification (Fig. 14-5): those having two parts, a shaft and an operative head (group II), and those in which the shaft and operative head are of one piece (group III). Common examples of single-part rotary instruments used in the United States are the Peeso and Gates-Glidden drills (Fig. 14-18). These are primarily used in the coronal third of the canal for enlarging the orifice, preparing post spaces, and as auxiliary instruments for flaring the canal.[1]

Group II instruments are similar in design to conventional endodontic hand instruments to which a latch-type attachment has been added to the shaft for use in slow handpieces. These are seldom used for root canal preparation but are more frequently employed to remove gutta-percha in making post space. Historically, engine-driven instruments have not been extensively advocated in the United States, principally because of the hazards of root perforation and instrument breakage. Caution should be exercised by both the novice and experienced clinician to avoid the excessive removal of root structure, which can occur rapidly with these instruments.

Reciprocal Endodontic Handpieces

To overcome the inflexibility of conventional endodontic hand instruments (group I) the Giromatic, a quarter-turn endodontic handpiece, was introduced in 1964. This handpiece operates by rotary reciprocal action through a 90-degree (quarter turn) arc. The Giromatic received much attention in spite of data that indicates it is significantly less effective in cleaning canals than conventional hand-operated instruments.[83] As with most power driven instruments, the loss of tactile sensation creates additional risks of instrument breakage, overinstrumentation, and penetration of the apical foramen.

Barbed broaches have been used in engine-driven contraangle handpieces designed for endodontics without significant incidents of instrument fracture.[63] They were selected for use in the Giromatic rotary reciprocal handpieces principally because of their flexibility. Investigations have revealed that they are ineffective as root canal–cleaning instruments when used in endodontic contraangle handpieces because the rotary action of the instrument compresses the barbs against the core of the instrument and burnishes them in place after a very few minutes.[109]

Another automated handpiece system, the Canal Finder, has been reported to be of some assistance in penetrating severely curved and constricted canals without causing perforation or ledging.[35,47,86] This device operates by reciprocal rotation of

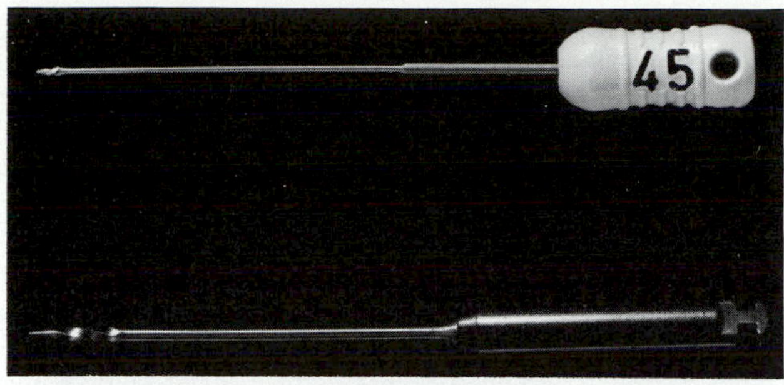

FIG. 14-19 Canal Master instruments (Brassler). Hand instrument *(top)*, engine reamer *(bottom)*.

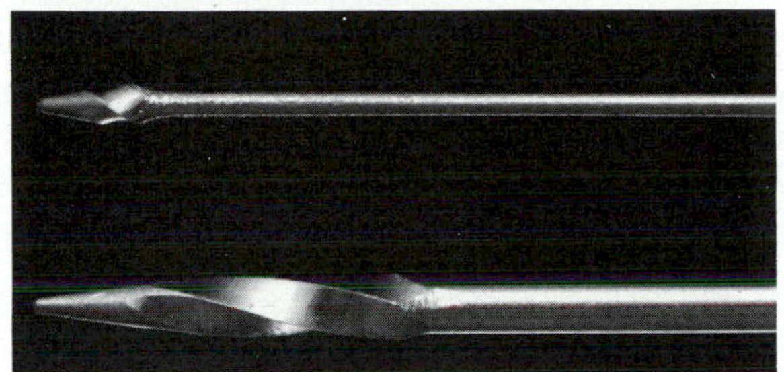

FIG. 14-20 Comparison of tip lengths of Canal Master hand- and engine-driven instruments. Hand instrument (0.75 mm), engine reamer (2.0 mm).

the shaft but also produces a filing motion that is controlled by an automatic clutch mechanism to prevent file breakage. Specially designed files are used with this system.

One of the most revolutionary concepts in root canal preparation has been presented by Drs. Senia and Wiley.[166] The Canal Master system employs both hand- and engine-driven instruments of unique design, which reportedly facilitates instrumentation of curved canals (Fig. 14-19). The instruments are not unlike the Gates-Glidden reamer, which has been used for some decades for enlargement of the coronal portion of root canals. Close inspection, however, reveals subtle differences between the two that make possible use of a hand-manipulated version of the newer instrument for apical preparation and an engine-driven version for flaring the coronal section of the canal. The noncutting pilot tip varies in length between 0.75 mm for hand-operated and 2 mm for engine-driven instruments (Fig. 14-20). According to its designers,[166] the Canal Master instruments incorporate three major features:

1. They replace the usual cutting tip with a noncutting pilot. The pilot helps limit transportation of the canal and guides the instrument to the foramen (Fig. 14-21).
2. The cutting segment of the instrument (cutting head) is reduced from the standard 16 mm to 1 to 2 mm. Unlike standard instruments that are capable of cutting anywhere on the entire 16 mm of cutting surface, the cutting head of the Canal Master instrument has a minimum cutting surface for maximal control.
3. The diameter of the instrument's smooth round shaft remains constant and is reduced to increase its flexibility.

The purpose of an instrument so designed is to combine a noncutting pilot tip with a reduced cutting surface at the head,

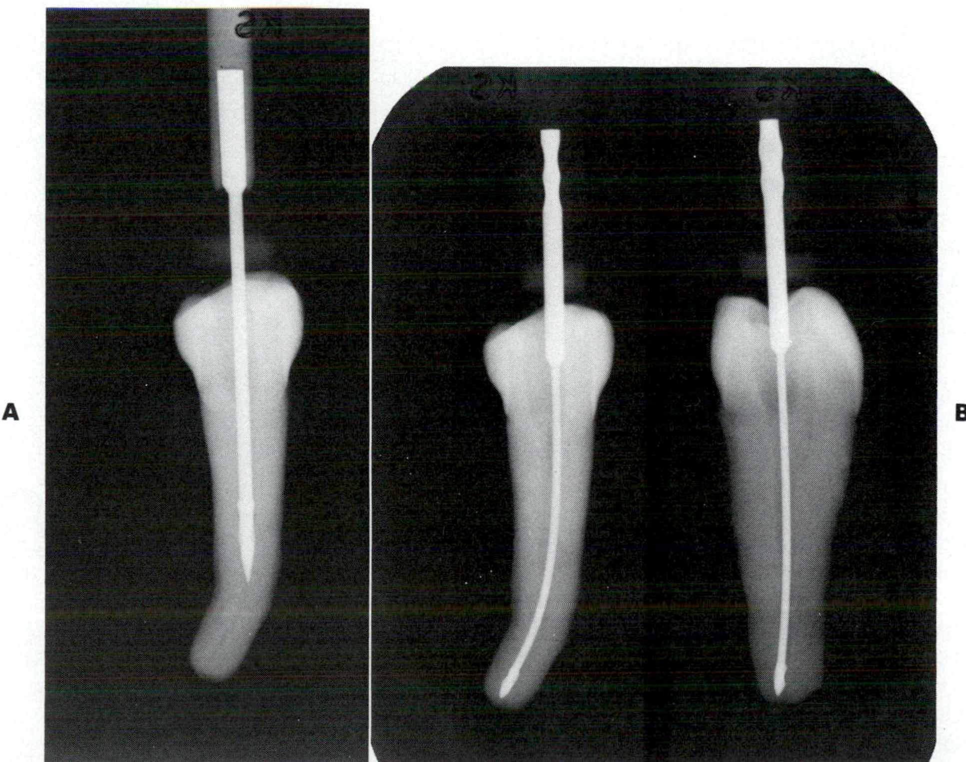

FIG. 14-21 A, No. 100 Canal Master engine reamer used for coronal flaring to the canal curvature. **B,** Canal Master no. 70 hand instruments shown in curved canal. Facial view *(left)*, proximal view *(right)*.

attached to a flexible shaft of reduced diameter that can better follow the original canal curvature and reduce transportation.

It has been illustrated that transportation occurs during preparation and enlargement of the root canal because of indiscriminate cutting of dentin at the tip and along the entire 16-mm cutting surface of instruments.[73] This has been attributed to previous design modifications that created sharper and more aggressive cutting instruments. The net result is a tendency for deviation from the original canal space, ledging, or perforation of curved roots, which further complicates or prohibits débridement and enlargement of the apical segment of the canal.[61,136]

Hand-operated Canal Master instruments have a 0.75-mm noncutting pilot tip with color-coded handles corresponding to standardized instrument sizes 20 through 80. The rotary version (sizes 50, 60, 70, 80, 90, 100) have color-coded latch-type attachments and a 2-mm noncutting tip for greater safety. The cutting head is approximately 1 mm long for the hand version and 2 mm for the rotary instruments. The recommended method for using the hand instruments is 60 degrees reciprocal rotation (reaming) of the instrument. It is said that the narrow shaft for both hand and rotary instruments facilitates debris removal and irrigation. Evaluation of the Canal Master system has revealed that it reduces the incidence of transportation within the root canal but has a greater tendency toward instrument breakage.[50,97]

Other examples of instruments with noncutting tips are illustrated in Figures 14-22 through 14-24. Potentially, these types of instruments may be of benefit in specific clinical applications. The Endosonic Diamond, Rispi, and Shaper files, a new variety of endodontic instruments, are described below.

Ultrasonic and Sonic Instrument Systems

A new generation of instrumentation has evolved that depends on the vibrational action of energized instruments in the root canal. Generally, two categories of devices have been developed, based on the frequency of vibration imparted to the instruments and the source of power. The ultrasonic systems that generate vibration above the audible range are powered by means of electric currents passing through a lamellar arrangement of metal plates. Alternating attractive and repulsive forces between the plates affect the mechanical vibratory movements, which are then transferred to the instrument. Sonic systems produce vibrations in the audible frequency range by means of compressed air, which activates a rotor and shaft assembly as a source of vibration.

Sonic and ultrasonic instrumentation differs from rotary or hand procedures since the cutting of dentin is facilitated by a mechanical device that imparts a sinusoidal motion to the instrument by the transfer of vibrational energy along the shaft. The term *ultrasonic instrumentation* has been used to describe these types of systems.[67] The first use of ultrasonics in root canal therapy and root resection has been credited to Richman.[122] The phrase *endosonic ultrasonic synergistic system* has also been applied to describe the combined effects of ultrasound on instrumentation and irrigation achieved with these devices.[36]

The Cavi-Endo ultrasonic unit was the first system of its type commercially available in the United States. Its development resulted from the extensive research performed at the Naval Research Center in Bethesda by Drs. Howard Martin and Walter Cunningham. Their original intention was to introduce ultrasonics to the root canal for the purpose of sterilization by sonication of bacteria.[94] The Endosonic 3000 is a sonic endodontic handpiece, similar to sonic air-driven scalers, that has been modified for use as a vibratory endodontic instrumentation device.

Length control during instrumentation differs for the various systems. Some employ a section of plastic tubing as a movable marker or gauge around the instrument shaft for visual reference. Endodontic rubber stoppers may interfere with the flow of irrigant down the instrument shaft. With other systems length control is provided by means of a metal guide bar or stop that limits the depth of instrument insertion, thus mechanically preventing overinstrumentation.

Another major difference between these systems is the method of irrigation and the type of irrigant employed. Both sonic and ultrasonic systems allow the clinician to adjust the rate or level of irrigation. The ultrasonic systems, however, permit the use of either an inert sterile or chemically active irrigant selected by the clinician. Irrigation with the sonic units is limited to filtered water as delivered through the dental unit cooling system.

Instruments provided for use in these systems have for the most part been modifications of either K-type or R-type hand

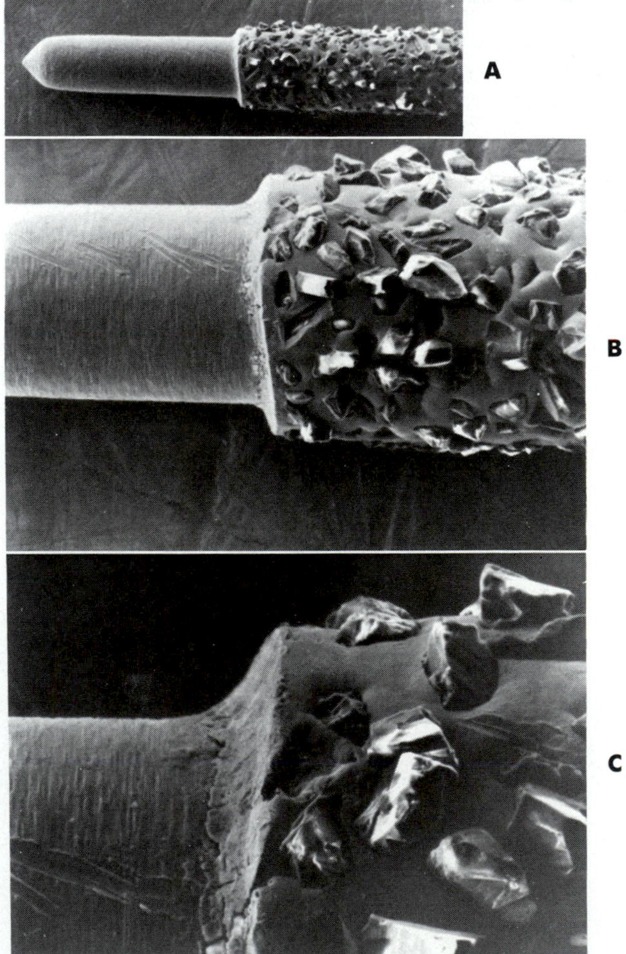

FIG. 14-22 A, Endosonic diamond file (L.D. Caulk). (Original magnification, ×30.) **B,** Endosonic diamond file. (Original magnification ×100.) **C,** Endosonic diamond file. (Original magnification, ×300.)

instruments. The Endosonic Diamond file (Fig. 14-22), on the other hand, has been designed specifically for use as an energized vibrational instrument and represents a considerable departure from previous types of instruments. Diamond particles bonded to a metal shaft provide the cutting edges for dentin removal. Cutting of dentin by abrasion occurs from contact of the instrument with the canal wall by vibrational movement imparted by the mechanical device and by manual filing movement. Use of the Endosonic Diamond file, however, is limited to coronal enlargement within the straight portion of canals, since it is relatively inflexible as compared to other types of instruments.

Greater cutting efficiency, as reported by the developers of this system,[95,96] might be expected because of automated debris removal from the cutting surface of the instrument. By combining the effects of irrigation with instrumentation, dentin chips and debris are removed simultaneously with cutting procedures. Before this, instrumentation, irrigation, and removal of debris from the canal and instrument surfaces would necessarily be performed as separate manipulations.

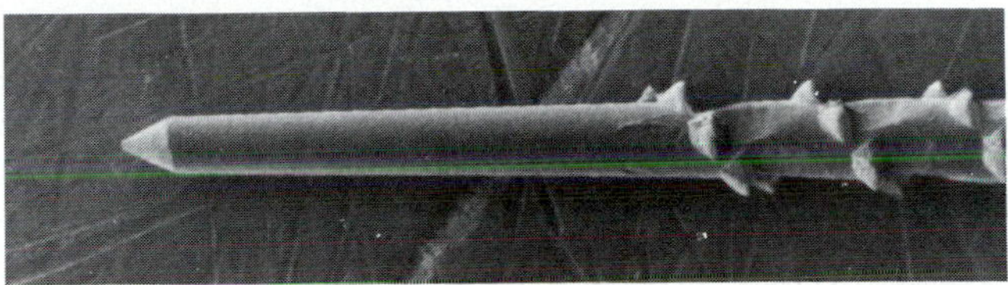

FIG. 14-23 Sonic Rispi file (Micro Mega). (Original magnification, ×30.)

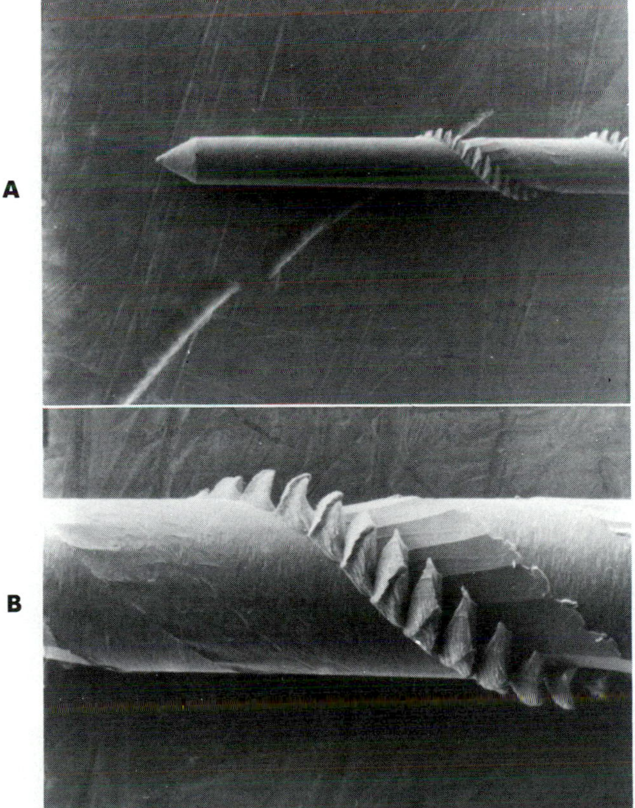

FIG. 14-24 A, Sonic Shaper file (Micro Mega). (Original magnification, ×30.) **B,** Sonic Shaper file (Micro Mega). (Original magnification, ×100.)

Vibratory instruments belonging to the R-type (rattail) category are typified by the Rispi and, with some modification, the Shaper files (Figs. 14-23, 14-24). As in the barbed broach or rasp-type hand instruments, cutting edges are created along the instrument shaft by a series of incisions that become elevated during the manufacturing process to form a roughened surface. Like the diamond file, it abrades rather than cutting per se. Both the ultrasonic diamond file and the sonic R-type instruments display much improved cutting efficiency over the K-type designs when employed in these systems[105] and when compared to hand instrumentation (Fig. 14-25).[106]

Other factors have been attributed to variations in the cutting performance of endodontic instruments. Stenman and Spangberg have reported differences in cutting performance as much as forty times for several brands and designs of instruments. Another significant factor is the use of a lubricant, which has been shown to improve the cutting ability of instruments by 200%.

The recommended technique for the use of vibratory instruments is circumferential filing. The effect of instrumentation procedures on the shape of the root canal preparation has been reported with various results.[29,30,148,167] With ultrasonic instrumentation the ability to maintain the original canal curvature appears to be similar to that with hand instrumentation for smaller sizes (no. 15),[29] but the occurrence of ledging and a tendency toward perforation have been reported for larger-sized files.[29,30,167] Other researchers have observed that sonic instrumentation is superior to either hand or ultrasonic devices in avoiding transportation in curved canals.[73,167]

The customary tactile sense experienced in hand instrumentation is much altered with the energized systems, and since greater cutting efficiency is claimed for these devices, caution must be exercised in their use, to avoid perforations.[80] Although the biologic effects of overinstrumentation on the periapical tissues have not been reported, some manufacturers have elected to include instruments with a noncutting tip, presumably to avoid this potential complication.

INSTRUMENTS FOR SEALING THE ROOT CANAL

Obturation of the root canal space would necessarily involve the introduction of a suitable biologically compatible filling material to prevent the egress of microorganisms or toxic products into the vital periapical tissues. A discussion of instruments or devices intended for use in the process of obturation will therefore require some mention of the filling materials themselves. A more detailed discussion of the physical and biologic properties of endodontic filling materials is presented later in this chapter.

Hand- and Finger-Held Instruments

Several varieties of specialized endodontic pliers and forceps are available for the handling and placement of silver point and gutta-percha cones (Fig. 14-26). The pliers generally have a tapered groove along the beak for firmly grasping the ridged silver cone, whereas the forceps may have either grooved or serrated beaks for holding gutta-percha cones. Endodontic forceps differ from common college or cotton forceps in that they have a latch mechanism for locking the instrument in the closed position. This mechanism allows for

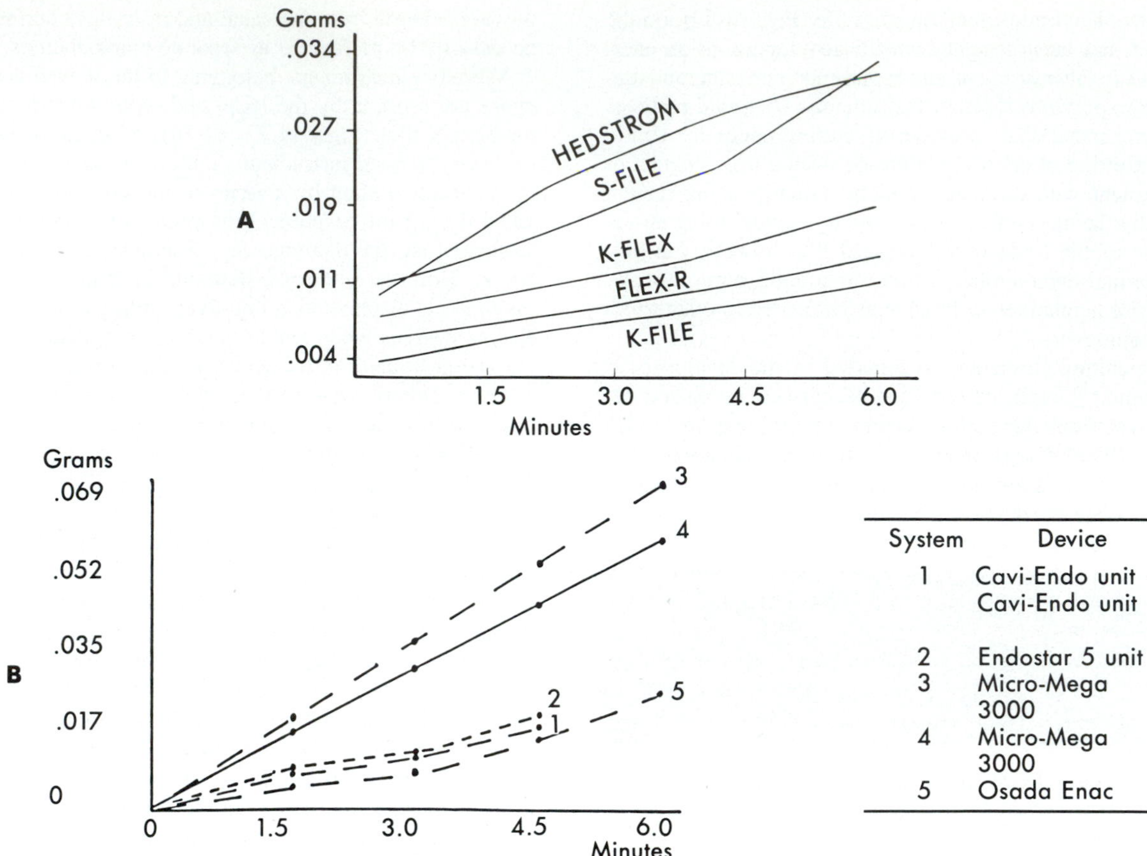

System	Device
1	Cavi-Endo unit Cavi-Endo unit
2	Endostar 5 unit
3	Micro-Mega 3000
4	Micro-Mega 3000
5	Osada Enac

FIG. 14-25 A, Cutting efficiency comparison of endodontic hand instruments. **B,** Cutting efficiency of endodontic vibratory instruments. System: Cavi-Endo *(1),* Endostar-5 *(2),* MM-3000 Rispi *(3),* MM-3000 Shaper *(4),* Enac *(5).*

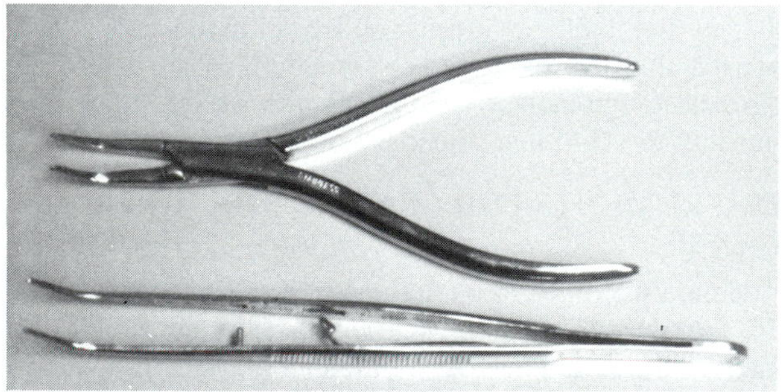

FIG. 14-26 Endodontic forceps. Gutta-percha locking forceps *(bottom),* silver point pliers *(top).*

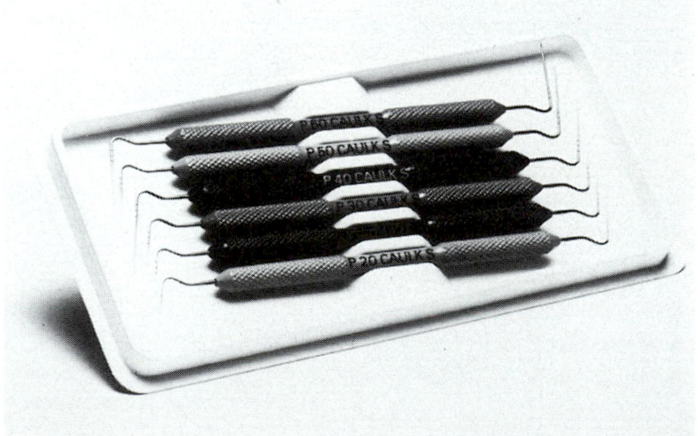

FIG. 14-27 M Series (Martin) plugger/spreaders in standardized sizes.

easier transfer of instrument and material from assistant to operator during treatment.

Endodontic condensers (pluggers) and spreaders are smooth tapered metal instruments used to compress and compact the gutta-percha material either laterally or vertically within the prepared root canal space according to either the lateral or vertical condensation of gutta-percha filling techniques. Condensers or pluggers have blunt or flat-ended tips for compression, whereas spreaders are generally more tapered and have pointed tips for lateral packing of the material. Long-handled spreaders and condensers are formed of chrome-plated or stainless steel with the operative head at various angles to the shaft, similar to instruments used in operative dentistry. M series plugger-spreaders are double-ended long-handled instruments that correspond to the standard sizing and taper of K-type files and reamers. The handles are color coded for easy identification (Fig. 14-27). Finger-held spreaders and condensers are similar in design to K-type files and reamers with either plastic or metal handles bonded to the shaft.

Specialized heat carriers are similar in design to condensers, spreaders, and explorers, used for softening or removal of gutta-percha. These instruments are made of metal alloys capable of withstanding the effects of high temperature cycling without causing alteration of their physical properties. The reader is warned against the use of condensers, spreaders, and explorers made from high carbon alloys for this purpose. Heating and rapid cooling of these instruments results in increased brittleness, which may cause fracture with the root canal.

Standardization of Endodontic Filling Instruments

To those familiar with the history and development of endodontic instruments, the adoption of specifications 28, 57, and 58 may represent some of the most significant advancements toward achieving the objectives of endodontic treatment. The effects of dimensional uniformity between brands of instruments and solid core filling materials have simplified and improved the profession's ability to effectively cleanse, prepare, and seal the complex anatomic system of the root canal. Recently, the standardization of endodontic auxiliary (conventional) gutta-percha cone sizes also represents a further advancement along these lines. The advantage of dimensional uniformity in filling materials can be realized only if filling instruments are similarly standardized to conform in both sizing and dimensions. In a survey of endodontic hand and finger spreaders,[100] it was found that instrument nomenclature (spreader size) provided no indication of the corresponding auxiliary cone size for most brands tested. Designations of instruments such as "D-11" or "D-11T" provide no information about the appropriate auxiliary cone size and, so, necessitate a trial-and-error method for selection of a suitably sized filling. In addition, instruments with the same nominal size designation were found to differ markedly in diameter and taper between brands. It would seem logical that instruments intended to prepare a space for the placement of a filling material having a uniform taper and dimension should likewise be dimensioned and sized to facilitate that placement.[69]

A specification for spreaders and condensers is currently being developed as the ANSI standard. The proposed method for size designation of these instruments is a five-digit number. The first two digits represent the diameter of the instrument at the tip, and the remaining three digits designate the taper in hundredths of millimeters.

Devices for Softening and Placement of Gutta-Percha

The most recent developments related to endodontic filling instruments and devices have been those directed toward facilitating the placement of either semisolid or plasticized gutta-percha into the root canal space. The desirability of injectable materials or materials that have the ability to accurately conform to the anatomic irregularities of the root canal system is evidenced by the introduction of a number of synthetic polymers as endodontic filling materials over the past few years.[15,71,169] Other attempts to utilize the thermoplastic properties of gutta-percha to produce root canal fillings that form a homogeneous mass and seal the canal in three dimensions may also have been the impetus for the development of delivery systems and devices for this same purpose.[130]

Heated Spreaders and Condensers

Two electrical devices are available for softening gutta-percha within the canal space during condensation. The Endoteck (Fig. 14-28) is a battery-operated portable unit that has a heating element within the handle for warming the gutta-percha once it is placed within the canal space. Various spreader tips can be inserted into the handle, which becomes warm when the unit is activated. The Touch' N Heat system (Analytic Technologies) employs a variety of plugger-condensers that are connected to the control unit by an insulated cable (Fig. 14-29). The temperature of the condenser tips can be varied from 400° F to 1200° F for softening and removal of gutta-percha material from the canal. Interchangeable tips are available for bleaching discolored teeth and thermal pulp testing. Figure 14-29 illustrates typical power and temperature settings for specific applications.

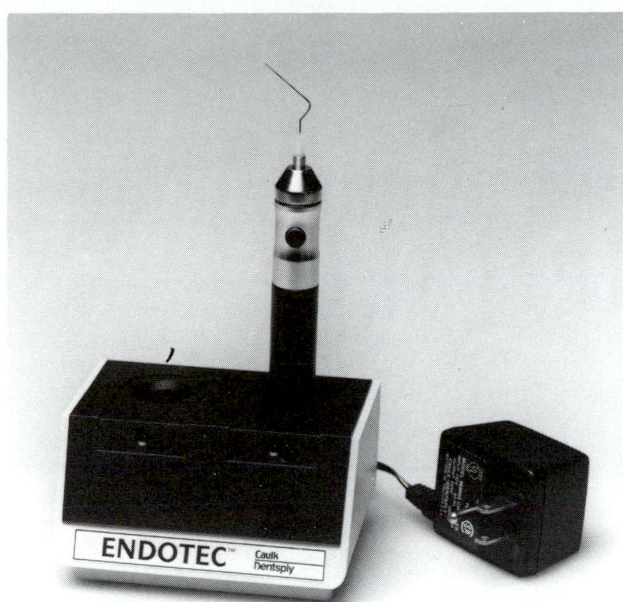

FIG. 14-28 Endotec rechargeable heated spreader for warm lateral condensation of gutta-percha (Caulk/Dentsply).

Thermoplastic Injection of Warmed Gutta-Percha

Two pressurized syringe systems for injection of warmed gutta-percha for the purpose of root canal obturation have been developed. The Obtura II (Fig. 14-30) consists of a pistol-like delivery unit for introduction of thermoplasticized gutta-percha into the root canal through either 20- or 23-gauge silver injection tips. The delivery unit is connected to a precision electrical control unit that features a digital temperature display for regulation and control of the viscosity of the extruded gutta-percha. The maximum internal temperature of the heating element with this system is 204° C. The temperature of the gutta-percha material, as expressed, is 160° C and has a reported working time of 3 to 5 minutes in root canal. Gutta-percha pellets loaded into a chamber in the delivery unit become soft enough within approximately 2 minutes to be extruded through the silver applicator tips by means of a ratchet plunger mechanism. It is recommended that, once placed in the chamber, the gutta-percha should be injected within 15 minutes, the best results being achieved within 4 minutes. Disposable polystyrene cones are used to insulate the delivery unit adjacent to the applicator tip. A special tool is provided for bending the tips for easier insertion into areas of difficult access. The applicator tips are reusable and may be resterilized.

A

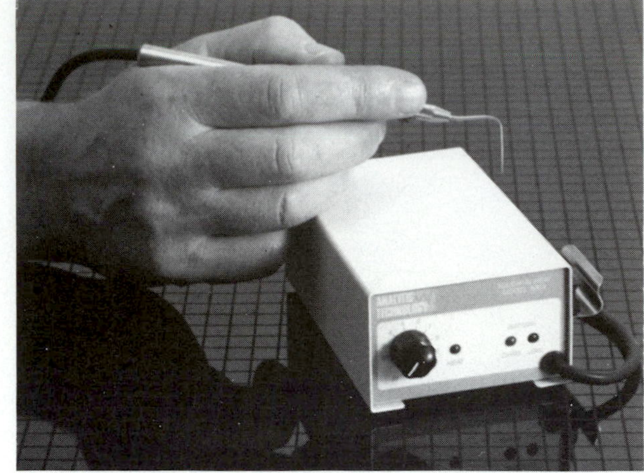

B

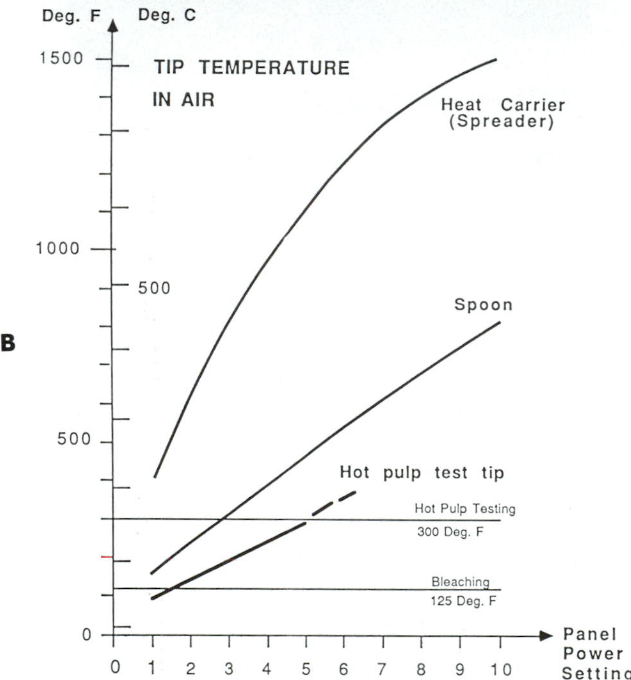

FIG. 14-29 A, Touch 'N Heat heated instrument system (Analytic Technology). **B,** Recommended power/temperature settings for application of Touch 'N Heat system.

The Ultrafil system (Fig. 14-31) for delivery of thermoplasticized gutta-percha differs from the Obtura II in that the temperature of the gutta-percha as extruded is 70° C; thus, it has been termed the *low-temperature injection system*. Other major differences are that the Ultrafil system consists entirely of three separate components; (1) preloaded gutta-percha–filled canules with 22-gauge stainless steel needles, (2) a heating/holding unit, and (3) an autoclavable injection syringe.

Three forms of gutta-percha material are available with this system for use in specific clinical applications and operator preferences. The setting time and consistency of each form of the material varies and is designated by the color of the canules. "Regular set" (coded white) material has greater flow and an approximate setting time of 30 minutes. "Firm set" (blue) has intermediate flow and a 2-minute setting time. "Endoset" (green) has greater resistance to condensation and a faster setting time of 2 minutes. The preloaded canules are individually packaged and are disposable. The stainless steel needles may be preshaped for easier insertion before tempering in the heating unit, which holds as many as four canules for storage. The proper temperature for injection is achieved within 15 minutes, and the canules may be held within the heated unit as long as 4 hours. Obturation is performed by inserting the prewarmed canules into the injection syringe and slowly squeezing the ratchet mechanism to express the plasticized material.

Specialized preparation techniques are also required for insertion of the injection tip or needle into the body of the canal, so that the material may flow to the apical constriction. The body of the canal should be enlarged from a no. 40 to no. 60 instrument when using the 23-gauge injection needle and to a size no. 70 to no. 100 for the 22- and 20-gauge, respectively. Filling may be accomplished by either passive injection of the material into the canal or with vertical condensation by hand instruments once placed. Reportedly a single canal may be obturated easily in less than 30 seconds with these systems.[72] The quality of the apical seal and adaptation of the filling produced by thermoplastic injection-molding techniques has been evaluated by the developers of these systems and by other investigators. In a scanning electron micrographic comparison of thermoplastic injection of gutta-percha to conventional techniques, investigators found that the adaptation of gutta-percha to the dentin wall surface of the root canal was comparable to that achieved with the traditional methods.[153] Leakage studies, as measured by both dye penetration and with radioisotope tracers, have indicated that sealing by thermoplastic injection-molding of gutta-percha with sealer cement is as effective as obturation by other conventional methods.[41,72,114] Other investigators have found the quality of the apical seal to be acceptable, though they reported a high occurrence of overextension of the filling material[77] when the apices were intentionally overinstrumented or when vertical condensation was used. The incidence of overfilling was reduced from 75% to 12.5% when passive injection was used without vertical condensation.[41] In another study the clinical success of injection-molded thermoplasticized gutta-percha obturation following biomechanical instrumentation was evaluated for 125 cases based on clinical and radiographic findings.[92] They reported an average success rate of 97% over a 12-month period for cases presenting either with or without periapical radiolucent areas.

A number of auxiliary applications have been proposed for these systems in the repair of perforations, as a retrograde filling material,[42] in the treatment of internal resorption, and for treatment of the open apex. It may be advisable to avoid using these systems to treat large open apices, since a high incidence of overfilling has been observed in the absence of a verifiable apical constriction. Various techniques have been recommended to overcome these specific clinical problems.

Gutta-Percha Carrier Devices

Systems designed for the delivery of warm, semisolid gutta-percha may also be beneficial as time-saving devices. Thermafil is an endodontic obturator delivery system for placement of softened gutta-percha into the prepared canal (Fig. 14-32). This device (delivery system) employs alpha phase gutta-percha and an endodontic file to seal the root canal. The first devices of this sort consisted of a cylinder of gutta-percha with an endodontic file as the central core carrier. More recently,

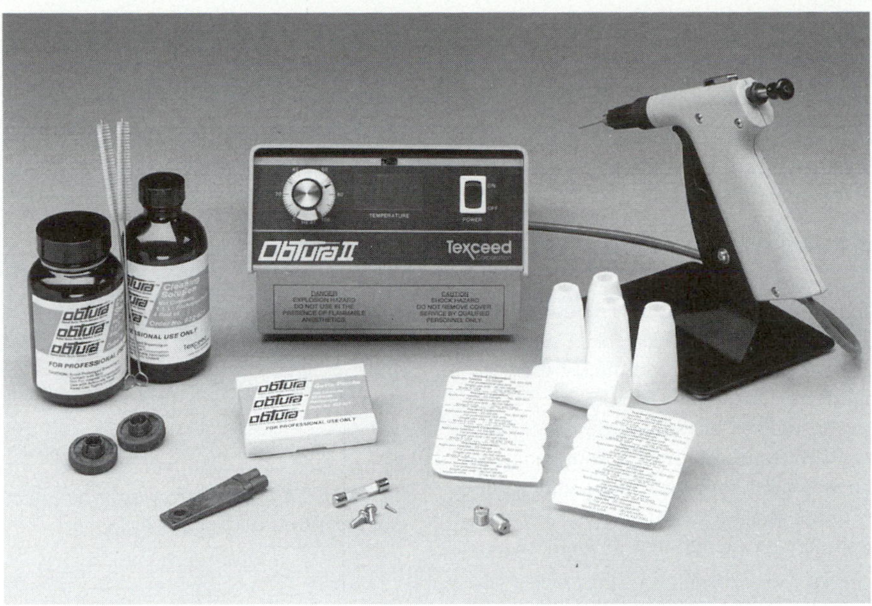

FIG. 14-30 Obtura II thermoplastic injection-molded gutta-percha delivery system (Texceed).

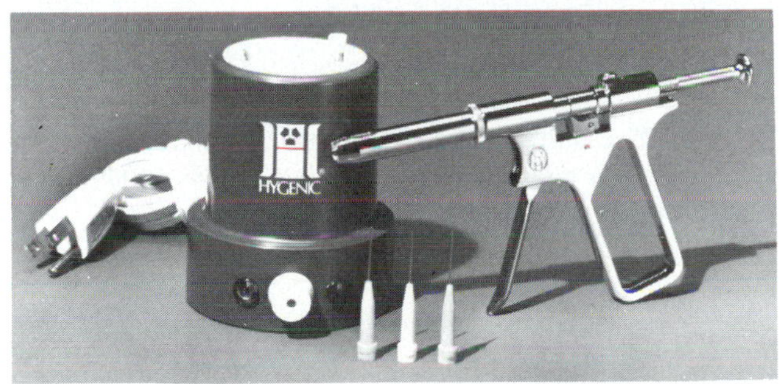

FIG. 14-31 Ultrafil thermoplastic injection-molded gutta-percha delivery system (Hygenic).

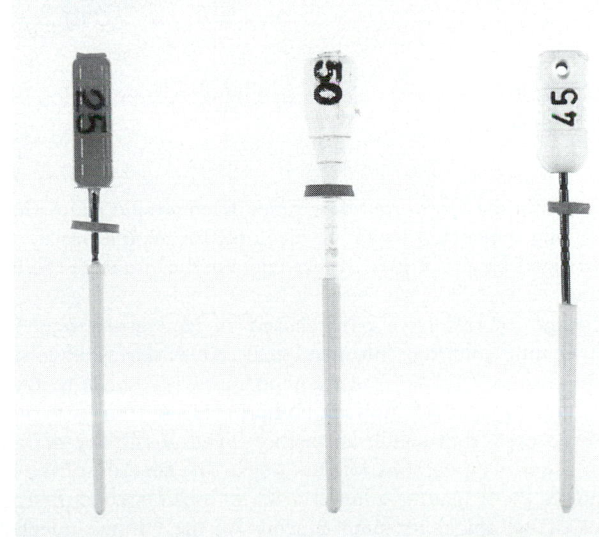

FIG. 14-32 Thermafil gutta-percha delivery system. *Left to right,* no. 25 titanium carrier, no. 50 plastic carrier, and no. 45 stainless steel carrier (Tulsa Dental Products).

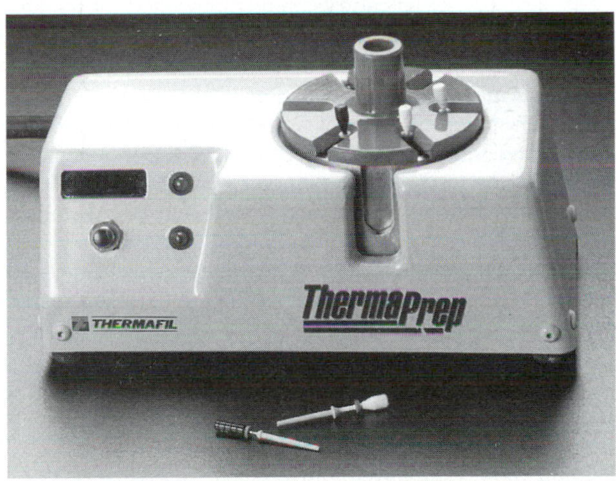

FIG. 14-33 Thermaprep oven for warming of the obturation device showing instrument carrier (foreground).

titanium metal and polysulfon plastic carriers have become available as core materials, possibly because of their excellent biocompatibility. Carriers range from size no. 20 to no. 140 with calibrated markings on the shaft to assist in measuring the depth of placement of the material on insertion. The gutta-percha material is softened by passing it over the flame of a Bunsen burner for the metal carriers or placing it into a special heating unit (Fig. 14-33) for the plastic carriers. A small amount of sealer cement is coated onto the canal walls before the device is inserted. Metal carriers may be prenotched, leaving the apical segment of the instrument as part of the filling material when post space is needed, or the instrument may be sectioned at the canal orifice to remove the file handle. Specialized friction burs are also available from the manufacturer for removal of the plastic core carriers.

Other systems of similar design have evolved for the placement of softened gutta-percha into the root canal space which employ a rigid core carrier as a feature of the obturation procedure. Some systems require that the carrier remain as part of the filling material whereas others provide a method for removing the carrier during obturation. The potential difficulty in removing core carriers for the purposes of retreatment is central to the question of whether or not they should remain as a permanent part of the filling material.

Delivery Systems for Polymeric and Paste-Type Materials

Paste root canal fillings and sealers present somewhat different clinical problems, and instruments have been designed specifically for use with them. The most commonly used instrument is the root canal paste carrier, or Lentulo spiral (Fig. 14-5). Mounted in either a straight or a contraangle handpiece, it is dipped into paste and rotated slowly into a root canal, at first to the length of the prepared root and then, with additional amounts of paste, to successively more occlusal levels, until the canal is filled. Filling a root canal by this method does *not* produce a densely compacted root canal filling, and much reliance is placed on adherence of the paste to the walls of the canal. The pastes used with the paste carrier to fill a canal often contain very radiopaque additives to give the illusion of a filling much denser than it actually is.

The paste carrier has also been recommended for the placement of root canal sealers into a prepared tooth before cementation of cones of silver or gutta-percha. Pastes or sealers are mixed to a readily flowing consistency if they are to be used with the paste carrier. Thicker mixes of zinc oxide–eugenol paste are recommended for obturation of the root canal system in surgical cases or for primary teeth, where the consequences of extruding filler beyond the apical foramen are not as serious.

In selected cases the Pulpdent pressure syringe (Fig. 14-34) has been adapted for use in the permanent dentition, particularly in cases involving immature roots, fine and tortuous root canals, and retrograde root canal fillings.[16,56,57] The device consists of an internally threaded octagonal syringe barrel; one end is machined to receive blunt-tipped needles with threaded hubs. The other end contains a screw-type plunger with a knurled handle. Filling paste or sealer is placed in the hub of a needle selected to suit the size of the root canal to be obturated; that is, a 30-gauge needle corresponds to root canal instrument sizes 15 to 30, a 25-gauge needle to a size 50 instrument, and an 18-gauge needle to approximately size 100 to 110. Seven sizes of needles (from 30- to 19-gauge) are available for the device.

Other preloaded syringe systems are available for placement of root canal dressings such as calcium hydroxide, chelating agents or disinfecting preparations prior to permanent sealing. Illustrated in Figures 14-35 and 14-36 are two preparations for use as interappointment medications and treatment of immature roots (see Chapter 15). Calasept, a calcium-hydroxide dressing, comes preloaded in 1.8-ml cartridges and large-gauge needles for use in standard local anesthetic injection syringes. Temp canal by Pulpdent is a calcium hydroxide–methyl cellulose combination that can be expressed through small-gauge disposable needles by means of a threaded plunger/tube mechanism.

Several syringes have been either proposed or marketed for use with endodontic irrigation needles. They provide for aspiration of irrigating solution as well as deposition of the solution within the tooth, and they range from simple adaptations of tubing connected to saliva ejectors (for aspiration) to sophisticated patented devices that inject and aspirate as the clinician wishes.

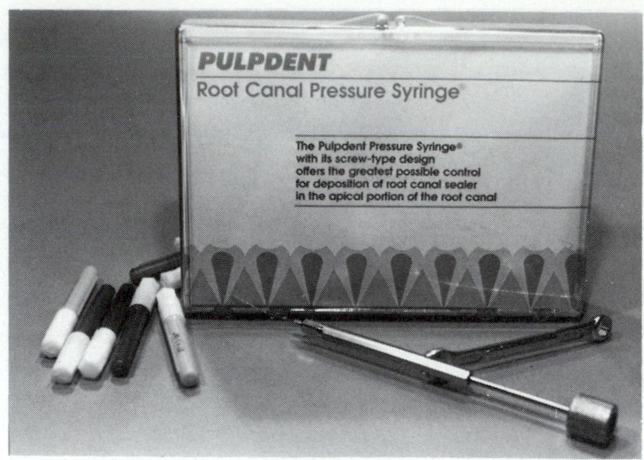

FIG. 14-34 Pressure syringe for injection of paste-type endodontic filling materials (Pulpdent).

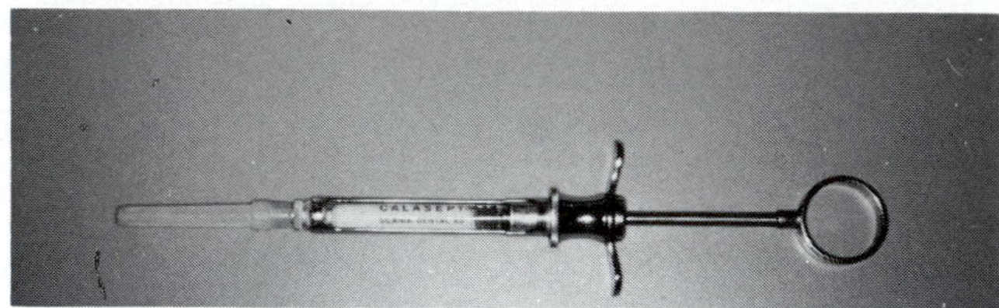

FIG. 14-35 Calasept calcium hydroxide root canal dressing and injection needles shown in standard dental anesthetic syringe (J.S. Dental).

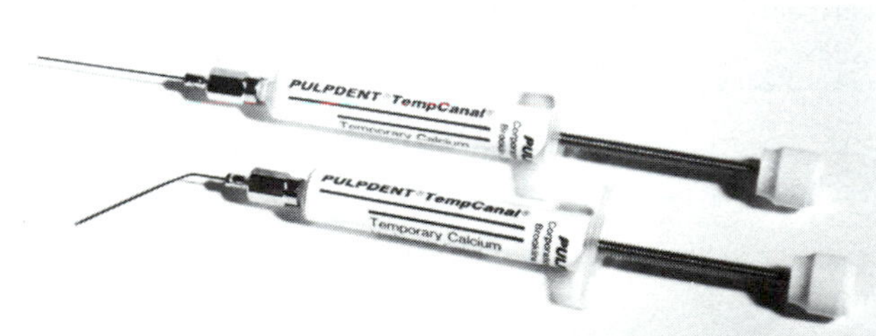

FIG. 14-36 Tempcanal calcium hydroxide paste injection system (Pulpdent).

Severe injuries have been caused by inadvertent injection of irrigating solutions into periapical tissues during endodontic procedures.[13,19,62,160] Air embolism has also been reported as a consequence of blowing compressed air from a syringe into the open root canals of teeth.[124] The possibility of fatal results has been demonstrated in dogs. The severity of the reaction to the irrigating solution's being forced beyond the confines of the apical foramen depends on the volume injected, the toxicity of the solution itself, and the location of the periapical tissues. In experimental situations[158] instrumentation of teeth flooded with irrigating solution by larger instruments (size 45 and larger) has been shown to increase the potential for extruding debris and irrigant beyond the apical foramen. Selection of the type of irrigating solution, the device for using it, and the safest method for a particular clinical procedure involving irrigants should be made with these hazards clearly in mind.

Other specialized injection syringes for endodontic use are available for placement of irrigants and lubricants during instrumentation. Investigators report that the depth of needle placement, volume, and type of irrigant have significant effects on the effectiveness of débridement by irrigation.[168]

Agents and Devices for Canal Irrigation

In current endodontic practice, sodium hypochlorite is generally recognized as the irrigant of choice. However, a commercial disodium ethylenediamine-tetraacetate (EDTA) preparation containing cetyl trimethylammonium bromide, sodium hydroxide solution, and distilled water (REDTA) is the most effective agent discovered to date for chemically cleaning the walls of a root canal.[98] Other types of EDTA solutions and lubricating gels or pastes are often recommended because of their chelating effects. RC Prep is a gellike commercial preparation that also contains urea peroxide, an antibacterial agent, as an active ingredient. Both agents appear to be less caustic than sodium hypochlorite and equal to it in every respect except for their tissue solvent and antibacterial effects (Fig. 14-37).

Scanning electron microscopic investigations[11] indicate that the particular irrigating solution or lubricating agent used may not be as important in removing root canal debris as the volume of the irrigating agent. Since the removal of debris seems to be a function of the quantity of irrigant used rather than the type of solution, physiologic saline may well suffice in many instances, and it is certainly less toxic to viable tissues. However, other histologic and electron microscopic investigations show NaOCl to be essential for removing organic components associated with root canal cleaning and shaping; and solutions of EDTA are essential for removal of the inorganic debris produced.[51,110,151,161,168]

Several technical problems are associated with endodontic irrigation: getting sufficient volume of the solution to the working area of the instrument, particularly in fine or tortuous root canal systems; aspirating the expended fluid and debris from the tooth and operating field; and preventing the extrusion of either irrigating solution or debris beyond the apical confines of the tooth.[128]

Devices have been developed to help the clinician overcome these problems. The endodontic irrigating syringe is the simplest approach. It consists of a disposable 3-ml syringe with a specially designed disposable irrigating needle. The needle is blunted and slit 4 to 5 mm along one side from the tip toward the hub to provide an escape for fluids should the needle inadvertently bind in a canal. Patented needles with an occluded tip and a series of perforations along the sides have been developed especially for endodontics[51,53]; however, the hydraulic pressure necessary to force liquid through the minute perforations of these needles may render the design impractical in clinical use.

Absorbent (Paper) Points

Following irrigation and before obturation of the root canal, residual moisture is removed with sterile absorbent points.

Absorbent points are uniformly tapered (0.2 mm/mm), smooth-sided paper cones to which a binder such as starch has been added to prevent unraveling and for stiffness. Absorbent points are packaged in boxes of 100 or more (bulk) or in cell packs of five or six points. Both cell packs and bulk absorbent points are presterilized as packaged. Sterilization is usually accomplished by irradiation prior to shipment. Individual cell packs are preferred because of the reduced risk of contamination.

Sizing for absorbent points, according to the developing specification (no. 73), corresponds to that for standardized and conventional gutta-percha cones. Other requirements proposed in specification no. 73 relate to the biocompatibility of the materials and binders used in their fabrication, and that they should not disintegrate upon immersion in liquid during use.

In the past, when medication of canals was popular, placement of medication-soaked absorbent points as interappointment dressings was common. This practice should be avoided, since the medicated absorbent point will act as a wick, drawing the cytotoxic liquid to the periapical tissues and causing an acute inflammatory reaction. Overextension of the absor-

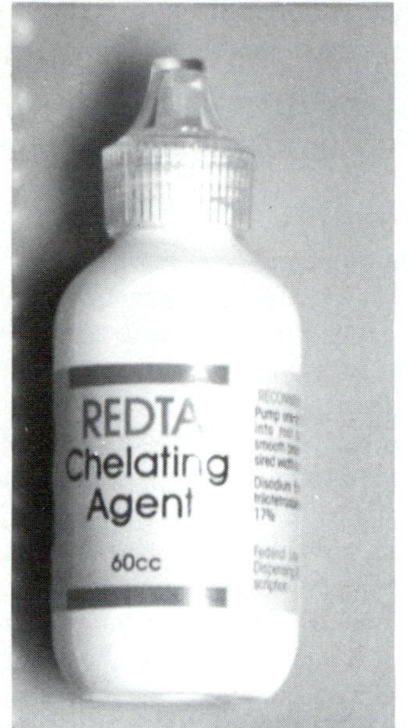

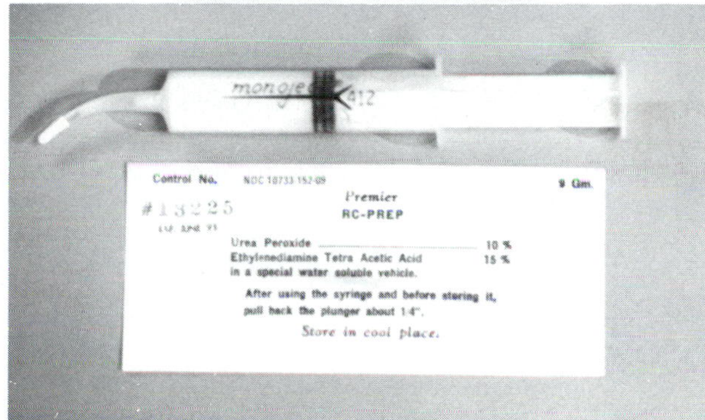

FIG. 14-37 A, Redta (Roth Drug), a commercial irrigating solution containing ethylene-diamine-tetraacetic acid (EDTA), a chelating agent. **B,** RC-Prep, an intracanal lubricant with chelating and disinfectant properties (Premier Dental Products). Composition: EDTA 15%, urea peroxide 10%, in a water-soluble glycol base.

bent point beyond the apex may also induce a foreign body reaction if it is sealed in the canal between appointments.

AUXILIARY INSTRUMENTS AND DEVICES

Removal of Foreign Objects and Broken Instruments

A bite of the cutting edge of a K-type file or reamer that is too deep into the root canal wall during rotatory movement of the instrument can lock the instrument into the tooth. If continued torque is applied in a clockwise cutting motion, the spirals will first elongate and then twist on themselves as the elastic limits of the metal are exceeded. Endodontic instruments with uneven spacing of the spirals or flutes of their working blades are subjected to these forces and are liable to fracture. Two types of fracture of K-type instruments have been observed in laboratory testing.[81] The first is splintering of the instrument as continued clockwise torque is applied; the second, a sudden clean break of the instrument, is usually seen when counterclockwise torque is applied to a locked instrument. The minimum values for torque, as required by the American specification, are shown in Figure 14-38. These are values for a clockwise instrument fracture and are significantly higher than those for a counterclockwise instrument fracture.

Two types of instrument failures have been observed under clinical use.[146] Filing has been shown to produce fatigue failures due to repeated bending of the instrument. Many thousands of cycles are required to break an instrument. Reaming, on the other hand, can cause low cycle instrument failure (clockwise and anticlockwise) when excessive torque is applied to the instrument. Deformation or surface splintering often precedes instrument fracture in low-cycle (reaming) failures (Table 14-3). High-cycle failures occur more quickly in instruments of smaller diameter, but they offer no detectable signs as a warning.

To avoid instrument breakage in clinical practice one should (1) discard files after a period of use, depending upon size; (2) develop a fine tactile sense using low levels of force (torque) when reaming; and (3) be aware of changes in the cross-sectional shape of various instrument sizes.

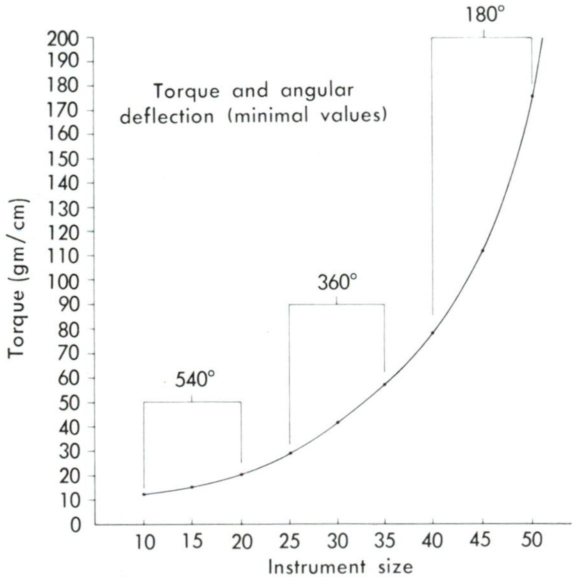

FIG. 14-38 Minimal torsional strength requirements for K-type files and reamers according the ANSI specification no. 28.

TABLE 14-3. Classification of file damage

Type I	Bent instrument
Type II	Unraveling without bending the instrument
Type III	Tearing off of metal at the edges of the instrument
Type IV	Reverse twisting of the instrument
Type V	Cracking along the file axis
Type VI	Fracture of the instrument

Measuring and Maintaining Accurate Root Length

Determining and remaining within the confines of the working length of the root canal during instrumentation is a recurrent problem in endodontics. Several devices are available to help solve the problem. Historically, the method of choice for determining the working length of a tooth in endodontics was to expose a radiograph of the tooth with a radiopaque instrument placed into the canal to an estimated working length as measured from a pretreatment radiograph for verification.

The method of determining the working length of a root canal as proposed in 1962 by Sunada[150] (Fig. 14-39) does not require radiographs. Sunada's work was based on the experimental studies of iontophoresis by Suzuki in 1942; in these studies the electrical resistance between the mucous membrane of the oral cavity and the periodontium was considered to be constant. Electrical resistance between the oral mucous membrane and the periodontal ligament supposedly would also register a constant reading when a measuring probe reached the periodontium via the pulp canal. This resistance to the passage of an electric current when a metal instrument introduced into the root canal reaches the apical area has been found to be consistent and equal to approximately 6.5 ohms. Other methods using voltage gradient measurements have also been tested for this purpose.[157] Several electronic devices based on this principle are currently available. Some use dials or gauges to indicate the electrical resistance relationships of the oral mucosa and the periodontal ligament at the tooth apex; others use audible tones or signals.

Evaluations of the various means and devices used for determining root length indicate that the radiographic methods still may be the most consistently accurate.[24,45,115] Difficulties may be encountered when using electrical resistance measurements to locate the anatomic apex. Contact of the probe with the periodontal ligament at perforation sites gives a false indication of working length. Likewise, contact of the probe with metallic restorations gives erroneous readings. One model of apex locator, the Endocator (Fig. 14-40), has modified, insulated probes to solve this problem.[68]

Clinical reports on the accuracy of electronic locators of the apical foramen are conflicting. Some indicate a rather high degree of accuracy (94%),[99] whereas others report the level of accuracy to be much lower (55% to 75%).[45] Radiographic determination of the location of the apical foramen would appear to be no more accurate in most instances.[33]

To control the working length of an instrument while it is being used once the working length has been determined, several varieties of instrument markers or stops are available. The simplest, and perhaps most common, are little pieces of sili-

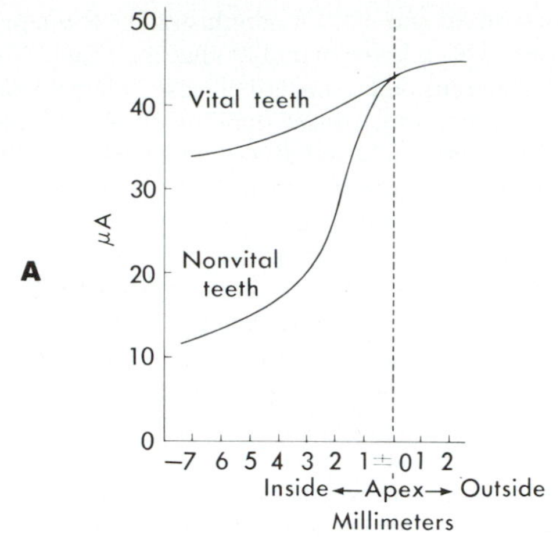

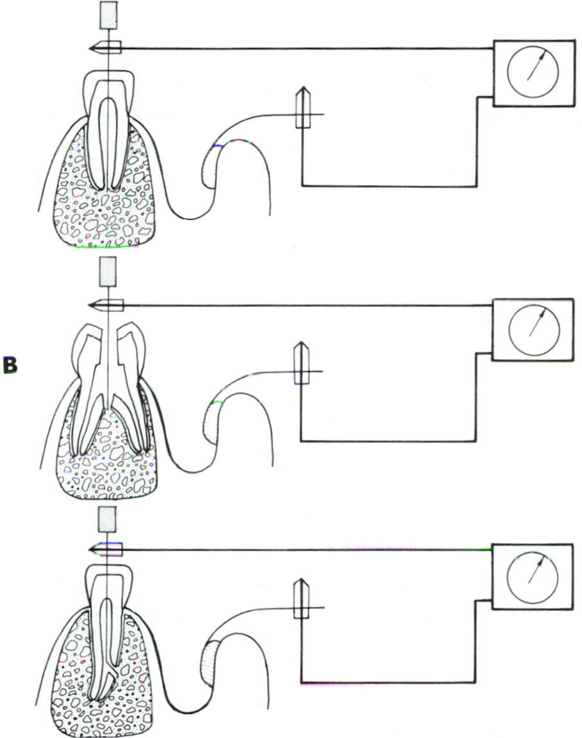

FIG. 14-39 A, Electrical resistance of teeth. (From Sunada IJ: Dent Res 41:375, 1962.) **B,** Principle of electric tooth length measurement.

cone rubber of various sizes and colors. Small, multicolored markers made of nylon or soft plastic are available commercially from several sources. These rubber or plastic markers are placed around the instrument shaft by passing the instrument through them, and they may be positioned along the shaft for visual reference when inserting the instrument to the predetermined working length.

Also available commercially (Hygenic Corp.) are cylindrical instrument stops made of colored silicone that slip onto the base of the instrument handle after the working blade has been passed through them. In effect they limit the extension of the instrument into the canal by creating a mechanical barrier to overextension. Various combinations of color-coded cylinders may be used to produce the desired working length.

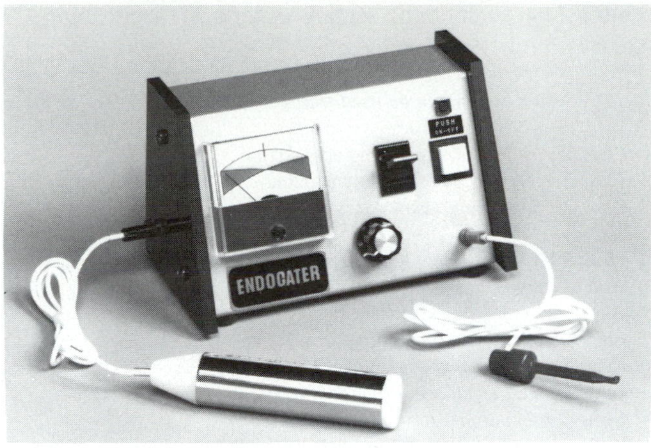

FIG. 14-40 Endocator canal measuring device (Hygenic). Insulated probe not shown.

ENDODONTIC MATERIALS

Several varieties of materials have been used in endodontic practice over the past two centuries. Although there is little information on the types of materials used for filling the root canal prior to the mid-1800s, numerous materials and compounds have been described for placement into the canal space since the latter half of the 19th century. A partial list includes gold foil, lead, silver amalgam, wood points soaked in various solutions, paraffin mixed with antiseptics, ivory, human or animal dentin, and a multitude of medicated pastes.

Since its introduction by Bowman in 1867, gutta-percha has emerged as the most widely used endodontic filling material to date. Gutta-percha is the purified exudate from "mazer wood trees" indigenous to Indonesia, South America, and the islands of Malaysia. At first, gutta-percha as a pure substance was found to be useless in dentistry; but the discovery that its innate hardness could be altered by the addition of zinc oxide, zinc sulfate, alumina, whiting, precipitated chalk, lime, or Silex in various combinations increased its potential as a restorative material. Attempts to use composites of gutta-percha as a permanent restorative material proved futile, but its use in temporary restorations continued unabated for more than 100 years.

Classification

For simplicity, the materials currently used in endodontics can be grouped into one of the following three categories, based upon their intended application: (1) intracanal filling materials, (2) permanent and temporary coronal restorative materials, and (3) retrograde filling materials.

In an effort to provide guidelines and to establish minimum standards for the various types of filling materials manufactured for use in endodontics, the Committee on Dental Materials of ANSI and corresponding council of the ADA adopted specification no. 57 for endodontic filling materials in 1984. Currently this document sets the requirements for the physical, dimensional, and biologic properties of both filling materials and sealer cements to be used in root canal obturation.

Owing to the broad scope of this specification, and in order to achieve harmony with developing international standards, a major revision of the specification is under way. The current proposal is to establish a separate specification no. 78 for solid-

TABLE 14-4. Endodontic sealing materials (specification no. 57)

Type I: ***Sealer cements to be used with core materials***

- Class 1 Powder and liquid nonpolymerizing
- Class 2 Paste and paste nonpolymerizing
- Class 3 Polymer and resin systems

Type II: ***Filling materials to be used without either core materials or sealer cements***

- Class 1 Powder and liquid nonpolymerizing
- Class 2 Paste and paste nonpolymerizing
- Class 3 Metal amalgams
- Class 4 Polymer and resin systems

core materials (obturating points) and to revise specification no. 57 to include endodontic sealing materials (sealer cements, pastes, polymers, and metal amalgams). Significant progress has already been achieved in the reorganization and development of these standards. A classification of endodontic materials based upon the proposed specifications is presented in Table 14-4.

Obturating Points

By definition, type I core (standardized) points should have a uniform taper of 0.02 mm/mm of length for all sizes of points. It is intended that nominal sizing and dimensioning of type I standardized points should correspond to those of standardized endodontic preparation instruments (files and reamers) to facilitate their placement in sealing of the root canal. Core-standardized points are used to seal the prepared root canal space by cementation of the core in conjunction with type II auxiliary (conventional) points. Conventional points, on the other hand, have various tapers that depend on their size. They are intended to be used as accessory points in conjunction with a central standardized core. Work is in progress (specifications no. 71 and 78) to provide uniformity in sizing and dimensions between type II auxiliary points and endodontic condensers (pluggers and spreaders). Once this uniformity is achieved selection of appropriate filling instruments and placement of materials will be simplified.

SEALING MATERIALS

Endodontic sealing materials include both sealer cements to be used in conjunction with core filling materials and sealing materials to be used alone, as the sole filling material. Both type I and type II sealing materials consist of pastes or fluidlike materials that are intended to flow into canal irregularities and voids when inserted in the unset state. Setting of the materials is achieved either by a chemical reaction of the materials once mixed or by polymerization of the material within the canal. Generally, these materials may take the form of powder and liquid mixtures, such as the zinc oxide–eugenol–based sealer cements, or two paste polymer systems. Also included in type II sealing materials are the metal amalgams that are used as retrofilling materials.

Physical Properties

Specification no. 57 sets out the requirements for the physical properties of type I (sealer cements) and type II filling materials (pastes, polymers, metals). The tests to be utilized have been standardized and call for administration at a temperature of 23° C and 50% relative humidity after the materials or components have been conditioned for at least 24 hours before testing. Setting time, dimensional stability, solubility, and disintegration tests are conducted at a temperature of 37° C and a relative humidity of not less than 95%, in addition to bench testing at room temperature and humidity.

The physical characteristics of the materials with which the specification is concerned are working time, flow, film thickness, setting time, dimensional stability, solubility, and disintegration. Specifications no. 57 and no. 78 do not require testing of either the compressive or tensile strength of root canal filling materials. It is questionable whether this information is truly applicable to the clinical circumstances in which these materials are used, and whether performance requirements for strength would add to the safe and effective use of the materials.

All types of endodontic filling materials, as covered by specifications nos. 57 and 78, must exhibit suitable radiopacity.[18] Since dentin and cortical bone have radiopacity equivalents of approximately 1100 aluminum alloy, endodontic materials must be more radiopaque than this. A 2-mm differential in the thickness of aluminum has been shown to produce a reasonable differential of radiopacity when applied to clinical endodontics, and most if not all commercially available materials meet this criterion.

Biologic Properties

The biocompatibility of endodontic filling materials has been a concern to dentistry for many decades, since in clinical use the materials are placed in direct apposition to the connective tissues of either the pulp or the periapex. These concerns have consumed a great deal of time and effort on the part of endodontic researchers and have been extended to all types of materials used in dentistry. Until recently no standard protocol existed for the biologic evaluation of dental materials. Then, in 1971, the Council on Dental Materials and Devices of the ADA approved protocols for circulation and use in an interim period (from 1972 until 1975) and recommended standard practices for toxicity tests of dental materials as developed by a Subcommittee of ANSI and later in 1978 for clinical evaluation.[64]

ANSI/ADA Document No. 41 ("Recommended Standard Practices for Biological Evaluation of Dental Materials") contains procedures for the assessment of the biological effects of two classes of endodontic materials. Class 1 materials are those medications and lining materials used in pulp capping and pulpotomy procedures. Class 2 materials are those used as endodontic filling materials. Under the document type I and II endodontic sealing materials are designated as root canal filling materials, for which cytotoxicity, hemolysis, Ames, cell transformation, subcutaneous implantation, sensitization, and endodontic use tests are described.

In general the following statements may be made regarding the biologic effects of endodontic filling materials:

1. All endodontic filling materials are cytotoxic when freshly mixed; the degree of cytotoxicity is directly related to the ingredients contained in the material. For example, eugenol, eucalyptol, chloroform, iodoform, paraformaldehyde, and acids are all very tissue toxic.
2. The sooner and more completely an endodontic filling material sets or becomes chemically stable, the greater is its biocompatibility. Not only do endodontic sealers

TABLE 14-5. Identification and dimensions of endodontic core (standardized) points*

Size designation	Projected diameter at tip (mm)	Diameter D_3 (3 mm from tip) (mm)	Diameter D_{16} (16 mm from tip) (mm)	Color
10	0.10	0.16	0.42	Purple
15	0.15	0.21	0.47	White
20	0.20	0.26	0.52	Yellow
25	0.25	0.31	0.57	Red
30	0.30	0.36	0.62	Blue
35	0.35	0.41	0.67	Green
40	0.40	0.46	0.72	Black
45	0.45	0.51	0.77	White
50	0.50	0.56	0.82	Yellow
55	0.55	0.61	0.87	Red
60	0.60	0.66	0.92	Blue
70	0.70	0.76	1.02	Green
80	0.80	0.86	1.12	Black
90	0.90	0.96	1.22	White
100	1.00	1.06	1.32	Yellow
110	1.10	1.16	1.42	Red
120	1.20	1.26	1.52	Blue
130	1.30	1.36	1.62	Green
140	1.40	1.46	1.72	Black

**Notes:* All dimensions must be measured to an accuracy of 0.005 mm. A tolerance of ±0.02 mm for class 1 core points and ±0.05 mm for class 2 core points applies to D_1, D_3, and D_{16}. Taper proportion is 0.02 mm/mm of uniform taper. Overall length is not less than 30 ± 2.0 mm unless otherwise specified.

with a large eugenol content have retarded setting times, but the leakage of free eugenol into tissue effects long-term tissue irritation (chronic inflammation). N-2 and some of the other "therapeutic cements" are deceptive because the initial inflammatory response appears to be delayed owing to the rapid setting of the material and the addition of antiinflammatory agents. There is a steady increase in tissue reaction, however, as the "therapeutic" agents leak out to compromise the supporting periodontium, or eventually lose their potency.

3. The more effective the filling material is in sealing the root canal system, the more biocompatible it is likely to be. A material with a low degree of solubility in tissue fluids that is biologically inert is better tolerated and provides a more lasting seal.

By being aware of information on the physical as well as the biologic properties of endodontic filling materials, responsible clinicians should be able to select materials that are best suited to their patients' needs and to their own.

CORE-FILLING MATERIALS

The dimensional requirements, nominal size designation, and color coding for type I (standardized) and type II (auxiliary) core filling materials are listed in Tables 14-5 and 14-6. A proposed system for inclusion of the variations in taper and a new size designation for type II (auxiliary) points based on the current draft of specification no. 78 is presented for future reference. As proposed, a five-digit code will be used to replace the current size designation. The first two digits would be the diameter of the tip (D_0) and the remaining three the taper as measured from (D_3) to (D_{16}) for each nominal size (Figs. 14-41, 14-42).

Gutta-Percha

Before the addition of waxes, fillers, and opacifiers, gutta-percha is a reddish tinged, gray translucent material that is rigid and solid at normal temperatures. It becomes pliable at 25° C and is a soft mass above 65° C; it melts and partially decomposes at 100° C.

TABLE 14-6. Identification and dimensions of endodontic auxiliary (conventional) points*

Normal size designation	Diameter D_3 (3 mm from tip) (mm)	Diameter D_{16} (16 mm from tip) (mm)
XF (extra-fine)	0.20	0.45
FF (fine-fine)	0.24	0.56
MF (medium-fine)	0.27	0.68
F (fine)	0.31	0.80
FM (fine-medium)	0.35	0.88
M (medium)	0.40	1.10
ML (medium-large)	0.43	1.25
L (large)	0.49	1.55
XL (extra-large)	0.52	1.60

**Notes:*
All dimensions must be measured to an accuracy of 0.005 mm.
A tolerance of ±0.05 mm applies to D_3 and D_{16}.
Taper proportion is variable dependent upon nominal size but is uniform.
Overall length is not less than 30 ± 2.0 mm unless otherwise specified.

Chloroform, carbon disulfide, and benzene are the best solvents for gutta-percha, as they are for most hydrocarbons. Exposed to light and air, gutta-percha changes crystalline form and may oxidize, becoming brittle and resinous. Ozone and sulfur cause similar reactions. Gutta-percha is 60% crystalline at ordinary temperatures; the remainder of the mass is amorphous. It exhibits a property common to some polymers, viscoelasticity being elastic and viscous simultaneously.

Natural rubber and gutta-percha represent an interesting example of isomerism. Both are high–molecular weight polymers structured from the same basic building unit, the isoprene monomer (Fig. 14-43). Natural rubber, *cis*-polyisoprene, exists with its CH_2 groups on the same side of the double bond; gutta-percha, *trans*-polyisoprene, exists with its chain of CH_2 groups on opposite sides of the double bond. The *trans* form of polyisoprene is more linear and crystallizes more readily;

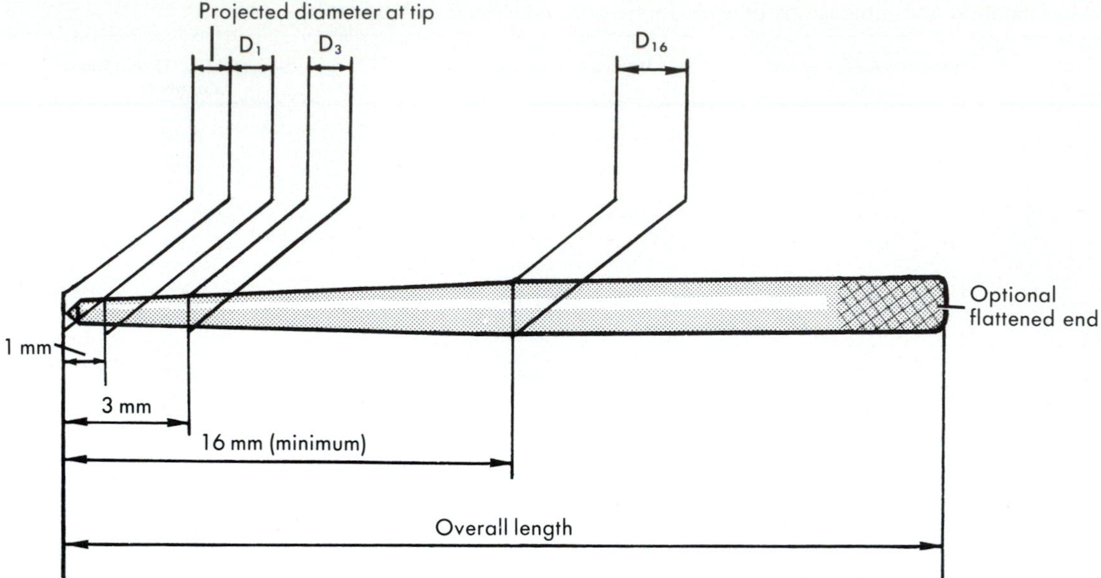

FIG. 14-41 Diagrammatic formula for core standardized points in accordance with current ANSI specification no. 57. Taper and sizing is equivalent to that of corresponding standardized instrument size (see Table 14-4 for dimensions.)

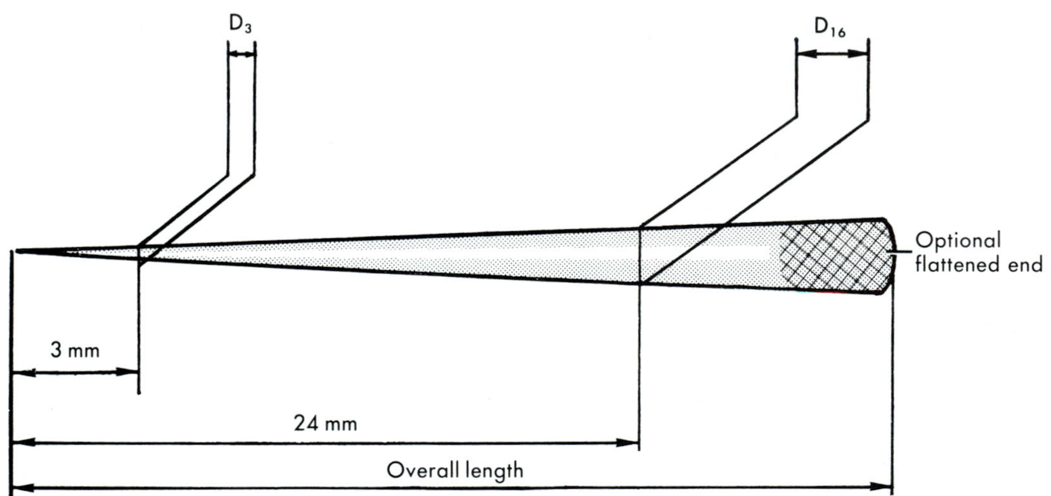

FIG. 14-42 Diagrammatic formula for auxiliary (conventional) points in accordance with current ANSI specification no. 57. Dimensions and taper vary according to nominal size.

consequently gutta-percha is harder, more brittle, and less elastic than natural rubber. Two crystalline forms of *trans*-polyisoprene exist that differ only in the configuration about their single bonds and their molecular repeat distance.

If the naturally occurring alpha crystalline gutta-percha is heated above 65° C, it becomes amorphous and melts. If the amorphous material is cooled extremely slowly (0.5° C or less per hour), then the alpha form will recrystallize. Routine cooling of the amorphous melted material, however, results in crystallization of the beta form. This occurs in most commercial gutta-percha, which becomes more amorphous when reheated at lower temperatures than does the naturally occurring material.

The reversion of the beta-crystalline form to the naturally occurring, more stable alpha form is the primary reason that the gutta-percha cones used in endodontics become brittle with age.[113] Gutta-percha aging can be delayed by storing it frozen or refrigerated and can be reversed by tempering the brittle cones in hot tap water for 1 minute.[145]

The complex admixture of alpha- and beta-crystalline forms (crystalline and amorphous states in the same mass) as well as the purity, molecular weight, and mechanical history of the batch, all affect the related volume changes and physical properties of commercial gutta-percha.[54,131,132] Chemical analysis of five brands of endodontic points has revealed the content of gutta-percha to be from 18.9% to 21.8%, of zinc oxide from 56.1% to 75.3%, of heavy metal sulfates from 1.5% to 17.3%, and of waxes and resins from 1% to 4.1%. The ratio of gutta-

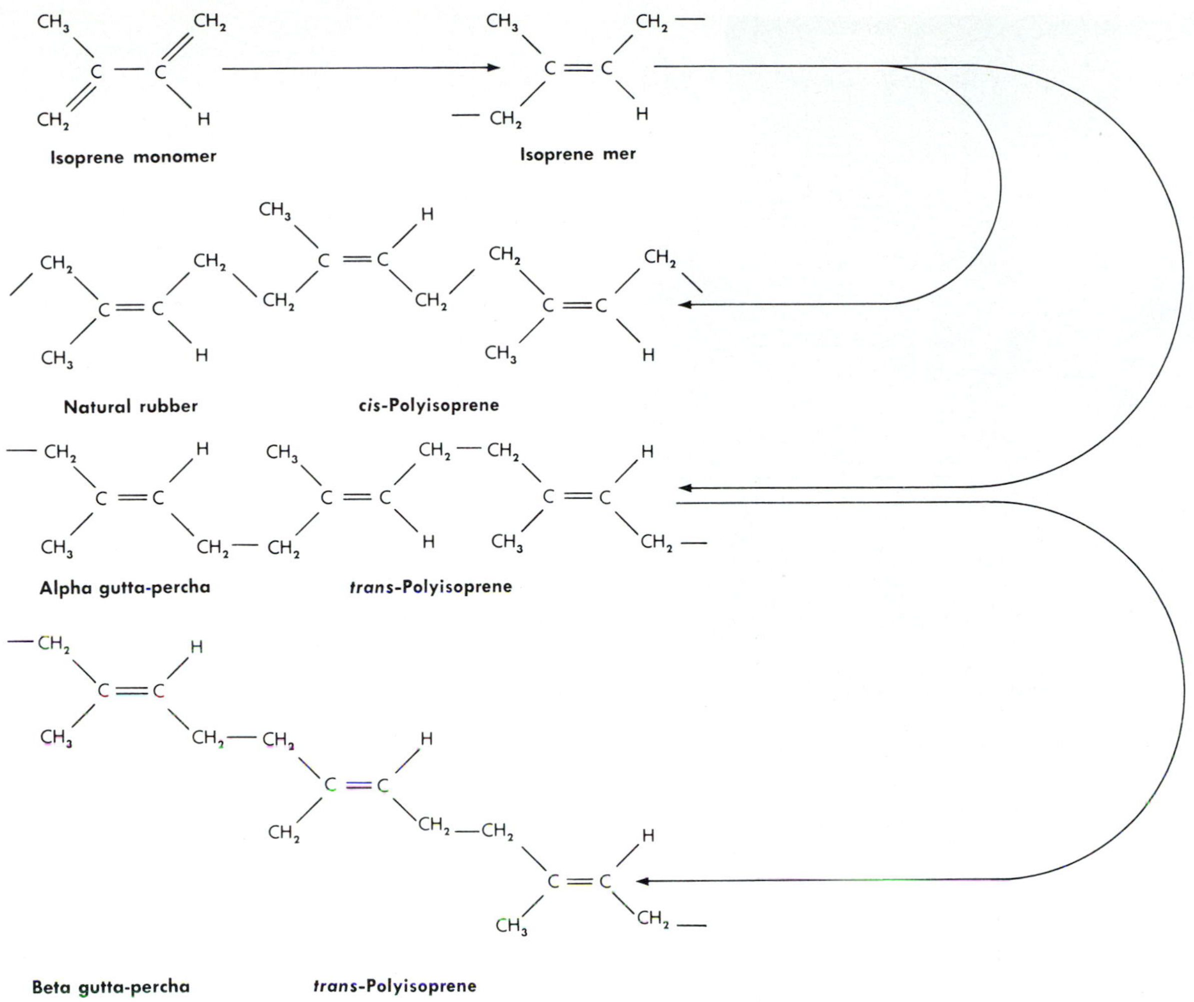

FIG. 14-43 Stereoisomers of polyisoprene. Note the more linear alpha form of gutta-percha is more stable owing to lower crystal latice energy.

percha and organic waxes to zinc oxide and heavy metal sulfates appears to be fairly constant despite variations in the specifics of either the organic or inorganic components of the material.

Deformation of gutta-percha endodontic points under tension (Fig. 14-44) and plots of the resultant stress-strain curves reveal the plastic and elastic characteristics of the material.[46] The mechanical properties demonstrated correspond to those of a typical viscoelastic, partially crystalline material. This is a substance that is extremely strain rate–sensitive, demonstrating a linear relationship between load and elongation up to the yield point, followed by a precipitous decrease in load tolerance. Comparison of these stress-strain data with the composition of the material reveals an inverse relation between the zinc oxide concentration and the percentage of elongation, possibly indicating that zinc oxide acts like a vulcanizing agent.

Testing of compounded dental gutta-percha by the application of compression reveals some of the same characteristics (Fig. 14-45). Unrestrained uniaxial testing prevents the development of stress levels sufficient to produce any molecular compression. Compressibility values obtained for dental gutta-percha in triaxial testing have proved to be less than those for water, which, for all practical purposes, is considered to be incompressible.[131] Below these levels of pressure, there is compaction of the material owing to consolidation and collapse of the internal voids, as could be predicted from scanning electron microscopic examinations. Contrary to empirical clinical claims, no molecular compression or expansion recovery of the material can be expected to assist in sealing the root canal by the methods of condensation used in clinical practice.

Several other parameters of the physical properties of gutta-percha have been reported.[59] The resistance of the material to penetration is affected by the temperature of the material. There is a uniform rate of increase in resistance as well as in hardness with decreasing temperature. Gutta-percha also undergoes linear expansion with alterations in temperature. A gutta-percha point cooled to 15° C undergoes three fourths of its expansion by the time it reaches body temperature (37° C).

The most recent developments related to endodontic filling materials and devices have been those directed toward the placement of either semisolid or plasticized gutta-percha into the root canal space. Gutta-percha softens when it is heated above 65° C. This is the result of overcoming the crystal lattice energies between the molecular chains of the polymer. To

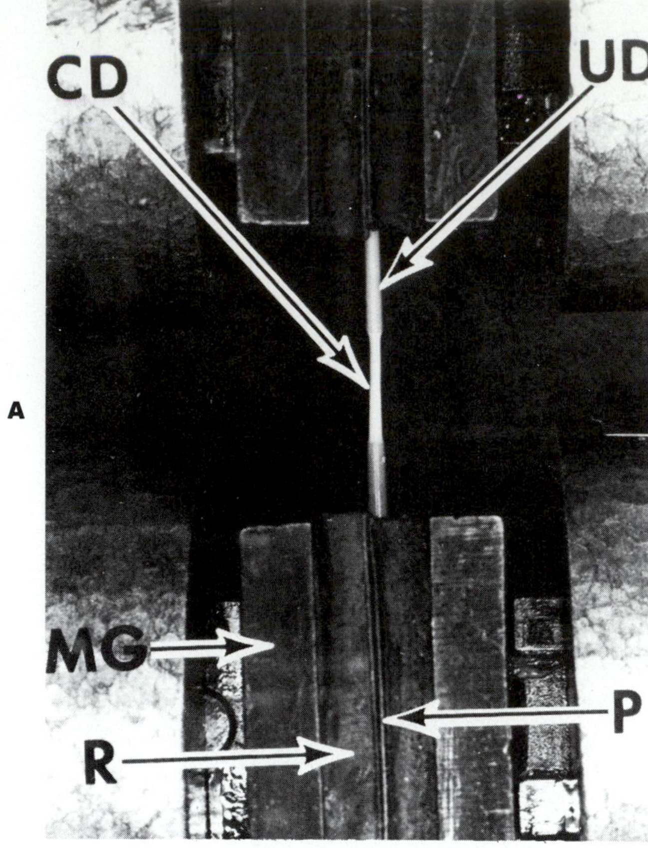

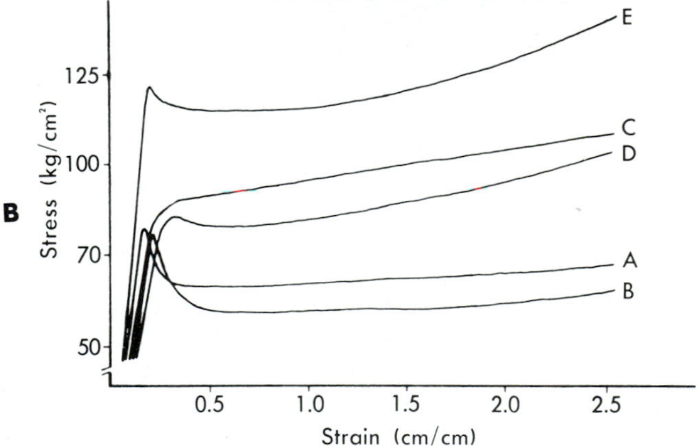

FIG. 14-44 A, Gutta-percha point being deformed under tension.[46] Key: *UD,* undeformed point; *CD,* deformed point under stress; *MG, R,* and *P,* clamping apparatus. **B,** Tensile stress-strain curves for five brands of gutta-percha.[56]

achieve sufficient fluidity for the beta form of the gutta-percha to flow through needles fine enough for injection into the root canal, the temperature must be raised to approximately 160° C.

One manufacturer has been able to alter the melting point of its gutta-percha by a special milling process that mechanically shortens the polymer chains, thus reducing the average molecular weight of the polymer. The shorter chains act as plasticizers which decrease intermolecular forces, thus lowering the melting temperature. By controlling the length of the polymer molecule, the melting point and flow characteristics of the gutta-percha material can be adjusted as desired. Shortening the length of the molecular chains not only affects the melting point and flow properties of the material but reduces the volumetric shrinkage observed on cooling.[55]

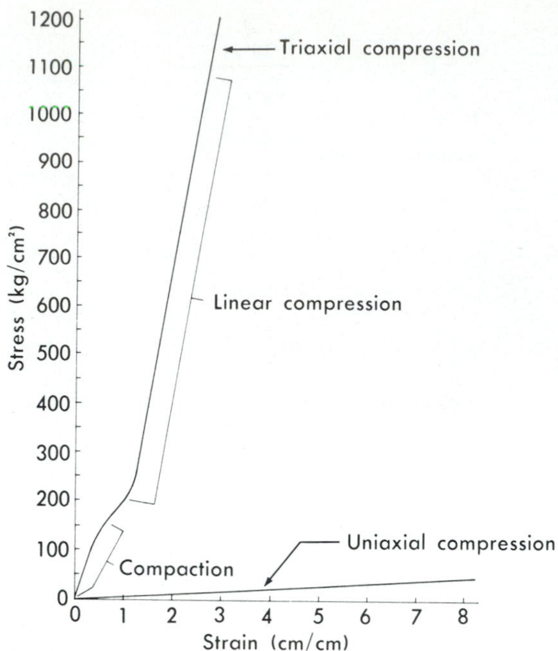

FIG. 14-45 Physical behavior of gutta-percha under various test conditions.[131]

Silver Cones

Silver points (cones), once favored as solid core filling materials for their ease of manipulation in the sealing of curved or constricted canals, are no longer used in contemporary endodontics because of the potential cytotoxicity of pure silver when used as an endodontic filling material.

ROOT CANAL SEALER CEMENTS

In almost all clinical situations core materials are used with a root canal sealer cement. The bond between the sealer and the core material is nonadhesive.[17,79] The core-and-sealer root canal filling techniques therefore involve two interfaces: one between the core and the sealer, and the other between the sealer and the dentin. One of the objectives of obturation is to maximize the amount of core material, which has greater dimensional stability than the sealer. The critical relationship of core material to sealer has been demonstrated in several cases when the adherence of sealing material to the tooth structure was at variance with the adherence to the core.[12,25,129] Investigations of the physical and chemical properties of root canal sealers and cements are therefore of prime importance to our understanding of endodontics.

Eugenol Sealer Cements

Several types of sealers have been formulated for use in endodontics. The most common ones in current use are based on zinc oxide–eugenol formulations. Some of the most widely used sealers are listed in Table 14-7. Richert's formula was

TABLE 14-7. Zinc oxide–eugenol sealers

Sealer	Content	Percent
CRCS (Hygenic) 1982		
Powder	Zinc oxide	
	Hydrogenated rosin ester	
	Barium sulfate	
	Calcium hydroxide	
	Bismuth subcarbonate	
Liquid	Eugenol	
	Eucalyptol	
Grossman's sealer (Grossman, 1974)		
Powder	Zinc oxide (reagent)	42.0
	Staybelite resin	27.0
	Bismuth subcarbonate	15.0
	Barium sulfate	15.0
	Sodium borate (anhydrous)	1.0
Liquid	Eugenol	100.0
Kerr sealer (Rickert, 1931)		
Powder	Zinc oxide	34.0-41.2
	Silver (precipitated-molecular)	25.0-30.0
		30.0-16.0
	Oleoresins (white resin)	11.0-12.8
	Thymol iodide	
Liquid	Oil of cloves	78.0-80.0
	Canada balsam	20.0-22.0
ProcoSol nonstaining cement (Grossman, 1958)		
Powder	Zinc oxide (reagent)	40.0
	Staybelite resin	27.0
	Bismuth subcarbonate	15.0
	Barium sulfate	15.0
Liquid	Eugenol	80.0
	Sweet oil of almond	20.0
ProcoSol radiopaque silver cement (Grossman, 1936)		
Powder	Zinc oxide USP	45.0
	Silver (precipitated)	17.0
	Hydrogenated resin	36.0
	Magnesium oxide	2.0
Liquid	Eugenol	90.0
	Canada balsam	10.0
Tubliseal (Kerr, 1961)		
Base	Zinc oxide	59.0-57.4
	Oleoresins	18.5-21.25
	Bismuth trioxide	7.5
	Thymol iodide	5.0-3.75
	Oils and waxes	10.0-10.1
Catalyst	Eugenol	
	Polymerized resin	
	Annidalin	
Wach's paste (Wach, 1925-1955)		
Powder	Zinc oxide	61.0-61.4
	Calcium phosphate tribasic	12.0-12.2
	Bismuth subnitrate	21.0-21.4
	Bismuth subiodide	2.0-1.9
	Magnesium oxide (heavy)	4.0-3.1
Liquid	Canada balsam	74.0-76.9
	Oil of clove USP	22.0-23.1
	Eucalyptol	2.0
	Beechwood creosote	2.0

developed in 1931 as an alternative to the gutta-percha–based sealers (chloropercha and eucapercha) of that period.[39] Several versions of Richert's formula have been introduced, and the range of ingredients in the powder component has varied slightly. Because of the relatively rapid setting time of Richert's sealer, Grossman's formula appeared in 1936, with the purpose of developing a sealer that afforded more working time.

Both Richert's and Grossman's formulas were criticized for including precipitated silver for radiopacity.[58] Grossman's formula was subsequently revised to exclude silver (Procosol nonstaining sealer). Grossman's formula was modified again by the addition of sodium borate to the powder and the elimination of all ingredients except eugenol from the liquid. Kerr Pulp Canal Sealer (Richert's formula) remains largely unchanged since its introduction nearly 45 years ago.

Wach's paste, introduced originally in 1925, is a variation of zinc oxide–eugenol cements with added beechwood creosote as a medicinal component. It did not receive widespread adoption until its reintroduction circa 1955. It is now marketed with minor variations in formulation.

Tubliseal by Kerr was introduced in 1961 as an alternative to the powder-liquid formula sealers that preceded it. It is a two-paste variation of a zinc oxide–eugenol system that displays the unique property of expansion on setting. Though the exact formula is a proprietary secret, an approximation is presented in Table 14-7.

Zinc oxide–eugenol sets because of a combination of chemical and physical reactions, yielding a hardened mass of zinc oxide embedded in a matrix of long, sheathlike crystals of zinc eugenolate $[C_{10}H_{11}O_2]_2Zn$. Excess eugenol is invariably present and is absorbed by both zinc oxide and the eugenolate. The presence of water, particle size of the zinc oxide, the pH, and additives are all important factors in the setting reaction.[34,112] Hardening of the mixture is due to the zinc eugenolate formation. Unreacted eugenol remains trapped and tends to weaken the mass.[144] The comparative hardness of fresh dentin to that exposed to zinc oxide–eugenol sealers is increased in direct proportion to the amount of free eugenol available.[20] The significance of free eugenol is most apparent in increased cytotoxcity rather than through alteration of the physical properties of dentin.

TABLE 14-8. Sealers without eugenol

Sealer	Content	Percent
Kloroperka N-O (Nygaard-Østby, 1939)		
Powder	Canada balsam	19.6
	Rosin	11.8
	Gutta-percha	19.6
	Zinc oxide	49.0
Liquid	Chloroform*	100.0
Diaket (Schmitt, 1951)		
Powder	Zinc oxide	98.0
	Bismuth phosphate	2.0
Liquid	2.2′-Dihydroxy-5,5′-dichlorodiphenylmethane	
	Propionylacetophenone	
	Triethanolamine	
	Caproic acid	
	Copolymers of vinyl acetate, vinyl chloride, and vinyl isobutyl ether	
AH-26 (Schroeder, 1957)		
Powder	Silver powder	10.0
	Bismuth oxide	60.0
	Hexamethylene tetramine	25.0
	Titanium oxide	5.0
Liquid	*bis*-Phenol diglycidyl either	100.0
Chlorapercha (Moyco)		
	Gutta-percha composition	9.0
	Chloroform*	91.0

*Although chloroform has been banned by the Food and Drug Administration because of its carcinogenic properties, it is mentioned here for thoroughness of the subject matter and not necessarily as a recommended solvent.

The method of preparation of the zinc oxide is closely related to the setting time. Increases in temperature or humidity decrease setting time. The longer and more vigorously the mixture is spatulated, the shorter the setting time. Setting time can be increased by decreasing the particle size of the zinc oxide.

Noneugenol Sealer Cements

Table 14-8 gives the formulas of some of the most popular root canal sealers other than the zinc oxide–eugenol types. Kloraperka was first introduced circa 1939 from Norway. It is similar to several empirical formulas dating back to the early 1900s. Chlorapercha (Moyco) is a direct descendant of materials used for nearly a century. Diaket is an organic polyketone compound introduced in Europe by Schmitt (1951). It enjoyed some popularity in the United States following reports of its superior strength and physical properties. The material consists of a very fine powder and a thick viscous liquid. The resin resulting from the mixture is very tacky in texture, adheres to tooth structure, and is often difficult to manipulate. As a polyvinyl resin, Diaket is essentially a keto complex in which basic salts and metal oxides react with neutral organic agents, forming polyketones. The polyketones thus formed unite with metallic substances in the material to form cyclic complexes that are insoluble in water but soluble in organic solvents. Used commercially as an industrial adhesive and insulator, AH-26, introduced in Europe by Schroeder, is an epoxy resin for use as an endodontic sealer. The addition of a hardener, hexamethylene tetramine, renders the cured resin chemically and biologically inert. Several proponents have advocated AH-26 as an endodontic sealer.

Therapeutic Sealer Cements

The biologic activity of calcium hydroxide in both vital pulp therapy and in apexification has been documented extensively in the literature. A number of calcium hydroxide preparations have also been tested experimentally as root canal filling materials or sealer cements in leakage and histologic studies.[49,65,66,138] Two commercial preparations are available as endodontic sealer-cements to be used in conjunction with core filling materials. The calciobiotic root canal sealer (CRCS) represents the first of the calcium hydroxide–based sealers. Sealapex, another calcium hydroxide–based preparation, appeared soon afterward. The two differ in that CRCS consists of a powder-liquid combination, whereas Sealapex is in the form of a two-tube–two-paste preparation. Both may be classified as biologically active sealers intended to promote periapical healing, calcium hydroxide being the active ingredient. Holland and de Souza have reported the ability of Sealapex and calcium hydroxide filling material to induce apical closure by cementum deposition in histologic studies of both primates and dogs.

An extensive study of the physical properties of two calcium hydroxide–based sealers (CRCS and Sealapex) has been reported by Caicedo and Fraunhofer.[26] They compared the setting time, solubility, compressive strength, and other properties of these two calcium hydroxide–containing sealers to Procosol, a zinc oxide–eugenol sealer based on Grossman's original formula. They observed that of the three sealers tested, Sealapex showed atypical behavior based on its pronounced volumetric expansion, water absorption, and change in radiopacity with time.

Temporary Canal Dressings

In the past, highly cytotoxic intracanal medications were used for disinfection of the root canal between appointments. Agents such as Formocresol and paraformaldehyde, for example, are no longer considered suitable for this purpose due to their potential carcinogenic effects.[88] The desire for less irritating dressing materials has led to the evaluation of calcium hydroxide, chlorhexidine, and potassium iodide as possible alternatives.[127,141,149]

Calcium hydroxide pastes have been advocated for use as temporary canal filling materials when continued root end development is desired, osseous repair, control of exudate, to create an apical barrier following overinstrumentation, and in the prevention of external root resorption following traumatic injuries to teeth.[84,85] Pastes of calcium hydroxide powder (USP) and sterile water or other vehicles have been proposed by several authors for their antibacterial effects, with reports of remarkable success.[82] Evaluation of an experimental timed-release delivery system of chlorhexidine as an intracanal antimicrobial agent has been performed, with promising results.[28]

Two premixed commercial preparations are currently available that may be of benefit as time-saving products and delivery systems. Calasept contains calcium hydroxide (56%) as the active ingredient, with trace amounts of sodium, potassium, and calcium chloride in a sterile water vehicle. The material is packaged in 1.8-ml carpules to be dispensed through 21-gauge blunt needles using a standard dental injection syringe. The carpules may be resterilized at 120° C for 20 minutes. Tempcanal is a suspension of calcium hydroxide in methylcellulose. The material is preloaded into a disposable pressure syringe that uses a threaded plunger mechanism to express the material.

Paraformaldehyde Pastes

This discussion of paraformaldehyde pastes should not be interpreted as an endorsement of their acceptability or usefulness. On the contrary, the reader must be aware of their shortcomings and hazards. Currently, neither the materials nor the techniques for their use have been advocated by any dental school in North America, the ADA, or the Food and Drug Administration.[5] *Use of these materials, therefore, constitutes substandard care in endodontic treatment.*

Sargenti paste (N-2), Endomethasone, and Reibler's paste are a group of root canal cements for which therapeutic properties are claimed. These materials are used either with or without core materials; thus, they are introduced into the root canal by means of either a Lentulo spiral or some type of injection device. The claim is made, particularly for the formulas containing either paraformaldehyde or iodoform, that failure of the materials to provide a compact root canal filling is compensated by their prolonged or permanent therapeutic properties. Riebler's paste is the most extreme example of this type of agent, whereas Mynol cement and iodoform paste are somewhat similar in their composition and usage as cements or as sealers with core materials. Endomethasone and N-2 (Sargenti, 1970) are similar insofar as they contain, besides paraformaldehyde, corticosteroids. Both these materials contain lead as an oxide, which by increasing radiopacity not only gives the illusion of the material's compactness once inserted but also, at least in the case of N-2, may contribute to the extreme hardness and slow solubility of the final set. Apparently, lead oxide reacts and binds with eugenol in a more permanent manner than does zinc oxide. Some current formulations of N-2 contain neither corticosteroids nor lead tetroxide but do contain paraformaldehyde.

Paraformaldehyde-containing pastes may be clinically successful in vital pulpotomy and pulpectomy procedures, but their limitations must be recognized. Formaldehyde causes necrosis of vital tissue; this is why formalin is used to fix tissues for histologic examination. Since tissue fixation with formaldehyde is a slow, low-grade process, pain is seldom a problem (unless the material is deposited beyond the apical foramen) and "clinical success" may appear to have been achieved. The consequences of accidentally extruding these materials beyond the confines of the tooth are often severe. Iodoform is somewhat less toxic, but it presents a similar hazard even though it does not achieve its antibacterial activity by cell fixation, as does paraformaldehyde.

The inclusion in root canal sealers of heavy metal ions (e.g., mercury or lead) is potentially dangerous because these ions are disseminated throughout the body, posing particular problems for target organs remote from the teeth.[32,116] Corticosteroids used in conjunction with these materials to suppress clinical symptoms may pose hazards that are as yet unsuspected.

Temporary Restorative Materials

Occasionally, conventional endodontic treatment procedures are performed in multiple appointments. Placement of interim restorations to prevent contamination of the root canal system by organisms in the oral environment is therefore a common practice. A great variety of temporary filling materials are available for this purpose. To be effective as a temporary coronal restoration, a material should be capable of maintaining its seal within the range of adverse conditions experienced in the oral cavity. The necessary properties of temporary restorative materials used in endodontics have been described by Deveaux and colleagues[38]: (1) good marginal seal, (2) minimal porosity, (3) dimensional stability, (4) resistance to abrasion and compression, (5) ease of insertion and removal, (6) compatibility, and (7) aesthetics.

Maintenance of an adequate coronal seal depends on a material's marginal adaptability and compressive strength. Masticating forces and temperature variations in the mouth may also adversely affect a material's ability to maintain its marginal seal. In addition to these physical requirements, ease of manipulation and time required for placement are important considerations when selecting a temporary restorative material.

Cavit is perhaps one of the most widely used endodontic temporary restorative materials. Despite its relatively low compressive strength, it has been favored for its easy placement and excellent sealing properties. Cavit is composed of zinc oxide, calcium sulfate, glycol acetate, polyvinyl acetate, polyvinyl chloride, triethanolamine, and red coloring. It is dispensed as a single tube paste that acts in the presence of moisture by absorbing water. The linear expansion observed on setting may contribute to its ability to effectively seal cavity margins. Laboratory tests have demonstrated its superior sealing properties and its ability to withstand thermal changes that may be experienced in the oral cavity.[8,117,152]

Other materials have been advocated for use as temporary endodontic restorations, based on their greater compressive strength. IRM is a zinc oxide–eugenol–based cement to which reinforcing particles have been added to improve the strength and toughness of the set material. Used as an interim restoration its longevity can extend a year or longer. TERM is a light-activated particle-filled composite resin for which the manufacturer does not recommend acid etching prior to placement. Marginal leakage with these two materials compares favorably with Cavit when initially placed, though leakage may be expected to increase with time (especially following thermal stresses) to levels greater than observed with Cavit.

Future Directions

Technologic advancements in endodontics generally have developed, not through primary investigative research, but rather by application of materials or devices borrowed from other fields. One may classify such progression by either its application (i.e., root canal–enlarging instruments versus filling materials) or by composition (i.e., metals, polymers, ceramics). Materials are often categorized by composition, whereas instruments and devices are more readily described according to intended use. The following is speculation about what may lie ahead in endodontic technology.

Materials

Corrosion behavior of various metals, mercury toxicity, strength, and elasticity are several properties of metallic materials that can significantly affect compatibility with the biologic environment in which they are used or the performance of instruments as they relate to the physical demands involved in root canal preparation.

Many materials used in other aspects of dentistry or biomaterials science have been tested for use as replacements for current endodontic filling and restorative materials. For example, titanium, Teflon, hydroxyapatite, tantalum, and various other materials have been experimentally applied in endodontics as retrofilling agents, implant stabilizers, and intracanal filling materials. These types of materials may offer some advantage in endodontics, owing to their excellent biocompatibility.

Future improvements in decreasing the solubility and reducing the tissue toxicity of dentin-bonding agents may also provide the clinician better materials for orthograde and retrograde sealing of the apex. Glass ionomer cements, synthetic polymers, resins, and low-fusing ceramics may at some point replace existing permanent and temporary restorative materials as they are used in endodontics.

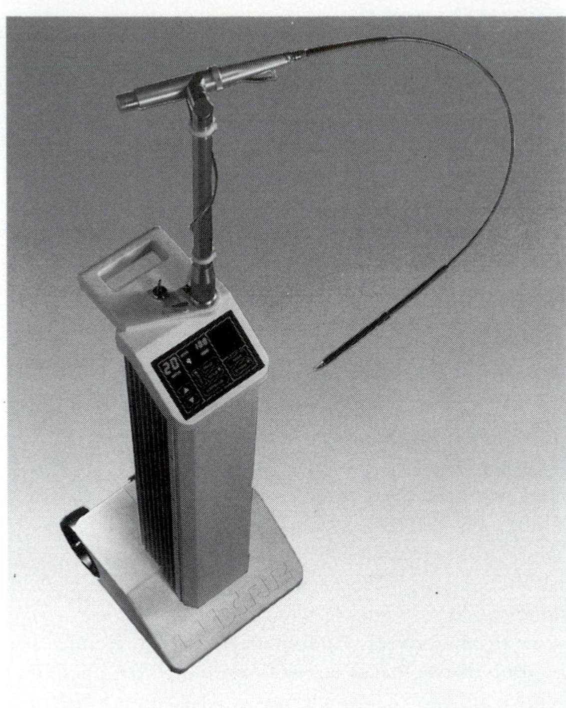

FIG. 14-46 Carbon dioxide laser unit (Luxar, Bothell, Wash.) with flexible waveguide for intraoral use.

Instruments

Tougher, more flexible alloys of carbon or stainless steel and nickel titanium may potentially improve the ability of tomorrow's practitioner to prepare constricted and or curved canals with reduced risk of instrument failure or perforation. Continued progress in the design of instruments such as noncutting tips, more efficient cutting surfaces, combined with innovative techniques for preparation and sealing of the root canal will inevitably lead to safer and more effective methods for delivery of endodontic treatment to growing numbers of patients.

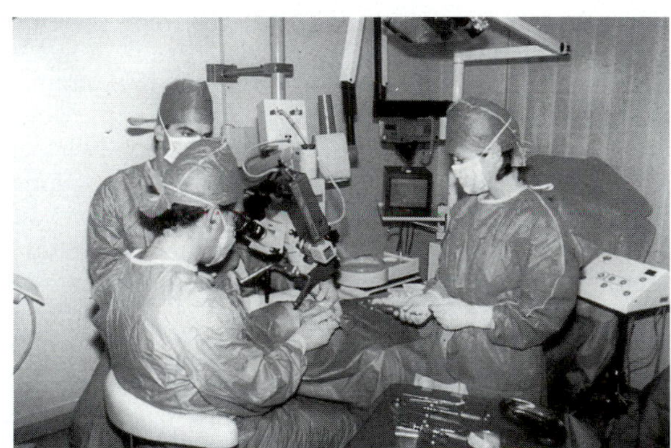

FIG. 14-47 Dental operating microscope as used in periapical surgery. (Courtesy G. Pecora and S. Adreana.)

New Technology

Endodontic applications of lasers

According to Zakariasen and others,[170] lasers will have a definite place in the future of dentistry and will have an equally significant role in the practice of endodontics. The dental profession is already well-prepared with the technical skills required, and may well benefit from the precision afforded by lasers. The unique properties of lasers provide the means for precise tissue removal, sterilization, and instant hemostasis.[107,108]

Clinical application of carbon dioxide laser (Fig. 14-46) for periapical surgery has already been demonstrated.[103] Fiber delivery systems, wave guides, and dental operating microscopes (Fig. 14-47) make plausible less invasive periapical surgery with added benefits of decreased postoperative pain and reduced scarring and treatment time, as has been reported with laser surgery. In addition to the benefit of sterilization of the contaminated root apex and root surface dentin,[104] laser apicoectomy has the potential to reduce the risk of bacterial contamination of the surgical wound and eliminates the hazards associated with blood-borne aerosols by replacing rotary air-driven instruments for this purpose.

Development of fiberoptic delivery systems for intracanal application of the neodymium-YAG laser (Fig. 14-48) has opened the door for a number of endodontic and pulpal treatments. Attempts to utilize lasers for vaporization of pulp tissue, canal enlargement, and for their antibacterial effects have thus far been promising.[87,119] The sterilizing and coagulating abilities of lasers for vital pulp procedures such as pulpotomy and pulp capping are also being pursued.

Development of newer laser systems capable of vaporizing dental hard tissue such as enamel, dentin, and bone will inevitably lead to broader applications of the laser in dental practice (Fig. 14-49). Practical and effective methods for repairing cracked teeth by recrystallization of enamel or fusion of ceramic restorative materials lie ahead.

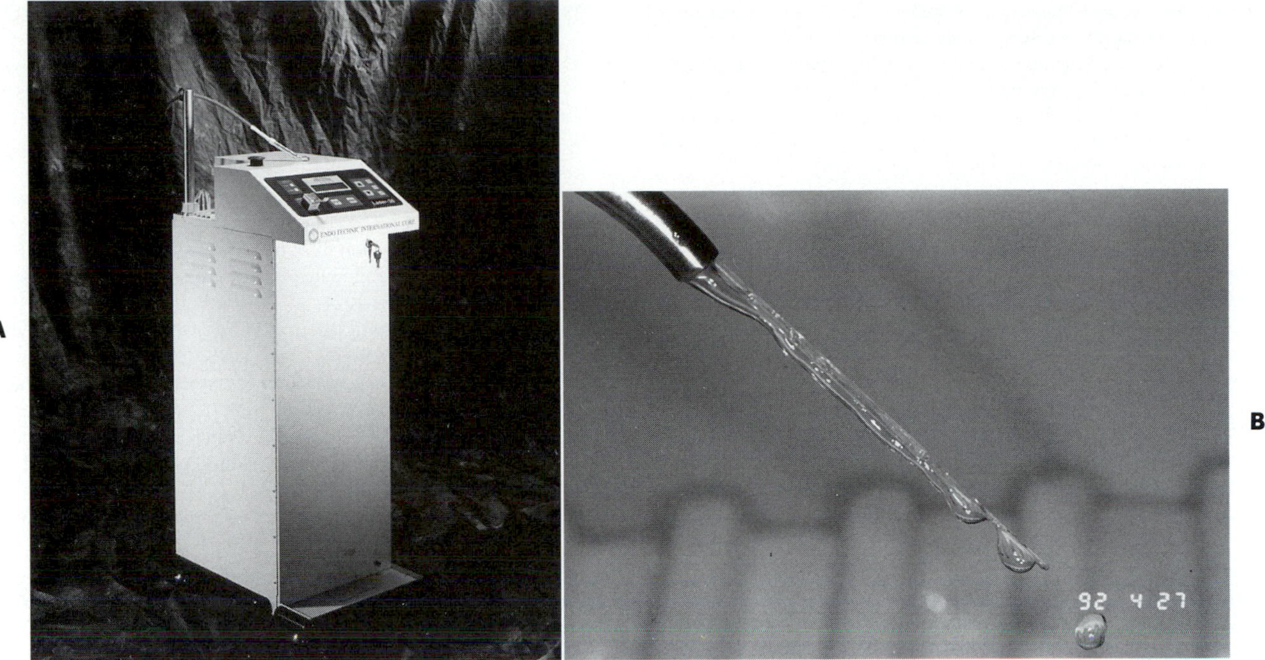

FIG. 14-48 A, Neodymium-YAG laser unit. (Courtesy Medical Laser Technology, San Clemente, Calif.) **B,** Water-cooled optical fiber delivery system.

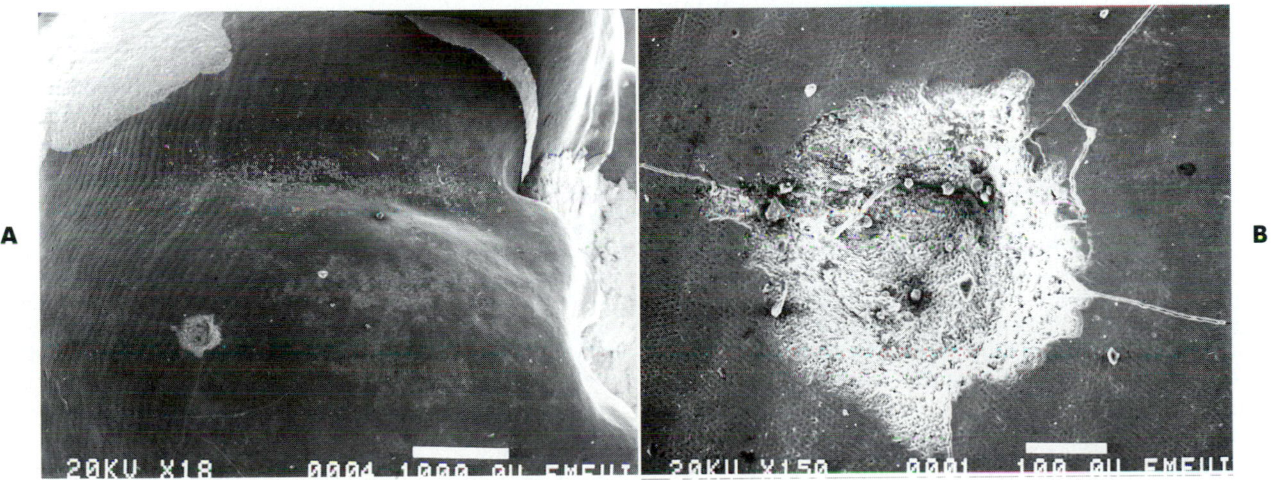

FIG. 14-49 Thermal fracture lines and fusion of enamel surface. (Original magnification, ×150). (Courtesy Electron Microscope Facility of RRC, University of Illinois at Chicago.)

REFERENCES

1. Abou-Rass M, and Jastrab RJ: The use of rotary instruments as ancillary aids to root canal preparation of molars, J Endod 8:78, 1982.
2. Ahmad M, Pitt Ford TR, and Crum LA: Ultrasonic debridement of root canal: an insight into the mechanisms involved, J Endod 13:93, 1987.
3. Ahmad M, et al: Ultrasonic debridement of root canal: acoustic cavitation and its relevance. J Endod 14:486, 1988.
4. Al-Nayhan S, Saporinas G, and Spangberg L: In vitro study of cytotoxicity of a composite resin, silver amalgam and cavit, J Endod 14:236, 1988.
5. American Dental Association, Council on Dental Materials, Instruments, and Equipment: Council on the use of root canal filling materials containing paraformaldehyde: a status report, J Am Dent Assoc 114:95, 1987.
6. American Dental Association, Council on Dental Therapeutics: (Resolution) JADA 123:18, 1992.
7. Anderson J, Corcoran J, and Craig R: Cutting ability of square versus rhombus cross-sectional endodontic files, J Endod 11:212, 1985.
8. Anderson RW, Powell BJ, and Pashly DH: Microleakage of three temporary endodontic restorations, J Endod 14:497, 1988.
9. Bahcall J, et al: Preliminary investigation of the effects of laser endodontic treatment on the periradicular tissue in dogs. J Endod 18:47, 1992.

10. Baker MC, et al: Ultrasonic compared with hand instrumentation: a scanning electron microscope study, J Endod 14:435, 1988.
11. Baker NA, et al: Scanning electron microscope study of the efficacy of various irrigating solutions, J Endod 1:127, 1975.
12. Barry GN, Heyman RA, and Fried IL: Sealing quality of instruments cemented in root canals with polycarboxylate cements, J Endod 1:112, 1975.
13. Becker GL, Cohen S, and Borer R: The sequelae of accidentally injecting sodium hypochlorite beyond the root apex, Oral 38:633, 1974.
14. Becker SA, and Von Fraunhofer JA: The comparative leakage behavior of reverse filling materials, J Endod 15:246, 1989.
15. Benkel BH, et al: Use of a hydrophillic plastic as a root canal filling material, J Endod 2:196, 1976.
16. Berk H, and Krakow A: Efficient endodontic procedures with the use of the pressure syringe, Dent Clin North Am :387, 1965.
17. Bernatti O, Stolf WC, and Ruhnke LA: Verification of the consistency, setting times, and dimensional changes of root canal filling materials, Oral Surg 46:107, 1987.
18. Beyer-Olsen EM, and Orstavik D: Radiopacity of root canal sealers, Oral Surg 51:320, 1981.
19. Bhat KS: Tissue emphysema caused by hydrogen peroxide, Oral Surg 38:304, 1974.
20. Biven GM, Bapna RJ, and Heuer MA: Effect of eugenol and eugenol-containing root canal sealers on the microhardness of human dentin, J Dent Res 51:1602, 1972.
21. Blackman R, Gross M, and Seltzer S: An evaluation of the biocompatibility of a glass ionomer-silver cement in rat connective tissue, J Endod 15:76, 1989.
22. Bondra DL, et al: Leakage in vitro with IRM, high copper amalgam, and EBA cement as retrofilling materials, J Endod 15:157, 1989.
23. Brady JM, and del Rio CB: Corrosion of endodontic silver cones in humans: a scanning electron microscope and x-ray microprobe study, J Endod 1:205, 1975.
24. Bramante CM, and Berbert A: A critical evaluation of some methods of determining root canal length, Oral Surg 37:463, 1974.
25. Brayton SM, Davis SR, and Goldman M: Gutta percha root canal fillings: an in vitro analysis, Oral Surg 35:226, 1973.
26. Cacedo R, and Von Fraunhofer JA: The properties of endodontic sealer cements, J Endod 14:527, 1988.
27. Callis PD, and Santini A: Tissue response to retrograde root fillings in the ferret canine: a comparison of a glass ionomer cement and gutta-percha with sealer, J Oral Surg 64:475, 1987.
28. Cervone F, Tronstadt L, Hammond B: Antimicrobial effect of chlorhexidine in a controlled release delivery system, Endod Dent Traumatol 6:33, 1990.
29. Chenail B, and Teplitsky P: Endosonics in curved root canals, J Endod 11:369, 1985.
30. Chenail BL, and Teplitsky PE: Endosonics in curved root canals—II, J Endod 14:214, 1988.
31. Chivian N: Endodontics: an overview, Dent Clin North Am 28:637, 1984.
32. Chong R, and Senzer J: Systemic distribution of 210 PbO from root canal fillings, J Endod 2:381, 1976.
33. Chunn CB, Zardiakas LP, and Menke RA: In vivo root canal length determination using the Forameter, J Endod 7:515, 1981.
34. Copeland HI, Brauer GM, and Forziati A: The setting mechanism of zinc oxide and eugenol mixtures, J Dent Res 34:740, 1955.
35. Compos JM, and del Rio C: Comparisons of mechanical and standard hand instrumentation techniques in curved root canals. J Endodont 16:230, 1990.
36. Cunningham WT, Martin H, and Forrest W: Evaluation of root canal debridement by the endosonic ultrasonic synergistic system, Oral Surg 53:401, 1982.
37. Davis MS, Joseph SW, and Bucher JF: Periapical and intracanal healing following incomplete root canal filling in dogs, Oral Surg 31:662, 1971.
38. Deveaux E, et al: Bacterial microleakage of Cavit, IRM, and TERM. Oral Surg Oral Med Oral Pathol 74:634, 1992.
39. Dixon CM, and Rickert UG: Histologic verification of results of root canal therapy in experimental animals, Am Dent Assoc J 25:1781, 1938.
40. Dolan DW, and Craig RG: Bending and torsion of endodontic files with rhombus cross sections, J Endod 8:260, 1982.
41. El Deeb M: The sealing ability of injection-molded thermoplasticized gutta-percha. J Endod 11:84, 1985.
42. Escabar C, et al: J Oral Surg 61:504-507, 1986.
43. Feldman G, et al: Retrieving broken endodontic instruments, J Am Dent Assoc 88:588, 1974.
44. Finne K, et al: Retrograde root filling with amalgam and cavit, J Oral Surg 43:621, 1977.
45. Fouad AF: A clinical evaluation of five electronic apex locators, J Endod 15:174, 1989.
46. Friedman CE, et al: The chemical composition and mechanical properties of gutta-percha endodontic filling materials, J Endod 3:304, 1977.
47. Fuchs C, et al: Statistical model for evaluating the penetrating ability of endodontic instruments. J Dent Res 69:1617, 1990.
48. Gercin MY: Root resection, J Can Dent Assoc 8:126, 1942.
49. Goldberg F, and Garfinkel J: Analysis of the use of Dycal with gutta-percha points as an endodontic filling techniques, Oral Surg 47:78, 1979.
50. Gilles JA, and del Rio CE: A comparison of the Canal Master endodontic instrument and K-type files for enlargement of curved root canals. J Endodont 16:561, 1990.
51. Goldman LB, et al: Scanning electron microscope study of a new irrigation method in endodontic treatment, Oral Surg 48:79, 1979.
52. Goldman M, and Pearson AH: A preliminary investigation of the "hollow tube" theory in endodontics: studies with neotetrazolium, J Oral Ther Pharmacol 1:618, 1965.
53. Goldman M, et al: New method of irrigation during endodontic treatment, J Endod 2:257, 1976.
54. Goodman A, Schilder H, and Aldrich W: The thermomechanical properties of gutta percha. II. The history and molecular chemistry of gutta percha, Oral Surg 37:954, 1974.
55. Grassi MD: A determination in the physical properties of low temperature (70° C) thermoplasticized gutta-percha systems, master's thesis, Pittsburgh, 1988, University of Pittsburgh.
56. Greenberg M: Filling root canals of deciduous teeth by an injection technique, Dent Dig 67:574, 1961.
57. Greenberg M: Filling root canals by an injection technique, Dent Dig 69:61, 1963.
58. Grossman LI: An improved root canal cement, J Am Dent Assoc 56:381, 1958.
59. Gurney BF, Best EJ, and Gervasio G: Physical measurements of gutta percha, Oral Surg 32:260, 1971.
60. Gutiérrez JH, and Garcia J: Microscopic and macroscopic investigation on results of mechanical preparations of root canals, Oral Surg 25:108, 1968.
61. Haikel Y, and Allemann C: Effectiveness of four methods for preparing root canals: a scanning electron microscopic evaluation, J Endod 14:340, 1988.
62. Harris WE: Unusual endodontic complication: report of a case, J Am Dent Assoc 83:358, 1971.
63. Harty FJ, and Stock CJR: The Giromatic system compared with hand instrumentation in endodontics, Br Dent J 137:239, 1974.
64. Heuer MA: Clinical evaluation of endodontic materials, J Endod 7:105, 1981.
65. Holland R, and de Souza V: Ability of a new calcium hydroxide root canal filling material to induce hard tissue formation, J Endod 11:535, 1985.
66. Holland R, et al: Reaction of the human periapical tissue to pulp extirpation and immediate root canal filling with calcium hydroxide, J Endod 3:63, 1977.
67. Horton JE, Tarpley TM, and Jacoway JR: Clinical applications of ultrasonic instrumentation in the surgical removal of bone, Oral Surg 51:236, 1981.

68. Hosegawa K, et al: J Nihon Univ School Dent 117, 1986.
69. Jerome CE, Hicks ML, and Pelleu GB: Compatibility of accessory gutta-percha cones used with two types of spreaders, J Endod 14:428, 1988.
70. Johnson WB, and Beatty RG: Clinical technique for removal of root canal obstructions, J Am Dent Assoc 117:473, 1988.
71. Jones G: The use of Silastic as an injectable root canal obturating material, J Endod 6:552, 1980.
72. Kerstein HW: Evaluation of three thermoplasticized gutta-percha filling techniques using a leakage model in vitro, Int Endod J 21:353, 1988.
73. Kielt LW, and Montgomery S: The effect of endosonic instrumentation on simulated curved root canals, J Endod 13:215, 1987.
74. Kirmura JT: A comparative analysis of zinc and nonzinc containing alloys used in retrograde endodontic surgery. II. Optical emission spectrographic analysis for zinc precipitation, J Endod 8:407, 1982.
75. Kim S, et al: Comparison of pulpal blood flow in dog canine teeth determined by the laser Doppler and 133 xenon washout methods. Arch Oral Biol 35:411, 1990.
76. Krupp J, Brantley W, and Gerstein H: An investigation of the torsional and bending properties of seven brands of endodontic files, J Endod 10:372, 1984.
77. La Combe JS, et al: A comparison of the apical seal produced by two thermoplasticized injectable gutta-percha techniques, J Endod 14:445, 1988.
78. Lado EA, Richmand AF, and Marks RG: Reliability and validity of a digital pulp tester as a test standard, for measuring sensory perception, J Endod 14:352, 1988.
79. Langeland K: Root canal sealants and pastes, Dent Clin North Am 18:309, 1974.
80. Langeland K, Liao K, and Pascon EA: Work-saving devices in endodontics: efficacy of sonic and ultrasonic techniques, J Endod 11:499, 1985.
81. Lautenschlager WP, et al: Brittle and ductile torsional failures of endodontic instruments, J Endod 3:175, 1977.
82. Laws AJ: Calcium hydroxide as a possible root filling material, NZ Dent J 58:199,1 962.
83. Laws AJ: Preparation of root canals—an evaluation of mechanical aids, NZ Dent J 64:156, 1968.
84. Lengheden A, Blomlof L, and Lindskog S: Effect of immediate calcium hydroxide treatment and permanent root-filling on periodontal healing in contaminated replanted teeth. Scand J Dent Res 99:139, 1990.
85. Lengheden A, Blomlof L, and Lindskog S: Effect of delayed calcium hydroxide treatment on periodontal healing in contaminated replanted teeth. Scand J Dent Res 99:147, 1991.
86. Levy G, and Abou-Ross M: Endodontic file design and dynamics in automated root canal preparation. Alpha Omegan 83:68, 1990.
87. Levy G. Cleaning and shaping the root canal with a Nd:YAG laser beam: a comparative study, J Endodon 18:123, 1992.
88. Lewis BB, and Chester SB: Formaldehyde in dentistry: a review of mutagenic and carcinogenic potential. J Am Dent Assoc 103:429, 1981.
89. Lilley JD, and Smith DC: An investigation of the fracture of root canal reamers, Br Dent J 120:364, 1966.
90. Lim KC, McCabe JG, and Johnson MR: SEM evaluation of sonic and ultrasonic devices for root canal preparation, Quintessence Int 18:793, 1987.
91. MacPherson MG, et al: Leakage in vitro with high-temp thermoplasticized gutta-percha high copper amalgam, and warm gutta-percha when used as retrofilling materials, J Endod 15:212, 1989.
92. Marlin J, et al: Clinical use of injection-molded thermoplasticized gutta-percha for obturation of the root canal system, J Endod 7:277, 1981.
93. Martin LR, et al: Histologic response of rat connective tissue to zinc-containing amalgam, J Endod 2:25, 1976.
94. Martin H: Ultrasonic disinfection of the root canal, Oral Surg 42:92, 1976.
95. Martin H, Cunningham WT, and Norris JP: A quantitative comparison of the ability of diamond and K-type files to remove dentin, Oral Surg 50:566, 1980.
96. Martin H, et al: Ultrasonic vs hand filing of dentin: a quantitative study, Oral Surg 49:79, 1980.
97. Massa GR, Nichols JI, Harrington GW. Torsional properties of the Canal Master instrument. J Endod 18:222, 1992.
98. McComb D, and Smith DC: A preliminary scanning electron microscopic study of root canals after endodontic procedures, J Endod 1:238, 1975.
99. McDonald NJ, and Hovland EJ: An in vivo evaluation of the apex locator endocator, J Endod 15:171, 1989 (abstract).
100. Miserendino LJ: Report submitted to ADA/ANSI Committee on Endodontists Instruments and Materials at the 42nd annual meeting of the American Association of Endodontics, San Diego, 1985.
101. Miserendino LJ, et al: Cutting efficiency of endodontic instruments. 1. A quantitative comparison of the tip and fluted regions, J Endod 11:435, 1985.
102. Miserendino LJ, et al: Cutting efficiency of endodontic instruments. 2. An analysis of the design of the tip, J Endod 12:8, 1986.
103. Miserendino LJ: The laser apicoectomy: endodontic application of the CO_2 laser for periapical surgery, Oral Surg 66:615, 1988.
104. Miserendino LJ: Sterilization of bacterially contaminated root apices by CO_2 laser irradiation, 1988.
105. Miserendino LJ, et al: Cutting efficiency of endodontic instruments. 3. Comparison of sonic and ultrasonic instruments systems, J Endod 14:24, 1988.
106. Miserendino LJ, Brantley WA, and Gerstein H: Cutting efficiency of endodontic hand instruments. 4. Comparison of hybrid and traditional instrument designs, J Endod 14:451, 1988.
107. Miserendino LJ, Neiberger EJ, and Pick RM: Current status of lasers in dentistry, Illinois Dent J 56:254, 1987.
108. Miserendino LJ, Pick RM, and Kos W: In vitro sterilization of dental caries by CO_2 laser irradiation, J Amer Soc Laser Med Surg 8:142, 1988.
109. Molven O: Engine- and hand-operated root canal exploration, Odontol Tidskr 76:61, 1968.
110. Moodnik RM, et al: Efficacy of biomechanical instrumentation: a scanning electron microscope study, J Endod 2:261, 1976.
111. Newman JG, Brantley WA, and Gerstein H: A study of the cutting efficiency of seven brands of endodontic files in linear motion, J Endod 9:316, 1983.
112. Norman RD, et al: The effect of particle size on the physical properties of zinc oxide eugenol mixtures, J Dent Res 43:252, 1964.
113. Oliet S, and Sorin SM: Effect of aging on the mechanical properties of hand-rolled gutta percha endodontic cones, Oral Surg 43:954, 1977.
114. Olson AK, Hartwell GR, and Weller RN: Evaluation of the controlled placement of injected thermoplasticized gutta-percha, J Endod 15:306, 1989.
115. O'Neill LJ: A clinical evaluation of electronic root canal measurement, Oral Surg 38:469, 1974.
116. Oswald RJ, and Cohen SA: Systemic distribution of lead from root canal fillings, J Endod 1:59, 1975.
117. Paris L, et al: The effect of temperature change on the sealing properties of temporary filling materials, Oral Surg 17:771, 1964.
118. Parkins DJ, Harrison JW, and Coltmore JM: An evaluation of the cytotoxcity potential of cavity varnish for use in endodontic surgery, J Endod 13:170, 1987.
119. Pini R, et al: Laser dentistry: a new application of eximer laser in root canal therapy, Lasers Surg Med 9:352, 1989.
120. Powell SE, Wong PD, and Simon JHS: A comparison of the effect of modified and non-modified instrument tips on apical canal configuration. II, J Endod 14:224, 1988.
121. Reynelds MA, et al: An invitro histologic comparison of the step-back, sonic, and ultrasonic instrumentation techniques, in small, curved root canals, J Endod 13:307, 1987.
122. Richman MJ: The use of ultrasonics in root canal therapy and root resection, J Dent Med 12:12, 1957.
123. Rickert UG, and Dixon CM: The controlling of root surgery. In

Transactions, Eighth International Dental Congress, sect. IIIa, Paris, 1931.
124. Rickles NH, and Joshi BA: Death from air embolism during root canal therapy, J Am Dent Assoc 67:397, 1963.
125. Roane J, Sabala C, and Duncanson M: The balanced force concept for instrumentation of curved canals, J Endod 11:203, 1985.
126. Safavi KE, et al: In vitro evaluation of biocompatibility and marginal adaptation of root retrofilling materials, J Endod 14:538, 1989.
127. Safavi KE, Spangberg LS, and Langland K: Root canal tubule disinfection. J Endodont 16:207, 1990.
128. Salzgeber RM, and Brilliant JD: An in vivo evaluation of the penetration of an irrigating solution in root canals, J Endod 3:394, 1977.
129. Sanders SH, and Dooley RJ: A comparative evaluation of polycarboxylate cement as a root canal sealer utilizing roughened and nonroughened silver points, Oral Surg 37:629, 1974.
130. Schilder H: Filling root canals in three dimensions, Dent Clin North Am 11:723, 1967.
131. Schilder H, Goodman A, and Aldrich W: The thermomechanical properties of gutta-percha. I. The compressibility of gutta-percha, Oral Surg 37:946, 1974.
132. Schilder H, Goodman A, and Aldrich W: The thermomechanical properties of gutta-percha. III. Determination of phase transition temperatures for gutta-percha, Oral Surg 38:109, 1974.
133. Schneider SW: A comparison of canal preparations in straight and curved root canals, Oral Surg 32:271, 1971.
134. Schwartz SA, and Alexander JB: A comparison of leakage between silver-glass ionomer cement and amalgam retrofilling, J Endod 14:385, 1988.
135. Seltzer S, et al: A scanning electron microscope examination of silver cones removed from endodontically treated teeth, Oral Surg 33:589, 1972.
136. Sepic AO, et al: A comparison of Flex-R files and K-type files for enlargement of severely curved root canals, J Endod 15:240, 1989.
137. Serene TP, Vesely J, and Boackle RJ: Complement activation as a possible in vitro indication of the inflammatory potential of endodontic materials, Oral Surg 652:354, 1988.
138. Shiveley J, et al: An in vitro autoradiographic study comparing the apical seal of uncatalyzed dycal to Grossman's sealer, J Endod 11:62, 1985.
139. Shoji Y: Studies on the mechanism of the mechanical enlargement of root canals, Nihon Univ Sch Dent J 70:71, 1965.
140. Shoji Y: Systematic endodontics, Berlin, 1973, Buch- und Zeitschriften-Verlag.
141. Sjogren U, et al: The antimicrobial effect of calcium hydroxide as a short-term intracanal dressing, Int Endodont J 24:119, 1991.
142. Skinner RL, and Himel VT: The sealing ability of injection-molded thermoplasticized gutta-percha with and without use of sealers, J Endod 13:315, 1987.
143. Smee G, et al: A comparative leakage study of P-30 resin bonded ceramic, Teflon, amalgam and IRM as retrofilling seals, J Endod 13:117, 1987.
144. Smith DC: The setting of zinc oxide-eugenol mixtures, Br Dent J 105:313, 1958.
145. Sorin SM, Oliet S, and Pearlstein F: Rejuvenation of aged (brittle) endodontic gutta percha cones, J Endod 5:233, 1979.
146. Sotokawa T: An analysis of clinical breakage of root canal instruments, J Endod 14:75, 1988.
147. Stamos DG, et al: Endosonics: clinical impressions, J Endod 11:181, 1985.
148. Stamos DE, et al: An in vitro comparison study to quantitate the debridement ability of hand, sonic, and ultrasonic instrumentation, J Endod 13:434, 1987.
149. Stuart K, et al: The comparative antimicrobial effect of calcium hydroxide. Oral Surg Oral Med Oral Pathol 72:101, 1991.
150. Sundada I: New method for measuring the length of the root canal, J Dent Res 41:375, 1962.
151. Svec TA, and Harrison JW: Chemomechanical removal of pulpal and dentinal debris with sodium hypochlorite and hydrogen peroxide vs normal saline solution, J Endod 3:49, 1977.
152. Teplitsky PE, and Meimaris IT: Sealing ability of Cavit and Term as intermediate restorative materials, J Endod 14:278, 1988.
153. Torabinejad M, et al: Scanning electron microscopic study of root canal obturation using thermoplasticized gutta-percha, J Endod 4:245, 1978.
154. Torneck CD: Reaction of rat connective tissue to polyethylene tube implants. I, Oral Surg 21:379, 1966.
155. Torneck CD: Reaction of rat connective tissue to polyethylene tube implants. II, Oral Surg 24:674, 1967.
156. Tuggle ST, et al: A dye penetration study of retrofilling materials, J Endod 15:122, 1989.
157. Ushiyama J, Nakamura M, and Nakamura Y: A clinical evaluation of voltage gradient method of measuring root canal length, J Endod 14:283, 1988.
158. Vande Visse JE, and Brilliant JD: Effect of irrigation on the production of extruded material at the root apex during instrumentation, J Endod 1:243, 1975.
159. Vessey RA: The effect of filing versus reaming on the shape of the prepared root canal, Oral Surg 27:543, 1969.
160. Walker JE: Emphysema of soft tissues complicating endodontic treatment using hydrogen peroxide: a case report. Br J Oral Surg 13:98, July 1975.
161. Walker TL, and del Rio CE: Histologic evaluation of ultrasonic and sonic instrumentation of curved root canals. J Endod 15:49, 1989.
162. Walton RE: Histologic evaluation of different methods of enlarging the pulp canal space, J Endod 2:304, 1976.
163. Weine FS, Kelly RF, and Brag K: Effect of preparation with endodontic handpieces on original canal shape, J Endod 2:298, 1976.
164. Weine FS, Kelly RF, and Lio PS: The effect of preparation procedures on canal shape and apical foramen shape. J Endod 8:255, 1975.
165. Wilder-Smith PE: A new method for the non-invasive measurement of pulpal blood flow. Int Endodont J 21:307, 1988.
166. Wildey WL, and Sevia ES: A new root canal instrument and instrumentation technique: a preliminary report, J Oral Surg 67:198, 1989.
167. Yahya AS, and El Deeb ME: Effects of sonic ultrasonic instrumentation on canal preparation. J Endod 15:235, 1989.
168. Yamada RS, et al: A scanning electron microscope comparison of high volume flush with several irrigating solutions. III, J Endod 9:137, 1983.
169. Yee FS, Lugassy AA, and Peterson JN: Filling of root canals with adhesive materials, J Endod 1:145, 1975.
170. Zakariasen KL, Boran T, MacDonald R: The emerging role for lasers in endodontics and other areas of dentistry. AD 83:65, 1990.

Self-assessment questions

1. The endodontic broach is used to
   a. locate the orifices of the root canals.
   b. remove pulp tissue from the pulp spaces.
   c. smooth the walls of root canals.
   d. enlarge the root canal spaces.
2. The basic difference between K-type files and reamers is
   a. the number of spirals or flutes per unit length.
   b. the geometric cross section.
   c. the depth of the flutes.
   d. the direction of the spirals.
3. The major determining factor that influences the efficacy of root canal débridement is the
   a. type of hand instrument used.
   b. irrigating solution.
   c. internal pulp space anatomy.
   d. instrumentation technique.

4. The working portion of an endodontic condenser (plugger) is
   a. smooth, tapered, and pointed.
   b. smooth, tapered, and flat-ended.
   c. smooth, of uniform width, and pointed.
   d. smooth, of uniform width, and flat-ended.
5. Modification of the cross-sectional design of K-type files from square to rhomboid has resulted in significantly greater
   a. torsional strength.
   b. tensile strength.
   c. stiffness.
   d. flexibility.
6. Significant deviations from circular canal preparations will occur when using a
   a. K-type reamer with a reaming action.
   b. K-type reamer with a filing action.
   c. K-type file with a reaming action.
   d. K-type file with a filing action.
7. The Hedström file is most commonly used to
   a. flare the canal.
   b. establish a circular preparation.
   c. prepare post space.
   d. locate canal orifices.
8. The temperature of the gutta-percha extruded from the "low-temperature," thermoplastic injection system is
   a. 160° C.
   b. 100° C.
   c. 70° C.
   d. 40° C.
9. Some studies have reported that the most important aspect of irrigation is the
   a. quantity of irrigant.
   b. chelating action of the solution.
   c. size of the needle.
   d. type of irrigant.
10. Hardening of zinc oxide–eugenol is due to the
   a. formation of zinc eugenolate.
   b. presence of water.
   c. evaporation of eugenol.
   d. heat generated during the chemical reaction.
11. With time and with exposure to light and air, gutta-percha
   a. does not change its physical properties significantly.
   b. will decompose and lose mass.
   c. becomes more brittle.
   d. alters, but can be restored by freezing.
12. Temporary canal medications are of various types. Which of the following seems to satisfy more criteria as to desirable properties?
   a. Formocresol.
   b. Chlorhexidine.
   c. Potassium iodide.
   d. Calcium hydroxide.
13. A disadvantage of Cavit as compared to IRM as a temporary restoration is that Cavit
   a. does not have as much compressive strength.
   b. does not seal as well with time.
   c. is more susceptible to thermal changes.
   d. shrinks while setting.
14. An inherent disadvantage of the gutta-percha/carrier systems is
   a. the carrier corrosion or disintegration products are toxic.
   b. difficulty in insertion.
   c. potential problems in retreatment.
   d. no means are available to prepare the post space.
15. The Canal Master intracanal instrument has some disadvantages over conventional instruments in that the Canal Master
   a. will enlarge the canal unevenly.
   b. will result in more transportation if not precurved.
   c. is more susceptible to breakage.
   d. cannot be utilized in all canal shapes.
16. Thinking in terms of design, which of the following size-50 endodontic instruments made from the same steel would be most susceptible to fracture (separation)?
   a. Triangular shaft file.
   b. Square shaft reamer.
   c. Rhomboid file.
   d. Hedström file.

Chapter 15

Pulpal Reaction to Caries and Dental Procedures

Syngcuk Kim
Henry O. Trowbridge

At the dental centenary celebration held in Baltimore in 1940, Bodecker commented on the current state of dentistry: "Operative procedures in the reconstruction of teeth have always been governed by engineering principles."[112] Although this is still true today, more than 50 years later, many other basic concepts of restorative dentistry have been changed drastically since then. One fundamental change in dental treatment in the past 40 years has been preservation of dentition and the pulp. Unfortunately, however, greater dental preservation all too often results in damage to the pulp. Of the various forms of dental treatment, operative procedures by far are the most frequent cause of pulpal injury. It is accepted that trauma to the pulp cannot always be avoided, particularly when the tooth requires extensive restoration. Nonetheless, the competent clinician, by recognizing the hazards associated with each step of the restorative process, can often minimize if not prevent trauma and thus preserve the vitality of the tooth.

In the past, pulpal responses to various dental procedures and materials have been discussed almost exclusively from a histologic perspective. Fortunately, active physiologic investigations in the last decade have shed new light on the dynamic changes in the pulp in response to dental procedures and materials. It is the purpose of this chapter to discuss new knowledge together with the old to understand pulpal responses to caries and to various restorative procedures and materials.

Supported in part by NIDR grants DEO-5605 and DEO-0121.

DENTAL CARIES

Dental caries is a localized, progressive destruction of tooth structure and the most common cause of pulp disease. It is now generally accepted that for caries to develop, specific bacteria must become established on the tooth surface. Products of bacterial metabolism, notably organic acids and proteolytic enzymes, cause the destruction of enamel and dentin. Bacterial metabolites are also capable of eliciting an inflammatory reaction. Eventually, extensive invasion of the dentin results in bacterial infection of the pulp. Basic reactions that tend to protect the pulp against caries involve (1) a decrease in the permeability of the dentin, (2) the formation of new dentin, and (3) inflammatory and immune reactions.

Inward diffusion of toxic substances from carious lesions occurs mainly through the dentinal tubules. Therefore, the extent to which toxins permeate the tubules and reach the pulp is of critical importance in determining the extent of pulpal injury. *The most common response to caries is dentin sclerosis.* In this reaction the dentinal tubules become partially or completely filled with mineral deposits consisting of apatite as well as whitlockite crystals.[31,110] Researchers[96] reported finding dentin sclerosis at the periphery of carious lesions in 95.4% of 154 teeth examined. Studies using dyes, solvents, and radioactive ions have shown that dentin sclerosis has the effect of decreasing the permeability of dentin, thus shielding the pulp from irritation.[4,9,29,62] Evidence suggests that in order for sclerosis to occur, vital odontoblast processes must be present within the tubules.[11,43]

The ability of the pulp to produce reparative dentin beneath a carious lesion is another mechanism for limiting the diffusion of toxic substances to the pulp (see Fig. 11-43). Researchers[96] reported the presence of reparative dentin in 63.6% of teeth with carious lesions and found that it often occurred in combination with dentin sclerosis. The characteristics of reparative dentin have already been discussed (see Chapter 11). In general, the amount of reparative dentin formed is proportional to the amount of primary dentin destroyed. The rate of carious attack also seems to be an influencing factor, since more dentin is formed in response to slowly progressing chronic caries than to rapidly advancing acute caries. For this reason, carious exposure of the pulp is likely to occur earlier in acute caries than in chronic caries.

Research has shown that along the border zone between primary and reparative dentin, the walls of dentinal tubules are thickened and the tubules are frequently occluded with material resembling peritubular dentin.[85] Thus the border zone appears to be considerably less permeable than ordinary dentin and may serve as a barrier to the ingress of bacteria and their products.

The formation of a dead tract in dentin is yet another reaction that may occur in response to caries. Unlike dentin sclerosis and the formation of reparative dentin, this response is not considered to be a defense reaction. A dead tract is an area in dentin within which the dentinal tubules are devoid of odontoblast processes. The origin of these tracts in dental caries is uncertain, but most authorities are of the opinion that they are formed as a result of the early death of odontoblasts. Dead tracts are most often observed in young teeth affected by rapidly progressing lesions. Because dentinal tubules of dead tracts are patent, they are highly permeable,[88] and therefore they are a potential threat to the integrity of the pulp. Fortunately, the healthy pulp responds to the presence of a dead tract by depositing a layer of reparative dentin over its surface, thus sealing it off.[29]

Dentin is demineralized by organic acids (principally lactic acid) that are products of bacterial fermentation. These acids also play a role in degrading the organic matrix of enamel and dentin. While very few oral bacteria possess collagenases, the collagenous matrix of dentin can be degraded by bacterial proteases if the collagen is first denatured by acid.

There is some controversy as to when caries first elicits an inflammatory response in the underlying pulp. One study observed an accumulation of chronic inflammatory cells in the pulp beneath enamel caries that had not yet invaded dentin.[16] Another study,[60] however, did not observe pulpal inflammation until the caries had penetrated beyond the enamel. There is general agreement that by the time caries has invaded the dentin some changes are occurring in the pulp. These changes represent a response to the diffusion of soluble irritants and inflammatory stimuli into the pulp. Such substances include bacterial toxins, bacterial enzymes, antigens, chemotaxins, organic acids, and products of tissue destruction. Substances also pass outward from the pulp to the carious lesion. Researchers reported finding plasma proteins, immunoglobulins, and complement proteins in carious dentin.[1,2,69-71] It is conceivable that some of these factors are capable of inhibiting bacterial activity in the lesion.

Unfortunately, diagnosis of the extent of pulpal inflammation beneath a carious lesion is difficult. Many factors play a role in determining the nature of the caries process, so the individuality of each carious lesion should be recognized. The response of the pulp may vary depending on whether the caries process is progressing rapidly or slowly or is completely inactive (arrested caries). Moreover, caries tends to be an intermittent process with periods of rapid activity alternating with periods of quiescence.[60] The rate of attack may be influenced by any or all of the following:

- Age of the host
- Composition of the tooth
- Nature of the bacterial flora of the lesion
- Salivary flow
- Buffering capacity of the saliva
- Antibacterial substances in the saliva
- Oral hygiene
- Cariogenicity of the diet and frequency with which acidogenic food is ingested
- Caries-inhibiting factors in the diet

Early morphologic evidence of a pulpal reaction to caries is found in the underlying odontoblast layer. Even before the appearance of inflammatory changes in the pulp there is an overall reduction in the number and size of odontoblast cell bodies.[102] Although normally tall, columnar cells, odontoblasts affected by caries appear flat to cuboidal in shape (Fig. 15-1). Electron microscopic examination of odontoblasts beneath carious lesions has revealed signs of cellular injury in the form of vacuolization, ballooning degeneration of mitochondria, and reduction in the number and size of other cytoplasmic organelles, particularly the endoplasmic reticulum.[59] These findings are in accord with biochemical studies[47,48] in which a reduction in the metabolic activity of odontoblasts was noted.

Concomitant with changes in the odontoblastic layer, a hyperchromatic line (calciotraumatic response) may develop along the pulpal margin of the dentin (Fig. 15-2). Formation of this line is thought to represent a disturbance in the normal equilibrium of the odontoblasts.[55] It may also delineate the point at which the primary odontoblasts succumbed to the caries process and were replaced by odontoprogenitor cells arising from the cell-rich zone. In either event, as new dentin is formed the hyperchromatic line persists and becomes permanently embedded in the dentin.

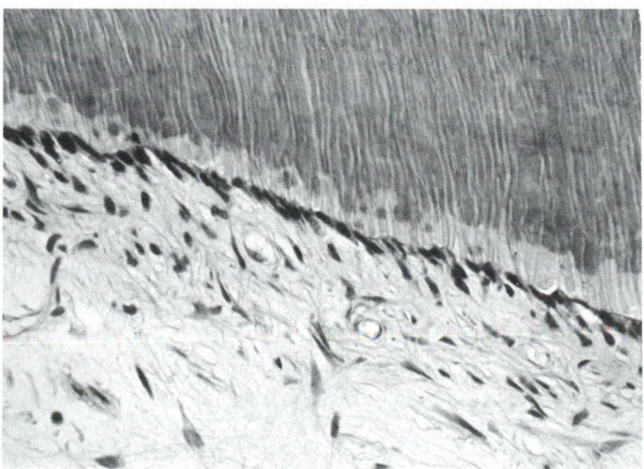

FIG. 15-1 Low cuboidal odontoblasts beneath a carious lesion. Compare the appearance of these cells with normal odontoblasts in Figure 11-16.

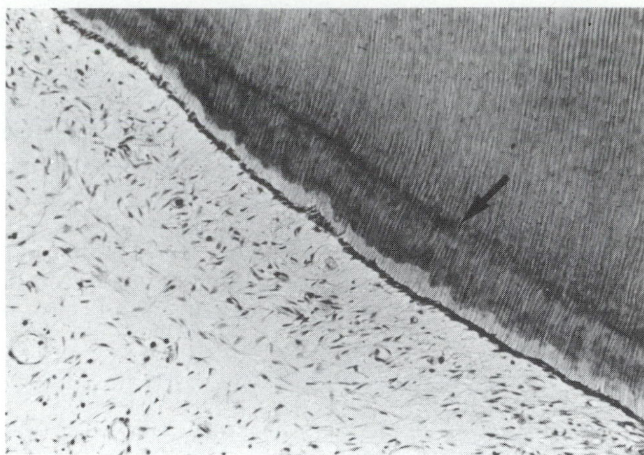

FIG. 15-2 Hyperchromatic line *(arrow)* in dentin beneath a carious lesion. (From Trowbridge H: J Endod 7:52, 1981. © by American Association of Endodontists, 1981.)

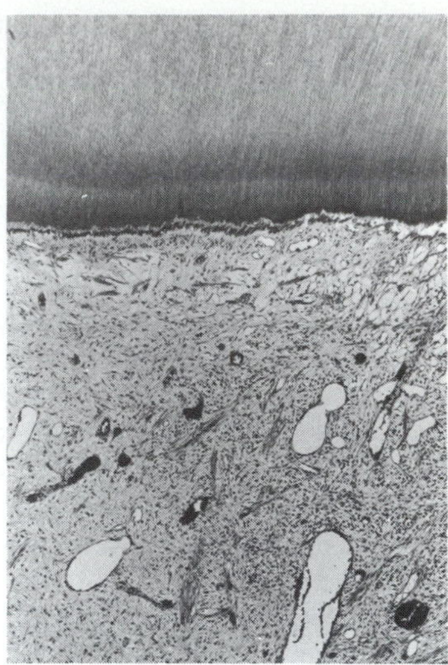

FIG. 15-3 Chronic inflammatory response evoked by a carious lesion in the overlying dentin.

Dental caries is a protracted process and lesions progress over a period of months or years. One investigator found that the average time from the stage of incipient caries to clinically detectable caries in children is 18 ± 6 months. Consequently, it is not surprising that pulpal inflammation evoked by carious lesions begins insidiously as a low-grade, chronic response rather than an acute reaction (Fig. 15-3). The initial inflammatory cell infiltrate consists principally of lymphocytes, plasma cells, and macrophages.[18] Within this infiltrate are immunologically competent cells responding to antigenic substances diffusing into the pulp from the carious lesion.[96] Additionally, there is a proliferation of small blood vessels and fibroblasts and the deposition of collagen fibers. This pattern of inflammation is regarded as an inflammatory-reparative process. It is wise to remember that not all injuries result in permanent damage. Should the carious lesion be eliminated or become arrested, connective tissue repair would ensue.

The extent of pulpal inflammation beneath a carious lesion depends on the depth of bacterial invasion as well as the degree to which dentin permeability has been reduced by dentinal sclerosis and reparative dentin formation. In a study involving 46 carious teeth, investigators found that if the distance between the invading bacteria and the pulp (including the thickness of reparative dentin) averaged 1.1 mm or more, the inflammatory response was negligible.[84] When the lesions reached to within 0.5 mm of the pulp, there was a significant increase in the extent of inflammation, but it was not until the reparative dentin that had formed beneath the lesion was invaded by bacteria that the pulp became acutely inflamed.

As bacteria converge on the pulp, the characteristic features of acute inflammation become manifest. These include vascular and cellular responses in the form of vasodilation, increased vascular permeability, and the accumulation of leukocytes. Neutrophils migrate from blood vessels to the site of injury in response to certain split products of complement that are strongly chemotactic. These products are formed when complement is activated in the presence of antigen-antibody complexes.

Pulpal Abscess

Carious exposure of the pulp results in progressive mobilization of neutrophils and eventually to suppuration, which may be diffuse or localized in the form of an abscess. The exudate associated with this reaction is called pus. Pus is formed when neutrophils release their lysosomal enzymes and the surrounding tissue is digested (a process known as liquefactive necrosis). The digested tissue has a greater osmotic pressure than the surrounding tissue, and this pressure differential is one of the reasons that abscesses are often painful and why drainage provides relief.

Few bacteria are found in an abscess, because bacteria entering the lesion are promptly destroyed by the antibacterial products of neutrophils. In addition, many bacteria cannot tolerate the low pH resulting from the release of lactic acid from neutrophils. However, as the size of the exposure enlarges and an ever-increasing number of bacteria enter the pulp, the defending forces are overwhelmed. It must be remembered that the pulp has a finite blood supply. Therefore when the demand for inflammatory elements exceeds the ability of the blood to transport them to the site of bacterial penetration, the bacteria become too numerous for the defenders and are able to proliferate without constraint. This ultimately leads to pulp necrosis.

Chronic Ulcerative Pulpitis

In some cases an accumulation of neutrophils may produce surface destruction (ulceration) of the pulp rather than an abscess. This is apt to occur when drainage is established through a pathway of decomposed dentin. The ulcer represents a local excavation of the surface of the pulp resulting from liquefactive necrosis of tissue. Because drainage prevents the buildup of pressure, the lesion tends to remain localized and asymptomatic. The base of the ulcer consists of necrotic debris and a dense accumulation of neutrophils. Granulation tissue infiltrated with chronic inflammatory cells is found within the deeper layers of the lesion. Eventually a space is created between the area of suppuration and the wall of the pulp chamber, giving the lesion the appearance of an ulcer (Fig. 15-4).

Hyperplastic Pulpitis

Hyperplastic pulpitis occurs almost exclusively in primary and immature permanent teeth with open apices. It develops

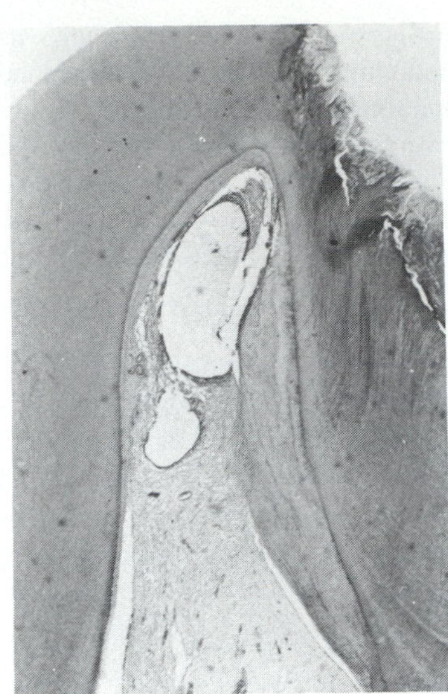

FIG. 15-4 Chronic ulcerative pulpitis.

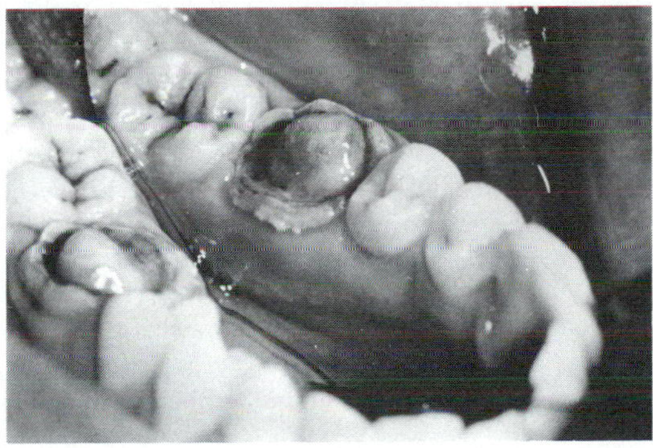

FIG. 15-5 Hyperplastic pulpitis (pulp polyp) in a lower first permanent molar. (Courtesy Dr. A. Stabholz, Jerusalem.)

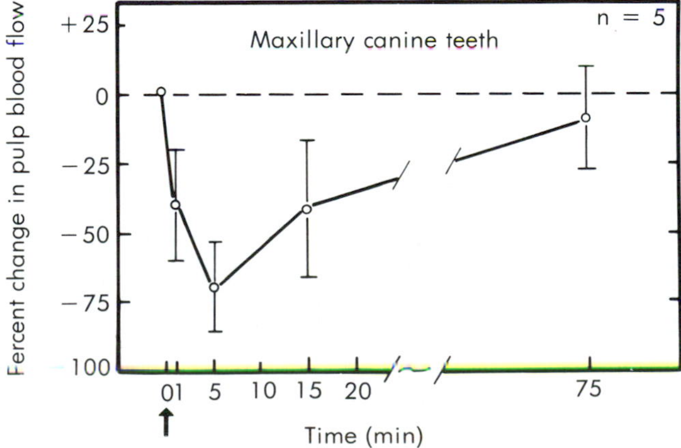

FIG. 15-6 Effects of infiltration anesthesia (2% lidocaine with 1:100,000 epinephrine) on pulpal blood flow in the maxillary canine teeth of dogs. There is a drastic decrease in pulpal blood flow soon after the injection. The arrow indicates the time of injection. The bars depict standard deviation. (From Kim S: J Dent Res 63[5]:650, 1984.)

in response to carious exposure of the pulp when the exposure enlarges to form a gaping cavity in the roof of the pulp chamber. This opening provides a pathway for drainage of the inflammatory exudate. Once drainage is established, acute inflammation subsides and chronic inflammatory tissue proliferates through the opening created by the exposure from a "pulp polyp" (Fig. 15-5). Presumably the young pulp does not become necrotic following exposure because its natural defenses and rich supply of blood allow it to resist bacterial infection. Clinically the lesion has the appearance of a fleshy mass that may cover most of what remains of the crown of the tooth.

EFFECTS OF LOCAL ANESTHETICS ON THE PULP

The purpose of adding a vasoconstrictor to local anesthetics is to potentiate and prolong the anesthetic effect by reducing blood flow in the area in which the anesthetic is administered. Although this enhances anesthesia, a recent study has shown that an anesthetic such as 2% lidocaine with epinephrine 1:100,000 is capable of significantly decreasing pulpal blood flow.[53] This reduction in blood flow may place the pulp in jeopardy for reasons explained later. Both infiltration and mandibular block injections cause a significant decrease in pulpal blood flow, although the flow reduction lasts a relatively short time (Fig. 15-6). With the ligamental injection, pulpal blood flow ceases completely for about 30 minutes when 2% lidocaine with 1:100,000 epinephrine is used (Fig. 15-7). With a higher concentration of epinephrine the cessation of pulp flow lasts even longer. There is a direct relationship between the length of the flow cessation and the concentration of the vasoconstrictor used.[52] Because the rate of oxygen consumption in the pulp is relatively low, the healthy pulp can probably withstand a period of reduced blood flow. Researchers reported that pulpal blood flow and sensory nerve activity returned to normal levels after 3 hours of total cessation of blood flow.[72] Recently, it has been demonstrated that little histologic change takes place in the pulp following ligamental injection of an anesthetic solution containing a vasoconstrictor.[57] However, a prolonged reduction in oxygen transport could interfere with cellular metabolism and alter the response of the pulp to injury. Irreversible pulpal injury is particularly apt to occur when dental procedures such as full crown preparations are performed immediately following a ligamental injection. At least four documented cases have occurred in which the mandibular anterior teeth were devitalized as a result of crown preparation following ligamental injection.[52] Presumably irreversible pulp damage resulting from tooth preparation is caused by the release of substantial amounts of vasoactive agents, such as substance P, into the extracellular compartment of the underlying pulp.[71] Under normal circumstances these vasoactive substances are quickly removed from the pulp by the bloodstream. However, when blood flow is drastically decreased or completely arrested, the removal of vasoactive substance from the pulp is greatly delayed. Accumulation of these substances as well as other metabolic waste products may thus result in permanent damage to the pulp. One investigator has shown that the concentration of substances diffusing across the dentin into the pulp depends in part on the rate of removal via the pulpal circulation.[75] Thus a significant reduction in blood flow during a restorative procedure could lead to an increase in the concentration of irritants accumulating within the pulp. *Therefore, whenever possible, it is advisable to use vasoconstrictor-free local anesthetics for restorative proce-*

dures on vital teeth. Since the addition of epinephrine at a concentration of 1:100,000 to local anesthetics appears to provide adequate vasoconstriction, stronger concentrations should be avoided during routine restorative procedures.

For dental treatments where clinicians need not be concerned about the vitality of the pulp, such as endodontic therapy and extractions, the use of a vasoconstrictor-containing local anesthetic is recommended. When used with an epinephrine-containing anesthetic, the ligamental injection is effective in obtaining anesthesia (Fig. 15-8). Over 80% of the problem teeth were successfully anesthetized with epinephrine 1:100,000 containing anesthetic. Endodontists have found the ligamental injection to be an important tool to obtain profound anesthesia when treating so-called hot mandibular molars.

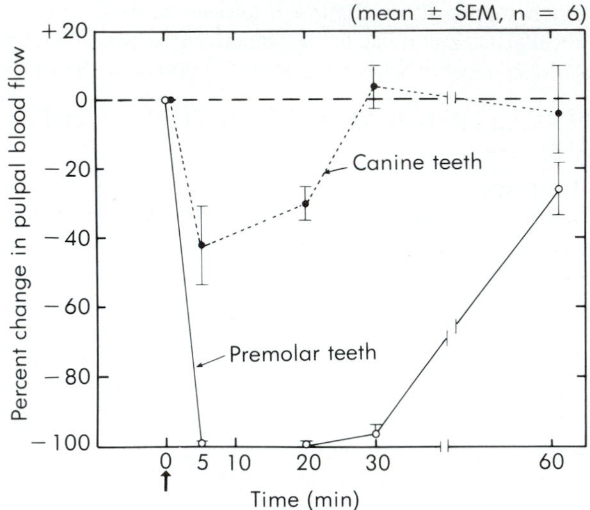

FIG. 15-7 Effects of ligamental injection (2% lidocaine with 1:100,000 epinephrine) on pulpal blood flow in the mandibular canine and premolar teeth of dogs. The injection was given at the mesial and distal sulcus of the premolar teeth. The injection caused total cessation of pulpal blood flow, which lasted about 30 minutes in the premolar teeth. The arrow indicates the time of injection. (From Kim S: J Endod 12[10]:486, 1986. © by American Association of Endodontists, 1986.)

CAVITY AND CROWN PREPARATION

"Cooking the pulp in its own juice" is how Bodecker described tooth preparation without proper coolant.[87] As shown in Figure 15-9, pulpal responses to cavity and crown preparation depend on many factors. These include thermal injury, especially frictional heat; transsection of the odontoblastic processes; vibration; desiccation of dentin; pulp exposure; smear layer; remaining dentin thickness; and agents for cavity cleansing, drying, sterilization, and acid etching.

Thermal Injury

Cutting of dentin with a rotating bur or stone produces a considerable amount of frictional heat. The amount of heat produced is determined by speed of rotation, size and shape of the cutting instrument, length of time the instrument is in contact with the dentin, and amount of pressure exerted on the handpiece. If high temperatures are produced in deep cavities by continuous cutting without proper cooling, the underlying pulp may be severely damaged.[93] According to one investigator,[112] the production of heat within the pulp is the most severe stress that restorative procedures impart to the pulp. If damage is extensive and the cell-rich zone of the pulp is destroyed, reparative dentin may not form.[68]

The thermal conductivity of dentin is relatively low. Therefore heat generated during the cutting of a shallow cavity preparation is much less likely to injure the pulp than a deep cavity preparation. One study found that temperatures and stresses

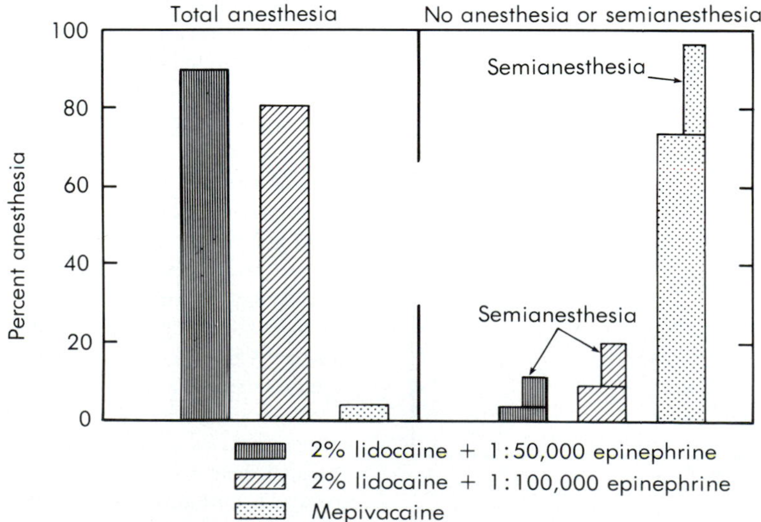

FIG. 15-8 Ligamental injection was effective in obtaining anesthesia in about 90% of cases with 2% lidocaine with 1:50,000 epinephrine and in about 80% of cases with 2% lidocaine with 1:100,000 epinephrine. The injection with mepivacaine (Carbocaine) practically failed to achieve anesthesia. The criteria for total anesthesia is no pain to pulp extirpation and canal instrumentation; semianesthesia is characterized by discomfort as a file approaches the apex.

developed during dry cutting of dentin were sufficiently high to be detrimental to tooth structure.[20] These investigators found that the greatest potential for damage was within a 1- to 2-mm radius of the dentin being cut.

The importance of the use of water-air spray during cavity preparation has been well established. For example, more than 15 years ago it was reported that high-speed cutting with an adequate coolant caused cooling of the pulp to subambient level.[112] Without a coolant the pulpal temperature rose to a critical level, 11° F above the ambient temperature. The same is true in the case of slow-speed cutting (11,000 rpm). The reaction of the pulp to cavity preparation with and without a water spray has been studied histologically (Figs. 15-10 to 15-12).[94] When water-air spray was used, there was a negligible response, providing the remaining dentin thickness was greater than 1 mm (Fig. 15-10). However, when the same procedure was performed without using a water spray, severe damage was found underneath the cutting site (Fig. 15-13). Recently a physiologic investigation[51] revealed that a full crown preparation without water spray in dog canine teeth leaving 1 mm remaining dentin resulted in a drastic reduction in pulpal blood flow. The flow was further reduced 1 hour after the completion of the crown preparation, suggesting irreversible damage. In a similar experiment utilizing a water spray, only minor changes in pulpal blood flow were observed (Fig. 15-14).

Other researchers[68] investigated the effects of heat on the pulps of anesthetized young premolar teeth scheduled for orthodontic extraction. Class V cavities were prepared in the teeth, leaving an average of 0.5 mm remaining dentin thickness. Subsequently, a constant heat of 150° C was applied to the surface of the exposed dentin for 30 seconds. Following this procedure the teeth remained asymptomatic for a month, following which the teeth were extracted. Histologic examination of the pulps revealed varying degrees of pathosis, which included development of a homogenized collagenous zone along the dentin wall, disappearance of the "cell-rich" zone, and generalized cellular degeneration. Localized abscesses were observed in some of the teeth.

"Blushing" of teeth during or after cavity or crown preparation has been attributed to frictional heat. Characteristically the coronal dentin develops a pinkish hue very soon after the dentin is cut. This pinkish hue represents vascular stasis in the subodontoblastic capillary plexus blood flow. Under favorable conditions, this reaction is reversible and the pulp will survive. However, a dark purplish color indicates thrombosis, and this is associated with a poorer prognosis. Histologically, the pulp tissue adjacent to the blushed dentinal surface is engorged with extravasated red blood cells, presumably as a result of the rupture of capillaries in the subodontoblastic plexus.[64] The incidence of dentinal blushing is greatest beneath full crown preparations in teeth that were anesthetized by ligamental injection using 2% lidocaine plus 1:100,000 epinephrine.[52] In such cases, the cessation of pulpal blood flow following ligamental injection may be a contributing factor. Tooth preparation may lead to the release of various vasoactive substances such as substance P, and accumulation of such agents as a result of cessation of pulpal blood flow following ligamental injection may cause the tooth to blush.

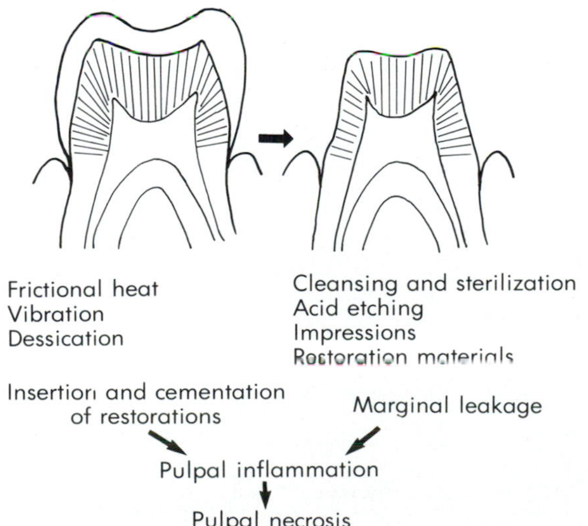

FIG. 15-9 Schematic illustration of factors that might cause pulpal reaction.

Transection of the Odontoblastic Processes

The length of the odontoblast process in fully formed teeth is still a matter of controversy. For many years it was believed that the process is confined to the inner third of the dentin. However, recent scanning electron microscopic studies have provided evidence suggesting that many of the processes extend all the way from the odontoblast layer to the dentinoenamel junction.[50] In any event, amputation of the distal seg-

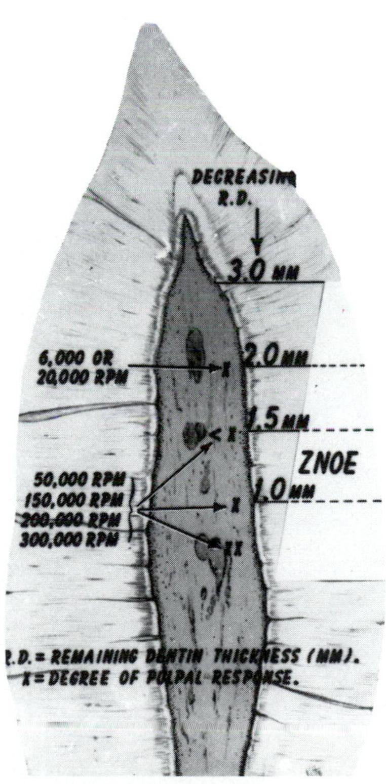

FIG. 15-10 With adequate water coolant, the same cutting tools, and a comparable remaining dentin thickness, the intensity of the pulpal response with high-speed techniques (decreasing force) is considerably less traumatic than with lower-speed techniques (increasing force). (From Stanley HR, and Swerdlow H: J Prosthet Dent 14:365, 1964.)

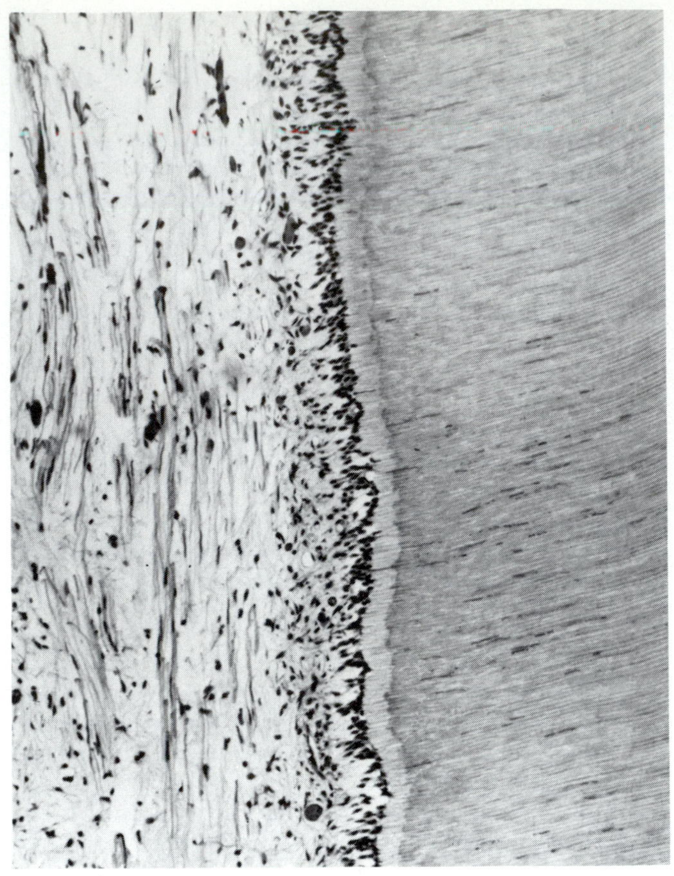

FIG. 15-11 Two-day specimen, high speed with air-water spray. The superficial layers lack infiltrating inflammatory cells. Some odontoblast displacement is present. Pulp architecture is generally intact. (From Swerdlow H, and Stanley HR: J Prosthet Dent 9:121, 1959.)

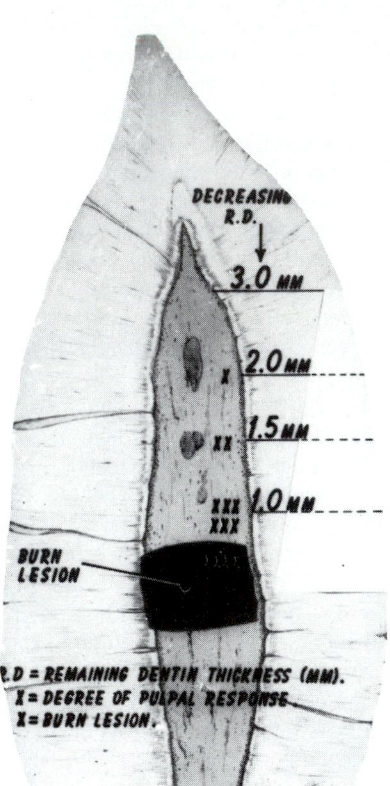

FIG. 15-12 Without adequate water coolant, larger cutting tools (e.g., a No. 37 diamond point) will create typical burn lesions within the pulp when the remaining dentin thickness becomes less than 1.5 mm. (From Stanley HR, and Swerdlow H: J Prosthet Dent 14:365, 1964.)

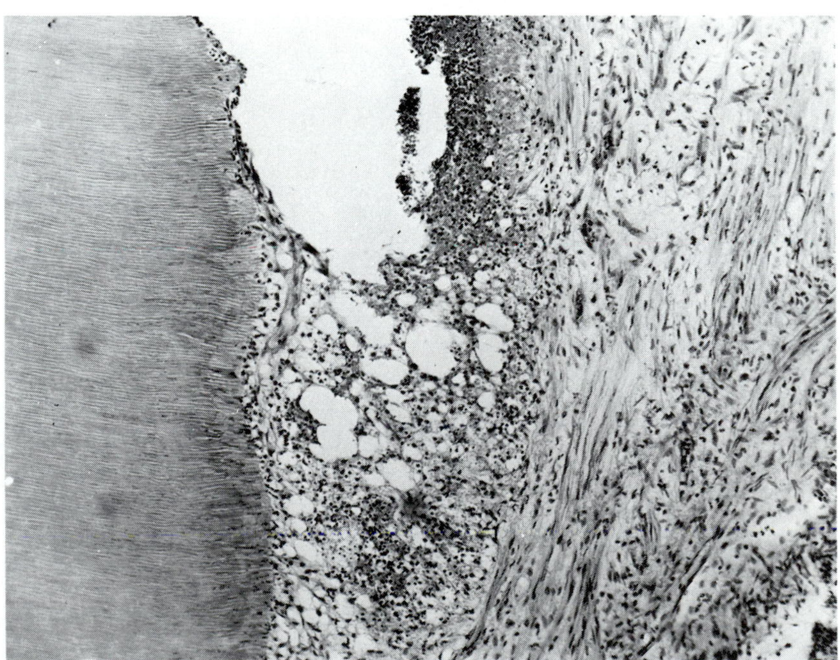

FIG. 15-13 Burn lesion with necrosis and expanding abscess formation in a 10-day specimen. Cavity prepared dry at 20,000 rpm with remaining dentin thickness is 0.23 mm. (From Swerdlow H, and Stanley HR: J Am Dent Assoc 56:317, 1958.)

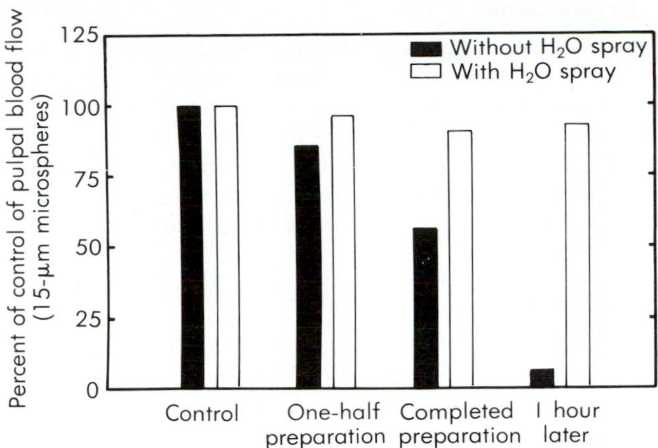

FIG. 15-14 Effects of crown preparation, in dogs, with and without water-air spray (at 350,000 rpm) on pulpal blood flow. The tooth preparation without water spray caused a substantial decrease in pulpal blood flow, whereas that with water spray caused insignificant changes in the flow.

ment of odontoblast processes is often a consequence of cavity or crown preparation. Histologic investigation would indicate that amputation of a portion of the process does not invariably lead to death of the odontoblast. We know from numerous cytologic studies involving microsurgery that amputation of a cellular process is quickly followed by repair of the cell membrane. However, it would appear that amputation of the odontoblast process close to the cell body results in irreversible injury.[86]

It is not always possible to determine the exact cause of death when odontoblasts disappear following a restorative procedure, since these cells may be subjected to a variety of insults. Frictional heat, vibration, amputation of processes, displacement as a result of desiccation, exposure to bacterial toxins, and other chemical irritants may each play a role in the demise of odontoblasts.

Investigators[21] studied the effects of class V cavity preparation on rat molar odontoblasts and observed a significant decrease in the amount of rough endoplasmic reticulum and number of mitochondria. There was also a loss of tight junctions between adjacent odontoblasts. Under the conditions of this experiment, these changes were reversible. Tight junctions provide a semipermeable barrier that prevents the passage of macromolecules from the pulp into the predentin. It has been shown that cavity preparation disturbs this barrier, thus increasing the permeability of the odontoblast layer.[106] The disruption of tight junctional complexes in the odontoblast layer could increase the potential for entry of toxic substances into the subjacent pulp tissue.

Recently, Taylor and associates[99] observed an extensive increase in calcitonin gene–related peptide (CGRP) immunoreactive nerve fibers in the odontoblast layer beneath superficial dentinal cavities in rat molars. It was postulated that this increase represented nerve sprouting. The greatest number of nerve endings was observed at a postoperative interval of 4 days, but within 21 days these fibers had disappeared. The function of nerve sprouting in tissue injury is still unclear.

Crown Preparation

Researchers[28] studied the long-term effects of crown preparation on pulp vitality and found a higher incidence of pulp necrosis associated with full crown preparation (13.3%) as compared with partial veneer restorations (5.1%) and unrestored control teeth (0.5%). The placement of foundations for full crown restorations was associated with an even greater incidence of pulp morbidity (17.7%).

Vibratory Phenomena

Surprisingly little is known about the vibratory agitation that may be produced by high-speed cutting procedures. One study[39] demonstrated violent disturbances in the pulp chambers of teeth beneath the point of application of the bur as well as at other points remote from the cavity preparation. According to the observations, the shock waves produced by vibration were particularly pronounced when the cutting speed was reduced; therefore, stalling of the bur by increased digital pressure on the hand piece should be avoided. Obviously this problem deserves further study.

Desiccation of Dentin

When the surface of freshly cut dentin is dried with a jet of air, there is a rapid outward movement of fluid through the dentinal tubules as a result of the activation of capillary forces within.[15] According to the hydrodynamic theory of dentin sensitivity, this movement of fluid results in stimulation of the sensory nerve of the pulp. Fluid movement is also capable of drawing odontoblasts up into the tubules. These "displaced" odontoblasts soon die and disappear as they undergo autolysis. However, desiccation of dentin by cutting procedures or with a blast of air does not injure the pulp.[12,15] Although one might expect that death of odontoblasts would evoke an inflammatory response, probably too few cells are involved to evoke a significant reaction. Moreover, since death occurs within the dentinal tubules, dentinal fluid would dilute the products of cellular degeneration that might otherwise initiate an inflammatory response. Ultimately, odontoblasts that have been destroyed as a result of desiccation are replaced by new odontoblasts that arise from the cell-rich zone of the pulp, and in 1 to 3 months reparative dentin is formed.[12]

Pulp Exposure

Exposure of the pulp during cavity preparation occurs most often in the process of removing carious dentin. Accidental mechanical exposure may result during the placement of pins or retention points in dentin. In both types of exposure, injury to the pulp appears to be due primarily to bacterial contamination. Investigators demonstrated that surgical exposure of the pulps of germ-free rats was followed by complete healing with no appreciable inflammatory reaction.[46,109] Another investigator has shown that pulps exposed during the removal of carious dentin become infected by bacteria that are carried into the pulp by dentin chips harboring microorganisms.[22] It is safe to state that carious exposure results in much more bacterial contamination than does mechanical exposure.

Smear Layer

The smear layer is an amorphous, relatively smooth layer of microcrystalline debris whose featureless surface cannot be seen with the naked eye.[76] Although the smear layer may interfere with the adaptation of restorative materials to dentin, it may not be desirable to remove the entire layer, since its removal greatly increases dentin permeability. By removing most of the layer but leaving plugs of grinding debris in the apertures of the dentinal tubules, dentin permeability is not increased, yet the walls of the cavity are relatively clean. Whether or not the smear layer should be removed is a matter of controversy. One view is that microorganisms present in the smear layer may irritate the pulp. Initially few bacteria are present in the smear layer, but if conditions for growth are favorable these will multiply, particularly if a gap between the restorative material and the dentinal wall permits the ingress of saliva.[14] Brännström believes that most restorative materials do not adhere to the dentinal wall.[14] Consequently, contraction gaps form between such materials and the adjacent tooth structure, and these gaps are invaded by bacteria either from the smear layer or from the oral cavity. As a result, bacterial metabolites diffuse through the dentinal tubules and injure the pulp.

Remaining Dentin Thickness

As discussed in Chapter 10, dentin permeability increases almost logarithmically with increasing cavity depth due to the difference in size and number of dentinal tubules. In short, permeability of the dentin is of great importance in determining the degree of pulpal injury resulting from restorative procedures and materials. Stanley[94] found that the distance between the floor of the cavity preparation and the pulp (i.e., the remaining dentin thickness) greatly influences the pulpal response to restorative procedures and materials. He suggested that a remaining dentin thickness of 2 mm would protect the pulp from the effects of most restorative procedures, provided that all other operative precautions are observed.

Agents for Cavity Cleansing, Drying, Sterilization, and Acid Etching

Cleansing agents are used to reduce microorganisms on the cut surface of dentin and to remove the smear layer that remains on the dentin after cavity preparation. It is believed that if this superficial smear layer were removed, a liner or cement would adapt better to the cut surface of dentin. Cleansing agents contain either an acid or a chelating agent such as ethylenediamine-tetraacetic acid (EDTA). In one study it was found that the incidence of pulpal inflammation increased significantly when cavities were treated with an acid cleansing agent (50% citric acid) before being filled as compared with controls where the cleanser was omitted.[23] Another study[95] reported that Epoxylite Cavity Cleaner intensified and prolonged the severity of pulpal reactions when used in conjunction with a composite resin filling material. It has also been demonstrated that by removing the smear layer and enlarging the orifices of the dentinal tubules, acid cleansing agents greatly increase the permeability of dentin, thus enhancing penetration of the dentin by irritating substances.[80] It follows that if bacteria grow beneath a restoration, the toxins they produce will more readily diffuse through dentin that has been cleansed with acid. Another product, Cavilax, was developed to eliminate residual eugenol after removal of temporary fillings. The ingredients are 50% methylethyl ketone and 50% ethyl acetone. Investigators[25] found that use of this cleanser resulted in only a very mild pulpal response and some odontoblast displacement.

Drying agents

Cavity drying agents generally contain organic solvents such as ether and acetone. Solvent-containing drying agents should not be used in very deep cavities, since these agents are capable of damaging odontoblast processes and cells of the pulp. Apparently when used in shallow to moderately deep cavities they produce no significant pulpal inflammation, but because of their desiccating effect, they are apt to cause odontoblast displacement.

Cavity sterilization

At one time cavity-sterilizing agents such a phenol, silver nitrate, and their germicidal agents were used routinely. However, it became obvious that agents capable of efficiently destroying bacteria are also highly irritating to pulp tissue, and today such caustic agents are seldom used. Recently, disinfectants such as benzalkonium chloride, chlorhexidine, and 9-aminoacridine have been employed to reduce the risk of bacterial contamination beneath restorations. One researcher[15] advocates the use of a cavity cleanser that contains a low concentration of EDTA (0.2%) to remove the superficial smear layer and benzalkonium chloride to disinfect the walls of the cavity.

Acid etching

Although acid etching of cavity walls is cleansing, acid etching is specifically designed to enhance the adhesion of restorative materials. In the case of dentin, however, the ability of acid etching to improve long-term adhesion has been questioned.[40] Acid cleansers applied to dentin have been shown to widen the openings of the dentinal tubules, increase dentin permeability, and enhance bacterial penetration of the dentin.[108] One study showed that in deep cavities, pretreatment of the dentin with 50% citric or 50% phosphoric acid for 60 seconds is capable of significantly increasing the response of the pulp to restorative materials.[95] Results of a recent physiologic investigation have shown that acid etching a small class V cavity having a remaining dentin thickness of 1.5 mm has little effect on pulpal blood flow.[92] Thus direct effect of the acid on the pulpal microvascular vessels appears to be negligible, possibly due to a rapid buffering of the acid by the dentinal fluid. However, it is possible that in very deep cavities acid etching may contribute to pulpal injury.

TAKING OF IMPRESSIONS

Heated modeling compound has been reported to produce significant injury to the pulp when applied to cavity or full crown preparations. Presumably this is due to the combination of heat and pressure exerted on the pulp.[87] Investigators demonstrated intrapulpal temperatures of up to 52° C during impression taking with modeling compound in copper bands.[35] Other investigators[113] have shown that an intrapulpal temperature increase of this magnitude may result in severe pulpal injury. Another[58] also observed vascular and odontoblastic changes. Crown preparation and impression taking with modeling compound caused an arteriolar dilation and formation of an irregular odontoblastic layer. A drastic increase in pulpal blood flow was seen immediately after heated modeling compound was placed on crown preparations in canine teeth in dogs.[52] Pulpal blood flow then decreased significantly when acrylic temporary material contacted the prepared tooth sur-

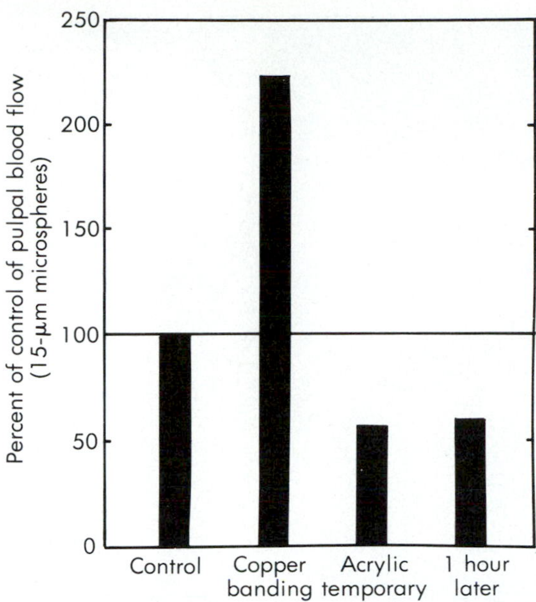

FIG. 15-15 Effects of impression taking using modeling compound with copper banding on pulpal blood flow in dogs.

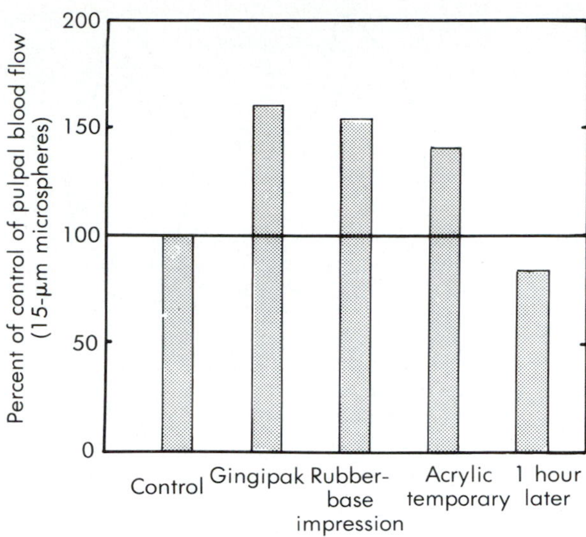

FIG. 15-16 Effects of impression taking using rubber-based material on pulpal blood flow in dogs.

face (Fig. 15-15). The use of modeling compound with a copper band poses two hazards to the pulp: heat generation and hydraulic force, since the copper band tightly fits the prepared tooth. Thus Lindholm's observation on the irregular odontoblastic layer and our observation on the changes in pulpal blood flow suggest that this impression technique may damage the pulp.

In contrast, histologists have found that *rubber-based and hydrocolloid impression materials are well tolerated by the pulp*.[56] Recent physiologic evidence supports this finding. Pulpal blood flow changed insignificantly when an impression was taken with a rubber-based material (Fig. 15-16).

INSERTION OR CEMENTATION OF RESTORATIONS

Strong hydraulic forces may be exerted on the pulp during cementation of crowns and inlays, as the cement is driven toward the pulp, thus compressing the fluid in the dentinal tubules. In extreme cases this may actually cause a separation of the odontoblast layer from the dentin. This will not occur if the exposed dentin is first covered by a liner or base. In addition to hydraulic forces, chemical effects of cementing materials seem to occur. There is experimental evidence that cementation of a crown with zinc phosphate cement causes inflammatory reactions in the pulp. In view of other reports[81] that chemical ions of the luting agent have no effect on the pulp, there is obviously a need for additional research in this area.

RESTORATIVE MATERIALS

How do restorative materials evoke a response in the underlying pulp? For many years it was believed that toxic ingredients in the materials were responsible for pulpal injury. However, pulpal injury associated with the use of these materials could not be correlated with their cytotoxic properties. Thus irritating materials such as zinc oxide–eugenol (ZOE) produced a very mild pulpal response when placed in cavities, whereas less toxic materials such as composite resins and amalgam produced a much stronger pulp response. Besides chemical toxicity, some of the properties of materials that might be capable of producing injury include:

1. Acidity (hydrogen ion concentration)
2. Absorption of water during setting
3. Heat evolved during setting
4. Poor marginal adaptation resulting in bacterial contamination

Investigators[81] found that the pulpal response beneath a material is not associated with the material's hydrogen ion concentration. The acid percent in restorative materials is probably neutralized by the dentin and dentinal fluid.[18] As the superficial dentin is demineralized, phosphate ions are liberated, thus producing a buffering effect. However, placement of an acidic material such as zinc phosphate at luting consistency in a deep cavity may have a toxic effect on the pulp since the diffusion barrier is extremely thin. In a study conducted in our laboratory, zinc phosphate cement of luting consistency placed on a deep (0.5 mm remaining dentin layer) and large class V cavity on canine tooth caused a moderate decrease in pulpal blood flow as measured with the 15 μm microsphere method. After the cement had hardened for about 30 minutes blood flow had again increased, suggesting that the cement had a temporary and transitory effect on the pulpal circulation (Fig. 15-17). The changes in pulpal blood flow may have been due to chemical and/or exothermal effects of the cement. One study found that of all materials studied, zinc phosphate cement was associated with the greatest temperature rise—an increase of 2.14° C.[81] This amount of temperature increase, however, is not sufficient to produce tissue injury.[112] In a microcirculatory study using hamster cheek pouch, a drop of zinc phosphate liquid caused stasis, followed by hemolysis, resulting in total cessation of blood flow in the vessels that were in contact with the liquid. Thus there seems to be a real possibility of pulpal dam-

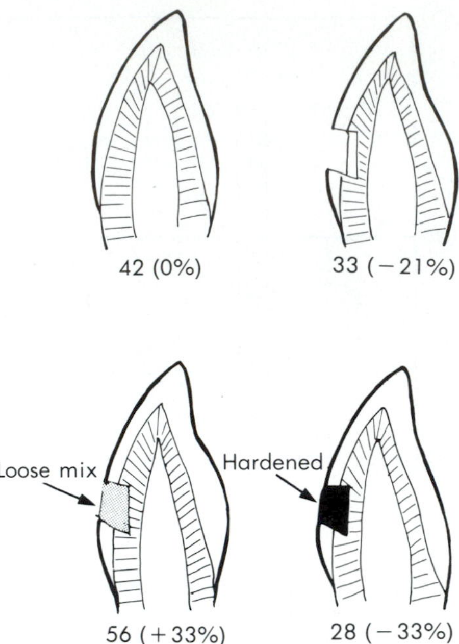

FIG. 15-17 Effects of zinc phosphate cement on pulpal blood flow (ml/min/100 g). A cement of luting consistency was placed in a deep and large class V in the canine teeth of dogs and pulpal blood flow was measured. A 33% increase was observed initially, but the hardened cement caused a decrease in pulpal blood flow.

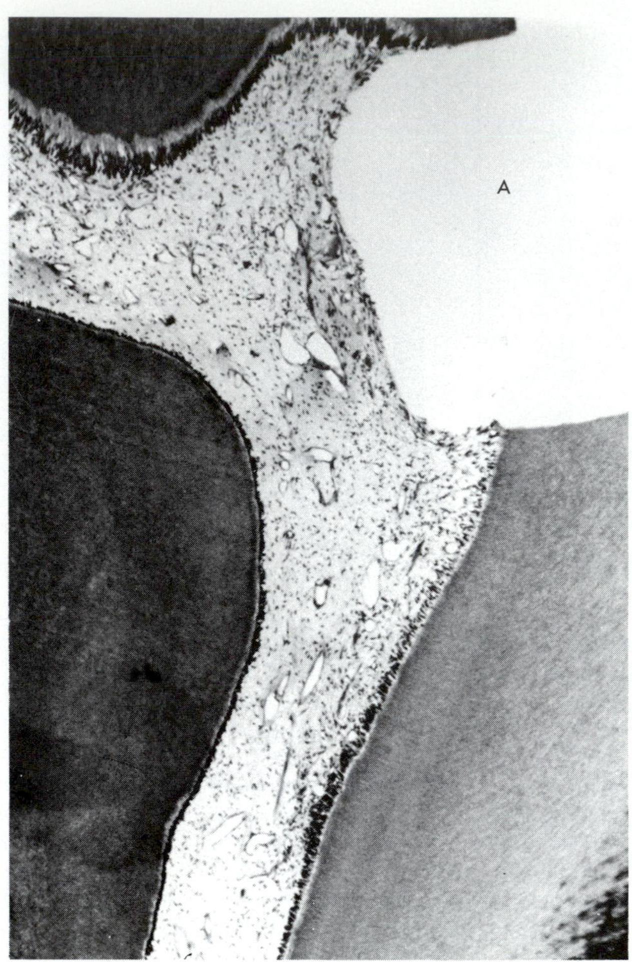

FIG. 15-18 Appearance of pulp 7 days following placement of amalgam restoration *(A)* directly against pulp tissue. Note absence of inflammatory response. (From Cox CF, et al: J Prosthet Dent 57:1, 1987.)

age if the pulp is in close contact with the liquid portion of the cement. Absorption of water during the setting of a material can also be ruled out as a cause of pulpal injury. Compared with the removal of fluid from dentin by an airstream during cavity preparation (which produces no inflammatory response in the pulp), absorption of water by a material is insignificant. Researchers[81] found no relationship between the hydrophilic properties of materials and their effect on the pulp.

This brings us to bacterial contamination. It has long been recognized that, in general, dental materials do not adapt to tooth structure well enough to provide a hermetic seal. Thus it has been acknowledged that bacteria may penetrate the gap between the restored material and the cavity wall. Presumably, bacteria growing beneath restorations create toxic products that can diffuse through the dentinal tubules and evoke an inflammatory reaction in the underlying pulp. Converging evidence suggests that *products of bacterial metabolism are the major cause of pulpal injury resulting from the insertion of restorations*. Let us briefly review some of that evidence. One investigator showed that material such as composite resins, zinc phosphate, and silicate cements produced only a localized tissue reaction when placed directly on exposed pulps in germ-free animals.[109] The same procedure in conventional animals resulted in total pulp necrosis. Employing bacterial staining methods, researchers[18] demonstrated that the growth of bacteria under restorations was correlated with the degree of inflammation of the adjacent pulp tissue. They also found that bacteria did not grow when the outer portions of restorations were replaced with ZOE, thus producing a surface seal (Fig. 15-18). When bacterial growth was thus inhibited, pulpal inflammation was negligible. Similar studies[8] showed that colonies of bacteria become established under restorative materials that do not provide an adequate marginal seal. Of the materials they tested—Dispersalloy amalgam (Johnson & Johnson Products Co., East Windsor, N.J.), Concise composite resin (3M Co., St. Paul, Minn), Hygienic gutta-percha (The Hygienic Corp., Akron, Oh), MQ silicate cements (White Dental Products, Philadelphia, Pa), and ZOE—only ZOE consistently prevented bacteria from becoming established beneath the restoration. Using ZOE as a surface seal, Cox and associates[24] found that materials such as amalgam, composites, silicate cement, zinc phosphate cement, and ZOE produced only a thin zone of contact necrosis and no inflammation when placed directly on primate pulps (Fig. 15-19).

In vitro and in vivo studies on marginal adaptation of restorative materials have often yielded conflicting results. Obviously it is difficult to duplicate clinical conditions in the laboratory. Two important factors affecting marginal adaptation are temperature changes and masticatory forces. Nelson and associates[65] were the first to study the opening and closing of the margin of restorations that were subjected to temperature changes. If a material has a different coefficient of thermal expansion than tooth structure, temperature change is likely to produce gaps between the material and the cavity wall. An-

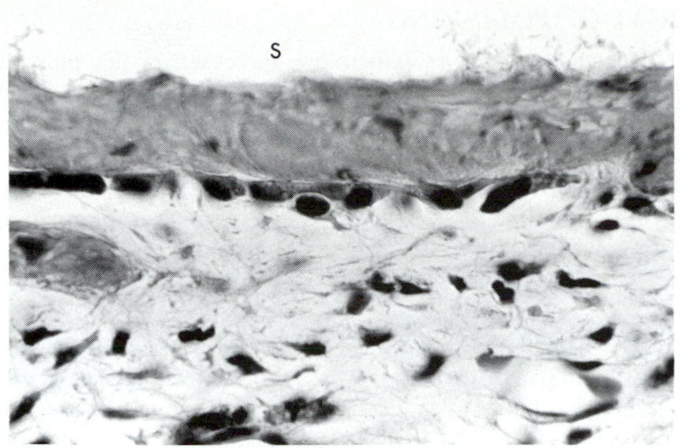

FIG. 15-19 Pulpal response 21 days following placement of silicate cement *(S)* directly against the pulp. Silicate was surface-sealed with zinc oxide–eugenol. Note formation of hard tissue and new odontoblasts. (From Cox CF, et al: J Prosthet Dent 57:1, 1987.)

other investigator[83] demonstrated a marked effect of functional mastication on marginal adaptation of composite restorations. He found gap formation along 71% of the restorations in teeth that were in functional occlusion, whereas leakage occurred in only 28% of teeth with no antagonist.

As yet no permanent filling material has been shown to consistently provide a perfect marginal seal, so leakage and bacterial contamination are always a threat to the integrity of the pulp. Consequently, an adequate cavity liner or cement base should be employed to seal the dentinal tubules before inserting restorative materials. Despite these findings, it must be acknowledged that pulps frequently remain healthy under restorations that leak. Factors that determine whether bacterial growth beneath a restoration will injure the pulp probably include pathogenicity of the microorganisms, permeability of the underlying dentin (i.e., degree of sclerosis, number of tubules, thickness of dentin), and the ability of the irritated pulp to produce reparative dentin.

Since there is convincing evidence that bacterial growth beneath restorations is the primary cause of pulpal injury, the antibacterial properties of filling materials may be of considerable importance. Not all materials have been studied, but there is evidence that ZOE, calcium hydroxide, and polycarboxylate cement have some ability to inhibit bacterial growth. Zinc phosphate cement, the restorative resins, and silicate cements lack antibacterial ingredients, and it is these materials that are most often associated with injury to the pulp.

Zinc Oxide–Eugenol

ZOE is used for a variety of purposes in dentistry. In addition to being a popular temporary filling material, it is used for provisional and permanent cementation of inlays, crowns, and bridges, as a pulp-capping agent, and as a cement base. Eugenol, a phenol derivative, is known to be toxic, and it is capable of producing thrombosis of blood vessels when applied directly to pulp tissue.[82] It also has anesthetic properties and is used as an anodyne in relieving the symptoms of painful pulpitis. This presumably results from its ability to block the transmission of action potentials in nerve fibers.[104] Experimentally, ZOE has been shown to suppress nerve excitability in the pulp when applied to the base of a deep cavity.[103] This effect is obtained only when a fairly thin mix of ZOE (e.g., powder-liquid ratio 2:1 w/w) is used. Presumably it is the free eugenol in the cement that is responsible for the anesthetic effect. ZOE has two important properties that explain why it is such an effective base material: (1) it adapts very closely to dentin, thus providing a good marginal seal, and (2) its antibacterial properties inhibit bacterial growth on cavity walls. However, because eugenol injures cells, some authorities question whether ZOE should be used in very deep cavity preparations where there is a risk of pulp exposure.

Zinc Phosphate Cement

One study[41] found that when a liner was omitted, severe pulpal reactions (principally abscess formation) occurred in all teeth in which deep class V cavities were restored with zinc phosphate cement. The pulpal response was attributed to the phosphoric acid contained in the cement. In retrospect, however, it is likely that irritation to the pulp was due primarily to marginal leakage rather than to acidity.[17] Because of its high modulus of elasticity, zinc phosphate is the cement base of choice for amalgam restorations. This results from the fact that it is better able to resist the stresses of mastication than other cements.[27]

Zinc Polycarboxylate Cements

Polycarboxylate cement is well tolerated by the pulp, being roughly equivalent to ZOE cements in this respect.[41] This may be due to its ability to adapt well to dentin. Also, it has been reported that this cement has bacteriocidal qualities.[5]

Restorative Resins

The original unfilled resins were associated with severe marginal leakage, caused by dimensional changes that resulted from a high coefficient of thermal expansion. This in turn resulted in marked pulpal injury. The development of sulfinic acid catalyst systems and the nonpressure insertion techniques have improved the performance of resins considerably. The epoxide resins with a benzoyl peroxide catalyst that are 75% filled with glass or quartz (the so-called composite resins) represent another group of resins. These have much more favorable polymerization characteristics and a lower coefficient of thermal expansion than the original unfilled resins. The marginal seal has been further improved by acid etching of beveled enamel and the use of a bonding agent or primer. This reduces the risk of microbial invasion but does not eliminate bacteria that may be present on cavity walls. However, it has been shown that the initial marginal seal tends to deteriorate as the etched composite restoration ages.[45] Furthermore, one study showed that functional mastication is capable of producing gaps that result in increased leakage.[83] Many investigators[18,90] have shown that unlined composite resins are harmful to the pulp, primarily because of bacterial contamination beneath the restoration. Thus the use of a cavity liner is strongly recommended. Since copal varnish is not compatible with the restorative resins, the use of a polystyrene liner has been advocated.[19] Bases containing calcium hydroxide have also been shown to provide good protection against bacteria.

Glass-Ionomer Cement Restorations

Studies on glass-ionomer cements indicate that they are well tolerated by the pulp.[49,67] However, researchers[3] have shown that leakage may occur around ionomer cement fillings, so this material should be used in conjunction with a liner or base. There have been reports of postcementation tooth sensitivity following the use of glass-ionomer cements to cement gold castings, but the cause of this sensitivity has not been determined. It appears that sensitivity is not the result of marginal leakage, because the results of an in vitro leakage study demonstrated that glass-ionomer luting cements provide a good marginal seal.[36]

Dental Amalgam

Dental amalgam, first used for the restoration of carious teeth in the sixteenth century, is still the most popular restorative material in dentistry. Unvarnished amalgam restorations leak severely when they are first inserted, but within a period of 12 weeks a marginal seal develops that resists dye penetration beyond the dentinoenamel junction.[42] Investigators[38] found that pulp responses to unlined amalgams—Sybraloy (Kerr Mfg. Co., Romulus, Mich.), Dispersalloy (Johnson & Johnson, East Windsor, N.J.), Tytin (S.S. White Dental Products, Philadelphia, Pa.) and Spheraloy (Kerr Mfg. Co., Romulus, Mich.) consisted of slight to moderate inflammation. The inflammation tended to diminish with time, and within a few weeks reparative dentin was deposited. Other investigators[82] theorized that the high mercury content of amalgam may exert a cytotoxic effect on the pulp, as they found that mercury penetrates into the dentin and pulp beneath an amalgam restoration. They have also reported that rubbing the bottom of the cavity with a calcium hydroxide/water mixture protects the pulp from the irritating effects of amalgam. Bacteria were found beneath unlined amalgams, while the pulps of teeth in which a ZOE liner was used exhibited a milder response and no bacteria was present. In vitro bacterial tests indicated that amalgam has no inhibitory effect on bacterial growth.

It is well known that insertion of amalgam restorations may result in postoperative thermal sensitivity, even when amalgam is placed in a shallow cavity. Brännström[13] is of the opinion that such sensitivity results from expansion or contraction of fluid that occupies the gap between the amalgam and the cavity wall. This fluid is in communication with fluid in the subjacent dentinal tubules, so variations in temperature would cause axial movement of fluid in the tubules. According to the hydrodynamic theory of dentin sensitivity, this fluid movement would stimulate nerve fibers in the underlying pulp, thus evoking pain.[103] The use of a cavity varnish or base is recommended in order to seal the dentinal tubules and prevent this form of postoperative discomfort.

Cavity Varnish

The effectiveness of cavity varnish in providing protection for the pulp is highly controversial. One study[30] has called attention to the fact that in vivo surfaces are wet and therefore the application of liners or varnishes may not result in an impervious coating. Even the application of two or three coats of varnish may not prevent gaps from occurring in the lining. Furthermore, other investigators[19] have reported that a double layer of Copalite did not prevent bacterial leakage and growth of bacteria on the cavity walls. Nonetheless, several reports indicate that varnish can act as a barrier to the toxic effects of restorations.[26,32,91,111] One study[66] assessed the ability of several commercial varnishes to decrease microleakage beneath a high-copper spherical alloy restorative material and found Copalite to be the most effective.

HEAT OF POLISHING

One study reported temperature increases in the pulp of more than 20° C when amalgam restorations were polished continuously with prophylactic cups.[34] This is sufficient to cause severe pulpal injury. They found that polishing appliances made of rubber created higher temperatures than cup brushes. Continuous polishing using high speeds of rotation was associated with greater heat than intermittent polishing using low speeds.

POSTOPERATIVE SENSITIVITY

Postoperative discomfort, though usually transient, indicates that the restorative procedure has inflicted trauma on the tooth or the supporting structures. Severe persistent pain almost certainly signifies that pulpal inflammation has resulted in hyperalgesia. Researchers[89] examined 40 patients who had received dental treatment involving insertion of amalgam and composite restorations. They found that 78% of the patients experienced some degree of postoperative discomfort. Sensitivity to cold was the most frequent complaint, whereas sensitivity to heat occurred much less often. Another study[44] found that there was a positive correlation between heat sensitivity and pulpal inflammation. The significance of sensitivity to cold has not been fully established. Since the response occurs very soon after stimuli such as ice, cold water, and cold air come into contact with the tooth, it is believed that pain is caused by the stimulation of sensory nerve fibers of the pulp by hydrodynamic forces.[105] Because these fibers have a relatively low excitability threshold, they will respond to low-level stimuli that do not necessarily produce tissue injury. However, the presence of hyperalgesia associated with inflammation produces an exaggerated response to cold. Sensitivity that develops soon after a restoration is placed may also be due to poor marginal adaptation, resulting in leakage of saliva under the filling.

Mechanisms and Management of Hypersensitive Teeth

Tooth sensitivity to various stimuli is a persisting problem that affects as many as one of seven adult dental patients.[33] Although the clinical features of tooth hypersensitivity are well described, the exact causes and their physiologic mechanisms are only beginning to be understood.

Mechanisms

The enamel and cementum covering the dentin, and thus the dentinal nerves, are protective layers. When these protective layers are removed and the dentin tubules are exposed by various means (e.g., scaling, caries, fracture, restorative procedures), often the teeth become hypersensitive. Dentin sensitivity is the result of activation of Aδ type nerve fibers located in the dentinal tubules. Hypersensitivity is characterized as sharp, transient, and well-localized, and two mechanisms account for the pain, stimulation of the dentinal *nerves* and dynamics of *exposed dentin*. These two mechanisms are interrelated.

According to the hydrodynamic theory, dentin sensitivity should be proportional to the hydraulic conductance of dentin. According to Pashley,[77] the most important variable related to hydraulic conductance in dentin is the condition of the tubule aperture. Anything or any agent that makes the dentin hypoconducting by blocking the aperture will alleviate the hypersensitive teeth syndrome.

Another mechanism involves the intradental nerves. Although the nerves themselves are unaffected, the environment surrounding them might be changed so that the normal stimuli, which under normal conditions do not evoke sensation, now evoke the sensation. The causes in the environment may be due to changes in ionic concentration (e.g., excessive sodium or potassium around the nerve terminals in the tubules as the result of pulpal inflammation or exposed dentin).

Hypersensitive teeth and inflamed pulps in many ways present the same symptoms, such as sensitivity to cold, air, and heat. Hypersensitivity due to inflammation of the pulp is the result of excitation of C fibers, which release neuropeptides (e.g., CGRP and substance P) in the pulp. These neuropeptides play a key role in neurogenic inflammation by increasing blood flow and capillary permeability. In the dental pulp, in its low-compliance environment, the increase in flow and permeability causes a dramatic increase in tissue pressure, which can lower the excitatory threshold level of the intradental nerves, resulting in hypersensitivity.

Agents that block exposed dentinal tubules

As previously discussed, one of the two possible causes of hypersensitive teeth is exposed dentin. To block the exposed tubules would be a simple solution, but finding agents or instruments to do just that has turned out to be not that simple. After many years of experimentation we still do not have an agent or agents that completely block the tubules. Nevertheless, there has been substantial progress in discovering an agent that blocks dentinal tubules sufficiently to reduce hypersensitivity. Pashley and coworkers,[77] using dentin permeability techniques and scanning electron microscopic examination of the dentin surface, discovered that oxalate salts are effective agents to block dentinal tubules. Figure 15-20 shows a dentin surface that was treated with oxalate salts for 2 minutes. When applied to the exposed dentin, potassium oxalate solution forms a microcrystal consisting of calcium oxalate. The calcium oxalate crystals are small enough to block the tubules, and thus reduce hydraulic conductance. According to Pashley[77] the oxalate salts reduced dentin permeability by over 95%. Results of the clinical studies also agree with experimental results.

Agents that reduce intradental nerve excitability

The electrophysiologic method has been used to assess the function of the sensory nerves in response to various potentially useful chemical agents.[54] Sodium, lithium, and aluminum compounds have insignificant effects on reducing sensory nerve activity. Potassium compounds, however, were most effective ingredients for sensory nerve activity reduction. Important potassium compounds were potassium oxalate, -nitrate, and -bicarbonate. This finding lends credence to the hypothesis that reduction in sensory nerve activity is caused by the increase in potassium concentration around the nerve terminals in the dentin tubules.

Figure 15-21 provides the summary diagram illustrating the mechanisms and solutions to these problems. The far left-hand slice represents the sensitive dentin with open tubules. The second slice represents a smear layer covering the exposed dentin surface and occluding the dentinal tubules. However, this smear layer is extremely acid fabrile and is easily removed and therefore can not be considered an effective way of managing the problem. The third slice represents other ways of occluding the dentin tubules. CaOxalate is the crystalized product of the chemical reaction between potassium oxalate and dentinal calcium, and is very effective in occluding the tubules. CaF_2 and Ag-nitrate are other agents that showed reasonable effectiveness. Tubular occlusion can also occur from the pulp side, mainly by plasma protein, especially fibrinogen, which is released from blood vessels.[78] The right-hand slice represents desensitization by altering nerve excitability by potassium, and possibly by eugenol.

CURRENT THINKING ON THE CAUSE OF PULPAL REACTION TO RESTORATION

In the past, pulp reactions to dental procedures were thought to be due to mechanical insults, such as frictional heat, and generally this is true. The reaction to dental materials, on the other hand, has been attributed to chemical effects, such as acidity of the restorative materials. Although the chemical effects cannot be entirely discounted, especially in a deep cavity where only a very thin layer of dentin remains, in current thinking *pulpal injury is primarily due to microleakage*

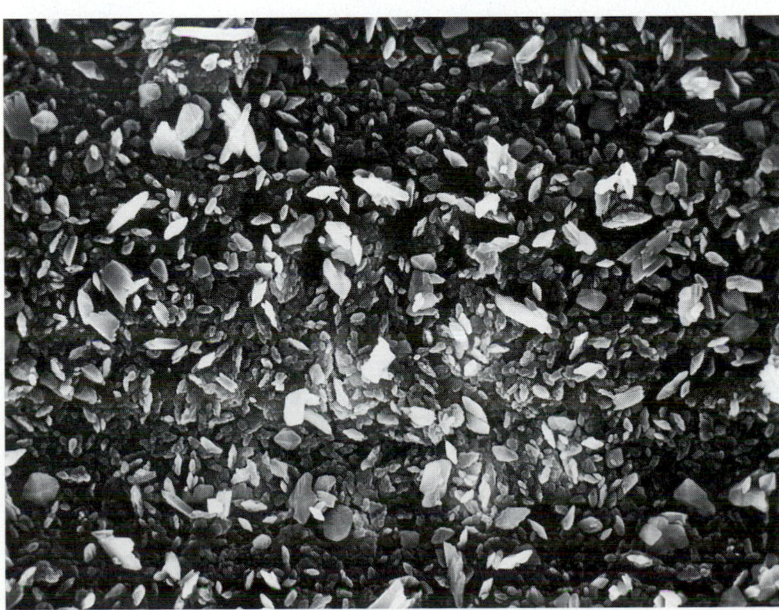

FIG. 15-20 Smear layer treated with 30% dipotassium oxalate for 2 minutes plus 3% monopotassium–monohydrogen oxalate for 2 minutes. The dentin surface is completely covered with calcium oxalate crystals. (Original magnification, × 1900.) (From Pashley DH, and Galloway SE: Arch Oral Biol 30:731, 1985.)

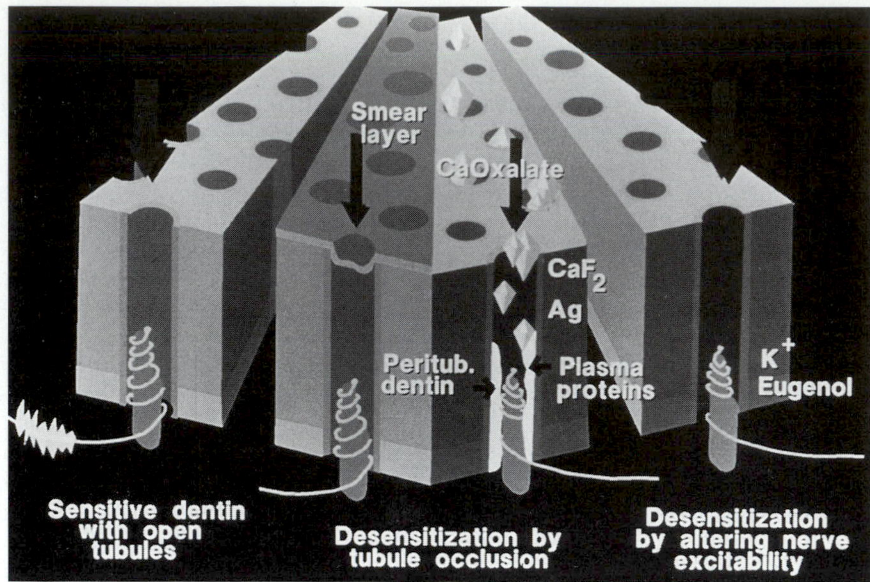

FIG. 15-21 Summary diagram illustrates the mechanisms and solutions to hypersensitivity problems. (Courtesy Dr. D.H. Pashley.)

TABLE 15-1. Surface area of dentin available for diffusion at various distances from the pulp

Distance from pulp	Number of tubules (million/cm^2)		Tubular radius (cm × 10^4)		Area of surface (Ap) (%)*	
(mm)	Mean	Range	Mean	Range	Mean	Range
	4.5	3.0–5.2	1.25	2.0–3.2	22.1	9–42
0.1–0.5	4.3	2.2–5.9	0.95	1.0–2.3	12.2	2–25
0.6–1.0	3.8	1.6–4.7	0.80	1.0–1.6	7.6	1–9.0
1.1–1.5	3.5	2.1–4.7	0.60	0.9–1.5	4.0	1–8.0
1.6–2.0	3.0	1.2–4.7	0.55	0.8–1.6	2.9	1–9.0
2.1–2.5	2.3	1.1–3.6	0.45	0.6–1.3	1.5	0.3–6
2.6–3.0	2.0	0.7–4.0	0.40	0.5–1.4	1.1	0.1–6
3.1–3.5	1.9	1.0–2.5	0.40	0.5–1.2	1.0	0.2–3

Modified from Garberoglio and Brännström (1976); from Pashley DH: Operative Dent (suppl) 3:13, 1984.
*$Ap = nr^2$, where n is the number of tubules/cm^2; Ap represents the percentage of the total area of the physical surface available for diffusion.

through gaps between the filling material and the walls of the cavity. It is believed that bacteria growing in these gaps elaborate products that diffuse through the dentinal tubules and irritate the pulp. It must be recognized that all permanent filling materials may allow these gaps to form! It is a miracle that all restored teeth do not show some degree of pulpal inflammation. On the other hand, it is not surprising that many teeth that have been restored require endodontic therapy. One study[8] reported that the quantity of bacterial toxins filtered from the base of a class V cavity depends on the type of restorative material used. The greatest amount of leakage occurred with silicate cements, followed by composite resins and amalgam fillings. Little or no leakage occurred when ZOE was used. Even full crown restorations have been found to leak.

It is impossible to examine pulpal reactions without understanding structural and functional properties of the dentin. Pulp reactions begin when irritants make contact with the surface of the dentin. As the dentin's thickness decreases, the danger of pulpal reaction increases dramatically. A simple physiologic law of diffusion states that the rate of diffusion of substances depends on two factors: (1) the concentration gradient of the substances and (2) the surface area available for diffusion. Of importance in determining the extent of pulp reactions is the surface area of dentin available for diffusion. Because the dentinal tubules vary in diameter and density across the thickness of the dentin, the surface area (i.e., product of tubular area and density) available for diffusion varies from one region of the dentin to the other. Table 15-1 demonstrates the available dentinal surface for diffusion at various distance from the pulp. For example, the diffusible surface area is 1% of the total dentin surface area at the dentinoenamel junction, whereas it is 22% at the pulp. Thus the harmful effects of an insult increase significantly as the thickness of dentin over the pulp decreases.

The natural defense mechanisms of the tooth should be recognized. In some situations the dentinal tubules may become blocked by hydroxyapatite and other crystals, a condition known as dentin sclerosis. Another reaction resulting in a de-

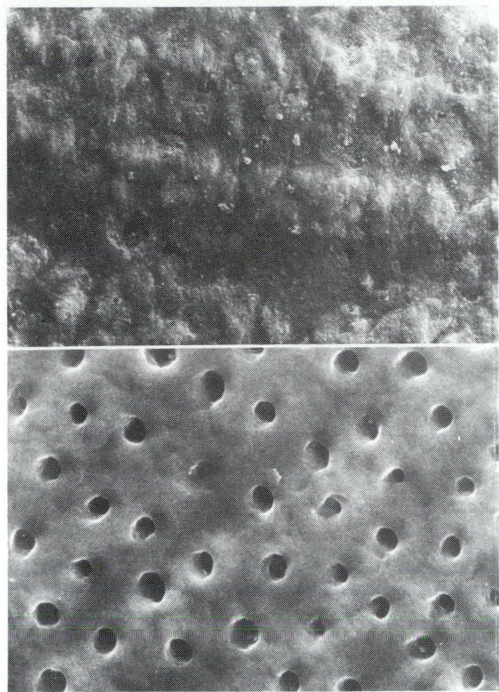

FIG. 15-22 SEM photomicrographs of smear layer intact and smear layer removed. Notice the patent dentinal tubules. (Courtesy Dr. D.H. Pashley.)

crease in dentin permeability is reparative dentin formation.

The smear layer also influences the permeability of dentin and thus protects the pulp by hindering the diffusion of toxic substances through the tubules. According to one investigation, the smear layer accounts for 86% of the total resistance to flow fluid.[74] Thus acid etching, which removes the smear layer, greatly increases permeability by increasing the diffusable surface area (Fig. 15-22). The question arises of what to do with the smear layer. Should it be removed or left alone? Some authorities are of the opinion that it should be removed, since the smear layer may harbor bacteria. Yet the presence of a smear layer constitutes a physical barrier to bacterial penetration of the dentinal tubules.[61,108] However, another investigator demonstrated that the presence of the smear layer cannot prevent diffusion of bacterial products, although it effectively blocks actual bacterial invasion.[6] It has been shown that bacterial products reaching the pulp are capable of evoking an inflammatory response.[7] It follows that the best way to solve the problem is to remove the smear layer and replace it with a "sterile, nontoxic" artificial smear layer. Research in the field has yielded some agents that look promising, two of which are potassium oxalate[37] and 5% ferric oxalate.[10]

Since at the present time there is no material that can bond chemically to dentin and thus prevent leakage, the use of a cavity liner to seal dentin is highly recommended. According to one investigator, there are three possible routes for microleakage: (1) within or via the smear layer, (2) between the smear layer and the cavity varnish or cement, and (3) between the cavity varnish or cement and the restorative material (Fig. 15-23).[76]

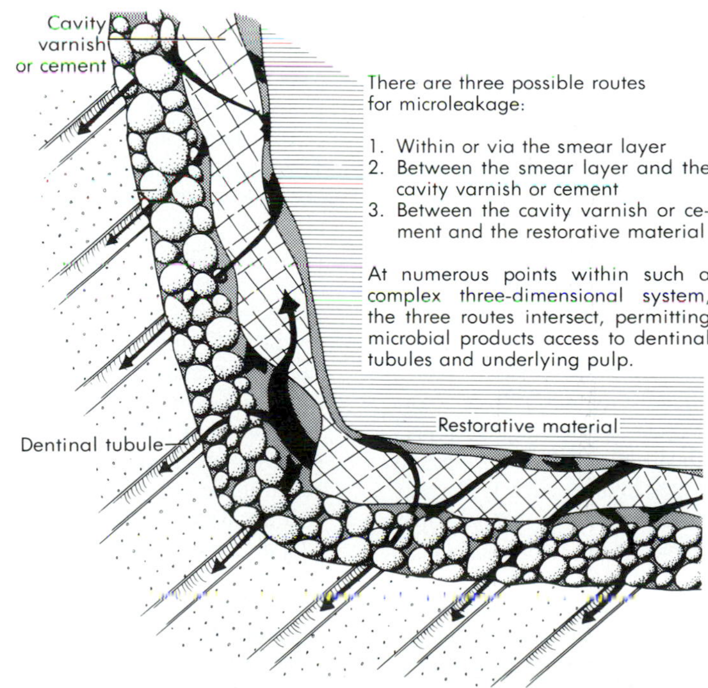

FIG. 15-23 Schematic representation of the interface of dentin and restorative material in a typical cavity. The granular constituents of the smear layer have been exaggerated out of their normal proportion for emphasis. Three theoretical routes for microleakage are indicated by arrows. (Reprinted with permission from Pashley DH, et al: Arch Oral Biol 23:391, 1978. Copyright 1978, Pergamon Press, Ltd.)

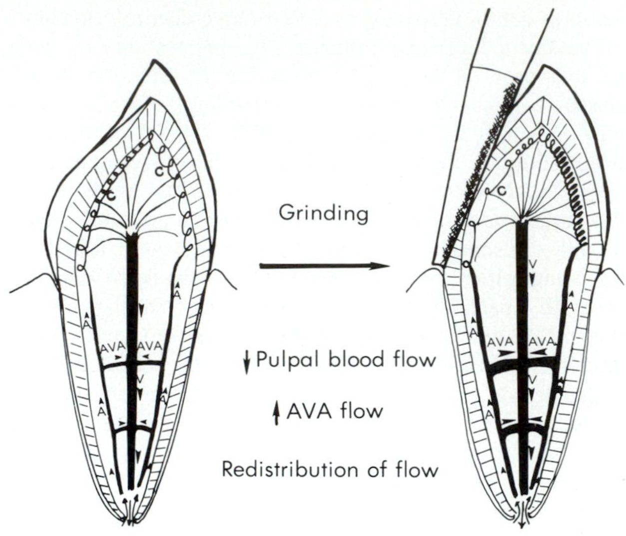

FIG. 15-24 Schematic representation of the changes in pulpal blood flow distribution in response to dry preparation. Notice that there is an increase in flow through the AVAs.

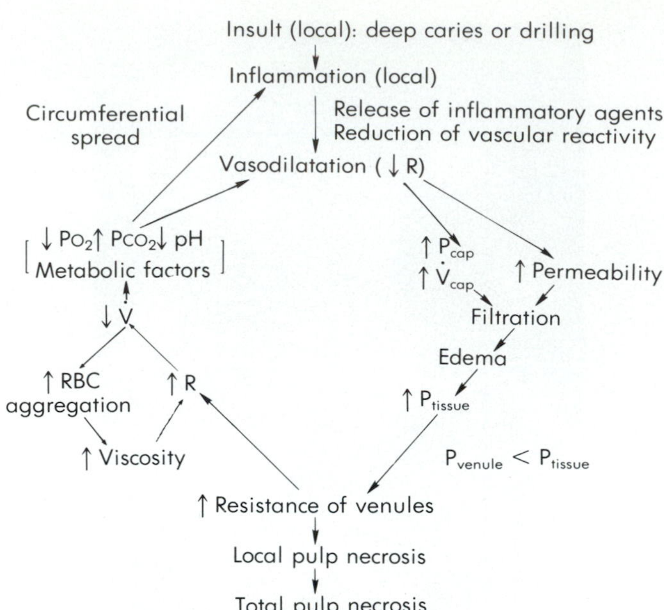

FIG. 15-25 Pathophysiologic mechanism of pulp inflammation and necrosis. This hypothetical mechanism is constructed from the results of many structural and functional investigations.

Compensatory Pulpal Reaction to Outside Insults

Mechanisms exist by which the pulp is able to ward off insults. The ability of the pulp to deposit reparative dentin beneath a restoration is an excellent example. In addition, the vascular system is able to respond to mechanical insults. For example, it has been shown that deep drilling without proper water coolant causes a profound decrease in pulpal blood flow in the area of injury. Blood is shunted away from the area by an abrupt increase in the flow of blood through arteriovenous anastomoses (AVAs) or U-turn loops located in the root canal (Fig. 15-24). It is possible that opening of the previously closed AVAs occurs as pulpal tissue pressure increases to critical levels. The opening of the AVAs is a compensatory mechanism of the pulp to maintain blood flow within physiologically normal limits (Fig. 15-24).

It should be remembered that the pulp is a very resilient tissue and that is has a great potential for healing. It is only when all compensatory mechanisms fail that the pulp becomes necrotic. Figure 15-25 depicts the current thinking on the pathophysiologic mechanisms involved in pulp necrosis. Since the pulp is rigidly encased in mineralized tissues, it is protected from most forms of trauma to which the tooth is exposed. Nevertheless, insults such as dental caries and restorative procedures are capable of producing localized inflammatory lesions in the pulp. The tissue adjacent to the inflammatory lesion may show no sign of inflammation and physiologic analysis may reveal no abnormalities. Thus investigators found that pulpal tissue pressure near a site of localized inflammation was almost normal.[100] This indicates that tissue pressure changes do not spread rapidly. Similar findings have been reported by another researcher.[107] Local insults cause inflammation by triggering the release of various inflammatory mediators and reducing vascular reactivity. These mediators produce vasodilation and decrease the flow resistance in the resistance vessels. Vasodilation and decreased flow resistance cause an increase in both intravascular pressure and blood flow in the capillaries, which in turn precipitate an increase in vascular permeability, favoring filtration of serum proteins and fluid from the vessels. As a result, the tissue becomes edematous. This results in an increase in the tissue pressure. Since the pulp is encased in mineralized tissue, it is in a low compliance environment. As the tissue pressure increases it may exceed that of the venules, in which case the venules will be compressed, thus producing an increase in flow resistance. This in turn results in a decrease in blood flow since the venous drainage is impeded. The sluggish flow of blood flow causes the red blood cells to aggregate, resulting in an elevation of blood viscosity. This vicious cycle leads to even greater problems by producing hypoxia and thus suppressing cellular metabolism in the affected area of the pulp. The stagnation of blood flow not only causes rheologic changes (i.e., RBC aggregation and increased blood viscosity), it also causes an increase in carbon dioxide and a decrease in pH levels in the blood. The increase in P_{CO_2} results from impaired removal of waste products from the tissue. These changes in local metabolism lead to vasodilation in the adjacent area and the gradual spread of inflammation. The spread of inflammation is circumferential as was demonstrated in an elegant experiment by Van Hassel.[107] Thus, total pulp necrosis is the gradual accumulation of local necroses.

It has been shown that the pulp has tremendous healing potential. This raises the question as to how the pulp recovers from the adverse effects of localized inflammation. Although the exact physiologic mechanisms are not yet known, recent research findings suggest the following: First, as the tissue pressure increases as a result of an increase in blood flow, the AVAs or the U-turn loop vessels open and shunt the blood before it reaches the inflamed region of the coronal of the pulp. This prevents a further increase in blood flow and tissue pressure. Also, the increase in tissue pressure pushes macromolecules back into the bloodstream via the venules in the adjacent healthy region (Fig. 15-26). Once the macromolecules and

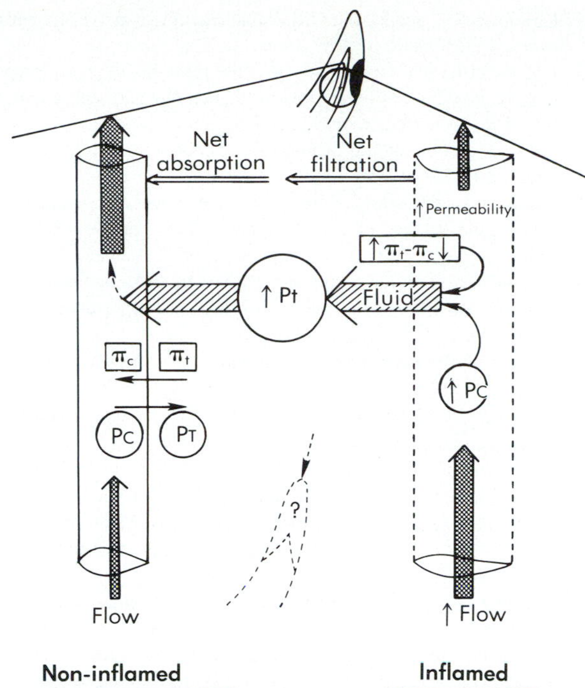

FIG. 15-26 Schematic representation of the compensatory mechanism of the pulp during inflammation. Key: P_C and P_T, hydrostatic pressure of capillary and tissue, respectively; π_c and π_t, osmotic pressure of capillary and tissue, respectively.

accompanying fluid leave the extracellular tissue space through the venule, the tissue pressure decreases and normal blood flow is restored.

Prevention

To preserve the integrity of the pulp, the dentist should observe certain precautions while rendering treatment. The following is a list of *do's* and *dont's* that should prevent or minimize injury to the pulp.

- Cutting procedures: use light, intermittent cutting, an efficient cooling system, and high speeds of rotation.
- Avoid desiccating the dentin: do not overdry the cavity preparation.
- Do not apply irritating chemicals to freshly cut dentin.
- Choose restorative materials carefully, considering the physical and biologic properties of the material.
- Do not use caustic cavity sterilizing agents.
- Assume that all restorative materials will leak. Use a cavity liner or base to seal the openings of exposed dentinal tubules.
- Do not use excessive force when inserting a restoration.
- Employ polishing procedures that do not subject the pulp to excessive heat.
- Establish a patient recall system that ensures periodic evaluation of the status of pulps that have been exposed to injury.

REFERENCES

1. Ackermans F, Klein JP, and Frank RM: Ultrastructural localization of immunoglobulins in carious human dentine, Arch Oral Biol 26:879, 1981.
2. Ackermans F, Klein JP, and Frank RM: Ultrastructural localization of *Streptococcus mutans* and *Streptococcus sanguis* antigens in carious human dentine, J Biol Buccale 9:203, 1981.
3. Alperstein KS, Graver HT, and Herold RCB: Marginal leakage of glass-ionomer cement restorations, J Prosthet Dent 50:803, 1983.
4. Barber D, and Massler M: Permeability of active and arrested carious lesions to dyes and radioactive isotopes, J Dent Child 31:26, 1964.
5. Beagrie GS, and Smith DC: Development of a germicidal polycarboxylate cement, J Can Dent Assoc 44:409, 1978.
6. Bergenholtz G: Effect of bacterial products on inflammatory reactions in the dental pulp, Scand J Dent Res 85:122, 1977.
7. Bergenholtz G, and Reit C: Reactions of the dental pulp to microbial provocation of calcium hydroxide treated dentin, Scand J Dent Res 88:187, 1980.
8. Bergenholtz G, et al: Bacterial leakage around dental restorations: its effect on the dental pulp, J Oral Pathol 11:439, 1982.
9. Berggren H: The reaction of the translucent zone to dyes and radioisotopes, Acta Odontol Scand 23:197, 1965.
10. Bowen RL, Cobb EN, and Rapson JE: Adhesive bonding of various materials to hard tooth tissues: improvement in bond strength to dentin, J Dent Res 61:1070, 1982.
11. Bradford EW: The dentine, a barrier to caries, Br Dent J 109:387, 1960.
12. Brännström M: The effect of dentin desiccation and aspirated odontoblasts on the pulp, J Prosthet Dent 20:165, 1968.
13. Brännström M: A new approach to insulation, Dent Pract 19:417, 1969.
14. Brännström M: Dentin and pulp in restorative dentistry, London, 1982, Wolfe Medical Publications Ltd.
15. Brännström M: Communication between the oral cavity and the dental pulp associated with restorative treatment, Operative Dent 9:57, 1984.
16. Brännström M, and Lind PO: Pulpal response to early dental caries, J Dent Res 44:1045, 1965.
17. Brännström M, and Nyborg H: Pulpal reaction to polycarboxylate and zinc phosphate cements used with inlays in deep cavity preparations, J Am Dent Assoc 94:308, 1977.
18. Brännström M, Vojinovic O, and Nordenvall KJ: Bacterial and pulpal reactions under silicate cement restorations, J Prosthet Dent 41:290, 1979.
19. Brännström M, et al: Protective effect of polystyrene liners for composite resin restorations, J Prosthet Dent 49:331, 1983.
20. Brown WS, Christensen DO, and Lloyd BA: Numerical and experimental evaluation of energy inputs, temperature gradients, and thermal stresses during restorative procedures, J Am Dent Assoc 96:451, 1978.
21. Chiego DJ Jr, Wang RF, and Avery JK: Ultrastructural changes in odontoblasts and nerve terminals after cavity preparations, J Dent Res 68 (special issue): 1023, 1989 (abstract 1251).
22. Cotton WR: Bacterial contamination as a factor in healing of pulp exposures, Oral Surg 38:441, 1974.
23. Cotton WR, and Siegel RL: Human pulpal response to critic acid cavity cleaner, J Am Dent Assoc 96:639, 1978.
24. Cox CF, et al: Biocompatibility of various surface-sealed dental materials against exposed pulps, J Prosthet Dent 57:1, 1987.
25. Eames WB, Hedrix K, and Mohler HC: Pulpal response in rhesus monkeys to cementation agents and cleaners, J Am Dent Assoc 98:40, 1979.
26. Edwards DL: The response of the human dental pulp to the use of a cavity varnish beneath amalgam fillings, Br Dent J 145:39, 1978.
27. Farah JW, Hood JA, and Craig RG: Effects of cement base on the stresses in amalgam restorations, J Dent Res 54:10, 1975.
28. Felton D: Long term effects of crown preparation on pulp vitality, J Dent Res 68 (special issue):1009, 1989 (abstract 1139).
29. Fish EW: An experimental investigation of the enamel, dentine and dental pulp, London, 1933, John Bale Sons, and Danielson, Ltd.

30. Frank RM: Reactions of dentin and pulp to drugs and restorative materials, J Dent Res 54:176, 1975.
31. Frank RM, and Voegel JC: Ultrastructure of the human odontoblast process and its mineralization during dental caries, Caries Res 14:367, 1980.
32. Going RE, and Massler M: Influence of cavity liners under amalgam restorations or penetration by radioactive isotopes, J Prosthet Dent 2:298, 1961.
33. Graf H, and Galasse R: Mobidity, prevalence and intraoral distribution of hypersensitive teeth, J Dent Res, special issue A, 162:2, 1977.
34. Grajower R, Kaufman E, and Rajstein J: Temperature in the pulp chamber during polishing of amalgam restorations, J Dent Res 53:1189, 1974.
35. Grajower R, Kaufman E, and Stern N: Temperature of the pulp during impression taking of full crown preparations with modeling compound, J Dent Res 54:212, 1975.
36. Graver T, Trowbridge H, and Alperstein K: Microleakage of castings cemented with glass ionomer cements, Oper Dent (in press).
37. Greenhill JD, and Pashley DH: The effects of desensitizing agents on the hydrodynamic conductance of human dentin in vitro, J Dent Res 60:686, 1981.
38. Heys DR, et al: Histologic and bacterial evaluation of conventional and new copper amalgams, J Oral Pathol 8:65, 1979.
39. Holden GP: Some observations on the vibratory phenomena associated with high-speed air turbines and their transmission to living tissue, Br Dent J 113:265, 1962.
40. Hoppenbrouwer PMM, Driessens FCM, and Stadhouders AM: Morphology, composition and wetting of dentinal cavity walls, J Dent Res 53:1255, 1964.
41. Jendresen M, and Trowbridge H: Biologic and physical properties of a zinc polycarboxylate cement, J Prosthet Dent 28:264, 1972.
42. Jodaikin A, and Austin JC: The effects of cavity smear layer removal on experimental marginal leakage around amalgam restorations, J Dent Res 60:1861, 1981.
43. Johnson NW, Taylor BR, and Berman DS: The response of deciduous dentine to caries studied by correlated light and electron microscopy, Caries Res 3:348, 1969.
44. Johnson RH, Daichi SF, and Haley JV: Pulpal hyperemia—a correlation of clinical and histological data from 706 teeth, J Am Dent Assoc 81:108, 1970.
45. Jones JCG, Grieve AR, and Kidd EAM: An in vitro comparison of marginal leakage associated with three resin based filling materials, Br Dent J 145:299, 1978.
46. Kakehashi S, Stanley HR, and Fitzgerald RJ: The effects of surgical exposures of pulps in germ-free and conventional rats. Oral Surg 20:340, 1965.
47. Karkalainen S, and LeBell Y: Odontoblast response to caries. In Thylstrup A, Leach SA, and Qvist V, (eds): Dentine and dentine reactions in the oral cavity, Oxford, 1987, IRL Press.
48. Karjalainen S, and Soderling E: The autoradiographic pattern of the in vitro uptake of proline by the coronal areas of intact and carious human teeth, Arch Oral Biol 24:909, 1980.
49. Kawahara H, Imanishi Y, and Oshima H: Biological evaluation of glass ionomer cement, J Dent Res 58:1080, 1979.
50. Kelley KW, Bergenholtz G, and Cox CF: The extent of the odontoblast process in rheusus monkeys *(Macaca mulatta)* as observed by scanning electron microscopy, Arch Oral Biol 26:893, 1981.
51. Kim S: Dynamic changes in the dental pulp circulation in response to dental procedures and materials. In Rowe NH (ed): Dental pulp reactions to restorative materials in the presence or absence of infection, Ann Arbor, 1982, University of Michigan.
52. Kim S: Ligamental injection: a physiological explanation of its efficacy, J Endod 12:486, 1986.
53. Kim S, et al: Effects of local anesthetics on pulpal blood flow in dogs, J Dent Res 63:650, 1984.
54. Kim S: Hypersensitive teeth: desensitization of pulpal sensory nerves. J Endod 12:482, 1986.
55. Kuwabara RK, and Massler M: Pulpal reaction to active and arrested caries, J Dent Child 33:190, 1966.
56. Langeland K, and Langeland LK: Pulp reactions to crown preparation, impression, temporary crown fixation and permanent cementation, J Prosthet Dent 15:129, 1965.
57. Lin L, et al: Periodontal ligamental injection: effects on pulp tissue, J Endod 11:529, 1985.
58. Lindholm K: The effect of crown preparation and compound impressions on the diameter of the pulp arteriole, Proc Finn Dent Soc 71:10, 1975.
59. Magloire H, et al: Ultrastructural alterations of human odontoblasts and collagen fibers in the pulpal border zone beneath early caries lesions, Cell Molec Biol 27:437, 1981.
60. Massler M: Pulpal reaction to dentinal caries, J Dent Res 17:441, 1967.
61. Michelich VJ, Schuster GS, and Pashley DH: Bacterial penetration of human dentin in vitro, J Dent Res 59:1398, 1980.
62. Miller WA, and Massler M: Permeability and staining of active and arrested lesions in dentine, Br Dent J 112:187, 1962.
63. Möller B: Reaction of the human dental pulp to silver amalgam restorations: the modifying effect of treatment with calcium hydroxide, Acta Odont Scand 33:233, 1975.
64. Mullaney TP, and Laswell HR: Iatrogenic blushing of dentin following full crown preparation, J Prosthet Dent 22:354, 1969.
65. Nelson RJ, Wolcott RB, and Paffenbarger GC: Fluid exchange at the margins of dental restorations, J Am Dent Assoc 44:288, 1952.
66. Newman SM: Microleakage of a copal rosin cavity varnish, J Prosthet Dent 51:499, 1984.
67. Nordenvall K-J, Brännström M, and Torstensson B: Pulp reactions and microorganisms under ASPA and Concise composite fillings, J Dent Child 46:449, 1979.
68. Nyborg H, and Brännström M: Pulp reaction to heat, J Prosthet Dent 19:605, 1968.
69. Okamura K, et al: Plasma components in deep lesions of human carious dentin, J Dent Res 58:2010, 1979.
70. Okamura K, et al: Serum proteins and secretory component in human carious dentin, J Dent Res 58:1127, 1979.
71. Okamura K, et al: Dentinal response against carious invasion: localization of antibodies in odontoblastic body and process, J Dent Res 59:1368, 1980.
72. Olgart L, and Gazalius B: Effects of adrenaline and felypressin (Octapressin) on blood flow and sensory nerve activity on the tooth, Acta Odontol Scand 35:69, 1977.
73. Olgart L, et al: Localization of substance p-like immunoreactivity in nerves in the tooth pulp, Pain 4:153, 1977.
74. Parfitt GJ: The speed of development of the carious cavity, Br Dent J 100:204, 1956.
75. Pashley DH: The influence of dentin permeability and pulpal blood flow on pulpal solute concentrations, J Endod 5:355, 1979.
76. Pashley DH: Smear layer: Physiological consideration, Operative Dent 3:13, 1984.
77. Pashley DH: Dentin permeability, dentin sensitivity and treatment through tubule occlusion, J Endod 12:465, 1986.
78. Pashley DH, Galloway SE, and Stewart F: Effects of fibrinogen in vivo on dentin permeability in the dog, Arch Oral Biol 29:725, 1984.
79. Pashley DH, and Livingston MJ: Effect of molecular size on permeability coefficients in human dentine, Arch Oral Biol 23:391, 1978.
80. Pashley DH, Michelich V, and Kehl T: Dentin permeability: effects of smear layer removal, J Prosthet Dent 46:531, 1981.
81. Plant CG, and Jones DW: The damaging effects of restorative materials. I. Physical and chemical properties, Br Dent J 140:373, 1976.
82. Pohto M, and Scheinin A: Microscopic observations on living dental pulp. IV. The effects of oil of clove and eugenol on the circulation of the pulp in the rat's lower incisor, Dent Abstr 5:405, 1960.
83. Qvist V: The effect of mastication on marginal adaptation of composite restorations in vivo, J Dent Res 62:904, 1983.

84. Reeves R, and Stanley HR: The relationship of bacterial penetration and pulpal pathosis in carious teeth, Oral Surg 22:59, 1966.
85. Scott JN, and Weber DF: Microscopy of the junctional region between human coronal primary and secondary dentin, J Morphol 154:133, 1977.
86. Searls JC: Light and electron microscope evaluation of changes induced in odontoblasts of the rat incisor by high-speed drill, J Dent Res 46:1344, 1967.
87. Seltzer S, and Bender IB: The dental pulp, ed 3, Philadelphia, 1984, JB Lippincott Co.
88. Silverstone LM, et al: Dental caries: aetiology, pathology and prevention, London, 1981, Macmillan Press, Ltd.
89. Silvestri AR, Cohen SN, and Wetz JH: Character and frequency of discomfort immediately following restorative procedures, J Am Dent Assoc 95:85, 1977.
90. Skogedal O, and Ericksen HM: Pulpal reactions to surface-sealed silicate cement and composite resin restorations, Can J Dent Res 84:381, 1976.
91. Sneed WD, Hembree JH, and Welsh EL: Effectiveness of three varnishes in reducing leakage of a high-copper amalgam, Operative Dent 9:32, 1984.
92. Son HG, Kim S, and Kim SB: Pulpal blood flow and bonding, IADR Abstract for The Hague Meeting, 1986.
93. Stanley HR: Pulpal response to dental techniques and materials, Dent Clin North Am 15:115, 1971.
94. Stanley HR: Pulpal response. In Cohen S, and Burns R, editors: Pathways of the pulp, ed 3, St. Louis, 1984, Times Mirror/Mosby College Publishing.
95. Stanley HR, Going RE, and Chauncey HH: Human pulp response to acid pretreatment of dentin and to composite restoration, J Am Dent Assoc 91:817, 1975.
96. Stanley HR, et al: The detection and prevalence of reactive and physiologic sclerotic dentin, reparative dentin and dead tracts beneath various types of dental lesions according to tooth surface and age, J Pathol 12:257, 1983.
97. Swerdlow H, and Stanley HR: Reaction of human dental pulp to cavity preparation. I. Effect of water spray at 20,000 rpm, J Am Dent Assoc 56:317, 1958.
98. Swerdlow H, and Stanley HR: Reaction of human dental pulp to cavity preparation, J Prosthet Dent 9:121, 1959.
99. Taylor PE, Byers MR, and Redd PE: Sprouting of CGRP nerve fibers in response to dentin injury in rat molars, Brain Res 461:371, 1988.
100. Tönder K, and Kvinnsland I: Micropuncture measurement of interstitial tissue pressure in normal and inflamed dental pulp in cats, J Endod 9:105, 1983.
101. Torneck CD: Changes in the fine structure of the dental pulp in human caries pulpitis. II. Inflammatory infiltration, J Oral Pathol 3:83, 1974.
102. Trowbridge HO: Pathogenesis of pulpitis resulting from dental caries, J Endod 7:52, 1981.
103. Trowbridge HO, Edwall L, and Panopoulos P: Effect of zinc oxide–eugenol and calcium hydroxide on intradental nerve activity, J Endod 8:403, 1982.
104. Trowbridge H, Scott D, and Singer J: Effects of eugenol on nerve excitability, IADR Prog Abstr 56:115, 1977.
105. Trowbridge HO, et al: Sensory response to thermal stimulation in human teeth, J Endod 6:405, 1980.
106. Turner DF, Marfurt CF, and Sattleberg C: Demonstration of physiological barrier between pulpal odontoblasts and its perturbation following routine restorative procedures: horseradish peroxidase tracing study in the rat, J Dent Res 68:1261, 1989.
107. Van Hassel HJ: Physiology of the human dental pulp. In Siskin, editor: The biology of the human dental pulp, St. Louis, 1973, Times Mirror/Mosby College Publishing.
108. Vojinovic O, Nyborg H, and Brännström M: Acid treatment of cavities under resin fillings: bacterial growth in dentinal tubules and pulpal reactions, J Dent Res 52:1189, 1973.
109. Watts A: Bacterial contamination and toxicity of silicate and zinc phosphate cements, Br Dent J 146:7, 1979.
110. Yamada T, et al: The extent of the odontoblast process in normal and carious human dentin, J Dent Res 62:798, 1983.
111. Yates JL, Murray GA, and Hembree JH: The effect of cavity varnishes on certain insulating bases: a microleakage study, Operative Dent 5:43, 1980.
112. Zach L: Pulp liability and repair: effect of restorative procedures, Oral Surg 33:111, 1972.
113. Zach L, and Cohen G: Pulp responses to externally applied heat, Oral Surg 19:515, 1965.

Self-assessment questions

1. The most common dentin response in the zone deep to caries is
   a. increased permeability.
   b. alteration of collagen.
   c. dissolution of peritubular dentin.
   d. dentin sclerosis.
2. Although each carious lesion is individual and influenced by multiple factors, the caries process is generally
   a. continuous.
   b. rapid.
   c. intermittent.
   d. slow.
3. Relatively few bacteria are found in a pulp abscess because of the
   a. immune response of pulp tissue.
   b. high tissue pH in the adjacent inflammation.
   c. mechanical blockage of sclerotic dentin.
   d. antibacterial products of neutrophils.
4. Hyperplastic pulpitis
   a. occurs only in permanent molars.
   b. occurs when there is no damage.
   c. is not invaded by bacteria.
   d. is predominantly acute inflammation.
5. A periodontal ligament injection of 2% lidocaine with 1:100,000 epinephrine will cause the pulp circulation to
   a. cease for about 30 minutes.
   b. remain the same.
   c. increase markedly.
   d. decrease slightly.
6. Of the following, the highest incidence of pulp necrosis is associated with
   a. class V preparations on root surface.
   b. inlay preparations.
   c. partial veneer restorations.
   d. full crown preparations.
7. According to the hydrodynamic theory of dentin sensitivity, the movement of fluid through dentinal tubules
   a. stimulates the sensory nerve fibers of the underlying pulp.
   b. displaces odontoblasts into the pulp tissue.
   c. has minimal effect on the odontoblasts.
   d. results in the death of many odontoblasts.
8. Acid etching of dentin before insertion of the restorative material
   a. protects the pulp from bacterial invasion.
   b. enhances bacterial penetration of the dentin.
   c. destroys odontoblastic processes in the tubules.
   d. decreases the pulp response to the restorative material.

9. Pulpal blood flow is most increased by
   a. impression taking using modeling compound with copper banding.
   b. fabrication of acrylic temporary restoration.
   c. rubber base impression.
   d. hydrocolloid impression.
10. Dental tubules should be sealed before placement of restorations to
    a. allow a calcium bridge to form in the pulp.
    b. reduce the pathogenicity of the microorganisms.
    c. decrease the number of dentinal tubules.
    d. decrease the permeability of underlying dentin.
11. The smear layer on dentin walls acts to prevent pulpal injury by
    a. reducing diffusion of toxic substance through the tubules.
    b. resisting the effects of acid etching of the dentin.
    c. eliminating the need for a cavity liner or base.
    d. its bactericidal activity against oral microorganisms.
12. A common histologic change in the pulp in response to moderately deep dentin caries is
    a. chronic inflammation.
    b. acute inflammation.
    c. vasoconstriction.
    d. increased numbers of odontoblasts.
13. Application of frictional heat to exposed dentin may result in
    a. severe postoperative symptoms.
    b. vascular stasis or intrapulpal hemorrhage.
    c. proliferation of cells in the cell-rich zone.
    d. invariably chronic inflammation.
14. Hypersensitivity is best relieved or controlled by
    a. opening tubules to permit release of intrapulpal pressure.
    b. root planing to remove surface layers that are hypersensitive.
    c. applying antiinflammatory agents to exposed dentin.
    d. blocking exposed tubules on the dentin surface.
15. Deeper cavity preparations have more potential for pulp damage because
    1. tubule diameter and density increase; therefore, there is increasing permeability.
    2. there is more vibration to pulp cells.
    3. odontoblastic processes are more likely to be severed.
       a. 1 only.
       b. 3 only.
       c. 1 and 3.
       d. 2 and 3.
16. The pulp generally begins to show histologic changes of inflammation as soon as caries has entered
    a. the dentin.
    b. the enamel.
    c. the pulp.
    d. the reparative (irregular secondary) dentin.
17. Of the following, which is the *best* way to prevent pulp damage during cavity preparation?
    a. Retain the smear layer.
    b. Use diamond burs with a brush stroke.
    c. Use adequate air coolant.
    d. Use adequate water coolant.
18. Which is the major reason why class II restorations with composite is damaging to the pulp?
    a. Microleakage at the occlusal.
    b. Microleakage at the gingival margin.
    c. Toxic chemicals are released from the composite and diffuse into the pulp.
    d. Polymerization shrinkage distorts the material at the occlusal and opens gaps which results in recurrent caries.
19. A pulp has been damaged and is inflamed because of deep caries and cavity preparation. What material placed on the floor of the cavity aids the pulp in resolving the inflammation?
    a. $Ca(OH)_2$
    b. ZnOE base.
    c. Steroid formulations.
    d. There is no medication or material that actively promotes pulp healing.
20. A cusp fractures and exposes dentin but not the pulp. What is the probable response in the pulp?
    a. Severe damage with irreversible inflammation.
    b. Mild-to-moderate inflammation.
    c. Pain but no inflammation.
    d. No pulp response.

PART THREE

RELATED CLINICAL TOPICS

Chapter 16

Traumatic Injuries

Stuart B. Fountain
Joe H. Camp

Hindsight explains the injury that foresight would have prevented.

Author Unknown

In considering dental traumatic injuries, it becomes quickly apparent that the majority of them are minor, consisting of cracked and chipped teeth. As such they could have been prevented by a little foresight on the part of each patient. However, dentists must be prepared to treat not only the minor cracked and chipped tooth injuries but also the more traumatic broken crowns, roots, bones, and missing teeth.

This chapter will discuss the epidemiology of traumatic injuries, the multiplicity of therapies available for the injuries, and a few preventive measures to lessen the incidence and severity of the injuries.

INCIDENCE

Although dental injuries occur at any age, one of the more likely times is ages 2 to 5 years. During this developmental period children are learning to walk and then to run. Because their coordination and judgment are not keenly developed, falls are common. Approximately 30% of these young children suffer injuries to their primary teeth, generally fractured or displaced maxillary incisors.[15,31,39]

As children gain confidence and coordination, the incidence of dental injuries decreases; it then rises again during the very active 8- to 12-year age range, as a result of bicycle, skateboard, playground, or sports accidents.[11,172,181]

By the time students complete high school it is estimated that as many as one out of three boys and one out of four girls will have suffered a dental injury.[181] This seemingly high incidence of injuries to the permanent teeth is the result of the collective activities of young people throughout their school years. During high school the increased participation of boys and girls in sports creates a high risk of injury.

Prior to the 1960s, boys had three times as many injuries as girls. The rapid increase in women's athletics during the 1970s has reduced this ratio, however, to one and one half injuries to boys for each injury to girls.[127,226]

In the teen and young adult years dental injuries result from motor vehicle accidents, sports, and accidental falls. A study of military personnel[136] showed the largest number of dental injuries to young male enlisted men occurring after hours as a result of fistfights. A fourth of the dental injuries in the public schools have been observed to be due to fighting and pushing.[69]

The place in which tooth injuries are most likely to occur is the home. Injuries at home or indoors account for 49% to 60% of tooth injuries.[83,93,156]

The dental injuries are predominantly enamel only or enamel and dentin fractures of the maxillary incisors. Approximately 90% of dental injuries are chipped teeth,[127,224,226] the remainder being severe crown fractures involving the pulp, tooth displacement, or avulsion.

The number of teeth injured in an accident varies, depending on the force, the size, and the resiliency of the object hitting the teeth. A fall in which a tooth hits a table corner will probably result in a crown fracture of one tooth. But an automobile accident in which the face hits a padded dash could result in multiple teeth being displaced and no crown fracture.[167]

A blow to a tooth creates stresses throughout its length and into the surrounding alveolus. If the bone is resilient, the tooth will be displaced. But if the bone is thick and rigid, the tooth will fracture because of its being more brittle than the bone.[31]

The most vulnerable tooth is the maxillary central incisor, which sustains approximately 80% of dental injuries, followed by the maxillary lateral and the mandibular central and lateral incisors.[127,224]

A major predisposing factor in dental injuries is incisal overjet of the maxillary incisors. As the dimension of incisal overjet increases from a normal 0 to 3 mm to a distinct 3 to 6 mm range, the incidence of injury to the maxillary incisors doubles. The severity of injury also increases with the overjet dimension. Children with an extreme overjet (6 mm) are twice as likely to injure two or more incisors.[126] A possible reason for this increase in severity of injury is the lack of lip closure over the overjet incisors, thereby reducing the impact-absorbing protection of the lips.

Unfortunately, dental injuries are a common finding among battered children. The abused child is generally very young (prekindergarten) and is injured by an enraged parent who resorts to force to silence the crying or screaming child. The symptoms include multiple bruises all over the body as well as oral lacerations and fractured teeth.[210] For the protection of the child it is the responsibility of clinicians to report these suspicious symptoms to the proper authorities.

HISTORY AND CLINICAL EXAMINATION

Dental injuries are never convenient for either the patient or the clinician. Consequently, the emergency visit often consists of a distraught patient and/or parent meeting a hurried clinician. It is one of the challenges that face clinicians to control the scene, calm the patient and parents, and take the necessary time to conduct a qualitative evaluation of the patient's injuries. Without such control by the clinician, significant injuries can be easily missed in the haste of the moment.

The medical history (Fig. 10-2) is fundamental to all other evaluation and treatment of the patient. Local anesthesia cannot be administered safely without the completion of a standard medical questionnaire.

History of the Accident

The *how, when,* and *where* of the accident are significant.[31]

Understanding *how* it occurred will assist the clinician in locating specific injuries. A blow to the lips and anterior teeth could possibly cause crown, root, or bone fractures to the anterior region and is less likely to injure the posterior regions. A blow under the chin or jaw could cause fractures to any tooth in the mouth. A padded blow (fall against a covered chair arm) could cause a root fracture or tooth displacement, whereas a hard blow (concrete walk) would tend to cause coronal fractures.

When the accident occurred is most important. With the passage of time blood clots and collagen fibers begin to form, periodontal ligaments and teeth dry out, saliva contaminates the wound, and all these become factors in making decisions about the sequence of treatment.

Where the trauma occurred becomes significant for prognosis. A tooth avulsed on the bottom of a swimming pool has a much better chance for successful replantation than one found lying in a pool of gasoline and oil following an automobile accident. The necessity for prophylactic tetanus toxoid is influenced by the location of the accident. Where the trauma oc-

SAMPLE OF A PREPRINTED FORM TO BE GIVEN TO THE PATIENT WITH INJURY OF THE HEAD OR NECK OR TO THE PERSON ACCOMPANYING THE PATIENT

Attention!

When oral structures are injured, there can be additional injury that may not be evident immediately.

If any of these symptoms occur within 48 hours, please call your physician immediately for further examination:

- Difficulty with breathing
- Difficulty with vision
- Dizziness
- Pain in the region of the neck or inability to turn the head normally
- Numbness of any area of the body
- Ringing in the ears
- Lethargy (unusual sleepiness)
- Nausea or vomiting
- Change in ability to function normally

If you do not have a physician whom you regularly see, please contact our office, and we will refer you for medical consultation.

Dentist's name
Address
Telephone

From Croll TP et al: J Am Dent Assoc 100:530, 1980.

curred may also be significant because of insurance and possible litigation.

Another important question to ask is whether treatment, of any kind, has been given for this injury by a parent, coach, physician, school nurse, teacher, or ambulance attendant. A normal-appearing tooth may have been replanted or repositioned 2 days previously by any of these or by the patient himself, and this will influence the prognosis for treatment and the sequence of treatment. See box on page 437.

Clinical Examination

Chief complaint

Aside from pain and bleeding, there may be a specific uncomfortable sensation. If the complaint is that the teeth "don't fit together now," the clinician must consider possible displacements or a bone fracture. Pain that occurs *only* when the patient closes the teeth together could indicate crown, root, or bone fractures or displacement.

Neurologic examination

While the clinician is obtaining the history of the accident and chief complaint, the patient should be observed for neurologic or other medical complications. See box below. Dental injuries may occur simultaneously with other head and neck injuries. Note should be made of whether the patient is communicating coherently. Does the patient have difficulty focusing or rotating the eyes, or in breathing? Airway obstruction by dental appliances must be considered.

Can the patient turn the head from side to side? Is there any paresthesia of the lips or tongue? Does the patient complain of ringing in the ears? Have there been persistent headaches, dizziness, drowsiness, or vomiting since the accident?

Before analgesics are prescribed or sedation by inhalation of nitrous oxide/oxygen is used, the clinician must be satisfied that there are no neurologic injuries.[73,137] If there is any question about this, the patient should be referred for to appropriate medical treatment.

External examination

Before having the patient open his mouth for an intraoral examination, the clinician should first look for external signs of injury. Lacerations of the head and neck are easily detected. However, deviations of normal bone contours must be closely observed. The temporomandibular joint should be palpated externally while the patient opens and closes. Does the patient's opening and closing pattern deviate to either side? If so, this could indicate a unilateral mandibular fracture. Similarly the zygomatic arch, angle, and lower border of the mandible should be bilaterally palpated and note made of any areas of tenderness, swelling, or bruising of the face, cheek, neck, or lips. They could be clues to possible bone fractures.

Intraoral soft tissue examination

One next looks for lacerations of the lips, tongue, cheek, palate, and floor of the mouth. The facial and lingual gingivae and oral mucosa are palpated, with note made of areas of tenderness, swelling, or bruising. The anterior border of the ramus of the mandible is palpated. Any abnormal findings suggest possible tooth or bone injuries or fractures, and further radiographic examination of the area is indicated. Lacerations of the lips and tongue must be felt for embedded foreign objects.[60,114]

Hard tissue examination

One of the best examinations for evidence of traumatic injuries is simply to look carefully. Each tooth and its supporting structures must be examined with an explorer and periodontal probe. Basic questions such as Is the occlusal plane

OUTLINE OF INITIAL NEUROLOGIC ASSESSMENT FOR THE PATIENT WITH TRAUMATIC DENTAL INJURIES

Notice unusual communication or motor functions.

Look for normal respiration without obstruction of the airway or danger of aspiration.

Replant avulsed teeth as indicated.

Obtain a medical history and information on the accident.

Determine blood pressure and pulse.

Examine for rhinorrhea or otorrhea.

Evaluate function of the eyes—Is diplopia or nystagmus apparent? Are pupillary activity and movement of the eyes normal?

Evaluate movement of the neck—Is there pain or limitation?

Examine the sensitivity of the surface of the facial skin—Is paresthesia or anesthesia apparent?

Confirm that there is normal vocal function.

Confirm patient's ability to protrude the tongue.

Confirm hearing—Is tinnitis or vertigo apparent?

Evaluate the sense of smell.

Assure follow-up evaluation.

From Croll TP, et al: J Am Dent Assoc 100:530, 1980.

disturbed? and Are there any missing teeth? must be answered before any thermal or electric tests are begun.

The examiner looks for gross evidence of injury initially. If several teeth are out of alignment, a bone fracture is the most reasonable explanation. The mandible should be examined for fractures by placing the forefinger on the occlusal plane of the posterior teeth with the thumbs under the mandible and then rocking the mandible from side to side and from anterior to posterior. A mandibular fracture will cause discomfort with these motions and the grating sound of broken fragments might be heard.[60] Gentle but firm pressure should be used to prevent possible additional trauma to the inferior alveolar nerve and blood vessels.

Also one can try to move the individual teeth with finger pressure in the maxilla and mandible. Any looseness is indicative of displacement from the alveolar socket. Movement of several teeth together is evidence of an alveolar fracture. Mobility of the crown must be differentiated from the mobility of the tooth. In instances of crown fractures the crown will be mobile but the tooth will remain in position. Occasionally root fractures can be felt by placing a finger on the mucosa over the tooth and moving the crown.

Any freshly fractured cusps or incisal edge fractures should be recorded. Incomplete cusp fractures can be noted by using the tip of a dental explorer as a wedge in the occlusal grooves of the posterior teeth to elicit movement of any cusps. The patient may be asked to bite on a rubber polishing wheel with each tooth in succession to help locate tenderness that could mean an incomplete cusp fracture or displaced tooth.

Each incisal edge and cusp can be gently percussed with the mirror handle to locate incomplete fractures or teeth that have been slightly displaced from the alveolar socket. Accumulation of extravasated fluid and tearing of periodontal fibers around a minimally displaced tooth will make the tooth tender to percussion.

Hemorrhage in the gingival sulcus may indicate a displaced tooth. Any discoloration of the teeth should be noted; viewing from the lingual surface of anterior teeth with a reflected light will help.

Obvious pulp exposures should be noted. Crown fractures with minute pulp exposures can be detected with a cotton pellet soaked in saline and pressed against the area of the suspected exposure.[31] The mechanical pressure of the cotton against an exposure will elicit a response. A dry cotton pellet can confuse the diagnosis by dehydrating dentinal tubules in a near exposure, causing a pain sensation, and should not be used.

When the visual examination is complete and all abnormal findings are noted, radiographs of the injured area should be exposed. These can be processed while additional tests are being conducted.

Thermal and electric tests

For decades controversy has surrounded the validity of thermal and electric tests on traumatized teeth. Only generalized impressions may be gained from these tests subsequent to a traumatic injury. They are, in reality, sensitivity tests for nerve function and do *not* indicate the presence or absence of blood circulation within the pulp. It is assumed that subsequent to traumatic injury the conduction capability of the nerve endings and/or sensory receptors is sufficiently deranged to inhibit the nerve impulse from an electric or thermal stimulus. This makes the traumatized tooth vulnerable to false negative readings from these tests.

The reader is referred to Chapter 1 for specific descriptions of pulp tests, but a few general statements in regard to pulp tests on traumatized teeth may be helpful in trying to interpret the results.

Thermal and electric pulp tests of teeth in the traumatized area should be done at the time of the initial examination and carefully recorded to establish a base line for comparison with subsequent repeated tests in later months. These tests should be repeated at 30-, 90-, and 180-day intervals and 1 year following the accident. The purpose of the tests is to establish a trend as to the physiologic status of the pulps of these teeth.

Teeth that give a positive response at the initial examination cannot be assumed to be healthy and continue to give a positive response. Teeth that yield a negative response or no response cannot be assumed to have necrotic pulps, because they may give a positive response later. It has been demonstrated that it may take as long as 9 months for normal blood flow to return to the coronal pulp of a traumatized fully formed tooth. As circulation is restored, the responsiveness to pulp tests returns.[95]

The transition from a negative to a positive response at a subsequent test may be considered a sign of a healthy pulp. The repetitious finding of positive responses may be taken as a sign of a healthy pulp. The transition from a positive to a negative response may be taken as an indication that the pulp is probably undergoing degeneration. The persistence of a negative response would suggest that the pulp has been irreparably damaged, but even this is not absolute.[51]

In testing teeth for response to cold, the dry ice pencil (carbon dioxide stick described in Chapter 1) gives more positive responses than does a water ice pencil. The intense cold (−78° C) seems to penetrate the tooth and covering splints or restorations and reach the deeper areas of the tooth. In addition, dry ice does not form ice water, which could disperse over adjacent teeth or gingiva to give a false-positive response.

Radiographic examinations

Radiographs are essential to the thorough examination of traumatized hard tissue. They may reveal root fractures, subgingival crown fractures, tooth displacements, bone fractures, or foreign objects.

However, the fracture line may run in a mesial-distal direction in the tooth and not be evident on the radiograph. Also the fracture line may be diagonal in a facial-lingual direction and not obvious on the film. Similarly, a hairline fracture may not be evident on the radiograph at the initial examination but later become obvious as tissue fluids and mobility spread the broken parts.

In instances of soft tissue laceration it is advisable to radiograph the injured area prior to suturing to be sure that no foreign objects have become embedded. A soft tissue radiograph with a normal-sized film briefly exposed at a reduced kilovoltage should reveal the presence of many foreign substances, including tooth fragments.

In reviewing the films of traumatized teeth, special attention should be directed to the dimension of the root canal space, the degree of apical closure of the root, the proximity of fractures to the pulp, and the relationship of root fractures to the alveolar crest. Whereas conventional periapical films are generally useful, an occlusal or Panorex film can supplement them when the examiner is looking for bone fractures or the presence of foreign objects.

In summary, the examination of traumatic injuries must be thorough and meticulously recorded. Most injuries are covered by some type of insurance, and many will eventually be involved in litigation. When asked to describe the condition of the patient at the time of the initial examination, months or years after the accident, the dentist will find a completely documented patient record, including quality radiographs, to be of immense assistance. These records form the basis for the justification of subsequent treatment and the associated professional fees. In addition, the rapid increase in professional liability claims against dentists further emphasizes the need for complete and accurate patient records (described in greater detail in Chapter 9).

CLASSIFICATIONS AND TREATMENT

Over the years various authors[31,45,87] have used a formal classification of traumatic injuries. While attempting to simplify discussion of traumatic injuries these authors were well intended; however, the result has been a confusing system of classes and subdivisions of classes that do not correspond from author to author. Therefore, to get back to basics, we have studiously avoided references to classes of traumatic injuries.

Crown Fractures

The reported incidence of crown fractures varies from 26% to 92% of all traumatic injuries to the permanent dentition[88,103] and from 4% to 38% of injuries to the primary dentition.[15,39] The wide variation in reported incidence is due to the diversity of sampling techniques and classifications of injuries.

Emergency treatment

All fractures of tooth structure must be treated as dental emergencies; thus the patient should be seen as soon as possible after injury. With crown fractures the immediate concern is pulpal protection. Rarely does a crown fracture occur without accompanying concussive or displacement injury. Therefore restoration of the tooth for esthetic purposes is not desirable or necessary at this time. Procedures involving mechanical preparation of the tooth, the application of forces such as wedge placement, and the seating of a stainless steel crown are contraindicated at this time unless necessary for pulpal protection because of the possibility of inflicting further damage to the pulpal or periodontal tissues.

The acid etch composite restoration is recommended whenever possible to maintain a protective pulpal dressing since it can be utilized without tooth preparation or the application of any forces, which might further damage the traumatized tooth (Fig. 16-1).

Since the introduction by Buonocore[62] of acid etching to increase the adhesion of resin to enamel, this technique has become widely accepted as the treatment of choice for restoring fractured teeth in children.[63,130,186] It does not adversely affect the pulp if proper protective measures are taken.[31,111] To protect the pulp adequately, a calcium hydroxide liner (e.g., Dycal or Life) must be placed on the exposed dentin before application of the phosphoric acid (Fig. 16-1). Eugenol-containing compounds (like zinc oxide–eugenol, or ZOE) must be avoided when resin or composite restorations are being utilized since these interfere with the setting reaction of the restorations.

Because preparation of the tooth is usually necessary when a temporary crown is to be the emergency restoration, this technique should not be considered unless the fracture is so extensive that the acid etch composite cannot be utilized. Preparation of the tooth will further damage the already traumatized tooth. Likewise, stainless steel crowns at this stage of treatment are contraindicated because of the forces necessary to fit them properly except as outlined below.

One of the prerequisites for using the acid etch composite restoration is maintenance of a dry field during the application and curing of the composite. Although the application of a rubber dam is usually not advisable at the emergency appointment, it may be helpful if it can be done without further trauma to the teeth. Rubber dam clamps must not be applied to the traumatized teeth. Most injuries occur in the mixed dentition phase, when the teeth are not fully erupted and application of the rubber dam is difficult under ideal conditions. Therefore use of the rubber dam at the emergency appointment is usually not possible. Isolation is achieved by cotton rolls or sponges.

When gingival tissue seepage or hemorrhage prevents a dry working field, the use of a welded stainless steel or preformed orthodontic band is advocated. The tooth is momentarily dried, and a protective base of calcium hydroxide or ZOE is placed over the exposed dentin. A loose-fitting band is fabricated or selected from an assortment of preformed bands. A strip of stainless steel is welded across the incisal to close the opening and prevent the loss of the protective base. The band is checked to ensure that it does not interfere with the occlusion. It is then cemented to the tooth with zinc phosphate or polycarboxylate cement. A permanent-type cement is used because retention of the band is derived exclusively from the cementation. The enamel may be acid etched before cementation to improve retention where necessary (Fig. 16-2).

An alternative to the band is the use of the incisal end of a stainless steel crown. The crown is trimmed to remove all undercuts and the incisal portion is fitted over the end of the tooth like a thimble. The crown should be large enough that it can be seated without any pressure. Otherwise, the technique is the same as for the band. When materials of this type are to be used, the patient and parents should be advised of the temporary nature of the restoration and that esthetics will be a more important consideration after healing has occurred.

Difficulty is encountered when proximal contacts with adjacent teeth are present and the acid etch composite restoration cannot be utilized because of inadequate moisture control. In these cases it may be necessary to relieve the proximal contact slightly with a thin diamond bur. However, this rarely happens since most injuries occur during the mixed dentition phase and in individuals with prognathic maxillary incisors.

It is crucial that the occlusion be checked after placement of any form of temporary restoration. If the injured tooth is left high in occlusion, it will receive additional trauma and be prevented from healing properly.

Crown infraction

Crown infraction is an incomplete fracture or crack of enamel without loss of tooth structure. It results from traumatic impact to the enamel and appears as craze lines running parallel with the direction of the enamel prisms and terminating at the dentin-enamel junction (Fig. 16-3). Infraction lines are often associated with luxation injuries.[31]

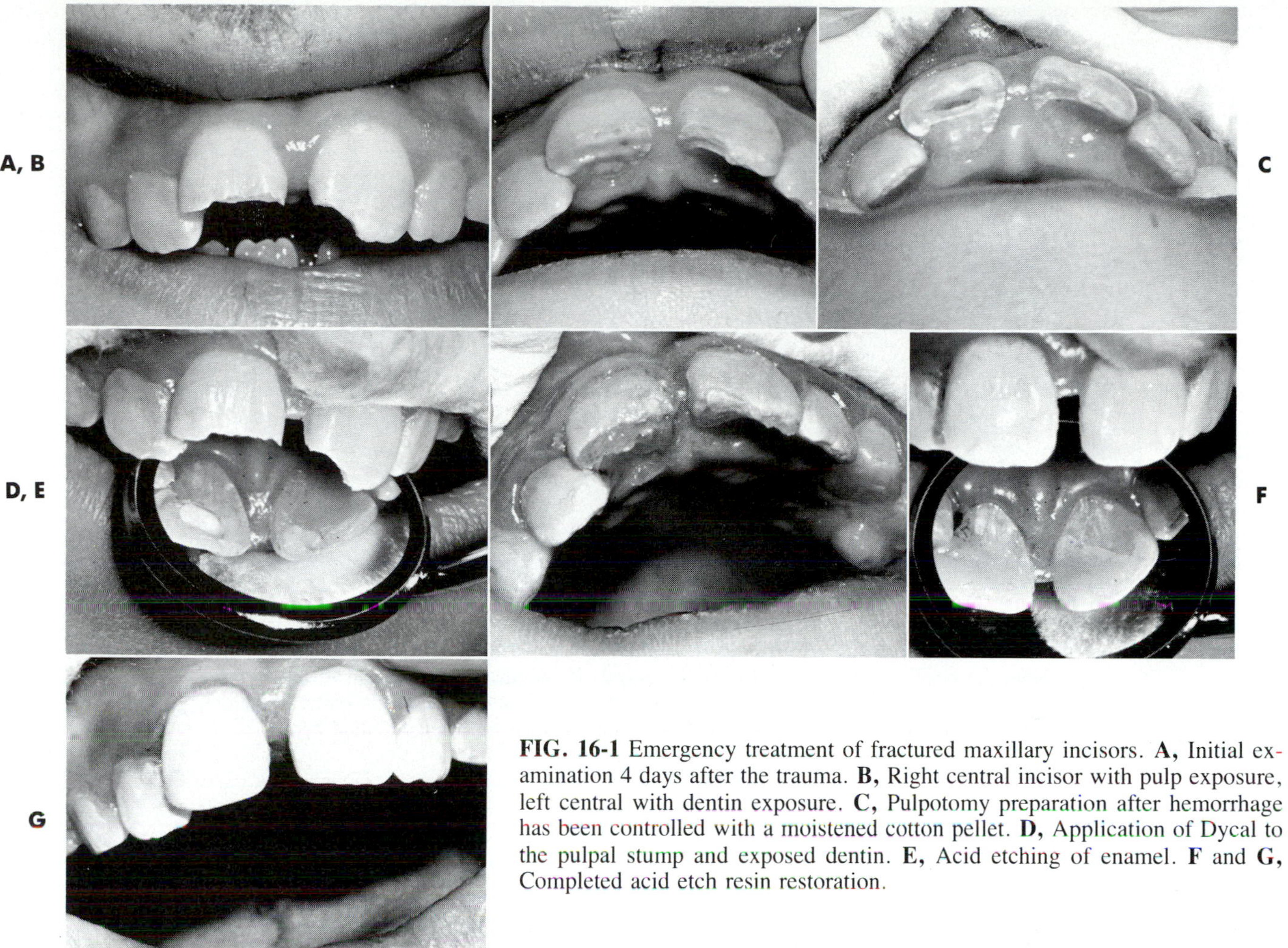

FIG. 16-1 Emergency treatment of fractured maxillary incisors. **A,** Initial examination 4 days after the trauma. **B,** Right central incisor with pulp exposure, left central with dentin exposure. **C,** Pulpotomy preparation after hemorrhage has been controlled with a moistened cotton pellet. **D,** Application of Dycal to the pulpal stump and exposed dentin. **E,** Acid etching of enamel. **F** and **G,** Completed acid etch resin restoration.

The severest pulpal reaction is often seen in teeth with the least apparent injury. Andreasen has shown that blows of low velocity, such as striking a tooth against the ground or with an elbow, are less apt to fracture the crown but cause the greatest damage to the supporting tissues. Crown fractures are more apt to occur as a result of a high-velocity impact against the tooth. The force of the blow is dissipated in creating the fracture, with less resulting damage to the supporting tissues.[15,31] Frequently teeth sustaining fracture retain their vitality while the adjacent traumatized teeth, which remained intact, undergo pulpal necrosis.

Crown infraction injuries do not require treatment, but vitality tests are necessary to determine the extent of pulpal damage. These tests should be conducted at the emergency appointment and recorded for future reference. The patient must be periodically recalled to check for vitality of the involved teeth. Pulpal problems arising from these types of injury will be discussed in the section on concussion injuries.

Crown fracture involving enamel only

Emergency treatment after a crown fracture involving only enamel (Fig. 16-4, *A*) is confined to removal of the sharp edges to prevent injury to the lips and tongue and the performance of vitality tests. Shaping of the tooth and adjacent teeth for esthetic purposes should be postponed several weeks until the pulp and periodontal tissues have had adequate time to recover. Whereas most of these fractures can be corrected by selective grinding and recontouring of the adjacent teeth, if this is not possible the treatment of choice is an acid etch composite restoration. The patient must be periodically recalled for vitality testing.

Crown fracture involving dentin

Crown fractures involving dentin expose large numbers of dentinal tubules through which bacteria and other harmful substances have a direct pathway to the pulp (Fig. 16-4, *B*). Emergency treatment consists of the application of a protective material over the exposed dentin to allow the pulp to form a protective barrier of reparative dentin. The restoration of choice to hold the protective dressing is the acid etch composite. The exposed dentin should be covered with a layer of calcium hydroxide product (e.g., Dycal or Life) before application of the phosphoric acid (Fig. 16-1, *D*).

Although esthetics is an ultimate concern, it is of little importance at the emergency appointment. The tooth should not be prepared at this time to receive the final acid etch compos-

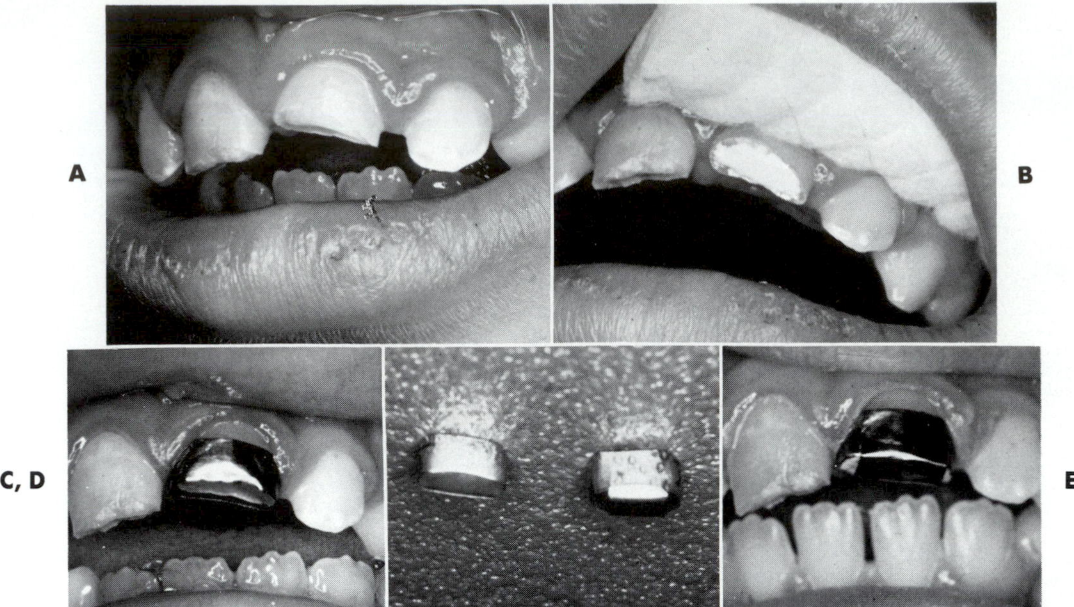

FIG. 16-2 Placement of a temporary stainless steel band to maintain a protective dressing over exposed dentin. Today, gloves are required. **A,** Crown fracture of the left central incisor. Note the previous fracture of the right central. **B,** Application of Dycal to all exposed dentin. **C,** Selection of a loose-fitting band. **D,** Strip of stainless steel matrix material welded across the incisal edge to prevent loss of the protective dressing. **E,** Cemented band.

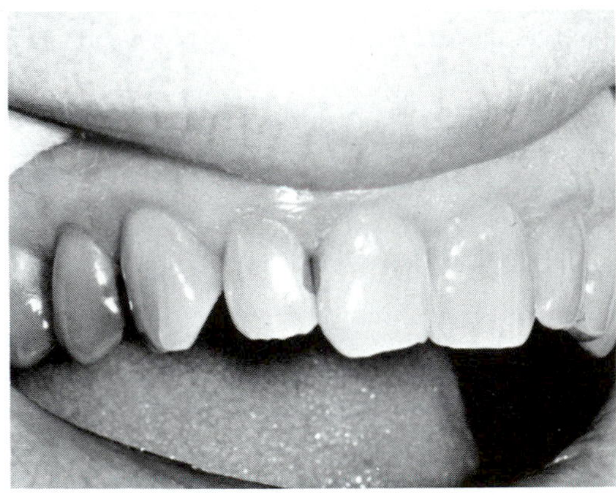

FIG. 16-3 Crown infraction lines resulting from trauma to the maxillary canine and lateral incisor.

ite. The use of rotary instruments will only further aggravate the injured tooth. Care should also be taken in placing the composite so that finishing of the restoration is not necessary. As little manipulation of the tooth as possible is desirable at this time. The tooth should not be restored to occlusion but left just out of occlusion.

Permanent restoration of the tooth may begin 6 to 8 weeks after the injury. This will allow sufficient time for pulpal healing, since it has been demonstrated that reparative dentin formation occurs primarily during the first month after injury to the dentin and then decreases markedly after 48 days.[205] Also during this period any injury to the periodontal tissues will have completely healed.[24,46]

The acid etch composite has been widely accepted as the restoration of choice for fractured crowns. In some cases, because of the extent of the fracture or for esthetic reasons, it may be necessary to restore the tooth with a crown.

The patient should be recalled at periodic intervals for vitality checks. These should be at 1, 3, and 6 months after the injury and every 6 months thereafter for several years. At each visit the tooth is examined, pulp tests are carried out, and a radiograph is made and compared with previous radiographs. Caution must be exercised in interpreting pulp tests since it is not uncommon for injured teeth to give abnormal responses for several months following injury.[187,195] If pulpal necrosis is determined, appropriate endodontic therapy should be provided.

Crown fracture exposing the pulp

In fractures involving exposure of the pulp when maintenance of vitality is desirable, the *best* prognosis is achieved if treatment is rendered as soon as possible after the injury (Fig. 16-4, *C*). Exposure of the pulp left untreated ultimately leads to pulpal necrosis from bacterial infection. Experiments in germ-free (gnotobiotic) animals have shown the importance of bacterial contamination in the healing of exposed pulps; healing occurred in germ-free animals, regardless of the severity of the exposure, but failed in the presence of microorganisms.[135]

According to Cvek,[78,79] after traumatic exposure of the pulp there is immediate hemorrhage into the underlying tissue followed by a superficial inflammatory response to breakdown products and bacteria. Clotting subsequently occurs. In the ensuing days tissue changes can be either destructive (e.g., abscess formation or necrosis) or proliferative (hyperplasia). Up

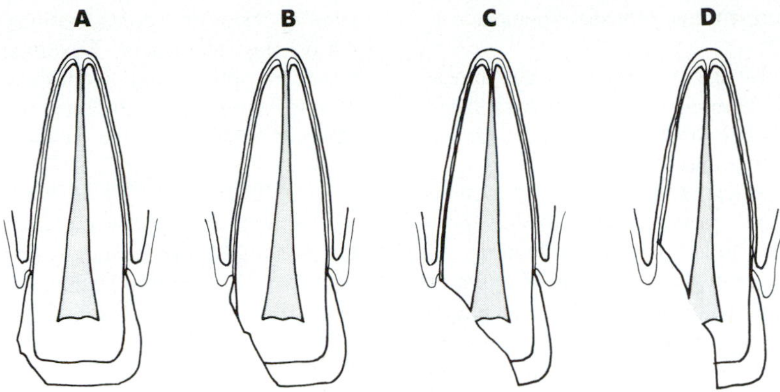

FIG. 16-4 Variations of crown fractures. **A,** Enamel only. **B,** Enamel and dentin. **C,** Enamel and dentin with pulpal exposure. **D,** Enamel, dentin, pulp, and root surface.

to 2 weeks, pulp exposure by mechanical means in teeth free of inflammation usually results in only a proliferative response, with inflammation extending no more than 2 mm from the exposure site.[78,82] When superficial necrosis does occur, healthy pulp tissue is usually found several millimeters deeper within the pulp.[104,105,198] Therefore, if superficial layers of the pulp are removed, healthy pulp tissue is usually encountered that will respond to vital conservative pulp procedures (Fig. 16-1).

Maintenance of pulpal vitality is especially important in the tooth with an incompletely developed root. In these teeth the treatment of choice should always be the procedure with the most favorable prognosis for retention of pulpal vitality so that completion of root development can be achieved.

After pulp exposure, when the objective of treatment is maintenance of vitality, this may be achieved by pulp capping or pulpotomy. When maintenance of vitality is not possible or practical, endodontic treatment should be performed.

Factors other than time affecting the outcome of pulp capping and pulpotomy procedures are (1) the accompanying injuries, (2) degenerative changes in the pulp, (3) the method of amputation of the coronal pulp, and (4) the type of dressing used for pulpal coverage.

Mature teeth with displacement injuries are poor candidates for pulp capping and pulpotomy procedures because of the impaired blood supply and the inflammation caused by the injury. However, this is not true for displaced teeth with immature roots.

Teeth with partial calcific pulpal obliteration indicative of degenerative and inflammatory changes within the pulp tissues resulting from caries or previous injuries are not candidates for pulp capping or pulpotomy.

The effects of tissue amputation and the type of capping agents used will be discussed later.

In practice, most clinicians reserve the pulpotomy procedure for treatment of teeth with incompletely formed roots. In mature teeth, if pulp capping is not feasible, a pulpectomy and root canal filling is usually the treatment of choice.

If fracture is so extensive that a post will be required for restoration of the tooth, a pulpectomy is the treatment of choice as long as the root is fully developed. If root formation is incomplete, a pulpotomy should be utilized, with a temporary post and crown until the root completes its development; then a pulpectomy and permanent post placement can be provided.

Pulp capping

Pulp capping is recommended for small traumatic exposures of the pulp that are treated within a few hours after the injury. Although pulp capping has been shown to be successful many days after exposure,[78] the maximum time at which this procedure will succeed has not been established. With longer times it has been shown[79] that more extensive tissue damage minimizes the chance for success especially when inflammation has resulted from contamination or debris at the exposure site.

Prior to placement of the dressing on the exposure site, the fractured tooth surface is cleaned with a moist cotton pellet and dried. Blowing of air directly on the exposure site should be avoided. The exposed dentin and pulp exposure are covered with a hard-setting calcium hydroxide material (e.g., Dycal or Life). The tooth is then acid etched and a covering of composite resin placed following the criteria outlined in the previous section on fractures involving dentin.

For a complete discussion of pulp capping procedures and agents, please refer to Chapter 23.

Pulpotomy

In the pulpotomy procedure a portion of the pulp is removed to allow the application of a dressing in an area of healthy tissue. It may be desirable to remove the superficial pulp tissue to reach tissue free of inflammation, or as has been shown,[78] the removal of a small amount of tissue will form a preparation to receive the pulpal dressing and thereby simplify the retention of the dressing during subsequent restorative procedures (Fig. 16-1, *C*). Cvek has achieved 96% success with utilization of this procedure.

It is usually necessary to remove only a few millimeters of pulp tissue. However, the depth to which tissue is removed is determined by the dentist's clinical judgment. Traditionally the term *pulpotomy* has implied removal of tissue to the cervical line. This is neither mandatory nor advisable. All tissue judged to be inflamed should be removed so the pulpal dressing can be placed against healthy uninflamed pulp tissue.

Cvek[78] has shown that *the time between the accident and treatment is not critical so long as the superficially inflamed tissue is removed prior to treatment*. In exposures of long duration, where surface abscess formation or surface necrosis has occurred, it may be necessary to go quite deep. Obviously the deep pulpotomy would be attempted only in teeth with incompletely developed roots where further root development was desirable.

The instrument of choice for tissue removal in the pulpotomy procedure is an abrasive diamond bur utilizing high speed and adequate water cooling. This technique has been shown to create the least damage to the underlying tissue.[96]

All tissue coronal to the application of the dressing must be removed since this tissue would be deprived of blood supply and undergo necrosis, resulting in failure of the pulpotomy.[203] The amputation site must be clean with no shreds of tissue or dentin debris remaining. Copious amounts of water or physiologic saline lavage are necessary to clean the amputation site.

Hemorrhage is controlled by the application of wetted cotton pellets thoroughly blotted to remove most of the moisture. The use of dry cotton pellets is contraindicated since clotting will occur on the dry fibers and when removed stimulate further hemorrhage.

When hemorrhage is controlled, a dressing of calcium hydroxide is placed over the amputation site (Fig. 16-1, *D*). If the pulpal amputation extends into the tooth only a few millimeters, the use of a hard-setting material (e.g., Dycal or Life) is usually easiest. However, for deeper amputations, we have found calcium hydroxide powder carried to the tooth in an amalgam carrier to be easiest method of application. *Care must be exercised to avoid packing the calcium hydroxide into the pulp tissue.* A round-ended plastic instrument is used to tease the calcium hydroxide powder gently against the pulp stump. If calcium hydroxide powder is utilized for the dressing, one of the hard-setting bases must be applied over the dressing and the remaining dentin. The tooth is then acid etched and restored with a composite resin according to the steps outlined in the section on fractures involving dentin.

For a complete discussion of the pulpotomy technique and other materials used as pulp dressings, please refer to Chapter 23.

Follow-up after pulp capping and pulpotomy

After pulp capping and pulpotomy the patient should be recalled periodically for 2 to 4 years to determine success. Although the normal vitality tests such as electric and thermal sensitivity are reliable after pulp capping and shallow pulpotomy, they are usually not helpful in the deeper pulpotomized tooth. Although histologic success cannot be determined, clinical success is judged by the absence of any clinical or radiographic signs of pathosis, the verification of a dentin bridge both radiographically and clinically, and the presence of continued root development in teeth with incompletely formed roots.

Controversy exists as to whether the pulp should be reentered after the completion of root development in the pulpotomized tooth. Many authors believe that pulp-capping and pulpotomy procedures invariably lead to progressive calcification of the root canal; however, it has been our experience and the experience of others[78,92,105,139] that when careful techniques and good case selection are used this seldom happens. When pulps of clinically successful pulpotomies were removed 1 to 5 years following treatment, researchers reported histologically normal findings. They concluded on the basis of the histologic evidence that routine pulpectomy following pulpotomy of accidental pulp exposure is not warranted.[82] Thus the routine reentry to remove the pulp and place a root canal filling after completion of root development is contraindicated unless dictated by restorative considerations such as the necessity for retentive post placement. Nevertheless, canal calcification, internal resorption, and/or pulp necrosis are potential sequelae of pulp capping and pulpotomy procedures. Although unlikely, they are possible and the patient should be clearly informed.

Treatment of primary crown fractures

Fractures of primary crowns not involving the pulp are treated in the same manner as those in permanent teeth. For a complete description of pulpal treatment in the primary dentition, please refer to Chapter 23.

Root Fractures

In the overall scope of traumatic injuries to teeth, root fractures are relatively uncommon, occurring in 7% or less of injuries to permanent teeth.[15,31] In primary and developing permanent teeth, root fractures are rare. These teeth, with very short roots, are more likely to be displaced or avulsed than to have fractured roots.

The diagnosis of a fractured root is based on the clinical mobility of the tooth, the displacement of the coronal segment, palpation tenderness over the root, and the radiographic appearance. Careful examination is frequently necessary to differentiate a root fracture from a subgingival crown fracture or a displaced tooth.

By placing the forefinger of one hand on the gingiva over the facial surface of the root of the affected tooth and gently moving the crown with the other hand, the clinician can often feel the location of the fracture. Also the arc of movement of the crown will aid in differentiating the injury. The closer the fracture is to the gingival crest, the longer will be the arc of movement of the crown; and the further the fracture is toward the apex, the shorter the arc of movement (Fig. 16-5).

The radiographic diagnosis of a root fracture requires careful review of radiographs of the site of injury, preferably with the aid of a magnifying glass. If the injury has caused a separation of the broken parts, the diagnosis is easy. If the central radiographic beam does not follow the direction of the fracture (Fig. 16-6), if the fracture runs in an oblique direction (Fig. 16-6), or if there has not been any separation of the broken segments of the root, then diagnosis becomes difficult at best or the fracture may be missed entirely. Fractures radiographed at an angle greater than ±15 or 20 degrees vertical to the fracture line have been shown to be of poor diagnostic quality.[31,84]

Andreasen has shown that an occlusal film exposure is best for diagnosing root fractures in the apical third of the root, and bisecting angle exposures are best for diagnosing fractures in the cervical third of the root. The occlusal films are exposed while the patient gently bites on the film packet and the central radiographic beam is at a moderately steep angle.[8,10]

As the clinician runs through the sequence of tests, the tooth with a fractured root generally will be noted to be tender to percussion; there may be bleeding from the gingival sulcus, and frequently the tooth will not respond to thermal or electric pulp testing procedures.

The variable response of the traumatized tooth to pulp tests brings the clinician into the realm of the art of dentistry rather than the science.

There is a tendency for root-fractured teeth to remain vital. It is believed that the fractured area provides an avenue of escape for fluid pressure from edema and allows for possible col-

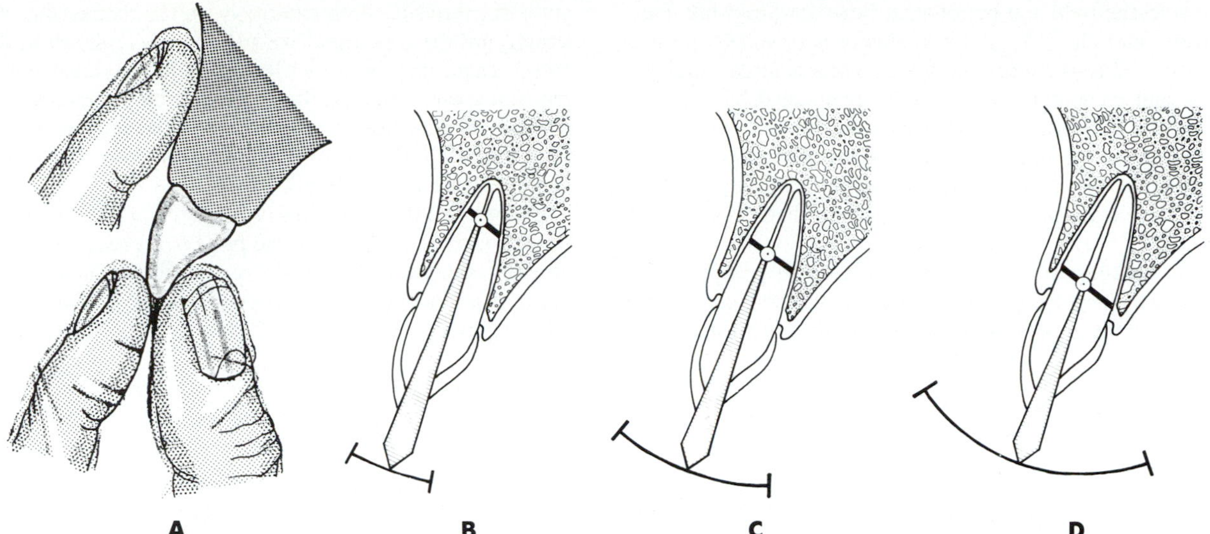

FIG. 16-5 Diagnosis of the location of a root fracture. **A,** Palpating the facial mucosa. By placing the forefinger of one hand on the mucosa and gently moving the crown of the injured tooth with the thumb and forefinger of the other hand, the dentist can often feel movement of the incisal segment of the root. **B** to **D,** Arc of mobility of the incisal segment of a tooth with a fractured root. As the location of the fracture moves incisally, the arc of a facial-lingual mobility of the incisal segment increases. (**B,** apical third fracture; **C,** middle third; **D,** incisal third.)

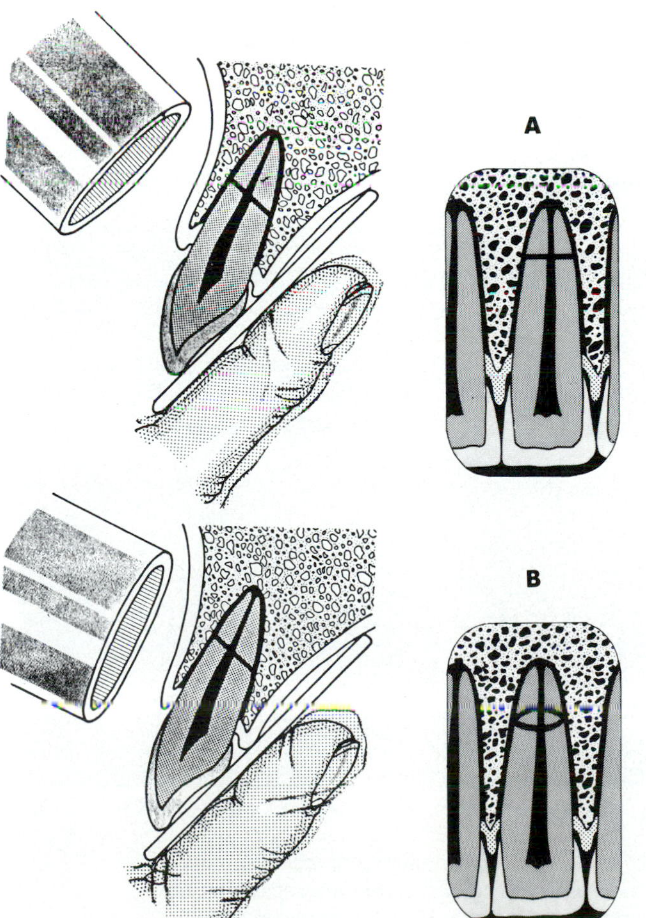

FIG. 16-6 Varying radiographic views of a root fracture depending on angulation of the central radiographic beam. **A,** Beam parallel with the fracture. **B,** Beam oblique to the fracture. This view gives an incorrect impression of an elliptical double fracture of the root.

lateral circulation from the periodontal ligament to assist in maintaining vitality of the traumatized pulp.[31,176,225] It has been shown that *only* 20% to 40% of teeth with fractured roots eventually undergo pulpal necrosis.[31,36,225]

If the fractured root is not apparent initially, it may become apparent days or weeks later as the patient continues to complain of sensitivity to biting pressure. This can be confirmed by percussion sensitivity. A follow-up radiograph may reveal a distinct fracture line at this later date due to separation of the broken root segments by edema and masticatory forces.[31]

Healing of fractured roots

Before beginning discussion of treatment of root fractures, it is essential that a basic understanding of the healing potentials of the fractured root be established. Given the background of these biologically normal healing patterns, the clinical decisions in regard to treatment become logical efforts to enhance the healing capacity of the tooth root. It is not our intent to describe the day-by-day histopathologic changes that occur at the fracture site but rather to present a general overview as a broad frame of reference. For a more detailed histopathologic description and references, the reader is referred to Andreasen.[31]

In the mechanism of root repair and separation of the broken segments in the alveolar socket, hemorrhage from broken capillaries in the pulp and periodontal ligament flows into the fracture site and clots. This clot gradually is organized by fibroblasts into fibrous connective tissue. The fractured surfaces of dentin and cementum are gradually remodeled by surface resorption and apposition of calcific tissue.

Depending on the amount of separation of the fragments, the severity of the injury, and the healing capacity of the pulp,[8,11] four alternative forms of repair have been classically described.[31,36]

Calcific healing. If the fragments are in close apposition with little mobility of the parts, and the tooth has a large root canal space,[8,11] it is possible to get a calcific callus formation at the fracture site, both externally on the root surface and internally on the root canal wall (Figs. 16-7, *A*, 16-8, *D*, and 16-9). There may be a thin layer of fibrous connective tissue remaining in the fracture line and seen on the radiograph as a delicate fracture line across the root. The pulp will likely be vital but at a reduced level of responsiveness. Mobility will be within physiologic limits.

Connective tissue healing. If the broken parts are separated further or some mobility of the parts is present, the formation of a calcified callus is impeded and a fibrous attachment similar to a periodontal ligament may develop between the fractured segments (Fig. 16-10, *D* and *E*). The fractured dentin

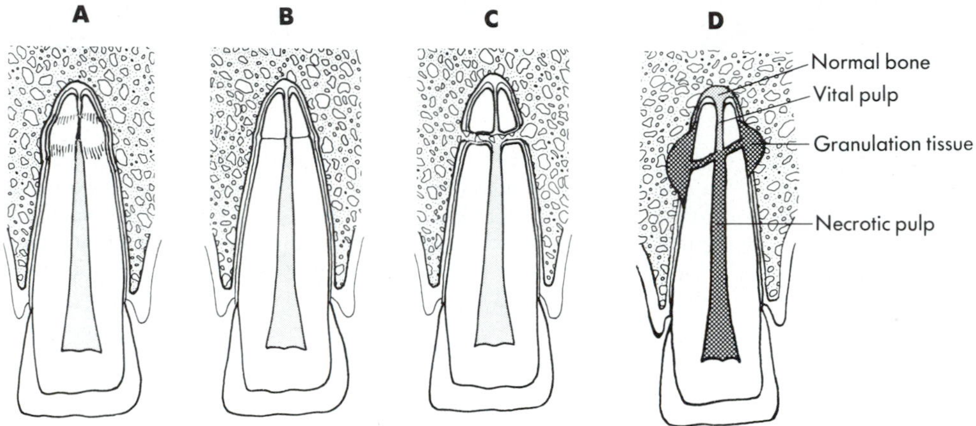

FIG. 16-7 Varying patterns of healing of a root fracture. **A,** Calcific callus union. **B,** Connective tissue union. **C,** Combination bone and connective tissue healing. **D,** Nonunion and granulation tissue formation. The apical pulp segment frequently remains vital.

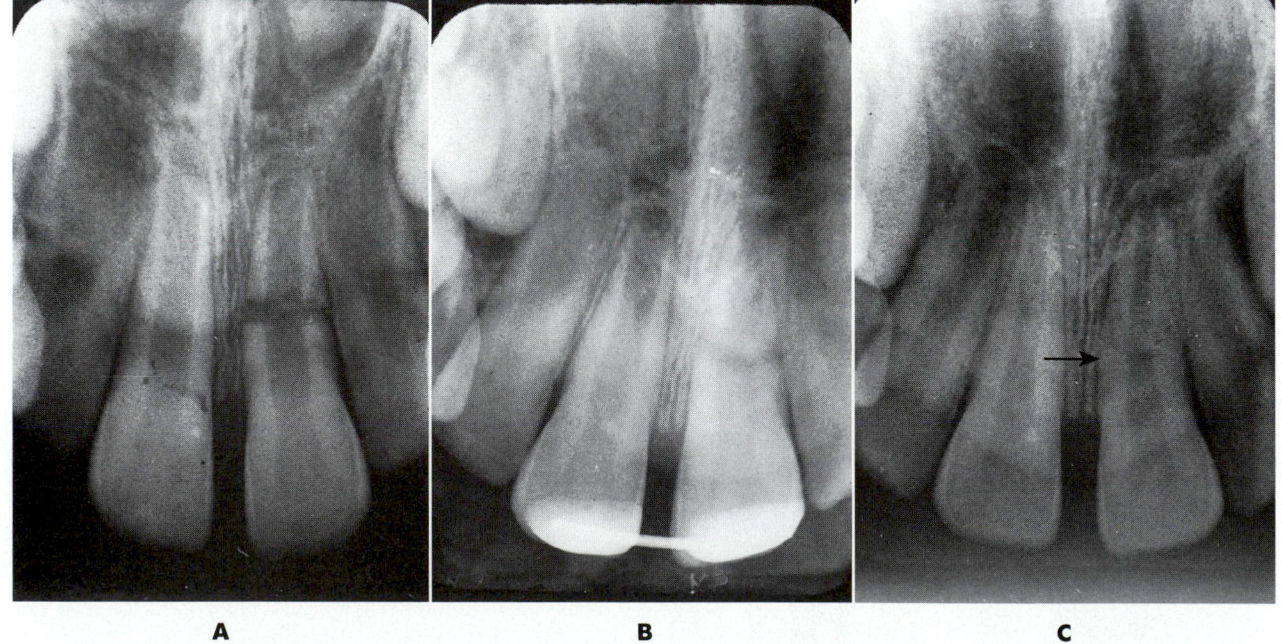

FIG. 16-8 Fracture in the middle third of a root treated by repositioning and splinting only. **A,** Initial examination of the central incisor an hour after the trauma. Note the separation of segments. **B,** Wire and acrylic splint. **C,** One-year follow-up. Both central incisors are equally responsive to pulp testing. Note the callus formation *(arrow)* and reduced pulpal lumen.

surfaces may be lined by cementum, and the sharp edges of the fracture may be rounded by surface resorption. The tooth will have little mobility after healing and pulp tests will be essentially normal. The connective tissue will be seen on the radiograph as a definite fracture line.

Combination bone and connective tissue healing. With further separation of the fragments and possible mobility of the broken parts, there may be growth of new bone between the fracture segments (Fig. 16-7, *C*). The fractured surfaces will be lined by cementum with a periodontal ligament between the tooth and the new bone. The tooth will be quite firm and the pulp will be vital to test procedures.

Healing with nonunion and granulation tissue formation. When there is severe dislocation of the fractured root, a constricted root canal space,[8,11] and/or possible contamination of the pulpal tissues by oral fluids, the pulp may be sufficiently injured or infected to undergo necrosis. Generally the incisal portion of the pulp will undergo necrosis and the apical segment will remain vital.[36,225] The necrotic pulp will stimulate inflammation and granulation tissue formation in the fracture lines. The inflammation will spread to the alveolar bone adjacent to the fracture line, causing resorption of bone in this area. Radiographically the widening of the fracture line and the loss of alveolar bone adjacent to the fracture will be evident. The tooth will be loose, sensitive to percussion, perhaps turning dark, and slightly extruded (Fig. 16-7, *D*).

Treatment philosophy of teeth with fractured roots

Studies[31,176,225] have shown that the *majority of teeth with root fractures will maintain vitality of the pulpal tissues.* This has had a direct effect on the philosophy of treating root fractures. Given the tendency for the pulpal tissues to remain vital, the primary purpose of treatment is to enhance this natural tendency for healing.

It is obvious that a tooth root with a calcific callus formation reuniting the broken fragments is stronger than one without union of broken parts. The ultimate goal of the clinician faced with a broken tooth root problem should be to attempt to gain reunion of the broken root by calcified callus formation. Preservation of the vitality of the pulp will certainly enhance the prognosis for achieving that ultimate goal as opposed to immediately proceeding with root canal treatment, with the strong possibility of extruding cement or sealer into the fracture site. Although the pulpal tissues are not essential to healing of the root fracture,[158] they are preferable to a foreign material in the fracture site. Therefore *the fracture should be reduced as soon as possible and the broken tooth firmly immobilized.* To avoid possible tearing of the pulpal tissues, excessive lateral pressure on the incisal portion of the fractured root should be avoided during repositioning of the broken parts. Contamination of the pulp through the fracture line with saliva or other contaminants should be carefully avoided. If necrosis of the incisal portion of the pulp occurs, reunion of the calcified tissues is not likely to occur. Every effort must be made to enhance healing of the delicate pulpal tissues.

With this philosophy of treatment as a basis, it becomes logical to divide root fractures into two types: those not communicating and those communicating with the oral cavity.

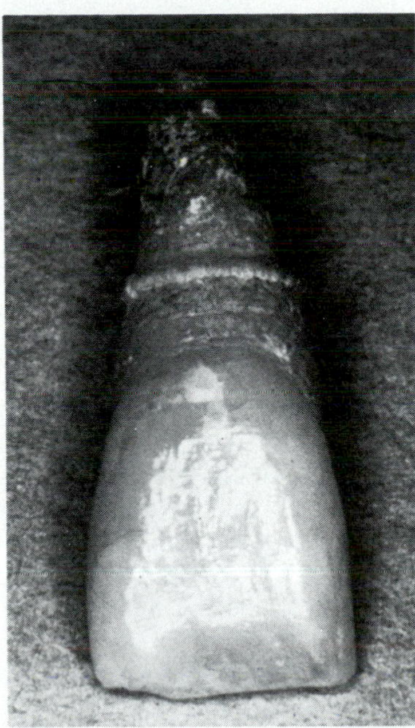

FIG. 16-9 Extracted tooth exhibiting callus formation of the root.

TREATMENT OF THE FRACTURED ROOT NOT COMMUNICATING WITH THE ORAL CAVITY

The noncommunicating fracture is generally in the apical or the middle third of the root. Diagnosis is dependent on possible mobility or displacement of the tooth, percussion sensitivity, and a correct angulation of the radiographic exposure.

The customary electric and thermal pulp tests should be done and carefully recorded. The degree of mobility and displacement as well as any tooth discoloration should also be noted on the chart. If the pulp is determined to be vital to clinical tests, the only treatment necessary is repositioning of the tooth to proper alignment and immobilizing by splinting to the adjacent teeth. The sooner the fracture is reduced prior to organization of a fibrin clot, the easier the fragments can be repositioned. If bone fragments interfere, they will have to be molded into position, permitting realignment of the tooth. A radiograph should be taken after repositioning the fractured parts to confirm realignment.

The time for leaving the splint in position varies from 1 week to 3 months or more depending on the location of the fracture and the degree of mobility of the tooth. If the fracture is in the apical third of the root and there is minimal displacement or mobility, a splint may not be necessary. At the other end of the spectrum, if the fracture is at the crest of the alveolar bone with moderate displacement and mobility of the crown the splint may have to remain in position for 3 months. The clinician must exercise judgment in each instance. No good clinical studies of a sizable number of cases have been documented to determine the relationship between the time of splinting and the healing of fractured roots. A suggested rule of thumb for midroot fractures is 2 to 3 months. The tooth with the fractured root will need to be reevaluated as to the stability of the splint at 30 to 60 days following the accident.

When the splint is removed, the clinical status of the traumatized area must be determined. The degree of mobility, color of the crown, and percussion and palpation sensitivity need to be recorded as well as the responsiveness to electric and thermal tests. The depth of the gingival sulcus must be determined and recorded. Root fractures that retain vitality of

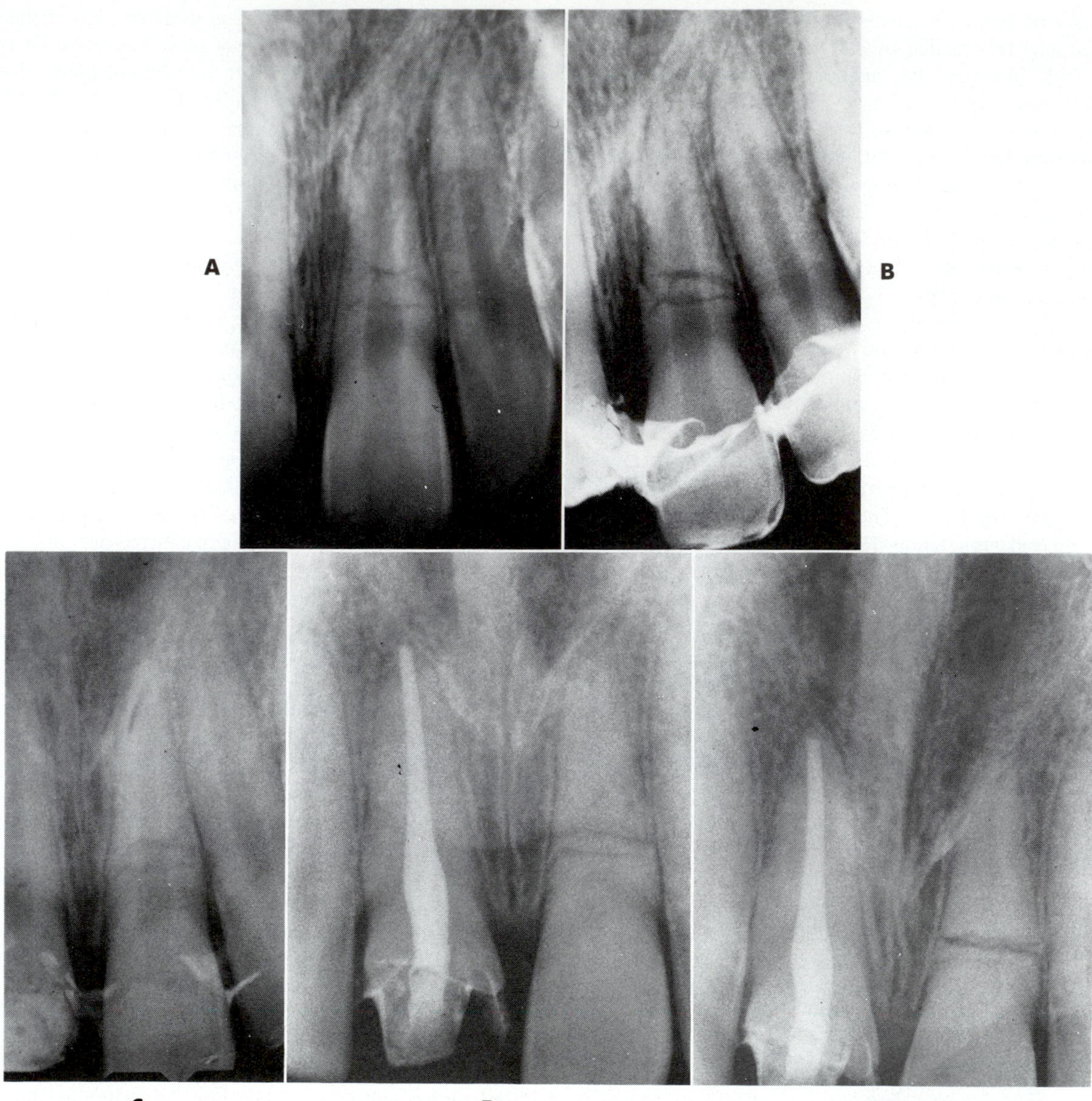

FIG. 16-10 Fractured incisal third of a root. **A,** Left central incisor with a fracture of both crown and root. **B,** Splinted with acrylic and cemented with zinc oxyphosphate. **C,** Three months after injury. **D,** Nine years after injury. Endodontic treatment was necessary on the right central incisor as well. Note the pulpal obliteration of the left central. **E,** Same as **D** but with a 10-degree variation in radiographic vertical angulation. Note the difference in appearance of the fracture. (Compare with Fig. 16-6.)

the pulp have been shown to heal 77% of the time.[225] Closure of the root canal is an indicator of a vital pulp.

If the periodontal attachment has failed to heal and the probe penetrates the periodontal ligament space to the depth of the fracture site, the prognosis for healing of the fracture and retaining vitality of the pulp diminishes drastically.

If there is minimal mobility, the tooth responds positively to pulp tests and has not darkened in color, the patient is comfortable, and the radiograph indicates that healing is progressing, then no further treatment is necessary except to repeat the evaluation at 6-month and 1-year intervals. Any variations from this list of indicators of healing will indicate that complications are occurring.

If mobility is present, the splint must be reapplied and the occlusion adjusted to eliminate stress on the tooth. If after 4 to 6 months the tooth continues to be mobile and the fracture site cannot be probed through the gingival sulcus, the tooth should be permanently splinted to the adjacent teeth.

All root fractures that do not communicate with the oral cavity after repositioning of the broken fragments should be treated as if the pulp is vital regardless of the results of the pulp tests at the initial emergency visit. If complications occur subsequently, indicating pulp necrosis, endodontic treatment should be instituted at that time.[123,125]

Root Fractures with Evidence of Pulpal Necrosis

The radiographic appearance of bone destruction in or adjacent to the fracture site is the best indicator of pulpal necro-

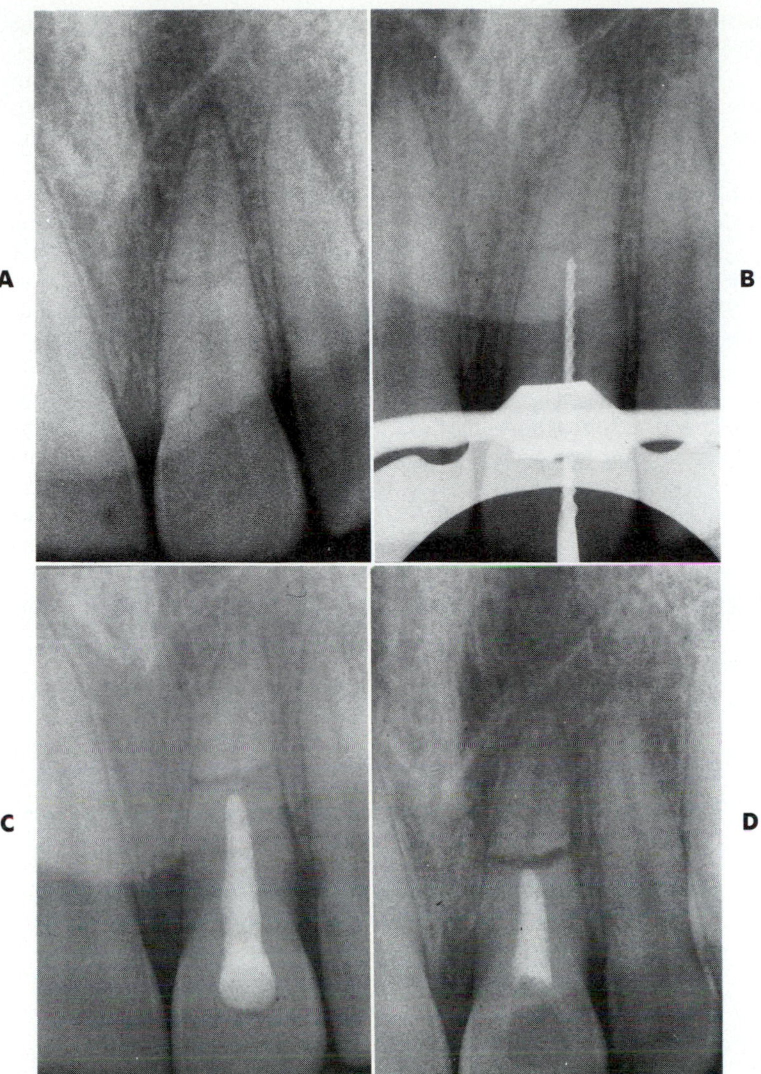

FIG. 16-11 Necrosis of the incisal segment of a pulp, with subsequent endodontics on the coronal segment only. **A,** Initial injury. **B,** Three months later the coronal pulp necrosed, and endodontic treatment was initiated. Vital tissue was noted in the apical segment. **C,** Treatment completed. **D,** Two years after treatment of the coronal segment.

sis,[123] and may take several months to develop. Lack of response to electric and thermal pulp tests without radiographic evidence of bone destruction adjacent to the fracture site does not warrant instituting endodontic therapy.[225] Darkening of the tooth and sensitivity to percussion and palpation are more reliable than electric and thermal pulp tests as indicators of pulpal necrosis.

Pulpal necrosis subsequent to root fractures has been shown to occur from 20% to 44% of the time. The occurrence of necrosis of the pulp seems to be related not to the location of the root fracture in the apical, middle, or incisal third but rather to communication with the oral cavity and the severity of displacement of the incisal segment.[31,32,225] If there is evidence of pulpal necrosis of the coronal portion of the pulp, it is generally believed that the apical segment will remain vital.[11,36,123] Endodontic treatment is therefore usually confined to the coronal segment of the root canal (Fig. 16-11).

Cvek[77,79] made the interesting observation that the displaced coronal segment of the root-fractured tooth should be treated similarly to a displaced intact tooth.

The coronal portion of the tooth with a fractured root and necrotic pulp can be filled with gutta-percha after routine endodontic instrumentation of the coronal segment (Fig. 16-11) if it meets the following criteria:

1. There is no evidence of a periapical radiolucency at the end of the apical segment.
2. The space between the two fragments at the fracture site is minimal.
3. The root canal space is sufficiently constricted at the apical end of the coronal segment to permit creation of a mechanical stop for condensation of gutta-percha.
4. The apical segment of the pulp bleeds when touched with a paper point, indicating that vascularity is intact and permitting healing of the apical segment.

Filling the coronal portion of the pulpal space with calcium hydroxide seems to be indicated with the following criteria.[77,79,123]

1. There is no evidence of a periapical radiolucency at the end of the apical section.
2. The apical segment of the pulp seems vital as evidenced by bleeding on a paper point.
3. A radiolucent space is evident between or adjacent to the fractured segments.
4. A widened space can be detected between the broken fragments.
5. There is evidence of internal or external resorption of the coronal segment.
6. A wide root canal space makes a filling of the root canal with gutta-percha difficult, with a strong possibility of extrusion of the gutta-percha or cement into the fracture site.

Because pulp tests are not reliable in determining the vitality of the coronal pulp, endodontic treatment is generally not instituted until a radiolucency is visible at the fracture site. Therefore most teeth with fractured roots requiring endodontics in the coronal segment are treated with calcium hydroxide. When healing of the fracture site is evident after 6 months to a year, the calcium hydroxide can be replaced with gutta-percha.

If the periodontal attachment is intact, preventing leeching of calcium hydroxide from the fracture site, and mobility is minimized, the prognosis for healing is excellent.[77,79,225]

If a radiolucency is present at the apex of the apical segment, this indicates pulpal necrosis in that segment as well. Root canal treatment of both the coronal and the apical fragments is indicated (Fig. 16-12, *A*). This is feasible if both fragments are well approximated and access to the root canal of the apical fragment can be obtained through the coronal segment.

Various authors[97,161,223] have advocated the use of rigid filling materials to tie the two fragments together. The rigid filling materials may be necessary in instances of persistent mobility, generally in fractures involving the coronal third of the root. However, these concepts have slowly begun to change with the advent of the more esthetic acid etch resin splint and greater documentation of healing capacity of root fractures that do not communicate with the oral cavity.[36,122,125] The prognosis is markedly reduced, with persistent mobility, and healing that utilizes the rigid internal splint is questionable.

It has also been suggested[91] that the greater sealing capac-

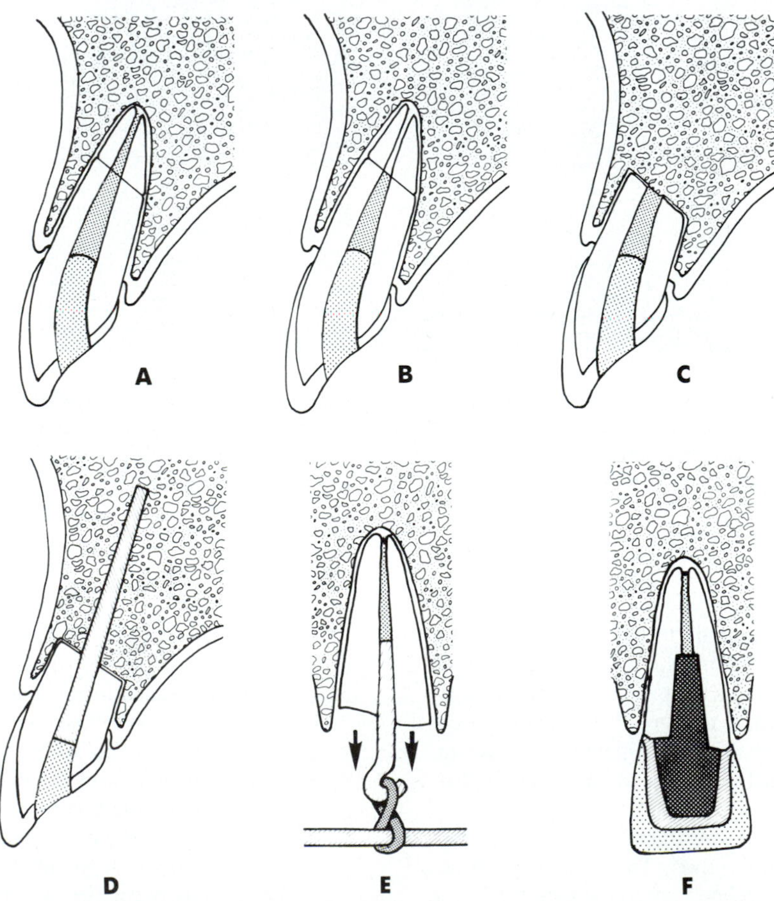

FIG. 16-12 Configurations of endodontic treatment of a fractured root. **A,** Coronal and apical segments. **B,** Coronal segment only. The apical segment pulp remains vital. **C,** Coronal segment with surgical removal of the abscessed apical segment. **D,** Endosseous implant for stabilization of the tooth with an excessively short root. **E,** Orthodontic extrusion of the apical segment after a fracture of the incisal third. **F,** Restoration of the orthodontically extruded apical segment.

ity of gutta-percha makes it more appropriate as the filling material of choice. Furthermore, healing without a rigid internal splint has been documented.[158] Recent research has shown calcific union of the incisal and apical segments following complete pulpal necrosis, utilizing $Ca(OH)_2$ therapy and long-term splinting for a year.[177]

Adequate studies have not been done comparing the healing of teeth with fractured roots and pulpal necrosis of the coronal and apical segments utilizing gutta-percha, calcium hydroxide, or a rigid filling material as an internal splint. Less than 1% of dental injuries are of this type, making clinical studies difficult.

If pathosis exists in the apical segment and endodontic treatment is not possible, the apical segment must be removed surgically (Figs. 16-12, *C*, and 16-13). Frequently loss of the apical fragment does not create mobility problems.

The loss of the apical segment occasionally creates problems of an unfavorable crown root ratio. With improvements in the acid etch composite resin techniques, it is possible to achieve permanent splinting for a tooth with minimal root structure. Placement of a "Maryland bridge" type of framework or direct interproximal bonding may be utilized for permanent splinting to the adjacent teeth.

The placement of an endodontic endosseous implant has been advocated to improve the stability of the coronal segment[31,90,91] (Fig. 16-12, *D*). However, in addition to the experimental status designation by the American Dental Association (ADA), recent studies[31,192] have shown corrosion of the implants and persistent inflammation around them. The Council of Dental Materials, Instruments, and Equipment of the ADA[72] has recently stated that it does *not* currently recommend endosseous implants for routine clinical practice. Unfortunately the endodontic endosseous implant, which has the advantage of utilizing a natural tooth with its periodontal attachment, has been grouped with implants for replacement of missing teeth that do not develop a periodontal attachment. However, in view of this official position of the ADA, it is advisable that the clinician obtain written informed consent from the patient before utilizing the endodontic endosseous implant for tooth stabilization.

Root Fractures with Pulpal Obliteration

After reduction of the fracture site and splinting and adjustment of the occlusion, the fracture will generally heal. One of the manifestations of healing is heavy calcification of the pulpal space, which has been reported in 69% to 86% of cases.[31,125] The obliteration seems to take two different patterns: partial obliteration occurs in the apical root canal space and the fracture site extending 1 or 2 mm into the coronal fragment, or the entire pulpal space becomes progressively obliterated.

The type of repair seems to be influenced by the severity of the fragment dislocation and the healing capacity of the pulp.[8,11] With moderate displacement of the fragments and a large root canal space, the likelihood of total pulpal obliteration increases,[8,11,125] Studies[123] have shown that 21% of root-fractured teeth undergoing total pulpal obliteration also have pulpal necrosis. Since there are four out of five chances that the pulp will not necrose in the presence of heavy pulpal calcification, intervention with endodontic treatment to prevent calcific pulpal obliteration does not appear to be justified.[122,152]

Tooth Color

After traumatic injuries a tooth may undergo a variety of color changes. These are frequently subtle and difficult to compare from one evaluation appointment to another. Lighting, adjacent restorations, dryness of the tooth, stains, and normal variations in tooth color all create errors in using color as a diagnostic criterion. Subjective judgment, varying from clini-

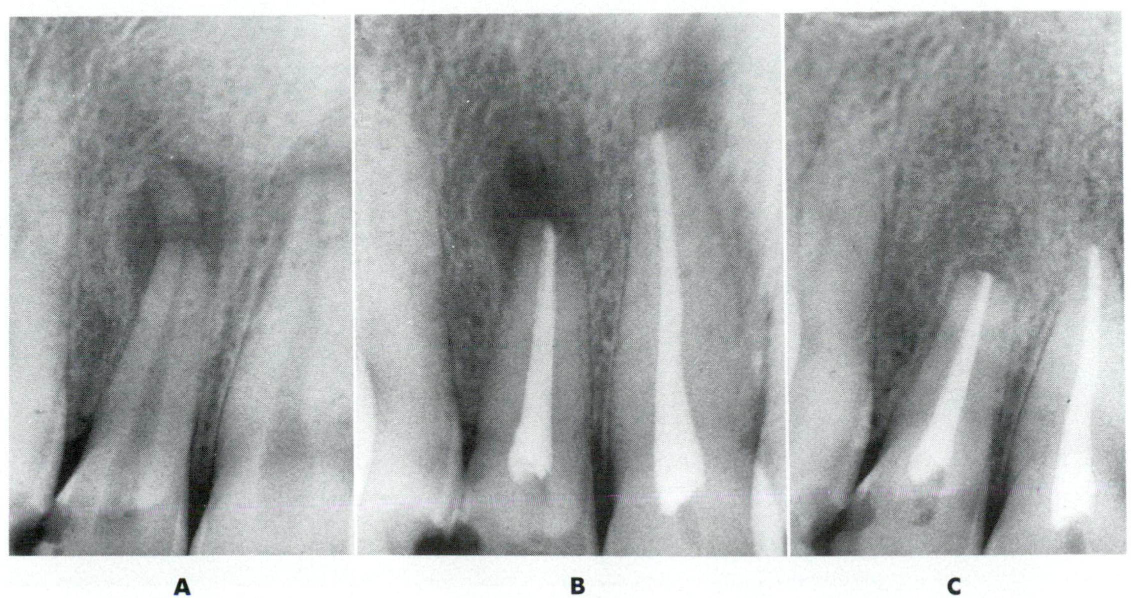

FIG. 16-13 Root fracture with pulpal necrosis and periapical pathosis. **A,** Initial examination. The patient reported a history of trauma approximately 1 year earlier. **B,** Endodontic treatment and surgical removal of the apical segment. **C,** Nine months subsequent to treatment. The periapical lesion is healing.

cian to clinician, and different descriptive phrases also create inaccuracies.

In the face of these realistic variables, it may be stated that a dramatic change from normal tooth color to a distinct strong pink, purple, or dark gray can be taken as indicative of pulp necrosis when combined with tenderness to percussion and radiographic changes. A change to yellow or yellow-brown may indicate calcification of the pulp chamber as confirmed on the radiograph. Caution must be used in determining pulpal status by color. We have seen teeth with discoloration and no response to vitality tests in which the pulps were found to be vital.

Root fractures in permanent anterior teeth with incompletely developed roots are relatively unusual because of the tendency of these short-rooted teeth to be displaced rather than fractured. In these rare instances the large apical foramen seems to enhance healing. If the periodontal attachment is intact and adequate immobilization is attained, the tooth root will probably continue to develop normally.[121] However, obliteration of the pulp is more likely to occur in these teeth.

ROOT FRACTURES COMMUNICATING WITH THE ORAL CAVITY

Fractures of any part of the root coronal to the periodontal attachment have a poor prognosis for healing. There is periodontal breakdown along the fracture line with subsequent pulpal necrosis from the microbial contamination of the pulp through the fracture (Fig. 16-14).

The typical situation is the fractured maxillary incisor with the fracture on the labial surface 2 to 3 mm supragingival but tapering obliquely to 2 to 5 mm subgingivally on the lingual. A similar fracture can occur with premolar and molar cusps. The emergency visit will require anesthetizing the patient facially and lingually and teasing off the broken crown from the residual periodontal attachment on the lingual. Endodontic treatment should be completed in one visit. Frequently the natural crown can be recemented on the tooth root with the aid of a temporary post or splinted to the adjacent teeth with acid etch resin. It makes an excellent temporary covering and tends to prevent invagination of the lingual gingiva into the fracture site.

When the emergency has been resolved, plans must be made for restoring the tooth. In this instance clinical judgment becomes very important. The choices are (1) periodontal gingival and osseous surgery to expose an adequate amount of tooth structure for a crown margin, (2) extrusion of the root until all the fracture site is supragingival sufficient for restoring the tooth (Fig. 16-12, *E* and *F*), (3) combined orthodontic extrusion and periodontal gingival and osseous recontouring for adequate margination, and (4) removing the clinical crown segment and retaining the submerged root with its vital pulp followed by placement of a fixed bridge across the space (Fig. 16-15). If the root pulp is necrotic, endodontic treatment must be accomplished. At the emergency appointment, removing the crown permits evaluation of the depth of the fracture. If the deepest aspect of the fracture is greater than approximately 2 mm below the bone level, extrusion of the tooth seems preferable to periodontal surgery. If less than 2 mm below bone on the lingual, periodontal gingival and osseous surgery seems indicated. The reason for this arbitrary distinction is that a minimal periodontal surgical procedure on the lingual will not compromise the support of the tooth, will not involve adjacent teeth, can be maintained hygienically, and will not alter the appearance of the tooth.

Periodontal procedures on the facial create an esthetic problem, and extrusion is preferable. When periodontal healing has occurred the tooth is restored with a post and crown. The reader is referred to Chapter 22 for these procedures.

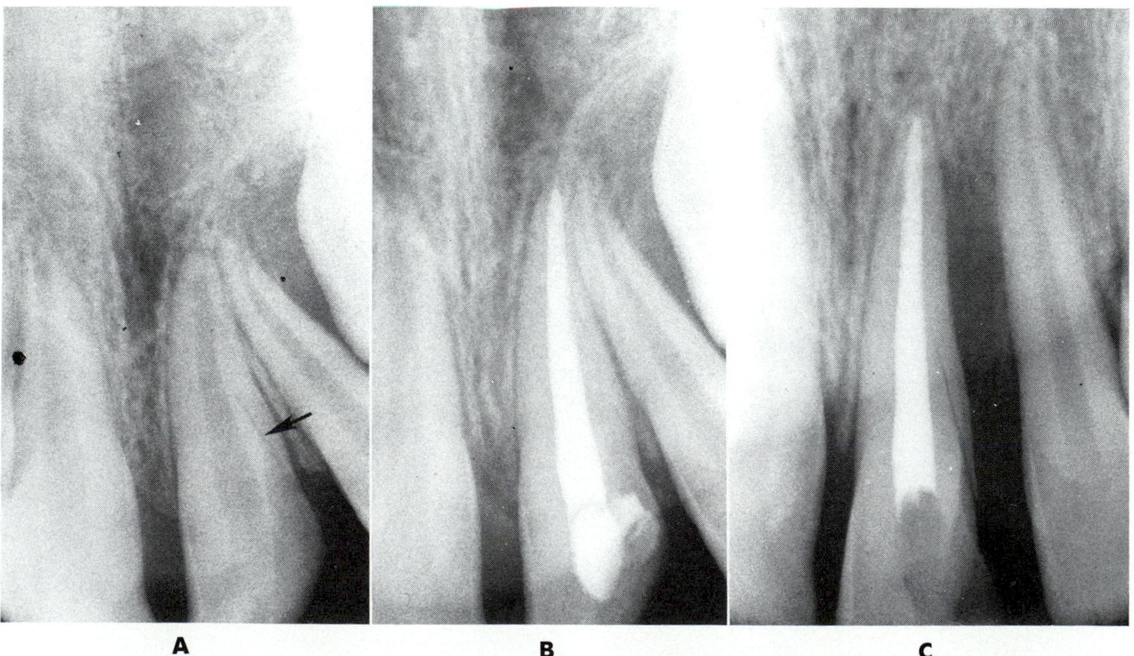

FIG. 16-14 Vertical root fracture communicating with the oral cavity. **A,** Immediately after the trauma. Note the vertical root fracture *(arrow)*. **B,** Root canal filled with gutta-percha. **C,** Two years later a severe periodontal defect developed adjacent to the vertical root fracture.

Extrusion of the root is preferable if excessive periodontal surgery will be required to expose the fracture site. Heithersay[109,110] added the concept of combined endodontic-orthodontic treatment of fractured teeth to the treatment options (Fig. 16-12, *E, F*). Since then the technique has become a standard in the treatment of subcrestal defects.[85,154,165] A recent variation[76] suggests cementing the permanent post and core prior to beginning orthodontic treatment, thus eliminating the need for repeated post preparations.

Ingber[120] introduced an interesting concept into the treatment of cervical third root fractures. By utilizing small tattoo marks he showed that the marginal gingiva will follow the root as it is extruded orthodontically. The fractured root is extruded until the marginal gingiva and underlying bone have moved coronally beyond the level of the gingival crest of the adjacent teeth. Then the tooth is stabilized in the new position for 4 to 6 weeks to permit reorientation of the gingival fibers. During this stabilization period, the gingiva may migrate apically[52] and minimize the gingival and osseous surgical contouring required to align the height of the bone and gingiva with that of the adjacent teeth. However, periodontal surgery is almost invariably required before crown construction. This combined endodontic-orthodontic-periodontal technique has several advantages. By the surgical exposure of the root a better margin is obtained for restoring the tooth with less orthodontic movement. In contrast to a strictly periodontal surgical approach, the Ingber technique does not leave a residual periodontal defect on the broken tooth and does not affect adjacent teeth. When the periodontal and the orthodontic approaches are combined, the crown/root ratio of the result is stronger than with either technique alone. The coronal movement of bone requires less extrusion and less periodontal recontouring.

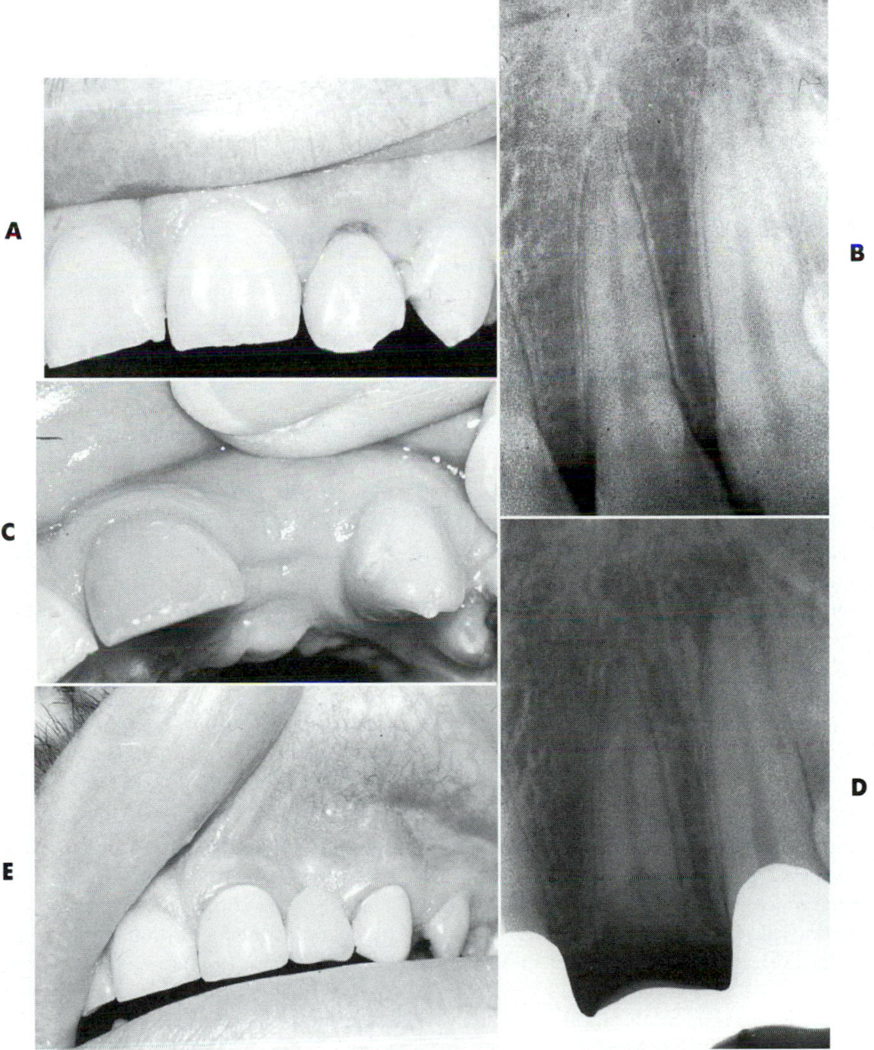

FIG. 16-15 Root fracture at the alveolar crest. The root was retained to preserve the alveolar ridge. **A,** Clinical view of a fractured lateral incisor with slight displacement of the crown. **B,** Radiographic view of the root fracture. The patient refused the opportunity for root extrusion but was willing to retain the root to preserve the alveolar ridge. **C,** Healed alveolar ridge after crown removal. **D,** Eighteen-month follow-up radiograph of the retained root after placement of a fixed bridge. Note the developing periapical lesion on the canine abutment. **E,** Clinical view of the bridge.

To prevent the coronal migration of bone and gingiva, it has been shown that repeated intrasulcular incisions through the supracrestal attachment apparatus every 2 weeks stops the migration and eliminates the need for osseous surgery. It also reduces the stabilization period because the crestal periodontal fibers no longer have a tendency to relapse.[138]

If for some reason the patient objects to wearing an orthodontic appliance, an "immediate" surgical extrusion of the tooth may be done. This requires careful, intentional extrusive displacement of the tooth with elevators until an adequate amount of tooth is available supragingivally for a crown margin. The tooth is stabilized in its extruded position with multiple sutures and periodontal dressing.[132-134,211] It has been suggested, in instances of diagonal fractures, with the apical extent of the fracture line on the lingual, that the tooth root be rotated so that the longer facial surface of the crown can cover the more extensive fracture defect.[133,212]

Endodontic treatment may be delayed a week after the tooth has been repositioned and stabilized. This facilitates a more accessible and aseptic endodontic procedure.[221] After 6 weeks the tooth can be restored with a post and crown.

Primary Teeth with Fractured Roots

Primary teeth with root fractures are unusual, since they are short rooted and therefore are generally displaced.[16]

When root fractures occur, the primary root will heal if there is little dislocation of the coronal fragment and normal physiologic resorption will occur.[31]

If the coronal fragment is severely dislocated, the primary tooth should be extracted. Similarly a fracture that communicates with the oral cavity is an indication for extraction. Any small root fragments remaining in the socket should be left there, for they will be resorbed.[36]

Displaced Teeth

Some authors[31,97,218] have referred to traumatized teeth as having concussions, subluxations, and partial or total luxations. There is confusion as to the differences among these terms. Different authors have used varying definitions. In the discussions to follow, concussion, displacement, and avulsion will be used since they seem to be adequate for clinical differentiation and treatment of traumatic conditions.

Concussion is an injury to a tooth and its attachment apparatus without displacement from its position in the alveolus. The most noticeable clinical finding is a markedly increased sensitivity to percussion. While there is no visible displacement, mobility may be present.

Displacement refers to an injury in which the tooth is moved from its position in the socket. If there is any movement of the tooth from its customary position, it has been displaced. The displacement may be lateral (facial, lingual, mesial, distal), extrusive (out of the socket), or intrusive (deeper into the alveolar bone) (Fig. 16-16).

Avulsion is the complete dislocation of the tooth from its socket.

Traumatic injuries to the tooth apparently cause obstruction of the major pulpal vessels at the apex. Subsequently there is diffusion of blood with dilation of the pulpal capillaries. The congestion of the capillaries is followed by capillary degeneration with release of erythrocytes and edema of the pulp. Because of the lack of collateral circulation in the pulp, there is little inflammatory response to the injury and the pulp may undergo partial or complete ischemic infarction. With little or no circulation the pulp persists in this fashion for months or years. A transient bacteremia may penetrate small vessels at the apex and eventually become established in the infarcted pulpal tissues.

The infection that follows may be the first clinical indication of pulpal necrosis. Stanley and associates[204] noted that in some cases the infarction process is not total. A few vessels may remain functioning and transport fresh blood to parts of the pulp.[95] These parts will remain vital. If pulp tests indicate negative responses but the pulp chamber has sensitive tissue and bleeding in the deeper parts, a persistent blood supply is supporting some nerve fibers.[7] Apparently the thermal-mechanical receptors in the pulp are obstructed by the infarcted tissue, preventing transmission of a stimulus received through the enamel and dentin.[204]

It is inferred that if the trauma to the tooth and enclosed pulp is minimal, the brief pulpal ischemia may cause reversible superficial infarcts. This might account for the return of positive pulpal responses weeks later.[187]

A transient apical breakdown of the periapical bone and periodontal ligament has been described following moderate displacement injuries to fully formed teeth. It is suggested that this is part of the healing process. As the periapical areas heal for a period of months, responsiveness to electric pulp tests often returns.[6,8]

Concussion

In concussion injuries the blow to the tooth may be sufficient to cause bleeding in the periodontal ligament and pulpal edema.[31] The increased fluid in the periodontal ligament apparently increases the pressure of masticatory forces on the tooth and is uncomfortable to the patient because of the preexisting intraligamentary pressure.

The pulp may not respond to tests initially, but positive responses can return weeks or months later. Teeth that test vital immediately after the trauma tend to remain vital. At 3 months there is a high correlation between teeth testing vital and those remaining vital indefinitely.[48,187]

In concussion injuries the only treatment required is adjusting the tooth slightly out of occlusion. Pulp tests for vitality should be repeated and compared with the initial appointment base line at 1-, 3-, 6-, and 12-month intervals (Fig. 16-16). If the tooth initially responds positively and then responds negatively, this is a strong indicator of pulpal necrosis.

Displacement

If a tooth is displaced from its socket minimally, it will be slightly mobile and sensitive to percussion and biting pressure. There may be some bleeding from the gingival sulcus because of injury to the periodontal ligament. A slight thickening of the periodontal ligament may be noted radiographically. This tooth probably will not require splinting. If there is *any* doubt as to the necessity for a splint, one should be placed on the tooth.

It has been shown that tooth mobility in conjunction with other injuries significantly increases the incidence of pulpal necrosis. Coronal fractures without concussion or mobility produced a 3% incidence of pulpal necrosis. However, coronal fracture with concussion and mobility increased the incidence of pulpal necrosis to over 30%.[182-184]

Teeth with obvious clinical or radiographic displacement

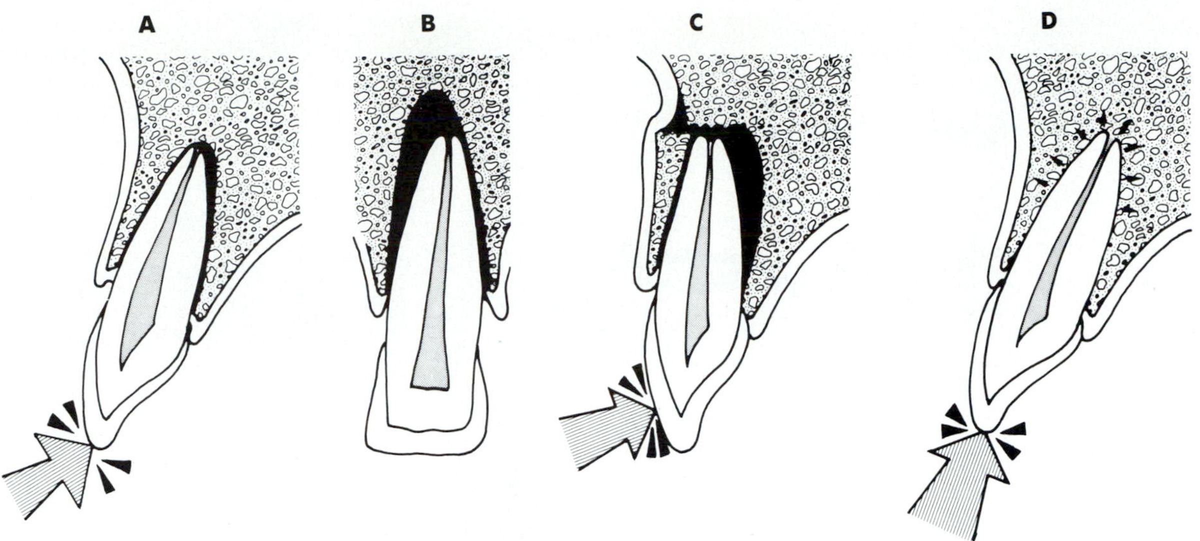

FIG. 16-16 Configurations of displaced teeth. **A,** Lateral displacement. In this instance the crown is forced lingually and the root facially. The same relationship would apply to mesial-distal lateral displacements. **B,** Extrusive displacement. **C,** Major lateral displacement with fracture of the alveolar bone. **D,** Intrusive displacement.

must be repositioned and splinted. Teeth with minor displacement are not routinely endodontically treated; however, approximately half of these will ultimately undergo pulpal necrosis and require root canal therapy.[188] Therefore these teeth must be followed clinically to determine pulpal status.

Major displacements

Teeth with major displacements (over 5 mm) from their position in the socket have sustained severe injuries. These injuries may be accompanied by alveolar bone fractures (Fig. 16-16, *D*). Diagnosis is obvious by extrusion of the tooth or facial-lingual displacement.

If multiple teeth are involved, as in an automobile accident, several teeth may be displaced and their normal positions may be confused. These teeth will have to be repositioned to occlude with the opposing arch.

An occlusal radiograph has been shown to be the best exposure for disclosing extrusive and lateral displacements, and occlusal and periapical exposures are equally good for disclosing intrusive displacements.[9]

Radiographically, an extruded tooth will exhibit a markedly increased periodontal ligament space apically. If the root has been displaced in a mesial or distal direction, the widened space will be evident on the mesial or distal surface of the root (Fig. 16-17). If the root has been forced in a facial or lingual direction, the widened space may be masked by the tooth root in its new position.

Thermal and electric pulp tests are unpredictable in displaced teeth. The problem of reliable pulp tests with traumatized teeth has been discussed. Generally, the more severe the displacement and the greater the mobility the less likely the pulp will survive.[187]

Lateral and extrusive displacements. In detecting severe lateral displacements when the root is forced facially and the crown lingually, it is helpful to palpate the facial mucosa at the level of the root apex. With marked displacement the root end can be forced through the cortical plate of bone and can be felt with digital pressure. The tooth may be locked into the bone in the displaced position and will not be mobile. In repositioning the tooth it may be necessary to apply finger pressure on the root apex in a coronal direction to move it back through the fenestration into the socket. The fractured cortical bone can be molded back into place with fingers (Fig. 16-18).[31] The teeth should be radiographed immediately prior to splinting to confirm their correct repositioning.

Teeth with major lateral displacements or those extruded from the socket are repositioned in the socket and splinted for 7 to 14 days. They must be adjusted out of hyperocclusion. The time interval in repositioning displaced teeth is important because of the possibility of root resorption. Teeth repositioned in 90 minutes from the time of injury have less root resorption. There is also a greater possibility of loss of periodontal support with delayed repositioning.[16]

Teeth that have been displaced long enough for blood to be thoroughly clotted around them should not be repositioned forcefully, because of possible induction of root resorption. It is preferable to move them into their normal position orthodontically after healing has occurred. If a tooth is severely displaced and interfering with closure of the mouth, it should be adjusted to allow normal occlusion. When closure cannot be achieved by occlusal adjustment, it will be necessary to extract and replant the tooth. The socket should be irrigated with saline or water and aspirated to remove the blood clot. If curettage is necessary to remove the clot, care must be taken to prevent damage to the periodontal ligament. In this instance the tooth must be treated as one that has been avulsed.

Intrusive displacements. The intruded tooth is severely traumatized and requires special attention. This injury is second only to avulsion in severity. Depending upon the strength of the blow the intruded tooth may look short and be confused with a fractured crown. Sometimes it will be completely intruded into the bone and mistakenly assumed to be lost. The

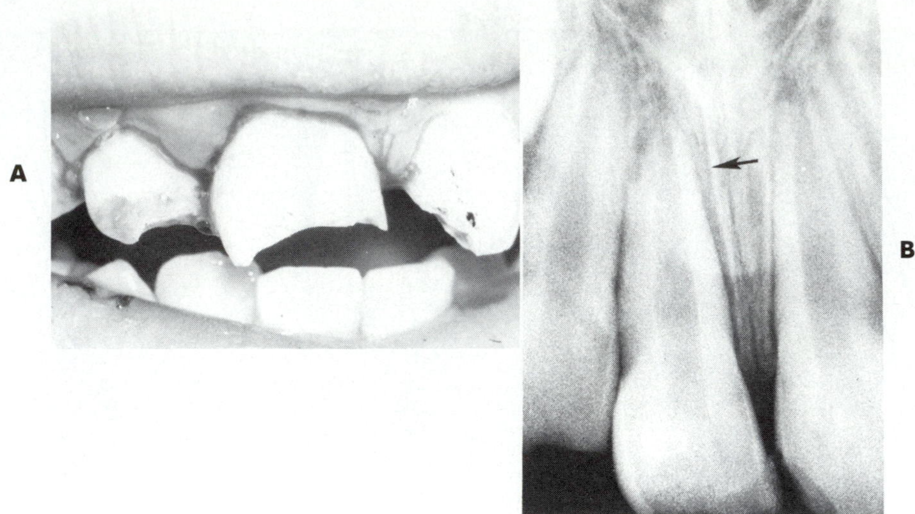

FIG. 16-17 Lateral displacement of a maxillary central incisor. **A,** Clinical view of the injury. Note the gingival sulcular hemorrhage and the crown fractures. **B,** Radiographic view of the injury. The periodontal ligament space is widened on the mesial of the right central incisor *(arrow)*.

tooth is so firmly wedged in the bone that it is not mobile. Percussion will sound hard and harsh as compared to that of a normal tooth. If a permanent central incisor is completely intruded, it may have penetrated the floor of the nose and may even be seen in the nostril[17] (Fig. 16-19). The radiograph may show a loss of the periodontal space around a minimally intruded tooth. With a severe intrusive displacement the radiograph will show the location of the tooth and the severity of the intrusion.

Treatment of the intruded tooth is variable. A minimally intruded tooth will frequently reerupt spontaneously, particularly one with incomplete root formation. If the intrusion injury is severe, it will be necessary to retrieve the tooth with forceps and to splint it (Fig. 16-19) or move it into position orthodontically. The least complications of root resorption and loss of crestal bone support occur when the intruded tooth is moved into position orthodontically over 3 to 4 weeks.

Ankylosis may occur as a sequel to root resorption. Recent evidence has shown that ankylosis occurs in as few as 5 to 6 days in experimental animals subjected to intrusive forces.[216] Orthodontic extrusion should be initiated promptly following injury in order to move the tooth into proper position prior to the onset of possible ankylosis.[201]

Another consideration is that pulpal necrosis will occur (seen in 96% of intruded teeth).[16] In addition, external root resorption increases in the presence of necrotic pulps.[31] *To prevent the onset of inflammatory resorption, the fully formed intruded tooth must have the pulp removed within 1 to 2 weeks of the time of injury.* Subsequently, calcium hydroxide therapy should be instituted soon after pulp removal. Andreasen[24] has shown that placement of calcium hydroxide should be delayed at least 7 days after an injury to allow for initial healing of the periodontal ligament. Therefore it must be in position to allow access to the root canal, which is another justification for proceeding with orthodontic treatment promptly rather than waiting for spontaneous eruption that might take several months. If the intrusion has not inhibited access to the pulp chamber, waiting for spontaneous eruption is a possibility; however, ankylosis may occur preventing movement of the tooth into its proper position. Sometimes gingival scar tissue will inhibit spontaneous eruption and will have to be surgically removed to speed eruption.[193]

Complications of displacement injuries. The major complications of displacement injuries have been described by Andreasen.[16] They are pulpal necrosis, pulpal obliteration, root resorption, and loss of marginal bone support (Fig. 16-20).

1. Pulpal necrosis, noted in 52% of displacement injuries, occurs in 96% of intrusive injuries. Reports vary concerning the incidence of pulpal necrosis following extrusive injury, from 64% to 98%. The risk of pulpal necrosis increases with the severity of the injury to the pulp and periodontal ligament and with the degree of constriction of the root canal space and apical foramen.[14,75] It is more likely to occur in teeth with fully developed roots than in those whose roots are incompletely developed.[8,12]

2. Pulpal obliteration with calcified tissue occurs approximately 20% to 25% of the time.[16,32] It is a response to a moderate injury such as minimal displacement. Severe displacement will probably lead to pulpal necrosis. The pulp is more likely to survive after trauma in teeth with incompletely formed roots, but these teeth are also more likely to have pulpal obliteration.[8,13] With intrusive injuries there is a high incidence of pulpal necrosis, so pulpal obliteration is uncommon.[16]

Pulpal necrosis subsequent to pulpal obliteration occurs in approximately 10% of traumatized teeth.[16,122] Therefore prophylactic pulp extirpation performed after evidence of pulpal obliteration with calcifications is not justified.[31,122,152] A successful rate of 80% in endodontically treated teeth with pulpal obliteration has been noted.[79]

3. Root resorption is usually seen after intrusive injuries; the next highest incidence follows extrusive injuries. Intrusions are also the injuries that have the higher incidence of pulpal necrosis. It is thought that the presence of the necrotic pulp contributes to root resorption.[31] Root resorption can be de-

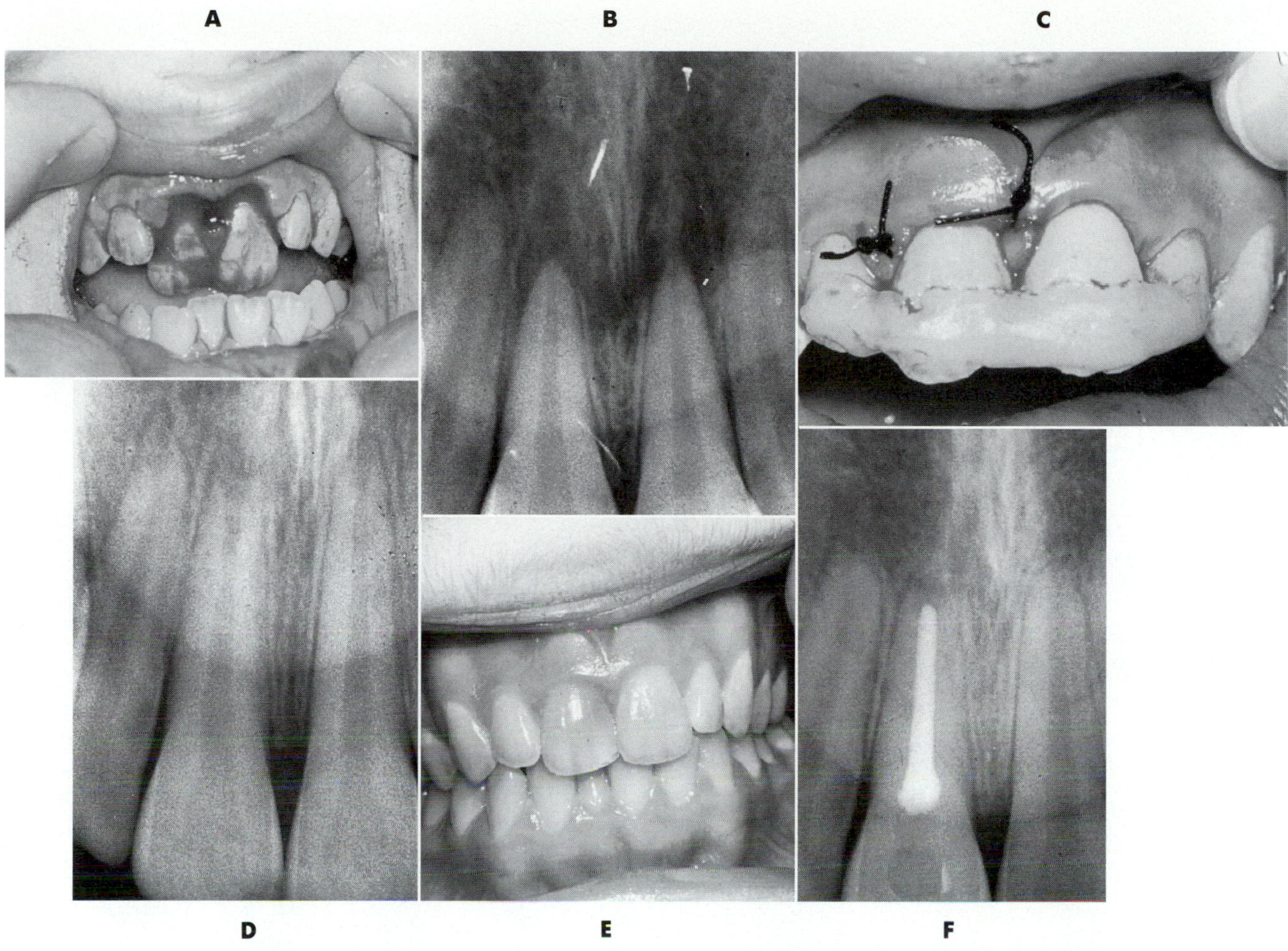

FIG. 16-18 Severe extrusive displacement of the maxillary central incisors. **A,** Clinical view of the injury. Note the extrusive and lingual displacement of both centrals, suggesting bone fracture because of segmental displacement. Today, gloves should be used. **B,** Radiographic view showing the displaced bone and teeth. Note the intact bone interproximally between the traumatized teeth. White marks are film scratches. **C,** Teeth and bone repositioned and splinted. Gingiva sutured. **D,** Six-month follow-up. A periapical lesion is developing around the right central. **E,** Clinical view at 6 months. Note the darkening of the crown of the right central. The left central responds normally to pulp testing. **F,** One year after the injury. The bone has healed, and the left central remains vital to pulp tests.

tected as early as 2 months after an injury, but it may also be delayed for several months.[16] An extended period of splinting is thought to contribute to root resorption.[171]

4. Loss of marginal bone support increases with the severity of the injury, particularly in intrusive and extrusive injuries. Delayed repositioning of the teeth also increases the risk of damage to the supporting periodontal tissues.[16]

Endodontic treatment of displaced teeth. Endodontic treatment of displaced teeth must be a clinical decision made on a case-by-case basis. Several factors may be helpful in deciding whether or not to enter the root canal. The primary determining factor for endodontic treatment is the diagnosis of pulpal necrosis. This is based on percussion sensitivity, marked discoloration, lack of pulpal responses to thermal and electric tests, and radiographic appearance (Fig. 16-18). Traumatized teeth are notoriously unreliable in responding to pulp tests.

In mature permanent teeth having severe displacement (over 5 mm) or intrusive injuries, pulpal necrosis is quite likely. Root canal treatment is therefore indicated in these teeth since the incidence of root resorption is particularly high. Applying calcium hydroxide as the temporary root canal filling material seems justified to prevent the onset of root resorption (Fig. 16-19).

Teeth with minimal displacement will require splinting and close monitoring of pulpal status and radiographic appearance at 1, 3, 6, and 12 months.[8] If a periapical radiolucency appears or inflammatory resorption becomes evident, endodontic treatment should be started promptly. A periapical radiolucency occurring without simultaneous inflammatory resorption in a completely developed tooth would warrant endodontic treatment with gutta-percha. Any evidence of inflammatory root resorption would be justification for using calcium hydroxide temporarily to assist in arresting the root resorption.[79]

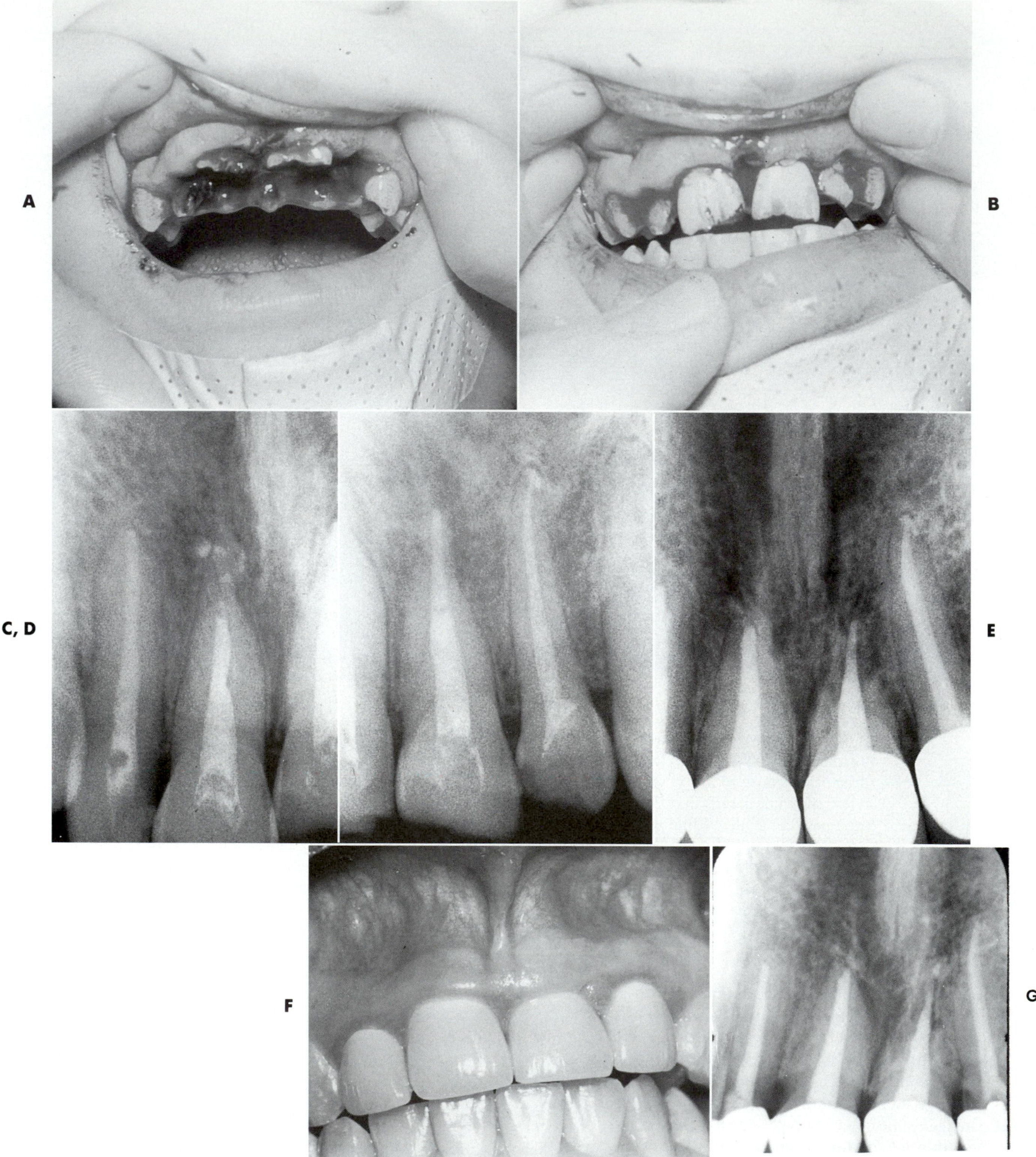

FIG. 16-19 Severe intrusion of the permanent central and lateral incisors. **A,** Clinical view of the traumatic injury. The roots of the teeth protruded into the nasal cavity. Today, gloves should be used. **B,** Teeth surgically repositioned. Note the minor crown fractures. **C** and **D,** Root canals filled with calcium hydroxide with barium sulfate added to improve radiopacity. **E,** Nine-year follow-up. The calcium hydroxide was removed 2 years after treatment, and the root canals were filled with gutta-percha. Note the minimal resorption of the apical third of the root of the left central incisor. **F,** Clinical view of the crowns placed on the teeth. **G,** Twenty-year follow-up showing very little change.

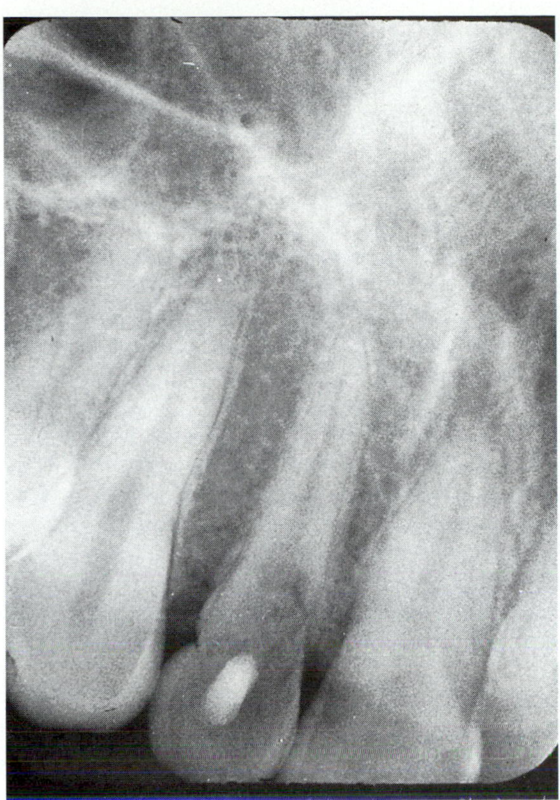

FIG. 16-20 Pulpal necrosis and resorption following a concussion injury. Maxillary central and lateral incisors were injured in a fall 4 months previous to radiograph. The maxillary central is pulpless; the lateral is vital but undergoing massive external resorption.

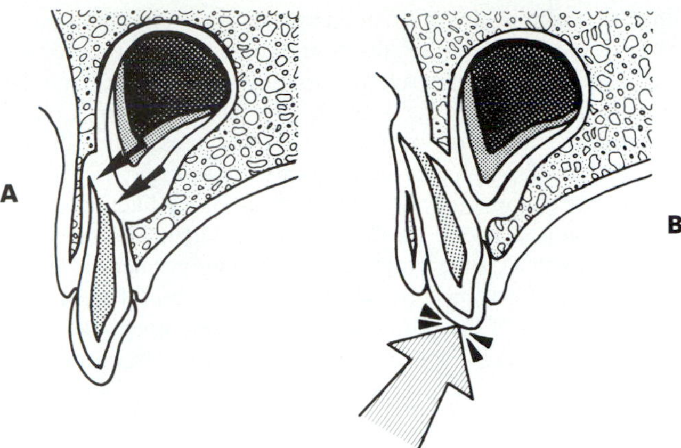

FIG. 16-21 Primary tooth displacement. **A,** Normal resorption of the primary root occurs on the lingual due to eruption of the permanent tooth. The apical portion of the primary root curves facially. **B,** Lateral displacement injuries to the primary tooth generally force the primary root facially with little injury to the erupting permanent tooth.

A displaced tooth with an incompletely developed root has a better prognosis for pulp survival.[14,16] Retention of the vital pulp is desirable to enhance normal development of the root. On the other hand, inflammatory root resorption in immature teeth progresses more rapidly.[31] Close monitoring of these teeth radiographically is therefore essential. When the decision is made that pulp necrosis has occurred or there is evidence of a periapical radiolucency or root resorption, endodontic treatment should begin promptly. Calcium hydroxide is used to fill the canal until the apex has closed and root resorption has been arrested. This is followed later by a permanent filling of gutta-percha.

In a retrospective study of 885 displaced nonvital incisors that were followed for up to 4 years after completion of endodontic therapy, Cvek[80] found that once periapical healing occurred or inflammatory resorption was arrested it was unlikely that deterioration would occur later. In those instances of cervical root fractures following treatment, there was a marked correlation with the stage of root development. If a cervical root fracture occurred, it was far more likely to occur in an incompletely developed and thin-walled root than in a thicker, more mature root.

Displaced primary teeth

In young patients displacement occurs more frequently than crown or root fracture because of the resiliency of the alveolar bone and the shorter tooth roots.[15]

Determining the angle of displacement is critical in diagnosing displaced primary teeth since the primary roots are so close to the developing permanent teeth. The most typical displacement injury results in the crown's being tilted lingually while the root is forced facially but the tooth remains intact. If the root of the primary tooth has been forced facially, there is less likelihood of damage to the underlying permanent tooth (Fig. 16-21) than if the primary tooth has been forced lingually or intruded. Then the possibility of damage to the permanent tooth is greatly increased.

It has been noted that about 10% of the enamel hypoplasias in permanent anterior teeth are the result of trauma to the primary tooth. The enamel hypoplasias were primarily white and yellow-brown. More serious injuries such as permanent crown or root malformations and sequestration of the permanent tooth germ are possible but not likely.[40]

Treatment of the concussed or minimally displaced primary tooth is confined to clinical and radiographic checkups.

Severe lateral or intrusive displacements will require radiographic ascertainment of the root position. An occlusal film held by the parent on the face of the child so that a lateral view of the traumatized tooth is obtained can be helpful in diagnosing the position of the root.[31,219]

If the root of the primary tooth has been displaced facially, the prevailing opinion[31,38,178] is that the tooth should be allowed to reerupt spontaneously. There seems to be no difference in complications for the permanent tooth if this is allowed to occur.[38] Furthermore, there is the possibility of increased damage to the permanent tooth by attempts to extract the traumatized primary tooth.[213] Reeruption will generally occur in 1 to 6 months.[31,180] If the intruded primary tooth does not reerupt in 2 to 3 months, it may be ankylosed and have to be extracted. Also, if cellulitis develops, the intruded primary tooth should be extracted.

If the primary root is displaced lingually into the developing permanent tooth, the primary tooth should be extracted.[31] The primary anterior tooth root is resorbed initially from the lingual. There is also a facial curvature to the remaining root. Since most traumatic accidents are from a frontal direction, we believe that primary anterior tooth displacements force the crown lingually and the root facially (Fig. 16-21). Consequently, the incidence of primary anterior teeth being driven into the developing permanent tooth is quite low.

The parent and child should be warned of the likelihood that serious damage to the developing tooth will occur when the primary tooth is driven into the developing permanent tooth. Insurance and litigation possibilities require careful records of the accident until the permanent teeth have erupted and have been carefully examined for developmental disturbances.

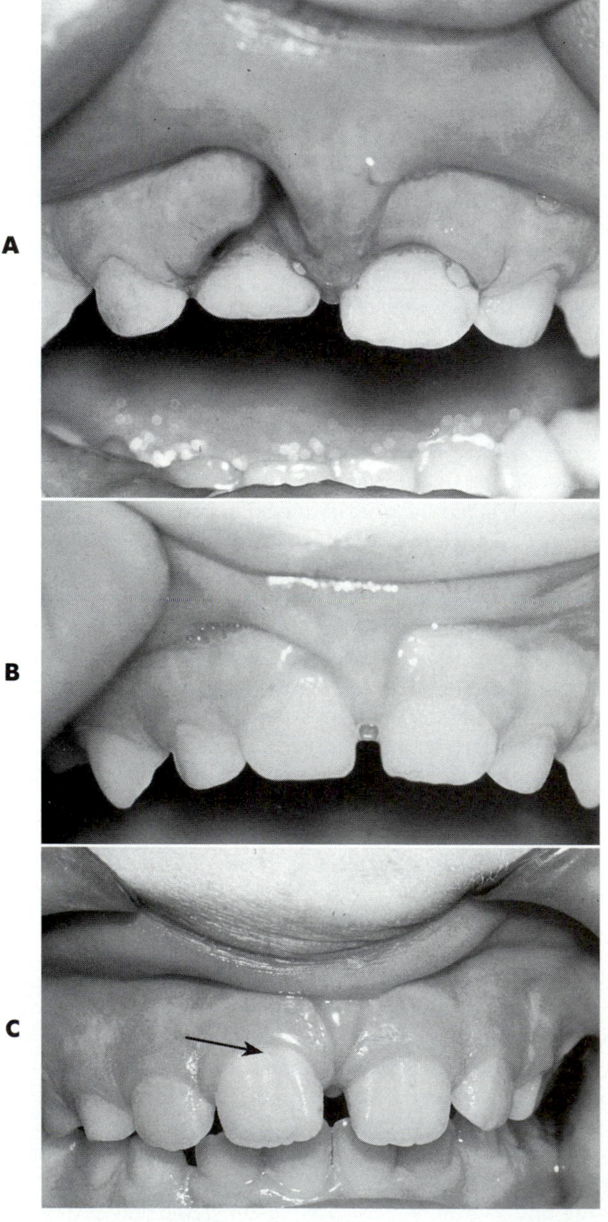

FIG. 16-22 Intruded primary tooth. **A,** Clinical view of the primary right maxillary central incisor. **B,** Six weeks later the tooth has reerupted spontaneously. **C,** Six-year clinical follow-up of the erupted permanent incisor. Note the very slight enamel hypoplasia defect at the gingival line *(arrow)*.

There is a distinct conflict of opinion concerning treatment of displaced primary teeth. One opinion is that these teeth should be extracted.[31,74,79] An opposing view, which we hold, is that displaced primary teeth should be retained (Fig. 16-22).[116]

The reasoning behind our view is that for primary teeth endodontic therapy is a successful procedure. If the primary tooth is displaced rather than avulsed, it generally has a sufficient root to reattach in the socket. Therefore, if it can be repositioned and stabilized, it should be retained just as a permanent tooth is retained. In our experience the facial curvature of the primary tooth enables it to be snapped back into position, often not even requiring a splint. If the tooth is mobile, an acid etch splint for 7 to 10 days is desirable.

The open apex of the primary tooth lends itself to revascularization.[124] Sometimes root canal treatment is not necessary. Discoloration of the primary tooth crown without evidence of periapical pathology is not likely to cause damage to the crown of the developing permanent tooth.[200] If signs of pulpal necrosis such as persistent percussion sensitivity, radiographic evidence of periapical radiolucency, or continuing darkening of the tooth occurs, endodontic treatment should be instituted.

Intruded primary teeth that have been permitted to reerupt will have pulpal necrosis in approximately one third of the cases.[180] The diagnosis of pulpal necrosis is based upon tenderness, periapical radiolucencies, and discoloration. One study[124] showed that 50% of graying discolorations were reversible in primary teeth. The gray discoloration subsequently turned yellow from pulpal obliteration. Caution in diagnosing pulpal necrosis should be exercised. Pulpal necrosis of 6 weeks' duration with associated periapical inflammation did not cause damage to the developing permanent tooth in monkeys.[41] When pulpal necrosis of the primary tooth has been diagnosed, endodontic treatment of the primary teeth should be initiated promptly to eliminate the periapical inflammation.

It is thought that the initial impact of injury to the primary tooth causes the greatest damage to the developing permanent tooth.[38,213,219] Consequently, if the decision has been made to retain a primary tooth with facial displacement of the root, routine pedodontic-endodontic therapy is justified to eliminate periapical inflammation of extended duration.

Minor Fractures of the Alveolar Process

If comminuted minor bone fractures occur simultaneously with trauma to the teeth, they should be molded back into place with the fingers (Fig. 16-18). No retained bone fragments should be discarded. The shorter the time interval between accident and repositioning of bone fragments, the greater will be the success rate.[16] This is due to the fact that the blood clot has not yet organized and exposure of bone to contamination has been minimized. If subsequent sequestration of bone occurs, the loss of periodontal support of involved teeth is permanent but the teeth may remain clinically functional.[16]

If the gingiva has been torn, it should be carefully sutured around the teeth at the cervical line. The teeth should be splinted for 7 to 10 days. However, if the fracture of bone is extensive, a longer splinting period may be required.

Complete Avulsion and Replantation

Complete avulsion or exarticulation occurs when a traumatic injury totally displaces a tooth from the socket. Variations in the reported incidence of complete avulsion range from 1% to

16% of all traumatic injuries to the permanent dentition and from 7% to 13% of traumatic injuries to the primary dentition.[15,185] Males experience complete avulsion three times as often as females; and the most frequently involved age groups are 7 to 11 years, as the permanent incisors are erupting.[34,98,145] According to Andreasen[31] the loosely structured periodontal ligaments surrounding erupting teeth favor complete avulsion.

The maxillary central incisors are the most frequently avulsed teeth in both the permanent and the primary dentition. Usually only one tooth is involved, and rarely are the mandibular teeth affected.

Factors affecting the success of replantation

Although there are reports of replanted teeth remaining in function for over 40 years,[34,49] most are ultimately lost because of progressive root resorption or problems associated with ankylosis in the growing child. Although reattachment usually occurs, approximately 75% to 85% of all replanted teeth are affected by progressive root resorption.[2,34,145] The rate of root resorption is age-related and progresses more rapidly in younger than in older patients.[2,3] A replanted tooth with a necrotic periodontal ligament in a young child will usually be resorbed within 3 to 7 years, whereas the same tooth in an older patient may remain functional for decades or throughout life.[2]

Many times the prognosis for the avulsed tooth is jeopardized by mismanagement of the situation. This is not surprising in light of the many conflicting techniques and philosophies contained in the replantation literature. Current techniques taught by various disciplines within dentistry differ greatly from those taught by other disciplines. Many of the previously accepted standards in treatment of avulsed teeth were based upon empiricism rather than scientific research, and numerous principles applied to the treatment of bony fractures had been erroneously adopted in the management of avulsed teeth. Although much remains to be discovered, the application of recent research has dramatically improved the prognosis for longer periods of retention of replanted teeth.

Extraoral time. Universal agreement exists that *the shorter the extraoral period the better the prognosis for retention of the replanted tooth*. Among the factors associated with root resorption, the length of extraoral time seems to be most critical.[15,20,81] The storage medium during extraoral time has also been shown to be critically related to the prognosis[25,56] (see below).

A well-documented clinical and radiographic study[34] with observation periods of 2 years or more showed that 90% of teeth replanted in less than 30 minutes exhibited no discernable resorption of the roots whereas 95% of teeth replanted after 2 hours demonstrated root resorption. These clinical findings have been substantiated by animal experiments.[1,25,151] The importance of extraoral time was summed up by Grossman and Ship,[98] who pointed out that success diminishes inversely with the length of time the tooth is out of the mouth; the longer the extraoral time, the less the success.

However, it should be noted that teeth may be replanted with success many hours or days after avulsion. Teeth replanted from 6 hours to 48 days after avulsion and treated endodontically were examined 1 to 7 years later and shown to be clinically functional. Although ankylosed and undergoing replacement resorption, there was no evidence of periapical infection.[107] Teeth replanted within a few minutes at the site where the injury occurred have the best prognosis for reattachment and prolonged retention. Consequently, when a parent or patient informs the dentist by telephone of an avulsed tooth, instructions should be given to replace the tooth in the socket. If the tooth is covered with debris, it can be cleaned by sucking on it or running cold tap water over it. The tooth should not be scrubbed or chemically cleansed in any manner. It is then teased into the socket and held in place until the patient reaches the dental office.

The education of allied professions as to the proper treatment to be rendered at the site of a dental injury is the responsibility of dentistry. Medical and allied personnel most likely to encounter injured persons after an accident should be able to render dental first aid and instruct patients as to the necessity of immediate dental care. Obviously medical injuries of a severe nature would take precedence over dental injuries. Individuals such as pediatricians, emergency room physicians and attendants, school nurses, athletic coaches and trainers, police officers, fire fighters, and other emergency personnel likely to be the first on the site of an injury or the first consulted following an injury should be instructed in proper first aid for dental injuries.[66]

Storage media and transportation of avulsed teeth. To prevent further damage to the periodontal ligament cells, whenever possible, the avulsed tooth should be replanted at the site of the accident. Since viability of these cells has been shown to be of utmost importance,[21,24,29] the storage medium is critical if immediate replantation is not feasible. When replantation is delayed the tooth should be stored in a physiologic medium to prevent further injury to the periodontal ligament cells.[57] Under no circumstances should the tooth be allowed to dry, because this accelerates cellular necrosis.[147,199] Extended storage in an unsuitable environment causes increased necrosis of cells, which leads to ankylosis and extensive root resorption.[2]

Because of its physiologic osmolality, composition, and markedly fewer bacteria, milk has been shown to be superior to saliva for the storage of the avulsed tooth.[54,59,146] Mitotic activity of periodontal cells has been maintained after storage in milk for up to 6 hours.[147] Storage in milk for longer than 6 hours has been proven unsatisfactory.[115,215] The nonphysiologic osmolality, less favorable composition, and presence of microorganisms makes saliva a less desirable storage medium for the avulsed tooth. However, it is preferable to dry storage for short periods.[56,147]

Andreasen[25] has shown that the storage medium may be more important than the extraoral time. Short periods of dry storage proved harmful, whereas prolonged storage in physiologic saline or saliva did not significantly impair periodontal healing. Surface resorption was found to be similar, regardless of the extraoral time or storage medium; however, inflammatory resorption was much more with dry storage. Replacement resorption was significantly increased with dry storage or storage in tap water. It was concluded that physiologic saline or saliva offers good protection against root resorption during the extraoral period.[25]

While physiologic saline is satisfactory, it is not as readily available as milk. When teeth were stored in milk, much less root resorption, especially inflammatory resorption, was observed than when they were stored in saliva. Storage of avulsed teeth in saliva for 2 to 3 hours causes swelling and membrane damage to periodontal ligament cells owing to saliva's nonphysiologic osmolality.[57,59]

Hank's balanced salt solution (HBSS) has been used for years to support and maintain various mammalian cells in tissue cultures. Clinical success[140] of 91% coupled with excellent results reported[115] in maintaining lip fibroblast vitality in tissue cultures have led to the recommendation to use HBSS as an extraoral transporting medium for avulsed teeth. Histologic study[215] has shown HBSS to be superior to milk and comparable to Viaspan, a new medium presently used for transplant organ storage. Storage times up to 12 hours showed repair of all resorption in 8-week specimens. Results at 72 and 96 hours were comparable to 6- and 12-hour results. Thus, in cases where medical complications preclude reimplantation of avulsed teeth for a few days, storage in HBSS preserves viability of the periodontal cells until it can be achieved.

A system has been developed to transport avulsed teeth that cannot readily be replanted at the site of the injury. SAVE-A-TOOTH (Biological Rescue Products, Conshohocken, Pa.) contains a basket in which the teeth are suspended in HBSS, thus providing an optimal storage and transport medium. These small containers may be purchased and kept at sites such as schools, gymnasiums, sports facilities, emergency vehicles, and homes to be used if the need arises (Fig. 16-23).

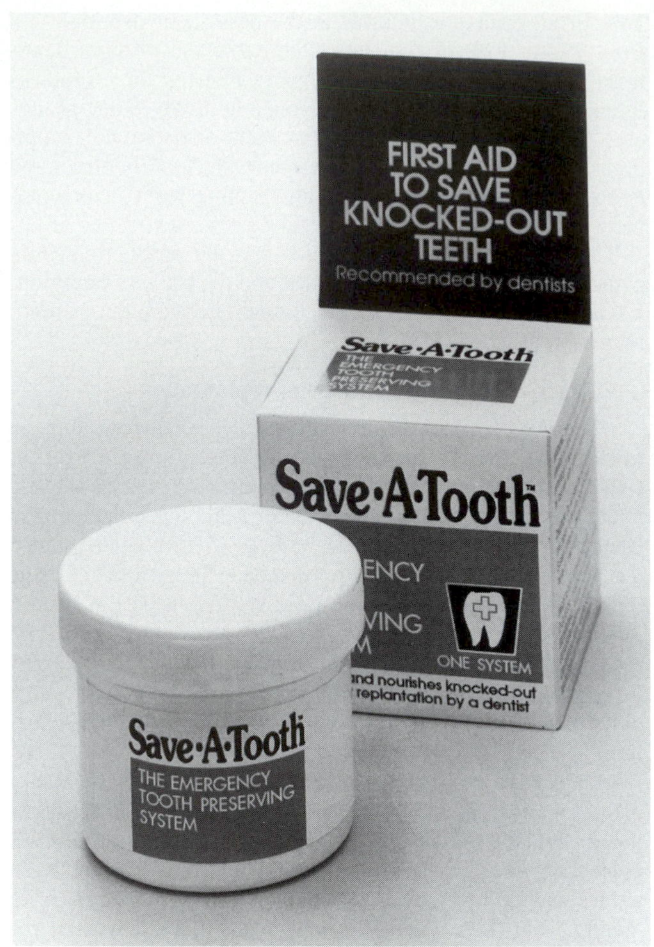

FIG. 16-23 Save-A-Tooth transport product. (Courtesy Biological Rescue Products, Conshohocken, Pa.)

Numerous investigations[27,58,202] have demonstrated the importance of keeping the avulsed tooth moist during the extraoral period. Allowing air drying of the periodontal ligament cells always increases resorption and ankylosis. While milk, HBSS and physiologic saline are the best storage media, these may not readily be available when immediate replantation is impossible.

It has been shown that periodontal ligament fibroblasts can survive 60 minutes of storage without culture medium if kept in a humid atmosphere. Storage of avulsed teeth in dry plastic foil for 60 minutes prior to replantation resulted in periodontal healing similar to that in teeth replanted immediately.[58] Thus, wrapping a tooth in plastic foil to prevent air drying seems advisable if it cannot be immediately replanted or stored in a physiologic medium such as milk.

The critical time of dry storage is about 30 minutes, after which irreversible damage to the periodontal ligament cells will occur, leading to a marked increase in root resorption following replantation.[25,42] Replantation after dry storage for 60 minutes resulted in inflammatory resorption over the entire root surface within 8 weeks.[58,100]

Using tissue-culturing techniques, Söder and associates[199] demonstrated that after 2 hours of dry extraoral time, periodontal ligament cells will not demonstrate cell viability. As time increases, the number of viable cells declines very rapidly.

Preservation of the periodontal ligament and resorption. When immediate replantation cannot be achieved and a more physiologic medium is not readily available, the tooth should be placed in the oral vestibule or under the tongue while the patient is transported to the dentist. If there is danger of aspiration because of the age of the patient or the extent of injury, the tooth may be placed in the mouth of the parent for transportation. Under no circumstances should the tooth be allowed to air dry. At the very least, storing it in a moist towel or in a cup of water is preferable to allowing the tooth to dry.

Andreasen[28] has concluded that the presence of an intact and viable periodontal ligament on the root surface is the *most* important factor in assuring healing without root resorption. He has also shown that resorption is more likely to occur on certain areas of the root surface of an avulsed tooth than on others. These are the surfaces of the root receiving the most trauma during the removal of the tooth because the periodontal ligament is forced against the alveolar process, damaging cementoblasts. Resorption takes place on the root surfaces directly beneath the areas of cementoblastic damage.[29]

Healing in a tooth with a normal periodontal ligament is not achieved when it is replanted with a necrotic periodontal membrane. Ankylosis will develop as the necrotic tissues are replaced by bone.[4,21,25] The presence of vital periodontal tissues has been shown to inhibit invasion of bone cells, whereas its absence has led to the opposite effect.[157] It has been postulated that the periodontal ligament and cementum contain a potent collagenase inhibitor which probably represents an antiinvasive factor that resists the invasion of bone.[149]

Extensive replacement resorption occurs when the periodontal tissues are removed before replantation.[28,31,37] It has been demonstrated that even after all the periodontal fibers are devitalized, a tooth replanted with the periodontal tissues still attached resorbs more slowly than one replanted with denuded roots.[151] Therefore, regardless of the extraoral time, the periodontal ligament should not be removed or treated with any caustic chemicals prior to replantation of an avulsed tooth.

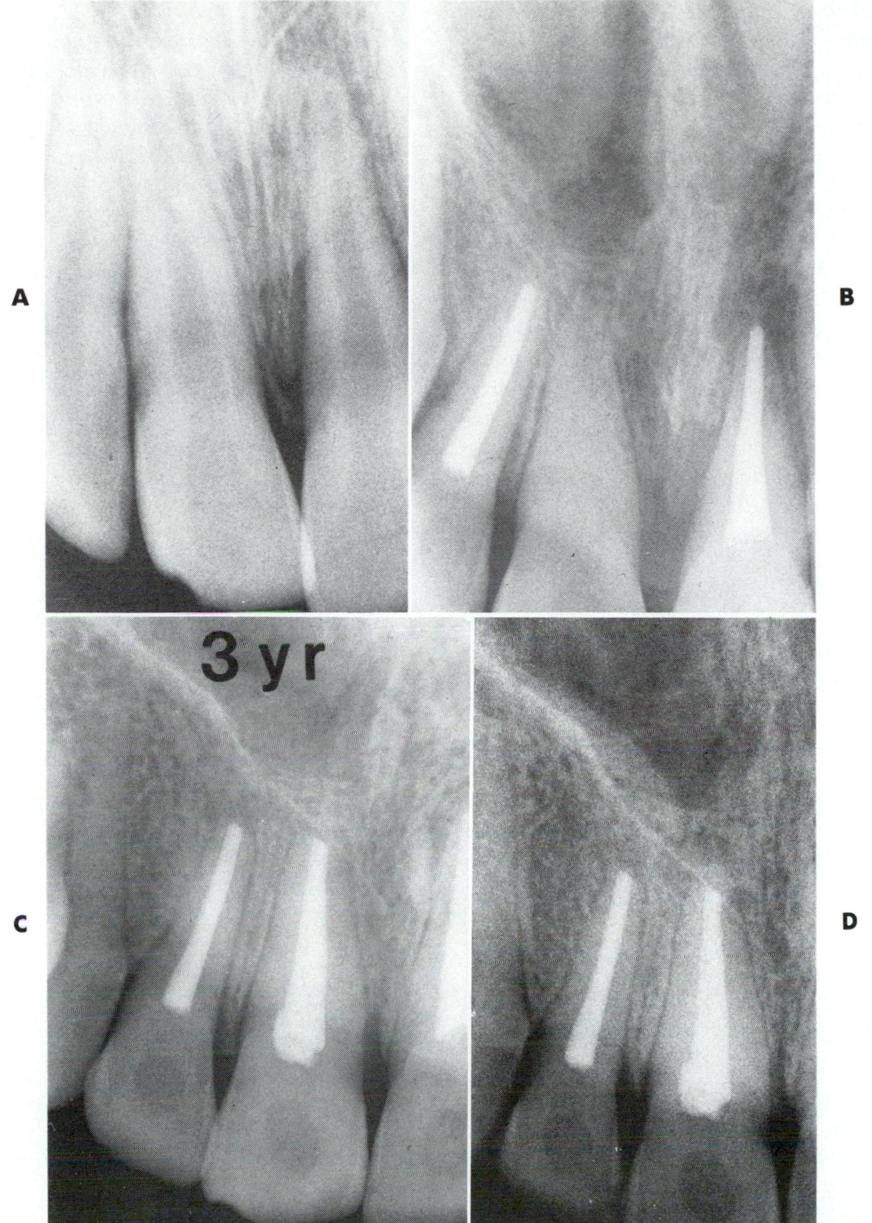

FIG. 16-24 Healing with a normal periodontal ligament after replantation. Extraoral time 30 minutes. **A,** Radiographic immediately after replantation of the left central incisor. **B,** Root canal of the replanted tooth filled with calcium hydroxide. Adjacent teeth required conventional root canal treatment due to pulpal necrosis. **C,** Three years after replantation. Calcium hydroxide was replaced with gutta-percha after 1 year. **D,** Seven years after replantation. Note the normal periodontal ligament space and the absence of root resorption.

Following replantation a clot is formed in the torn periodontal ligament. Soon afterward, healing of the periodontal ligament begins with the proliferation of the connective tissue cells. The continuity of the periodontal ligament and supracrestal connective tissue is reestablished at 1 week. At 2 weeks new collagen fibers extend from the cementum to the alveolar bone. Periodontal healing is complete in 2 to 4 weeks when assessed histologically and by mobility tests. Surface resorption of the root was first recognized at 1 week and became prominent at 2 weeks.[24,35,160]

On the basis of histologic examination of replanted human and animal teeth, Andreasen[31] and Andreasen and Hjorting-Hansen[35] have divided periodontal healing into three types:

Healing with a normal periodontal ligament. Complete repair of the periodontal ligament occurs with this type of healing. This takes place without significant inflammatory changes in the periodontal tissues. Small areas of resorption representing localized areas of damage to the periodontal ligament, termed *surface resorption,* are present on the root. These usually involve only cementum but occasionally involve dentin. A normal-appearing periodontal space is seen radiographically. The tooth is not ankylosed[22,25,29] (Fig. 16-24).

When dentin is resorbed, healing occurs with an altered root outline.[22] Surface resorption is not related to the contents of the root canal. However, if the resorption penetrates into dentinal tubules with infected pulpal tissue or a pus zone, it can quickly change into inflammatory resorption.[33]

Healing with ankylosis or replacement resorption. Ankylosis occurs when areas of root resorption are repaired by the deposition of bone, resulting in a fusion of the root surface and the alveolar bone (Fig. 16-25). Andreasen[21,29] showed that ankylosis develops as a response in the periodontium to areas of damage to the periodontal ligament or root surface occurring as the tooth is avulsed or because of storage conditions before replantation. It may be temporary in areas of minor damage and later cease. Andreasen has termed this type *transient replacement resorption*.[31]

The etiology of replacement resorption is related to the absence of a vital periodontal ligament on the root surface. Progenitor cells with osteogenic potential from the adjacent bone marrow migrate into the damaged areas and subsequently form an ankylosis as healing occurs.[33]

Replacement root resorption associated with ankylosis is initiated by osteoblasts and is hormonally regulated in contrast to inflammatory resorption, which is triggered by inflammatory cells.[101] Osteoblasts, unlike cementoblasts, respond to parathyroid hormone by exposing the underlying hard tissue to colonization by osteoclastic cells, which initiate resorption. As long as the protective covering of cementoblasts is intact, resorption will not occur. In ankylosis, the periodontal membrane and cementoblasts are lost and the root is covered by osteoblasts. Parathyroid hormone stimulation causes the osteoblasts to mediate root resorption.[148]

In more extensive injuries (i.e., denuded periodontal ligaments or teeth subjected to drying) the entire root is gradually resorbed and replaced by bone. Andreasen has termed this *progressive replacement resorption*.[31] (Fig. 16-25). This type of resorption is always elicited when the entire periodontal ligament is removed before replantation.[28,29]

Replacement resorption can be observed histologically in 2 weeks[24] and radiographically in 2 months.[34] Radiographically, the normal periodontal space is absent and radiolucencies are not present. Clinically, the tooth is immobile (Figs. 16-25, 16-26).

Ankylosis usually does not present a problem in the fully formed jaw of an adult. Ankylosed teeth can be maintained until replacement resorption leads to loosening and exfoliation of the tooth. In younger patients, in whom maturation of the alveolar processes has not occurred, ankylosis may interfere with normal growth and development. When infraocclusion occurs in these patients, the tooth must be extracted and replaced prosthetically to prevent malocclusion.

Investigators[153] have developed a surgical technique to preserve the alveolar ridge of ankylosed, infrapositioned incisors to improve subsequent prosthetic replacement. The crown and root filling are removed. The root is retained and covered with a mucoperiosteal flap. This allows maintenance of the alveolar ridge while continued resorption of the root through replacement by bone occurs. No pathologic changes were observed in the study. In children treated before or during the pubertal period of growth, no further infrapositioning of the alveolar segment was observed.

Inflammatory resorption. Granulation tissue in the periodontal ligament adjacent to large areas of root resorption char-

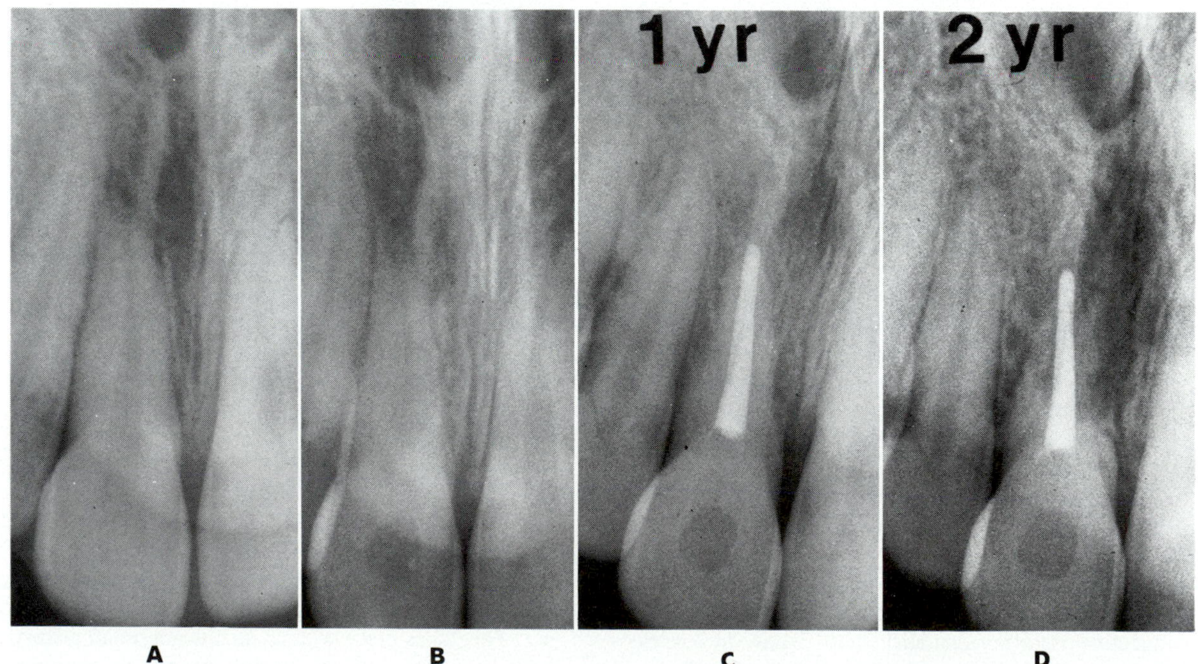

FIG. 16-25 Healing with replacement resorption and ankylosis. Extraoral time 90 minutes. **A,** Radiograph immediately after replantation of the right maxillary central incisor. **B,** Calcium hydroxide placement 1 month after replantation. **C,** Gutta-percha placed after removal of the calcium hydroxide 1 year after replantation. **D,** Two years after replantation. The tooth is resorbing and ankylosed. Note the lack of periodontal ligament space.

acterizes this type (Fig. 16-27).[35] Andreasen[22] has shown that these resorption defects occur on the root surface adjacent to areas of damage to the periodontal ligament during avulsion or extended drying before replantation. The etiology is communication between the surface resorption and the pulp via the dentinal tubules. The mechanism of action is toxic products and bacteria penetrating from the root canal, which contains necrotic tissue, into the periodontal tissues, causing the inflammatory process.[18] Resorption, in turn, is accelerated. Root resorption may progress rapidly, resulting in loosening and early loss of the tooth. Endodontics may lead to evidence of repair in some cases.

Inflammatory resorption can be demonstrated 1 week after replantation and is progressive if endodontics is not performed. According to Andreasen,[33] inflammatory resorption is dependent on four conditions:

1. Injury to the periodontal ligament.
2. Exposure of dentinal tubules.
3. Communication of the exposed tubules with necrotic pulp or with a leukocytic zone with bacteria.
4. The presence of a maturation factor (more frequent in immature than mature teeth).

Inflammatory resorption can also be caused by an inflammatory process originating in the marginal gingiva.

Inflammatory resorption is the mechanism of eliminating infected calcified tissue from the body. Osteoclasts acting as specialized macrophages actively participate in the healing process to repair traumatized tooth and bone.[33]

Endodontic treatment effectively prevents inflammatory resorption if the necrotic pulp is removed before the initiation of bacterial infection.[3,5,100] Inflammatory resorption is difficult to eliminate once it begins if endodontic treatment is delayed more than 3 weeks following replantation. Once bacterial infection is present in the dentinal tubules, it becomes more difficult to eradicate.[3] Andersson[2] cites this fact in emphasizing the importance of early endodontic treatment of avulsed

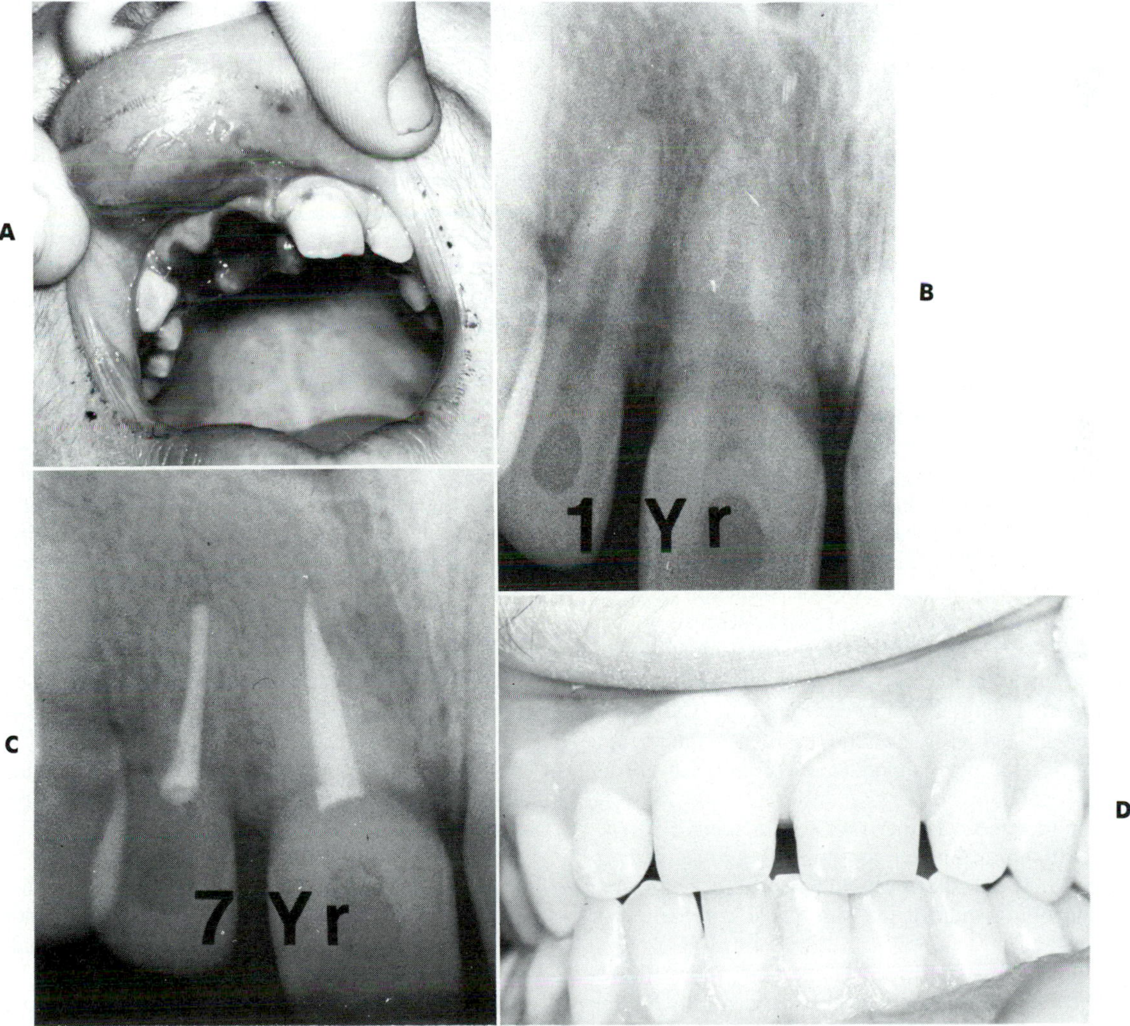

FIG. 16-26 Ankylosis subsequent to replantation 3½ hours after avulsion. **A,** Clinical view. Patient's fingers holding lip up. **B,** Radiograph at 1 year. Canals have been repacked several times with calcium hydroxide. Note the loss of periodontal ligament space and the minor root resorption. **C,** Seven-year follow-up showing progressive replacement, resorption, and ankylosis. **D,** Clinical view 7 years after replantation. Despite ankylosis, the teeth are functioning normally.

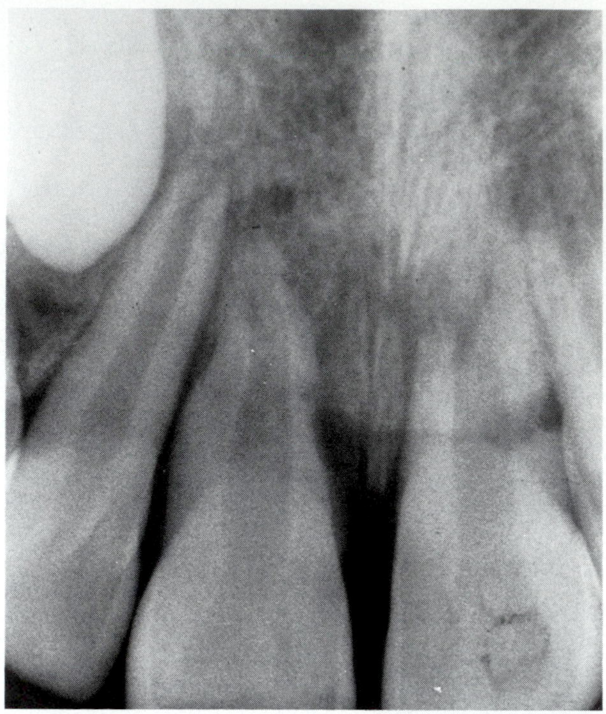

FIG. 16-27 Inflammatory root resorption after replantation. Root canal therapy was not instituted. Extensive root resorption has occurred within 3 months.

teeth, especially those with a compromised or necrotic periodontal ligament.

Endodontic treatment of replanted teeth

Teeth with incomplete root formation. In avulsed teeth with incomplete root formation, revascularization may occur following replantation. Chances for revitalization are improved if replantation is achieved immediately or within 30 minutes. Studies[34,145,166] have shown that *the pulp will not survive after an extraoral time of 2 hours.*

In avulsed teeth with incomplete root formation pulp removal should be delayed until signs of pulpal necrosis are evident (Figs. 16-28, 16-29). These teeth must be followed closely and, if signs of pulpal necrosis occur, endodontic treatment should immediately be instituted (Fig. 16-30). It is recommended that in such cases patients be seen monthly until continued root development is evident or pulpal necrosis confirmed.

It is possible to achieve further root development in the replanted tooth with an incomplete root following revascularization (Figs. 16-28, 16-29); however, in most cases root formation ceases and obliteration of the pulp canal with dentin or bone occurs[31,197] (Fig. 16-28).

The usual vitality tests are not very reliable following replantation. The radiograph should be checked carefully for any signs of developing pathosis. Vitality may be checked by oral examination for color changes by transillumination or tissue changes (e.g., inflammation or sinus tract formation) or by percussion sensitivity or mobility. Although functional repair of pulp nerve fibers has been shown to be reestablished in approximately 35 days following replantation,[166] the electric pulp tester is unreliable in teeth with incompletely formed roots.

If more than 2 hours has elapsed before replantation is achieved in the tooth with incomplete root development, the pulp will usually necrose. If pulpal necrosis is diagnosed, the treatment is with calcium hydroxide, the same as that outlined later for the avulsed tooth with a fully formed root. In our experience the prognosis for such teeth is poor.

Teeth with complete root formation. Although reported,[34,166] revascularization of the pulp following replantation of avulsed teeth with fully formed roots is rare. Researchers[142] have shown that revitalization was significantly related to the stage of root development, sometimes occurring in immature teeth and almost totally lacking in young mature or mature teeth. With fully formed roots, the usual sequelae are pulpal necrosis and accompanying inflammatory resorption. Therefore *all replanted teeth with complete root formation must be treated endodontically.*

Numerous investigations comparing fully developed replanted teeth both with and without endodontic treatment have shown more favorable results in the former.[18,46,81] Periapical abscess formation invariably formed when the pulp tissue was not removed (Fig. 16-27), whereas teeth with root canal fillings did not show such abscesses (Figs. 16-24 and 16-26).

Andreasen[26,30] has shown the mechanism of action to be communication with infected dentinal tubules under areas of surface resorption on the root adjacent to injury to the periodontal ligament. When the resorptive defect is deep enough to communicate with dentinal tubules, toxic elements enter the periodontal ligament through the exposed tubules and create an inflammatory response. Inflammatory root resorption was always related to either a leukocytic zone or necrotic pulp tissue adjacent to the dentinal tubules communicating with the resorption site. Vital pulp tissue was never found in relation to active inflammatory root resorption. When bacteria were present, inflammatory resorption was worse. If the resorptive defect is shallow and does not penetrate the cemental surface, inflammatory resorption does not occur since the toxic elements do not reach the periodontal ligament but are arrested by the cementum. If the pulp contains vital tissue or if root canal filling has been done, only surface resorption occurs irrespective of the depth of the resorptive cavities.[26,30] Therefore early removal of pulp tissue and placement of a root canal filling should be part of the replantation procedure.

When inflammatory resorption has begun, it can sometimes be arrested by removal of the necrotic pulp tissue and placement of a calcium hydroxide filling within the root canal.[17] (See the discussion that follows.)

In the past, controversy has existed over whether to perform endodontic treatment before or after replantation. It is now known that since root canal treatment would prolong the extraoral period it should be accomplished *after* replantation. Further damage to the periodontal ligament from handling the tooth or exposure to chemicals during the endodontic procedure can be avoided. Also, a source of bacterial contamination, which has been shown to be significantly related to resorption, may be eliminated by decreased manipulation of the avulsed tooth.[2]

Although some workers[53,71,194] have found that immersion of the roots of replanted teeth of experimental animals in 1% to 2% solutions of sodium fluoride or acidulated sodium fluoride before replantation decreased the amount and severity of root resorption, others[47] have found no significant reduction in resorption. Adequate research does not exist to warrant rec-

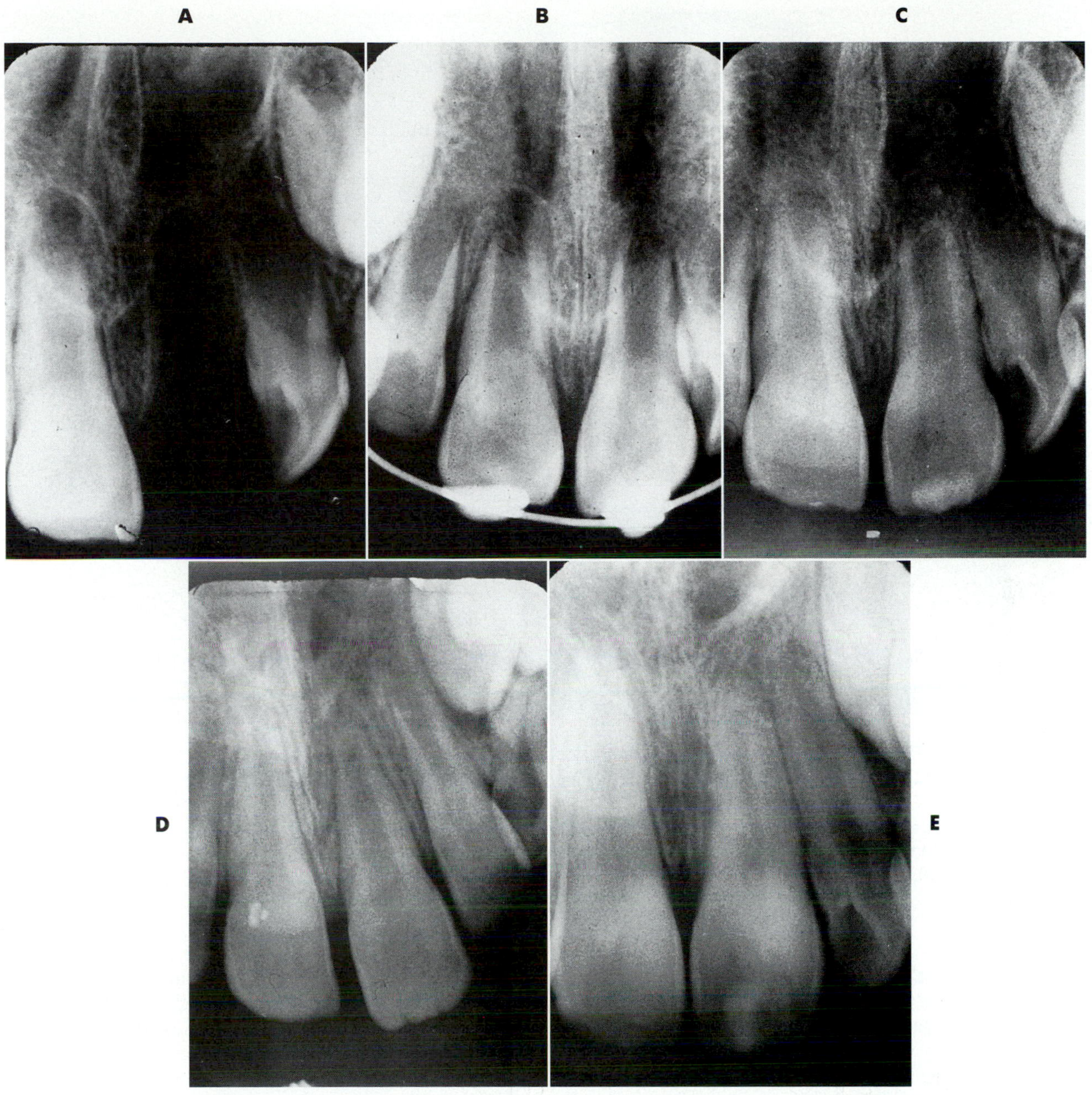

FIG. 16-28 Continued apical development following replantation of central incisor with incomplete root formation. **A,** Maxillary central incisor avulsed. **B,** Tooth replanted after 45 minutes extraoral time. Splint applied. **C,** Three months following replantation. **D,** One year following replantation. Apex has continued to form and tooth remains vital. **E,** Two years following replantation. Tooth remains vital while calcification of root canal is occurring.

ommending this procedure. Coating of the roots of avulsed teeth with a biodegradable compound, polylactic acid, in an attempt to inhibit resorption and ankylosis has also been shown to be ineffective.[102]

Replantation technique

The avulsed tooth must be replanted as soon as possible, preferably at the site where the injury occurred. Care must be taken to avoid further damage to the periodontal tissues. Obvious contamination with soil or foreign matter should be cleaned with physiologic saline or water. The periodontal ligament should not be removed or the root altered in any manner, and *no* attempt should be made to sterilize the tooth.

The pulp should not be removed, and alternative treatments such as apical seal of the root with alloy or other materials are contraindicated. Removal of the apex and creation of openings in the root surface to encourage revascularization have proved fruitless.[196]

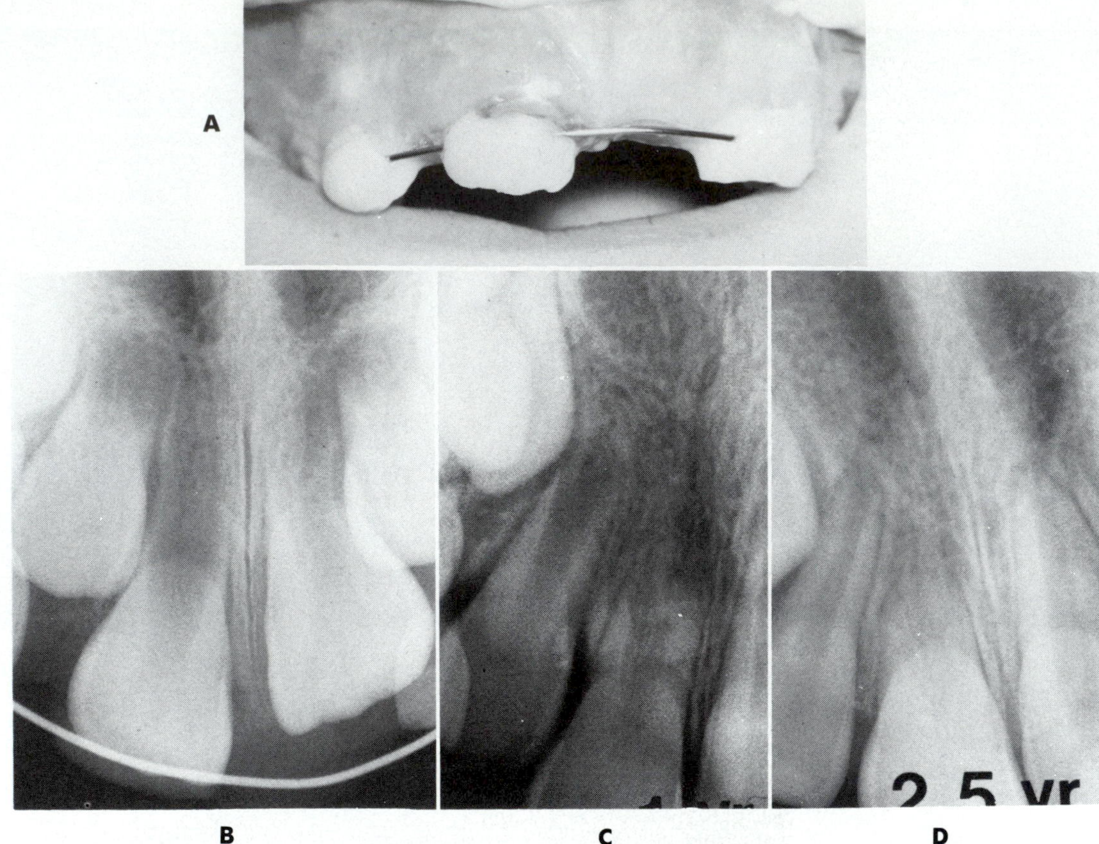

FIG. 16-29 Replantation of a tooth with incomplete root formation. Extraoral time 15 minutes. **A,** Clinical view with acid etch resin and wire splint immediately after replantation and splinting. **B,** Radiograph same day. **C,** Continued root development and pulpal obliteration 1 year later. **D,** Complete pulpal obliteration and blunting of root development 2 years after replantation.

Venting or raising a tissue flap for purposes of creating a vent through the cortical bone is unnecessary and only causes more tissue damage and inflammation.

The alveolar socket should be examined; and if fracture has occurred, it may be necessary to reposition the fractured bone prior to replantation. Fracture of the alveolar bone has been shown to lead to earlier and more rapid progression of root resorption in replanted teeth.[34] However, Andreasen has shown that vital periodontal ligament is able to induce the formation of new alveolar bone.[27] Therefore it is possible to obtain reattachment of replanted teeth if part of the alveolar socket is destroyed during the accident.

Maintenance of the periodontal tissues within the socket is important and has been shown to play a role in resorption and ankylosis.[159] Therefore, one must not curette the socket. If a blood clot is present, it should be removed by irrigation rather than curettage. Andreasen[23] found similar results in animals whether the coagulum was removed before replantation or the tooth was replanted with the coagulum in situ.

The use of local anesthetic is usually not necessary. Often the pain associated with the injection is more severe than the pain from replantation. Even when soft tissue lacerations necessitate the use of anesthetic, the tooth should be replanted immediately to minimize the extraoral time.

The tooth is replanted and repositioned with light finger pressure. A radiograph should be exposed to verify the adequacy of the repositioning. Any soft tissue lacerations are sutured to arrest seepage of hemorrhage prior to splinting of the tooth.

Antibiotics. The systemic administration of antibiotics at the time of and during the first week following replantation has been shown to prevent bacterial invasion of the necrotic pulp. Recent research[100,101] has demonstrated that inflammatory resorption did not occur following antibiotic therapy. The cementum layer was found to be basically intact. Antibiotic administration suppressed the initial resorption of cementum, probably by preventing infection in the traumatized and necrotic periodontal tissues while inhibiting ingrowth of bacteria from the periodontal membrane into the pulp. Systemic administration of antibiotics 3 weeks after replantation had no effect, although local application in the root canal was shown to stop inflammatory resorption. Consequently, systemic administration must be instituted immediately after replantation before infection of the pulp has begun. Because a hematogenous infection of the necrotic pulp tissue may occur later, the administration of antibiotics must not be regarded as a substitute for endodontic treatment in cases in which revascularization cannot be expected.[2] Considering this research, *it is now rec-*

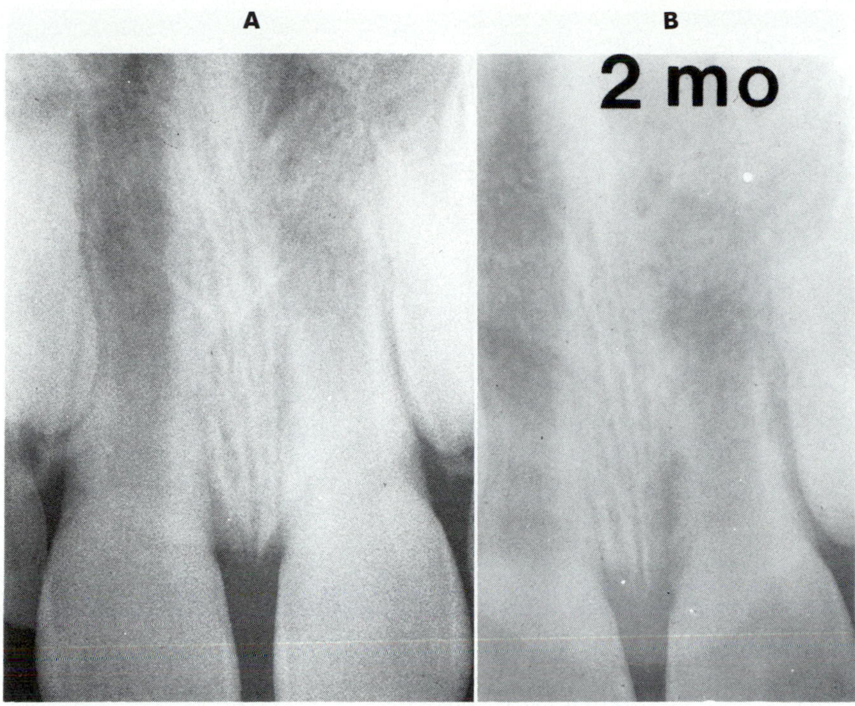

FIG. 16-30 Replantation of a tooth with incomplete root formation. Extraoral time 30 minutes. **A,** Immediately after replantation. **B,** Two months later root resorption is apparent. If root resorption is to be arrested, endodontic treatment with calcium hydroxide must be started immediately. However, the prognosis is poor due to advanced root resorption in an immature root.

ommended that systemic antibiotic therapy be instituted immediately following replantation.

Steroids and other drugs. Active preliminary research in the use of steroidal and nonsteroidal medications is under way at this time.[174,175,220] Application of a corticosteroid-antibiotic paste (Ledermix) has been shown to be an effective treatment for external inflammatory root resorption when placed in root canals. In a follow-up in vitro study, the authors[174] examined the effects of this medicament on dentinoclasts that were cultured in the presence of the antibiotic alone or in combination with the steroid. The steroid component of the combination directly inhibited the spread of the dentinoclasts, which suggests that the drug acts by detaching resorbing dentinoclasts from the root surface, thus preventing inflammatory resorption.

Oral administration of nonsteroidal antiinflammatory drugs has proven ineffective in preventing resorption. Indomethacin, a nonsteroidal, antiinflammatory analgesic, was given to dogs; it did not reduce resorption except in extremely high dosages, which caused severe or fatal gastric problems.[220]

Although systemic administration has been shown to be ineffective,[47] the intrapulpal application of calcitonin, a hormone with osteoclastic bone resorption inhibitor potential, stopped experimentally induced root resorption in monkeys. The authors[173] of this study concluded that calcitonin might be a useful therapeutic adjunct in difficult cases of external root resorption.

Routine administration of systemic antibiotics is recommended for avulsed teeth that have been replanted; however, the use of steroids and other drugs must await further research to verify their application.

Tetanus prophylaxis. If the avulsed tooth or wound has been contaminated with soil, the patient must receive a tetanus injection. In other situations clinical judgment must be used in making this determination. Consultation with the patient's physician is advised.

Pulp extirpation and calcium hydroxide root canal filling. The use of calcium hydroxide in the treatment of inflammatory root resorption was first reported by Andreasen.[18] The material was used in replanted teeth with incomplete root formation in which inflammatory root resorption had begun following pulp necrosis (Fig. 16-31). This technique evolved from the use of calcium hydroxide to promote apexification in pulpless teeth with undeveloped apices. Calcium hydroxide was later reported to inhibit root resorption when endodontic treatment was performed and the canals temporarily filled with calcium hydroxide paste.[81] Since that time the use of these pastes to inhibit root resorption has become the accepted treatment.[67] The exact mode of action of calcium hydroxide in inhibiting resorption is unknown. A number of theories have been proposed. Webber's report[222] on the expanded endodontic role of calcium hydroxide provides a thorough review of these theories.

Endodontics should be instituted within 1 or 2 weeks after replantation to prevent the development of inflammatory root resorption. As stated earlier, root canal treatment is achieved after replantation of the avulsed tooth to avoid further damage to the periodontal ligament and to minimize extraoral time.

Andreasen[26] has shown that there is increased replacement and surface root resorption when gutta-percha fillings are placed in avulsed teeth prior to replantation compared with

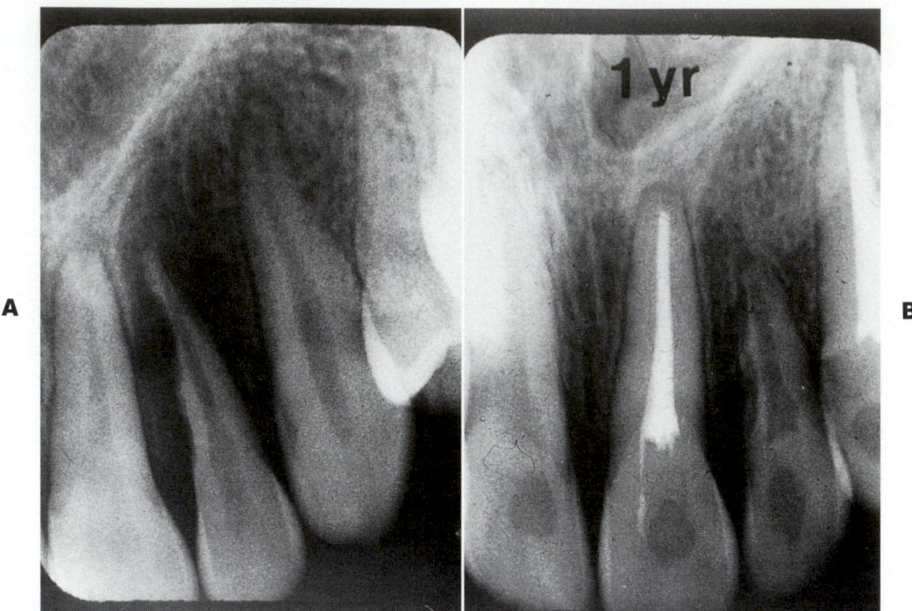

FIG. 16-31 Inflammatory root resorption in a replanted lateral incisor. **A,** Inflammatory resorption 6 weeks following replantation. The pulp was not removed. **B,** Repair of lesion and termination of inflammatory resorption was achieved by removal of necrotic pulp and placement of calcium hydroxide in the root canal. The central incisor and canine became pulpless, requiring root canal filling with gutta-percha.

those left untreated or those that have extirpated pulps. This is due to increased extraoral time and further damage to the periodontal ligament from handling and/or chemical contact. Pulp extirpation did not increase resorption in these teeth as compared with those with nonextirpated pulps.

To prevent inflammatory root resorption, the pulp must be extirpated within 1 or 2 weeks following replantation. This may be achieved through the splint placed during the emergency appointment. Since the tooth will not be firmly attached, extirpation should be done before the splint is removed. The presence of the splint may make use of the rubber dam difficult. As in all endodontic procedures, however, isolation of the tooth is essential; therefore, if placing the rubber dam is difficult, an alternative is to use sponges and cotton rolls with the patient seated upright.

When endodontic treatment is rendered without the rubber dam, strong precautionary measures must be taken to avoid the accidental swallowing or aspiration of endodontic instruments or irrigants. This is achieved by tying dental floss on the handles of the instruments. In cases of accidental dropping, the floss serves as a means of retrieval. A more desirable alternative is to prepare a large opening in the rubber dam that allows several teeth to fit through. A rubber dam clamp is placed on the teeth mesial and distal to the tooth undergoing endodontic treatment.

The usual access cavity is made, the pulp extirpated, and the access cavity sealed with a sterile cotton pellet and a temporary restoration placed. The tooth should *never* be left open to drain, as this will allow the ingress of bacteria and debris, leading to inflammatory root resorption.

Placement of calcium hydroxide in the root canal should be delayed 1 to 2 weeks following replantation. Andreasen[24] has shown that immediate insertion of the calcium hydroxide in replanted teeth causes noticeably more replacement resorption than is seen in teeth with extirpated pulps or gutta-percha fillings. He postulates that calcium hydroxide diffuses through the apical foramen, further injuring the periodontal ligament. He has also pointed out[24] that inflammatory resorption is initiated at around 2 weeks, about the time that periodontal healing is occurring[20]; therefore, this seems to be the ideal time for placement of the calcium hydroxide (Figs. 16-24 to 16-26).

Before the calcium hydroxide is placed, the root canal is thoroughly cleaned by routine endodontic treatment. As with any endodontic procedure, the use of the rubber dam is advisable. The working length is established radiographically or with the apex locator, care being taken to avoid overextension of instruments through the apex of the tooth into the periapical tissues. The canal is cleaned with endodontic instruments and frequently irrigated with sodium hypochlorite.

After mechanical debridement of the canal, it is thoroughly dried and filled with a thick paste of calcium hydroxide and water. Small amounts of barium sulfate may be added to aid in radiographic interpretation without altering the reaction of the calcium hydroxide[222] (Fig. 16-18, *C, D*). The paste is carried into the canal with an amalgam carrier and packed with blunt-ended pluggers until it reaches the apex. The addition of some dry calcium hydroxide powder within the canal will aid in condensing the material to the apex. The use of a Lentulo spiral, the McSpadden compactor, or syringes to carry the material into the canal is also an acceptable method of filling.

Vehicles other than water that have been used to form the paste with calcium hydroxide include camphorated parachlorphenol (CMCP), Cresanol, physiologic saline, and anesthetic solution. Although clinically the results with these agents seem to be the same, Cvek[79] has warned against combining calcium hydroxide with intracanal medicaments because of their proved damage to periapical tissues.

Commercial preparations of calcium hydroxide (e.g., Calasept, Pulpdent, Hypo-Cal, Calxyl) are acceptable as filling pastes. These products are injected into the canal. Multiple paper points are used to absorb the moisture while the material is packed into the canal. Additional compaction of the material is achieved with a blunt-ended plugger until the canal is totally filled. Calcium hydroxide preparations that set into a hard mass and have a short working time (e.g., Dycal) are *unacceptable* since the filling procedure cannot be completed before the material sets and they are more difficult to remove from the canal prior to final placement of gutta-percha. Small amounts of barium sulfate may be added to aid in radiographic interpretation without altering the reaction of the calcium hydroxide (Fig. 16-19, *C, D*).

The canal is generally filled without the use of local anesthetic. The patient's feeling is used as a guide in determining the depth of the filling paste. An attempt is made to fill the canal completely but to avoid overfilling. If overfilling occurs, no attempt is made to remove the excess since the material is absorbable.[117] Radiographic checks are made to verify the depth of the filling.

If conditions are not ideal for placement of the root canal filling after instrumentation (i.e., the canal cannot be dried thoroughly), the tooth may be temporarily closed again. Usually when these circumstances occur, the canal is medicated with calcium hydroxide paste and closed for a few weeks, after which the canal is recleaned and repacked.

When the canal is satisfactorily filled, the outer 3 to 4 mm of the access opening is sealed with a permanent filling material. Silicate cement or composite resin is the material of choice in anterior teeth, and amalgam for posterior teeth. It is necessary to place a permanent-type restoration in the access cavity since loss of the outer seal will quickly lead to loss of the root canal filling paste and the initiation of an infection with inflammatory root resorption.

Since calcium hydroxide is an absorbable material, it will eventually begin to dissipate out of the canal in some teeth. If this happens, the canal may become infected and an inflammatory resorption may be initiated. Therefore it is necessary to reclean and repack the canal periodically. The optimum time for this has not been established, and probably varies among individuals, but it is generally agreed that it should be done every 3 to 6 months until the decision is made to fill the canal with a permanent filling of gutta-percha.

We have noted that radiographically visible resorption terminates after the canals are filled with calcium hydroxide. In teeth treated endodontically within 2 weeks after replantation and filled with calcium hydroxide, there is usually no radiographic evidence of resorption as long as the calcium hydroxide filling remains intact. The mode of action of calcium hydroxide in inhibiting resorption is unknown. Investigators[214] have shown an increase in the pH of dentin in teeth in which the canals have been filled with calcium hydroxide. They have speculated that the rise in pH stimulates the repair processes of the tissues while reducing the resorptive process, since an acidic environment is necessary for osteoclastic activity.

While calcium hydroxide is present in the canal, the patient is recalled every 3 months and instructed to return immediately if any adverse symptoms occur before that time. If evidence of periapical involvement due to breakdown of the filling material exists, the canal is immediately recleaned and refilled. Otherwise, it is recleaned and refilled every 3 to 6 months. The optimum time for retention of the calcium hydroxide prior to placement of a permanent gutta-percha filling is unknown. Empirically the minimum time for retention has been established as 1 year.

It should be noted that recent research has called into doubt the long-term use of calcium hydroxide in replanted teeth with a compromised periodontal membrane. The researchers[143,144] reported that while calcium hydroxide prevents bacterial colonization, it also appears to necrotize the ingrowing cells that heal the periodontal tissue. This in turn allows ankylosis to develop, leading to increased replacement resorption. Teeth treated with gutta-percha root filling after 1 hour of dry extraoral time showed significantly less ankylosis than those filled with calcium hydroxide. The authors concluded that it appears likely that calcium hydroxide treatment of teeth with compromised periodontal membrane may harm the periodontal reparative process if left too long in the root canal or changed repeatedly, allowing replacement resorption to progress.[143,144] While this research is preliminary, it merits a close watch on further developments related to long-term use of calcium hydroxide in replanted teeth, and it points out the need for further study. Not enough evidence has been presented, however, to currently alter the accepted treatment regimen.

When a replanted tooth is adjacent to an erupting tooth, as in the case of a lateral incisor before eruption of the canine, there is acceleration of the resorptive process. In these cases it is advised that calcium hydroxide be left in the canal until the adjacent tooth has erupted (Fig. 16-32).

If orthodontic treatment is in progress, retention of the calcium hydroxide in the canal is recommended until active movement of the tooth is completed.

Permanent root canal filling with gutta-percha. Since calcium hydroxide is not a permanent root canal filling, the replanted tooth must ultimately be filled with gutta-percha (Figs. 16-24 and 16-26). As stated, the optimal time for retention of the calcium hydroxide filling has not been determined, but empirically a minimum of 1 year seems to be adequate in most cases.[222]

After calcium hydroxide is removed from the root canal and gutta-percha placed, replacement resorption begins in many replanted teeth. This may be followed by ankylosis, and, possibly, loss of the tooth. However, many teeth show little evidence of resorption, or very slow resorption, and the prognosis for long retention of these is excellent (Fig. 16-26).

Although much has been learned about the replanted tooth, many unanswered questions remain. Numerous areas of replantation have had little or no scientific investigation, among them the role of immunology. It is hoped that continued research will develop treatments that enable practitioners to retain these replanted teeth permanently.

Splinting

The development of the acid etch technique and the application of scientific research in the area of tooth-related injuries have revolutionized splinting. For years the principles and practice of treating bone fractures were erroneously applied to traumatized teeth. Many of the splinting techniques previously advocated were time consuming. Not only were the splints difficult to fabricate and difficult to remove, they also contributed to injury of the soft and hard supporting tissues.

Splinting techniques that cause gingival inflammation prevent the inflammatory response from resolving in the marginal gingiva and possibly around the replant. Splints that subject the teeth and alveolar bone to pressures and tensions in the

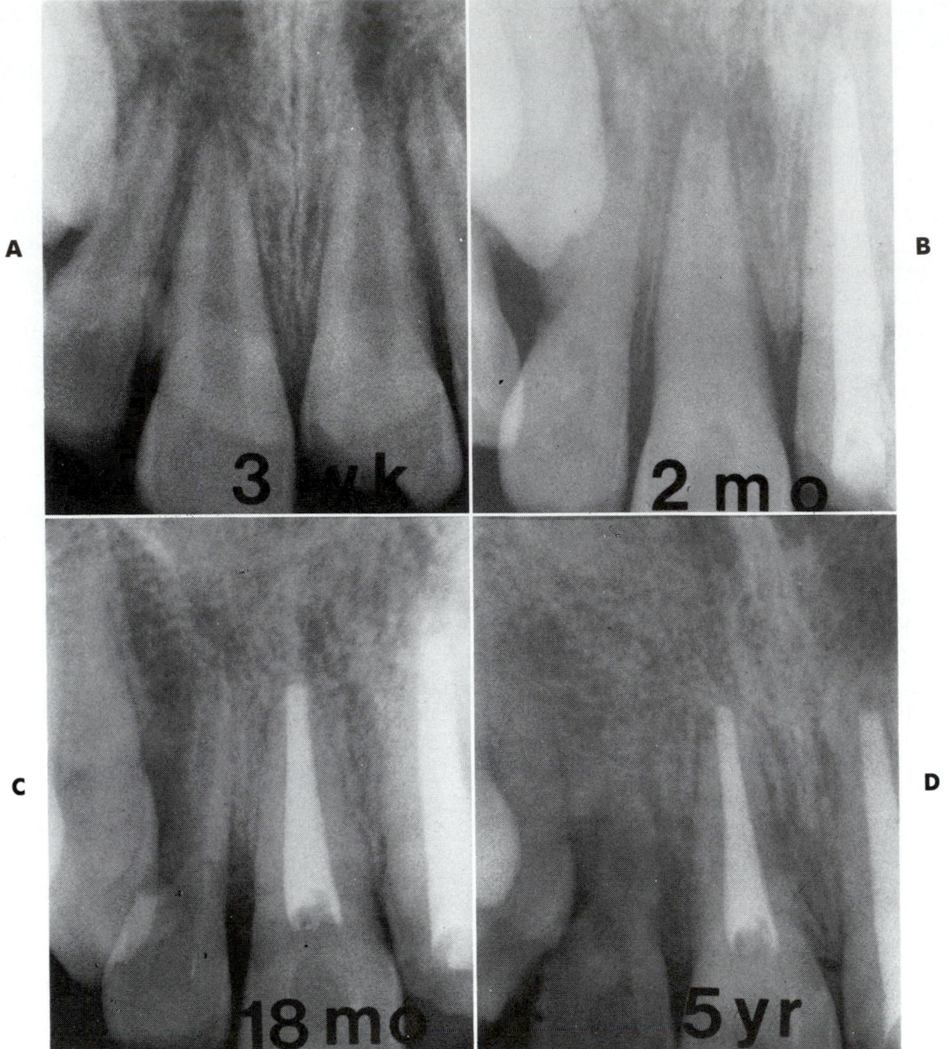

FIG. 16-32 Replantation of a permanent tooth adjacent to an erupting permanent tooth. **A,** Three weeks after replantation of the right maxillary central and lateral incisors adjacent to the erupting canine. **B,** Placement of calcium hydroxide in the replanted teeth. Routine endodontics has been completed on the left central incisor. **C,** Canine erupted. Note the advanced resorption of the lateral incisor. Calcium hydroxide was repacked every 3 months in the right lateral incisor. Gutta-percha has been placed in the right central. **D,** Massive root resorption of the right lateral incisor 5 years after replantation.

same manner as active orthodontic appliances cause inflammation and resorption. Interdental wiring and arch bars ligated to the teeth cannot be passively placed and therefore have no place in treating tooth trauma unless as techniques of last resort. Wire ligatures activate the resorptive mechanism, create gingival irritation, and are difficult to apply as well as to remove and clean (Fig. 16-33).

The exact value and influence of splinting on pulpal and periodontal healing have not been determined.[31] It has been shown that splinting failed to improve healing and exerted a harmful effect upon periodontal healing by increasing the extent of pulpal necrosis and inflammatory root resorption when compared to nonsplinting.[141]

Although it cannot be completely prevented, ankylosis can be partially overcome by using splinting techniques that allow the replanted tooth to be subjected to masticatory stimulation during the healing period. This stimulation facilitates an increase in the area of functional periodontal membrane in teeth with partially necrotic tissues.[5,31,168] A 0.3-mm wire-composite splint has been shown to act as a functional fixation while allowing slight vertical movement of the teeth during immobilization.[169]

Studies[2,19] have shown that rigid splinting of replanted teeth increases the amount of root resorption. Rigid splinting after replantation is a detriment rather than an asset. Poor formation of collagen fibers has been found with prolonged and rigid splinting and the postulation advanced that since little tension can be transmitted during rigid fixation this may cause atrophy and increased susceptibility to ankylosis.[119] However, some degree of mobility is desirable for proper regeneration,

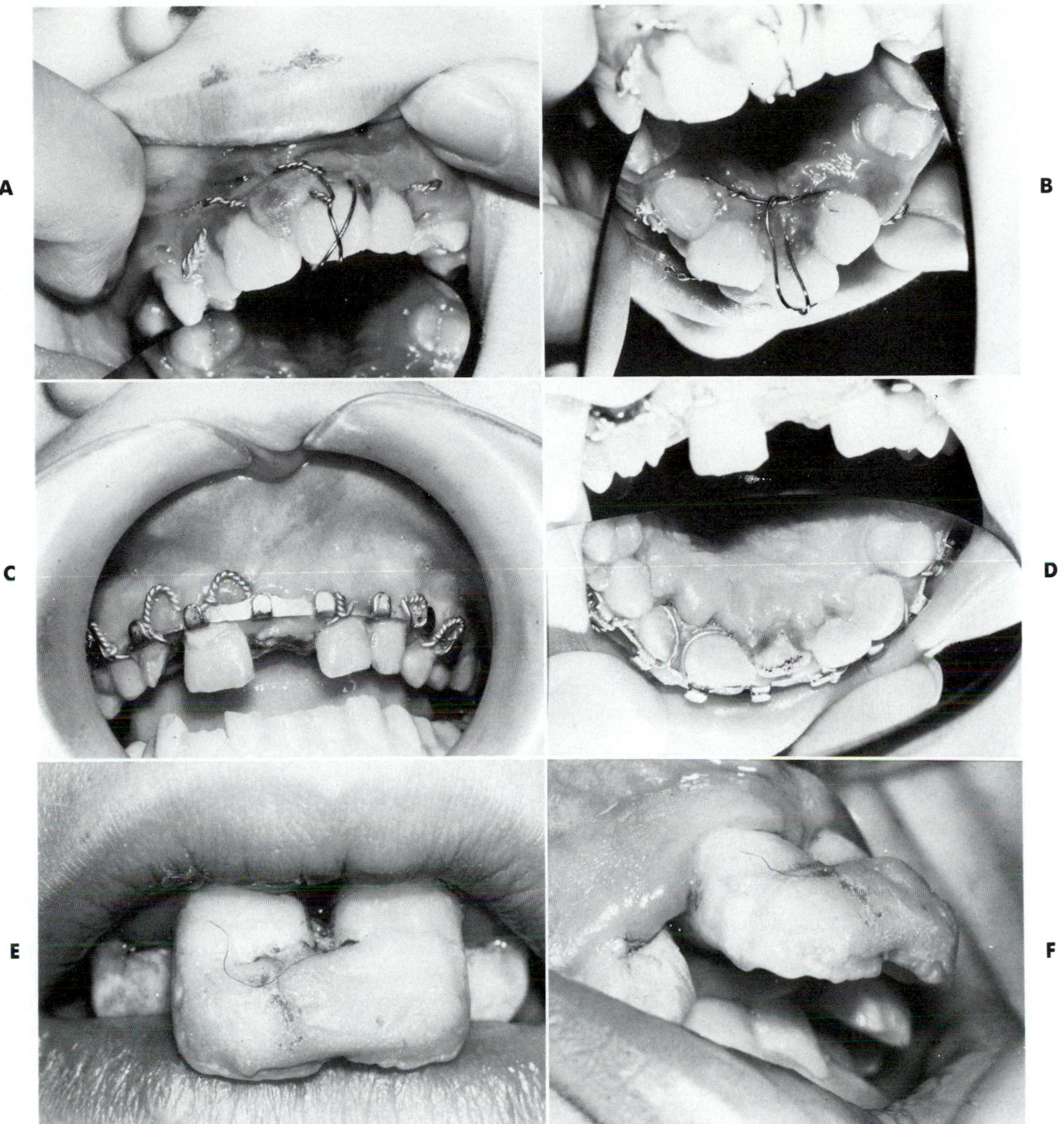

FIG. 16-33 Improper splinting. **A** and **B,** Maxillary left central incisor replanted. Note the inflammation of gingival tissues around the improperly placed wires. Today, gloves should be worn. **C** and **D,** Improper use of an arch bar. The wires caused gingival inflammation and pressures on the teeth, resulting in facial displacement. **E** and **F,** Splinting. Maxillary central incisors replanted and splinted without fixation to an adjacent sound tooth. Note the incorporation of hair in the resin.

functional orientation, and development after the initial attachment occurs.[119] Consequently Andreasen[31] has advised that replanted teeth be splinted for a minimum of 1 week since this time is sufficient to secure adequate periodontal healing.

The requirements for an acceptable splint are as follows:[66]

1. Is easy to fabricate directly in the mouth without lengthy laboratory procedures
2. Can be placed passively without causing forces on the teeth
3. Does not contact the gingival tissues, causing gingival irritation
4. Does not interfere with normal occlusion
5. Is easily cleaned and allows for proper oral hygiene
6. Should not traumatize the teeth or gingiva during application
7. Allows approach for endodontic therapy
8. Is easily removed

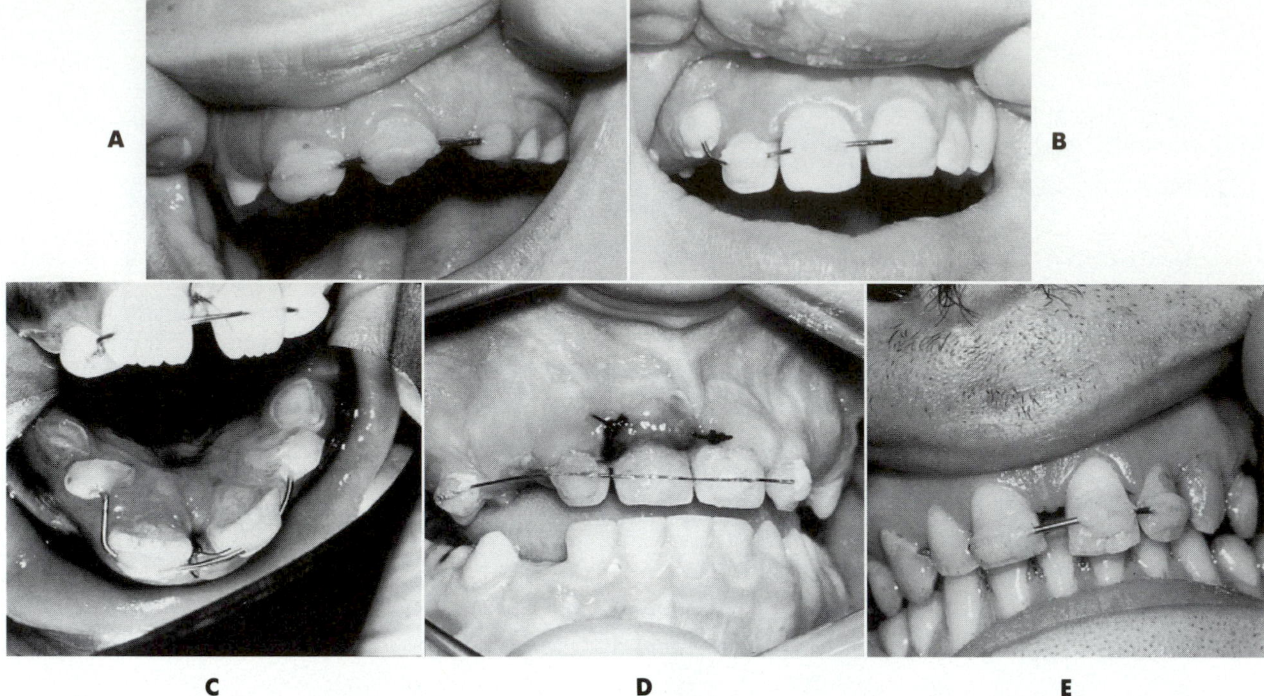

FIG. 16-34 Acid etch resin and arch wire splint. Today, gloves should be worn. **A,** Splinting in the mixed dentition utilizing primary and permanent tooth abutments. **B** and **C,** Splints attached to erupting teeth. **D,** Splinting across an edentulous space. **E,** Use of a paper clip for the arch wire.

The acid etch composite and arch wire splint, as advocated by Heiman and associates,[106] usually satisfies all the above requirements (Fig. 16-34).

Also, the flexible wire-composite splint has been shown to provide horizontal support while allowing greater vertical flexibility than other splints.[170] Restoration of vertical movement of luxated teeth has been reported both clinically and experimentally to promote healing and may remove small ankylotic areas on the tooth root.[19,20] The use of a 20- or 30-pound test monofilament nylon line as a substitute for the arch wire has been advocated[43] since this would allow a degree of physiologic movement; however, no difference in resorption was noted when compared with the use of a wire[50] (Fig. 16-34).

In this technique an orthodontic wire is bent to passively conform to the facial surfaces of the teeth, encompassing at least one sound tooth on each side of the injured tooth or teeth. Any shape of the wire is acceptable as long as it is between 0.015 and 0.030 in size. The middle third of the facial surfaces of the crowns is etched with phosphoric acid for 1 minute. The etching gels work better than liquids, since tissue seepage is generally a problem. After the teeth are thoroughly washed and dried, the arch wire is attached to the facial surfaces with resin. Any form of resin or composite is acceptable for attaching the wire to the teeth.

The wire is attached to the uninjured teeth first and the resin allowed to cure. Only a small amount of resin in the middle third of the exposed crown is necessary to hold the splint. The injured teeth are then attached to the wire with resin, care being taken to ensure that they are in the proper position. A radiograph is taken for verification.

An alternative to this technique is the use of direct-bonded orthodontic brackets and the application of an arch wire.[118] However, this is more time consuming and requires measures to ensure that the arch wire is totally passive.

Although it is possible that some injuries are so extensive that this type of splint cannot be utilized to treat traumatized teeth, we have not encountered such a situation (Fig. 16-35). Extensive injuries in which tissue seepage prevents drying of the teeth may require fabrication of acrylic or cast metal splints that are cemented or held by interdental wiring. However, these types of splints are reserved for situations in which direct-bonding techniques are impossible or impractical.

When one is splinting in the primary dentition with acid-etch techniques, the bonding must be enhanced by roughening the facial surface of the teeth to be etched with a rough diamond stone prior to placing the etching gel. After splint removal the roughened teeth should be polished.

The use of the acid etch resin and arch wire splint does not interfere with the occlusion; therefore mastication on the posterior teeth is possible. On mandibular anterior splints, where the wire on the facial would interfere with occlusion, the arch wire is placed on the lingual surface. The patient is instructed not to bite on the injured tooth for several weeks. Food should be cut into bite-sized pieces and placed in the mouth rather than incised.

The patient is instructed in proper oral hygiene and the importance of keeping the area clean. It is usually possible to continue brushing and flossing immediately after the splint is placed.

Removal of the acid etch resin and arch wire splint is sim-

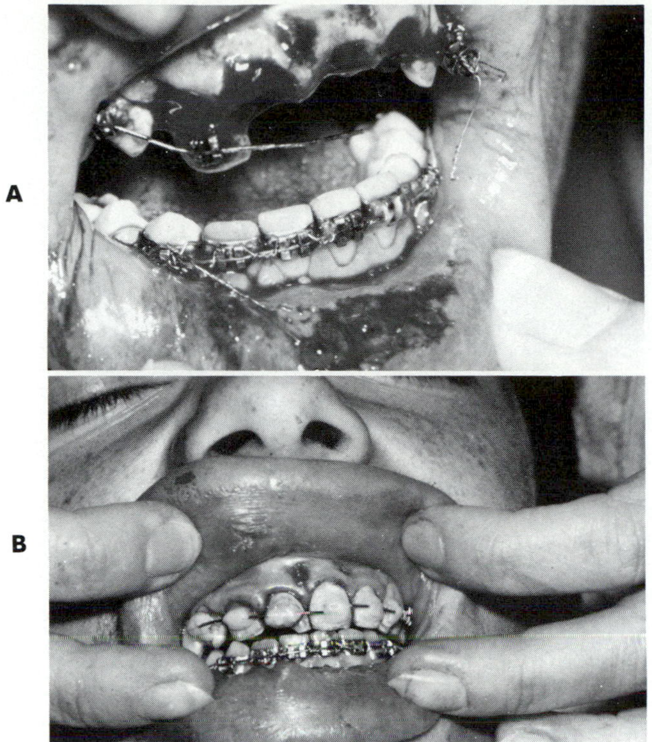

FIG. 16-35 Acid etch resin and arch wire splint of extensive injury. **A,** Three incisors were avulsed and one incisor was severely displaced. **B,** Teeth replanted and repositioned with splint in place. Fingers are those of patient's parent.

ple (Fig. 16-36). A high-speed diamond with copious water supply is used to grind through the resin to expose and free the wire. It is not necessary or advisable to remove all fragments of the resin at the time of splint removal. Since complete healing of the periodontal tissues has not occurred at 1 week, excessive manipulation may cause displacement of the teeth. When the wire is removed, the remaining resin is smoothed and left in place for several weeks. After healing is complete, the resin can be removed with a sharp scaler or carver.

Problems may be encountered in very young or retarded patients who will not tolerate a foreign material such as a splint in the mouth. Occasionally in the primary or early mixed dentition there are no adjacent teeth or not enough exposed tooth structure on which to attach acid-etch resin. In these cases a suture splint (as advocated by Rand[179] and modified by Camp[66]) is easily applied and provides good stabilization. After the injured tooth is repositioned, its facial surface is acid etched. Next a suture is passed through the gingiva above the facial surface, carried over the incisal edge of the tooth and into the lingual gingival tissue, and brought out again. The suture is then passed over the incisal edge and again into the facial gingival tissue, where it is drawn tight and tied. A small amount of resin is cured over the facial surface and the suture to assure retention of the suture on the incisal edge (Fig. 16-37).

Duration of splinting

There is confusion as to the optimum time that a splint should be left in place. This confusion is related to the diversity of situations requiring splinting.

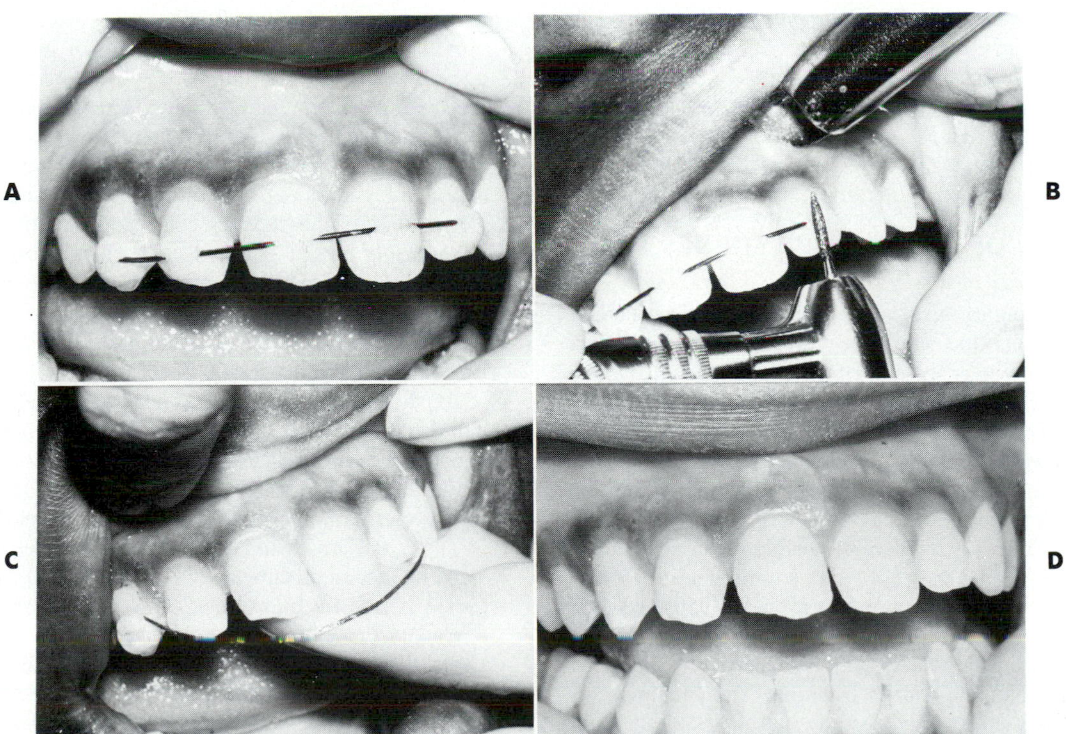

FIG. 16-36 Removal of acid etch resin and arch wire splint. **A,** Splint ready for removal. Today, gloves should be worn. **B,** High-speed diamond with copious water spray used to grind through the resin and free the arch wire. **C,** Wire removed. **D,** Resin smoothed. Remnants will be removed after healing is completed.

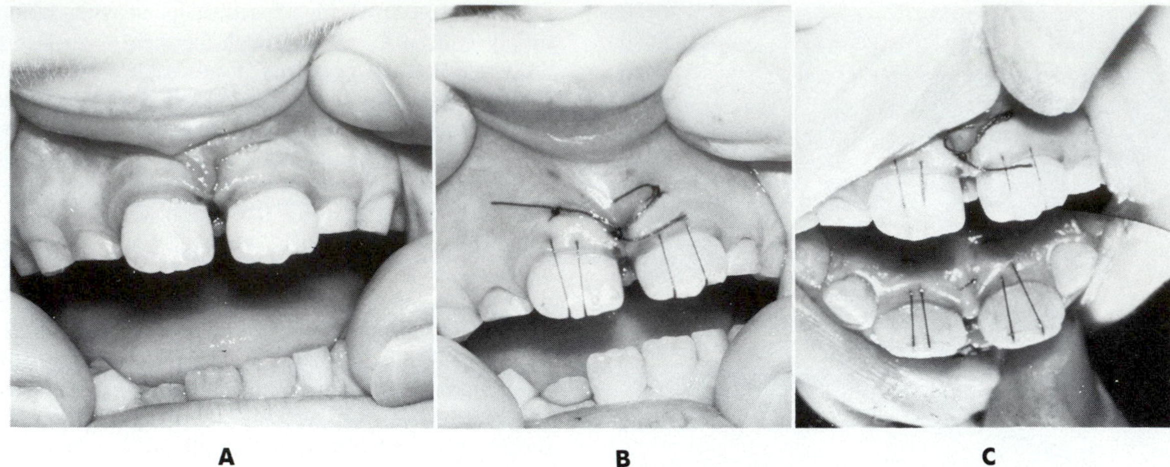

FIG. 16-37 Suture splint. **A,** The maxillary central incisors have been replanted. The short clinical crowns of the primary teeth make it difficult to place the acid etch resin and arch wire splint. The facial surfaces of the central incisors are acid etched. Today, gloves should be worn. **B** and **C,** A suture is placed in the facial tissue 5 to 6 mm above the gingival margin and is passed over the incisal of the tooth and into the lingual tissue. It then recrosses the incisal edge into the facial tissue and is tied. Resin is placed on the facial surface to maintain the suture in position.

Recent studies[19,31] have shown that rigid splinting of replanted teeth *increases* resorption and ankylosis. Therefore replanted teeth should be splinted for a minimum length of time. Andreasen[31] has pointed out that 1 week is sufficient to secure adequate periodontal support, since gingival fibers are healed during this time. The recommended splinting time for displaced and avulsed teeth is 7 to 10 days.

The optimum time for leaving a splint in place for displaced or avulsed teeth in combination with alveolar fracture has not been determined. We suggest 14 to 21 days. More extensive bone fractures may require longer splinting times. Root fractures require the longest splinting period (10 to 12 weeks) because of the time required for callus formation on the root.

PREVENTION OF TRAUMATIC INJURIES TO THE TOOTH

At the beginning of this chapter is the oft-quoted statement: "Hindsight explains the injury that foresight would have prevented." In all previous sections of the chapter we have looked at injuries that have already occurred (i.e., hindsight) and discussed methods of treating them. We must now use foresight and discuss ways to prevent some of these injuries. Because of the variety of ways they occur, however, it is unlikely that most of them can be prevented.

The remarkable story of prevention of dental injuries in football should encourage the profession to continue to look for ways to prevent traumatic oral injuries. In the 1940s and 1950s it was a source of pride among tough football players while talking to younger boys and girls to slip their "flipper" or "clicker" out of position with their tongue. The remaining gap-toothed grin was sufficiently startling that it invariably stimulated gasps of amazement among the boys and squeals of shock among the girls.

In those days of unprotected hard-nosed football, oral or facial injuries constituted 50% of football mishaps. There was a 10% chance each year that a player would have such an injury. However, with the introduction of the face guard and padded helmet, approximately half of these injuries have been eliminated.[108] In 1962 the National High School Alliance Football Rules Committee adopted a ruling requiring high school football players to wear mouth guards.[129] The incidence of dental injuries to high school football players has been reduced to a range of 0.3%[207] to 3.2%.[191]

After documentation of the benefits of mouth guards in reducing head and neck injuries[113,206] as well as dental injuries, the National Collegiate Athletic Association Football Rules Committee adopted a mouth protector requirement in 1973. In 1990 the NCAA adopted a refinement of this rule, requiring that mouth guards be colored, instead of clear or white, so that game officials and coaches can readily identify those players not wearing mouth guards.[162] The mandatory use of mouth guards has now extended to professional football.[61] It is estimated that over 200,000 injuries are being prevented annually[65] with a significant reduction in the expense of dental care for oral traumatic injuries.[190]

A particularly satisfying major side benefit of the mouth guard has been the reduction of head concussions and neck injuries requiring cervical traction.[206] One collegiate team reported elimination of head concussion injuries while players were wearing mouth guards during the season.[163]

The dental profession can take considerable pride in this outstanding accomplishment over the last 30 years. Football mouth guards for high school players have been fabricated as a voluntary public service by practicing dentists across the United States under the sponsorship of local dental societies at no cost, or perhaps minimal expense for materials, to the schools. A mouth guard program for the local high schools is an excellent project for a local dental society and enhances the stature of the profession of dentistry immeasurably.

The success of the football mouth guard program has not been duplicated in other sports. Although most boxers use mouth guards, not all ice hockey leagues require them. The rate of injury in ice hockey may be three to six times as great as that in football.[70,131] The use of mouth guards must be encouraged in basketball, wrestling, soccer, rugby, lacrosse, auto racing, karate, judo, field hockey, and baseball.[64,94]

With the enormous growth in female athletics, attention must be given to prevention of dental injuries in female athletes. Currently, mouth protectors are not mandatory for any organized female sports.[65] Similarly, there should be greater emphasis on wearing mouth guards in unorganized sports.[128]

There is an oft repeated quote from the late football coach Vince Lombardi, "Kissing is a contact sport, football is a collision sport."[207] If in a collision sport like football dental injuries can be reduced so dramatically, these other contact sports should also be able to enjoy a similar reduction in traumatic dental injuries. Individual sports like skiing, parachuting, gymnastics, hurdling, horseback riding, surfing, water skiing, and diving should also require mouth guards. Individuals who have mouth guards should be encouraged to use them in personal recreational activities, such as water sliding, in which dental injuries occur with significant frequency.[208]

It has been noted that currently more injuries occur from noncontact sports than from contact sports, because many contact sports participants are wearing mouth guards.[83]

Stevens[207] has described the functions of mouth guards as follows:

1. They hold the soft tissues of the lips and cheeks away from the teeth and prevent laceration and bruising of the lips and cheeks against the hard and irregular teeth during impact.
2. They cushion and distribute the forces from direct frontal blows that would otherwise cause fracture or dislocation of anterior teeth.
3. They prevent the teeth in opposing arches from violent contact, which might chip or fracture teeth or damage supporting structures.
4. They provide the mandible with resilient but braced support, which absorbs impacts that might fracture the unsupported angle or condyle of the mandible.
5. They help prevent concussions, cerebral hemorrhage, and possible death by holding jaws apart and acting as shock absorbers to prevent upward and backward displacement of the mandibular condyles against the base of the skull.
6. They give protection against neck injuries.
7. They are psychological assets to contact sport athletes by increasing confidence and aggressiveness.
8. They fill the space and support adjacent teeth so that removable partial dentures can be removed during contact sports, preventing possible swallowing or aspiration of loose appliances.

Acceptance of mouth guards by athletes is very important. Adolescents accept mouth guards more readily than adults.[86] The qualities of a good mouth guard are adequate retention, comfort, ease of speech, resistance to wear and tear, ease of breathing, and protection for the teeth, gingiva, and lips.

The three most common types of mouth protectors are stock, mouth formed, and custom made.

The *stock* mouth guards come in one size and supposedly fit everyone. Therefore they are likely to be loose and ill-fitting. The protection afforded by them is questionable and it has been recommended that they be withdrawn from use.[217]

The *mouth-formed* protectors come in a manufacturer's kit and consist of an outer shell of plastic and an inner liner that can be adapted to the teeth by biting into the material after warming in hot water. These are the most popular of the three types. They are readily accepted by players,[209] afford protection, and can be produced for an entire team in a short time at minimal expense (Fig. 16-38).

The *custom-fitted* mouth guards require an initial impression to make a stone model of the arches. The mouth guard is then individually custom made on the model. These offer the most protection but take more time and expense in preparation. A

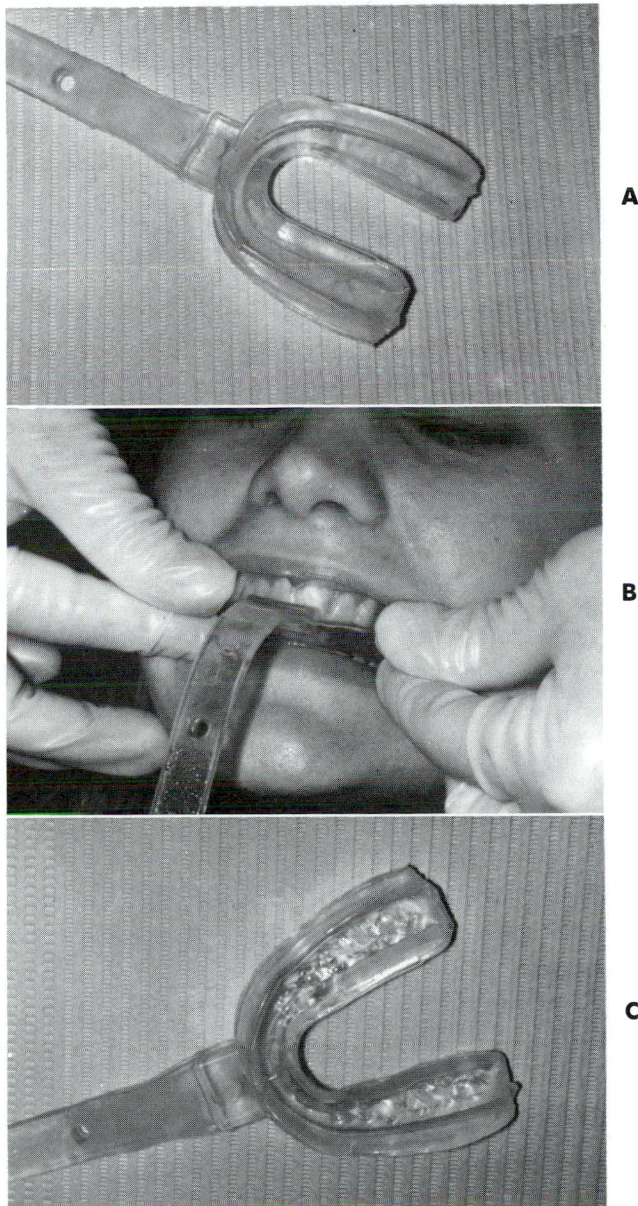

FIG. 16-38 Fabrication of mouth-formed protector. **A,** Preformed mouth guard from manufacturer. **B,** After softening in boiling water and momentarily chilling in room-temperature water, the mouth guard is placed in position and conformed to the occlusal anatomy of the maxillary arch, the cheek, and the lips. **C,** Completed mouth guard. Note the registration of the maxillary occlusal table.

EMERGENCY PROCEDURES FOR INJURED PERMANENT TEETH

Fractured anterior tooth

1. Pulp *not* exposed
   a. Cover exposed dentin with $Ca(OH)_2$ or ZOE.
   b. Place acid etch composite (composite will not set in contact with ZOE) or band over dressing to maintain seal.
   c. Restore tooth permanently in 6 to 8 weeks.
2. Pulp exposed in tooth with *open apex*
   a. Pulp cap with $Ca(OH)_2$ if treatment performed within 3 to 4 hours after injury.
   b. If massive pulp exposure or exposure over 3 to 4 hours, perform pulpotomy to maintain vitality and allow root completion. After root completion, perform root canal filling as necessary.
   c. If pulp necrotic, perform apexification procedure ($Ca(OH)_2$ powder) to induce apical closure. After root completion, fill canal with gutta-percha as permanent filling.
3. Pulp exposed tooth with fully formed root
   a. Perform root canal therapy, If you do not wish to try to preserve pulpal vitality with pulp capping.

Root fracture

1. Time critical
   a. Reposition segment as soon as possible and maintain vitality of pulp.
   b. Must achieve repositioning before blood clots.
2. Acid etch composite arch wire splint for 10 to 12 weeks
3. No root canal therapy *unless* evidence of pulpal pathosis
4. If root fracture communicates with oral cavity, prognosis is poor for reuniting segments

Displaced tooth

1. Time critical—reposition immediately (within 1 to 2 hours)
   a. Reposition the tooth correctly.
   b. Splint with acid etch composite arch wire for 7 to 10 days.
   c. Perform endodontic therapy if pulpal pathosis is confirmed during recalls.
      (1) Severe displacements (more than 5 mm) will usually require root canal therapy and $Ca(OH)_2$ powder filling. (See "$Ca(OH)_2$ root canal filling technique.")
      (2) Minor displacements should be followed closely to determine vitality. These teeth may not respond normally to electric pulp testing for several months.
   d. If bony involvement, see section on alveolar fractures.

Intruded tooth

1. Open apex, divergent canals
   a. If minor, leave alone.
   b. If severe, can surgically or orthodontically reposition.
      (1) May need to perform endodontic treatment.
      (2) Prognosis guarded.
2. Fully formed root
   a. Promptly reposition surgically or orthodontically.
   b. If surgically repositioned, splint with acid-etch composite arch wire for 7 to 10 days.
   c. Pulp must be removed during first 2 weeks.
   d. Clean canal and fill with $Ca(OH)_2$ powder.
   e. After 6 to 12 months, fill canal permanently with gutta-percha.

Minor fractures of the alveolar process associated with traumatized teeth

1. Bony fragments repositioned
2. Soft tissues sutured as necessary
3. Teeth splinted with acid etch composite arch wire, left in place 7 to 14 days
4. *More extensive fractures* of bone require longer splinting period

Avulsed, tooth out of mouth

1. Replantation immediately at time of injury, if possible
   a. Time critical. Prognosis deteriorates rapidly as extraoral time increases.
   b. Instruct patient or parent by telephone to replant tooth immediately at site of injury.
      (1) If tooth dirty, rinse under tap water. Do not scrub. Plug sink.

EMERGENCY PROCEDURES FOR INJURED PERMANENT TEETH—cont'd

(2) Gently tease tooth back into socket.
(3) Patient holds tooth in socket while being transported to dental office.

c. If replantation at site not possible.
(1) Place tooth in Hank's balanced salt solution (HBSS), a glass of milk, or physiologic saline, if available.
(2) If HBSS, milk, or physiologic saline is not available, hold tooth in buccal vestibule while coming to office. If danger of swallowing or if patient medically impaired from injury, place tooth in plastic wrap, wet towel, or glass of water. Do not allow tooth to air dry.
(3) As soon as patient arrives, replant tooth immediately.

d. For alveolar fracture, refer to section above.

e. Place acid etch composite and arch wire splint for 7 to 10 days.

f. Start antibiotic therapy and continue for 10 days.

2. Replantation of tooth with open apex (blunderbuss apex)
   a. Replant and do not perform endodontics.
      (1) Revitalization is desired.
      (2) During recalls, if pulp becomes necrotic clean root canal and fill with $Ca(OH)_2$ powder. (See "$Ca(OH)_2$ root canal filling technique.")
   b. If *longer* than 2 hours, pulp will likely necrose. Monitor pulpal status closely.
3. Replantation with completed root development
   a. Remove pulp and thoroughly cleanse canal during first 2 weeks.
   b. Fill canal with $Ca(OH)_2$ powder. (See "$Ca(OH)_2$ root canal filling technique.")
   c. Endodontic therapy must *always* be performed in tooth with completed root development.

$Ca(OH)_2$ root canal filling technique

4. Pulp extirpated, root canal thoroughly instrumented
5. $Ca(OH)_2$ to fill canal
   a. May use injectable $Ca(OH)_2$ preparations.
   b. Others use dry powder.
   c. Some prefer to make paste of $Ca(OH)_2$ with anesthetic solution or water.
   d. Others prefer a paste of $Ca(OH)_2$ with CMCP.
6. Canals recleaned and repacked with $Ca(OH)_2$ at 3-month intervals for *minimum* of 1 year
7. If resorption is arrested or nonexistent, canal filled with gutta-percha

The acid etch composite arch wire splint

1. Orthodontic wire bent to conform to facial surfaces of teeth to be splinted
   a. At least one sound tooth on each side of displaced tooth or teeth must be included.
   b. Size 0.015-0.030 wire.
   c. Shape of wire is unimportant.
   d. Monofilament nylon line acceptable.
2. Arch wire attached to teeth with acid etch composite
   a. Middle half of facial surfaces of teeth is etched with phosphoric acid gel or solution for 1 minute.
   b. Teeth are thoroughly washed and dried.
   c. Arch wire is attached to facial surfaces of teeth with composite.
      (1) Any form of resin or composite is acceptable.
      (2) Only a small amount of composite in facial half of crown is necessary to hold arch wire
      (3) Take care to avoid contact of composite with gingiva.
   d. During attachment of arch wire, one must ensure that injured tooth is in correct position.
      (1) Take radiograph following placement to verify correct position of injured tooth.
3. Instructions to patient
   a. Avoid biting on splinted teeth. Cut food into bite size and chew on posterior teeth.
   b. Remember to keep the area clean.
4. Removal of splint
   a. Composite and wire are drilled through and wire is freed.
   b. It is not advisable to remove all composite from injured teeth at time of splint removal.
      (1) Excessive manipulation of injured teeth may cause displacement.
      (2) Smooth composite and leave remnants for several months.
      (3) After teeth are firmly attached (2 to 3 months), fragments of remaining composite can be removed with sharp carver or scaler.

custom-fitted mouth guard has been estimated to cost 10 times as much as a mouth-formed one.[191] The additional expense and time are justified for those athletes who must talk or give clear instructions on the playing field, because speech is generally better with this type of protector. Athletes who wear orthodontic bands and wires should also have custom-fitted mouth guards.[191] A combination mouth guard and lip guard has been advocated for maximum oral protection.[99]

There have been many "spinoff" applications of mouth guards in extraathletic situations.[155] Mouth guards have been advocated for patients' use in the operating room during general anesthesia.[112,164,189] Anterior teeth are vulnerable to chipping or displacement during orotracheal or nasotracheal intubation procedures. With the increase in microlaryngoscopic and esophagoscopic procedures anterior teeth and fixed prostheses are more frequently at risk. Simple acrylic mouth guards can be prepared preoperatively if the operating room procedure is of a nonemergency nature. Anesthesiologists resist the use of mouth guards because the additional material in the patient's mouth reduces visibility, limits access, and in small mouths makes intubation more difficult or impossible.[44] However, it is felt that the acceptance of tooth protectors as a standard of care, combined with a thorough dental assessment before the administration of inhalation anesthetics, may prevent 90% of dental complications in general anesthesia.[150]

Custom-made mouth guards should be fabricated for handicapped children subject to frequent falls. Excellent retention is mandatory for these appliances.

Another preventive measure that can reduce traumatic injuries is prophylactic orthodontics. People with extreme overjet are two to five times as likely as other persons to suffer injury to their maxillary incisors.[126,207]

The use of seat belts, shoulder harnesses, and airbags in automobiles is another common sense precaution.

Education of the public is very important. It is the responsibility of dentists to educate all persons who might have the first contact with someone who has a dental injury as to the proper procedures for providing dental first aid until professional treatment can be obtained.[68] The North Carolina Dental Society has developed a public awareness campaign to educate coaches, teachers, industrial and school nurses, emergency medical personnel, and parents as to the proper procedures for handling dental emergencies, particularly the avulsed tooth. The boxed outline on pages 478 to 479 was distributed to all North Carolina dentists as a quick reminder of appropriate treatment.

REFERENCES

1. Anderson AW, Sharav Y, and Massler M: Periodontal reattachment after tooth replantation, Periodontics 6:161, 1968.
2. Andersson L: Dentoalveolar ankylosis and associated root resorption in replanted teeth. Experimental and clinical studies in monkeys and man, Swed Dent J 56(suppl):1, 1988.
3. Andersson L, Bodin I, and Sörensen S: Progression of root resorption following replantation of human teeth after extended extra-oral storage, Endod Dent Traumatol 5:38, 1989.
4. Andersson L, et al: Tooth ankylosis. Clinical, radiographic and histological assessments, Int J Oral Surg 13:423, 1984.
5. Andersson L, et al: Effect of masticatory stimulation on dentoalveolar ankylosis after experimental tooth replantation, Endod Dent Traumatol 1:13, 1985.
6. Andreasen FM: Transient apical breakdown and its relation to color and sensibility changes after luxation injuries to teeth, Endod Dent Traumatol 2:9, 1986.
7. Andreasen FM: Histological and bacteriological study of pulps extirpated after luxation injuries, Endod Dent Traumatol 4:170, 1988.
8. Andreasen FM: Pulpal healing after luxation injuries and root fracture in the permanent dentition, Endod Dent Traumatol 5:111, 1989.
9. Andreasen FM, and Andreasen JO: Diagnosis of luxation injuries: the importance of standardized clinical, radiographic and photographic techniques in clinical investigations, Endod Dent Traumatol 1:160, 1985.
10. Andreasen FM, and Andreasen JO: Resorption and mineralization processes following root fracture of permanent incisors, Endod Dent Traumatol 4:202, 1988.
11. Andreasen FM, Andreasen JO, and Bayer T: Prognosis of root-fractured permanent incisors: prediction of healing modalities, Endod Dent Traumatol 5:11, 1989.
12. Andreasen FM, and Vestergaard Pedersen B: Prognosis of luxated permanent teeth: the development of pulp necrosis, Endod Dent Traumatol 1:207, 1985.
13. Andreasen FM, et al: Occurrence of pulp canal obliteration after luxation injuries in the permanent dentition, Endod Dent Traumatol 3:103, 1987.
14. Andreasen FM, Zhijie Y, and Thomsen BL: Relationship between pulp dimensions and development of pulp necrosis after luxation injuries in the permanent dentition, Endod Dent Traumatol 2:90, 1986.
15. Andreasen JO: Etiology and pathogenesis of traumatic dental injuries: a clinical study of 1298 cases, Scand J Dent Res 78:329, 1970.
16. Andreasen JO: Luxation of permanent teeth due to trauma: a clinical and radiographic follow-up study of 184 injured teeth, Scand J Dent Res 78:273, 1970.
17. Andreasen JO: Treatment of fractured and avulsed teeth, J Dent Child 38:29, 1971.
18. Andreasen JO: Effect of pulpal necrosis upon periodontal healing after surgical injury in rats, Int J Oral Surg 2:62, 1973.
19. Andreasen JO: The effect of splinting upon periodontal healing after replantation of permanent incisors in monkeys, Acta Odontol Scand 33:313, 1975.
20. Andreasen JO: Periodontal healing after replantation of traumatically avulsed human teeth: assessment by mobility testing and radiography, Acta Odontol Scand 33:325, 1975.
21. Andreasen JO: Analysis of pathogenesis and topography of replacement root resorption (ankylosis) after replantation of mature permanent incisors in monkeys, Swed Dent J 4:231, 1980.
22. Andreasen JO: Analysis of topography of surface and inflammatory root resorption after replantation of mature permanent incisors in monkeys, Swed Dent J 4:135, 1980.
23. Andreasen JO: The effect of removal of the coagulum in the alveolus before replantation upon periodontal and pulpal healing of mature permanent incisors in monkeys, Int J Oral Surg 9:458, 1980.
24. Andreasen JO: A time-related study of periodontal healing and root resorption activity after replantation of mature permanent incisors in monkeys, Swed Dent J 4:101, 1980.
25. Andreasen JO: Effect of extra-alveolar period and storage media upon periodontal and pulpal healing after replantation of mature permanent incisors in monkeys, Int J Oral Surg 10:43, 1981.
26. Andreasen JO: The effect of pulp extirpation or root canal treatment on periodontal healing after replantation of permanent incisors in monkeys, J Endod 7:245, 1981.
27. Andreasen JO: Interrelation between alveolar bone and periodontal ligament repair after replantation of mature permanent incisors in monkeys, J Periodont Res 16:228, 1981.
28. Andreasen JO: Periodontal healing after replantation and autotransplantation of incisors in monkeys, Int J Oral Surg 10:54, 1981.
29. Andreasen JO: Relationship between cell damage in the periodontal ligament after replantation and subsequent development of root resorption: a time related study in monkeys, Acta Odontol Scand 39:15, 1981.
30. Andreasen JO: Relationship between surface and inflammatory resorption and changes in the pulp after replantation of permanent incisors in monkeys, J Endod 7:294, 1981.

31. Andreasen JO: Traumatic injuries of the teeth, ed 2, Philadelphia, 1981, WB Saunders Co.
32. Andreasen JO: Challenges in clinical dental traumatology, Endod Dent Traumatol 1:45, 1985.
33. Andreasen JO: External root resorption: its implication in dental traumatology, paedodontics, periodontics, orthodontics and endodontics, Int Endod J 18:109, 1985.
34. Andreasen JO, and Hjorting-Hansen E: Replantation of teeth. I. Radiographic and clinical study of 110 human teeth replanted after accidental loss, Acta Odontol Scand 24:263, 1966.
35. Andreasen JO, and Hjorting-Hansen E: Replantation of teeth. II. Histological study of 22 replanted anterior teeth in humans, Acta Odontol Scand 24:287, 1966.
36. Andreasen JO, and Hjorting-Hansen E: Intraalveolar root fractures: radiographic and histological study of 50 cases, Oral Surg 25:414, 1967.
37. Andreasen JO, and Kristensson L: The effect of limited drying or removal of the periodontal ligament: periodontal healing after replantation of mature permanent incisors in monkeys, Acta Odontol Scand 39:1, 1981.
38. Andreasen JO, and Ravn JJ: The effect of traumatic injuries to the primary teeth on their permanent successors, Scand J Dent Res 79:284, 1971.
39. Andreasen JO, and Ravn JJ: Epidemiology of traumatic dental injuries to primary and permanent teeth in a Danish population sample, Int J Oral Surg 1:235, 1972.
40. Andreasen JO, and Ravn JJ: Enamel changes in permanent teeth after trauma to their primary predecessors, Scand J Dent Res 81:203, 1973.
41. Andreasen JO, and Riis I: Influence of pulp necrosis and periapical inflammation of primary teeth on their permanent successors, Int J Oral Surg 7:178, 1978.
42. Andreasen JO, and Schwartz O: The effect of saline storage before replantation upon dry damage of the periodontal ligament, Endod Dent Traumatol 2:67, 1986.
43. Antrim DD, and Ostrowski JS: A functional splint for traumatized teeth, J Endod 8:328, 1982.
44. Aromaa U, et al: Difficulties with tooth protectors in endotracheal intubation, Acta Anaesthesiol Scand 32:304, 1988.
45. Bakland LK: Traumatic injuries. In Ingle JI, and Taintor JF (eds): Endodontics, ed 3, Philadelphia, 1985, Lea & Febiger.
46. Barbakow FH, Austin JC, and Cleaton-Jones PE: Experimental replantation of root-canal-filled and untreated teeth in the vervet monkey, J Endod 3:89, 1977.
47. Barbakow FH, Cleaton-Jones PE, and Austin JC: Healing of replanted teeth following topical treatment with fluoride solution and systemic admission of thyrocalcitonin: a histometric analysis, J Endod 7:302, 1981.
48. Barkin PR: Time as a factor in predicting the vitality of traumatized teeth, J Dent Child 40:188, 1973.
49. Barry GN: Replanted teeth still functioning after 42 years: report of a case, J Am Dent Assoc 92:412, 1976.
50. Berude JA, et al: Resorption after physiological and rigid splinting of replanted permanent incisors in monkeys, J Endod 14:592, 1988.
51. Bhaskar SN, and Rappaport HM: Dental vitality tests and pulp status, J Am Dent Assoc 86:409, 1973.
52. Bielak S, Bimstein E, and Eidelman E: Forced eruption: the treatment of choice for subgingivally fractured permanent incisors, J Dent Child 49:186, 1982.
53. Bjorvatn K, Selvig KA, and Klinge B: Effect of tetracycline and SnF_2 on root resorption in replanted incisors in dogs. Scand J Dent Res 97:477, 1989.
54. Blomlöf L, et al: Vitality of periodontal ligament cells after storage of monkey teeth in milk or saliva, Scand J Dent Res 88:441, 1980.
55. Blomlöf L, and Otteskog P: Viability of human periodontal ligament cells after storage in milk or saliva, Scand J Dent Res 88:436, 1980.
56. Blomlöf L, Lindskog S, and Hammarström L: Periodontal healing of exarticulated monkey teeth stored in milk or saliva, Scand J Dent Res 89:251, 1981.
57. Blomlöf L, Otteskog P, and Hammarström L: Effect of storage in media with different ion strengths and osmolalities on human periodontal ligament cells, Scand J Dent Res 89:180, 1981.
58. Blomlöf L, et al: Periodontal healing of replanted monkey teeth prevented from drying, Acta Odontol Scand 41:117, 1983.
59. Blomlöf L, et al: Storage of experimentally avulsed teeth in milk prior to replantation, J Dent Res 6:912, 1983.
60. Braham RL, Roberts MW, and Morris ME: Management of dental trauma in children and adolescents, J Trauma 17:857, 1977.
61. Brotman IN, and Rothschild HL: Report of a breakthrough in preventive dental care for a National Football League team, J Am Dent Assoc 88:553, 1974.
62. Buonocore MG: A simple method of increasing the adhesion of acrylic filling material to enamel surfaces, J Dent Res 34:849, 1955.
63. Buonocore MG, and Davila J: Restoration of fractured anterior teeth with ultraviolet-light polymerized bonding materials: a new technique, J Am Dent Assoc 86:1349, 1973.
64. Bureau of Dental Health Education, Council on Dental Materials and Devices: Mouth protectors: 11 years later, J Am Dent Assoc 86:1365, 1973.
65. Bureau of Health Education and Audiovisual Services, Council on Dental Materials, Instruments and Equipment: Mouth protectors and sports team dentists, J Am Dent Assoc 109:84, 1984.
66. Camp JH: Replantation of teeth following trauma. In McDonald RE et al, editors: Current therapy in dentistry, vol 7, St. Louis, 1980, The CV Mosby Co.
67. Camp JH, et al: Recommended guidelines for treatment of the avulsed tooth, J Endod 9:571, 1983.
68. Camp JH: Diagnosis and management of sports-related injuries to the teeth. Dent Clin North Am 35:733, 1991.
69. Carter AP, et al: Dental injuries in Seattle's public school children: school year 1969-70, J Public Health Dent 32:251, 1972.
70. Castaldi C: Injuries to the teeth. In Vinger PF and Hoerner EF (eds): Sports injuries: the unthwarted epidemic, Littleton, Mass, 1981, PSG Publishing Co., Inc.
71. Coccia CT: A clinical investigation of root resorption rates in reimplanted young permanent incisors: a five-year study, J Endod 6:413, 1980.
72. Council on Dental Materials, Instruments, and Equipment: Council reevaluates position on dental endosseous implants, J Am Dent Assoc 100:247, 1980.
73. Croll TP, et al: Rapid neurologic assessment and initial management for the patient with traumatic dental injuries. J Am Dent Assoc 100:530, 1980.
74. Croll TP, Pascon EA, and Langeland K: Traumatically injured primary incisors: a clinical and histological study, J Dent Child 54:401, 1987.
75. Crona-Larsson G, Bjarnason S, and Norén JG: Effect of luxation injuries on permanent teeth. Endod Dent Traumatol 7:199, 1991.
76. Cronin RJ: Prosthodontic management of vertical root extrusion, J Prosthet Dent 46:498, 1981.
77. Cvek M: Treatment of nonvital permanent incisors with calcium hydroxide, Odontol Rev 25:239, 1974.
78. Cvek M: A clinical report on partial pulpotomy and capping with calcium hydroxide in permanent incisors with complicated crown fractures, J Endod 4:232, 1978.
79. Cvek M: Endodontic treatment of traumatized teeth. In Andreasen JO: Traumatic injuries of the teeth, ed 2, Philadelphia, 1981, WB Saunders Co.
80. Cvek M: Prognosis of luxated nonvital maxillary incisors treated with calcium hydroxide and filled with gutta percha. A retrospective clinical study. Endod Dent Traumatol 8:45, 1992.
81. Cvek M, Granath LE, and Hollender L: Treatment of nonvital permanent incisors with calcium hydroxide. II. Variation of occurrence of ankylosis of reimplanted teeth with duration of extra-alveolar period and storage environment, Odontol Rev 25:43, 1974.
82. Cvek M, and Lundberg M: Histological appearance of pulps after exposure by a crown fracture, partial pulpotomy, and clinical diagnosis of healing, J Endod 9:8, 1983.

83. Davis GT, and Knott SC: Dental trauma in Australia, Aust Dent J 29:217, 1984.
84. Degering CI: Radiography of dental fractures, Oral Surg 30:213, 1970.
85. Delivanis P, Delivanis H, and Kuftinec MM: Endodontic-orthodontic management of fractured anterior teeth, J Am Dent Assoc 97:483, 1978.
86. deWet FA: The prevention of orofacial sports injuries in the adolescent, Int Dent J 31:313, 1981.
87. Ellis RG, and Davey KW: The classification and treatment of injuries to the teeth of children, ed 5, Chicago, 1970, Year Book Medical Publishers, Inc.
88. Ferguson FS, and Ripa LW: Prevalence and type of traumatic injuries to the anterior teeth of preschool children, J Pedod 4:3, 1979.
89. Flanagan VO, and Myers HI: Delayed reimplantation of second molars in the Syrian hamster, Oral Surg 11:1179, 1958.
90. Frank AL: Improvement of the crown-root ratio by endodontic endosseous implants, J Am Dent Assoc 74:451, 1967.
91. Frank AL: Resorption, perforations, and fractures, Dent Clin North Am 18:465, 1974.
92. Fuks AB, et al: Partial pulpotomy as a treatment alternative for exposed pulps in crown-fractured permanent incisors, Endod Dent Traumatol 3:100, 1987.
93. Galea H: An investigation of dental injuries treated in an acute care general hospital, J Am Dent Assoc 109:434, 1984.
94. Garon MW, Merkle A, and Wright T: Mouth protectors and oral trauma: a study of adolescent football players, J Am Dent Assoc 112:663, 1986.
95. Gazelius B, Olgart L, and Edwall B: Restored vitality in luxated teeth assessed by laser Doppler flowmeter, Endod Dent Traumatol 4:265, 1988.
96. Granath LE, and Hagman G: Experimental pulpotomy in human bicuspids with reference to cutting technique, Acta Odontol Scand 29:155, 1971.
97. Grossman LI: Endodontic practice, ed 10, Philadelphia, 1981, Lea & Febiger.
98. Grossman LI, and Ship II: Survival rate of replanted teeth, Oral Surg 29:899, 1970.
99. Guevara PA, and Ranalli DN: Techniques for mouthguard fabrication. Dent Clin North Am 35:667, 1991.
100. Hammarström L, et al: Replantation of teeth and antibiotic treatment, Endod Dent Traumatol 2:51, 1986.
101. Hammarström L, Blomlöf L, and Lindskog S: Dynamics of dentoalveolar ankylosis and associated root resorption. Endod Dent Traumatol 5:163, 1989.
102. Hardy LB, O'Neal RB, and del Rio CE: Effect of polylactic acid on replanted teeth in dogs, Oral Surg 51:86, 1981.
103. Hedegard B, and Stalhane I: A study of traumatized permanent teeth in children aged 7-15 years, Swed Dent J 66:431, 1973.
104. Heide S: Pulp reactions to exposure for 4, 48, or 168 hours, J Dent Res 59:1910, 1980.
105. Heide S, and Kerekes K: Delayed partial pulpotomy in permanent incisors of monkeys, Int Endod J 19:78, 1986.
106. Heiman GR, et al: Temporary splinting using an adhesive system, Oral Surg 31:819, 1971.
107. Heimdahl A, von Konow L, and Lundquist G: Replantation of avulsed teeth after long extraalveolar periods, Int J Oral Surg 12:413, 1983.
108. Heintz WD: Mouth protectors: a progress report, J Am Dent Assoc 77:632, 1968.
109. Heithersay GS: Combined endodontic-orthodontic treatment of transverse root fractures in the region on the alveolar crest, Oral Surg 36:404, 1973.
110. Heithersay GS, and Moule AJ: Anterior subgingival fractures: a review of treatment alternatives, Aust Dent J 27:368, 1982.
111. Helle A, Sirkkanen R, and Evalahti M: Repair of fractured incisal edges with UV-light polymerized and self-polymerized fissure sealants and composite resins: two-year report of 93 cases, Proc Finn Dent Soc 71:87, 1975.
112. Henry PJ, and Barb RE: Mouth protectors for use in general anesthesia, J Am Dent Assoc 68:569, 1964.
113. Hickey JC, et al: The relation of mouth protectors to cranial pressure and deformation, J Am Dent Assoc 74:735, 1967.
114. Hill FJ, and Picton JF: Fractured incisor fragment in the tongue: a case report, Pediatr Dent 3:337, 1981.
115. Hiltz J, and Trope M: Vitality of human lip fibroblasts in milk, Hanks balanced salt solution and Viaspan storage media. Endod Dent Traumatol 7:69, 1991.
116. Holan G, Topf J, and Fuks AB: Effect of root canal infection and treatment of traumatized primary incisors on their permanent successors. Endod Dent Traumatol 8:12, 1992.
117. Holland R, et al: Root canal treatment with calcium hydroxide. I. Effect of overfilling and refilling, Oral Surg 47:87, 1979.
118. Hovland EJ, and Gutmann JL: Atraumatic stabilization for traumatized teeth, J Endod 2:390, 1976.
119. Hurst RB: Regeneration of periodontal and transseptal fibers after autografts in Rhesus monkeys: a qualitative approach, J Dent Res 51:1183, 1972.
120. Ingber JS: Forced eruption. II. A method of treating nonrestorable teeth—periodontal and restorative considerations, J Periodontol 47:203, 1976.
121. Jacobsen I: Root fractures in permanent anterior teeth with incomplete root formation, Scand J Dent Res 84:210, 1976.
122. Jacobsen I, and Kerekes K: Long-term prognosis of traumatized permanent anterior teeth showing calcifying processes in the pulp cavity, Scand J Dent Res 85:588, 1977.
123. Jacobsen I, and Kerekes K: Diagnosis and treatment of pulp necrosis in permanent anterior teeth with root fracture, Scand J Dent Res 88:370, 1980.
124. Jacobsen I, and Sangnes G: Traumatized primary anterior teeth, Acta Odontol Scand 36:199, 1978.
125. Jacobsen I, and Zachrisson BV: Repair characteristics of root fractures in permanent anterior teeth, Scand J Dent Res 83:355, 1975.
126. Jarvinen S: Incisal overjet and traumatic injuries to upper permanent incisors: a retrospective study, Acta Odontol Scand 36:359, 1978.
127. Jarvinen S: Fractured and avulsed permanent incisors in Finnish children: a retrospective study, Acta Odontol Scand 37:47, 1979.
128. Jarvinen S: On the causes of traumatic dental injuries with special reference to sports accidents in a sample of Finnish children: a study of a clinical patient material, Acta Odontol Scand 38:151, 1980.
129. Johnsen DC, and Winters JE: Prevention of intraoral trauma in sports. Dent Clin North Am 35:657, 1991.
130. Jordan RE, et al: Restoration of fractured and hypoplastic incisors by the acid-etch resin technique: a three-year report, J Am Dent Assoc 95:795, 1977.
131. Josell SD, and Abrams RG: Traumatic injuries to the dentition and its supporting structures, Pediatr Clin North Am 29:717, 1982.
132. Kahnberg K-E: Intraalveolar transplantation of teeth with crown-root fractures, J Oral Maxillofac Surg 43:38, 1985.
133. Kahnberg K-E: Surgical extrusion of root-fractured teeth—a follow-up study of two surgical methods, Endod Dent Traumatol 4:85, 1988.
134. Kahnberg K, Warfvinge J, and Birgersson B: Intraalveolar transplantation, Int J Oral Surg 11:372, 1982.
135. Kakehasi S, Stanley HR, and Fitzgerald RT: The effects of surgical exposures of dental pulps in germ-free and conventional laboratory rats, Oral Surg 20:340, 1965.
136. Katz RV, et al: Epidemiologic survey of accidental dentofacial injuries among U.S. Army personnel, Community Dent Oral Epidemiol 7:30, 1979.
137. Kopel HM, and Johnson R: Examination and neurologic assessment of children with oro-facial trauma, Endod Dent Traumatol 1:155, 1985.
138. Kozlorsky A, Tal H, and Lieberman M: Forced eruption combined with gingival fiberotomy. A technique for clinical crown lengthening, J Clin Periodontol 15:534, 1988.

139. Krakow AA, Berk H, and Grøn P: Therapeutic induction of root formation in the exposed incompletely formed tooth with a vital pulp, Oral Surg 43:755, 1977.
140. Krasner P, and Person P: Preserving avulsed teeth for replantation. J Am Dent Assoc 123:80, 1992.
141. Kristerson L, and Andreasen JO: The effect of splinting upon periodontal and pulpal healing after autotransplantation of mature and immature permanent incisors in monkeys, Int J Oral Surg 12:239, 1983.
142. Kristerson L, and Andreasen JO: Influence of root development on periodontal and pulpal healing after replantation of incisors in monkeys, Int J Oral Surg 13:313, 1984.
143. Lengheden A, Blomlöf L, and Lindskog S: Effect of delayed calcium hydroxide treatment on periodontal healing in contaminated replanted teeth. Scand J Dent Res 99:147, 1991.
144. Lengheden A, Blomlöf L, and Lindskog S: Effect of immediate calcium hydroxide treatment and permanent root-filling on periodontal healing in contaminated replanted teeth. Scand J Dent Res 99:139, 1991.
145. Lenstrup K, and Skieller V: A follow-up study of teeth replanted after accidental loss, Acta Odontol Scand 17:503, 1959.
146. Lindskog S, and Blomlöf L: Influence of osmolality and composition of some storage media on human periodontal ligament cells, Acta Odontol Scand 40:435, 1982.
147. Lindskog S, Blomlöf L, and Hammarström L: Mitosis and microorganisms in the periodontal membrane after storage in milk or saliva, Scand J Dent Res 91:465, 1983.
148. Lindskog S, Blomlöf L, and Hammarstrom L: Comparative effects of parathyroid hormone on osteoblasts and cementoblasts. J Clin Periodontol 14:386, 1987.
149. Lindskog S, and Hammarström L: Evidence in favor of an anti-invasion factor in cementum or periodontal membrane of human teeth, Scand J Dent Res 88:161, 1980.
150. Lockhart PB, et al: Dental complications during and after tracheal intubation, J Am Dent Assoc 112:480, 1986.
151. Löe H, and Waerhaug J: Experimental replantation of teeth in dogs and monkeys, Arch Oral Biol 3:176, 1961.
152. Lundberg M, and Cvek M: A light microscopy study of pulps from traumatized permanent incisors with reduced pulpal lumen, Acta Odontol Scand 38:89, 1980.
153. Malmgren B, et al: Surgical treatment of ankylosed and infrapositioned reimplanted incisors in adolescents, Scand J Dent Res 92:391, 1984.
154. Malmgren O, Malmgren B, and Frykholm A: Rapid orthodontic extrusion of crown root and cervical root fractured teeth. Endod Dent Traumatol 7:49, 1991.
155. McWhorter AG, and Seale NS: Spin-off applications of mouthguards. Dent Clin North Am 35:683, 1991.
156. Meadow D, Needleman H, and Lindner G: Oral trauma in children, Pediatr Dent 6:248, 1984.
157. Melcher AH, and Turnbull RS: Inhibition of osteogenesis by periodontal ligament, J Periodont Res 10(suppl):16, 1972.
158. Michanowicz AE, Michanowicz JP, and Abou-Rass M: Cementogenic repair of root fractures, J Am Dent Assoc 82:569, 1971.
159. Morris ML, et al: Factors affecting healing after experimentally delayed tooth transplantation, J Endod 7:80, 1981.
160. Nasjleti CE, et al: Healing after tooth reimplantation in monkeys, Oral Surg 39:361, 1975.
161. Natkin E: Diagnosis and treatment of traumatic injuries and their sequelae. In Ingle JI (ed): Endodontics, Philadelphia, 1965, Lea & Febiger.
162. Nelson D: NCAA to adopt color standards for mouthguards, Amer Dent Assoc News 20:5, March 20, 1989.
163. News of dentistry: fitted mouthguards afford key protection, J Am Dent Assoc 84:531, 1972.
164. Noyek AM, and Winnick AN: An acrylic dental protector in perioral endoscopy, J Otolaryngol 5:1, 1976.
165. Oesterle LK, and Wood LW: Raising the root—a look at orthodontic extrusion, J Am Dent Assoc 122:193, 1991.
166. Ohman A: Healing and sensitivity to pain in young replanted human teeth: an experimental, clinical, and histological study, Odontol Tidskr 73:165, 1965.
167. Oikarinen K: Pathogenesis and mechanism of traumatic injuries to teeth, Endod Dent Traumatol 3:220, 1987.
168. Oikarinen K: Functional fixation for traumatically luxated teeth, Endod Dent Traumatol 3:224, 1987.
169. Oikarinen K: Comparison of the flexibility of various splinting methods for tooth fixation, Int J Oral Maxillofac Surg 17:125, 1988.
170. Oikarinen K, Andreasen JO, and Andreasen FM: Rigidity of various fixation methods used as dental splints. Endod Dent Traumatol 8:113, 1992.
171. Oikarinen K, Gundlach KKH, and Pfeifer G: Late complications of luxation injuries to teeth, Endod Dent Traumatol 3:296, 1987.
172. O'Mullane DM: Injured permanent incisor teeth: an epidemiological study, J Irish Dent Assoc 18:160, 1972.
173. Pierce A, Berg JO, and Lindskog S: Calcitonin as an alternative therapy in the treatment of root resorption, J Endod 4:459, 1988.
174. Pierce A, Heithersay G, and Lindskog S: Evidence for direct inhibition of dentinoclasts by a corticosteroid/antibiotic endodontic paste, Endod Dent Traumatol 4:44, 1988.
175. Pierce A, and Lindskog S: The effect of an antibiotic/corticosteroid combination on inflammatory root resorption *in vivo*, Oral Surg, Oral Med, Oral Pathol 64:216, 1987.
176. Pindborg JJ: Clinical, radiographic, and histological aspects of intra-alveolar fractures of upper central incisors, Acta Odontol Scand 13:41, 1955.
177. Rabie G, Barnett F, and Tronstad L: Long-term splinting of maxillary incisor with intra-alveolar root fracture, Endod Dent Traumatol 4:99, 1988.
178. Rakocz M, Keating J, and Croll TP: Traumatic impaction of a maxillary primary incisor into the nasal cavity, J Pedod 9:338, 1985.
179. Rand A: Suture splint for displaced teeth, J NJ Dent Assoc 46:30, 1975.
180. Ravn JJ: Sequelae of acute mechanical traumata in the primary dentition, J Dent Child 35:281, 1968.
181. Ravn JJ: Dental injuries in Copenhagen school children, school years 1967-1972, Community Dent Oral Epidemiol 2:231, 1974.
182. Ravn JJ: Follow-up study of permanent incisors with enamel cracks as a result of an acute trauma, Scand J Dent Res 89:117, 1981.
183. Ravn JJ: Follow-up study of permanent incisors with enamel-dentin fractures after acute trauma, Scand J Dent Res 89:355, 1981.
184. Ravn JJ: Follow-up study of permanent incisors with enamel fractures as a result of an acute trauma, Scand J Dent Res 89:213, 1981.
185. Ravn JJ, and Rossen I: Prevalence and distribution of traumatic tooth injuries among Copenhagen school children, 1967-68, Tandlaegebladet 73:1, 1969.
186. Roberts MW, and Moffa JP: Repair of fractured incisal angles with an ultraviolet-light-activated fissure sealant and a composite resin: two year report of 60 cases, J Am Dent Assoc 87:888, 1973.
187. Rock WP, et al: The relationship between trauma and pulp death in incisor teeth, Br Dent J 136:236, 1974.
188. Rock WP, and Grundy MC: The effect of luxation and subluxation upon the prognosis of traumatized incisor teeth, J Dent 9:224, 1981.
189. Salisbury PL, Curtis JW, and Kohut RI: Appliance to protect maxillary teeth and palate during endoscopy, Arch Otolaryngol 110:106, 1984.
190. Sane J: Comparison of maxillofacial and dental injuries in four contact team sports: American football, bandy, basketball, and handball. Am J Sports Med 16:647, 1988.
191. Seals RR, et al: An evaluation of mouthguard programs in Texas high school football, J Amer Dent Assoc 110:904, 1985.
192. Seltzer S, et al: Titanium endodontic implants: a scanning electron microscope, electron microprobe, and histologic investigation, J Endod 2:267, 1976.
193. Shapira J, Reger L, and Liebfeld H: Re-eruption of completely intruded immature permanent incisors, Endod Dent Traumatol 2:113, 1986.

194. Shulman LB, Kalis PJ, and Goldhaber P: Fluoride inhibition of tooth-replant root resorption in Cebus monkeys, J Dent Res 1968 (abstract 440).
195. Skieller V: The prognosis for young teeth loosened after mechanical injuries, Acta Odontol Scand 18:171, 1980.
196. Skoglund A: Pulpal survival in replanted and autotransplanted apicoectomized mature teeth of dogs with prepared nutritional canals, Int J Oral Surg 12:31, 1983.
197. Skoglund A, and Tronstad L: Pulpal changes in replanted and autotransplanted immature teeth of dogs, J Endod 7:309, 1981.
198. Smukler H, and Tagger N: Vital root amputation: a clinical and histological study, J Periodontol 47:324, 1976.
199. Söder PO, et al: Effect of drying on viability of periodontal membrane, Scand J Dent Res 85:164, 1977.
200. Sonis AL: Longitudinal study of discolored primary teeth and effect on succedaneous teeth, J Pedod 11:247, 1987.
201. Spalding PM, et al: The changing role of endodontics and orthodontics in the management of traumatically intruded permanent incisors, Pediatr Dent 7:104, 1985.
202. Stanley HR, Laskin J, and Broom CA: Moistness, more than temperature variations, prevents autolysis of pulp tissue in avulsed teeth, J Endod 9:360, 1983.
203. Stanley HR, and Lundy T: Dycal therapy for pulp exposures, Oral Surg 34:818, 1972.
204. Stanley HR, et al: Ischemic infarction of the pulp: sequential degenerative changes of the pulp after traumatic injury, J Endod 4:325, 1978.
205. Stanley HR, White CL, and McCray L: The rate of tertiary (reparative) dentin formation in the human tooth, Oral Surg 21:180, 1966.
206. Stenger JM, et al: Mouthguards: protection against shock to head, neck, and teeth, J Am Dent Assoc 69:273, 1964.
207. Stevens OO: Prevention of traumatic dental and oral injuries. In Andreasen JO: Traumatic injuries of the teeth, ed 2, Philadelphia, 1981, WB Saunders CO.
208. Stokes AN: Waterslide accidents, N Zealand Dent J 81:114, 1985.
209. Stokes ANS, Croft GC, and Gee D: Comparison of laboratory and intraorally formed mouth protectors, Endod Dent Traumatol 3:255, 1987.
210. Tate RJ: Facial injuries associated with the battered child syndrome, Br J Oral Surg 9:41, 1971.
211. Tegsjö U, Valerius-Olsson H, and Olgart K: Intra-alveolar transplantation of teeth with cervical root fractures, Swed Dent J 2:73, 1978.
212. Tegsjö U, et al: Clinical evaluation of intra-alveolar transplantation of teeth with cervical root fractures, Swedish Dent J 11:235, 1987.
213. Thylstrup A, and Andreasen JO: The influence of traumatic intrusion of primary teeth on their permanent successors in monkeys, J Oral Pathol 6:296, 1977.
214. Tronstad L: Root resorption—etiology, terminology and clinical manifestations. Endod Dent Traumatol 4:241, 1988.
215. Trope M, and Friedman S: Periodontal healing of replanted dog teeth stored in Viaspan, milk and Hanks balanced salt solution. Endod Dent Traumatol 8:183, 1992.
216. Turley PK, Joiner MW, and Hellstrom S: The effect of orthodontic extrusion on traumatically intruded teeth, Am J Orthod 85:47, 1984.
217. Turner CH: Mouth protectors, Br Dent J 143:82, 1977.
218. Vanek PM: Traumatic injuries. In Cohen S, and Burns RC (eds): Pathways of the pulp, ed 2, St. Louis, 1980, The CV Mosby Co.
219. Wald C: Consequences of intrusive injuries to primary teeth, J Pedod 3:67, 1978.
220. Walsh JS, Fey MR, and Omnell LM: The effects of indomethacin on resorption and ankylosis in replanted teeth, ASDC J Dent Child 54:261, 1987.
221. Warfvinge J, and Kahnberg KE: Intraalveolar transplantation of teeth. Swed Dent J 13:229, 1989.
222. Webber RT: Traumatic injuries and the expanded endodontic role of calcium hydroxide. In Gerstein H (ed): Techniques in clinical endodontics, Philadelphia, 1983, WB Saunders CO.
223. Weine FS: Endodontic therapy, ed 4, St. Louis, 1989, Mosby–Year Book.
224. York AH, et al: Dental injuries to 11-13 year old children, NZ Dent J 74:218, 1978.
225. Zacharisson BV, and Jacobsen I: Long-term prognosis of 66 permanent anterior teeth with root fracture, Scand J Dent Res 83:345, 1975.
226. Zadik D, Chosack A, and Eidelman E: A survey of traumatized incisors in Jerusalem school children, J Dent Child 39:185, 1972.

Self-assessment questions

1. If several teeth are out of alignment following trauma, the most reasonable explanation is
   a. luxation.
   b. subluxation.
   c. alveolar fracture.
   d. contusion.
2. Initial vitality testing of traumatized teeth is most useful to
   a. establish a baseline for comparison with future testing.
   b. determine whether or not root canal treatment is indicated.
   c. determine if the blood supply to the pulp is compromised.
   d. predict the prognosis.
3. Initial radiographic examination of dental injuries that include lip lacerations
   a. reveals hairline root fractures.
   b. reveals facial-lingual diagonal root fractures.
   c. may reveal foreign objects in the lips.
   d. should include occlusal views.
4. Rubber dam application for the placement of a restoration at the emergency appointment
   a. usually is not advisable.
   b. is absolutely essential.
   c. usually is possible.
   d. is dictated by the restorative material.
5. Which of the following radiographic film exposures is best for diagnosing root fractures in the apical third?
   a. Parallel.
   b. Bisecting angle.
   c. Occlusal.
   d. Panoramic.
6. The initial priority in treatment of a horizontal root fracture with significant mobility is
   a. preservation of the pulp.
   b. reduction and immobilization.
   c. root canal therapy.
   d. calcium hydroxide pulp therapy.
7. To prevent the onset of inflammatory resorption, the mature intruded tooth must
   a. be allowed to reerupt.
   b. have the pulp removed within 1 to 2 weeks.
   c. have the pulp removed after the tooth is in position.
   d. have an immediate root canal filling completed.
8. Inflammatory resorption is the mechanism of
   a. rejection of autogenous protein.
   b. eliminating infected calcified tissue.
   c. scar tissue formation.
   d. sequestration of bone.
9. Comparing dental trauma in boys and girls:
   a. The rate of trauma is increasing more rapidly in girls.
   b. Girls have more injuries as the result of fistfights.
   c. Boys have more injuries in the maxilla, girls in the mandible.
   d. Injuries are common in boys, rare in girls.

10. A direct facial "padded" blow to the incisors is more likely to cause
    a. enamel fracture.
    b. enamel-dentin fracture.
    c. dentin fracture-pulp exposure.
    d. luxation.
11. A pulpotomy (coronal pulp removal) is indicated when there is a crown fracture and pulp exposure and
    a. root formation is incomplete and the crown is fractured in the cervical one-third.
    b. the pulp has been exposed longer than 1 week.
    c. the pulp is hypersensitive to cold.
    d. any portion of the fracture extends to the root.
12. Nonunion of a root fracture and inflammatory response from pulp necrosis is indicated radiographically by
    a. a periapical lesion.
    b. marked separation of the segments.
    c. root resorption adjacent to the fracture.
    d. widening of the fracture and resorption of adjacent bone.
13. Displaced teeth that had pulp necrosis with root resorption and then had the appropriate endodontic treatment
    a. often had continued resorption.
    b. occasionally had ankylosis.
    c. had a high rate of success.
    d. usually developed apical pathosis.
14. Which medium of storage for an avulsed tooth is best for prolonged periods?
    a. Milk.
    b. Distilled water.
    c. Hank's balanced salt solution.
    d. Patient's saliva.
15. After replantation of an avulsed tooth that has air dried, comparing RCT with immediate gutta-percha obturation vs. treatment with intracanal calcium hydroxide, the research
    a. shows that both are doomed to failure.
    b. shows that RCT/immediate GP has the best success.
    c. shows that calcium hydroxide treatment first has the best success.
    d. as yet is inconclusive.
16. A primary tooth whose crown is displaced lingually and the root facially
    a. is likely to damage the permanent successor.
    b. should be extracted.
    c. often will ankylose, with resulting displacement of the erupting successor.
    d. generally requires no treatment and causes no damage to the successor.
17. If a fully formed tooth has suffered an intrusive injury and the crown is partially exposed, what is the recommended treatment?
    a. Leave alone and allow to erupt spontaneously.
    b. Splint for 7 to 10 days; watchful waiting.
    c. Orthodontically reposition into correct alignment within 3 to 4 weeks.
    d. Reposition with forceps.
18. If calcific metamorphosis (reduction in canal space) is observed radiographically following a displacement, the treatment is
    a. immediate root canal treatment.
    b. root canal treatment only if the tooth is unresponsive to pulp tests.
    c. root canal treatment only if the tooth discolors.
    d. nothing unless signs and symptoms of periapical pathosis develop in the future.
19. Alvused replanted teeth with incomplete root formation
    a. require pulp removal if the extraoral period is more than 2 hours.
    b. are prone to internal resorption.
    c. are tested for revascularization with the electric pulp tester.
    d. in most cases develop roots.
20. Which is most likely to result in severe pulp damage (necrosis)?
    a. Intrusion displacement.
    b. Lateral displacement.
    c. Enamel-dentin fracture.
    d. Cervical one-third root fracture.
21. In a tooth that has been injured, a dramatic or distinct color change to purple or dark gray after a few weeks is *usually* indicative of
    a. internal hemorrhage that is reversible.
    b. internal resorption that is irreversible.
    c. internal resorption that is reversible.
    d. pulp necrosis.
22. A nonmobile, asymptomatic root fracture with evidence of hypercalcification of the pulpal space of the coronal generally requires
    a. no further treatment.
    b. root canal therapy with gutta-percha.
    c. root canal therapy with calcium hydroxide initially.
    d. extraction because there is likely to be pathosis.
23. The best way to treat a mature root fractured in the middle one third with mobility and no response to pulp testing is
    a. to reposition segments, splint, and monitor.
    b. to splint, begin access, pack with $Ca(OH)_2$.
    c. to extract immediately, because restoration is impossible.
    d. to perform root canal therapy, anchor segments together with cast post, and restore.

Chapter 17

Root Resorption

Martin Trope
Noah Chivian

MECHANISMS

Unlike bone, which undergoes resorption and apposition as part of a continual remodeling process, the roots of permanent teeth are not normally resorbed. Only the resorption of deciduous teeth before they are shed can be considered physiologic.[47]

The osteoclast and osteocyte are the main cells involved in the resorption of hard tissues, but other cells such as the macrophage[117] and the monocyte[85] have been reported to have bone-resorbing capacity.[47] While the osteocyte resorbs bone osteoclasts are responsible for resorption of both bone and other hard tissues, including the root.[47] Currently it is accepted that osteoclasts originate from blood-borne leukocytes from the bone marrow and that precursor cells come from the monocyte cell line.[47,78] Slight morphologic differences have been described between bone-resorbing osteoclasts and the "odontoclasts," which are responsible for root resorption. Bone-resorbing osteoclasts are usually large with multiple nuclei. They contain filled vacuoles with two kinds of membranes: the clear zone, which attaches the cell to the hard tissue surface and seals the area from the surrounding environment, and, within it, the ruffled border involved in the resorption process.[42,47] The cells resorbing the root are usually smaller than the bone-resorbing osteoclasts, have fewer nuclei, and have very small clear zones, if any.[71] These cells are thought to be basically the same cell, and the morphologic differences reflect only the nature of the tissue being resorbed and the resorbing activity of the cells.[87,96]

The stimuli for resorption are enzymes, oxygen tension, hormones, locally produced chemical mediators, and electrical currents.[102] Under the influence of these stimuli bone is resorbed. The root is resistant to resorption both on its external surface and internally on its pulpal aspect, and generally would not be resorbed in response to these stimuli. The exact mechanisms by which the resorption process is inhibited is as yet unclear. The connective tissue of the periodontal ligament, the outermost layer (cementoblasts and cementoid), and the innermost intermediate layer of the cementum have been thought to play some role in the resistance of the external surface of the root to resorption, whereas the predentin and odontoblasts are accepted as the resorption inhibitors internally. The periodontal ligament is a specialized connective tissue that separates the alveolar bone and the cementum of the root. Included in the periodontal membrane are remnants of the epithelial root sheath, which surrounds the root like a net. This epithelial net has been thought to play a role in the resistance of the dental root to resorption and the fusion of root directly to bone.[75,90] A more recent study[14] did not support this theory. The cementum layers which cover the roots of the teeth are also thought to be essential elements in the resistance of the root to resorption. On the most external aspect of the cementum is a layer of cementoblasts covering a zone of nonmineralized cementoid. This cementoid layer is predominantly organic in nature, as is the predentin layer internally, and both are thought to be key in resisting resorption. Animal experiments support the theory that it is the outermost layers of the cementum that prevent resorption.[14,61,98] The resistance to resorption of uncalcified tissue on cemental surfaces has been demonstrated.[42] This phenomenon was also demonstrated in osteoid[30] and predentin.[115,123] It has also been demonstrated in cases of extensive idiopathic external root resorption that even though most of the dentin might have been resorbed the most pulpal part close to the predentin is spared, demonstrating this tissue's resistance to resorption.[47] The resorption resistance of these tissues has been postulated to be due to a resorption-inhibiting factor that has been demonstrated in hyaline cartilage. When purified, this factor inhibits the resorption of bone in vitro.[63] It is quite conceivable that a similar antiresorptive factor is present in the organic components of precementum and predentin. Another hypothesis is that the clastic cells are attracted only to or can attach only to mineralized tissue. Thus, if mineralized tissue is not present, the osteoclast will not be attracted to the surface. It is postulated that either removal or mineralization of the organic matrix of bone or the root covering will make it possible for the phagocytic cells to recognize the mineral component.[29,42] Thus, an injury that results in removal of the precementum or predentin, or any process that results in mineralization of the organic matrix, predisposes the root to resorption.

Another part of the cementum thought to play a role in resisting resorption is a highly calcified layer called the *intermediate cementum*.[58,104] The intermediate cementum is the innermost layer of the cementum and creates a barrier between the dentinal tubules and the periodontal ligament.[11,12] Under normal circumstances this barrier does not allow irritants to pass from an infected pulp space to stimulate an inflammatory response in the adjacent periodontal ligament, though, if this zone is lost or damaged, the toxins would pass from an infected pulp space into the periodontal ligament, setting up an inflammatory response and inflammatory root resorption could result.

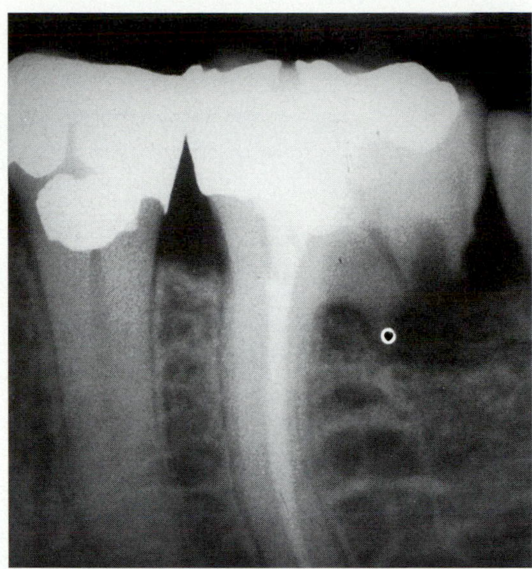

FIG. 17-1 Mandibular molar with idiopathic resorption of the distal root. Contralateral side showed no resorption. The patient was asymptomatic. No history could be elicited that pointed to a causative factor. Blood chemistry was normal. Pulp of the mesial canals appeared normal on extirpation.

Definitions

In this chapter we address the causes, and clinical, radiographic, and histologic appearance, and the treatment of root resorption.

The following definitions will be useful:[3]

Resorption A condition associated with either a physiologic or a pathologic process that results in loss of substance from a tissue, such as dentin, cementum, or alveolar bone.

Root resorption Resorption affecting the cementum or dentin of the root of a tooth. On the basis of the site of origin of the resorption, it may be referred to as *internal, external,* or *root end resorption*.

Idiopathic resorption Resorption without apparent cause.

External resorption Resorption initiated in the periodontium and affecting the external or lateral surfaces of a tooth.

Internal resorption Resorption initiated within the pulp cavity.

Idiopathic Resorption

Resorption of no apparent cause (Fig. 17-1) is often mentioned in the literature.[31,59,84] Commonly there is no apparent history of trauma or orthodontic treatment and blood chemistry is normal.[31,103] The term *idiopathic resorption* probably more accurately reflects our limited understanding of the causative factors in root resorption than the absence of a causative factor in these cases. It therefore remains a convenient diagnosis until our knowledge of root resorption expands.

Local Causes of Root Resorption

The root surface is resorbed (internal or external) by hard tissue resorbing cells. In order for this type of resorption to occur two conditions must be present. First, the *protective covering of the root must be missing or chemically altered* (i.e., the predentin and odontoblasts internally or the cementum and cementoblasts externally). This is usually due to physical damage after trauma or to diseases or procedures that result in an altered ratio of organic and inorganic component of these structures, making them more palatable to resorbing cells. Second, a stimulus for the resorbing cells must be present. As soon as this stimulus is removed (physiologically or by treatment) the resorption will stop and healing will follow. Thus, if additional stimulation is not present the resorption will be *transient*.[119] If the stimulus is sustained the resorption will be *progressive*.[119]

The major local causative factors of root resorption are *excessive pressure* and *inflammation* usually in response to infection.

Pressure

Pressure both damages the cementum and provides the continuous stimulus for the resorbing cells. The most common example of this type of pressure resorption is root resorption due to excessive forces of orthodontic tooth movement. Other examples are resorptions due to impacted teeth or from tumors or cysts.

Excessive forces of orthodontic tooth movement. Root resorption following orthodontic tooth movement has long been recognized.[35,46,69] Orthodontic literature usually states that the amount of tooth loss is clinically insignificant and that neither the stability nor the function of the teeth is affected by resorption. However, it is critical for the practitioner to be aware that in rare cases the resorption can be extensive enough to result in loss of the treated teeth (Fig. 17-2). In one study[35] it was found that 5 to 10 years after completion of the treatment 42.3% of the maxillary central incisors, 38.5% of the maxillary lateral incisors, and 17.4% of the mandibular incisors had undergone apical resorption. The overall incidence of resorp-

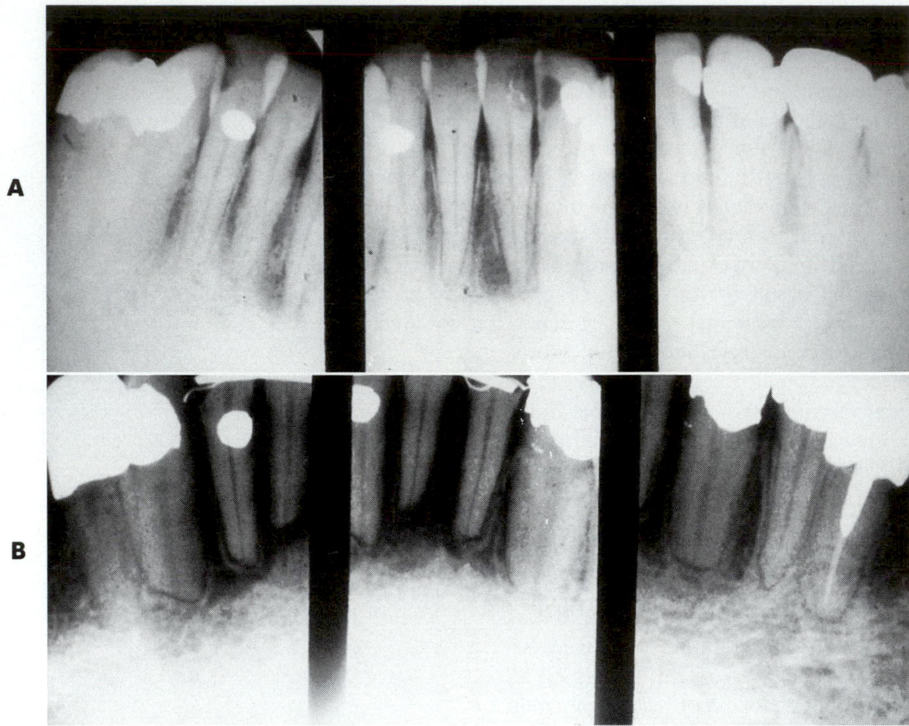

FIG. 17-2 Root resorption due to excessive forces of orthodontic tooth movement. **A,** Mandibular incisors at initiation of orthodontic treatment. **B,** Seven years later, extensive apical resorption of the mandibular incisors necessitates a permanent archbar to retain the incisor teeth.

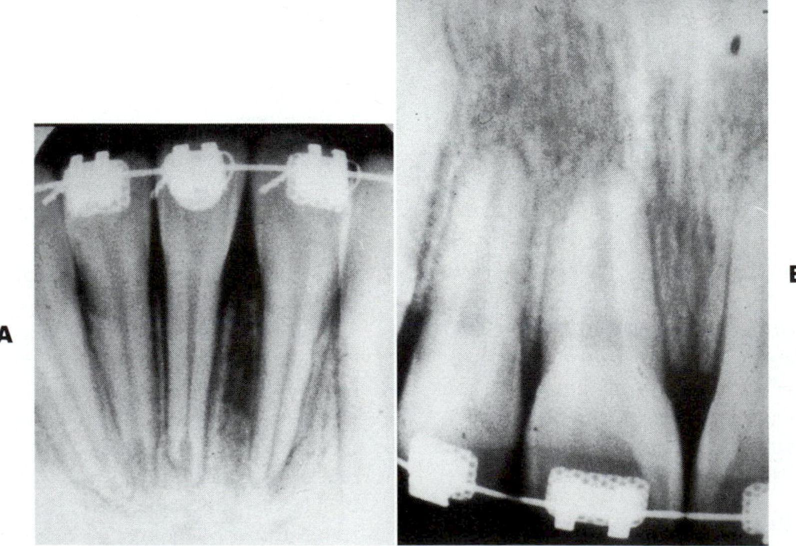

FIG. 17-3 Root resorption during active orthodontic tooth movement. **A,** Mandibular incisors show apical external and internal resorption. **B,** The maxillary incisors exhibit external apical resorption of approximately one third of the original root length.

tion was *28.8%* for the orthodontically treated incisors, compared to 3.4% for controls. Apical resorption was seen four times more often than lateral resorption (Fig. 17-3).[119]

Apical root resorption is a greater risk when orthodontic treatment is started after 11 years of age, and fixed appliances cause significantly more apical root resorption than removable ones.[74] There is no evidence that endodontically treated teeth are more susceptible to root resorption than vital teeth after orthodontic tooth movement.[81,126]

When the orthodontic treatment is both the cause and the stimulus for the root resorption, the removal of the forces will result in an immediate cessation of the resorption. There have been reports of continued resorption after the cessation of the orthodontic tooth movement[80]; however, *it would appear* that in these cases *pulpal disease* played some role in the continuation of the resorption process since *effective* endodontic treatment *stopped it!*

Orthodontic tooth movement has been implicated in other types of root resorption, including cervical resorption[42] and lateral external resorption.[37] In these cases the orthodontic movement is the cause of the damage or alteration of the cemental layer. The stimulus for the inflammation is something other than the orthodontic treatment and will be discussed under the appropriate headings.

Resorption due to impacted teeth. As impacted teeth attempt to erupt, resorption of the roots or crowns of adjacent teeth by pressure can occur (Fig. 17-4). Since the predentin and odontoblastic layer is the most resistant to this resorption the pulps of these teeth remain uninflamed.[99,127] As with other resorptions caused by pressure, if the impacted tooth is removed the resorption will stop.

Resorptions due to tumors or cysts. These pathologic lesions will cause resorption of roots by pressure in a way similar to that already mentioned. Again, if the cause is removed, the resorption ceases.

Inflammation

Inflammation in conjunction with injury to the root's protective covering is the major local cause of inflammatory root resorption. Infection stimulates an inflammatory response, resulting in resorption of a susceptible (unprotected) root surface. Inflammatory root resorption is traditionally divided into *external* and *internal* resorption.

External Root Resorption

For ease of discussion and explanation, external resorption is divided by site—in the apical, lateral, or cervical aspect of the root. Overlap between the areas is common.

Apical external root resorption

Practically all teeth exhibiting apical periodontitis exhibit apical resorption. The resorption can be minor and practically invisible radiographically or can be so extensive that a significant amount of the root tip is lost (Fig. 17-5).

Etiology. All the causes of apical periodontitis cause apical resorption. Thus, overinstrumentation of a root canal during endodontic therapy or, more commonly, an infected necrotic pulp are the main causes. The reason that the apex of the root is not as well protected as the other areas of the root from the resorbing factors produced during the inflammatory response is not obvious. A simple explanation might be that inflammation is confined to a small area at the apex of the root, so that the concentration of resorbing factors is so high that the resistance of the root to resorption is overcome. Another speculation is that the junction of the cementum and dentin (CDJ) at the apical foramen[64] provides an extremely thin protective

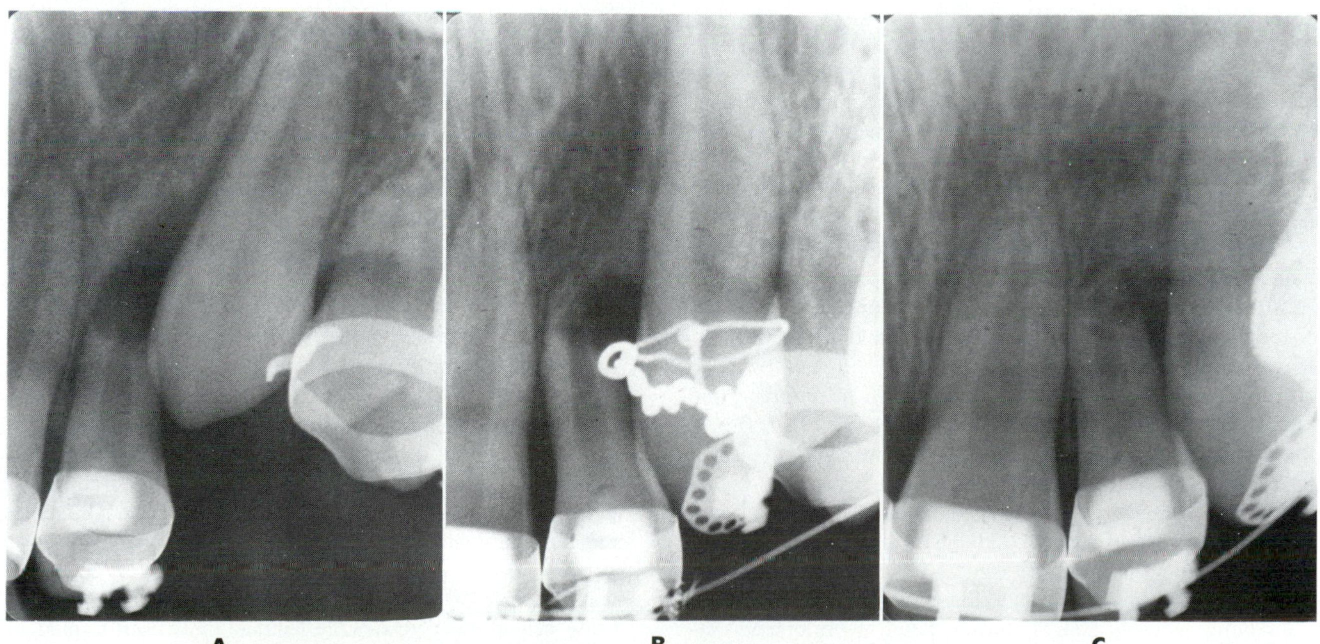

FIG. 17-4 External resorption due to an impacted canine. **A,** Resorption of the apex of the lateral incisor. **B,** The canine was surgically exposed and orthodontically moved away from the apex of the lateral incisor. Note that the predentin layer has survived. **C,** Repair of the apex. (Courtesy Dr. Isaac Post.)

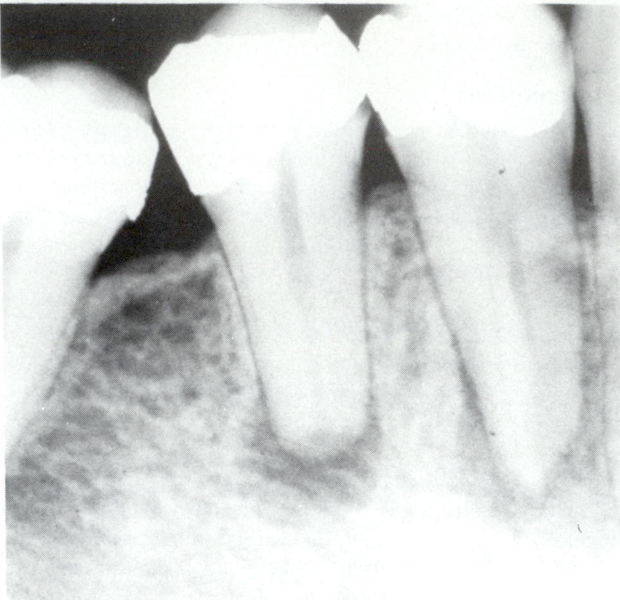

FIG. 17-5 Mandibular bicuspid with external apical resorption due to apical periodontitis. The pulp of the tooth is necrotic and infected.

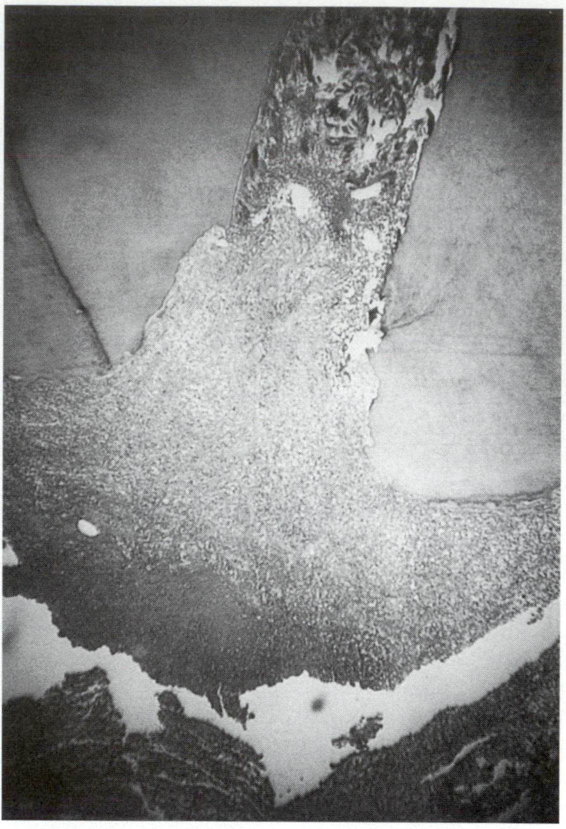

FIG. 17-6 Histologic appearance of apical resorption due to an infected root canal. Chronic inflammation is present apically. Resorption of the external and internal aspect of the root can be seen. (Hematoxylin and eosin stain.)

layer compared to the other areas of the root. It is also conceivable that the cementum and dentin might fail to meet in a certain percentage of cases, like the cementum and the enamel. Thus, the mineralized dentin would be exposed, attracting the clastic resorbing cells.

Clinical manifestations. Apical root resorption is asymptomatic. Symptoms that might lead to its diagnosis are associated with the periapical inflammation.

Radiographic appearance. Radiolucencies are apparent at the root tip and the adjacent bone. (Pathognomonic of root resorptions of inflammatory origin in any area of the root is the resorption of the adjacent bone as well.) Irregular shortening, stumping, or thinning of the root tip is sometimes seen (Fig. 17-4).

Histologic appearance. The periapical lesion can have the histologic appearance of a granuloma or a cyst.[21,66] On the root surface, resorption of the cementum and dentin is seen, resulting in a scalloped appearance of the root end (Fig. 17-6). Attempts at repair are often seen in the presence of the resorption lacunae, resulting in resorptive and mineralization processes observed adjacent to each other.[102]

Treatment. Treatment should be directed at removing the stimulus for the underlying inflammatory process. It had previously been believed that signs of apical resorption were a contraindication to nonsurgical endodontic treatment[45,52,56]; however, it is now accepted that nonsurgical treatment has a *fairly good* chance of success and should be attempted before surgical treatment is initiated (Fig. 17-7).[82,86,91] The clinician should be aware of the canal-altering pathologic process when establishing working length during canal débridement. Attempts should be made to instrument the full length of the remaining canal while creating a dentin shelf to create a stop for the gutta percha obturation. Apical closure techniques with long-term calcium hydroxide treatment can also be used to ensure a better prognosis for nonsurgical endodontic therapy.[62] Prevention of apical resorption when treating vital teeth can be obtained by confining the instrumentation to the root canal. Thus, the mechanical inflammation produced by overinstrumentation is avoided and resorption will not occur.

In the case of apical root resorption due to pulpal disease, adequate root canal therapy will resolve the apical inflammation, and healing of the bone defect and the root resorptive defect with cementum-like tissue will occur. If nonsurgical therapy has been unsuccessful in arresting the resorption, apical surgery should be attempted.

Lateral external root resorption

The external lateral aspects of the root (between the cementoenamel junction [CEJ] and the DEJ) are normally well protected by the periodontal ligament and a relatively uniform layer of cementum. If the periodontal ligament is absent, ankylosis will result (discussed later).[13,71] If, during a traumatic injury, mechanical damage to the cementum surface is sustained, a local inflammatory response and a localized area of root resorption results. If no further stimulation occurs, periodontal healing and root surface repair will occur within 14 days.[47] These healed small resorptive lacunae have been termed *surface resorption* (Fig. 17-8).[7,8] If a more severe injury results in damage to the deeper layers of cementum and further stimulation from the inflammatory response is present, the resorptive process of the root will continue. This process is termed *inflammatory root resorption* (Fig. 17-9).[10,15]

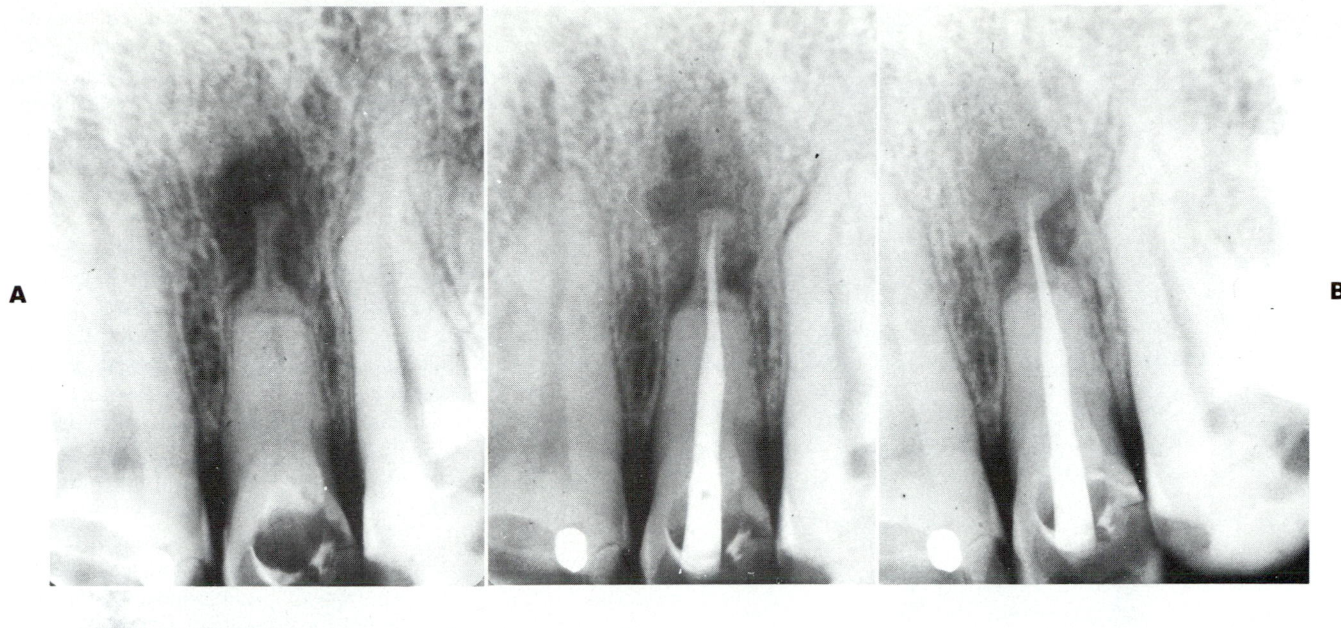

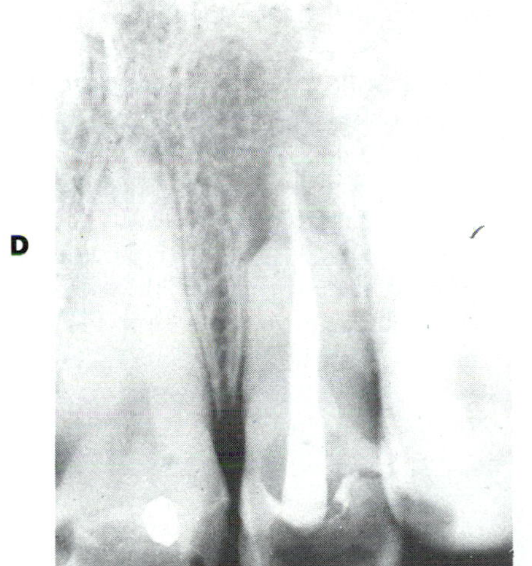

FIG. 17-7 Radiograph of maxillary central incisor with severe external apical resorption. Nonsurgical therapy. **A,** Pretreatment. Extensive resorption in the apical third, but the canal is intact. **B,** After instrumentation and disinfection, obturation with lateral condensation. **C,** Follow-up 6 months after treatment. There is some evidence of bone repair. **D,** Follow-up 5 years after treatment. Continued bone remineralization is evident.

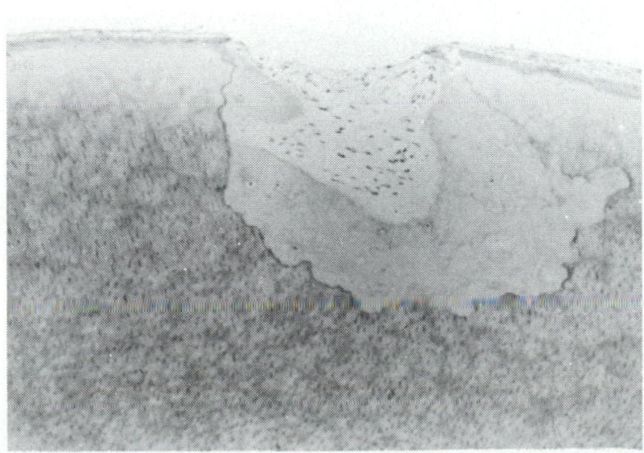

FIG. 17-8 Histologic appearance of surface resorption. Repair of the resorption lacuna with cementum-like tissue is evident. (Hematoxylin and eosin stain.) (Courtesy Dr. Leif Tronstad.)

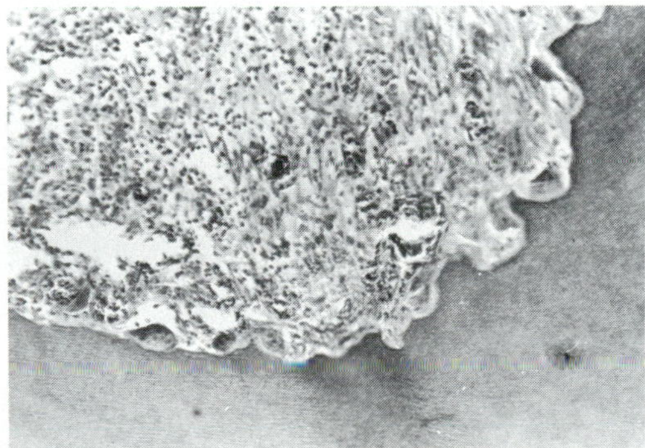

FIG. 17-9 Histologic appearance of inflammatory resorption. Granulation tissue in relation to the resorbed root surface. Multinucleated giant cells are present in the areas of active resorption on the root surface. Hematoxylin and eosin stain. (Courtesy Dr. Leif Tronstad.)

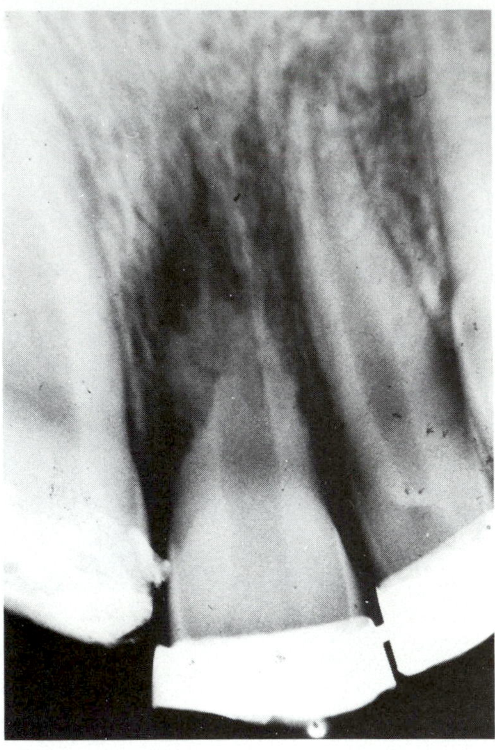

FIG. 17-10 Maxillary left incisor with inflammatory resorption 3 months after replantation without appropriate endodontic treatment. Resorption of the root and bone is apparent. The original root canal can still be traced radiographically.

Etiology. Minor injuries like traumatic occlusion, concussions, subluxations and minimal luxation injuries damage the root surface but are rarely extensive enough to cause necrosis of the pulp space. Thus, after the debris of the physical damage to the root surface has been removed by the inflammatory response, healing with new cementum and periodontal ligament (surface resorption) will occur because a stimulus for the continuation of the inflammatory response is absent. In cases of more serious injuries such as severe luxations or avulsions, displacement of the teeth leads to disruption of the blood vessels at the apical foramina and to ischemic pulp necrosis.[119] Microorganisms will then, in most instances, reach the root canal through enamel or dentin cracks and exposed dentinal tubules, and an infection is established in 2 to 3 weeks.[119] If the intermediate cementum has been penetrated either by the injury or by the ensuing inflammation, the biologically active substances of the bacteria in the root canal can move through the dentinal tubules and stimulate and sustain the inflammatory response and the resorbing cells. Progressive root resorption of this type has been classified as inflammatory root resorption (Fig. 17-10). The rate of progression of inflammatory root resorption is thought to be related to the ability of the bacterial toxins to reach the external surface of the root. Larger tubules of younger patients increase the rate of resorption (Fig. 17-11).[15]

Clinical manifestations. Resorption of the lateral root surface is asymptomatic. In the case of surface resorption, the pulp should be vital, resulting in normal findings on sensitivity tests. When inflammatory root resorption is present an abnormal response to sensitivity testing is expected and pain to percussion, although rare, might result from the inflammation in the periodontal ligament associated with the infected pulp. In the advanced stages of inflammatory root resorption, the tooth becomes mobile and sensitive to percussion and palpa-

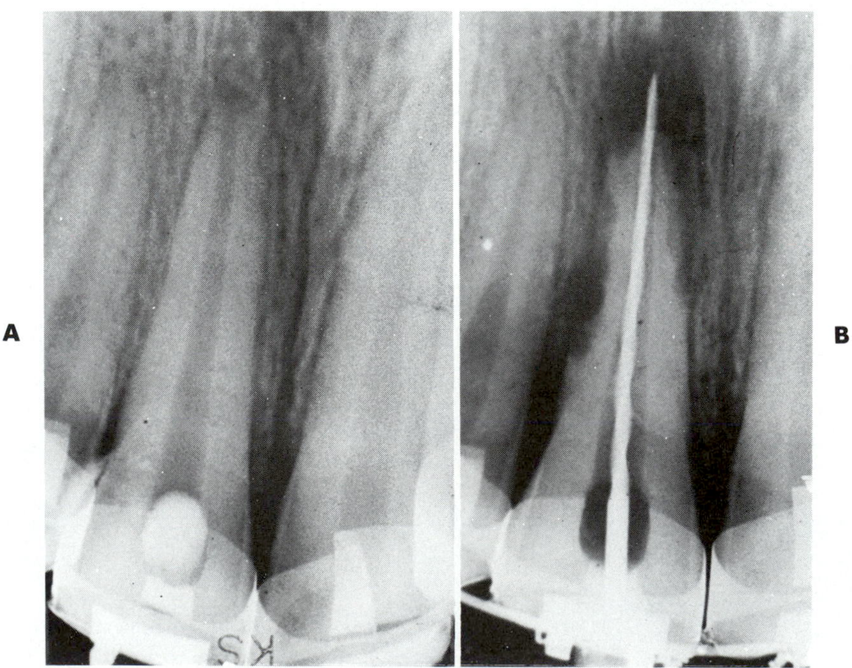

FIG. 17-11 Immature maxillary incisor at **(A)** replantation and **(B)** 3 weeks later. The rapid onset of inflammatory resorption is apparent with root and bone resorption.

tion. Abscess formation in the lateral periodontium is also possible.

Radiographic appearance. Surface resorption is not detectable radiographically. Inflammatory resorption presents with persistent or progressive radiolucent areas of the root *and* adjacent bone. Radiographically, the resorption does not penetrate into the root canal. The radiographic outline of the root canal is often apparent "within" the radiolucent area of resorption (Fig. 17-10). Radiographic changes appear 2 to 3 weeks after the injury (Fig. 17-11),[15] making sensitivity testing and radiographic controls of a traumatized tooth critical during this period.

Histologic appearance. Inflammation in the periodontal tissues is present in conjunction with bowl-shaped areas of resorption of the cementum and dentin (Fig. 17-9).[10,97] The periodontal infiltrate consists of granulation tissue with lymphocytes, plasma cells, and polymorphonuclear leukocytes. The bone is resorbed by multinucleated osteoclastic cells within Howship's lacunae. Similar resorption takes place on the root surface by action of clastic cells that are smaller, have fewer nuclei, and lack the clear zone of the bone-resorbing cells.[47]

Treatment. Surface resorption is self-limiting and requires no treatment. In the case of inflammatory root resorption, treatment is directed toward preventing or removing the stimulus for the inflammation (i.e., the bacterial toxins in the root canal and dentinal tubules). Systemic antibiotic therapy should be instituted immediately after the traumatic injury and before endodontic treatment, since it has been shown to be effective in preventing bacterial invasion and inflammatory root resorption.[49,50] Ideally, after a severe luxation injury or avulsion in which the assessment has been made that the pulp is necrotic, root canal therapy should be initiated in 10 to 14 days.[10] If treatment begins at this optimal point, the pulp should be involved by ischemic necrosis only or, at most, be minimally infected.[49,50] Any adequate endodontic treatment successfully prevents or treats inflammatory root resorption.[32] Therefore, endodontic therapy in addition to an effective antibacterial agent[27,109] over a relatively short time is sufficient to ensure obturation of a sterile canal.[122] For cooperative patients, long-term calcium hydroxide remains an excellent treatment method. The advantage is that this method allows the dentist to leave a temporary obturating material in place until an intact periodontal ligament space is confirmed. Long-term calcium hydroxide treatment should always be used when the injury occurred more than 2 weeks before the endodontic treatment was instituted or if radiographic evidence of resorption is present.[122]

The root canal is thoroughly instrumented and irrigated and then filled with a thick mix of calcium hydroxide and anesthetic solution (see Chapter 15). The calcium hydroxide is changed every 3 months within a range of 6 to 24 months.[4] The canal is obturated when a radiographically intact periodontal ligament can be followed around the root (Fig. 17-12). Calcium hydroxide is an effective antibacterial agent[27,109] and, in addition, has been reported to favorably influence the local environment at the resorption site, promoting healing.[119] It has also been shown to change the environment in the dentin to a more alkaline pH, which has been postulated to slow the action of the resorptive cells and promote hard tissue formation.[120] The calcium hydroxide should not be changed more often than every 3 months, since it has been shown to have a necrotizing effect on the cells attempting to repopulate the damaged root surface.[50,67,68] Though calcium hydroxide is considered the drug of choice for prevention and treatment of inflammatory root resorption, it is not the only medicament that has been recommended in these cases. Some attempts have been made not only to remove the stimulus for the resorbing cells but to affect them directly. The antibiotic corticosteroid paste *Ledermix* has been shown to be effective *in treating inflammatory root resorption by inhibiting the spread of dentinoclasts*[92,93,95] without damaging the periodontal ligament. Its ability to diffuse through human tooth roots has been demonstrated.[1] Its release and diffusion was enhanced when used in combination with calcium hydroxide paste.[2,116] Also, calcitonin, a hormone known to inhibit osteoclastic bone resorption, was shown to be an effective medication in the treatment of inflammatory root resorption.[94]

Occasionally, the resorptive defect is so extensive that the inflammatory exudate washes the calcium hydroxide away, not allowing it to stay in place and be effective. In a localized area this type of resorptive defect can be sealed by a surgical approach after obturation of the root canal has been completed (Fig. 17-13).

Cervical root resorption

Cervical root resorption is a progressive root resorption of inflammatory origin occurring immediately below the epithelial attachment of the tooth (usually but not exclusively the cervical area of the tooth).[10,77,119] It occurs as a delayed reaction after an injury, and its exact pathogenesis is not fully understood. The name *cervical root resorption* implies that the resorption must occur at the cervical area of the tooth. However, the periodontal attachment of teeth is not always at the cervical margin, leading to the same process occurring more apically on the root surface. The anatomic connotation of its name has led to confusion and misdiagnosis of this condition. Because of this confusion, many attempts have been made to rename this type of external resorption.[19,38,42]

Etiology. Since in its histologic appearance and progressive nature it is identical to other forms of progressive inflammatory root resorption, it appears logical that the pathogenesis would be the same (i.e., an unprotected or altered root surface attracting resorbing cells and an inflammatory response maintained by infection). Cervical root resorption occurs late after orthodontic tooth movement (Fig. 17-14), orthognathic surgery, periodontal treatment, or nonvital bleaching (Fig. 17-15).[34,51,119] It is assumed that these procedures are the cause of the denution or alteration of the root surface immediately below the epithelial attachment of the tooth. The pulp plays no role in cervical root resorption and is mostly normal in these cases. Because the source of stimulation (infection) is not the pulp, it has been postulated that it is bacteria in the sulcus of the tooth that stimulate and sustain an inflammatory response in the periodontium at the attachment level of the root.[42,119] The delayed nature (sometimes by many years) of this type of resorption is difficult to explain. It is possible that the inflammatory process does not reach the damaged root surface initially, and that only after years, with eruption of the tooth or periodontal recession, are the chemotactic factors of inflammation close enough to attract resorbing cells to the appropriate root surface. It would seem logical, however, that if a stimulus were not present immediately after the injury to the root surface, repair would take place and the root surface would no longer be susceptible to resorption. An alternate theory is

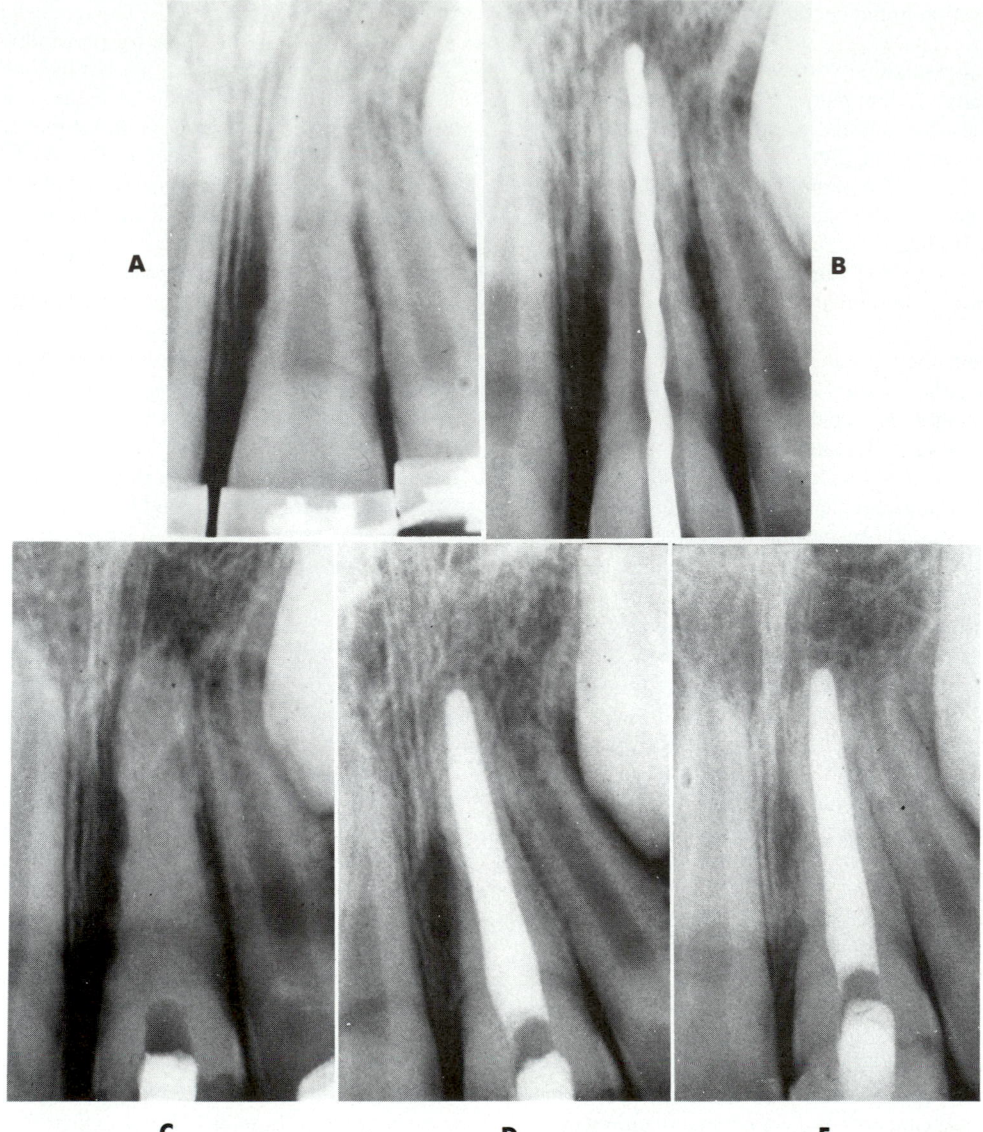

FIG. 17-12 Long-term calcium hydroxide therapy of lateral inflammatory root resorption. **A,** Maxillary central incisor shows radiographic signs of root resorption 1 month after a severe luxation injury. Sensitivity test result is negative. **B,** Root canal therapy is initiated. **C,** A thick mix of calcium hydroxide and anesthetic solution is packed into the canal. **D,** Nine-month recall. The resorption has abated and there is evidence of bone regeneration. The canal is obturated. **E,** One-year recall. Continued healing is apparent.

that the procedures mentioned above cause alteration in the ratio of organic and inorganic cementum,[100] making it relatively more inorganic and thus less resistant to resorption when challenged by inflammation. Also, it has been speculated that the altered root surface registers in the immune system as a different tissue and is attacked as a foreign body.[65] Thus, these root surfaces do not possess their original antiresorptive properties on healing and would be succeptible to resorption at all times. When, owing to periodontal recession or tooth eruption, the inflammation in the sulcular gingival area reaches the altered root surface, resorption takes place. Quite clearly, the *pathogenesis of cervical root resorption is not yet fully understood* and further research is required in this area.

Clinical manifestations. Cervical resorption is asymptomatic and usually is detected only through routine radiographs. As mentioned, the pulp is not involved in this type of resorption, and sensitivity test results would be within normal limits. On occasion, if the pulp is exposed by an extensive resorptive defect, abnormal sensitivity to thermal stimuli might be experienced; however, pain to percussion and palpation is not to be expected. When the predentin is reached the resorptive process is resisted and the resorption proceeds laterally and in an apical and coronal direction, to envelop the root canal (Fig. 17-16). When cervical root resorption is of long standing the granulation tissue can be seen undermining the enamel of the crown of the tooth, giving it a pinkish appearance (Fig.

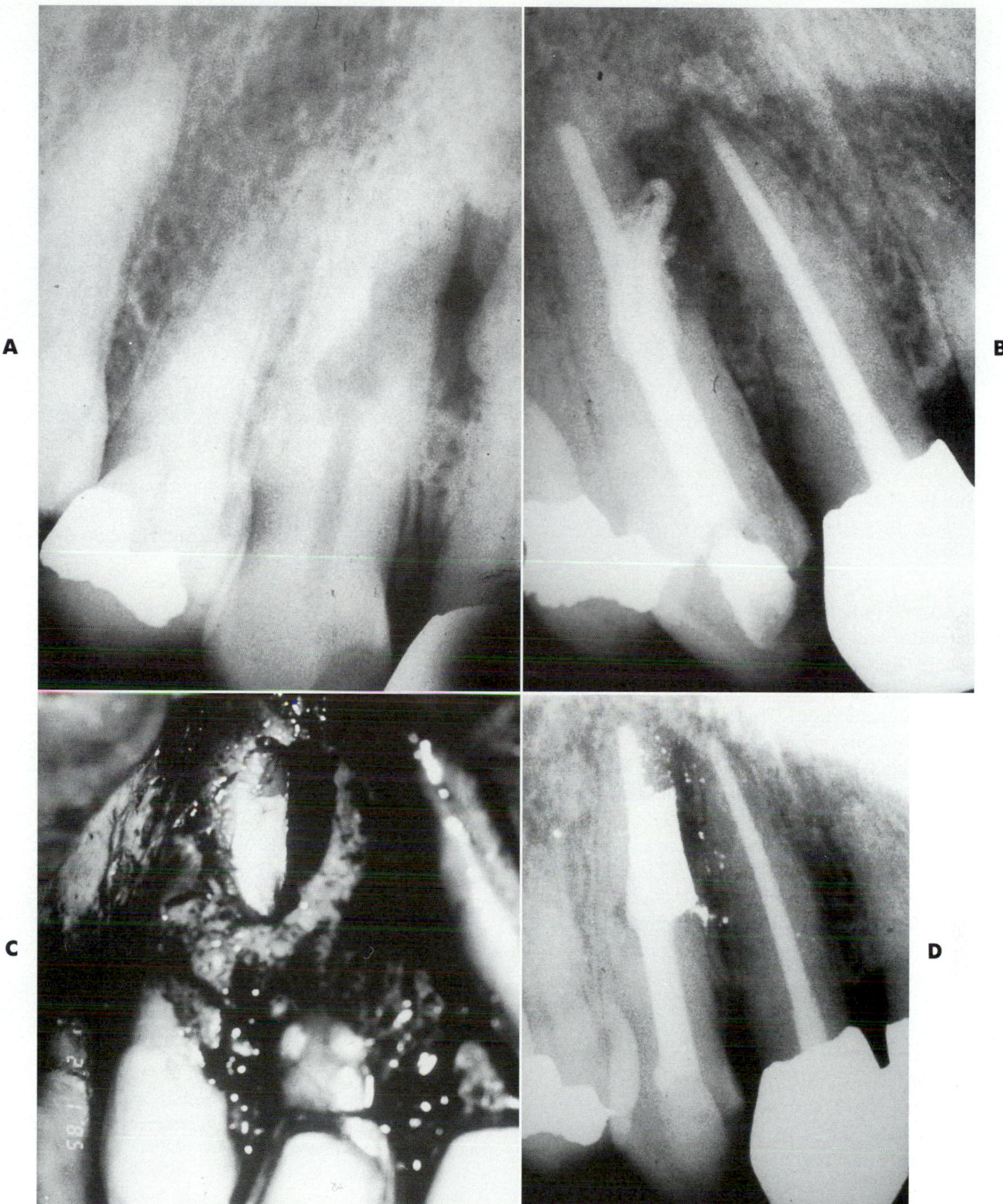

FIG. 17-13 A, Nonvital maxillary canine with a localized area of lateral inflammatory root resorption. **B,** After long-term $Ca(OH)_2$ failed due to washout of the medicament, the root canal was obturated and a surgical approach to treatment initiated. **C,** All granulation tissue was carefully curetted and the resorption defect was filled with amalgam. **D,** One-year follow-up shows bone remineralizing adjacent to the repaired resorption defect.

17-17). This "pink spot" has traditionally been used to describe the pathognomonic clinical picture of internal root resorption, resulting in many cervical root resorption cases being misdiagnosed and treated as internal root resorption.

Since, as with other inflammatory-type resorption, adjacent bone is resorbed as well as root, and in this type of resorption the bone loss is below the epithelial attachment, this condition is commonly misdiagnosed as an infrabony pocket of periodontal origin. However, when the "pocket" is probed copious bleeding and a spongelike feeling are observed when the granulation tissue of the resorptive defect is disturbed.

Radiographic appearance. The radiographic appearance of cervical root resorption can be quite variable. If the resorptive process occurs mesially or distally on the root surface, it is

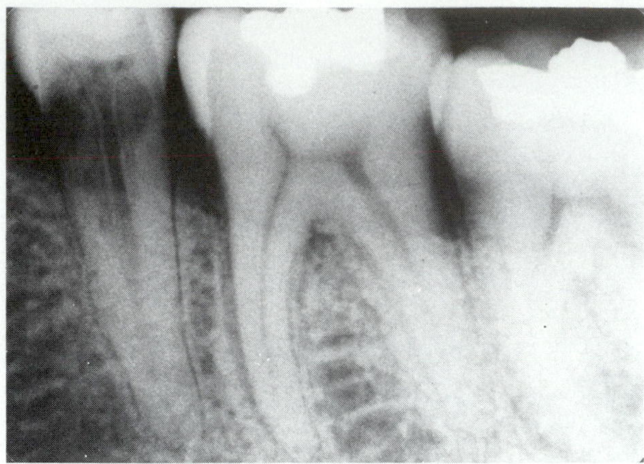

FIG. 17-14 Cervical root resorption on mandibular bicuspid 6 years after completion of orthodontic treatment. Note the mottled appearance of the resorptive defect and the outline of the root canal within the defect.

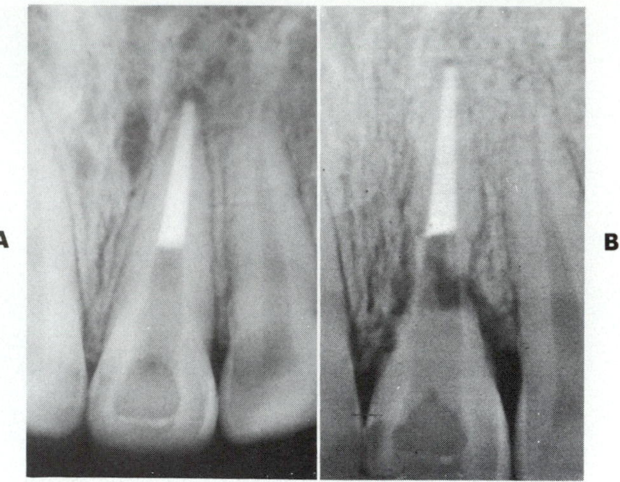

FIG. 17-15 A, Maxillary incisor after completion of root canal therapy and immediate bleaching procedure. **B,** Sixteen month follow-up showing severe cervical root resorption. (Courtesy Drs. William Goon and Stephen Cohen.)

common to see a small radiolucent opening into the root. The radiolucency expands coronally and apically in the dentin, and reaches, but usually does not perforate, the root canal (Fig. 17-18). Thus, the radiographic appearance is similar to that of deep caries. The bone resorption, which always accompanies inflammatory root resorption, mimics the radiographic appearance of an infrabony pocket (Fig. 17-18). If the resorptive process is buccal or palatal-lingual, the radiographic picture is dependent on the extent to which the resorptive process has spread in the dentin. Initially, a radiolucency near the attachment level (cervical margin) would be seen. However, if the process is long standing and extensive, the radiolucent area can extend a considerable way in a coronal and apical direction. The resorption site might have a mottled appearance owing to deposition of calcified reparative tissue within the resorptive lesion (Fig. 17-14).[106] Because the pulp in the root canal is not involved in this type of resorption, it is usually possible to clearly distinguish the outline of the canal through the radiolucency of the external resorptive defect (Fig. 17-14).

Histologic appearance. The histologic appearance of cervical root resorption is similar to that of other types of inflammatory root resorption (i.e., chronic inflammation and multinucleated resorbing cells). Also, it is very common to see histologic evidence of attempts at repair by cementum-like and bonelike material (Fig. 17-19). Union of bone and dentin (replacement resorption) sometimes occurs (Fig. 17-19).

Treatment. Treatment of this type of resorption poses many problems. In principle, the treatment requires removal of all the granulation tissue from the resorptive defects in the root and bone. The defect in the root is then filled with a restorative material, the bone shaped to be self-cleansing, and the periodontal tissues replaced. However, the pattern of expansion of this type of resorption makes application of these treatment principles very difficult. Often the resorptive process (filled with granulation tissue) has burrowed a considerable distance into the dentin in an apical direction. To thoroughly remove the granulation tissue, a considerable amount of bone must be removed, often leaving an unacceptable periodontal defect. Because of these difficulties, resorption cases are sometimes left untreated because treatment might lead to failure more quickly than not treating the defect at all. However, newly developed guided tissue regeneration procedures that promote new attachment onto previously denuded root surfaces[44,89] have resulted in hopeful treatment protocols for the treatment of these conditions.

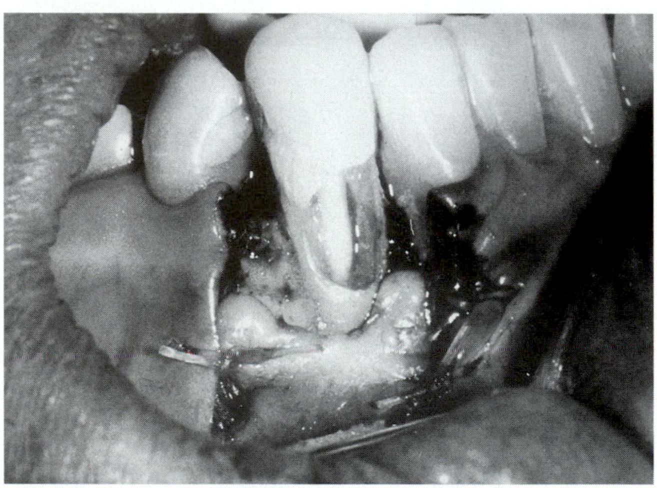

FIG. 17-16 Mandibular canine after removal of granulation tissue of a cervical resorption defect. Note the extensive nature of the defect in the dentin, but the root canal remains intact. (Courtesy Dr. Henry Rankow.)

In cervical root resorption the pulp is usually normal and therefore root canal therapy is not required; however, clinically the resorptive defect usually impinges on the predentin, making exposure of the pulp quite likely during removal of the granulation tissue. The dentist should be prepared to do root canal therapy at any time during the surgical procedure and if the resorption is extensive might elect to perform elective endodontic therapy before surgery. The following list of possi-

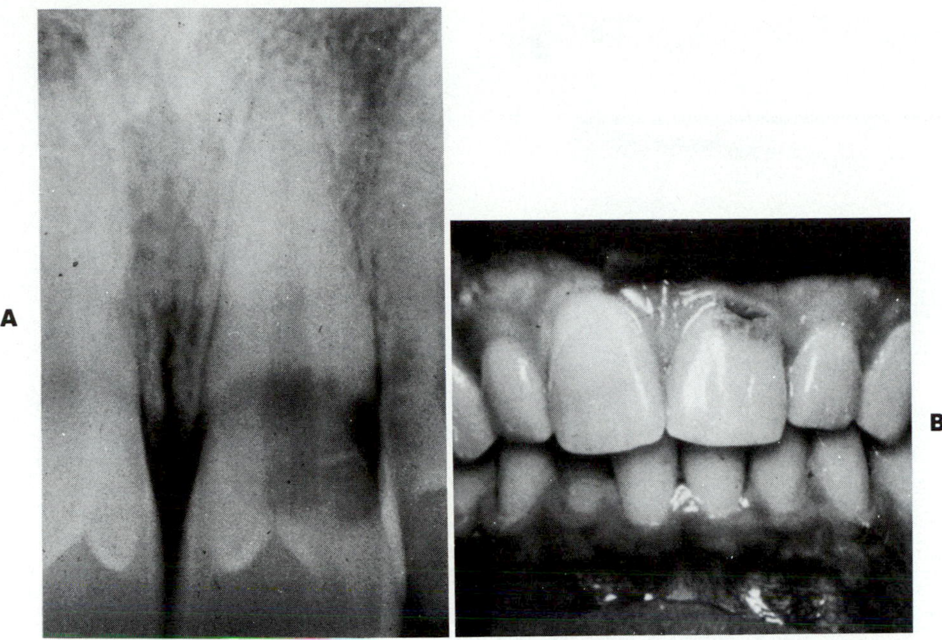

FIG. 17-17 A, Maxillary incisor with cervical root resorption extending coronally. **B,** The clinical appearance shows a pink spot on the labial surface of the tooth, close to the gingival margin.

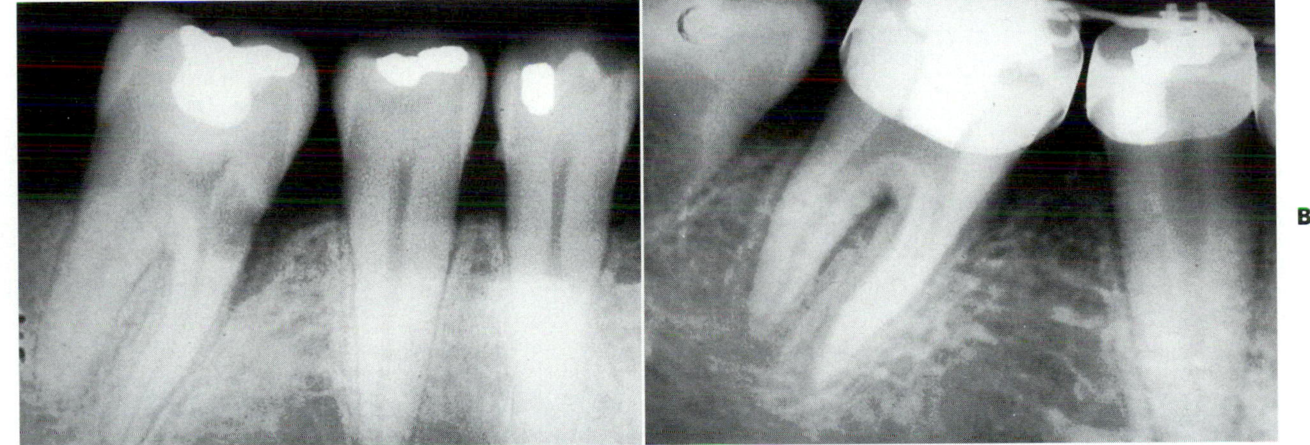

FIG. 17-18 A, Mandibular molar with cervical resorption on its mesial aspect. Note the small opening into the root, the extensive resorption in the dentin, but the pulp is not exposed. Also, a resorptive defect is present in the adjacent bone, appearing radiographically similar to an infrabony pocket. **B,** The apparent cause of the cervical resorption is the orthodontic uprighting performed 16 years earlier.

ble treatment approaches addresses the different clinical situations associated with cervical root resorption.

Localized defect close to the cervical margin (entirely within the coronal third). Angled radiographs are taken to determine by means of the buccal object rule the exact location of the defect (buccal or lingual-palatal; Fig. 17-33). Once the position has been determined, a full-thickness flap is raised and the granulation tissue is removed from the root and the bone defect. It is imperative that sound, healthy bone be reached, so that the blood supply of the granulation tissue is severed. The granulation tissue can be removed with a bur or by inducing necrosis with trichloroacetic acid.[53,54] The defect is filled with a restorative material and the flap replaced so that the periodontal defect is minimized (Figs. 17-20, 17-21). It is essential to remove all granulation tissue from the root and bone, leaving unaffected tissue behind (Fig. 17-21). Failure to do so will result in the continuation of the resorption surrounding the restorative material (Fig. 17-22).

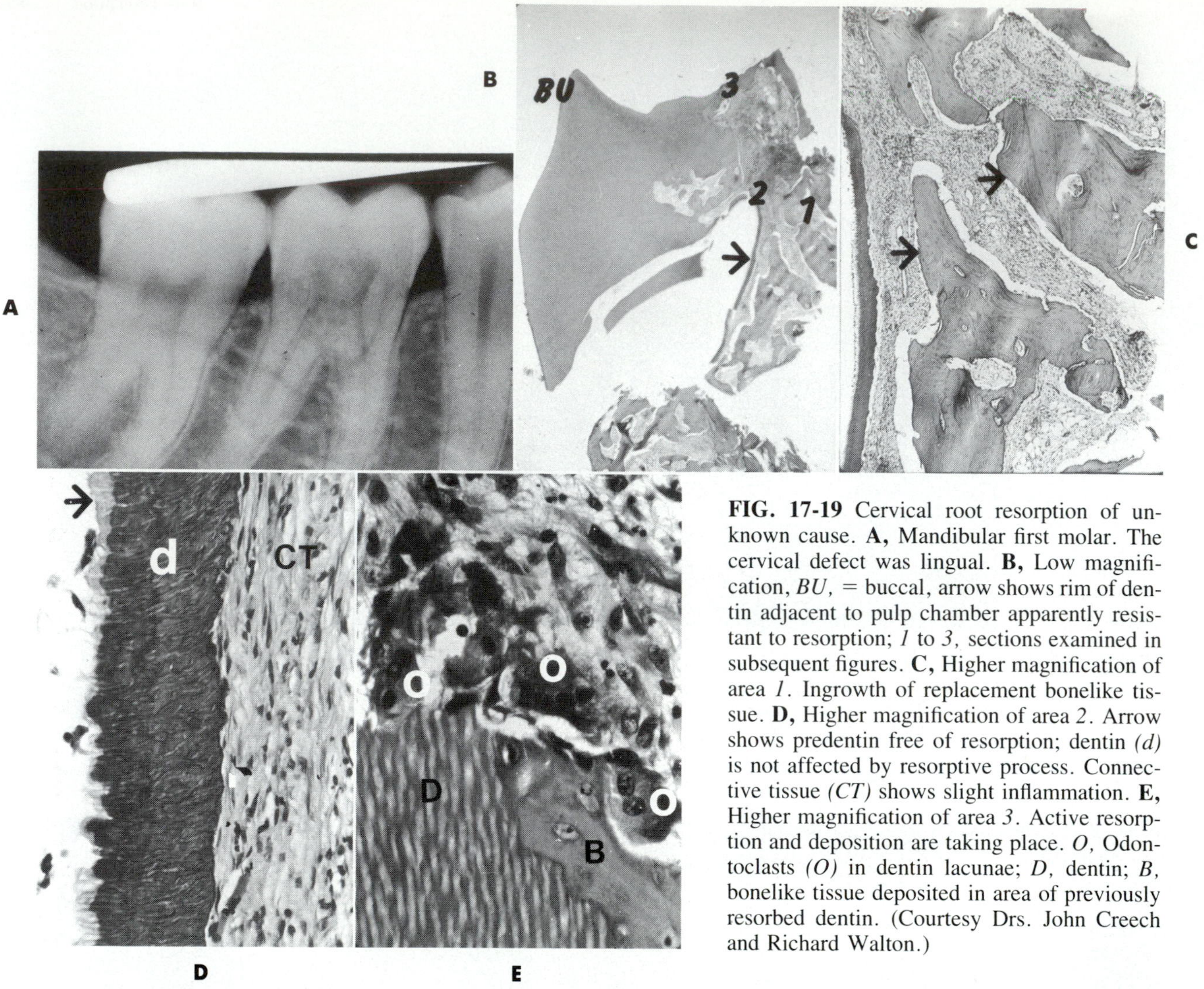

FIG. 17-19 Cervical root resorption of unknown cause. **A,** Mandibular first molar. The cervical defect was lingual. **B,** Low magnification, *BU,* = buccal, arrow shows rim of dentin adjacent to pulp chamber apparently resistant to resorption; *1* to *3,* sections examined in subsequent figures. **C,** Higher magnification of area *1*. Ingrowth of replacement bonelike tissue. **D,** Higher magnification of area *2*. Arrow shows predentin free of resorption; dentin *(d)* is not affected by resorptive process. Connective tissue *(CT)* shows slight inflammation. **E,** Higher magnification of area *3*. Active resorption and deposition are taking place. *O,* Odontoclasts *(O)* in dentin lacunae; *D,* dentin; *B,* bonelike tissue deposited in area of previously resorbed dentin. (Courtesy Drs. John Creech and Richard Walton.)

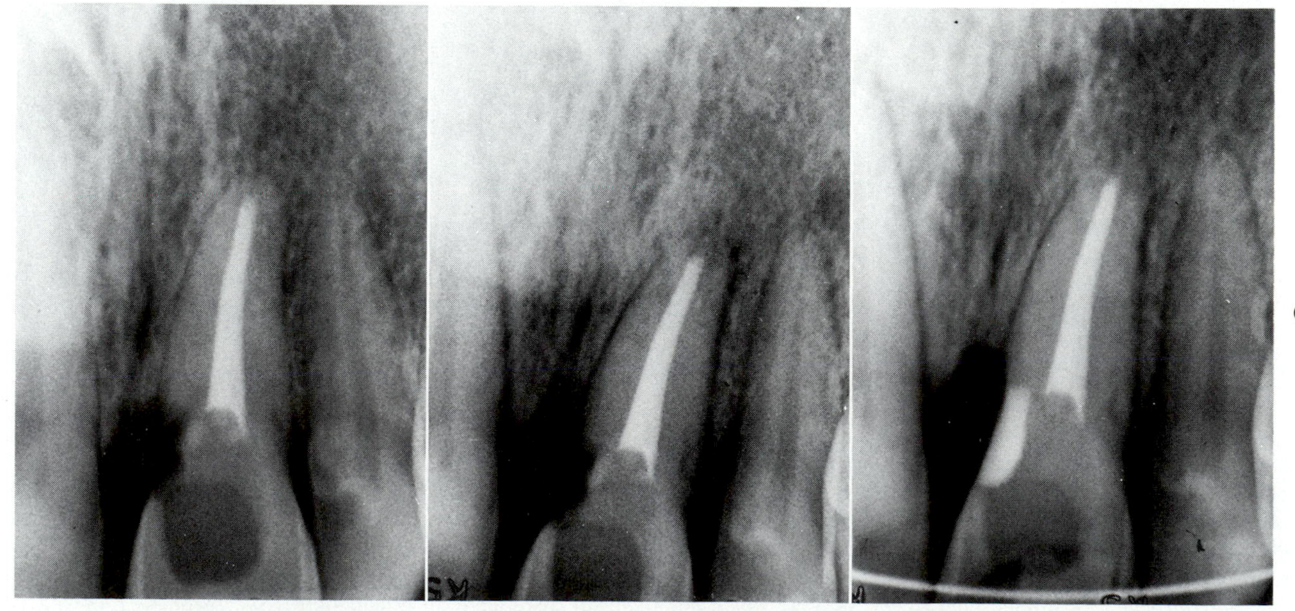

FIG. 17-20 A, Maxillary incisor with cervical root resorption 3 years after bleaching with superoxyl and heat. **B,** The defect is exposed and the granulation tissue removed from the root and bone. **C,** The defect is repaired with light-cured resin.

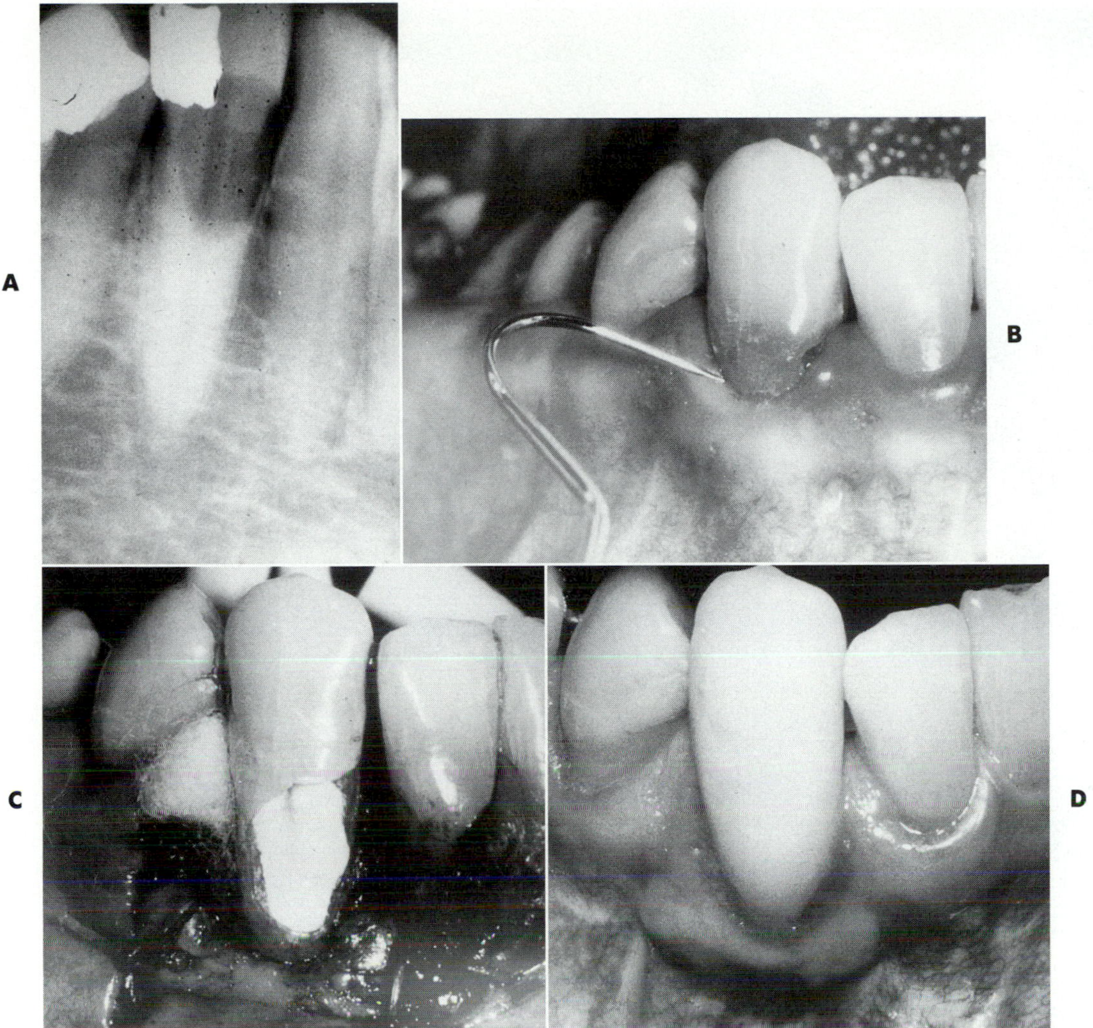

FIG. 17-21 A, Mandibular canine with cervical root resorption defect that is predominantly coronal. **B,** Clinical view shows the granulation tissue under the enamel appears as a pink spot. **C,** The granulation tissue has been removed from the root and bone. The unexposed pulp is covered with hard-setting calcium hydroxide. **D,** The defect is restored with light-cured resin and the flap replaced apical to it. (Courtesy Dr. Henry Rankow.)

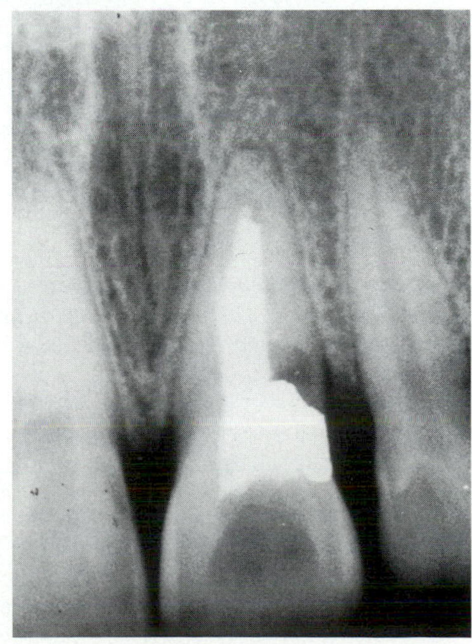

FIG. 17-22 Maxillary incisor 1 year after repair of distal cervical resorption defect. All the granulation tissue was not removed from the bone, resulting in continuation of the process around the restorative material.

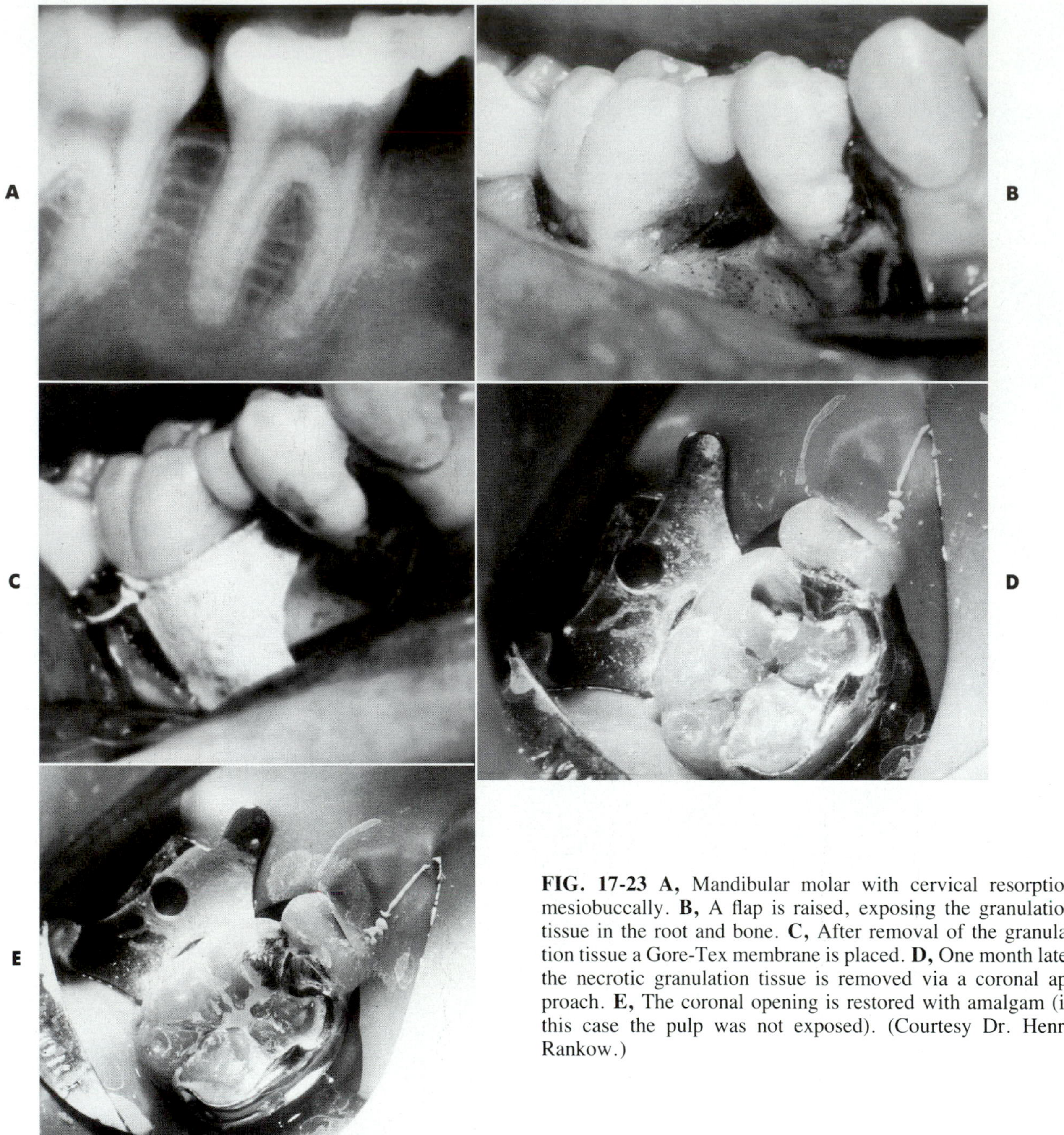

FIG. 17-23 A, Mandibular molar with cervical resorption mesiobuccally. **B,** A flap is raised, exposing the granulation tissue in the root and bone. **C,** After removal of the granulation tissue a Gore-Tex membrane is placed. **D,** One month later the necrotic granulation tissue is removed via a coronal approach. **E,** The coronal opening is restored with amalgam (in this case the pulp was not exposed). (Courtesy Dr. Henry Rankow.)

Localized, medium-sized defect located predominantly in the coronal dentin with a small subepithelial opening on the root. A flap is raised and the granulation tissue is removed from the bony defect only. Since the source of the blood supply to the root defect is the periodontal structures, removal of the granulation tissue in the bone results in necrosis of the resorbing tissue in the root. The small external opening into the root is sealed superficially with an *acid etch resin technique*. The flap is then replaced and sutured. An expanded polytetrafluoroethylene (Gore-Tex) membrane can be used if a considerable amount of bone is lost. After approximately a month, an opening is made coronally and the necrotic granulation tissue is removed (Fig. 17-23). The need for root canal therapy is assessed at this time.

Large defect extending apically. In these cases, removal of the granulation tissue would jeopardize the periodontal health of the tooth, almost definitely condemning the tooth to extraction and possibly affecting adjacent teeth. These cases can be treated in a number of ways.

(a) Forced eruption. If the remaining root apical to the resorption defect is long enough to maintain the tooth, erupting the tooth is a very effective treatment method. The resorption defect is moved to a position coronal to the adjacent attachment. The entrance of the defect into the root can now easily be found and the defect cleaned and restored. Reshaping of the "raised" bony contour now allows an ideal architecture to remain (Fig. 17-24). In cases where a poor crown-root ratio

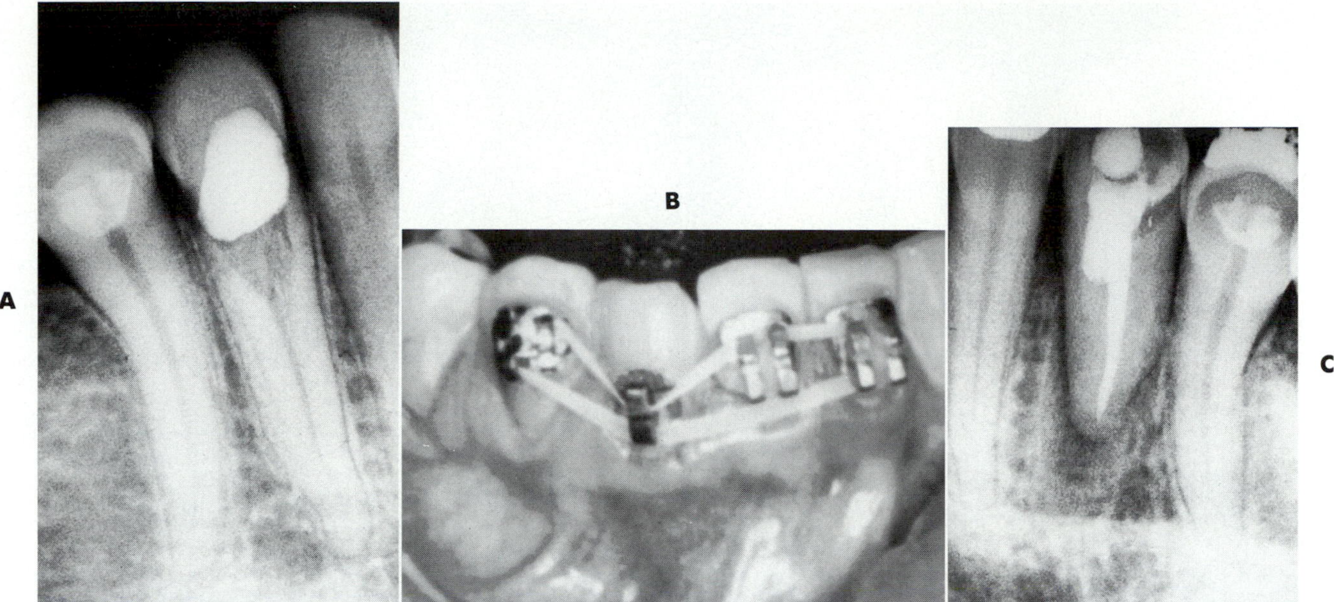

FIG. 17-24 A, Mandibular canine with cervical root resorption extending apically to the mid-root level. **B,** The tooth is erupted coronally so that the lesion is more coronal. **C,** The repaired lesion after bone recontouring. Note the acceptable bone level achieved by this procedure. (Courtesy Dr. Samuel Dorn.)

exists after eruption and repair of the defect, it would be possible to intrude the tooth after the repair is complete.

(b) Expanded polytetrafluoroethylene (Gore-Tex) membrane following removal of the granulation tissue. If the opening into the root is large, it theoretically is possible to create a new attachment on the sound unaffected root surface that remains after degranulation. Thus, the granulation tissue is completely removed, the defect and denuded root surface covered with a spacer (freeze-dried bone), and the entire area covered with a Gore-Tex membrane (Fig. 17-25). This procedure is too new to assess its prognosis but it still should be tried, since few if any alternatives exist.

Prevention. Since we know some of the indirect causes of cervical root resorption, it is possible to propose preventive measures that may prevent it.

Nonvital bleaching. Research suggests that 30% hydrogen peroxide activated with heat damages the cementum layer through the dentinal tubules.[41,51,76] To minimize these factors the following protective steps are suggested.

1. *Protection of the dentinal tubules.* Remove the gutta-percha apical to the cervical line to remove discolored dentin, but do not extend the preparation into the root. Use the crestal bone as a guide. Place a layer of cement (IRM, Cavit, glass ionomer) to prevent ingress of the bleaching agent apically and into the cervical dentinal tubules.

2. *Do not use heat.* Walking bleaches[88,112] have been effective for over a quarter of a century. Repeated treatments produce results equal to a one-sitting thermocatalytic procedure.[39,57]

3. *Avoid etching the dentin.* Some techniques suggest etching of the dentin before bleaching[26]; however, a recent study showed similar bleaching results with and without etching.[28] Etching the dentin opens the tubules leading to the gingival tissues and should therefore be avoided.

4. *Do not use Superoxol.* Superoxol is caustic. Some advocate sodium perborate (USP) and water for the walking bleach and report excellent results with no history of external resorption.[112,113] Others[101] showed in vitro the effectiveness of sodium perborate and water as a bleaching agent, though it took longer to work.

Orthodontic therapy. All orthodontic forces, and in particular tipping forces, should be as light as possible in order not to crush the attachment apparatus while a tooth is being uprighted.

Surgical procedures. Surgical procedures including *excessive* use of surgical elevators theoretically damage the attachment apparatus and should be avoided. Surgical procedures that could damage the cervical margin, for example the canine wire lasso before orthodontic movement of an impacted canine, should not be used; rather, surgical exposure and banding with acid etch and resin should be used to facilitate coronal movement.

Periodontal procedures. Procedures that leave the root surface denuded (i.e., without periodontal ligament or epithelium) should be avoided.

Internal Root Resorption

Internal root resorption is *rare* in permanent teeth. External resorption, which is much more common, is often misdiagnosed as internal resorption. Internal resorption is characterized by an oval-shaped enlargement of the root canal space.[10]

Etiology

Internal root resorption is characterized by resorption of the internal aspect of the root by multinucleated giant cells adjacent to granulation tissue in the pulp (Fig. 17-26). Chronic inflammatory tissue is common in the pulp, but only rarely does it result in resorption. There are different theories on the ori-

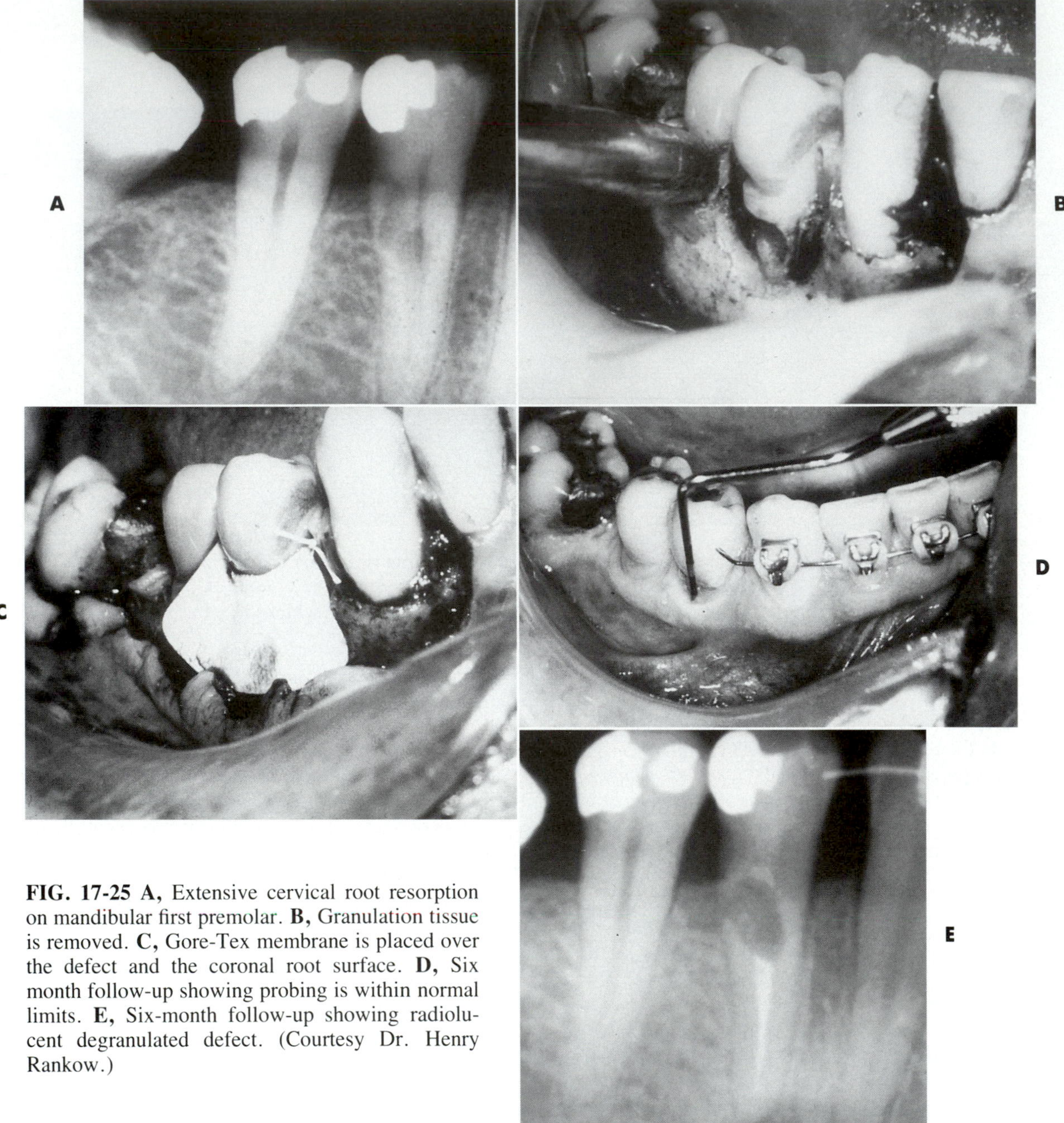

FIG. 17-25 A, Extensive cervical root resorption on mandibular first premolar. **B,** Granulation tissue is removed. **C,** Gore-Tex membrane is placed over the defect and the coronal root surface. **D,** Six month follow-up showing probing is within normal limits. **E,** Six-month follow-up showing radiolucent degranulated defect. (Courtesy Dr. Henry Rankow.)

gin of the pulpal granulation tissue involved in internal resorption. The most logical explanation is that it is pulp tissue that is inflamed owing to an infected coronal pulp space. Communication between the coronal necrotic tissue and the vital pulp is through appropriately oriented dentinal tubules (Fig. 17-27).[118,124] One investigator reports[114] that resorption of the dentin is frequently associated with deposition of hard tissue resembling bone or cementum and not dentin. He postulates that the resorbing tissue is not of pulpal origin but is "metaplastic" tissue derived from the pulpal invasion of macrophage-like cells.[47] Others[125] concluded that the pulp tissue was replaced by periodontium-like connective tissue when internal resorption was present. In addition to the requirement of the presence of granulation tissue, root resorption takes place only if the odontoblastic layer and predentin are lost or altered.[119,125] Reasons for the loss of predentin adjacent to the granulation tissue are not obvious. Trauma frequently has been suggested as a cause.[36,102] Some[124] report that trauma may be recognized as an initiating factor in internal resorption. They divided it into a transient type and a progressive type, the latter requiring continuous stimulation by infection. Another reason for the loss of predentin might be extreme heat produced when cutting on dentin without an adequate water spray (Fig. 17-28). The heat presumably would destroy the predentin layer, and if later the coronal aspect of the pulp became infected, the bacterial products could initiate the typical inflammation in conjunction with resorbing giant cells in the vital pulp adjacent to the denuded root surface. Internal root resorp-

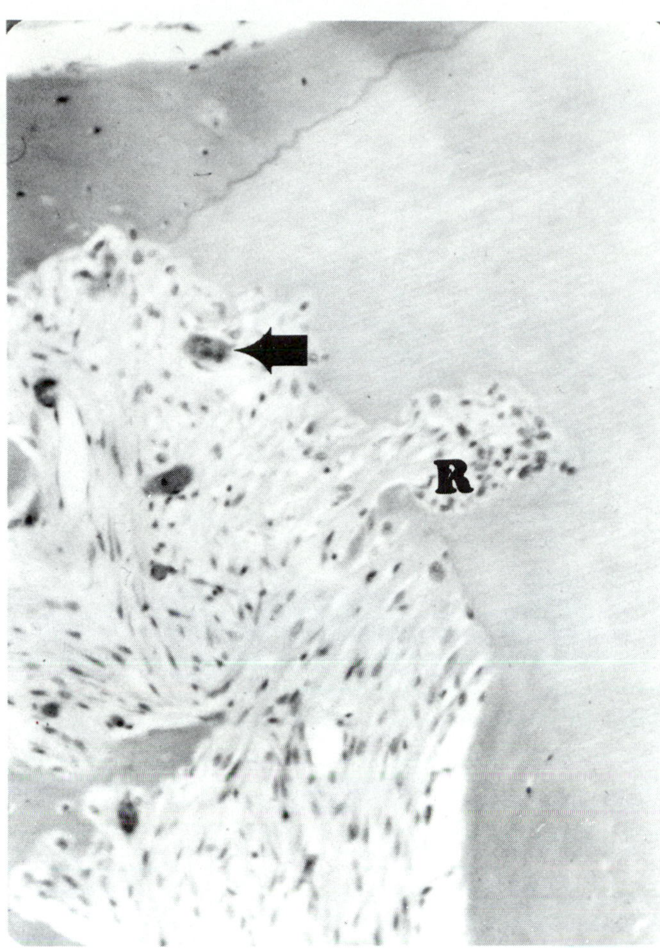

FIG. 17-26 Histologic appearance of internal resorption. Granulation tissue including multinucleated giant cells *(arrow)* is present. Resorptive lacunae *(R)* in dentin. Hematoxylin and eosin; original magnification, ×100.) (Courtesy Dr. Harold Stanley.)

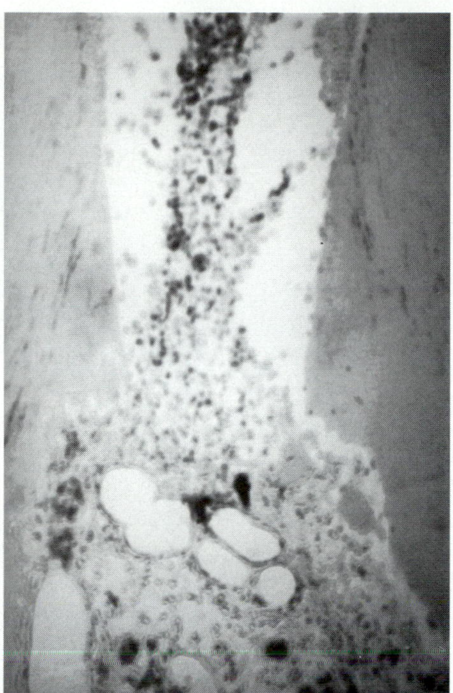

FIG. 17-27 Histologic section of internal resorption stained with Brown and Brenn. Bacteria are seen in the dentinal tubules communicating between the necrotic coronal segment and the apical granulation tissue and resorbing cells. (Courtesy Dr. Leif Tronstad.)

tion has been produced experimentally by the application of diathermy.[43] Strong chemical medicaments used in procedures like pulpotomies could theoretically also burn the predentin and predispose the canal to internal root resorption (Fig. 17-29).

Clinical manifestations

Internal root resorption is usually asymptomatic and is first recognized clinically through routine radiographs. Pain may be a presenting symptom if perforation of the crown occurs and the metaplastic tissue is exposed to the oral fluids. For internal resorption to be active, at least part of the pulp must be vital, so that a positive response to pulp sensitivity testing is expected. It should be remembered that the coronal portion of the pulp is often necrotic whereas the apical pulp, which includes the internal resorptive defect, can remain vital. Therefore, a negative sensitivity test result does not rule out active internal resorption. It is also possible that the pulp becomes nonvital after a period of active resorption, giving a negative sensitivity test, radiographic signs of internal resorption, and radiographic signs of apical inflammation (Fig. 17-30). Traditionally, the pink tooth has been thought pathognomonic of internal root resorption. The pink color is due to the granulation tissue in the coronal dentin undermining the crown enamel. The pink tooth can be a feature of cervical root resorption, which must be ruled out before a diagnosis of internal root resorption is made.

Radiographic appearance

Internal root resorption presents radiographically as a fairly uniform radiolucent enlargement of the pulp canal (Fig. 17-31). Because the resorption is initiated in the root canal, the resorptive defect includes the root canal space. Therefore, the original outline of the root canal is distorted. Only on rare occasions, when the internal resorptive defect penetrates the root and impacts the periodontal ligament, does the adjacent bone show radiographic changes.

Histologic appearance

Like that of other inflammatory resorptive defects, the histologic picture of internal resorption is granulation tissue with multinucleated giant cells (Fig. 17-26). An area of necrotic pulp is found coronal to the granulation tissue. Dentinal tubules containing microorganisms and communicating between the necrotic zone and the granulation tissue can sometimes be seen (Fig. 17-27).[119,124] Unlike external root resorption, resorption of the adjacent bone does not occur with internal root resorption.

Treatment

Treatment of internal root resorption is relatively easy. Once internal root resorption is diagnosed, endodontic treatment

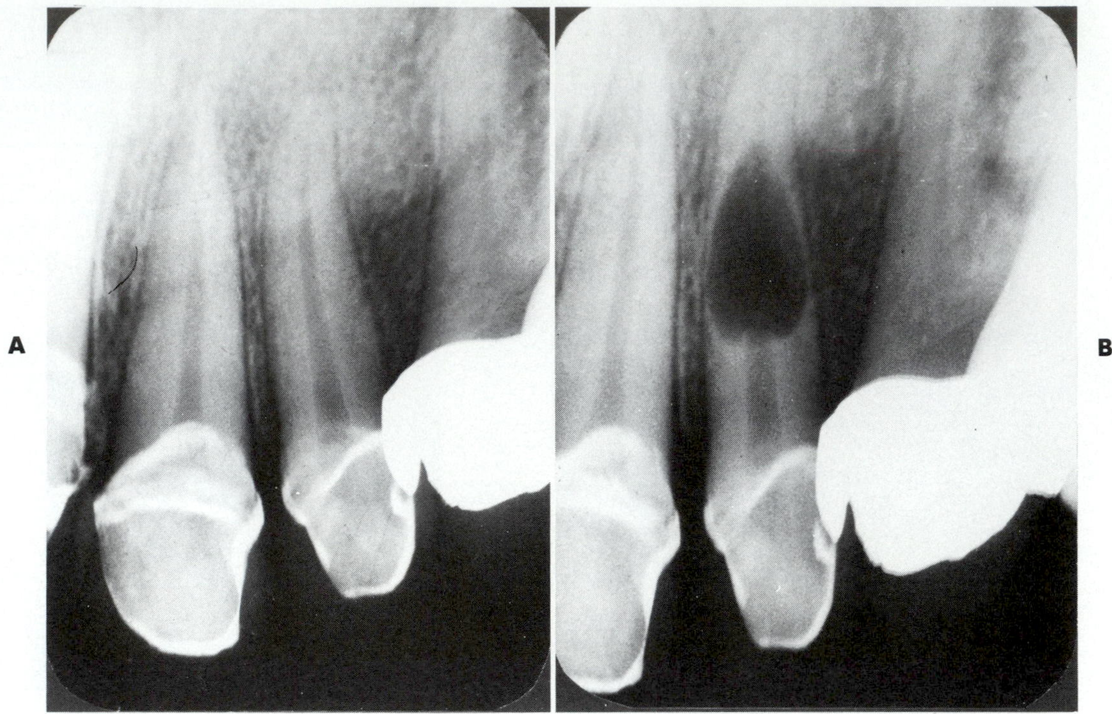

FIG. 17-28 Maxillary lateral incisor. **A,** At time of crown preparation. **B,** Four months later there is an extensive internal resorptive defect.

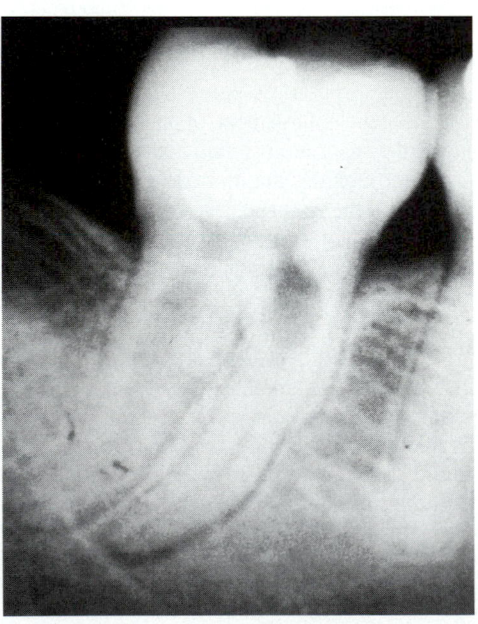

FIG. 17-29 Mandibular second molar. Internal resorptive defect in the mesial root three months after pulpotomy with formocreosol.

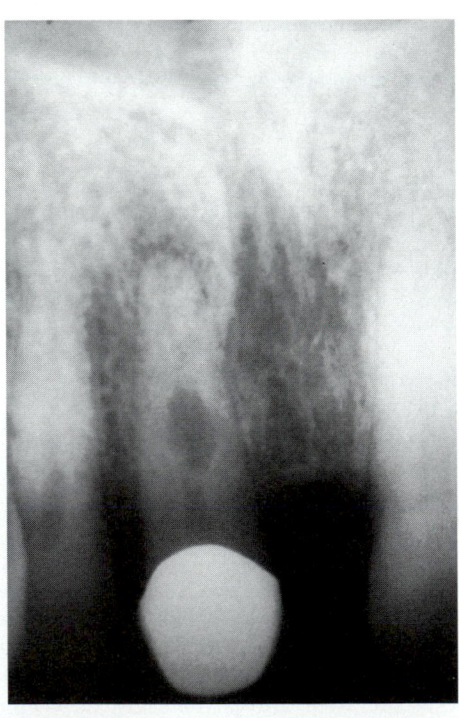

FIG. 17-30 Maxillary incisor with midroot radiolucency typical of internal resorption. Apical radiolucency is also present. The internal resorption must have occurred before the pulp became nonvital.

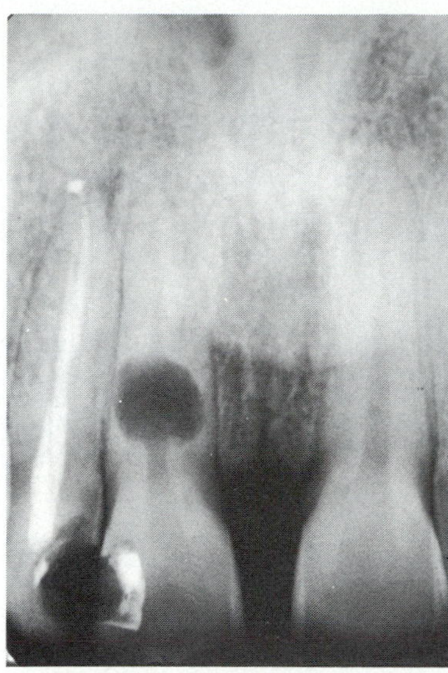

FIG. 17-31 Radiograph of maxillary incisor with internal root resorption. Uniform enlargement of the pulp space is apparent. Outline of the canal cannot be seen in the resorptive defect.

must be performed promptly. Full instrumentation to the root apex removes the blood supply to the resorptive defect. If the resorptive defect is extensive, it is usually not possible to remove all the granulation tissue initially. Calcium hydroxide placed for a period of time breaks down the remaining granulation tissue, which can then be washed out by copious rinsing with 5.25% NaOCl. If necessary the calcium hydroxide and NaOCl rinse can be repeated.

Once all the granulation tissue has been removed the defect can be treated in one of three ways: nonsurgically, by recalcification with calcium hydroxide, or surgically.

1. If the defect has not perforated the root to the periodontal ligament, obturation is completed with a warm gutta-percha technique in conjunction with a root canal sealer.
2. If the defect perforated the root below bone level, a hard tissue barrier can be produced with long-term calcium hydroxide treatment, after which obturation is carried out.
3. If the defect perforates coronal to the epithelial attachment, or if an extremely large perforation is present, a surgical approach is required to seal the perforation.

Diagnostic Features of External vs. Internal Root Resorption

It is often very difficult to distinguish external from internal root resorption, so misdiagnosis and incorrect treatment result. What follows is a list of typical diagnostic features of each resorptive type.

Radiographic features

A change of angulation of x-rays should give a fairly good indication of whether a resorptive defect is internal or external. A lesion of internal origin appears close to the canal whatever the angle of the x-ray (Fig. 17-32). On the other hand, a defect on the external aspect of the root moves away from the canal as the angulation changes (Fig. 17-33). In addition, by using the buccal-object rule it is usually possible to distinguish if the external root defect is buccal or lingual-palatal.

In internal resorption, the outline of the root canal is usually distorted and the root canal and the radiolucent resorptive defect appear contiguous (Figs. 17-31, 17-32). When the defect is external, the root canal outline appears normal and can usually be seen "running through" the radiolucent defect (Fig. 17-14).

External inflammatory root resorption is always accompanied by resorption of the bone as well (Figs. 17-12, *B*, 17-18). Therefore, radiolucencies are apparent in the root and the adjacent bone. Internal root resorption does not involve the bone, and as a rule the radiolucency is confined to the root (Fig. 17-28). On rare occasions if the internal defect perforates the root, the bone adjacent to it is resorbed and appears radiolucent on the radiograph.

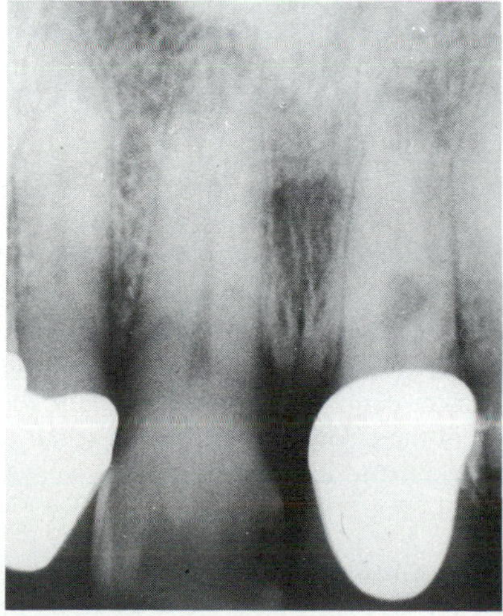

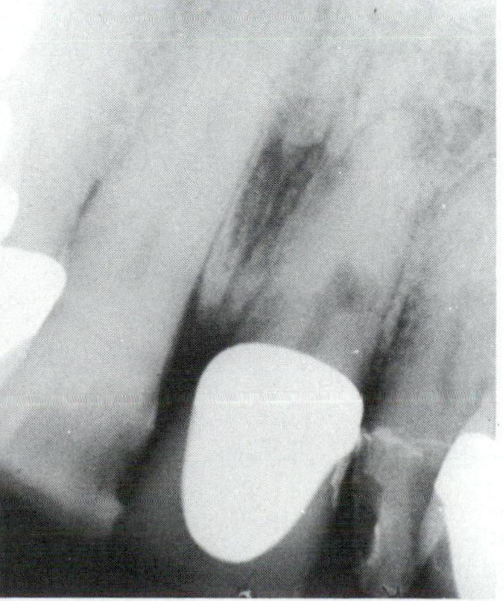

FIG. 17-32 Internal resorption. Radiographs from two different horizontal projections depict the lesion within the confines of the root canal on both views.

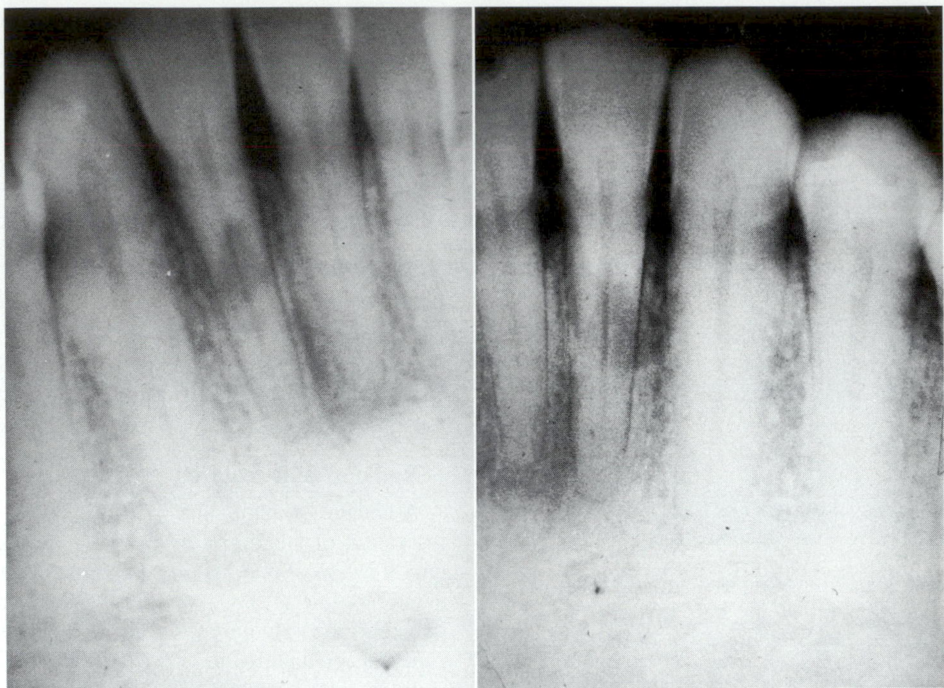

FIG. 17-33 External resorption. Radiographs from two different horizontal projections depict movement of the lesion to outside the confines of the root canal.

Vitality testing

External inflammatory resorption in the apical and lateral aspects of the root involves an infected pulp, so that a negative response to sensitivity tests is required to support the diagnosis. On the other hand, since cervical root resorption does not involve the pulp (the bacteria are thought to originate in the sulcus of the tooth) a normal response to sensitivity testing is usually associated with this type of resorption. Internal root resorption usually occurs in teeth with vital pulps and gives a positive response to sensitivity testing, though in teeth that exhibit internal root resorption it is not too uncommon to register a negative response to sensitivity testing, since often the coronal pulp has been removed (Fig. 17-29) or is necrotic and the active resorbing cells are more apical in the canal. Also, the pulp might have become necrotic after active resorption has taken place (Fig. 17-30).

Pink spot

With external root resorption apically and laterally the pulp is nonvital and therefore the granulation tissue that produces the pink spot is not present in these cases. For cervical and internal root resorption the pink spot due to the granulation tissue undermining the enamel is a possible sign.

Summary of possible diagnostic features

Inflammatory root resorption

Apical. Negative pulp sensitivity test, with or without a history of trauma.

Lateral. History of trauma, negative pulp sensitivity test, lesion moves on angled x-rays, root canal visualized radiographically overlying the defect, bony radiolucency also apparent.

Cervical. History of trauma (often forgotten by the patient), positive pulp sensitivity test, lesion located at the attachment level of the tooth, lesion moves on angled x-rays, root canal outline is undistorted and can be visualized radiographically, crestal bony defect associated with the lesion, pink spot possible.

Internal. History of trauma, crown preparation or pulpotomy; positive pulp sensitivity test, possible at any location along the root canal (not only attachment level); lesion stays associated with the root canal on angled x-rays, radiolucency contained in the root without an adjacent bony defect; pink spot possible.

The majority of misdiagnoses of resorptive defects are made between cervical and internal root resorptions. The diagnosis should always be confirmed while treatment is proceeding. If root canal therapy is the treatment of choice for an apparent internal root resorption, the bleeding within the canal should cease quickly after pulp extirpation since the blood supply of the granulation tissue is the apical blood vessels. If bleeding continues during treatment—and particularly if it is still present at the second visit—the source of the blood supply is external and treatment for external resorption should be carried out. Also, on obturation it should be possible to fill the entire canal from within in internal resorption. Failure to achieve this should make the operator suspicious of an external lesion. Finally, if the blood supply of an internal resorption defect is removed on pulp extirpation, any continuation of the resorptive process on recall radiographs should alert the dentist to the possibility that an external resorptive defect was misdiagnosed.

Dentoalveolar Ankylosis and Replacement Resorption

Dentoalveolar ankylosis describes the condition of ankylotic fusion between bone and the root cementum surface or between bone and shallow resorption lacunae (i.e., there is no periodontal ligament between these structures).[50] Replacement resorption is the process whereby the root dentin is replaced by bone.[9,10,13] Dentoalveolar ankylosis is thought to be a delayed form of replacement resorption in which the cementum layer significantly slows the resorption and replacement of the dentin with bone.[50]

Etiology

Dentoalveolar and replacement resorption occur if, after an injury, a necrotic periodontal membrane is present over a large area of the root.[73,75] This usually occurs after fairly severe dental injuries such as intrusive luxations, severe luxations, or exarticulation injuries complicated by a prolonged extraoral period, resulting in drying and death of the periodontal ligament cells. An inflammatory process removes the necrotic debris from the root surface. If infection is not present to sustain the inflammation, healing will follow by a competition between the remaining vital periodontal cells and ingrowth of alveolar bone across the periodontal space.[16] Replacement resorption can also occur after inflammatory root resorption has been reversed by removal of the inflammatory stimulating factor. Competition during healing occurs between the surrounding periodontal ligament cells and the bone-producing cells.[16] If the area affected by the inflammatory root resorption is large, it is extremely difficult for the periodontal ligament cells to populate the entire area before bone-producing cells move across the periodontal ligament space. If less than 20% of the root surface is involved, reversal of ankylosis may occur.[7,16,17] Since dentoalveolar resorption and replacement resorption occur after severe injuries it is quite common that the pulp subsequently becomes nonvital. However, these conditions occur independent of the status of the pulp, and treatment of the root canal does not affect the progression of replacement resorption.

Clinical manifestations

Replacement resorption is asymptomatic. Pathognomonic of ankylosis and replacement resorption is immobility of the affected tooth[7] and a distinctive metallic sound on percussion. Also, in time, teeth surrounding the affected tooth erupt normally, leaving the ankylosed tooth in infraocclusion. Eventually the root is resorbed completely and the crown of the tooth becomes undermined and breaks off, often leaving a gutta-percha point surrounded by bone. Although the condition of the root canal does not directly affect the progression of replacement resorption, the injuries that lead to replacement resorption are serious and often result in pulp death. Therefore root canal therapy is almost always required for these teeth.

Radiographic appearance

To radiographically diagnose dentoalveolar ankylosis and replacement resorption an attempt should be made to follow the lamina dura around the external surface of the root. In these conditions, the lamina dura is lacking. Generally, the root will have a moth-eaten appearance in the area affected by the replacement resorption (Fig. 17-34).[10,119] Unlike inflammatory resorption, the adjacent bone is not resorbed, so radiolucencies are not found in the bone adjacent to the affected root (Fig. 17-35).

Histologic appearance

Direct union of bone and the root substance is seen (Fig. 17-36).[10] Active resorption lacunae with osteoclasts can be seen in conjunction with the apposition of normal bone laid down by osteoblasts.

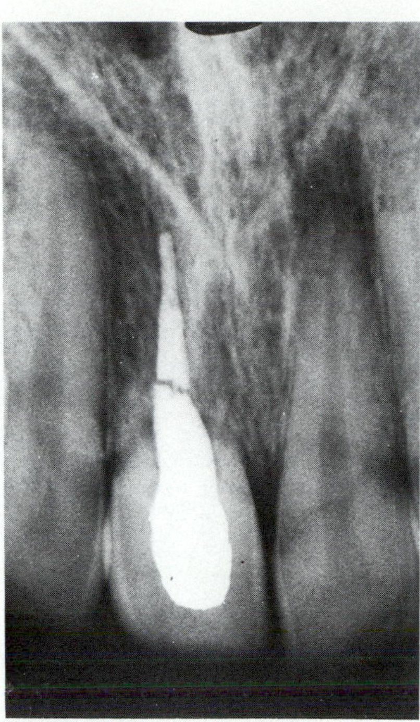

FIG. 17-34 Radiograph of maxillary central incisors with replacement resorption. Note the absence of lamina dura and the moth-eaten appearance of the roots.

Treatment

Once replacement resorption has developed there is no treatment known that will affect its progress. Therefore *prevention* of the development of the process is of utmost importance. Since nothing can be done about the extent of the initial injury to the attachment apparatus, the main emphasis is on (1) maintaining the health of the remaining periodontal ligament cells so that they are available to repopulate the denuded root surface and reestablish a normal periodontal ligament space and (2) removal of the irreversibly damaged periodontal ligament before replantation, to minimize inflammation afterward.

Intrusion injuries. An intrusion injury causes severe damage to the periodontal ligament; however, since the tooth is maintained in the mouth metabolic depletion by drying of the periodontal ligament is not a consideration. The objective in these cases is to minimize further injury when repositioning the teeth. In young intruded teeth, it is possible to wait for reeruption of the tooth, which occurs in approximately 2 to 3 weeks.[60] In older teeth, spontaneous eruption is not as predictable, and gentle repositioning with orthodontic forces is required. Extraction and repositioning is considered to cause too much damage to the periodontal ligament and to exacerbate rather than help prevent replacement resorption.

Severe extrusive luxation injuries. If replacement resorption will occur it is due to the initial injury, so very little can be done to prevent replacement resorption after severe extensive luxation injuries. The teeth must be repositioned as atraumatically as possible and physiologic splinting carried out for 10 to 14 days. The need for endodontic treatment should be assessed at this time. Luckily, the damage to the periodontal ligament is not as severe as that found in intrusion injuries, nor are the dehydration complications seen in exarticulations

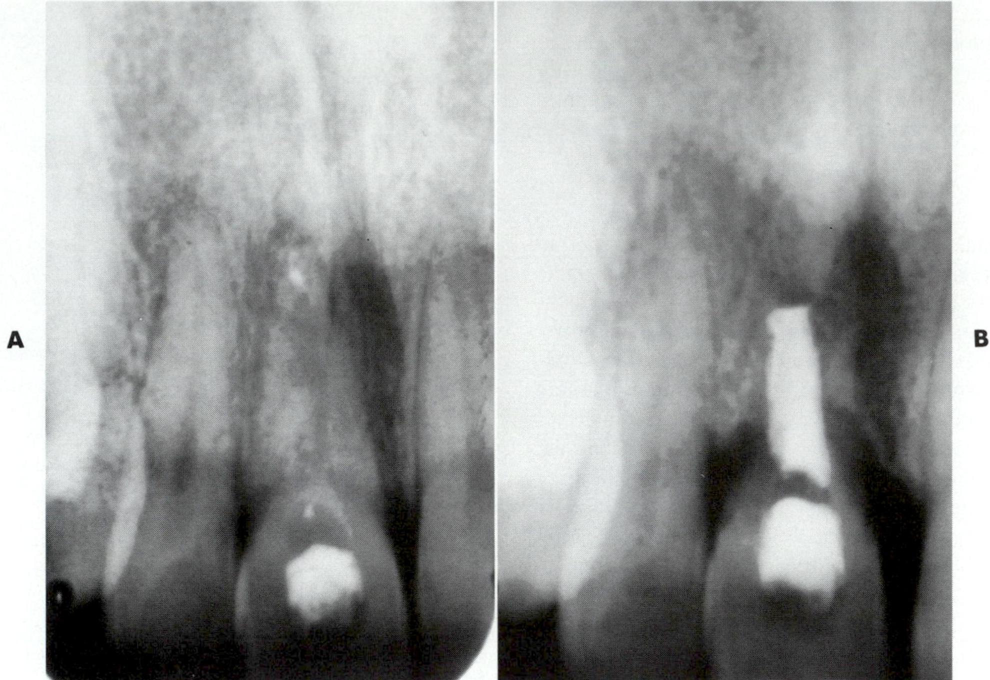

FIG. 17-35 A, Radiograph of maxillary central incisor 3 months after exarticulation. **B,** Seven years later the root has been replaced by bone.

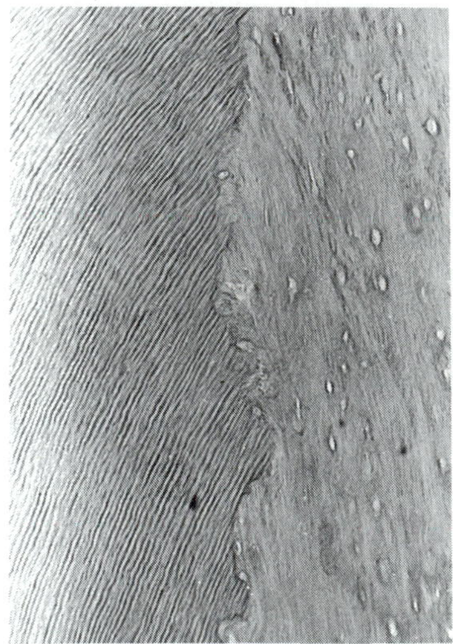

FIG. 17-36 Histologic appearance of dentoalveolar ankylosis with replacement resorption. Note the absence of the periodontal ligament and cemental layer and the direct union of the bone and root.

present. Therefore, the incidence of ankylosis and replacement resorption with these type of injuries is not as extensive.

Exarticulations. Again, nothing can be done about the damage to the attachment apparatus from the initial injury. All efforts are made to minimize necrosis of the periodontal ligament while the tooth is out of the mouth.

Treatment outside the dental office. Treatment outside the dental office is described in Chapter 16.

Treatment inside the office. To prevent or slow root resorption, the aim is to replant the tooth with the maximal number of periodontal ligament cells which have the potential to regenerate and repair the damaged root surface. Also, necrotic and irreversibly damaged cells should be removed if possible, before replantation. If it is not possible to maintain the periodontal ligament in a viable state, steps should be taken to treat the root, in order to slow the inevitable resorption. The following steps minimize root resorption.

1. *Preparation of the root.* If the tooth has not been dry for more than 20 minutes or was placed in an appropriate storage medium within this time frame, the root should be gently rinsed of debris with water or saline and replanted in as gentle a fashion as possible.[10] For drying periods of 20 minutes to 45 minutes there is some evidence that soaking the tooth in a replenishing medium can revitalize dying cells and reduce ankylosis.[79] Necrotic cells and debris float off the root during the soaking period. Thus, these teeth should not be replanted immediately but should be placed in a solution of Hanks' balanced salt solution for 30 minutes before replantation. When the root has been dry for 60 minutes or more all periodontal cells will have died[71,111,121] and soaking will be ineffective.[79] In these cases steps should be taken to prepare the root to be as resistant to resorption as possible, in order to slow the process. The teeth should be soaked in citric acid for 5 minutes followed by a 5-minute soak in 2% stannous fluoride, followed by another 5 minutes in doxycycline,[22,105] after which they are replanted.

2. *Splinting.* It is thought that movement of the tooth by semirigid splinting during the healing phase decreases the incidence of ankylosis.[5,6] Even though one group[20] found no difference in the incidence of resorption following physiologic

and rigid splinting, nevertheless, semirigid fixation for a minimal period (10 to 14 days) is recommended, as illustrated on page 474.

3. *Endodontic treatment*. Endodontic treatment should be initiated 10 to 14 days after avulsion in a closed-apex tooth (see Lateral Inflammatory Root Resorption). The treatment of the root canal does not directly influence the incidence of replacement resorption; however replacement resorption occurs subsequent to inflammatory resorption, and by minimizing the formation of inflammatory resorption the incidence of replacement resorption should decrease.[49,50]

4. *Antibiotics*. As with endodontic treatment, the systemic use of antibiotics immediately after the injury influences the incidence of inflammatory resorption, and therefore indirectly lowers the incidence of replacement resorption.[49]

SYSTEMIC CAUSES OF ROOT RESORPTION

The roots of teeth show a remarkable resistance to detectable resorption, even with systemic diseases that can cause significant bone resorption.[103] With hyperparathyroidism or osteitis deformans (Paget's disease), for example, radiographically apparent bone resorption is not accompanied by resorption of the roots.[108,110] However, hormonal disturbances and genetic factors have been shown sometimes to cause resorption of the root.[25,107] Renal dystrophy results in an increased oxylate concentration in the blood and precipitation in the hard tissues, which can cause root resorption.[42,83,103] Genetic linkage is likely, since external root resorption of no apparent cause has been found in members of the same family.[42,103] Resorption presently diagnosed as idiopathic root resorptions will in the future probably be increasingly found to be of systemic or genetic origin, as our knowledge and test procedures advance.

REFERENCES

1. Abbott PV, Heithersay GS, and Hume WR: Release and diffusion through human tooth roots in vitro of corticosteroid and tetracycline trace molecules from Ledermix paste, Endod Dent Traumatol 4:55, 1988.
2. Abbott PV, Hume WR, and Heithersay GS: Effects of combining Ledermix and calcium hydroxide pastes on the diffusion of corticosteroid and tetracycline through human roots in vitro, Endod Dent Traumatol 5:188, 1989.
3. American Association of Endodontists: Annotated glossary of terms used in endodontics, ed 4, Chicago, 1984, The Association.
4. American Association of Endodontists. Recommended guidelines for treatment of the avulsed tooth, J Endod 9:571, 1983.
5. Andersson L, Friskopp J, and Blomlof L: Fiber-glass splinting of traumatized teeth, J Dent Child 21-4, 1983.
6. Andreasen JO: The effect of splinting upon periodontal healing after replantation of permanent incisors in monkeys, Acta Odontol Scand 33:313, 1975.
7. Andreasen JO: Periodontal healing after replantation of traumatically avulsed human teeth. Assessment by mobility testing and radiography, Acta Odontol Scand 33:325, 1975.
8. Andreasen JO: Analysis of topography of surface and inflammatory root resorption after replantation of mature permanent incisors in monkeys, Swed Dent J 4:135, 1980.
9. Andreasen JO: Analysis of pathogenesis and topography of replacement root resorption (ankylosis) after replantation of mature permanent incisors in monkeys, Swed Dent J 4:231, 1980.
10. Andreasen JO: Traumatic injuries of the teeth, ed 2. Philadelphia, 1981, WB Saunders Co.
11. Andreasen JO: Relationship between surface and inflammatory resorption and changes in the pulp after replantation of permanent incisors in monkeys, J Endod 7:294, 1981.
12. Andreasen JO: The effect of pulp extirpation or root canal treatment upon periodontal healing after replantation of permanent incisors in monkeys, J Endod 7:245, 1981.
13. Andreasen JO: The effect of extra-alveolar period and storage media upon periodontal and pulpal healing after replantation of mature permanent incisors in monkeys, Int J Oral Surg 10:43, 1981.
14. Andreasen JO: Review of root resorption systems and models. Etiology of root resorption and the homeostatic mechanisms of the periodontal ligament. In Davidovitch (ed): The Biological Mechanisms of Tooth Eruption and Resorption, Birmingham, Ala, 1989, EBSCOP Media.
15. Andreasen JO, and Hjorting-Hansen E: Replantation of teeth. I. Radiographic and clinical study of 110 human teeth replanted after accidental loss, Acta Odont Scand 24:263, 1966.
16. Andreasen JO, and Kristersson L: The effect of limited drying or removal of the periodontal ligament. Periodontal healing after replantation of mature permanent incisors in monkeys, Acta Odont Scand 39:1, 1981.
17. Andreasen JO, and Kristersson L: Repair processes in the cervical region of replanted and transplanted teeth in monkeys, Int J Oral Surg :128, 1981.
18. Andreasen JO, et al: Periodontal and pulpal healing of monkey incisors preserved in tissue culture before replantation, Int J Oral Surg 7:104, 1978.
19. Antrim DD, Hicks ML, and Altaras DE: Treatment of subosseous resorption: a case report. J Endod 8:567, 1982.
20. Berude JA, et al: Resorption after physiologic and rigid splinting of replanted permanent incisors in monkeys. J Endod 14:592, 1988.
21. Bhaskar SN: Periapical lesions—types, incidence, and clinical features, Oral Surg 34:458, 1972.
22. Bjorvatn K, Selvig KA, and Klinge B: Effect of tetracycline and SnF_2 on root resorption in replanted incisors in dogs, Scand J Dent Res 97:477, 1989.
23. Blomlof L: Milk and saliva as possible storage media for traumatically exarticulated teeth prior to replantation, Swed Dent J 8(suppl):1, 1981.
24. Blomlof L, et al: Storage of experimentally avulsed teeth in milk prior to replantation, J Dent Res 62:912, 1983.
25. Bloom W: Resorption of bone metabolic interrelations, Trans Josiah Macy Jr Found 3:11, 1951.
26. Boksman R, Jordan RE, and Skinner DM: A conservative bleaching treatment for the nonvital discolored tooth, Compend Contin Educ 5:471, 1984.
27. Bystrom A, Claesson R, and Sundqvist G: The antibacterial effect of camphorated paramonochlorophenol, camphorated phenol and calcium hydroxide in the treatment of infected root canals, Endod Dent Traumatol 1:170, 1985.
28. Casey LJ, et al: The use of dentinal etching with endodontic bleaching procedures. J Endod 15:535, 1989.
29. Chambers TJ: Phagocytic recognition of bone by macrophages, J Pathol 135:1, 1981.
30. Chambers TJ, Pringle JAS, and Horton MA: The relationship between osteoclasts and cells of the mononuclear phagocyte system in rodents and man. A functional and antigenic assessment, Calcif Tiss Int 36(suppl 2):550, 1984.
31. Cowie P, and Wright BA: Multiple idiopathic root resorption, Can Dent Assoc J 47:111, 1981.
32. Cvek M: Treatment of non-vital permanent incisors. II. Effect on external root resorption in luxated teeth compared with the effect of root filling with gutta-percha, Odontol Revy 24:343, 1973.
33. Cvek M, Granath LE, and Hollander L: Treatment of nonvital permanent incisors with calcium hydroxide. III. Variations of occurrence of ankylosis of reimplanted teeth with duration of extraalveolar period and storage environment, Odontol Revy 25:43, 1974.
34. Cvek M, and Lindvall AM: External resorption following bleaching of pulpless teeth with oxygen peroxide, Endod Dent Traumatol 1:56, 1985.

35. Cwyk F, Saint-Pierre F, and Tronstad L: Endodontic implications by orthodontic tooth movement, J Dent Res 63:1984 (IADR abstr No. 1039).
36. Dargent P: A study of root resorption, Acta Odontostomatol 117:47, 1977.
37. Edmunds DH, and Beck C: Root resorption in autotransplanted maxillary canine teeth, Int Endod J 22:29, 1989.
38. Frank AL, and Bakland LK: Nonendodontic therapy for supraosseous extracanal invasive resorption, J Endod 13:348, 1987.
39. Freccia WF, et al: An in vitro comparison of non-vital bleaching techniques in the discolored teeth, J Endod 8:70, 1982.
40. Friedman S, et al: Incidence of external root resorption and esthetic results in 58 bleached pulpless teeth, Endod Dent Traumatol 4:23, 1988.
41. Fuss Z, Szajikis S, and Tagger M: Tubular permeability to calcium hydroxide and to bleaching agents, J Endod 15:362, 1989.
42. Gold SI, and Hasselgren G: Peripheral inflammatory root resorption, J Periodontol 19:523, 1992.
43. Gottlieb B, and Orban B: Veranderungen im Periodontium nach chirurgischer Diathermie, Z J Stomatol 28:1208, 1930.
44. Gottlow J, et al: New attachment formation in the human periodontium by guided tissue regeneration: case reports. J Clin Periodontol 13:604, 1986.
45. Grossman LI: Endodontic practice, ed 10, Philadelphia, 1981, Lea & Febiger.
46. Hall AM: Upper incisor root resorption during stage II of the Begg technique: two case reports, Br J Orthod 5:47, 1978.
47. Hammarstrom L, and Lindskog S: General morphologic aspects of resorption of teeth and alveolar bone, Int Endod J 18:293, 1985.
48. Hammarstrom L, et al: Effect of calcium hydroxide treatment on periodontal repair and root resorption. Endod Dent Traumatol 2:184, 1986.
49. Hammarstrom L, et al: Replantation of teeth and antibiotic treatment, Endod Dent Traumatol 2:1, 1986.
50. Hammarstrom L, et al: Tooth avulsion and replantation: a review, Endod Dent Traumatol 2:1, 1986.
51. Harrington GW, and Natkin E: External resorption associated with bleaching of pulpless teeth, J Endod 5:344, 1979.
52. Healy HJ: Endodontics: selection of case treatment procedures, J Am Dent Assoc 53:434, 1956.
53. Heithersay GS: Clinical endodontic and surgical management of tooth and associated bone resorption, Int Endod J 18:93, 1985.
54. Heithersay GS, and Wilson DF: Tissue responses with rat to trichloracetic acid—an agent used in the treatment of invasive cervical resorption, Aust Dent J 33:451, 1988.
55. Hiltz J, and Trope M: Vitality of human lip fibroblasts in milk, Hanks balanced salt solution and Viaspan storage media, Endod Dent Traumatol 7:69, 1991.
56. Hinman TP: The interpretation of x-ray pictures of apical granulations, giving differential diagnosis of cases favorable and cases unfavorable for treatment and root canal filling, J Natl Dent Assoc 8:83, 1921.
57. Ho S, and Goering AE: An in vitro comparison of different bleaching agents in the discolored tooth. J Endod 15:106, 1989.
58. Hopewell-Smith A: The process of osteolysis and odontolysis or so-called "absorption" of calcified tissues; a new original investigation, Dent Cosmos 72:323, 1903.
59. Hopkins R, and Adams D: Multiple idiopathic resorption of teeth, Br Dent J 146:305, 1979.
60. Jacobsen I: Traumatic injuries to the teeth. In Magnusson BO, Koch G, Poulson S (eds): Pedodontics, Copenhagen, 1981, Munksgaard.
61. Karring T, Nyman S, and Lindhe J: Healing following implantation of periodontitis affected roots into bone tissue, J Clin Periodont 7:96, 1980.
62. Kerekes K, Heide S, and Jacobsen I: Follow-up examination of endodontic treatment in traumatized juvenile incisors, J Endod 6:744, 1980.
63. Kuettner KE, and Pauli BU: Resistance of cartilage to normal and neoplastic invasion. In Horton JE, Tarpey TM, and Davis MF (ed): Mechanisms of localized bone loss, Calcif Tissue Res (suppl):251, 1978.
64. Kuttler Y: Microscopic investigation of root apexes, J Am Dent Assoc 50:544, 1955.
65. Lado EA, Stanley HR, and Weissman, MI: Cervical resorption in bleached teeth, Oral Surg 55:78, 1983.
66. Lalond ER, and Luebke RG: The frequency distribution of periapical cysts and granulomas, Oral Surg 25:861, 1968.
67. Lengheden A, Blomlof L, and Lindskog S: Effect of immediate calcium hydroxide treatment and permanent root-filling on periodontal healing in contaminated replanted teeth, Scand J Dent Res 99:139, 1990.
68. Lengheden A, Blomlof L, and Lindskog S: Effect of delayed calcium hydroxide treatment on periodontal healing in contaminated replanted teeth, Scand J Dent Res 99:147, 1991.
69. Levender E, and Malmgren O: Evaluation of the risk of root resorption during orthodontic treatment: a study of upper incisors, Eur J Orthodont 10:30, 1988.
70. Lindskog S, and Blomlof L: Influence of osmolality and composition of some storage media on human periodontal ligament cells, Acta Odontol Scand 40:435, 1982.
71. Lindskog S, Blomlof L, and Hammarstrom L: Repair of periodontal tissues in vivo and in vitro, J Clin Periodontol 10:188, 1983.
72. Lindskog S, Blomlof L, and Hammarstrom L: Cellular colonization of denuded root surfaces in vivo: cell morphology in dentin resorption and cementum repair, J Clin Periodontol 14:390, 1987.
73. Lindskog A, et al: The role of the necrotic periodontal membrane in cementum resorption and ankylosis, Endod Dent Traumatol 1:96, 1985.
74. Linge BO, and Linge L: Apical root resorption in upper anterior teeth, Eur J Orthodont 5:173, 1983.
75. Loe H and Waerhaug J: Experimental replantation of teeth in dogs and monkeys, Arch Oral Biol 3:176, 1961.
76. Madison S, and Walton R: Cervical root resorption following bleaching of endodontically treated teeth, J Endod 16:570, 1990.
77. Makkes PG, and Thoden Van Velzen SK: Cervical external root resorption, J Dent Res 3:217, 1975.
78. Marks SC, and Walker DG: The origin of osteoclasts: evidence, clinical implications and investigative challenges of an extra-skeletal source, J Oral Pathol 12:226, 1983.
79. Matsson L, et al: Ankylosis of experimentally reimplanted teeth related to extra-alveolar period and storage environment, Pediatr Dent 4:327, 1982.
80. Mattison GD, Gholston LR, and Boyd P: Orthodontic external root resorption—endodontic considerations, J Endod 9:253, 1983.
81. Mattison GD, et al: Orthodontic root resorption of vital and endodontically treated teeth, J Endod 10:354, 1984.
82. Maurice CG: Selection of teeth for root canal treatment, Dent Clin North Am 761, 1957.
83. Moskow BM: Periodontal manifestations of hyperoxaluria and oxalosis, J Periodont 60:271, 1989.
84. Mount GJ: Idiopathic internal resorption, Oral Surg 33:80, 1972.
85. Mundy Gr, et al: Direct resorption of bone by human monocytes, Science 196:1109, 1977.
86. Nichols E: An investigation into the factors which may influence the prognosis of root canal therapy. Master's thesis, Faculty of Medicine, University of London, 1960.
87. Nilsen R: Microfilaments in cells associated with induced heterotopic bone formation in guinea pigs, Acta Pathol Mund Scand A88, 85:1297, 1980.
88. Nutting EB, and Poe GS: A new combination for bleaching teeth, J South Calif Dent Assoc 31:289, 1963.
89. Nyman S, et al: New attachment following surgical treatment of human periodontal disease, J Clin Periodont 9:290, 1982.
90. Orban B: The epithelial network in the periodontal membrane, J Am Dent Assoc 44:632, 1952.
91. Penick EC: The endodontic management of root resorption, Oral Surg 16:344, 1963.

92. Pierce A: Experimental basis for the arrangement of dental resorption, Endod Dent Traumatol 5:255, 1989.
93. Pierce A, and Lindskog S: The effect of an antibiotic corticosteroid combination on inflammatory root resorption in vivo, Oral Surg Oral Med Oral Pathol 64:216, 1987.
94. Pierce A, Berg JO, and Lindskog S: Calcitonin as an alternative therapy in the treatment of root resorption, J Endod 14:459, 1988.
95. Pierce A, Heithersay G, and Lindskog S: Evidence for direct inhibition of dentinoclasts by a corticosteroid/antibiotic endodontic paste, Endod Dent Traumatol 4:44, 1988.
96. Pierce AM: Cellular mechanisms in bone and tooth resorption. Dissertation, Karolinska Institute, Stockholm, 1988.
97. Pinborg JJ, and Hansen J: A case of replantation of an upper lateral incisor: a histologic study, Oral Surg 4:661, 1951.
98. Polson AM, and Caton JM: Factors influencing periodontal repair and regeneration, J Periodont 53:617, 1982.
99. Rankow H, Croll TP, and Miller AS: Preeruptive idiopathic coronal resorption of permanent teeth in children, J Endod 12:36, 1986.
100. Rotstein I, Lehr Z, and Gedalia I: Effect of bleaching agents on inorganic components of human dentin and cementum, J Endod 18:290, 1992.
101. Rotstein I, et al: In vitro efficacy of sodium perborate preparations used for intracoronal bleaching of discolored non-vital teeth, Endod Dent Traumatol 1:177, 1991.
102. Seltzer S: Endodontology, Philadelphia, Lea & Febiger, 1988.
103. Seltzer S: Personal communication.
104. Selvig KA, and Zander HA: Chemical analysis and microradiography of cementum and dentin from periodontically diseased human teeth, J Periodont 33:303, 1962.
105. Selvig KA, Bjorvatn K, and Claffey N: Effect of stannous fluoride and tetracycline on repair after delayed replantation of root planed teeth in dogs, Acta Odontol Scand 48:107, 1990.
106. Seward GR: Periodontal disease and resorption of teeth, Br Dent J 34:443, 1963.
107. Sharawy AM, Mills PB, and Gibbons RJ: Multiple ankylosis occurring in rat teeth, Oral Surg 26:856, 1968.
108. Silverman S, et al: The dental structures in primary hyperparathyroidism, Oral Surg 15:426, 1962.
109. Sjogren M, et al: The antimicrobial effect of calcium hydroxide as a short term intracanal dressing, Int Endod J 24:119, 1991.
110. Smith BJ, and Eveson JW: Paget's disease of bone with particular reference to dentistry, J Oral Pathol 10:233, 1981.
111. Soder P-O, et al: Effect of drying on viability of periodontal membrane, Scand J Dent Res 85:167, 1977.
112. Spasser HF: A simple bleaching technique using sodium perborate, NY State Dent J 27:332, 1961.
113. Spasser HF: Personal communication, 1986.
114. Stanley HR: Diseases of the dental pulp. In Tiecke RW (ed): Oral Pathology, New York, 1965, McGraw-Hill Co.
115. Stenvik A, and Mjor IA: Pulp and dentin reaction to experimental tooth instrusion, Am J Orthodont 57:370, 1970.
116. Taylor MA, Hume WR, and Heithersay GS: Some effects of Ledermix paste and Pulpdent paste on mouse fibroblasts and on bacteria in vitro, Endod Dent Traumatol 5:266, 1989.
117. Teitelbaum SL, Stewart CC, and Kahn AJ: Rodent peritoneal macrophages as bone resorbing cells, Calcif Tissue Int 27:255, 1979.
118. Tronstad L: Pulp reactions in traumatized teeth. In Gutman JL, and Harrison JW: Proceedings of the International Conference on Oral Trauma. Chicago: 1984, American Association of Endodontists Endowment and Memorial Foundation.
119. Tronstad L: Root resorption—etiology, terminology and clinical manifestations, Endod Dent Traumatol 4:241, 1988.
120. Tronstad L, et al: pH changes in dental tissues following root canal filling with calcium hydroxide, J Endod 7:17, 1981.
121. Trope M, and Friedman S: Periodontal healing of replanted dog teeth stored in Viaspan, milk and Hanks balanced salt solution, Endod Dent Traumatol 8:183, 1992.
122. Trope M, et al: Effect of different endodontic treatment protocols on periodontal repair and root resorption of replanted dog teeth, J Endod 18:492, 1992.
123. Wedenberg C: Evidence for a dentin-derived inhibitor of macrophage spreading, Scand J Dent Res 95:381, 1987.
124. Wedenberg C, and Lindskog S: Experimental internal resorption in monkey teeth, Endod Dent Traumatol 1:221, 1985.
125. Wedenberg C, and Zetterqvist L: Internal resorption in human teeth—a histological, scanning electron microscope and enzyme histo-chemical study, J Endod 13:255, 1987.
126. Weiss SD: Root resorption during orthodontic treatment in endodontically treated and vital teeth, Master's thesis, Memphis, University of Tennessee, College of Dentistry, 1969.
127. Yaacob HB: The resistant dentine shell of teeth suffering from idiopathic external resorption, Aust Dent J 25:73, 1980.

Self-assessment questions

1. Internal resorption
   a. radiographically is often confused with external replacement resorption.
   b. is associated with systemic disease.
   c. is usually associated with trauma.
   d. usually results only if odontoblasts and/or predentin layer is lost or altered.
2. Studies of internal resorption have shown
   a. histologic differences in the process in primary and permanent teeth.
   b. no difference in rate of progression of the process in primary and permanent teeth.
   c. normal pulp is replaced by a periodontal-like connective tissue.
   d. resorption of dentin and no deposition of mineralized tissue.
3. External resorption may be found in which one of the following systemic diseases?
   a. Hypoparathyroidism.
   b. Diabetes.
   c. Leukemia.
   d. Parkinson's disease.
4. Apical external resorption, as related to periapical pathosis,
   a. requires surgical intervention (apicoectomy).
   b. is usually associated with a necrotic pulp.
   c. is initially treated with conventional root canal treatment, although this has a questionable outcome.
   d. is usually irreversible, has a poor prognosis, and requires extraction.
5. Resorption following bleaching
   a. is a reason not to treat tetracycline-stained teeth with root canal therapy and internal bleaching.
   b. may be due to erosion of dentin exposed at the cervical line.
   c. is related to the use of heat and 30% hydrogen peroxide.
   d. does not occur unless there is a history of trauma.
6. Orthodontic treatment resorption is most prevalent in
   a. maxillary incisors.
   b. mandibular incisors.
   c. maxillary premolars.
   d. mandibular premolars.
7. Avulsed teeth replanted without pulpectomy usually exhibit
   a. revascularization of pulp space.
   b. surface resorption.

c. inflammatory resorption.
d. ankylosis.

8. Cementum is more resistant than bone to resorption. A theory as to why this is true is that
a. cementum is more mineralized than bone.
b. cementum contains an antiresorptive factor.
c. bone is vascular; cementum avascular.
d. fiber patterns in cementum are different than in bone and tend to be more resistant to clast-type cells.

9. The two major local causes of root resorption are
a. inflammation and excessive pressure.
b. inflammation and cementoclast-activating factor.
c. excessive pressure and increased pH of ground substance.
d. cementoclast-activating factor and increased pH of ground substance.

10. As related to root resorption during orthodontic movement root canal–treated teeth are
a. more resistant to resorption.
b. less resistant to resorption.
c. no different than untreated teeth.
d. more prone to resorption if there is a history of apical root resorption as related to apical pathosis.

11. Lateral inflammatory root resorption is usually
a. related to a tooth injury that damages the PDL.
b. related to sterile pulp necrosis.
c. irreversible.
d. successfully treated only if calcium hydroxide is placed in the canal prior to obturation.

12. Clinical features of early stages of lateral inflammation root resorption include that usually it is
a. associated with normal pulp testing, visible radiographically.
b. asymptomatic, not visible radiographically.
c. associated with no (or abnormal) response to pulp testing, symptomatic.
d. symptomatic, not visible radiographically.

13. Cervical root resorption is in many (or most) cases
a. of unknown etiology.
b. related to a subluxation injury.
c. associated with a necrotic, infected pulp.
d. unrelated to inflammation in the cervical periodontium.

14. Treatment of medium depth cervical root resorption usually requires
a. root canal treatment alone.
b. root canal treatment followed by surgery.
c. surgery alone.
d. surgery, followed if necessary by root canal treatment.

15. These clinical features of internal resorption usually include
a. positive response to pulp testing, visible in the pulp space radiographically.
b. visible in both the pulp space and as a defect in the adjacent bone.
c. symptomatic, visible radiographically in the pulp space.
d. asymptomatic, visible radiographically in the pulp space, variable response to pulp testing.

16. In the treatment of nonperforating internal resorption, calcium hydroxide may be used in the canal *primarily* to
a. sterilize the canal space.
b. remineralize the resolved areas.
c. aid in breaking down inaccessible areas containing tissue.
d. lower pH in the tissue to counteract the dentinoblasts.

17. A common histologic feature of replacement resorption is
a. areas of fusion of bone with cementum/dentin.
b. inflammation in the adjacent periodontium.
c. pulp necrosis with bacteria deep into the tubules.
d. areas of necrotic bone and necrotic cementum.

18. A treatment approach that will generally arrest replacement resorption is
a. pulpectomy and placement of $Ca(OH)_2$.
b. surgery to expose and curette the defect.
c. pulpectomy and immediate obturation.
d. nonexistent. There is no known effective treatment.

Chapter 18

Endodontic-Periodontal Relations

James H. S. Simon
Leslie A. Werksman

No tooth is an island. The relationship of the pulp and the periodontium is dynamic. The astute diagnostician should be aware that endodontic and periodontal lesions arise from inflammation or degeneration of both tissues. *The function of a tooth depends on the health and vitality of the periodontium and not on the status of the pulp.* Thus, the tooth and its supporting structures form a biologic unit.

EFFECT OF PULPAL DISEASE ON ATTACHMENT APPARATUS

Endodontic disease is a bacterial disease. When pulpal disease progresses beyond the confines of the tooth, inflammation replaces the attachment apparatus. Several avenues exist for the extension of pulpal pathosis.

Apical Foramen

Inflammatory cells and the products of pulpal inflammation replace the periodontal ligament and surrounding bone. The resultant bone loss from pulpal infection is most apparent at the apical foramen. External resorption of cementum can occur concurrently if the infectious process persists. This inflammatory resorption can ultimately change the shape and location of the apical foramen of the affected tooth.

Lateral Canals

The same inflammatory response seen at the apical foramen also occurs through the lateral and accessory canals of the pulp. Inflammation associated with lateral canals may appear as a radiolucency or a notch on the side of the root surface.[38] (For purposes of this chapter *the terms "lateral" and accessory" are used interchangeably to designate those pulpal periodontal vascular communications other than the main canal.)*

In an extensive study of 7275 teeth,[33] the highest percentage of lateral canals occurs in the middle one third of the root and the maxillary central incisor is the tooth most frequently affected (11.9%, Figs. 18-1 through 18-4). The percentage of lateral canals in the furcation is 46% in first molars[49] and 50% to 60% in any multirooted tooth.[28] Other studies report that both maxillary and mandibular molars have at least two foramina in the furcation.[8]

Recently, histologic evaluations of hemisected or amputated roots with persistent periodontic and endodontic involvement[1] revealed untreated accessory canals containing remnants of pulp tissue, bacteria, and necrotic debris. They concluded that residual infected necrotic tissue in untreated canals can lead to periradicular pathosis and periodontal defects (Fig. 18-4).

Dentinal Tubules

The dentinal tubules are another potential pathway of communication between the periodontium and the pulp. As early as 1963 the hydrodynamic theory was proposed to explain the mechanism of dentin hypersensitivity. Experts believe that fluid movement in the tubules is responsible for stimulating nerve fibers in the pulp. Subsequently, when root surface treatment increases the number of exposed dentinal tubules, there is enhanced opportunity for fluid movement, resulting in pulpal sensitivity.[30,32] During pulpal death, however, degeneration of odontoblastic processes and collagen fibers occurs, further increasing the permeability of the tubules and easing transport of toxins from the pulp into the attachment apparatus (Fig.

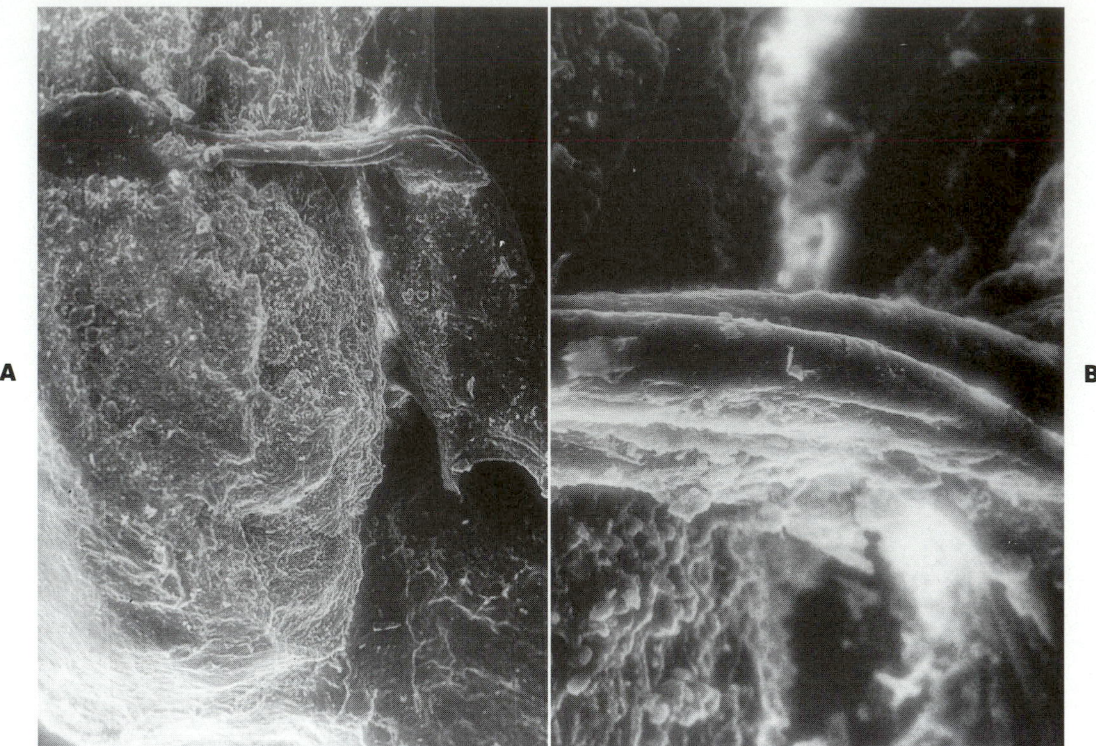

FIG. 18-1 A, Low-power scanning electron micrograph of pulp entering the apical foramen and small vessel branching into a lateral canal. **B,** High-power view of two vessels (capillary size) entering lateral canal.

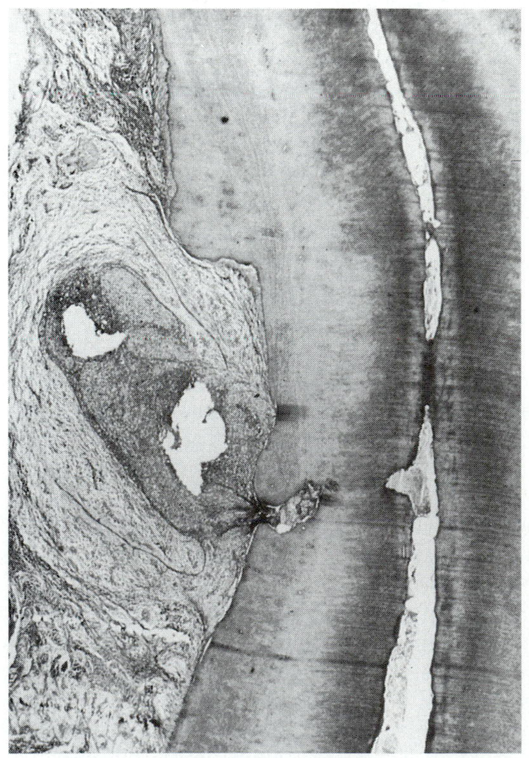

FIG. 18-2 Histologic section of lateral incisor with necrotic canal and lateral canal with inflammatory response in the periodontal ligament. Note proliferating epithelium.

18-5). Cementum removal or acid etching of dentin during periodontal procedures also enhances the ability of bacteria and products of pulpal or periodontal inflammation to penetrate the tubules.[11] Thus, the effect of pulpal disease on the periodontium is a direct inflammatory one.

EFFECT OF ENDODONTIC TREATMENT ON PERIODONTIUM

The pulpal inflammatory process results in replacement of the periodontal ligament by inflammatory tissue, with accompanying resorption of alveolar bone, cementum, and sometimes dentin. Therefore, periodontal inflammation of endodontic origin should heal following adequate endodontic treatment.[51]

Recently, researchers have investigated the periodontal response to different forms of endodontic treatment, including the perpetuation of pulpal infection.[5,6] Not only did the presence of pulp infection encourage clastic activity and aggravate a periodontal lesion, but high concentrations of calcium hydroxide and corticosteroid antibiotics can also irritate the attachment apparatus.

In his text on *Advanced Periodontal Disease*,[34] Prichard suggested that endodontically treated teeth may not respond as well as untreated teeth to periodontal procedures. To substantiate this hypothesis, researchers[39,42] found that after osseous regenerative procedures 60% of nonendodontically treated teeth healed but only 33% (5 of 15) of the endodontically obturated teeth did. The authors concluded that endodontic obturation of teeth may adversely affect the final result of osseous regenerative procedures. At this time it is not clear

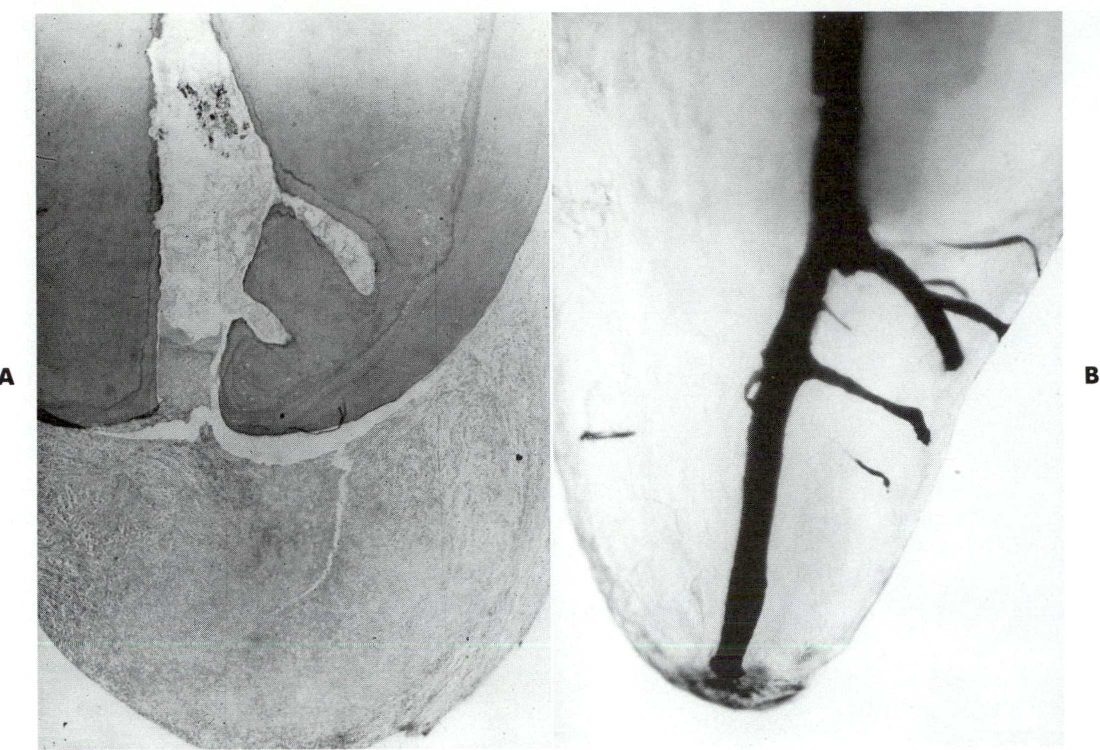

FIG. 18-3 A, Histologic section of lower bicuspid with two lateral canals. **B,** Cleared, decalcified lower bicuspid shows multiple lateral canals. (Courtesy Dr. Paul Fitzwalter.)

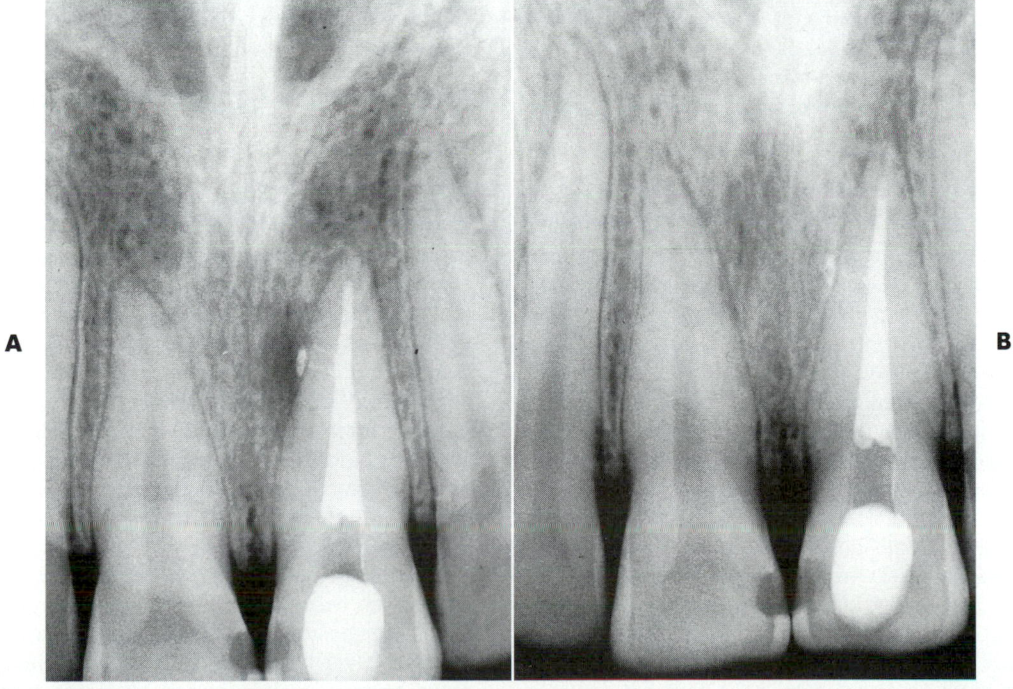

FIG. 18-4 A, Filled central incisor with two lateral canals opening into a lateral radiolucency. **B,** At 1-year recall, the lateral radiolucency has healed.

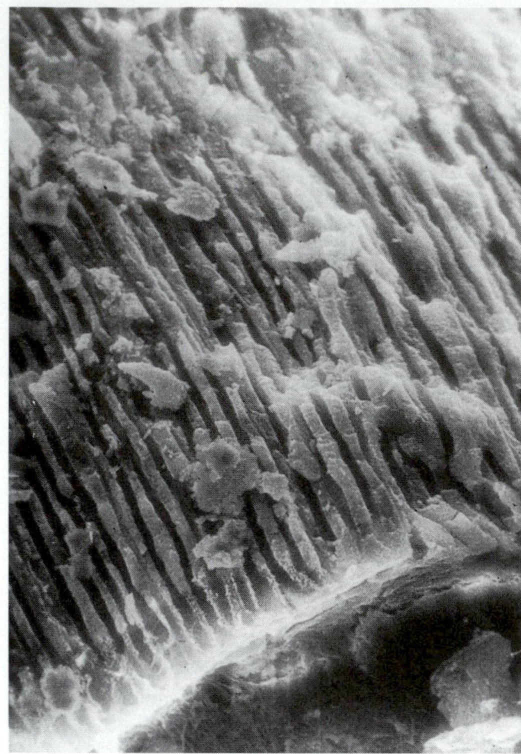

FIG. 18-5 Scanning electron micrograph of empty dentinal tubules. With the odontoblastic processes gone, these may act as empty channels.

whether the materials for obturation, the inadequacy of instrumentation or obturation, or other factors are responsible for failure of such periodontal procedures.

With proper endodontic treatment periodontal disease of pulpal origin should heal. If concomitant periodontal inflammation exists independent of pulpal pathosis, Prichard recommends delaying debriding and hermetically sealing the root canal system until after surgical treatment of the periodontal defect.[35]

EFFECT OF PERIODONTAL DISEASE ON PULP

Considerable controversy surrounds the effect of periodontal disease on the pulp. Periodontal disease may extend to the pulp through the accessory canals, the apical foramen, and open dentinal tubules.[13]

In 1963, Seltzer and coworkers[41] evaluated the status of the pulp of 85 periodontally diseased teeth. Thirty-seven percent of the periodontally involved teeth without caries or restorations had pulpal inflammation or necrotic pulps. Other researchers[25,36,46] have found that the greatest atrophic and inflammatory changes occur when teeth have many accessory canals or when the periodontal defect has progressed to the apex. Others[3,25] concluded that the cumulative effect of periodontal disease has a damaging effect on the pulp, as indicated by the presence of pulp calcification, inflammation, or resorption; but total pulp disintegration is a certainty only when the apical foramen is infected.

In contrast to these studies, others have found no pulpal changes in the presence of periodontal disease.[14] Mazur and Massler[29] compared periodontally involved and healthy teeth from the same mouth in 30 patients and could not correlate the extent of periodontal disease with the histologic status of the pulp. Czarnecki and Schilder[12] evaluated over 40 teeth and also concluded that periodontal disease had no effect on the pulp. The pulpal changes reported by previous researchers as pathologic were attributed instead to inadequate histologic fixation and varying degrees of normal between young and old pulps. They further noted that each of the teeth with a necrotic pulp had either extensive caries or massive restorations. Finally in their study of 34 asymptomatic teeth with periodontitis only six showed evidence of pulpal pathosis.

In an attempt to reproduce periodontal disease in monkeys and then to evaluate the histologic status of the pulp, researchers placed cotton floss ligatures around the necks of 92 permanent teeth.[3] After a period of 5 to 7 months, with 30% to 40% loss of periodontal support on the root, 57% of the teeth exhibited some pathologic pulp tissue alterations histologically. The effect was considered mild since the reaction consisted primarily of secondary dentin formation and localized inflammatory cell infiltrates. Overall, they concluded that the pulp tissue in the majority of roots subjected to periodontitis displayed no pulpal pathologic alterations.

Periodontal disease is an inflammatory and infective process; however, it does not appear to have a direct inflammatory effect on the pulp. The initial effect of periodontal inflammation may be degenerative. This is evident histologically as an increase in secondary dentin formation, dystrophic calcification, fibrosis, and collagen resorption.[40]

Confusion begins to mount as researchers note that pathologic pulpal changes occurred as often in teeth without periodontitis as in those with periodontitis. Teeth from the same patient showed no difference in the pulpal findings, regardless of the presence or severity of periodontal disease.[47]

Although there is a plethora of information on the effect of periodontal inflammation on the pulp, a concrete conclusion cannot be drawn. Aging, caries, and operative procedures complicate the interpretation of the effect of periodontal disease on the pulp.[4]

THE EFFECT OF PERIODONTAL TREATMENT ON PULP

All treatment modalities for periodontal disease have the potential to adversely affect the pulp. Increased hypersensitivity is one of the common sequelae of nonsurgical and surgical periodontal therapy. This hypersensitivity is caused by the complete removal of cementum and the subsequent exposure of dentinal tubules to the oral environment. At this point, dentinal tubules become an open avenue of communication between oral fluids and the pulp, leading to pulpal pain.[55]

Dentin hypersensitivity persists until formation of a smear layer, or until natural occlusion of the dentinal tubules.[50] Researchers have found the intentional creation of a smear layer, or application of low-pH solutions such as sodium chloride or potassium oxalate, can temporarily decrease patients' postoperative pain.[11,21]

For periodontal soft tissue reattachment therapy use of citric acid has become routine. The rationale for use of demineralizing agents concerns the removal of bacterial endotoxin.[37] There are two theoretical functions for citric acid: (1) to remove bacterial endotoxin and anaerobic bacteria, and (2) to expose collagen bundles to serve as a matrix for new connective tissue attachment to cementum.[24] Though beneficial in the treatment of periodontal disease, citric acid removes the smear layer, an important pulp protector.

The effects of citric acid on the pulp have been studied. The duration of citric acid contact on the root surface, and the length of time before histologic analysis, may be responsible for the conflicting results reported in the literature. Evidence from three dog studies indicates that, though pulpal inflammation does not occur after citric acid use, superficial changes in dentin peritubular and tubular structures do occur.[56] Root planing procedures increase reparative dentin formation, yet surprisingly use of citric acid did not worsen the pulp's status.[31] In one study the authors go so far as to conclude that the mechanical procedures on the pulp are more responsible for pulpal changes than the application of citric acid for 3 minutes.[24] In a study on cats,[18] standard procedures for citric acid application revealed no pulpal changes 3 days after treatment; but a human study revealed that citric acid cleanser was toxic to the pulp when applied to freshly prepared dentinal surfaces.[10]

Periodontal surgery affects the pulp to the extent that it is exposed to endotoxin or bacteria via lateral canals, dentinal tubules, or in extreme cases the apical foramen.[22] In addition, added stress and trauma in the form of restorative or prosthetic treatment further increases the incidence of pulpal necrosis.[4,12,41]

DIAGNOSIS

Most dentists call pulpal disease "combined periodontal-pulpal" disease if bone resorption is evident radiographically in the furcation or crestal area.[35] Another frequent mistake is to give the disease process a "combined" designation if bone resorption extends to the apex of an affected tooth.[15] Differential diagnosis of periodontic and/or endodontic disease requires insightful understanding and thorough methodology.

To obtain a correct diagnosis the dentist must utilize the full spectrum of pulpal and periodontal testing procedures. Since differential diagnosis is not always obvious, several factors need to be considered when determining the etiology.

A thorough patient history should be obtained. Be aware of previous periodontal and endodontic signs and symptoms. The patient may report a history of trauma or recent dental treatment. The character of pain will aid in the diagnosis. Sharp severe pain is of pulpal etiology.

Expose a new radiograph. Radiographs help evaluate bone loss of any source. However, when bony breakdown extends from the cementoenamel junction to the apex the radiograph alone is insufficient. Take more than one radiograph, especially where no clear diagnosis emerges.[35] A minor alteration in the angulation may reveal a tooth fracture or periodontal furcation involvement. Morphologic anomalies such as developmental grooves or dens invaginatus can cause a localized defect, especially on a virgin tooth (Fig. 18-6).[42]

The shape, location, and extension of a bony lesion also inform the diagnosis. If the borders of the lesion are not visible on a periapical radiograph the clinician must expose an occlusal or panoramic radiograph to visualize them. When multiple radiographs reveal generalized periodontal disease but the patient reports only isolated discomfort, the dentist must test the pulp status of the teeth to rule out a pulpal lesion.

Pulp status is probably the most important test for determining the extent of endodontic involvement.[53] Test the pulp with thermal and electrical stimulation, or perform a test cavity. Evaluate the periapex by percussion and palpation sensitivity test. Record any mobility or evidence of occlusal trauma seen as wear facets.

Look at the soft tissue carefully in order to detect swelling or fistula. Always track the fistula with a gutta-percha point or balled silver cone. Often, the fistula will not appear to be associated with the involved tooth.[19] By tracking the lesion and taking angled radiographs, the clinician can avert inappropriate treatment. Fistulas of endodontic or periodontic origin can exit through the gingival crevice, a gingival papilla, the attached gingiva, or the alveolar mucosa.[35] When a sinus tract of endodontic origin fistulates through the periodontal ligament space it can easily be mistaken for a periodontal abscess. This is further evidence for the need for pulp testing.

Owing to the paucity of diagnostic tests for discriminating between periodontic and endodontic lesions, the dentist needs to carefully perform periodontal probing. Conscientious probing around the external surface of the tooth may reveal the source of the lesion.

The presence of a radiolucency coupled with an intact, gingival sulcus that cannot be probed indicates the problem is not of periodontal origin.[17] If a pulpal cause has been demonstrated, endodontic treatment alone resolves the problem. If the pulp responds within normal limits and periodontal disease has been ruled out, a biopsy must be performed to determine the cause.[35]

An acute endodontic abscess that tracks through the periodontal ligament space of a tooth can easily be missed by a practitioner. The tooth usually probes within normal limits around the entire surface, except in one narrow area where the probe sinks to or near the apex. Usually no radiolucency is evident on the radiograph, but swelling may be present on the labial or buccal surface.[17] The track is about 1 mm wide; therefore, probing must be completely around the sulcus. If the patient is in distress and all other diagnostic tests are complete, then proper probing may necessitate anesthesia.

Occasionally probing indicates a sinus tract wider than 1 mm in a pulpless tooth. The sinus tract may disrupt the gingival sulcus for 4 to 5 mm. Some experts believe this is associated with a chronic endodontic lesion. Nevertheless, resolution depends on adequate endodontic treatment.

For a complete diagnostic assessment we cannot overemphasize the importance of careful probing of the involved tooth and adjacent ones. Just as probing depths are documented before periodontal treatment, any tooth evaluated for pulpal disease must also have its periodontal probings recorded.

Recently evidence shows that the spirochete concentration may differ in lesions of endodontic origin and in periodontal lesions.[20,48] In two difficult cases the percentage of spirochetes in the lesion was the only evidence that helped the clinician make the diagnosis. In both cases the lesions healed after appropriate treatment.[48]

Making the diagnosis of endodontic and periodontic lesions may be difficult, but establishing the correct diagnosis is necessary for devising an appropriate treatment plan and making a prognosis. Ignorance of the signs and symptoms of these disease processes may lead to needless loss of teeth.

CLASSIFICATIONS OF COMBINED ENDODONTIC PERIODONTAL DISEASE

To clarify the interrelationship of pulpal and periodontal disease states, a classification system was proposed[44] in 1972

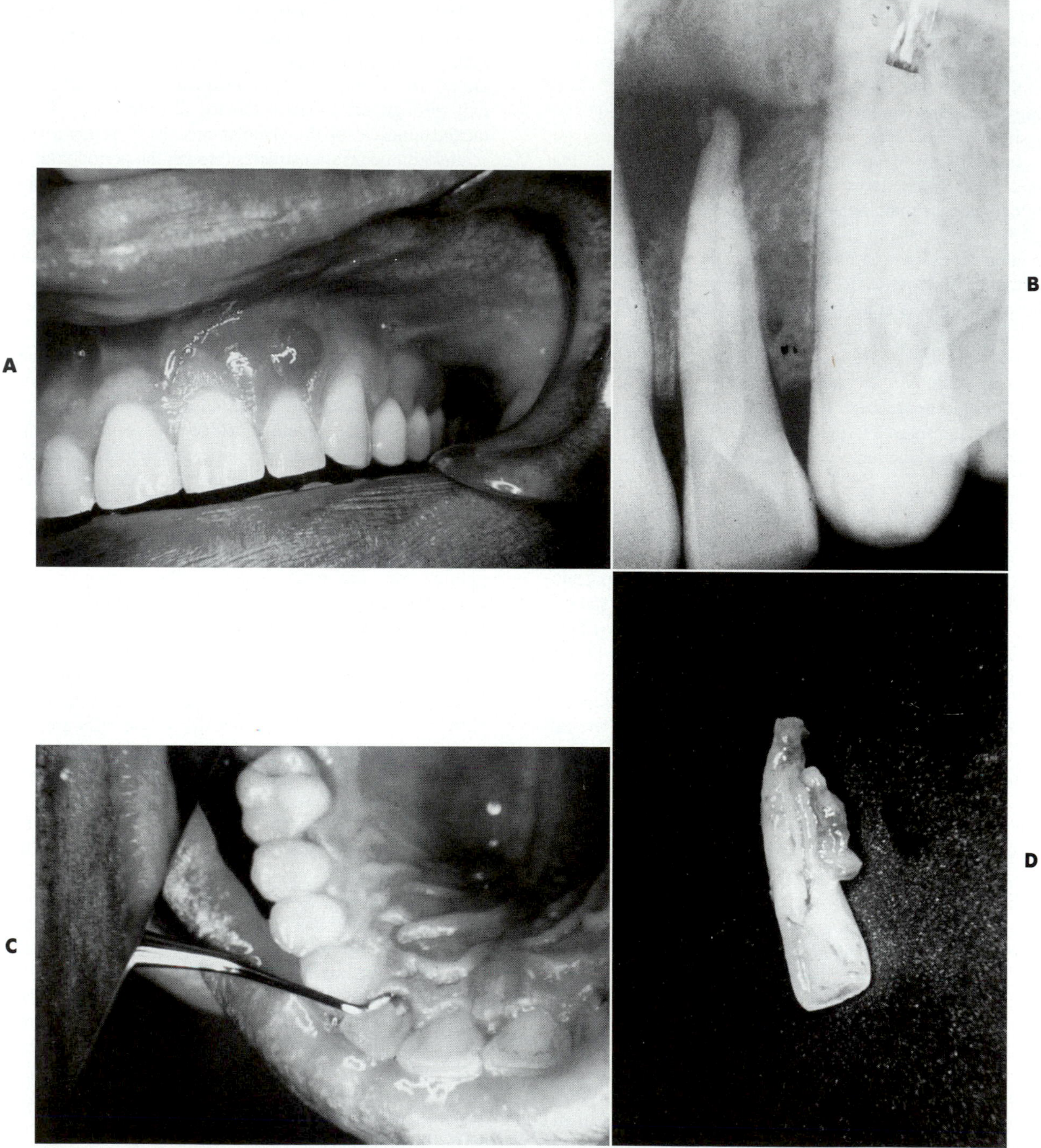

FIG. 18-6 A, Clinical photograph with swelling above upper lateral incisor. **B,** The upper lateral incisor shows a periapical radiolucency and no apparent cause. **C,** Clinical photograph with periodontal probe sunk to the apex. **D,** Extracted tooth with inflamed tissue removed to reveal palatogingival groove extending to the apex. This is a primary periodontal lesion. The pulp may be involved secondarily in long-standing disease. (Courtesy Dr. Stephen Schwartz.)

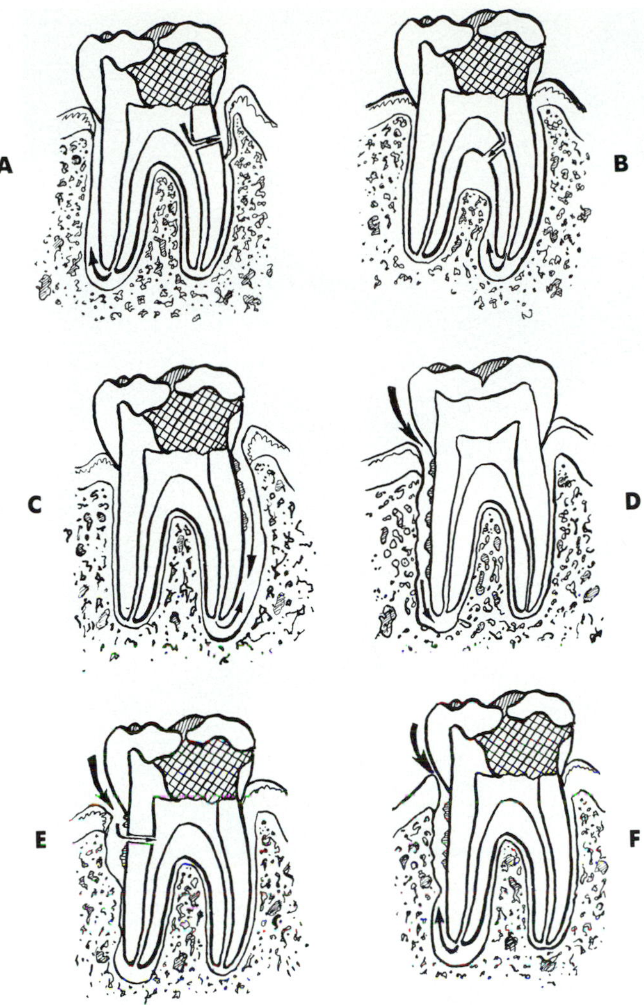

FIG. 18-7 A–C, Endodontic lesions. **A,** The pathway of fistulation is evident through the periodontal ligament from the apex or a lateral canal. **B,** Fistulation through the apex or a lateral canal, causing bifurcation involvement. **C,** Secondary periodontal involvement. The existing pathway, as in **A,** is shown; with the passage of time, however, periodontitis, with plaque and calculus formation, begins at the cervical area. **D–F,** Periodontal lesions. **D,** This is the progression of periodontitis to apical involvement. Note the vital pulp. **E,** Secondary endodontic involvement. The primary periodontal involvement at the cervical margin and the resultant pulpal necrosis once the lateral canal is exposed to the oral environment produce this picture. **F,** True combined lesions-coalescence.

(Fig. 18-7). This paper presented a feasible classification based on the theoretic pathways of lesion formation.

Primary Endodontic Lesion

Sinus tract formation through the periodontal ligament has been shown to be a part of the natural history of pulpal disease. A sinus tract originating from the apex or a lateral canal may form along the root surface and exit through the gingival sulcus (Fig. 18-8). This is not a true periodontal pocket but a fistula that, instead of opening on the buccal or lingual mucosa, drains along the periodontal ligament into the sulcus. This drainage through the sulcus often shows as a radiolucency along the mesial or distal root surface or in the bifurcation area (Figs. 18-9 to 18-12). The tract usually involves only one aspect of the tooth. For example, if the fistula goes through the bifurcation area, the mesial and distal crestal bone levels may be normal.

Clinically, drainage may be evident in the sulcus area and some swelling may be present, especially in the bifurcation area, simulating a periodontal abscess. This may be the only area of apparent periodontal involvement. The tract can usually be probed with a gutta-percha or silver cone or a periodontal probe that will go toward the source of irritation, generally the root apex or a lateral canal. This tract is usually more tubular and thinner than an infrabony periodontal pocket. Pain is not often present, though the patient may have some minor discomfort. Endodontic testing procedures should reveal a necrotic pulp or, in multirooted teeth, at least an altered response, indicating that at least one canal is necrotic. Because this lesion is an endodontic problem that has merely fistulated through the periodontal ligament, complete resolution is usually anticipated after routine endodontic treatment.

Primary Endodontic Lesion with Secondary Periodontal Disease

This condition occurs when pulpal disease is long standing and periapical drainage becomes chronic. As the drainage persists through the gingival sulcus, superimposition of plaque and calculus into the pocket results in a periodontal pocket and apical migration of the attachment. Radiographs may show generalized periodontal disease with angular defects at the initial site of endodontic involvement.

Resolution of the primary endodontic and the secondary periodontal lesion relies on treatment of both. One can expect bone loss of endodontic origin to heal if appropriate root canal treatment is performed. The periodontal bone loss depends on the efficacy of periodontal therapy (Fig. 18-13).

Primary Periodontal Lesion

Pulp of teeth with moderate to severe periodontal disease and no endodontic involvement tests within normal limits. Clinically, probing detects broad-based pocket formation and causes bleeding of the tissue. Examination may also find plaque, calculus, and soft tissue inflammation associated with a purulent exudate (Figs. 18-14, 18-15). Traumatic occlusion may be the cause of an isolated periodontal problem.

Treatment depends on the extent of the periodontal disease and on the patient's ability to comply with possible long-term treatment and maintenance therapy. Because the pulps of these teeth test within normal limits the prognosis depends on the outcome of periodontal therapy.

Primary Periodontal Lesion with Secondary Endodontic Involvement

This lesion differs from the primary endodontic lesion with secondary periodontal involvement only by the temporal sequence of the disease processes. The tooth with primary periodontal and secondary endodontic disease has deep pockets and a history of extensive periodontal disease, and possibly treatment. When the pulp becomes involved the patient reports accentuated pain and clinical signs of pulpal disease. Pulp tests confirm irreversible pulpal inflammation or necrosis. This situation exists when the apical progression of periodontal dis-

Text continued on p. 527.

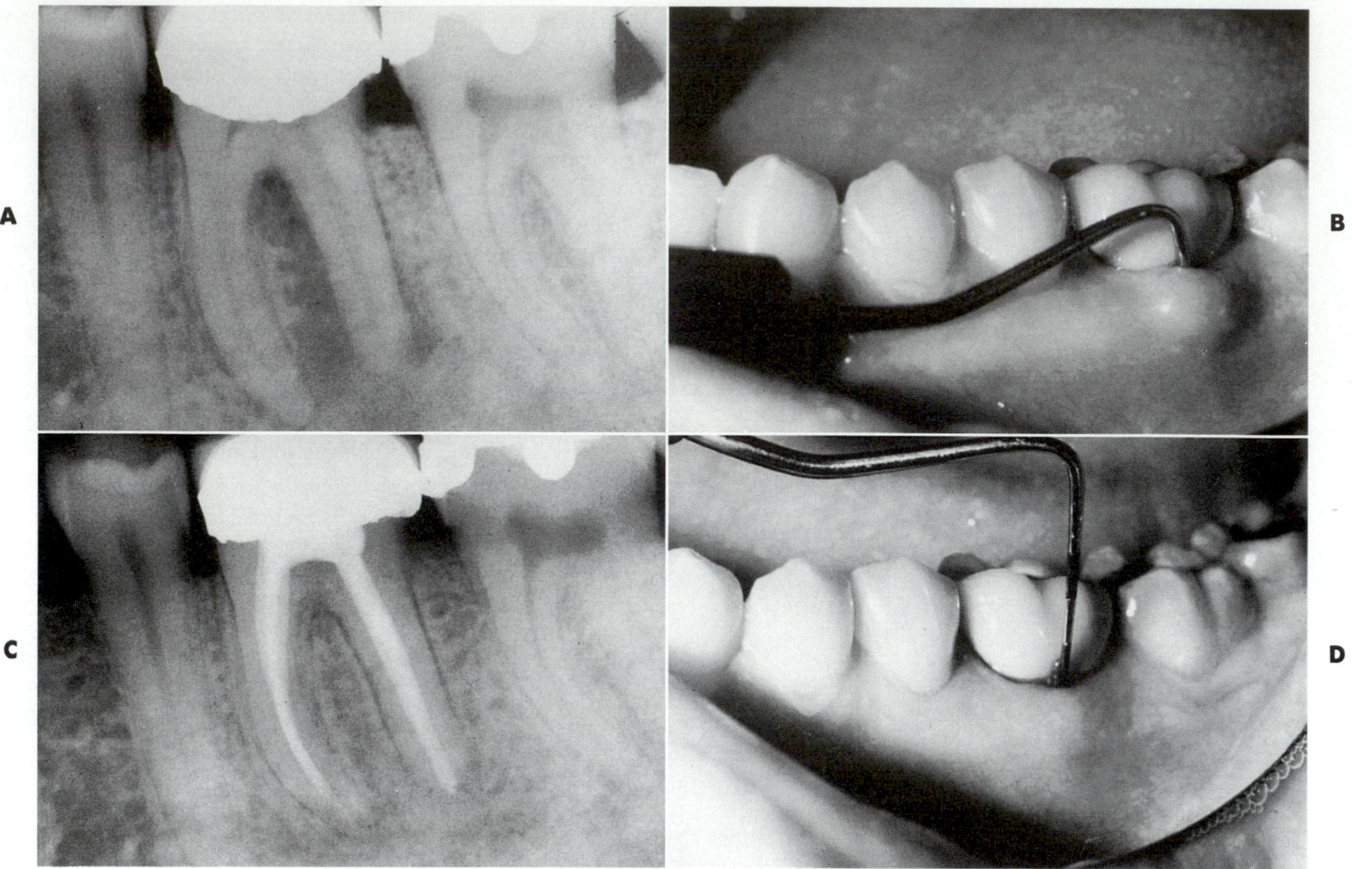

FIG. 18-8 Primary endodontic lesion. **A,** Preoperative radiograph with periapical and furcal radiolucency. **B,** Clinical photograph with periodontal probe in place. Note small gingival swelling that simulates a periodontal abscess. **C,** Only 6 months after endodontic treatment the lesion has healed. **D,** Clinical photograph shows healing with periodontal probe in place. (Courtesy Dr. Frank J. Wilkinson.)

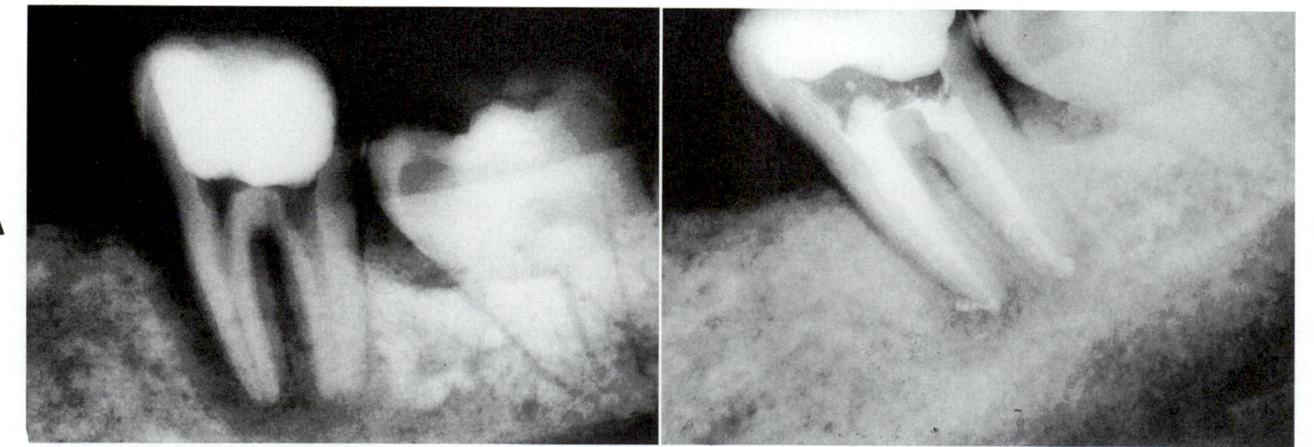

FIG. 18-9 Primary endodontic lesion. **A,** Preoperative radiograph with radiolucency along entire mesial root, giving the appearance of periodontal disease. **B,** Nine months after endodontic therapy the mesial bone appears to have remineralized almost completely.

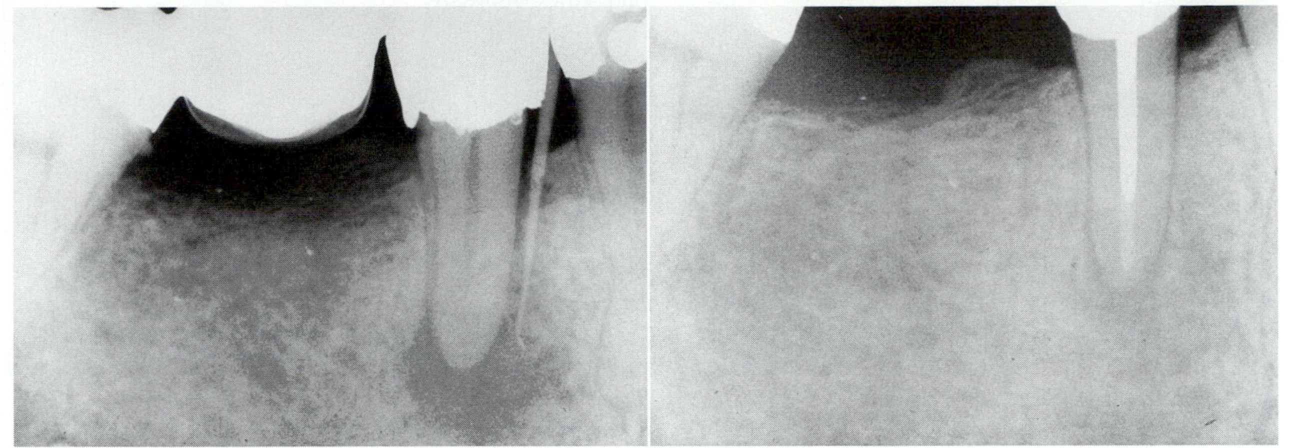

FIG. 18-10 A, Radiograph of lower necrotic bicuspid with periapical and lateral radiolucency. Gutta-percha cone is inserted through gingival sulcus, extending to the apex. **B,** Recall radiograph demonstrates almost complete healing with endodontic therapy. (Courtesy William H. Kelly.)

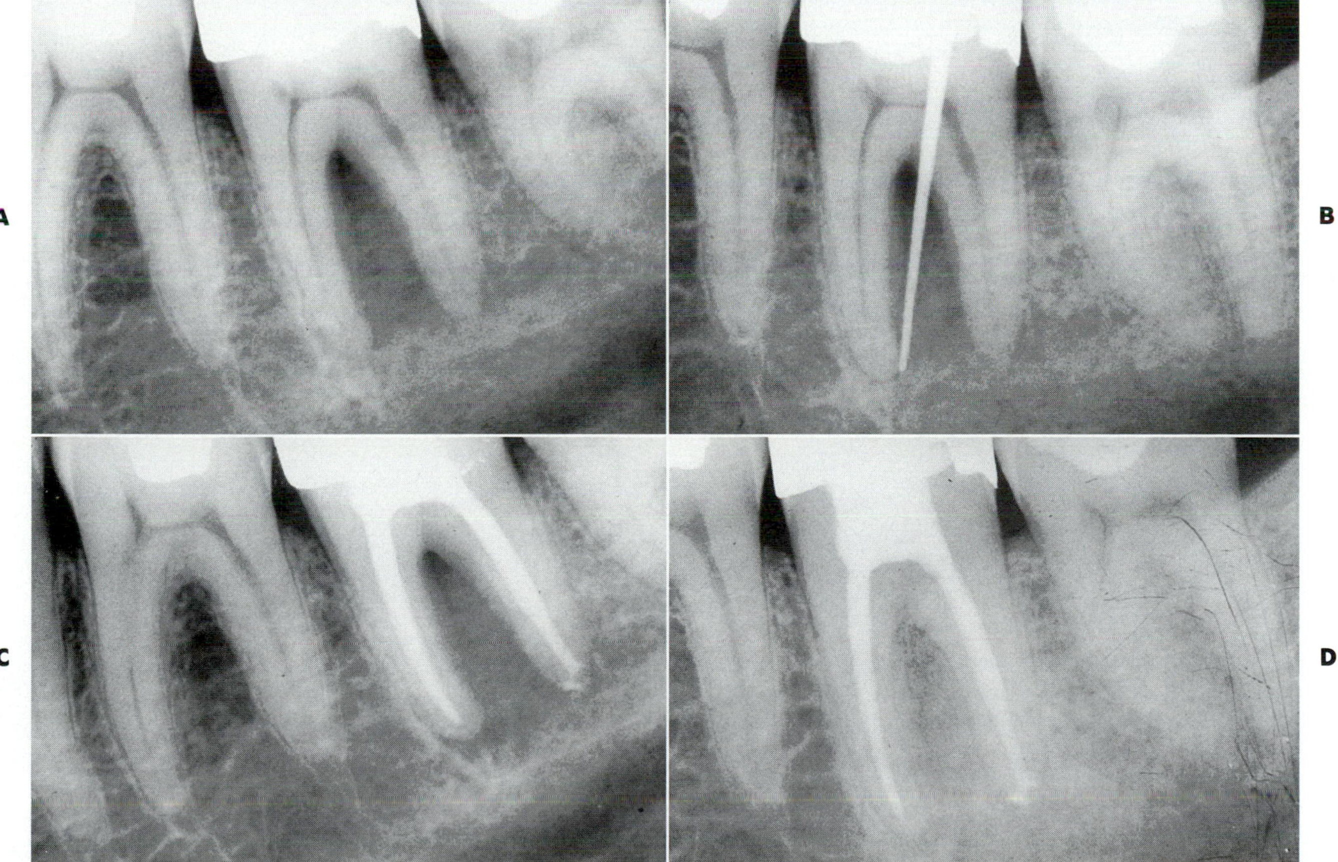

FIG. 18-11 A, Preoperative radiograph of lower second molar with furcal radiolucency. Note crestal bone level on mesial and distal. **B,** Radiograph with periodontal probe into furca extending to the apex of the mesial roots. **C,** Postoperative radiograph. **D,** Recall radiograph demonstrates complete furcal healing with endodontic therapy. (Courtesy Dr. Frank J. Wilkinson.)

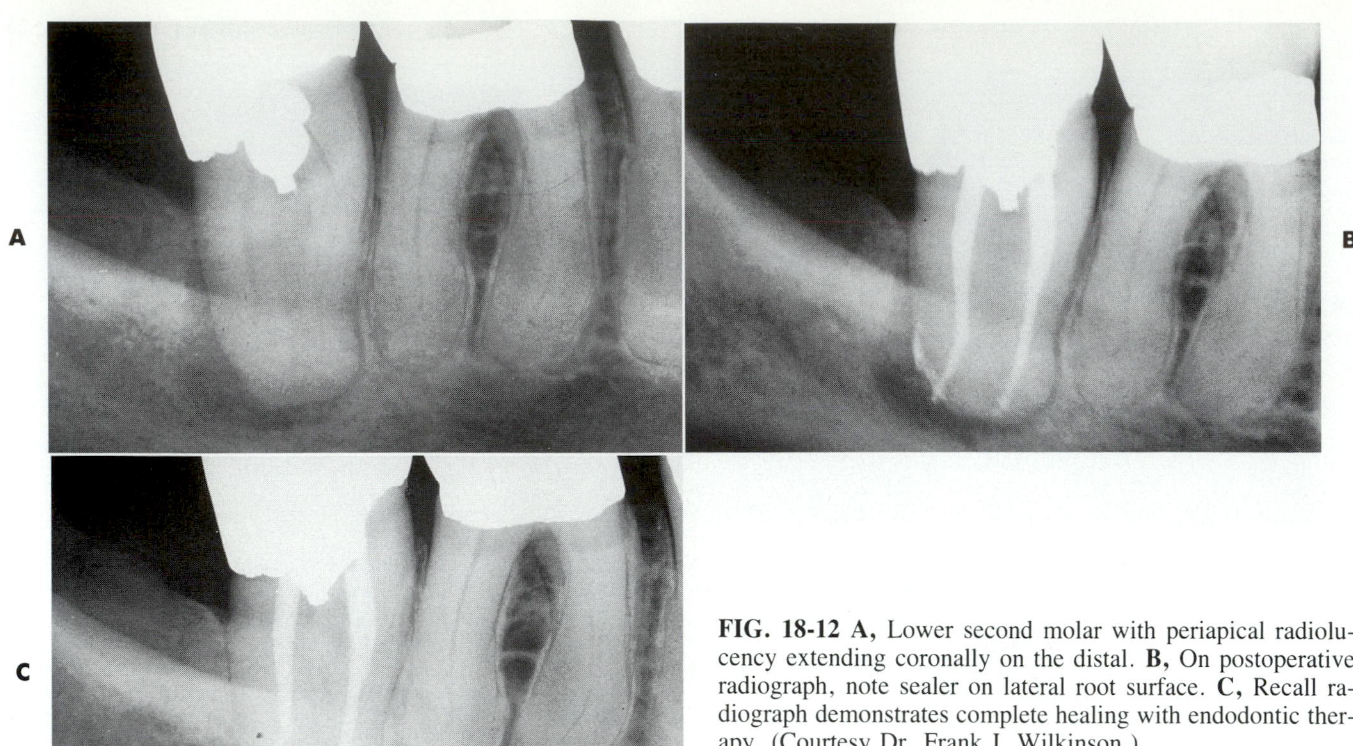

FIG. 18-12 A, Lower second molar with periapical radiolucency extending coronally on the distal. **B,** On postoperative radiograph, note sealer on lateral root surface. **C,** Recall radiograph demonstrates complete healing with endodontic therapy. (Courtesy Dr. Frank J. Wilkinson.)

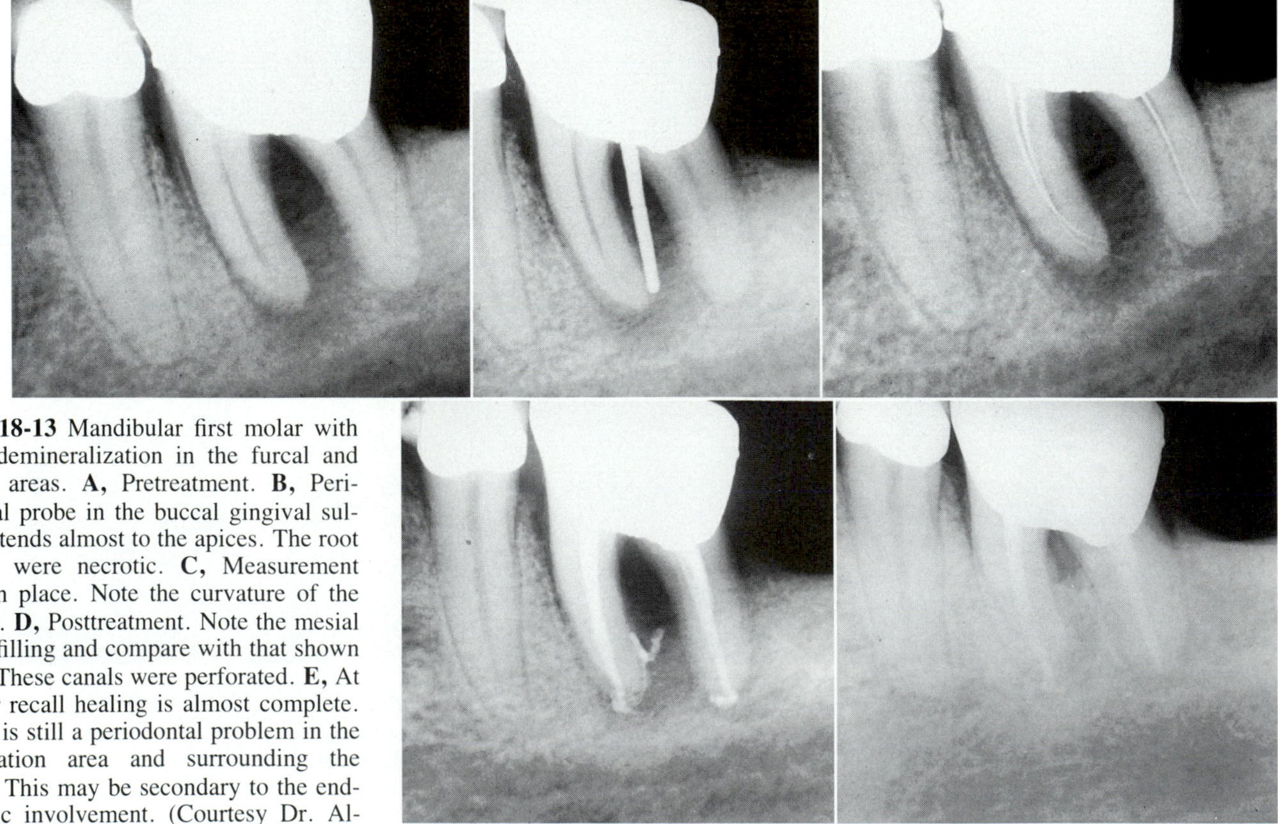

FIG. 18-13 Mandibular first molar with bone demineralization in the furcal and apical areas. **A,** Pretreatment. **B,** Periodontal probe in the buccal gingival sulcus extends almost to the apices. The root canals were necrotic. **C,** Measurement files in place. Note the curvature of the canals. **D,** Posttreatment. Note the mesial canal filling and compare with that shown in **C.** These canals were perforated. **E,** At 2-year recall healing is almost complete. There is still a periodontal problem in the bifurcation area and surrounding the tooth. This may be secondary to the endodontic involvement. (Courtesy Dr. Alfred L. Frank.)

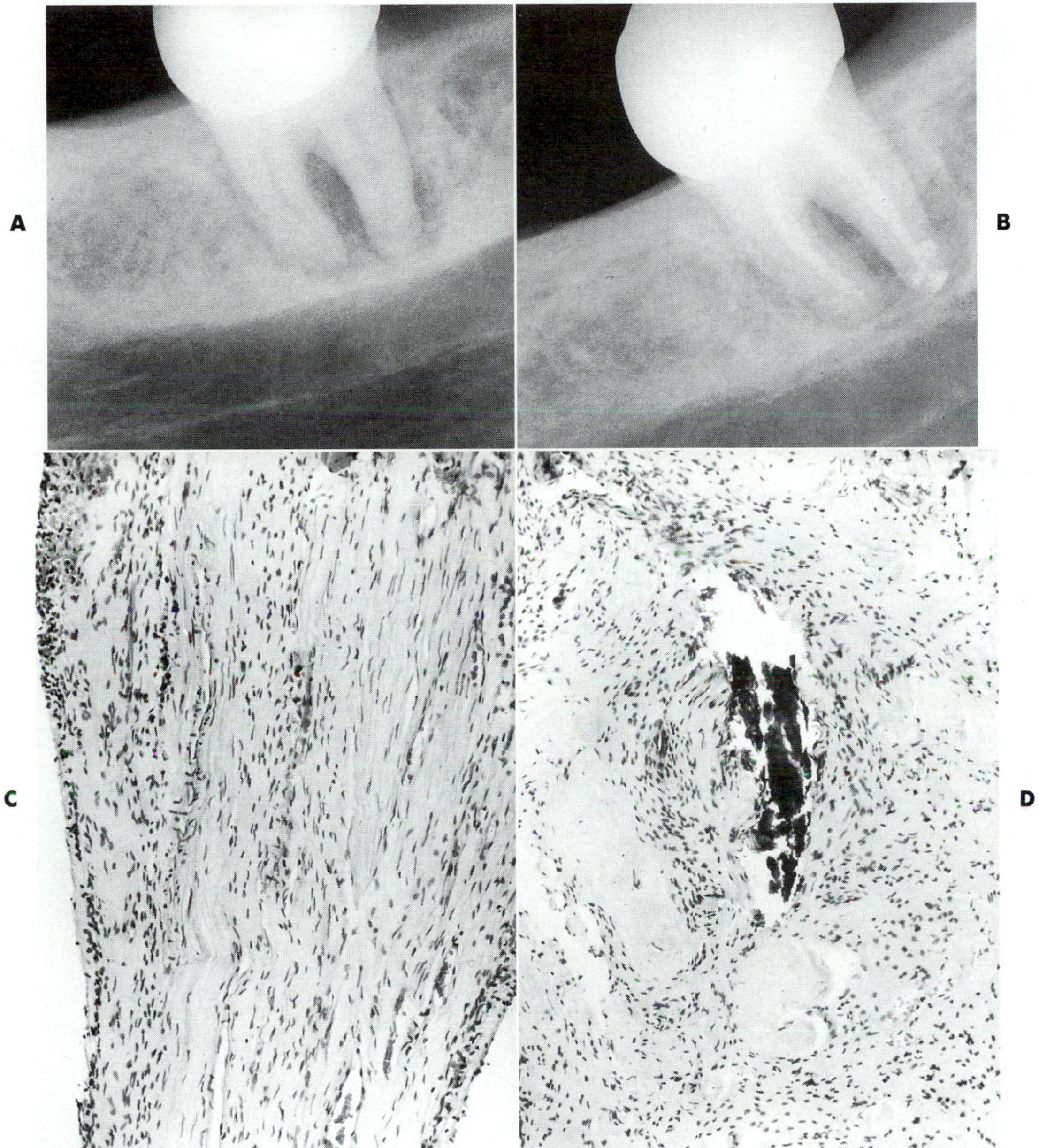

FIG. 18-14 A, A molar has an apparent periapical lesion. The tooth responded within normal limits to pulp testing procedures and could be probed on the distal aspect. The periodontist insisted it was an endodontic lesion and needed endodontic therapy. **B,** Postoperative radiograph. **C,** Low-power view of a section of vital pulp extirpated from this molar. **D,** High-power photomicrograph shows vital pulp tissue with calcification. The final diagnosis was normal pulp. The periapical lesion was a periodontal one. (Courtesy Dr. Charles K. Reince.)

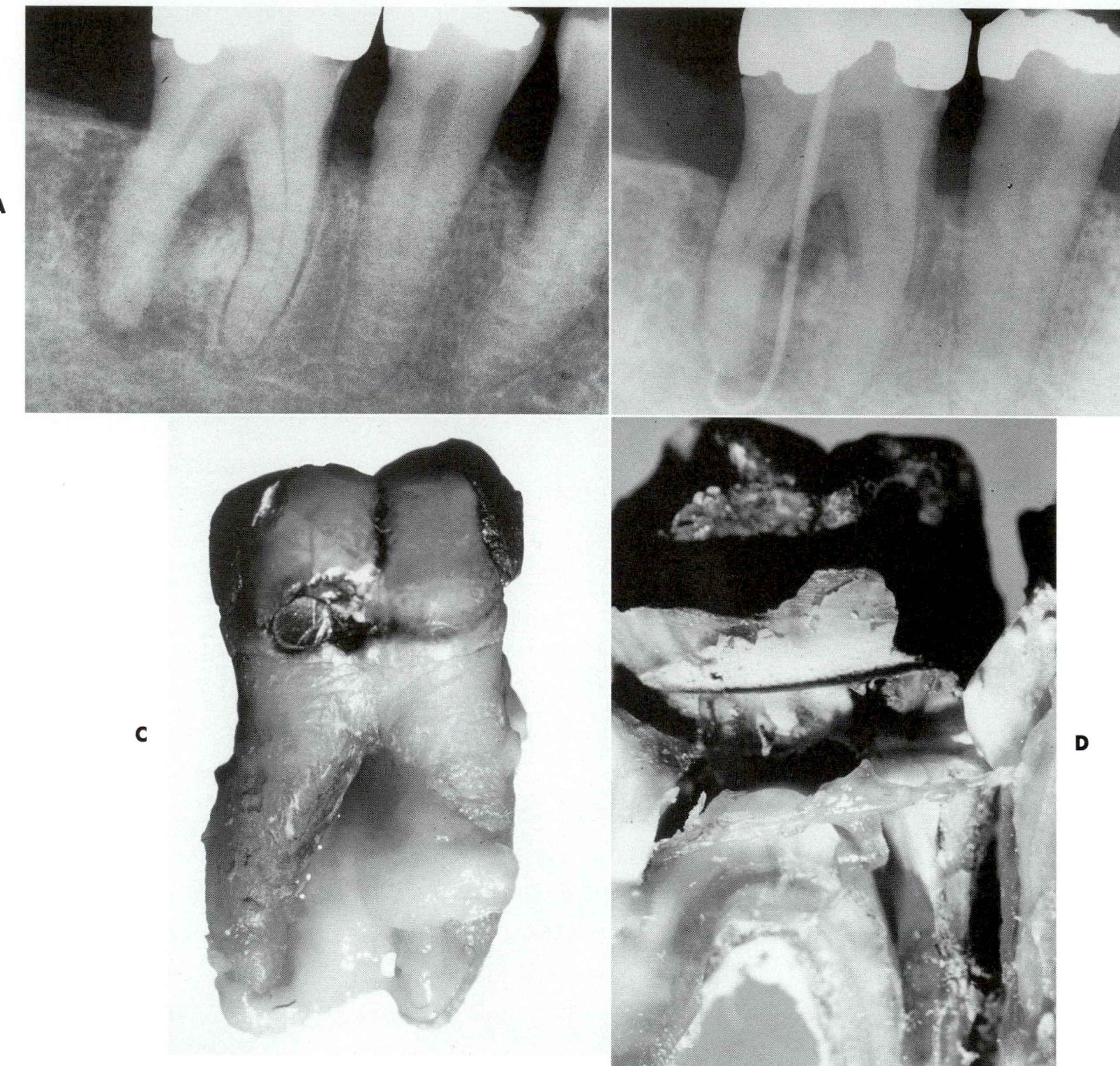

FIG. 18-15 A, A lower first molar with furcal and distal radiolucency, large MOD restoration, and recurrent M and D decay. **B,** Gutta-percha probe to the apex of the distal root. Pulp testing results were within normal limits. **C,** Diagnosis of periodontal periodontitis lesion. Note calculus on the root surface. **D,** Tooth fractured to reveal vital pulp tissue, confirming diagnosis of periodontitis.

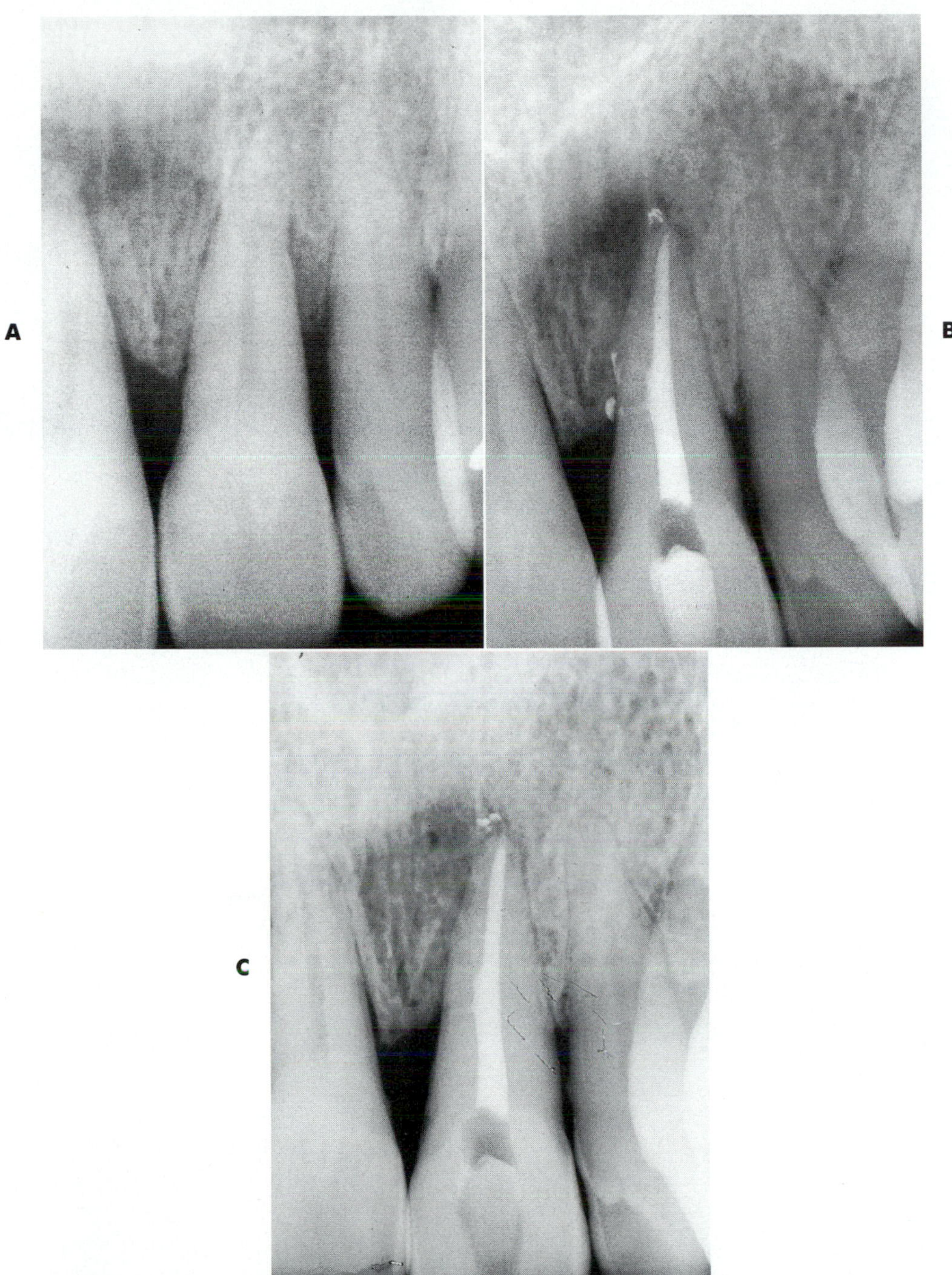

FIG. 18-16 A, Maxillary central incisor with severe periodontal disease. The canal is necrotic despite its being a virgin tooth. **B,** After endodontic therapy, two lateral canals were to the oral environment. This was interpreted as primary periodontal disease uncovering lateral canals to the oral cavity, allowing secondary endodontic disease. **C,** One-year follow-up.

A

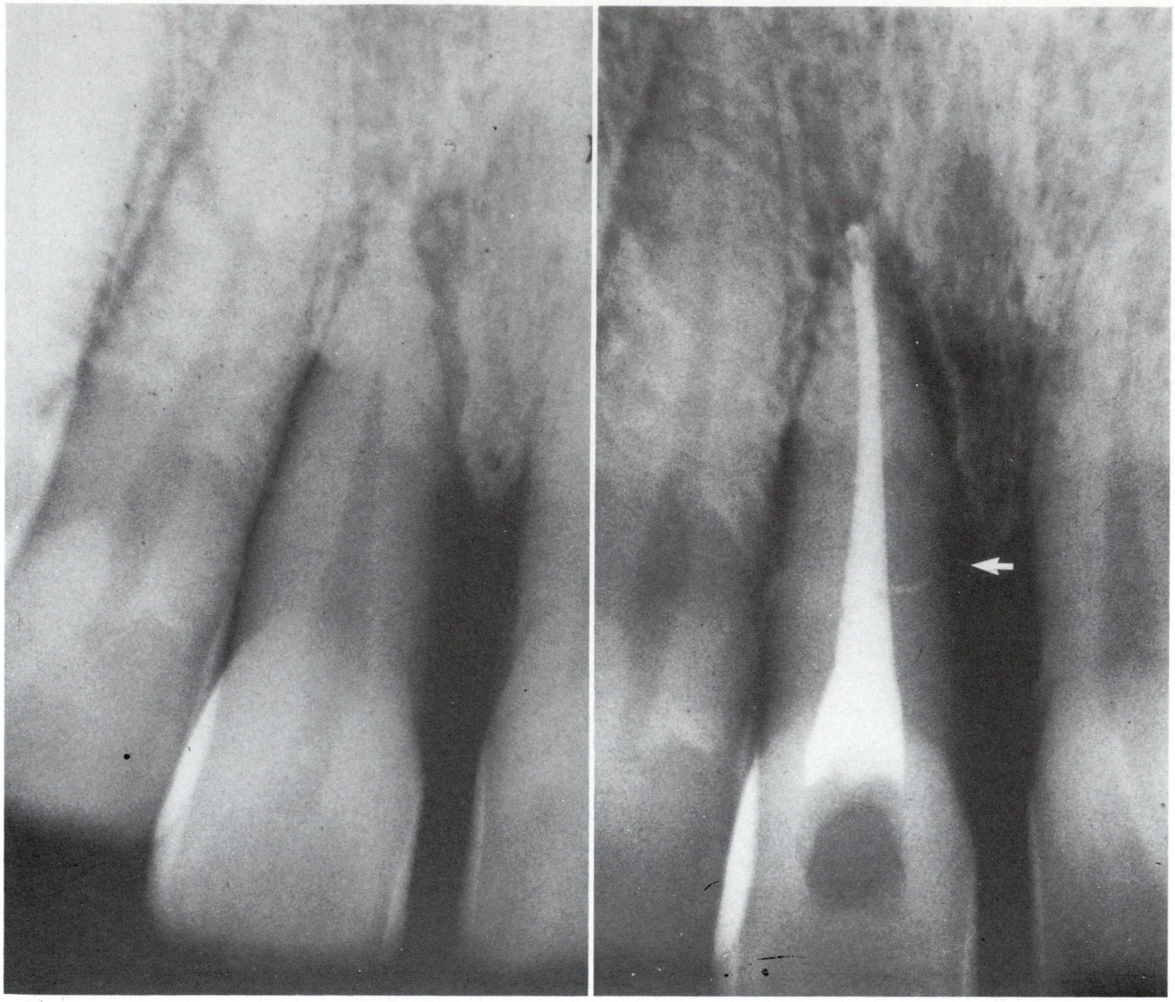

B

FIG. 18-17 A, Preoperative periodontal involvement. **B,** Postoperatively, lateral canal opening to the oral environment *(arrow)*.

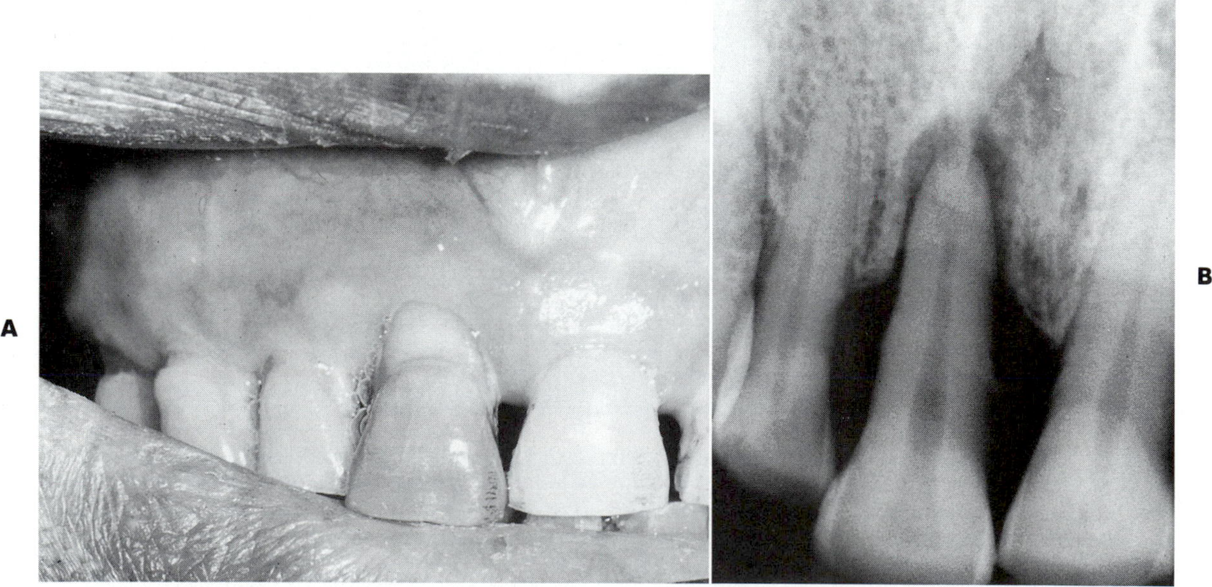

FIG. 18-18 A, Discolored incisor with gingival recession. **B,** Periapical radiolucency and evidence of periodontal bone disease. The tooth had a necrotic root canal. This is thought to show the formation of "true" combined lesions wherein separate endodontic and periodontic lesions may join.

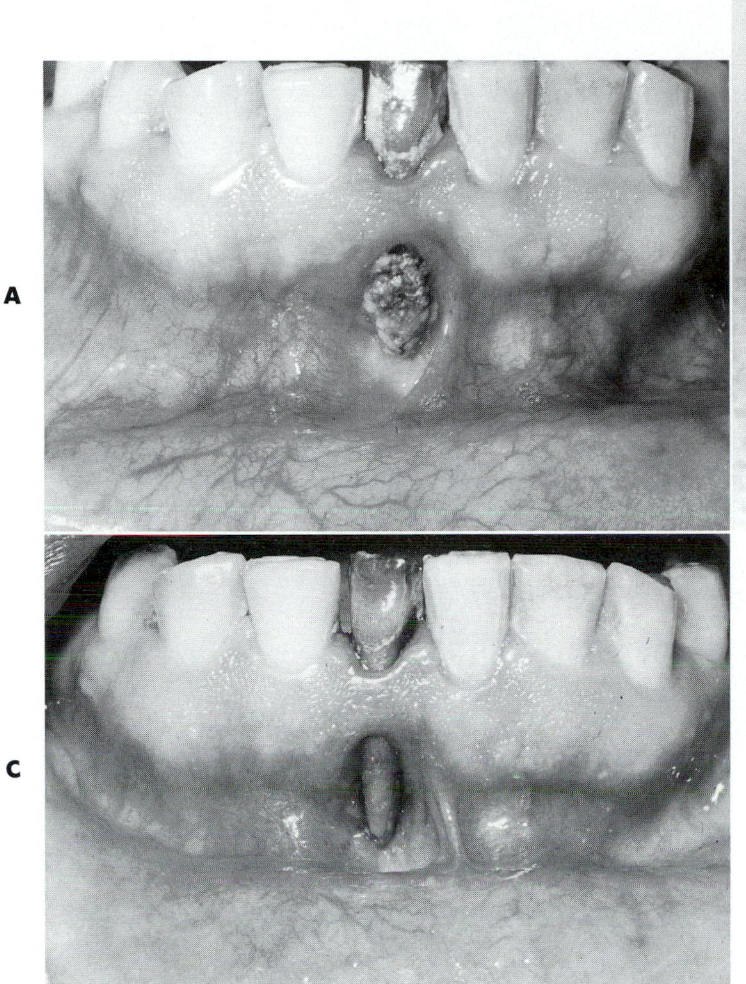

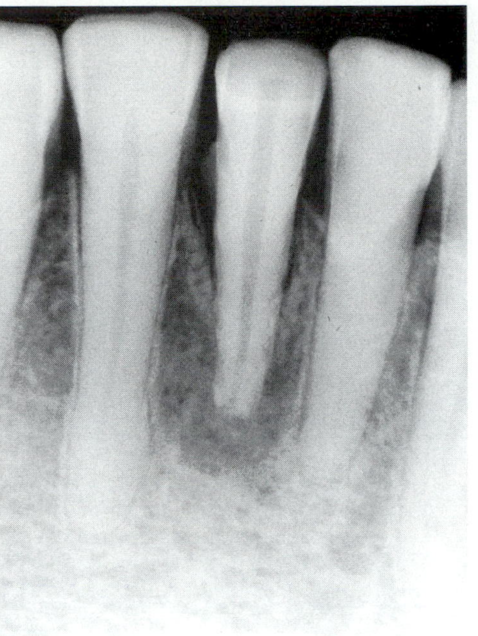

FIG. 18-19 A, Clinical photograph of lower central incisor with discolored crown and calculus on the root surface. **B,** Radiograph of necrotic central incisor. **C,** Scaled root reveals the root out of the alveolar housing with the apex exposed. Dramatic representation of combined endodontic and periodontal disease.

ease is sufficient to open and expose the pulp to the oral environment via lateral canals or dentinal tubules (Figs. 18-16, 18-17).

The prognosis depends on continuing periodontal treatment subsequent to endodontic therapy. It is important to evaluate the restorability of the tooth before beginning endodontic and periodontic treatment.

True Combined Endodontic and Periodontic Lesions

Teeth fit in this classification when independent endodontic and periodontal disease merge to form a combined lesion (Figs. 18-18, 18-19). Pulp tests indicate necrosis and periodontal probing reveals deep pockets. The character of the combined lesion may mimic a lesion of endodontic origin, or radiographically these lesions may simulate a vertical fracture with a teardrop bone defect.

A new term has been given to those teeth which have both disease processes occurring but do not communicate. This *concomitant pulpal-periodontal lesion* requires both periodontal and endodontic treatment. They are separate entities.

As with the other combined lesions the endodontic aspect heals with adequate root canal therapy, and the prognosis ultimately depends on the success of periodontal treatment. The outlook is poorer for combined lesions of long standing. While interpretation of which disease process came first may vary, thorough diagnosis and evaluation leads the practitioner to the most appropriate treatment sequence, and hopefully increases the longevity of the affected tooth.

ALTERNATIVE TREATMENT MODALITIES

When traditional endodontic and periodontic treatments prove insufficient to stabilize an affected tooth, the clinician must consider other treatment alternatives. After combined therapy, a patient has to maintain an impeccable level of oral hygiene. This may be virtually impossible where bifurcation or trifurcation bone loss exists. A localized periodontal defect, inability to perform adequate root canal therapy, or an iatrogenic problem are other reasons to explore other treatment options.

Root amputation procedures may ameliorate a furcation defect in maxillary molars, and a hemisection in mandibular mo-

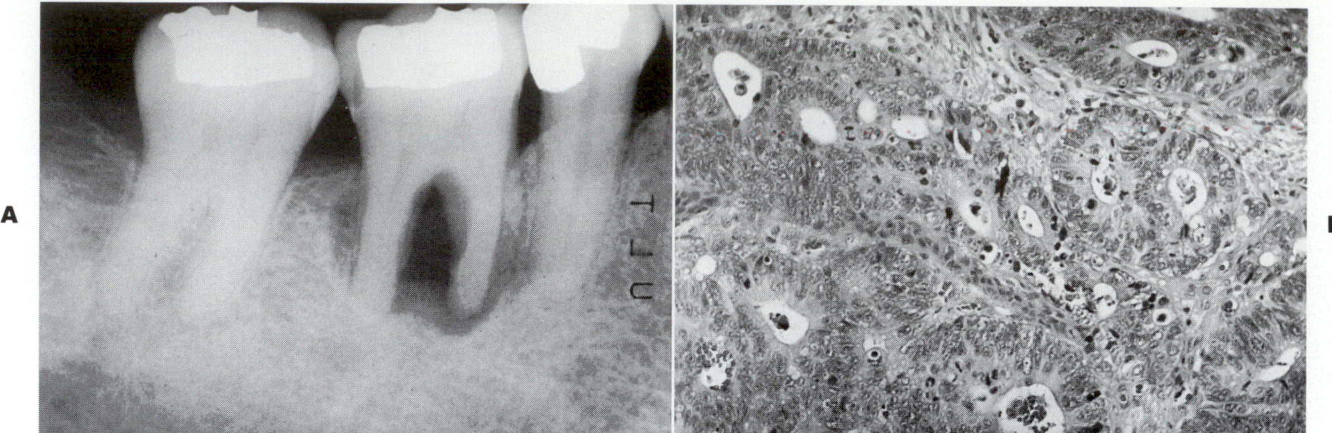

FIG. 18-20 A, A lower first molar with a furcal radiolucency. The pulp responded within normal limits and the periodontium could not be probed. **B,** Histologic section of biopsy reveals adenocystic carcinoma.

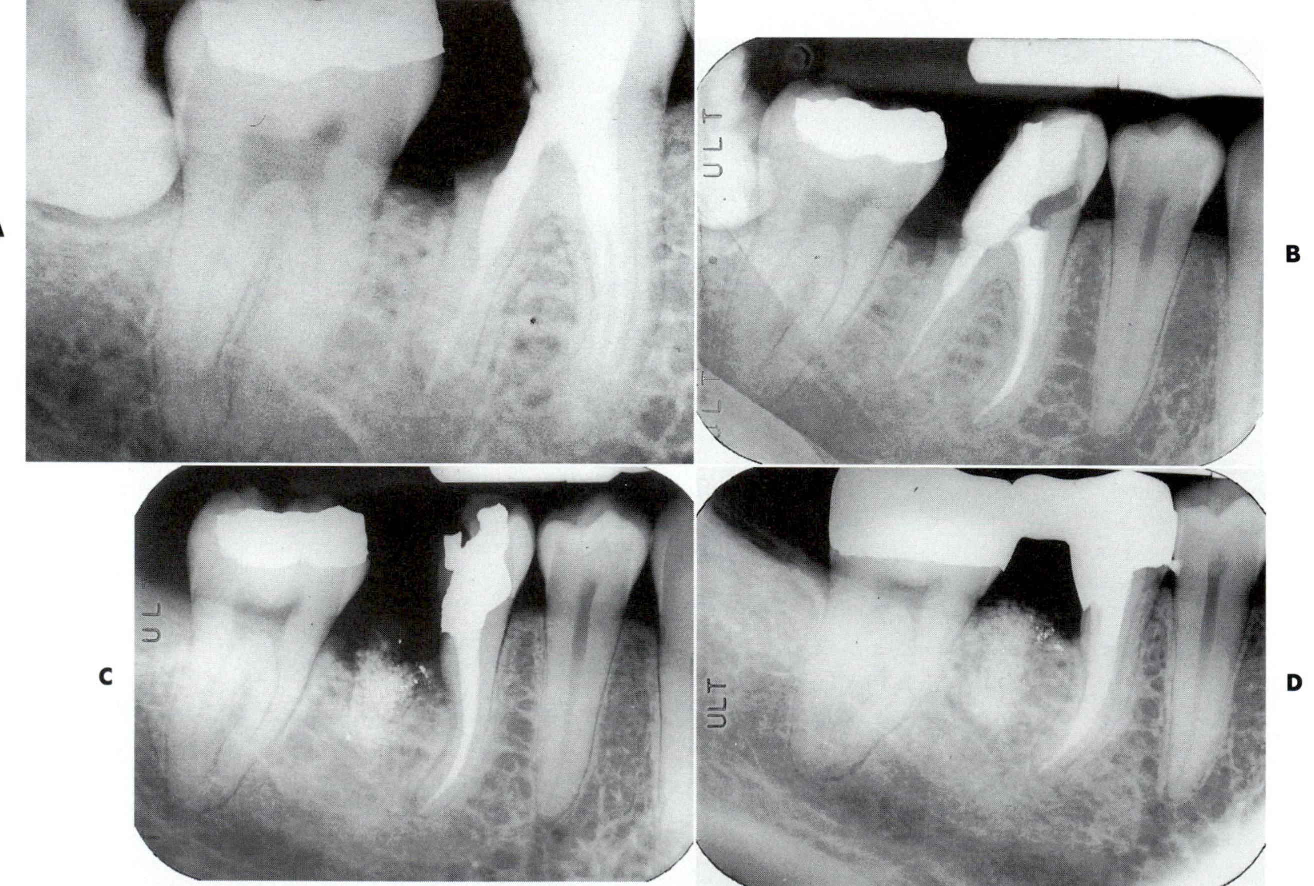

FIG. 18-21 A, Radiograph of lower molar with inadequate endodontic treatment and caries extending down distal root. **B,** Roots retreated endodontically. **C,** Distal root was resected and extracted. Note hydroxyapatite placed where buccal bone was lost during extraction. **D,** At 1-year recall, with restoration in place.

lars. Before carrying out such procedures the occlusal forces, the restorability, and the value of the remaining roots must be examined.[7] A carefully constructed treatment plan is crucial for the success of these procedures.[16] Proper reshaping and restoration of the clinical crown is essential. The root surface is recontoured to remove the root stump, thus avoiding formation of a potential food trap.[23]

According to a long-term retrospective study almost 40% of 100 teeth subjected to resection procedures failed after 10 years.[26] Most of the failures were due to root fractures, followed by progressive periodontal disease, recurrent endodontic pathosis, and cement washout of abutment teeth. Root extrusion procedures can also help save teeth if the periodontal defect is no greater than 4 mm from the alveolar crest.[43] Vertical extrusion replaces periodontal surgery when there is risk of creating an esthetic deformity on adjacent teeth in the anterior region.

There are cases that either do not fit a characteristic endodontic or periodontic lesion or do not respond to treatment as expected. A biopsy and histologic analysis may be necessary (Figs. 18-20, 18-21). A variety of systemic diseases can mimic endodontic-periodontal disease on a radiograph. The conscientious clinician must always be alert for lesions of nonendodontic or nonperiodontic origin, such as scleroderma, metastatic carcinoma, and osteosarcoma.

REFERENCES

1. Barkhordar RN, and Stewart GG: The potential of periodontal pocket formation associated with untreated accessory root canals, Oral Surg 70:769, 1990.
2. Belk CE, and Gutmann JL: Perspectives, controversies and directives on pulpal-periodontal relationships, J Can Dent Assoc 56:1013, 1990.
3. Bergenholtz G, and Lindhe J: Effect of experimentally induced marginal periodontitis and periodontal scaling on the dental pulp, J Clin Periodontol 5:59, 1978.
4. Bergenholtz G, and Nyman S: Endodontic complications following periodontal and prosthetic treatment of patients with advanced periodontal disease, J Periodontol 55:63, 1984.
5. Blomlof L, et al: Endodontic infection and calcium hydroxide treatment. Effects on periodontal healing in mature and immature replanted monkey teeth, J Clin Periodontol 19:652, 1992.
6. Blomlof L, Linskog S, and Hammarstrom L: Influence of pulpal treatments on cell and tissue reactions in the marginal periodontium, J Periodontol 59:577, 1988.
7. Buhler H: Evaluation of root resected teeth, results after 10 years, J Periodontol 59:805, 1988.
8. Burch JG, and Hulen S: A study of the presence of accessory foramina and the topography of molar furcations, Oral Surg 38:451, 1974.
9. Christie WH, and Holthuis AF: The endo-perio problem in dental practice: diagnosis and prognosis, J Can Dent Assoc 56:1005, 1990.
10. Cotton W, and Seigel R: Human pulpal response to citric acid cavity cleanser, J Am Dent Assoc 97:639, 1978.
11. Cuenin MF, et al: An in vivo study of dentin sensitivity: the relation of dentin sensitivity and the patency of dentin tubules, J Periodontol 62:668, 1991.
12. Czarnecki RT, and Schilder H: A histological evaluation of the human pulp in teeth with varying degrees of periodontal disease, J Endodontics 5:242, 1979.
13. Dongari A, and Lambrianidas T: Periodontally derived pulpal lesions, J Endod Dent Traumatol 4:49, 1988.
14. Gold SI, and Moskow BS: Periodontal repair of periapical lesions: the borderland between pulpal and periodontal disease, J Clin Periodontol 14:251, 1987.
15. Goldman HM, and Schilder H: Regeneration of attachment apparatus lost due to disease of endodontic origin, J Periodontol 59:609, 1988.
16. Green EN: Hemisection and root amputation, J Am Dent Assoc 112:511, 1986.
17. Harrington GW: The perio-endo question. Differential diagnosis, Dent Clin North Am 23:673, 1979.
18. Johnson WT, Johnson GK, and Goodrich JL: Pulpal response to the topical application of citric acid following root planing in cats, J Endodontics 11:389, 1985.
19. Kelly WH, and Ellinger RF: Pulpal-periradicular pathosis causing sinus tract formation through the periodontal ligament of adjacent teeth, J Endodontics 14:251, 1988.
20. Kerekes K, and Olsen I: Similarities in the microfloras of root canals and deep periodontal pockets, J Endod Dent Traumatol 6:1, 1990.
21. Kerns DG, et al: Dentinal tubules occlusion and root hypersensitivity, J Periodontol 62:421, 1991.
22. Kipioti A, et al: Microbiological findings of infected root canals and adjacent periodontal pockets in teeth with advanced periodontitis, Oral Surg 58:213, 1984.
23. Kirchoff DA, and Gerstein H: Presurgical occlusal contouring for root amputation procedures, Oral Surg 27:379, 1969.
24. Kitchings SK, et al: The pulpal response to topically applied citric acid, Oral Surg 58:199, 1984.
25. Langeland K, Rodriques H, and Dowden W: Periodontal disease bacteria and pulpal histopathology, Oral Surg 37:257, 1974.
26. Langer B, Stein SD, and Wagenberg B: An evaluation of root resections: a ten year study, J Periodontol 52:719, 1981.
27. Linskog S, Blomlof L, and Hammarstrom L: Evidence for a role of odontogenic epithelium in maintaining the periodontal space, J Clin Periodontal 15:371, 1988.
28. Lowman JV, Burke RS, and Pellen GB: Patent accessory canals incidence in molar furcation region, Oral Surg 36:580, 1973.
29. Mazur B, and Massler M: The influence of periodontal disease on the dental pulp, Oral Surg 17:598, 1964.
30. Michelich VJ, Schuster GS, and Pashley DH: Bacterial penetration of human dentin in vitro, J Dent Res 59:1393, 1980.
31. Nilveus R, and Selvig KA: Pulpal reactions to the application of citric acid to root planed dentin in beagles, J Periodont Res 18:420, 1983.
32. Pashley DH, Michelich VJ, and Kehl T: Dentine permeability: effects of smear layer removal, J Prost Dent 46:531, 1981.
33. Pineda F, and Kuttler U: Mesiodistal and buccolingual roentgenographic investigation of 7,275 root canals, Oral Surg 33:101, 1972.
34. Prichard JF: Advanced periodontal disease, ed 2, Philadelphia, 1972, WB Saunders Co.
35. Prichard JF: Diagnosis and management of vertical bony defects, J Periodontol 54:29, 1983.
36. Reeh ES, and Eldeeb M: Rapid furcation involvement associated with a devitalizing mandibular first molar, Oral Surg 69:95, 1990.
37. Register AA, and Burdick FA: Accelerated reattachment with cementogenesis to dentin, demineralized in situ I. Optimum range, J Periodontol 46:646, 1975.
38. Rubach WC, and Mitchell DF: Periodontal disease, accessory canals and pulpal pathosis, J Periodontol 36:34, 1965.
39. Sanders JJ: Clinical evaluation of freeze dried bone allografts in periodontal osseous defects-Part III, J Periodontol 54:1, 1983.
40. Seltzer S: Endodontology, ed 2, New York, 1988, McGraw-Hill Book Co.
41. Seltzer S, Bender IB, and Ziontz M: The interrelationship of pulp and periodontal disease, Oral Surg 16:1474, 1963.
42. Sepe WW, et al: Clinical evaluation of freeze-dried bone allografts in periodontal osseous defects-Part II, J Periodontol 49:9, 1978.
43. Simon JH: Root extrusion: rationale and techniques, Dent Clin North Am 28:909, 1984.
44. Simon JH, Glick DH, and Frank AL: The relationship of endodontic periodontic lesions, J Periodontol 43:202, 1972.
45. Simon JH, Glick DH, and Frank AL: Predictable endodontic and periodontic failures as a result of radicular anomalies, Oral Surg 31:823, 1971.

46. Simring M, and Goldberg M: The pulpal periodontal approach: retrograde periodontitis, J Periodontol 35:22, 1964.
47. Torabinejad M, and Kiger RD: A histologic evaluation of dental pulp tissue of a patient with periodontal disease, Oral Surg 59:198, 1985.
48. Trope M, Rosenberg E, and Tronstad L: Darkfield microscopic spirochete count in the differentiation of endodontic and periodontal abscesses, J Endodontics 18:82, 1992.
49. Vertucci FJ, and Williams RG: Furcation canals in the human mandibular first molar, Oral Surg 38:308, 1974.
50. Wallace JA, and Bissada NF: Pulpal and root sensitivity related to periodontal therapy, Oral Surg 69:743, 1990.
51. Weine FS: Endodontic therapy, ed 4, St. Louis, 1986, Times Mirror/Mosby College Publishing.
52. Weissman DP, Weine FS, and McGarry J: The interrelationship between periodontics and endodontics: report of a case, Compend Contin Educ Dent 10:130, 1989.
53. Whyman RA: Endodontic-periodontic lesions. Part 1: Prevalence aetiology and diagnosis, NZ Dent J 84:74, 1988.
54. Whyman RA: Endodontic-periodontic lesions, Part II: management, NZ Dent J 84:109, 1988.
55. Wong R, Hirsch RS, and Clarke NG: Endodontic effects of root planing in humans, Endod Dent Traumatol 5:193, 1989.
56. Yeung S, and Clarke N: Pulpal effect of citric acid applied topically to root surfaces, Oral Surg 56:317, 1983.

Self-assessment questions

1. The highest percentage of lateral canals occurs
   a. in the coronal third of the root.
   b. in the middle third of the root
   c. in the apical third of the root.
   d. anywhere along the root, depending on the tooth in question.
2. Treatment of pulpal diseases that cause periodontal diseases usually requires
   a. endodontic treatment alone.
   b. both endodontic and periodontal treatment.
   c. periodontal surgery and curettage.
   d. combined periradicular and periodontal surgery.
3. Studies on the effects of periodontal disease on the pulp have shown
   a. pathologic pulp changes.
   b. degenerative pulp changes.
   c. no pulp changes.
   d. all of the above.
4. Which of the following statements concerning a sinus tract of pulpal origin is *false?*
   a. The tract is usually thinner than an infrabony periodontal pocket.
   b. Vitality tests may evoke an unaltered, normal response.
   c. Pain is not often present.
   d. It can be traced to the source of irritation.
5. Which of the following statements concerning a primary endodontic lesion with secondary periodontal disease is *false*?
   a. This condition occurs with long-standing pulpal disease and chronic periapical drainage.
   b. Radiographs may show generalized periodontal disease with angular defects at the initial site of endodontic involvement.
   c. Resolution of the lesion requires both endodontic and periodontal therapy.
   d. If appropriate endodontic therapy is performed all bone loss will heal.
6. In a primary periodontic lesion with secondary endodontic involvement
   a. there is a history of extensive periodontal disease.
   b. the pulp always responds to vitality tests.
   c. pain is usually absent.
   d. periodontal therapy should precede endodontic therapy.
7. The concomitant pulpal-periodontal lesion
   a. is another name for the combined endodontic-periodontic lesion.
   b. requires either periodontal or endodontic treatment.
   c. radiographically may simulate a vertical fracture.
   d. depends for its prognosis on the success of periodontal treatment.
8. The most common cause of root resection failures is
   a. progressive periodontal disease.
   b. recurrent endodontic pathosis.
   c. root fracture.
   d. poor oral hygiene.

Chapter 19

Surgical Endodontics

Gary B. Carr

DEFINITION AND SCOPE

Surgical endodontic therapy is the treatment of choice when teeth have responded poorly to conventional treatment or when they cannot be treated appropriately by nonsurgical means. The skillful endodontic surgeon borrows techniques from the periodontist, the oral surgeon, and the restorative dentist and integrates those skills into the art of endodontic surgery. The goal of all endodontic surgery is to remove disease and to prevent it from recurring. Accordingly, our ultimate end is to facilitate healing so that affected teeth may be restored to function.

The endodontic surgeon must have comprehensive knowledge of anatomy and a clear understanding of the biologic principles underlying soft and hard tissue management, including an understanding of surgical wound healing. These requirements have made endodontic surgery a highly disciplined skill.

DIAGNOSIS

Skillful diagnosis in endodontic surgery requires accurate determination of the reasons for endodontic failure and the surgeon's certitude that this failure can be corrected by the appropriate surgical procedure. It is axiomatic that endodontic surgery is not a substitute for careless nonsurgical treatment.[51,79,143]

Many root canal systems do not easily lend themselves to surgical therapy. In fact, many systems become more difficult to treat when a surgical approach is employed (Fig. 19-1). (The important role of retreatment in endodontic failure is covered in Chapter 24.) Once the practitioner is certain that no better result can be achieved by using nonsurgical treatment, *then and only then* should the surgical option be considered.[48,79,145] If the root canal system is properly cleaned, shaped, and obturated, the endodontic failure rate is extremely low, and the need for surgical procedures is minimal.[36,51,80] In most cases, the surgical approach addresses the inability of the clinician to adequately seal the root canal system three dimensionally. Since research has consistently shown us that incompletely obturated canal systems have a markedly reduced surgical success rate,[59,100] the thoughtful clinician attempts to three-dimensionally clean, shape, and pack the entire root canal system. *Surgery should be the choice only when these attempts have failed* (Fig. 19-2).[51,80,143]

CONTRAINDICATIONS TO SURGICAL ENDODONTICS

The restorability and the periodontal prognosis of a tooth are important in choosing treatment, but the medical condition of the patient is paramount. Because a surgical entry obviously requires an incision into soft tissue and the removal of bone, the patient must be physically, mentally, and systemically healthy enough to permit uneventful healing. Thus, a thorough medical history (described in Chapter 1) should be recorded, reviewed, and discussed with the patient to determine if any potential health risks exist.

When doubt arises from an evaluation of the patient's health history, medical consultation with the attending family physician is indicated. Because the patient's welfare becomes the clinician's responsibility once treatment begins, all questions should be answered *before* the surgery. Failure to identify existing medical contraindications constitutes failure to meet the standard of care. Attention must also be given to the patient's daily pharmacotherapeutic regimen. To avert any adverse drug reaction, all medications must be appraised and proper precau-

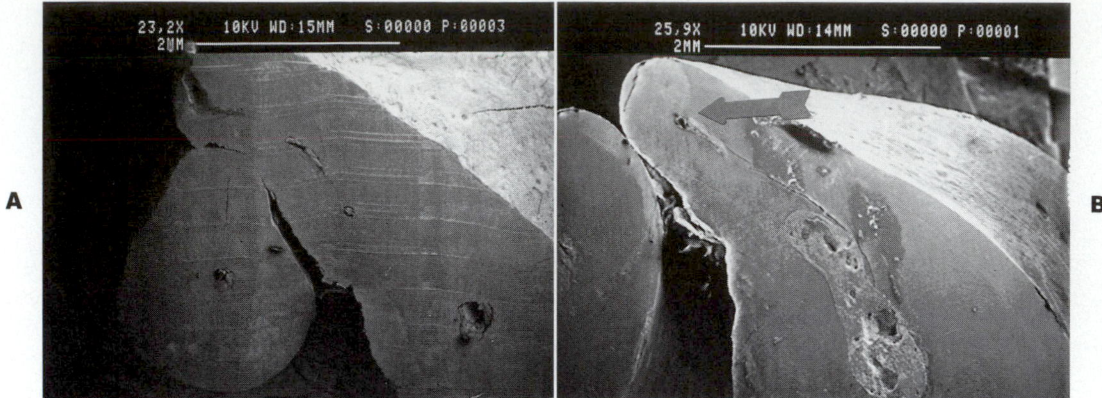

FIG. 19-1 A, Resected root of a maxillary first molar. Note the irregular ramifications between the MB-1 and the MB-2 canals and the difficult retropreparation this would require. **B,** Completed retrofilling material on mesial-buccal root of maxillary molar. Note the extreme lingual position of the missed MB-2 canal *(arrow)* and the connecting isthmus.

tions taken. (For appropriate antibiotic prophylactic therapy prior to surgery, see Chapter 4.)

Few overt medical conditions contraindicate endodontic surgery; however, since apical surgery is an invasive procedure, the practitioner should be extremely wary of treating patients with (1) clotting deficiencies or blood dyscrasias, (2) "brittle" diabetes, (3) kidney disease that requires dialysis, and (4) compromised immune systems.

Clotting Deficiencies

Good hemostasis is mandatory for apical surgery and uneventful healing; therefore, careful questioning of the patient regarding potential clotting deficiencies is indicated. The patient's experience with surgery or trauma wounds often reveals details that are unknown, even to the patient or the patient's current attending physician. Do you bruise easily, Ms. Jones? Did you experience prolonged bleeding after wisdom teeth extraction? Were there any bleeding complications during pregnancy?—These are essential questions to ask. Thus, the skilled clinician must be not only a meticulous historian but an adroit detective as well. If any doubt exists, a prothrombin time and bleeding time should be taken before the surgery.

Brittle Diabetes

Brittle diabetics are particularly poor risks for surgery as they suffer from multisystem organ disease. Since diabetes is essentially a disease of the terminal arterioles, these patients exhibit markedly reduced wound healing capability. Long-term "brittle diabetics" all manifest end-stage renal disease, so a serious infection can threaten their lives. Diabetics' leukocyte function is severely compromised because of decreased chemotaxis and phagocytosis.[34,44,125] These patients are always covered with antibiotics and monitored daily until they are out of danger. One study shows that supplemental vitamin A may enhance wound healing in brittle diabetics.[132]

Dialysis Patients

Dialysis patients are another high-risk group because they frequently suffer from a multitude of bleeding disorders, viral blood infections (e.g., hepatitis, human immunodeficiency virus [HIV] infection), altered drug metabolism, and impaired wound healing.[86] These patients are managed only after careful consultation with their nephrologist and after a thorough blood workup is analyzed (bleeding time, platelet count, hematocrit, hemoglobin). Since proteoglycan synthesis and ground substance metabolism of dialysis patients are diminished, they suffer from delayed or incomplete soft and hard tissue wound repair. All dialysis patients require prophylactic antibiotics because of the presence of arteriovenous shunts and the potential for fatal infective endarteritis.

Immunocompromised Patients

Immunocompromised patients are also at serious surgical risk. Frequently these patients take a combination of cytotoxic drugs and corticosteroids and suffer from poor wound healing and susceptibility to infection. Surgical procedures should be avoided unless the risk-benefit ratio is much in the patient's favor.

THE PRESURGICAL WORKUP

If surgery is necessary, a presurgical workup is in order. The surgeon must explain to the patient the proposed procedures and all available alternative treatments. A brief explanation, in lay terms, of what is to be done and what the patient can expect postsurgically is often neglected or delegated to auxiliary personnel. This is a mistake because the doctor misses the opportunity to assess the patient's psychological status, address concerns, and establish a bond that conveys the doctor's understanding, empathy, and skill. Nothing enhances a surgical result more than a patient's confidence in his surgeon. Whether the effect is psychological or physiologic dentists need to cultivate this bond more assiduously than other medical professionals, because theirs is one of the few surgical disciplines in which extensive invasive procedures are performed while patients are fully conscious and alert.

During the presurgical workup, the dentist must advise patients of any necessary changes in daily activities: drug regimen (i.e., no aspirin for 3 days before surgery); the need to begin chlorhexidene rinses two days before surgery; the need

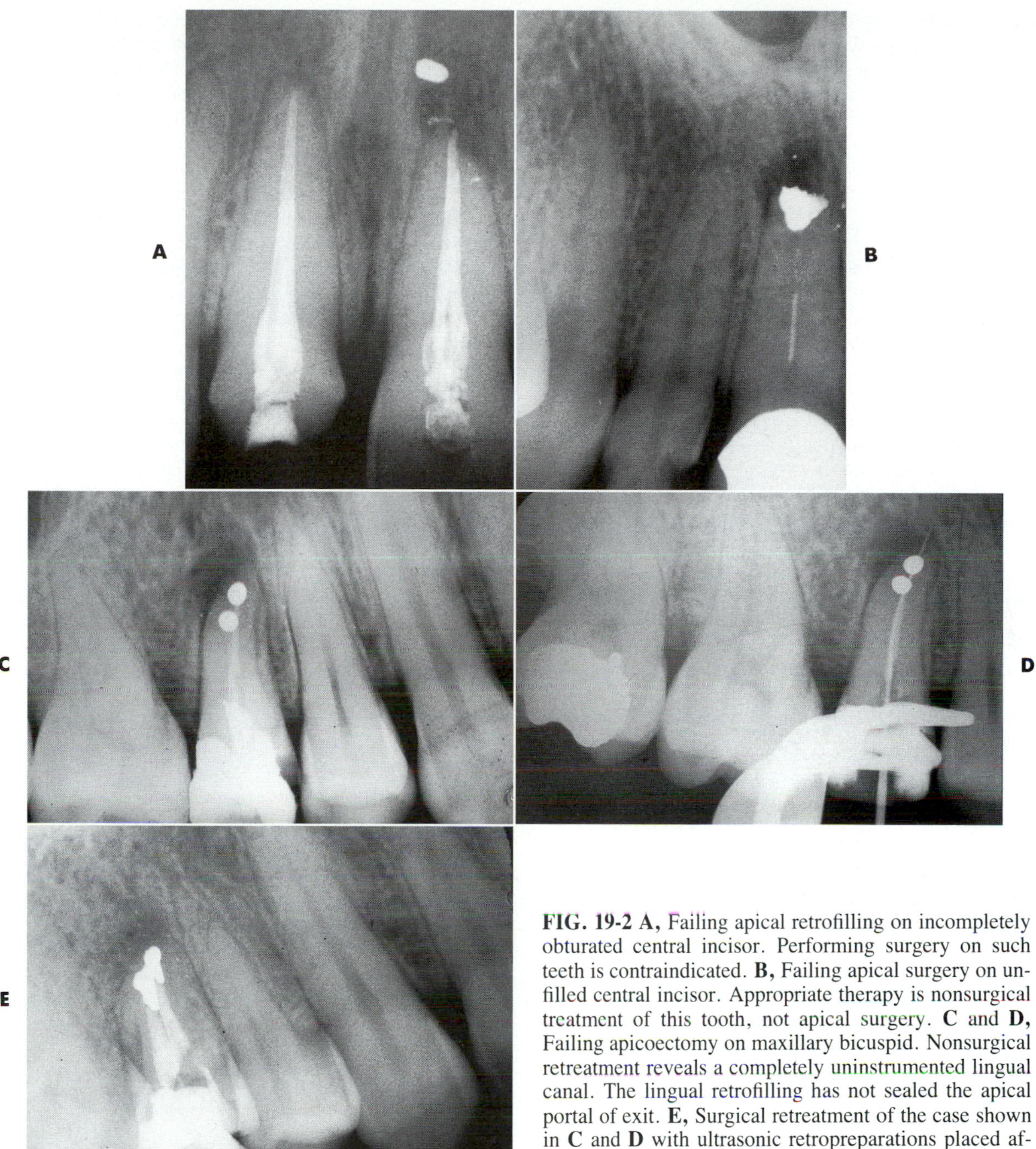

FIG. 19-2 A, Failing apical retrofilling on incompletely obturated central incisor. Performing surgery on such teeth is contraindicated. **B,** Failing apical surgery on unfilled central incisor. Appropriate therapy is nonsurgical treatment of this tooth, not apical surgery. **C** and **D,** Failing apicoectomy on maxillary bicuspid. Nonsurgical retreatment reveals a completely uninstrumented lingual canal. The lingual retrofilling has not sealed the apical portal of exit. **E,** Surgical retreatment of the case shown in **C** and **D** with ultrasonic retropreparations placed after the nonsurgical retreatment.

to arrange for transportation home following surgery; and the need to restrict activities following the procedure (i.e., no smoking or alcohol consumption for 3 days; no vigorous exercise that would dramatically increase blood pressure). These discussions have more impact at the presurgical workup than they would just before the procedure, as they involve changes in lifestyle and scheduling that the patient might not normally anticipate. It contributes to a nonstressful surgical environment if there are no surprises and if patients know exactly what to expect and what is expected of them. This professional bonding between doctor and patient minimizes, to a large extent, the anxiety and trepidation often observed in surgical endodontic patients.

The clinical presurgical workup should attempt to anticipate all possible complications. Medical history review, blood pressure check, and, if necessary, consultation with the patient's family physician should be conducted at this time and noted in the chart. It is important to observe the patient's crown contour, pocket depth, alveolar bone topography, zones of attached gingiva and alveolar mucosa, vestibular depth, muscle attachments, root eminences, furcal involvements, and the health and architecture of the interdental papilla. Additional radiographs are exposed, if needed, to better assess critical anatomic structures that may be endangered by the procedure (e.g., mental or mandibular nerve location and height of the maxillary sinus). After evaluating these factors, the dentist outlines the preliminary flap design and enters it in the patient's chart. Time spent in presurgical screening pays dividends by ensuring that the surgeon has anticipated and planned for all possible complications. The patient is dismissed with full knowledge of the procedure and of what is expected, and the doctor has entered a surgical treatment plan based on careful assessment of the patient's psychological and physiologic status.

SURGICAL PROTOCOL AND ANESTHESIA

At the surgical appointment the surgeon should again review the procedure with the patient and respond to any additional concerns. Blood pressure is taken, chlorhexidene rinse given, and a nonsteroidal antiinflammatory drug administered preoperatively. Research shows that it is easier to prevent pain than to reduce it after it occurs.[14,108] Techniques for administering anesthesia are explained in Chapter 20. Surgical anesthesia must be longer lasting than that for conventional endodontic treatment. One of our goals in surgical anesthesia is not only to provide profound anesthesia for the procedure itself but also to maintain analgesia for a prolonged period following the surgery. Additionally, the surgeon depends on the anesthesia for its hemostatic effect. Good surgical anesthesia involves a "piggyback" or dual-entry technique. The initial injection utilizes one of the longer-acting anesthetics (e.g., bupivacaine, etidocaine). These long-acting anesthetics provide 2 to 4 hours' profound surgical anesthesia and up to 4 to 10 hours' effective analgesia. After regional block anesthesia is confirmed, the surgeon administers 2% lidocaine with 1:50,000 epinephrine to achieve good hemostasis. Even in medically compromised patients, the slow administration (over 2 minutes) of 1:50,000 epinephrine poses no systemic risk. It is only rapid injection of 1:50,000 epinephrine that poses a risk. Inadvertent intravascular injection or too rapid an injection should be avoided.

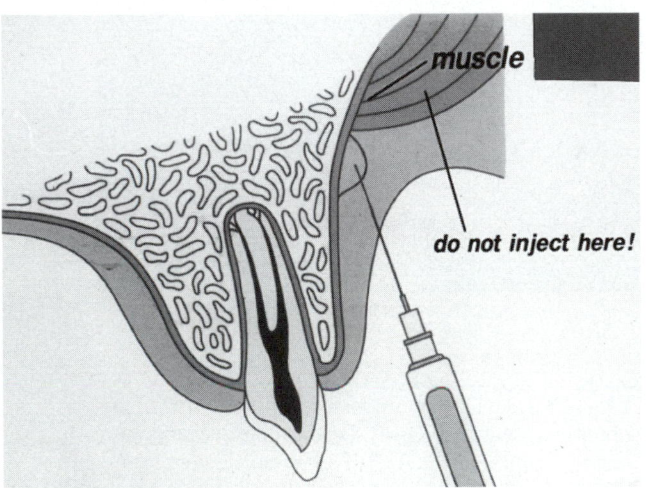

FIG. 19-3 Correct placement of anesthesia is at the root apices and not into the muscle attachments. Injection into the muscle results in increased bleeding.

The best injection technique to achieve maximum hemostasis involves depositing the solution near the apices of the root with the needle beveled toward the periosteum in the loose connective tissue of the alveolar submucosa.[7,124] Slow (2-minute), multiple injections ensure rapid diffusion without damaging the delicate collagen bundles that compose the alveolar submucosa (Figs. 19-3 and 19-4). Because the primary blood supply of the gingival tissues emanates from vertically oriented vessels in the alveolar mucosa (Fig. 19-5), enhanced hemostasis is achieved by depositing solution there, *not* by injecting it into the attached gingiva. The attached gingiva consists of dense fibrous connective tissue; its compartmentalized, collagenous nature impedes diffusion of anesthesia. Injections into attached gingiva, or worse yet into the papilla, to achieve hemostasis is contraindicated and causes unnecessary surgical trauma.[51] Additional injections apical to the root apices into the vestibular tissues are completely unnecessary. The aforementioned injections are sufficient to provide adequate hemostasis.

The hemostatic effect of the epinephrine is produced by its action on α_2-adrenergic receptors on vessels of the terminal microvasculature. Injection into the deeper vestibular tissues or near basal bone, with its muscle attachments, places the solution near tissues that have a much higher concentration of β_2- adrenergic receptors, causing vasodilatation.[41,101] For example, injection of 1:50,000 epinephrine near the buccinator muscle attachment or mentalis muscle attachment results in increased bleeding into the surgical site, compromising one of the surgeon's most vital resources: visibility.

After profound anesthesia is confirmed, the patient is cov-

A
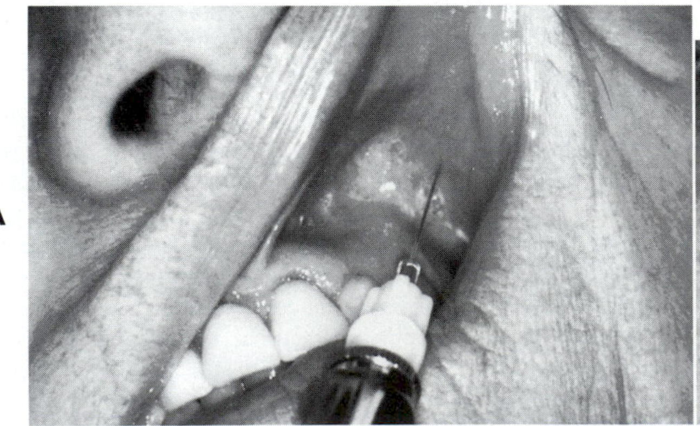

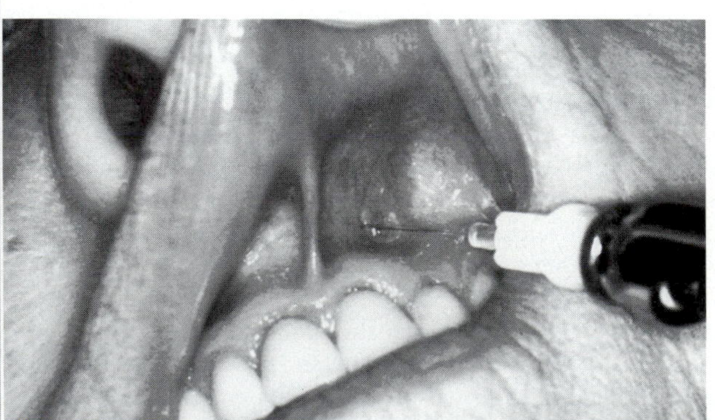
B

FIG. 19-4 A, Incorrect placement of anesthesia into the deep vestibular tissues. **B,** Correct placement of anesthesia in proximity to the root apices.

ered with a gown, the eyes protected by glasses or an eye drape (Fig. 19-6), and the perioral skin is cleansed with Betadine or iodine wash to remove skin bacteria, cosmetics, and other facial contaminants that can only complicate surgical wound healing. Facial hair (i.e., beard, mustache) is trimmed at this time if it appears that it could contaminate the surgical field. After the patient is draped, the surgery can begin.

SOFT TISSUE MANAGEMENT IN ENDODONTIC SURGERY

The first surgical trauma inflicted is the puncture wound from the anesthetic needle and the additional trauma produced by injecting the anesthetic. The next trauma is the actual incision. All flaps for endodontic apical surgery require a horizontal and a vertical component. *It is the site of the horizontal component that determines the type of flap.*[43,75,128] Previous classifications of flaps have complicated the present classifications somewhat. We recognize the two basic types as *sulcular* and *mucogingival* (Figs. 19-7, 19-8). The number of vertical releasing incisions determines whether the flap is rectangular or triangular.

Triangular/Rectangular Flap with Sulcular Incision

A triangular/rectangular flap with a sulcular incision provides the best access of all flaps. Of utmost concern when utilizing this design is the health of the gingival tissues. Using the triangular or rectangular flap with a sulcular incision on a diseased attachment apparatus is contraindicated. When sulcular incisions are made in healthy gingiva, every attempt should be made to preserve the integrity of the sulcular epithelium of the gingival crevice and to minimize trauma to the root-attached gingival fibers. Preservation of these soft tissues, especially in the interdental col area, is crucial for obtaining healing by primary intention. If the tissues that comprise the attachment apparatus are handled with skill during incision and elevation, healing by primary intention will occur, provided no other surgical principle is violated.[51]

Vertical releasing incisions are generally made one or two

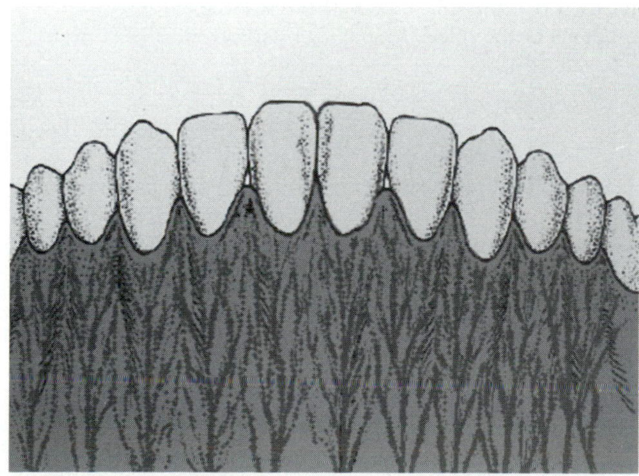

FIG. 19-5 Diagrammatic view of the vertical orientation of blood vessels in the alveolar gingival mucosa. This orientation means that flaps do not need to be broader at the base and the releasing incisions can be oriented vertically without endangering the vascular supply at the flap corners.

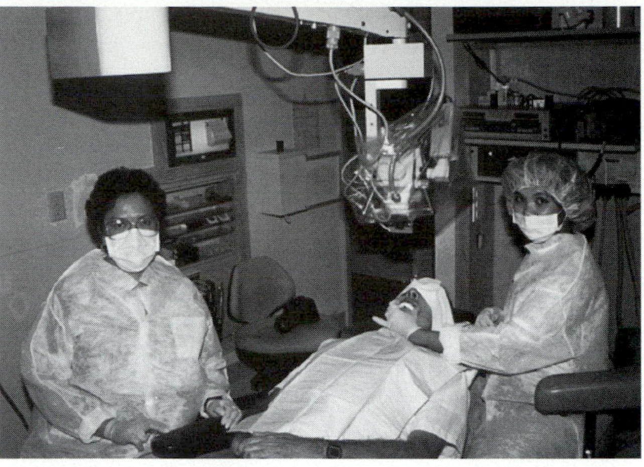

FIG. 19-6 The placement of an eye drape protects the patient's eyes from inadvertent injury and helps shield the patient from the intense dental light.

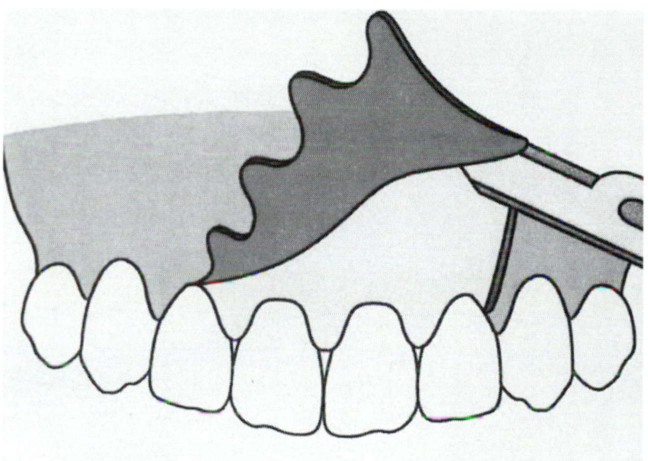

FIG. 19-7 Sulcular triangular/rectangular flap. This flap may have either one or two vertical releasing incisions.

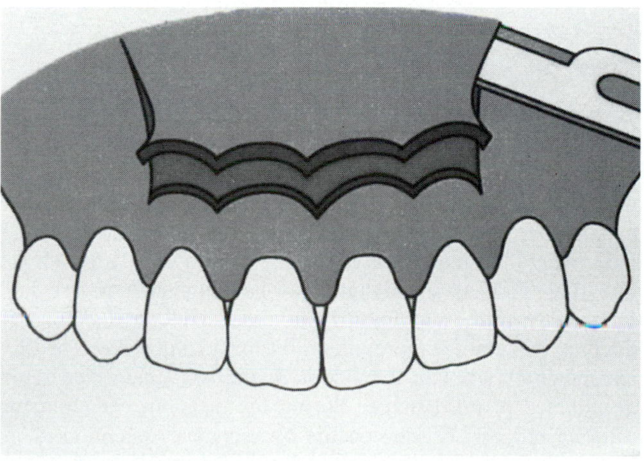

FIG. 19-8 Mucogingival flap with two vertical releasing incisions. The horizontal incision must be at least 2 mm apical to the attachment apparatus.

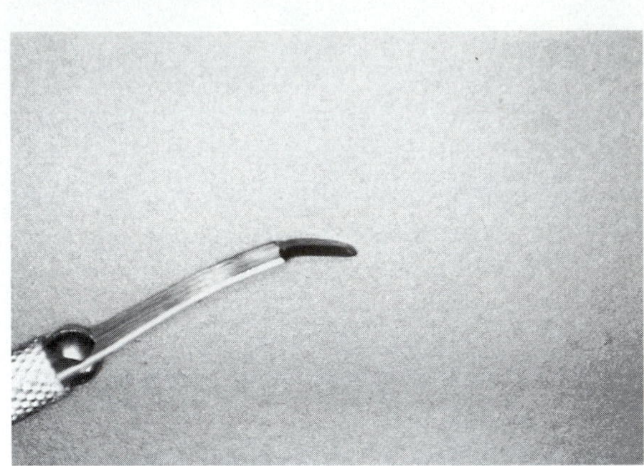

FIG. 19-9 Microsurgical scalpel curved to conform to the cervical convexity of the tooth.

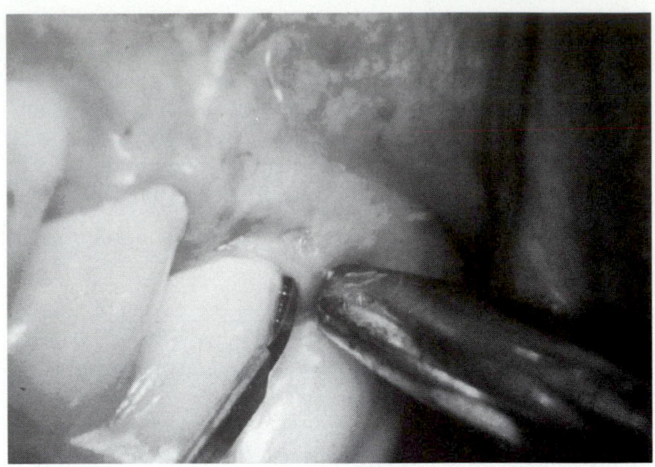

FIG. 19-10 Microsurgical incision using microsurgical scalpel blades permits very accurate and atraumatic incision into the sulcus and interdental papilla area.

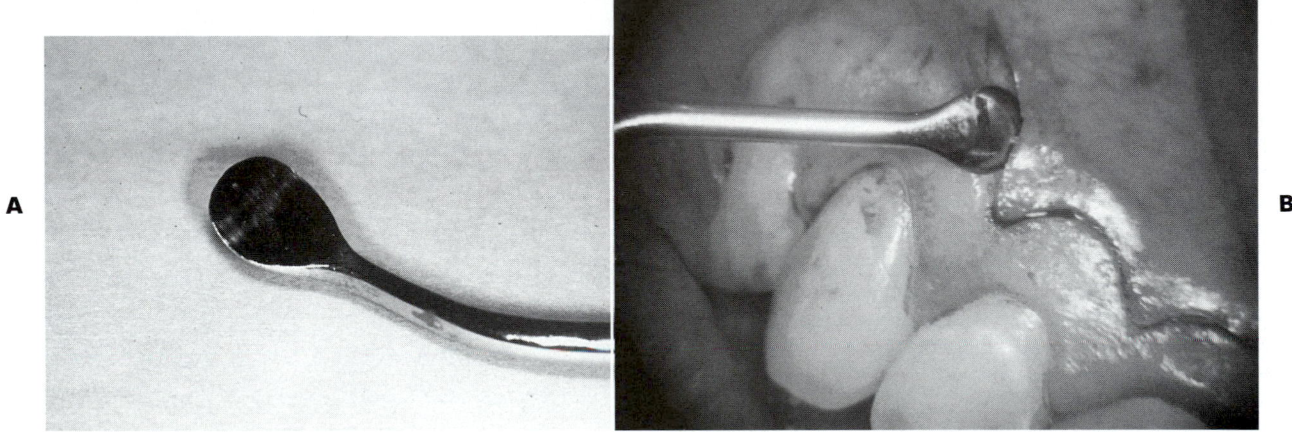

FIG. 19-11 A, Ruddle 30-degree curettes are exceptionally sharp and can be used like a scalpel to perform sharp dissection when elevating the flap. **B,** Correct placement of the Ruddle 30-degree curette. The correct elevation of the flap begins at the releasing incision and elevates the coronal margins of the flap from below.

teeth proximal to the involved tooth. The incision should be placed perpendicular to the horizontal sulcular incision, and the two should converge at the mesial or distal line angle of the tooth. Scrupulous care must be taken to place the vertical incision *between* the root eminences and not over the root surface, where the mucosa is thin and, therefore, difficult to suture. This flap has the advantage of having excellent vascularity because all the supraperiosteal vessels are contained within the flap. Accurate reapproximation is easy to achieve. The disadvantage of this flap is evident: If the attachment apparatus is inflamed or mismanaged during the incision, elevation, or suturing process, healing occurs by secondary intention. Secondary intention healing results in irreversible loss of crestal bone, increased pocket depth, and a prolonged healing period. Handled properly, this flap design can preserve the existing epithelial attachment with no loss of marginal gingiva.[58] Microsurgical scalpel blades (Figs. 19-9, 19-10) curved to conform to the cervical contour of the tooth are extremely helpful in preserving the sulcular epithelial lining and minimizing damage to the root-attached gingival fibers while making the interproximal incision in the col area easier to accomplish.

The elevation of this flap follows the principle of *undermining elevation*.[50] Such elevation respects and protects the delicate tissues of the attachment apparatus and preserves their structural integrity so that when they are reapproximated, reattachment begins almost immediately. This elevation technique always begins in the vertical releasing incision, utilizing a sharp Molt or Ruddle 30-degree curette (Fig. 19-11). Periosteum and alveolar mucosa are elevated apical to the attached and marginal gingiva. Then, using gentle sharp dissection, the surgeon frees up the attached gingiva and gently elevates the papilla and marginal gingiva from underneath

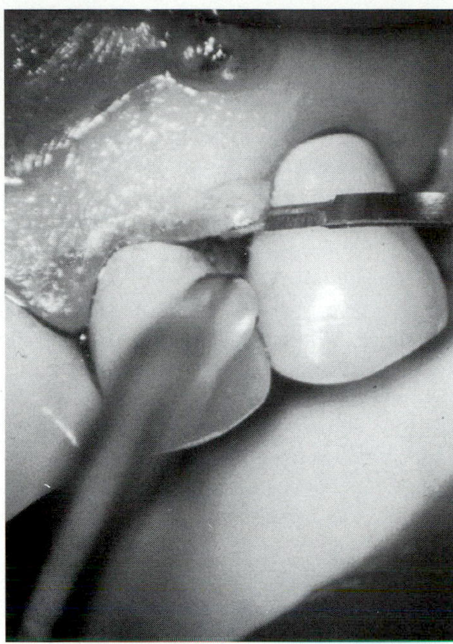

FIG. 19-12 Microsurgical dissection of the interdental col and papilla prior to elevation. Atraumatic management of this tissue results in primary intention healing. This papilla will be elevated from underneath by the Ruddle 30-degree curette. In this technique, no crushing or tearing injury is associated with the elevation of the flap.

(Fig. 19-12). This technique avoids the crushing and tearing trauma commonly associated with traditional methods of flap elevation.[119,121,146]

Triangular or Rectangular Flap with a Mucogingival Incision

This flap design, commonly referred to as a *Luebke-Ochsenbein flap,*[80] owes its popularity to the fact that the marginal gingiva and attachment apparatus remain undisturbed. If the mucogingival incision is scalloped, reapproximation is simplified (Fig. 19-13). The elevation of the flap follows the same principles as those for the sulcular flap, beginning at the vertical releasing incision and moving to the coronal margins from an apical direction. This technique protects the wound edges from traumatic crushing and ischemic injury. When reapproximated, the wound edges are ready to heal by primary intention. Since the horizontal incision of this flap severs the major blood supply to the remaining marginal gingiva, the survival of this tissue depends on the secondary blood supply from the alveolar bone, which can be highly variable and whose extent, unfortunately, is unknown to the surgeon. Another problem we encounter with this design is flap shrinkage, causing scar formation due to secondary intention healing. The mucogingival incision is contraindicated if there is limited attached gingiva, short roots, large periapical lesions, or when the cervical aspect of the root needs to be examined.

Additional Flap Designs

As the field of endodontic surgery becomes more refined, so too does our knowledge of other traditional techniques. A wide variety of other flaps—trapezoidal, gingival, semilunar—are no longer used in endodontic surgery, not only because they offer no additional advantages to those previously discussed, but also because serious disadvantages preclude their use.[51]

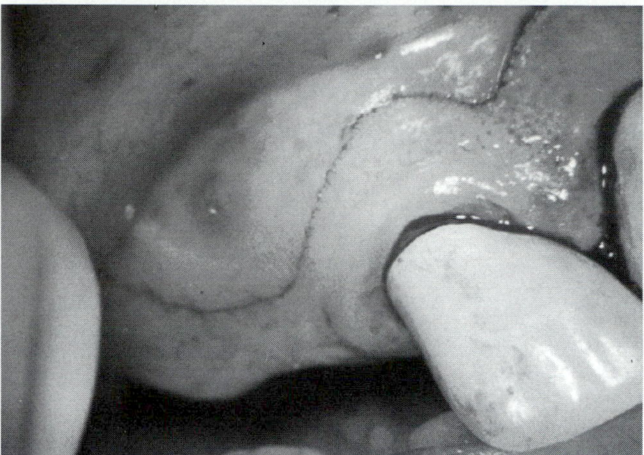

FIG. 19-13 A scalloped incision permits easy reapproximation of the flapped tissues.

Atraumatic Flap Management

Rapid and uneventful healing depends on the surgeon's deft, atraumatic handling of the flap throughout surgery and on accurate reapproximation of the wound edges at the conclusion of the procedure. Most flap injuries result from inadvertent crushing, tearing, or ischemic damage that occurs during incision, elevation, retraction, or suturing. The surgeon may avoid these multiple injuries if a flap design is developed that is appropriate for the bony manipulation that is required. Microsurgical incisions and undermining elevations reduce the crushing and tearing injury commonly associated with flap elevation. In cases where the lesion has perforated the buccal cortex and has subsequently attached itself to the periosteum, sharp dissection is needed to separate the flap from the lesion (Fig. 19-14).

After the flap has been elevated, the surgeon should ensure that minimum tension exists at all perimeters before commencing with the osteotomy. If tension exists, one or both releasing incisions may need to be extended.

Once the flap is passively reflected, the retractors are positioned. Since typically the surgeon holds one retractor and the assistant another, both operators must have unrestricted visibility of the bony architecture and *both* must be certain that the flap is not being impinged upon. *The most common cause for postsurgical swelling and ecchymosis is inadvertent crushing of the reflected flap by the retractor(s).*[57] Since the doctor's attention is focused on the root end procedure, he is frequently unaware of flap impingement until it is too late. This unnecessary trauma can be prevented by preparing two short, shallow grooves in the alveolar bone (Fig. 19-15, *top*) and letting the retractors rest in the grooves. This technique reduces the visual requirement on the part of the assistant and makes slippage of the retractors over the flap much less likely (Fig. 19-15, *bottom*).

Surgeons who follow this protocol for atraumatic flap management are rewarded with patients who experience remark-

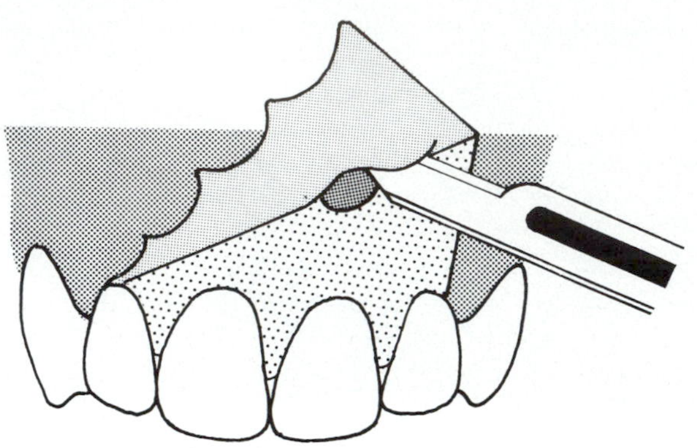

FIG. 19-14 Chronic lesions of long duration occasionally prevent elevation because the granulation tissue grows out of its bony crypt and becomes an integral part of the overlying mucoperiosteum. A scalpel is required to release the lesion from the mucoperiosteum.

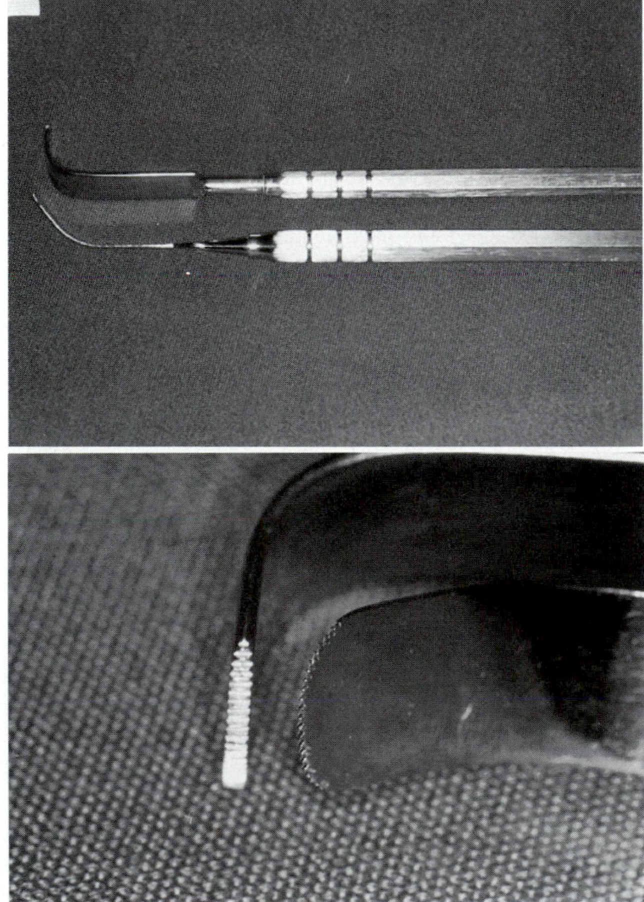

FIG. 19-15 Carr retractors No. 1 and 2 are notched at their ends to facilitate placement in grooves placed in the bone. These notches prevent slippage of the retractor and prevent impingement of soft tissue.

able healing rates, even when the surgical procedure takes 1 or 2 hours.

HARD TISSUE MANAGEMENT

The goal in developing a good flap design is to allow the surgeon and the assistant both visual and manual access. Once the flap is atraumatically reflected and both visual and manual access are obtained, the surgeon initiates bony access. Like manipulation of the mucoperiosteum, atraumatic surgical manipulation of bone depends on the surgeon's knowledge of bone and of how it responds to the various insults inherent in periradicular surgery. Injury to hard tissue in periradicular surgery involves trauma to bone, cementum, and dentin. Of these, dentin is the only tissue that does not repair itself. Bone heals more slowly than cementum and much more slowly than soft tissue, perhaps because the periostium does not survive the elevation process.[51,74] Bone, a very labile organ, sustains mechanical, thermal, and chemical insults during periradicular surgery.

Removal of bone with a rotary bur in an atraumatic manner requires dexterity, patience, and skill. The correct technique requires first positioning a bone-cutting bur (Fig. 19-16) or a No. 4 round bur at high speed (greater than 200,000 rpm), using very light, brushing strokes that minimize mechanical and thermal injury.[17,24,138] Because of the danger of air embolism using high-speed handpieces under a flap, handpieces have been devised that have no air output at the working end (Fig. 19-17). These have the added advantage of not spraying surgical debris into the bone and under the flap. Bone burs are designed to minimize clogging, and thereby to decrease frictional heat buildup. A new bur should be used for every procedure and discarded after use. A properly adjusted water spray is imperative to control generation of heat.

The location of the lesion may not be obvious if the buccal plate has not been perforated by the soft tissue lesion. Presurgical radiographs are helpful for estimating its location, and measurements taken from the radiograph can be transferred to the surgical site. The similar appearance of dentin and bone can further complicate entry; however, dentin is typically slightly yellower and smoother in texture than bone. Once the root outline is observed, cortical bone is removed in an intermittent, brushing-like circular action,[77,89,137] to allow appropriate manual access to the lesion and root end. When there are few external landmarks, an accurate osteotomy takes skill

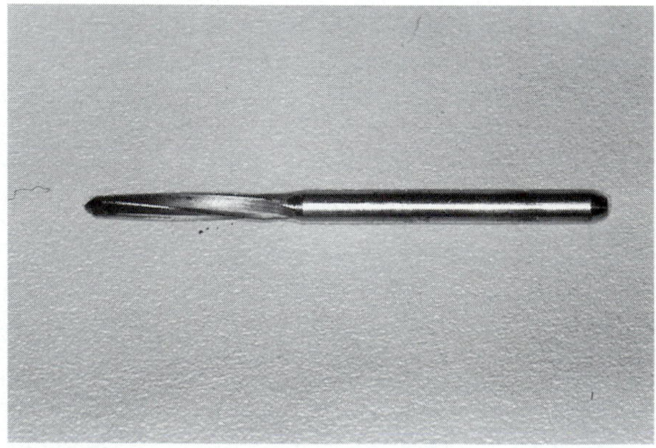

FIG. 19-16 The Lindemann bone-cutting bur is designed to reduce clogging and, therefore, minimize heat buildup.

and judgment. If after initial entry doubt remains about the location of the root, a piece of sterilized x-ray foil is placed at the entry point and a radiograph is taken to confirm its location. The bony access must be sufficient so that adequate visibility and proper illumination are achieved. Inadequate illumination and limited visibility severely handicap the surgeon, compromising the end result. Roots that are positioned more lingually require larger bone accesses.

When operating near vital anatomic structures such as the maxillary sinus or mental or mandibular nerve bundles, conservative osteotomy begins midroot and progresses apically after the surgeon has established landmarks. After achieving suitable bony access and identifying the root, the surgeon curettes the lesion and sends tissue for histologic examination.

No matter how benign the clinical appearance, ideally tissue from every lesion should be sent for pathologic examination. Although greater than 90% of all lesions are cysts, granulomas, or odontogenic abscesses, a small number are nonodontogenic neoplasms, which may require further medical or dental intervention.

The surgeon should attempt to remove the lesion in toto, using the techniques outlined in Figure 19-18. Whether it is necessary to remove every last remnant of tissue to ensure healing is unclear[48,55,133]; in all likelihood, simply disrupting the lining will lead to healing if the factors that caused the lesion have been eliminated. When complete removal of tissue would endanger neurovascular bundles (mental or mandibular nerves) or violate other anatomic structures (floor of the nose, maxillary sinus), aggressive curettement is contraindicated. Research has repeatedly shown that healing proceeds only after the contaminants within the root canal system have been eliminated or sealed from the periapical tissues.[50,96,120] The periapical lesion itself is simply a response to those irritants and is not the primary culprit. For this reason, apical curettage alone is not considered definitive treatment. Neglecting to rectify the causative factors within the root canal system invites failure.

ROOT RESECTION AND RETROPREPARATION

Once adequate osseous access has been made and the periradicular lesion removed, the surgeon is ready to address the cause of the problem: an incompletely cleaned and sealed root canal system. Close scrutiny of the root may reveal more than one possible cause of failure: multiple apical portals of exit, additional roots not seen in the radiograph, extruded filling materials or foreign bodies, apical root fractures, or accessory portals of exit on the lateral root surface. A doctor's knowledge of root canal system anatomy and root morphology is tested every time he makes an apical examination of a failed root canal. We should view these opportunities as privileged sites of learning that enhance our insight into endodontic failure.

After root inspection, the surgeon forms a three-dimensional mental image of the morphology of the root and its probable internal pulp system anatomy and plans an appropriate resection. For an upper anterior tooth close to the buccal cortex, this resection is simple and straightforward. For teeth that are multirooted or multicanaled and lingually inclined the task is more difficult (Fig. 19-19, *A, B*). Because the operator does not have knowledge about the true buccal or lingual inclination of the root, a resection that appears to cut directly through the root may in fact be an extreme oblique resection (Fig. 19-19, *C, D*). This is especially true in lower posterior teeth, where a thick buccal cortex is present or in lower anterior teeth where roots have a natural lingual inclination and the surgeon has limited manipulative access owing to the mentalis muscle attachment. Failure to cut completely through the root in a buccal-lingual direction is one of the most common errors in periradicular surgery. Even when the resection is complete, the bevel is frequently so oblique that the lingual apical ramifications are not eliminated. A good rule to follow is this: *Whatever the angle of the bevel is, it is almost always greater than it appears to be*. The experienced surgeon compensates for this distortion of perspective by reducing the angle of the bevel and positioning it more perpendicular to the longitudinal axis of the root. Another disadvantage of the extreme bevel is that, as the bevel angle increases, the surface area of the cut dentinal tubules likewise increases and the canal systems that must be sealed become elongated in a buccal-lingual direction (Fig. 19-20). This scenario places severe restorative demands on the surgeon, requiring extremely skillful retropreparations close to the lingual aspect of the root (Fig. 19-21).

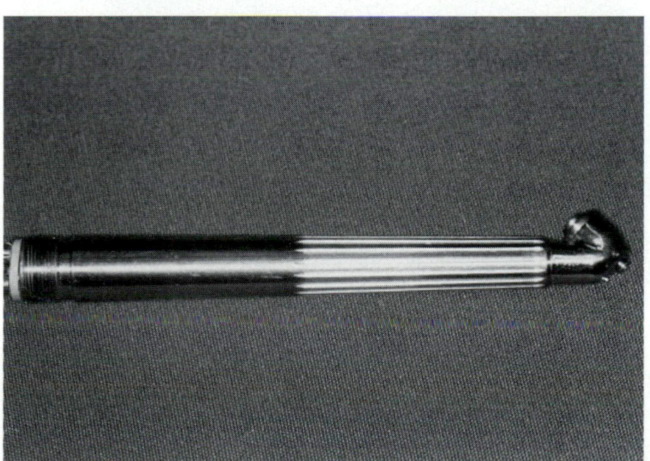

FIG. 19-17 The Impact-Air 45 handpiece has no air that exits from the working end, reducing the possibility of producing air emphysema or air embolism while operating under the flap.

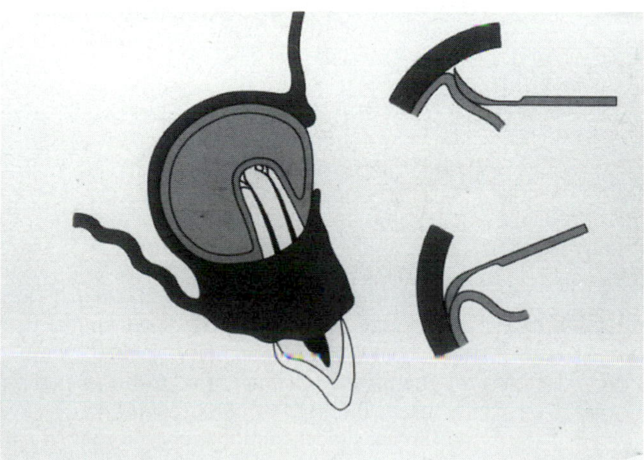

FIG. 19-18 Correct curettement of the soft tissue lesion, utilizing a sharp spoon in different positions in various locations in the crypt. Many lesions can be removed in one piece by careful curettement in the bony crypt.

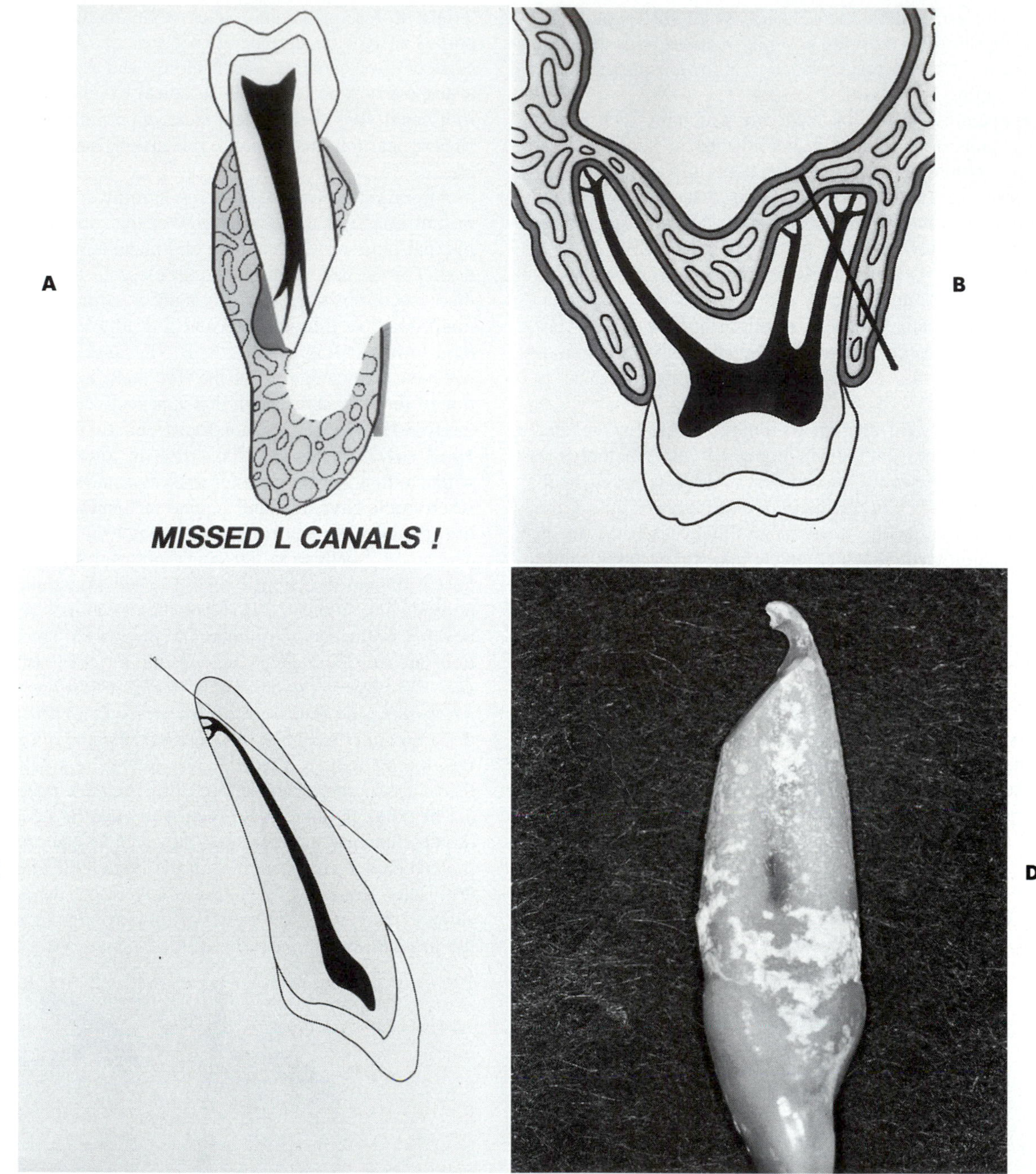

FIG. 19-19 A, An acute bevel on a lower bicuspid can entirely miss the lingual canal if the practitioner is not aware of the actual angle of the bevel. **B,** Acute bevel on a maxillary molar may miss the MB-2 canal or lingual ramifications that typically are present on mesial-buccal roots of maxillary molars. A more moderate bevel is recommended that will ensure complete resection through the lingual aspect of the root. **C** and **D,** Failure to completely resect through an upper canine may leave the lingual aspect of the root intact or leave the lingual apical ramifications present. Such acute bevels position the lingual ramifications so close to the lingual aspect of the root that the retropreparation becomes very difficult.

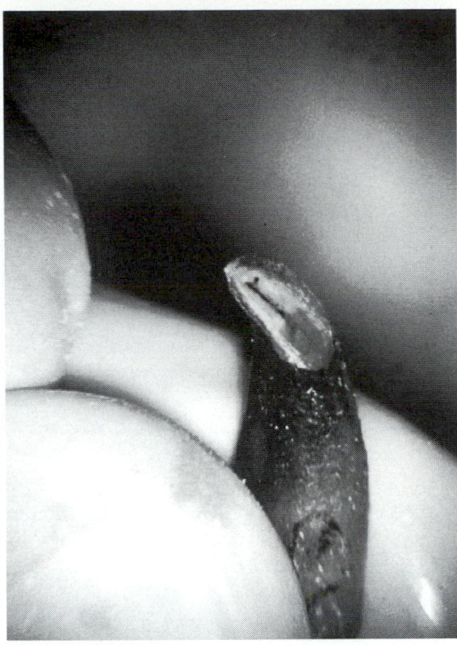

FIG. 19-20 A maxillary bicuspid with acute bevel demonstrating the additional surface area needed for an adequate retropreparation.

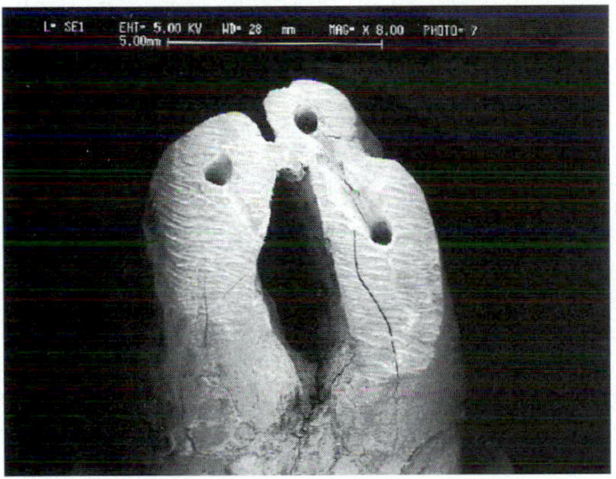

FIG. 19-21 Ultrasonic root end preparations placed very close to the lingual margin of the root because of a very acute bevel.

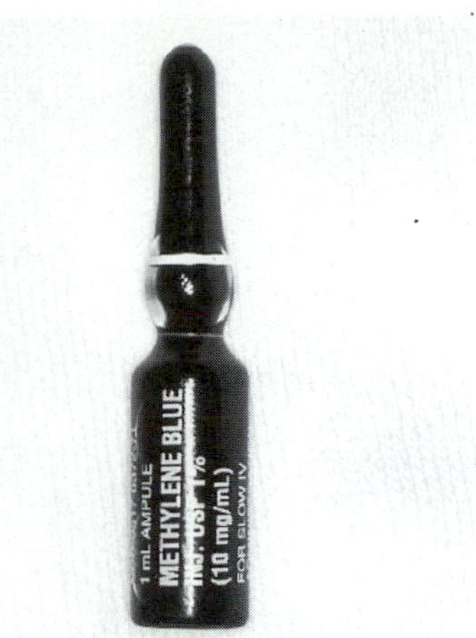

FIG. 19-22 Methylene blue dye can be used to stain vital tissue and can help delineate the root outline.

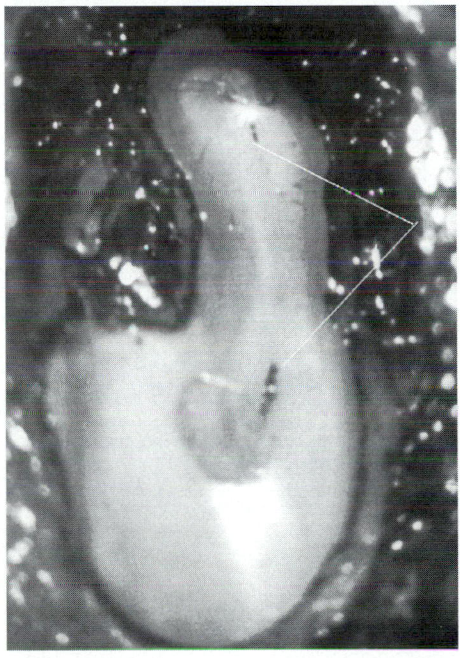

FIG. 19-23 Methylene blue dye stains the periodontal ligament and facilitates identification of the root and periodontal ligament. It also stains the vital pulp tissue, which can be seen lingual (lines) to the gutta-percha.

After the root has been beveled, the cut surface requires close inspection to verify that the root is completely sectioned, the cut smooth, and the bevel angle sufficient enough to provide manual access to perform the retropreparation.[48,60,110]

Frequently the osseous access needs to be enlarged at this juncture, especially if retropreparations are required in the lingual part of the crypt. To clearly identify the complete outline of the root, a small amount of methylene blue dye (Figs. 19-22, 19-23) can be painted on the root surface (Fig. 19-24). After preliminary inspection is complete and the surgeon feels no additional modifications will be needed, the crypt is packed with one of the many surgical dressings available. Collacote (Colla-Tec, Inc.; Fig. 19-25) and Avitene (Avicon, Inc.) are particularly efficacious dressings because they contain collagen, which is a primary activator of the intrinsic pathway for clotting. The retrofilling procedure must take place in a dry, sterile field, so hemostasis within the crypt is a significant concern. Adaptic (Johnson and Johnson), Melolite (Smith & Nephew), Gelfoam (Upjohn Company), Surgicel (Johnson and Johnson), and Telfa pads (Kendall Company; Fig. 19-26) are also useful adjuncts for this packing, as they contain no cotton fibers that could contaminate the field and retard wound healing.[21,53,93] Hemostasis within the crypt can also be achieved by using a solution of ferric subsulfate (Fig. 19-27), which has an extremely low pH and rapidly causes intravascular coagulation. Since ferric subsulfate is a necrosing

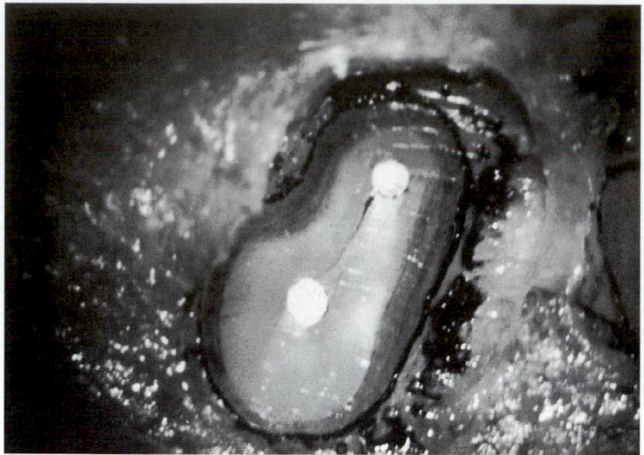

FIG. 19-24 Mesial-buccal root of maxillary molar stained with methylene blue demonstrating vital PDL and isthmus tissue.

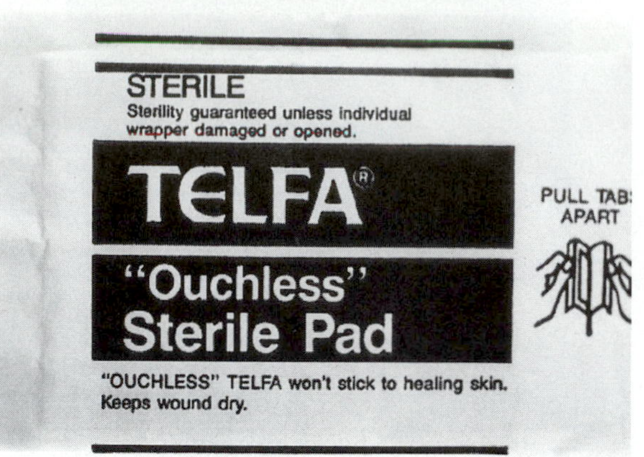

FIG. 19-26 Telfa pads can also be packed into the bony crypt, where they help with hemostasis and prevent contamination by foreign debris.

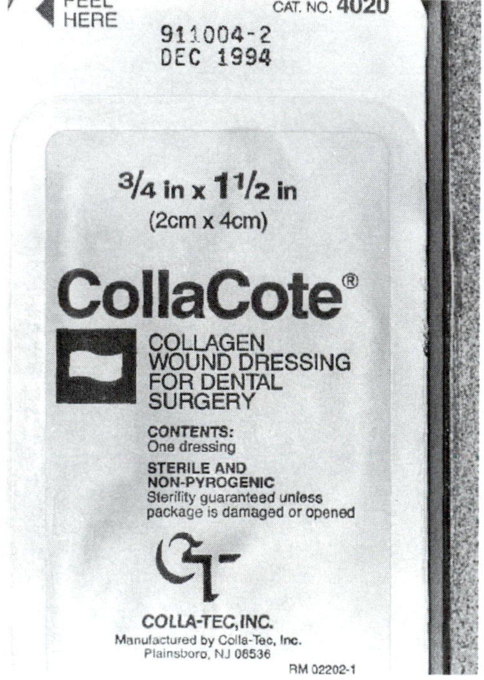

FIG. 19-25 Collacote can be placed in the bony crypt and aids in hemostasis by activating the intrinsic clotting mechanism.

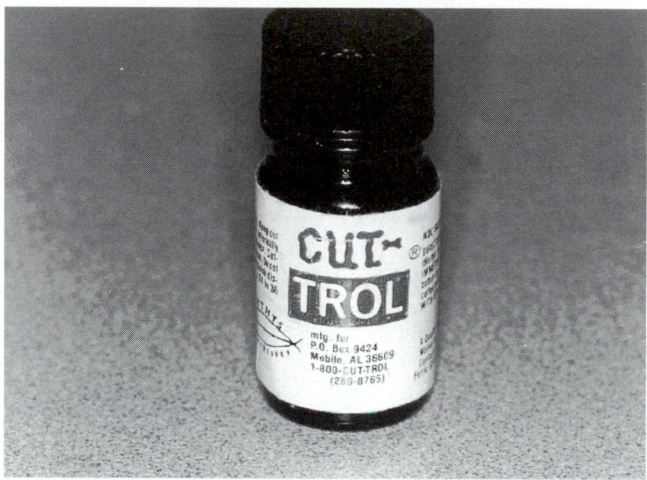

FIG. 19-27 Ferric subsulfate is a powerful hemostatic agent and should be used with caution in the bony crypt. Care needs to be taken to avoid having this solution contact any of the basal bone or any part of the flap.

agent,[78] it needs to be used judiciously and with caution. The proper technique is to place a drop on a Telfa pad, remove the excess by squeezing the pad, and then station it against the wall of the crypt for 5 minutes. It is imperative to keep this solution away from the buccal bone, the flap margins, the periodontal ligament, neurovascular bundles, sinus membranes and the floor of the nose. It is important to understand that the cells responsible for initial healing in the periradicular area originate from the periodontal ligament[66,95,97]; minimizing trauma to these cells is a high priority for the surgeon.

Apical Retropreparation Examination

After hemostasis is achieved and the crypt packed, the beveled root end is critically examined. This examination requires supplemental illumination and magnification.[20] Attempting a thorough assessment of the root end without appropriate magnification and illumination is inappropriate. Perhaps no area of endodontics is in greater need of improvement than the evaluation of the beveled root end. Since the operator is confronted with the problem of microscopic leakage, the more detailed the inspection that can be achieved, the more confidence we can have about our attempted seal. The simple act of root resection opens up the entire root canal system, with all its irregularities, to the periapex. Creating a hermetic seal of these systems requires a magnification system.[20]

Review of Retropreparation Technique

Retropreparation techniques have historically involved a cursory examination of the root end and an assessment of the adequacy of the existing root canal filling.[49,80,143] Evaluating such seals with the unaided eye is nothing more than a guess.

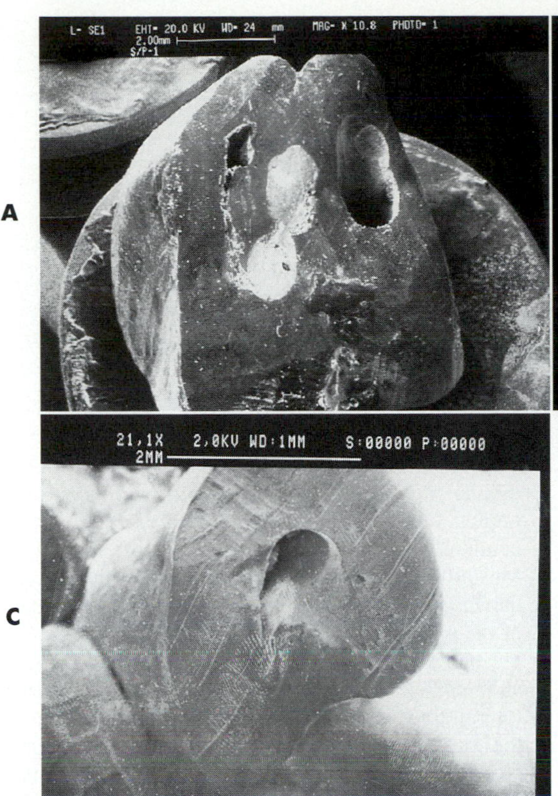

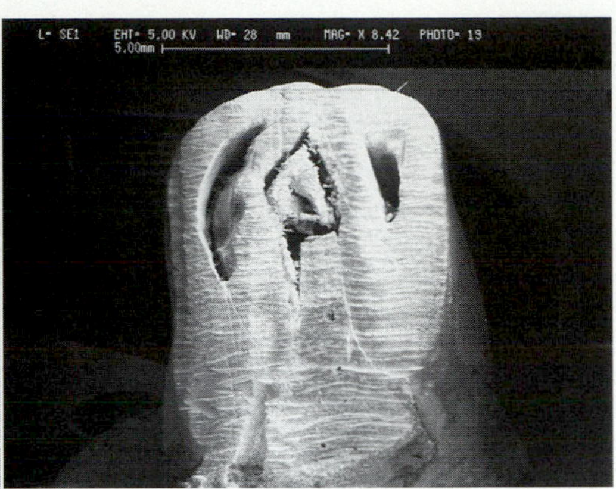

FIG. 19-28 A, Failed apicoectomy shows that the practitioner has mistaken the fusion line between the mesial and distal roots for the MB-2 canal. The MB-2 canal and isthmus are completely uninstrumented. **B,** Fused roots can present a confusing picture to the practitioner. Fusion lines and intrafurcal bone can resemble canal spaces. **C,** Incomplete ultrasonic root end preparation of maxillary bicuspid reveals incomplete instrumentation of the lingual ramifications. Failure to extend preparations lingually is a common mistake.

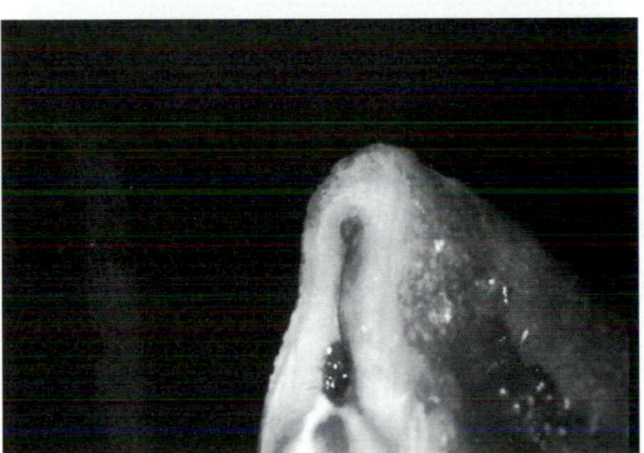

FIG. 19-29 Beveled root of No. 14 with communicating isthmus tissue.

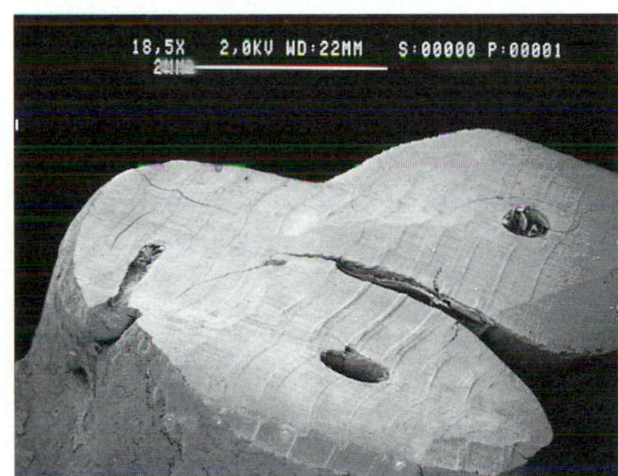

FIG. 19-30 Complex anatomy of maxillary molar shows the need to extend retropreparation to the lingual cementodentinal junction.

The best assessment of hermetic apical seals requires measurement tolerances on the order of microns, and we do not possess the technology today to confidently evaluate such a seal in a clinical setting. *Until such technology becomes available, prudence dictates that we assume that all beveled root canal fillings are leaking.* Independent SEM studies show that the simple act of resection disturbs the gutta-percha seal.[25,135] Therefore, the placement of a retrofill is essential unless there are extenuating circumstances.

The simple act of root resection exposes the periradicular tissues to the myriad complexities of the root canal system. Even a cursory examination of beveled roots on extracted teeth can reveal to the practitioner the infinite variety of pulpal configurations found in nature (Fig. 19-28, *A* and *C*). Interpreting these configurations in cross section at the time of surgery can be a daunting challenge. The practitioner can be confronted with a bewildering array of communicating anastomoses, lateral canals, fracture lines, cul de sacs (Figs. 19-29 and 19-30), fusion lines, etc. Additionally, since the root is usually much broader buccolingually than mesiodistally, these confusing arrays are elongated and distorted by the typically angled bevel. To say nothing of the restorative challenges presented, simply understanding what needs to be done to create a seal takes a great deal of skill, judgment, and experience. *The idea*

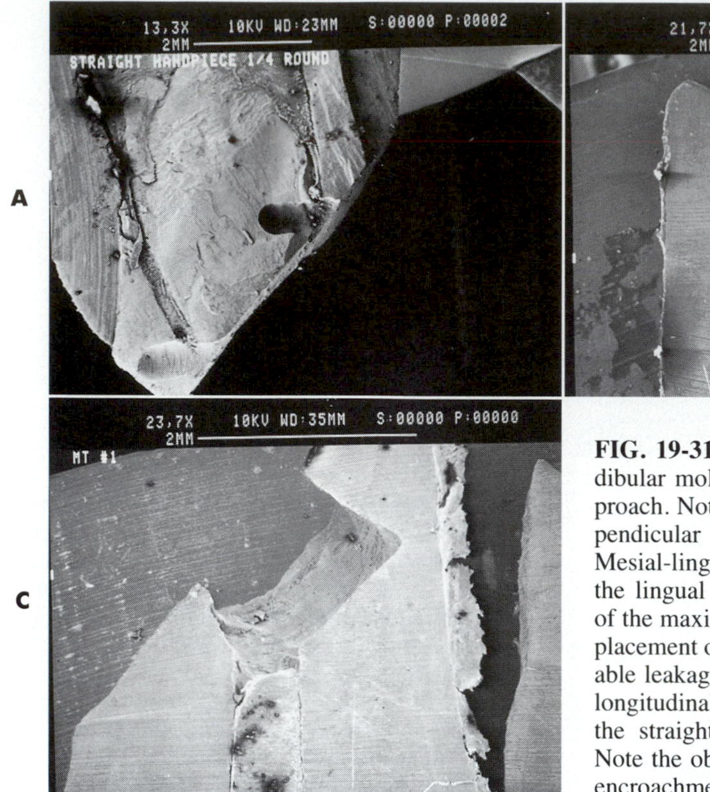

FIG. 19-31 A, Split longitudinal section of mandibular molar utilizing the straight handpiece approach. Note that the preparations are actually perpendicular to the longitudinal axis of the pulp. Mesial-lingual preparation has nearly perforated the lingual wall. **B,** Sectioned longitudinal view of the maxillary lateral incision shows the oblique placement of the retrofilling material and the probable leakage at the anterior margin. **C,** Sectioned longitudinal view of the retropreparation utilizes the straight handpiece with inverted cone bur. Note the oblique angle of the preparation and the encroachment upon the lingual wall of the root.

that the classic, round, ball bearing–type preparation is adequate is no longer valid because round preparations seldom conform to anatomic structures. In truth, retropreparations should rarely be round; rather they should be oval or slot shaped. Fortunately, the recent development of ultrasonic retropreparation has helped to standardize these preparations and increased the likelihood that they will be consistently well placed.

Traditional handpiece retropreparation technique utilizes either miniature contraangle rotary burs or a straight handpiece. Both devices are hindered by the limited access that apical surgery provides. Rarely can a contraangle microhandpiece or a straight handpiece with quarter-round bur be placed down the long axis of the root. These preparations are placed obliquely into the root, sometimes even at right angles to the long axis of the pulp canal (Fig. 19-31). Such a misplacement has the major disadvantage of having to rely on the axial wall of the preparation, instead of the pulpal floor, to effect a seal (Fig. 19-32). Since research has shown that we can expect all nonphysiologic retrofilling materials to undergo some degree of circumferential resorption, the marginal sealing capability will quickly be jeopardized with only minimal resorption.

Retropreparations should accept filling materials that predictably seal off the root canal system from the periradicular tissues. These preparations must fulfill the following requirements:

1. The apical 3 mm of the root is cleaned and shaped.
2. The preparation is parallel to the anatomic outline of the pulpal space.
3. There is adequate retention form.
4. All isthmus tissue is removed.
5. Remaining dentinal walls are not weakened.

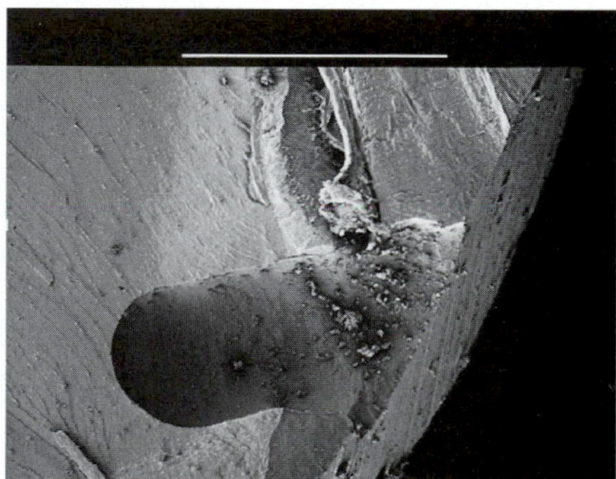

FIG. 19-32 Sectioned longitudinal view demonstrating how the pulp is sealed off by the axial wall of the preparation instead of the pulpal floor of the preparation.

An ideal retropreparation is placed so that its outline form is parallel to and coincident with the anatomic configuration of the pulpal space.

In posterior teeth, roots with dual canal systems routinely have multiple anastomoses between them. The complex nature of these systems has been well documented for more than 50 years.[22,62,111] Once the apex has been removed, the surgeon confronts a much more complex situation. If webbing or interstitial pulp harbors microorganisms or their toxic products, removing these irritants or sealing them off from the periapical tissues is necessary. The endodontic requirements for suc-

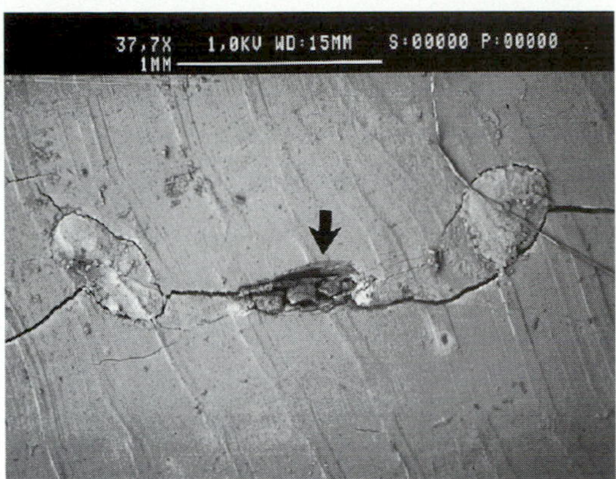

FIG. 19-33 Scanning electron micrograph of a failed apicoectomy with amalgam retrofills in the MB and ML canals and with no instrumentation or filling in the isthmus area connecting the two canals. (Microfractures are artifacts of specimen preparation.)

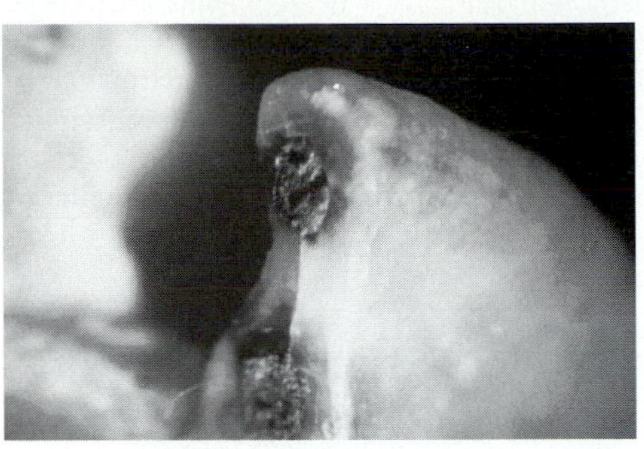

FIG. 19-34 Resected root of the mandibular molar clearly demonstrating the connecting anastomoses between the buccal and lingual canal.

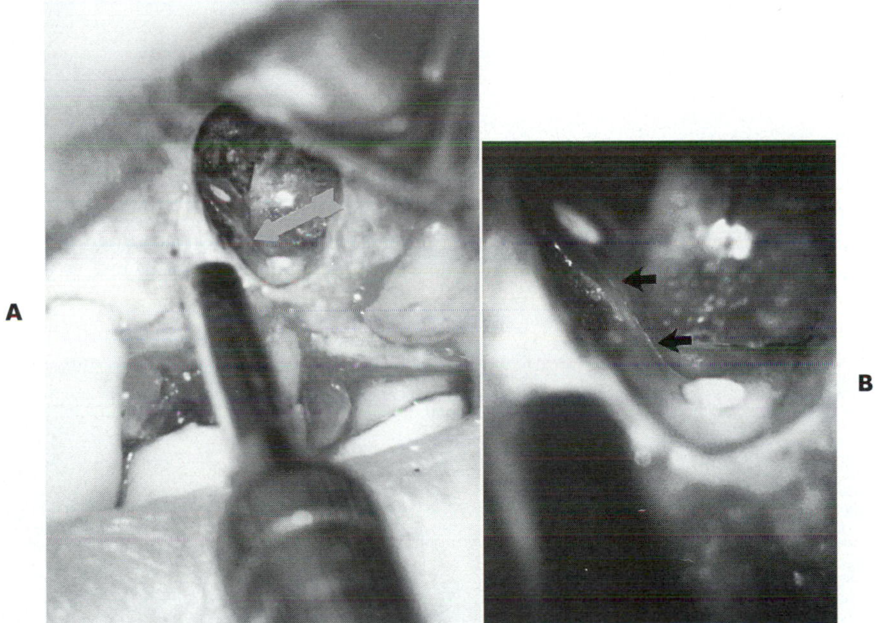

FIG. 19-35 A, Resected root of maxillary bicuspid with connecting isthmus area. Even at 6×, the isthmus can be difficult to visualize *(arrow)*. B, Same root seen at 22×. The connecting isthmus is more easily visualized *(arrows)*.

cessful healing are the same for surgical and nonsurgical treatment. Success depends on cleaning, shaping, and sealing all portals of exit. Failure to prepare and seal the isthmus areas or any of the anatomic variations (Figs. 19-33, 19-34) invites failure. The narrow isthmus areas between confluent canal systems can be difficult to see, even with a microscope (Fig. 19-35). As a general rule, *all roots with multiple canal systems contain isthmus tissue*. A brief consideration of the morphogenesis of these roots explains why (pulpal anatomy is discussed in Chapter 6). The retropreparation of these narrow isthmus areas presents the surgeon with a great challenge (Fig. 19-36). Since the margin of error is less than 1 mm, the surgeon must be especially careful to avoid inadvertent perforation (Fig. 19-37).

For successful retropreparation, the surgeon needs to be well versed, not only in root canal system anatomy, but also in root morphology. The kinds of cases that present for surgery are precisely those in which the anatomy is either aberrant or unusually complex. There are hundreds of anatomic studies documenting the infinite variation in tooth morphology and root canal anatomy (Figs. 19-38 and 19-39). The surgeon who lacks an appreciation of this anatomic diversity is likely to be disappointed in the surgical results. Of particular note is the high prevalence of fourth roots on maxillary molars (Fig. 19-40),[145] third roots on mandibular molars, and bifurcated roots on canines and bicuspids of both arches. The experienced endodontic surgeon will maintain a healthy "anatomic skepticism" at all times.

Another requirement for successful retropreparation is to provide adequate retention form without weakening the root. Silver amalgam, Super EBA, and IRM all require mechanical retention, in the form of either undercuts or parallel walls. Creating mechanical undercuts in already very thin dentinal walls is dangerous, especially in narrow isthmus areas. A parallel preparation avoids hollowing out the delicate root dentin while providing for mechanical retention.

ULTRASONIC RETROPREPARATIONS

The ultrasonic retropreparation technique was devised to address the major shortcomings of conventional rotary bur–type

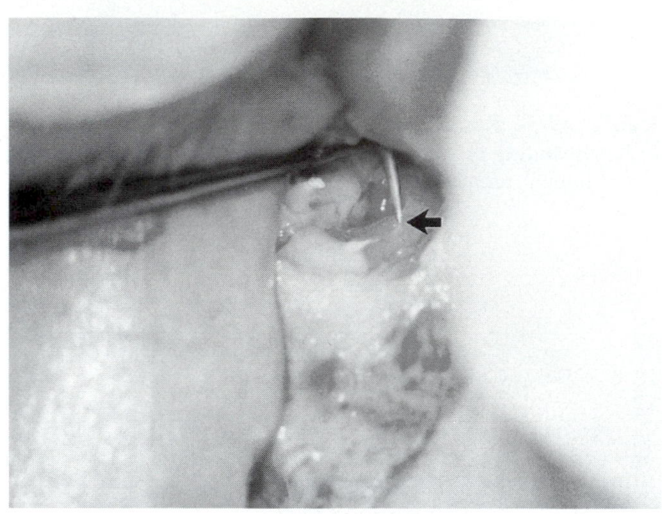

FIG. 19-36 Ultrasonic preparation of the MB-2 *(arrow)* and isthmus tissue on a maxillary first molar.

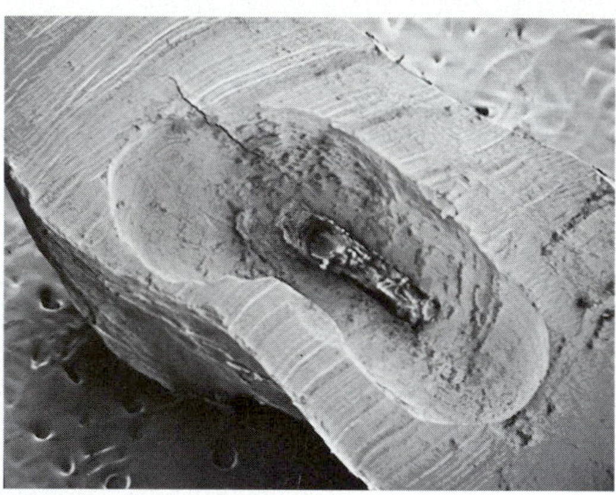

FIG. 19-37 Scanning electron micrograph of a microhandpiece preparation on a mandibular bicuspid. Note the near-perforation on the mesial wall.

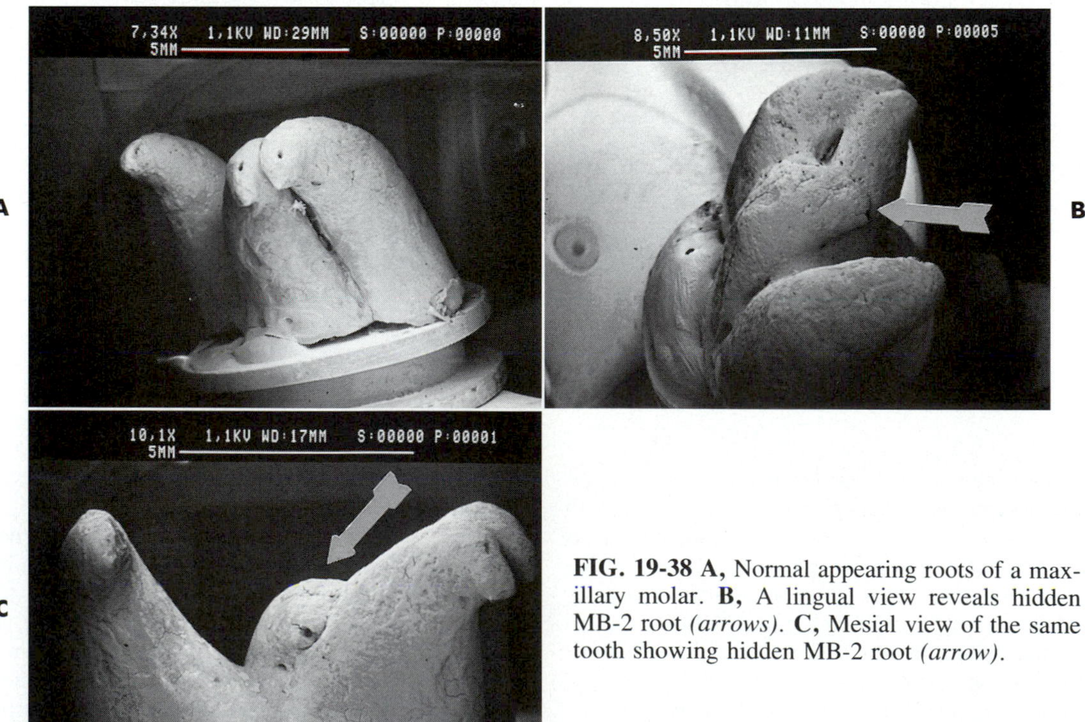

FIG. 19-38 A, Normal appearing roots of a maxillary molar. **B,** A lingual view reveals hidden MB-2 root *(arrows)*. **C,** Mesial view of the same tooth showing hidden MB-2 root *(arrow)*.

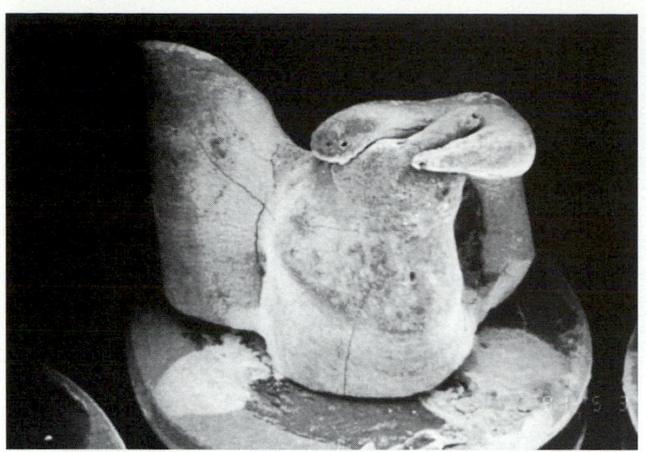

FIG. 19-39 Aberrant root morphology of a maxillary molar. Resection of this root would present the surgeon with an extremely complex restorative problem.

preparations.[19,20] Because of the much reduced size of the ultrasonic tip, it is easily placed into the crypt and down the long axis of the root, even in inaccessible areas. Ultrasonic units (Excellence in Endodontics, Inc., and Amadent) specifically designed for root end preparation are now commercially available, as are a wide variety of tip designs (Excellence in Endodontics, Inc.) that facilitate preparation in all areas of the mouth, even on buccal approaches to palatal roots of upper molars (Figs. 19-41, 19-42).[19]

Ultrasonic root end preparations should always be done with copious irrigation to avoid heat buildup around the tip. After the ultrasonic unit is activated at its lowest power, the tip is guided along the surface of the beveled root using very light pressure in an etching-type motion. After cutting a shallow tracking groove, the tip should be moved rapidly back and forth, utilizing minimal pressure until the entire preparation is 2.5 to 3 mm deep. This technique produces a very well-defined, conservative preparation 2 to 3 mm into the root with

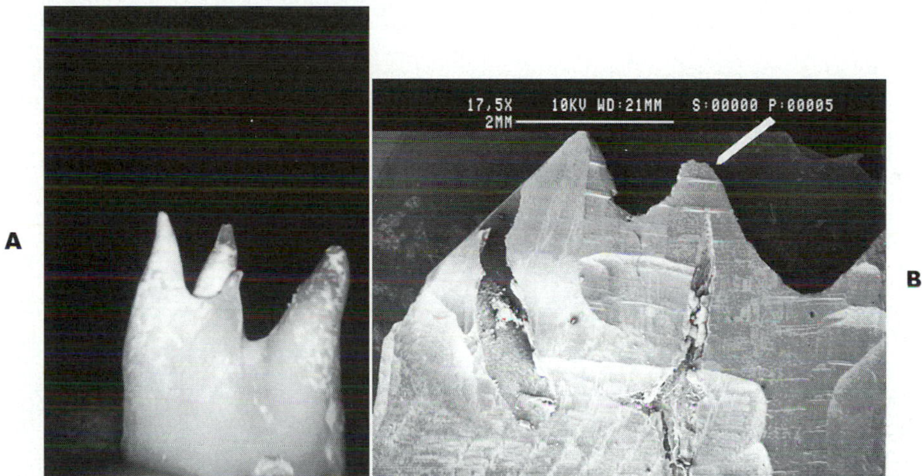

FIG. 19-40 A, Common MB-2 root of maxillary molar remains hidden from the surgeon even after beveling through the MB-1 root. **B,** Sectioned longitudinal view of ultrasonic root-end preparation on the MB root with a failure to detect a second MB-2 root *(arrow)*.

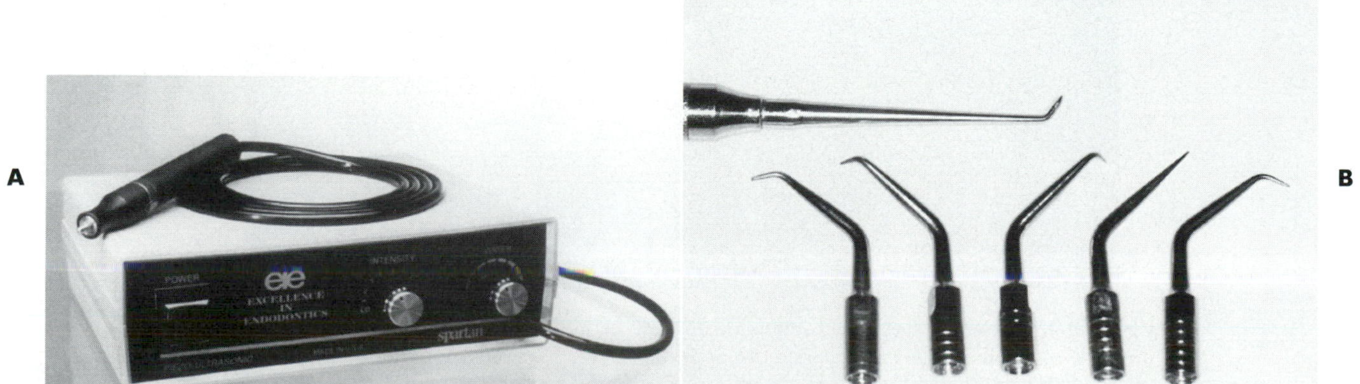

FIG. 19-41 A, Ultrasonic unit from Excellence in Endodontics, Inc., is designed specifically for ultrasonic root end preparation. **B,** Assortment of ultrasonic root end preparation instruments that facilitate placement of ultrasonic preparation in all areas.

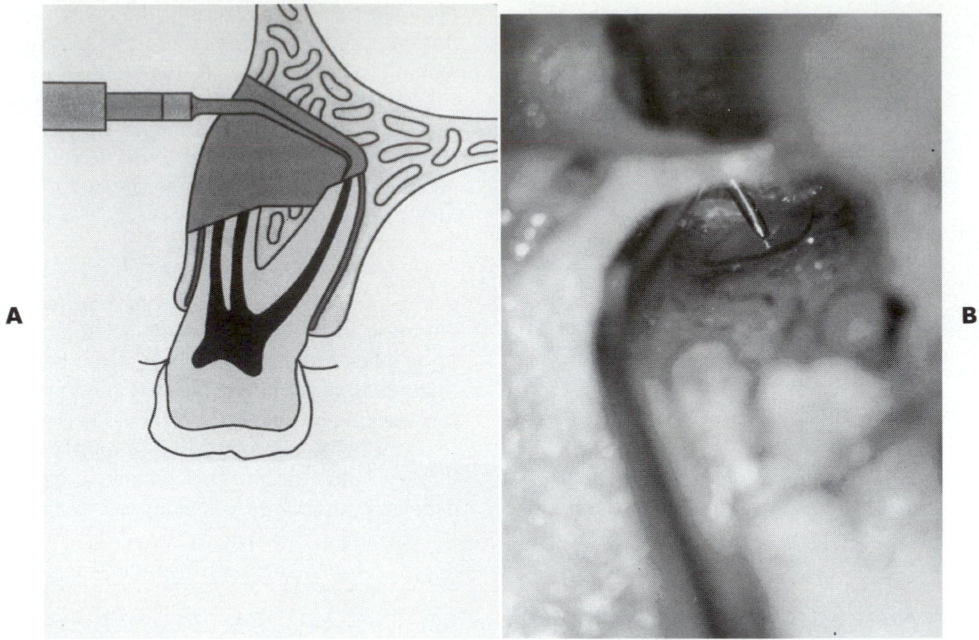

FIG. 19-42 A, Diagrammatic view of trans-sinus approach to the palatal root of a maxillary molar. **B,** High magnification view of the trans-sinus ultrasonic preparation of palatal root. Note the dark PDL from placement of methylene blue dye.

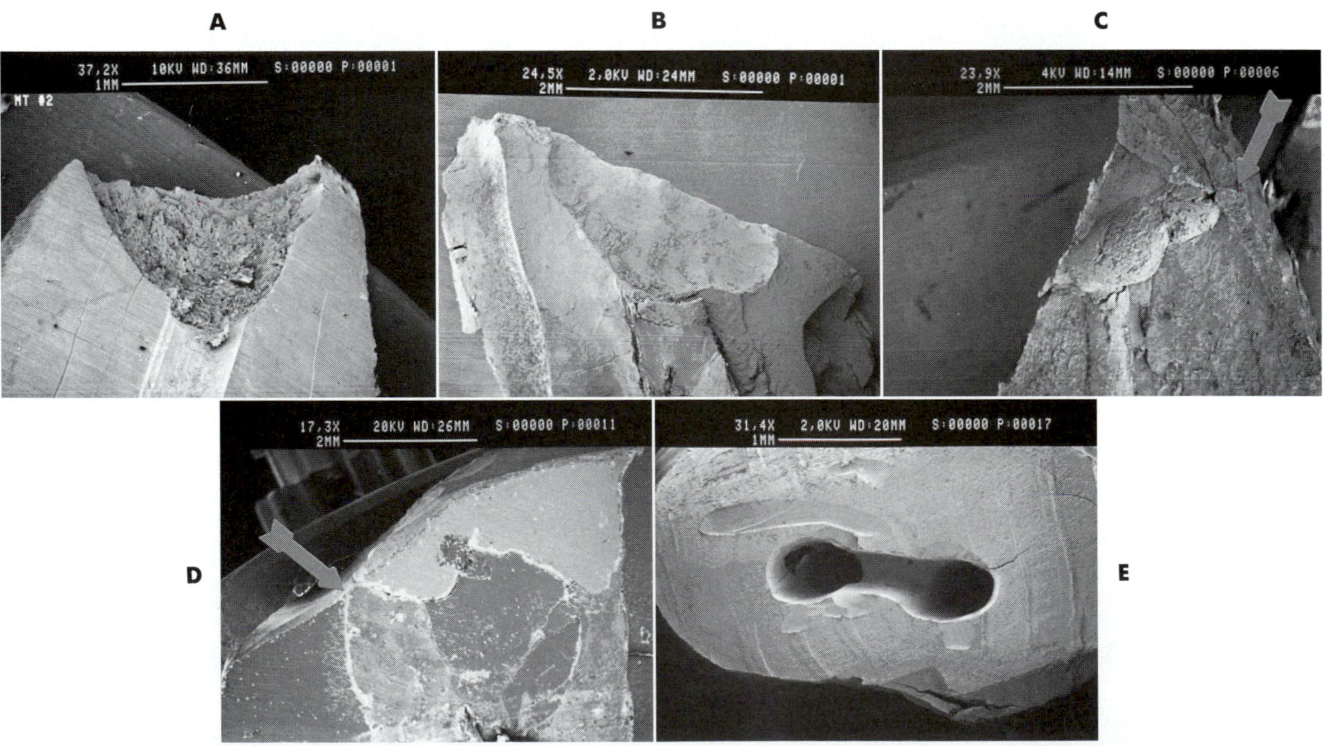

FIG. 19-43 A and **B,** Sectioned longitudinal view of the microhandpiece preparation. Note the lack of retention and the cupped-out appearance. **C,** Sectioned longitudinal view of the microhandpiece preparation. Note the oblique angle of the preparation and its encroachment on the lingual wall of the root *(arrow)*. **D,** Sectioned longitudinal view of amalgam retrofill in mesial root of maxillary molar. Note the oblique orientation of the amalgam retrofill and the failure to seal the buccal margin *(arrow)*. **E,** Ultrasonic root end preparation of a maxillary bicuspid. The preparation is conservative mesiodistally, courses down the long axis of the root, and has very parallel walls.

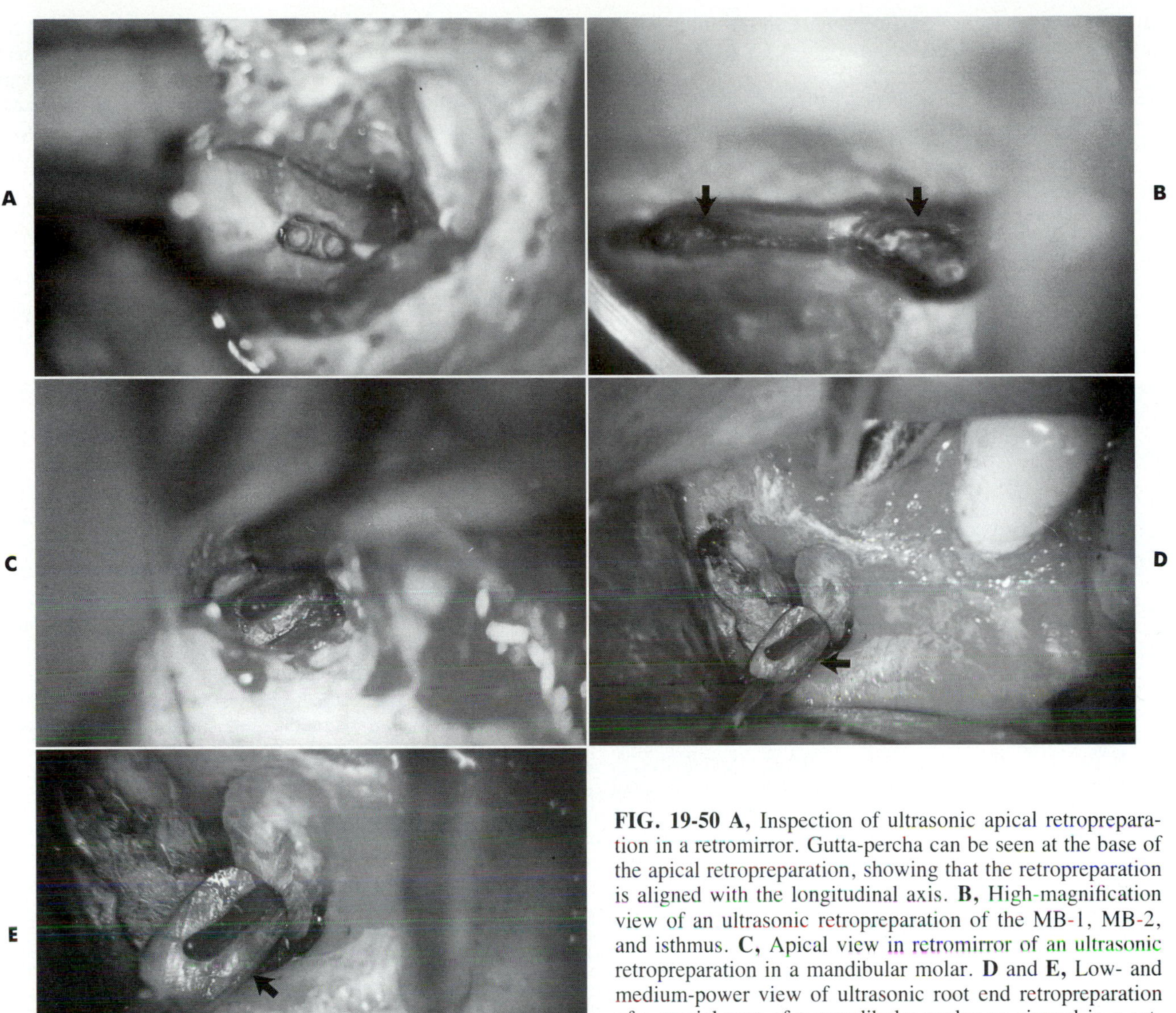

FIG. 19-50 A, Inspection of ultrasonic apical retropreparation in a retromirror. Gutta-percha can be seen at the base of the apical retropreparation, showing that the retropreparation is aligned with the longitudinal axis. **B,** High-magnification view of an ultrasonic retropreparation of the MB-1, MB-2, and isthmus. **C,** Apical view in retromirror of an ultrasonic retropreparation in a mandibular molar. **D** and **E,** Low- and medium-power view of ultrasonic root end retropreparation of a mesial root of a mandibular molar as viewed in a retromirror (arrow).

blasts into cementoblasts, leading to a cementogenic repair of the root apex and reconstruction of the periodontal ligament at the beveled surface.
3. Nonresorbable.
4. Easy to prepare and place.
5. Radiographically visible.
6. Unaffected by moisture.

The ideal physiologic retrofilling material will, in all likelihood, be composed of some form of calcium phosphate cement or hydroxyapatite mixture, perhaps bonded to tooth structure by plasma or laser energy. But until such a material is developed and tested with long-term follow-up, retrofilling materials will be imperfect.

Of these imperfect materials, silver amalgam has been used most often.[49,103,139] Recently, it has fallen out of favor because of concerns about its toxicity and its failure to provide long-term healing.[37,39,46] But additional factors also argue against its use. Silver amalgam expands on setting, especially in a wet environment.[68,131,140] Such expansion can fracture the delicate apical dentin. It has no adhesive capabilities; therefore, it requires substantial mechanical undercuts in an area of the root that can ill afford them. Whether zinc amalgam, zinc-free amalgam, or high-copper amalgam, each exhibits long-term marginal leakage.[70,82,92] Additional concerns about electrochemical reactions and tissue discoloration[54,73,102] have led to the gradual movement away from silver amalgam and to the search for alternative materials that do not have these limitations (Table 19-2). Of the materials listed in Table 19-2, Super EBA (Fig. 19-51) and IRM appear to offer the most advantages.[5,32,114] Both are ZOE cements. IRM is 80% zinc oxide, 20% polymethylmethacrylate, with the liquid being 99% eugenol. Super EBA is 60% zinc oxide, 30% alumina, 6% nat-

TABLE 19-2. Alternatives to silver amalgam retrofilling materials

Cavit
Composite resin
Daiket
Gold foil
IRM
Polycarboxylate cement
Super EBA
Zinc phosphate cement

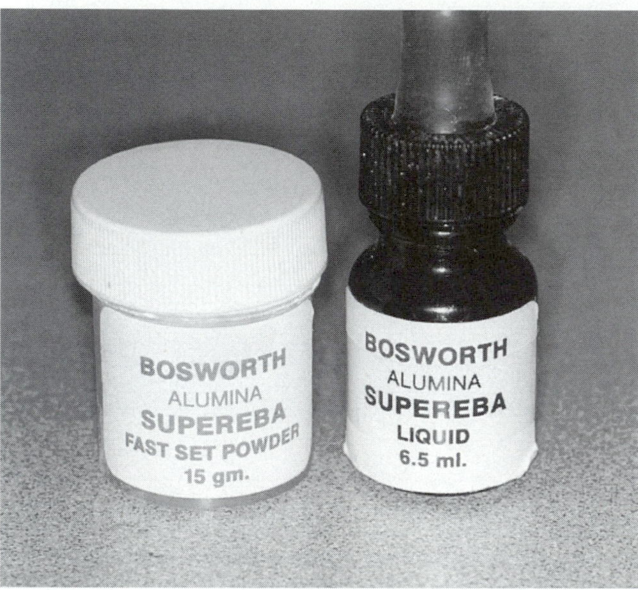

FIG. 19-51 Super EBA cement.

ural resin, with the liquid being 37.5% eugenol and 62.5% *ortho*-ethoxybenzoic acid. These cements have excellent sealing capability and are nontoxic after setting. Studies have compared 10-year success rates for IRM/EBA versus amalgam and found higher success rates for the former.[32] Until the ideal physiologic root end–filling material is developed, these retrosealing cements at this time appear to be best.

PLACEMENT AND FINISHING OF RETROFILLING MATERIALS

After the retropreparation has been dried and inspected, the retrofilling material is placed. IRM or EBA is mixed to a claylike consistency, shaped into a narrow cone, and attached to the end of a spoon or Hollenback carver (Fig. 19-52). The material can then be introduced into the surgical site and placed accurately into the retropreparation. It is compacted using miniature condensers. The material is overpacked (Fig. 19-53) on the root surface and allowed to set. The placement and condensation procedures should occur in a dry field. After the setting is complete, a sharp discoid carver can be used to carve away the excess retrofilling material. A 30-fluted composite finishing bur (Fig. 19-54) can be applied to the cut surface to achieve a highly polished surface without fear of ditching either the root surface or the retrofilling material. After finishing, the retrofilling is examined for completeness and marginal integrity (Fig. 19-55). A final radiograph is exposed at this time, to confirm correct placement of the retrofilling (Fig. 19-56).

Every step in this technique is critical for the successful completion of apical surgery. Each of these steps requires not only mastery of technique and a feel for dental materials but also refinement in the surgeon's visual acuity and an appreciation for the very close tolerances required. Performed on such a miniature scale these skills challenge even the most fastidious dentist. Time spent in perfecting these skills rewards the surgeon with a satisfying sense of professional accomplishment.

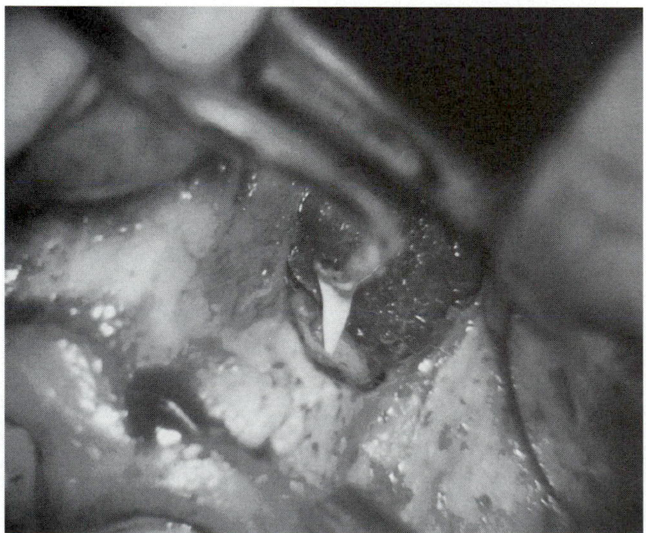

FIG. 19-52 After mixing to a claylike consistency, Super EBA is shaped into a cone, placed on the back edge of a spoon, and then placed into the dried retropreparation.

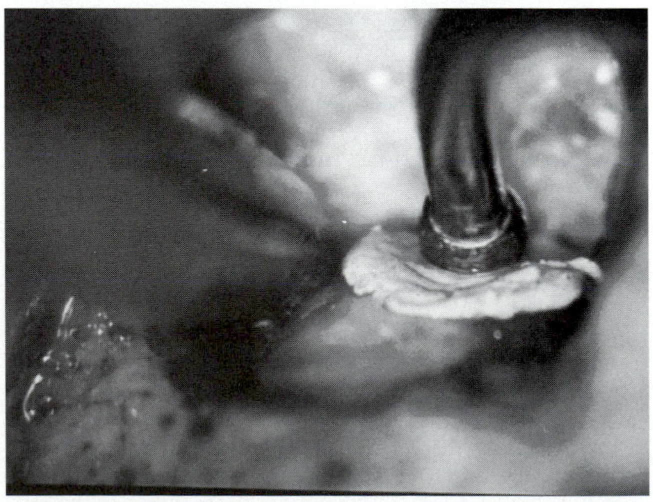

FIG. 19-53 Final condensation of Super EBA using a Buchanan condenser.

CLOSURE

After final inspection and appropriate radiographs, the crypt packing is removed and the entire surgical site examined for extraneous debris. After irrigation with sterile saline, the wound edges are reapproximated. Time spent in the accurate reapproximation of the wound edges aids in the initiation of primary wound healing.[136] The goal of reapproximation is to enable the wound edges to heal by primary intention. With sulcular incisions, the wound edges are located at the attachment apparatus near the cervical aspect of the crown and at the papilla and in the interdental col area. If the incision and elevation of these tissues have been atraumatic, primary intention healing should follow.[29,63,106] Mucogingival flap margins are easy to approximate if the incisions have been scalloped. After a brief period of compression, the flap is sutured.

The role of sutures is to hold the reapproximated tissues in place during the initial events in wound healing. The thickness of the clot between the opposed edges determines if the tissue heals by primary or secondary intention (Figs. 19-57 to 19-60).[9,10,105] For this reason, postsurgical compression of the wound site decreases the thickness of the coagulum and allows closer approximation of the wound edges.[51]

The placement of sutures creates another unavoidable wound. Suture wounds are longitudinal puncture wounds and can add significant trauma to the tissues. Sutures are very rapidly colonized by bacteria and can be a significant impediment to rapid wound healing.[13,83,113]

Skillful suturing requires practice and a deft touch. Most flaps reflected during apical surgery can be reapproximated with either interrupted, mattress, continuous, or sling sutures (Fig. 19-61). Suturing always proceeds from the unattached mucosal surface to the attached mucosal surface. Unnecessary tension on the suture will cause the tissue to tear, or possibly become ischemic. Vertically releasing incisions rarely require more than one suture, as the releasing incisions are predominantly in alveolar mucosa, which has many elastic fibers. These fibers cannot be approximated once they are cut, no matter how many sutures are used.

Various suture materials are commercially available and every surgeon quickly develops preferences for one or another. Silk has been favored by many practitioners because of its easy handling and low cost, but it is very quickly colonized by bacteria, owing to its wicking action, and can impede primary intention healing.[83] Supramid Extra has working characteristics very similar to those of silk (Figs. 19-62, 19-63), but it is colonized more slowly and, therefore, it is kinder to tissue. The removal time for sutures has progressively decreased as our understanding of surgical wound healing has progressed.[35,40,130] If no surgical principles have been violated and if healing has occurred by primary intention, suture removal is indicated after 48 hours.[61,90] With uneventful healing, after 48 hours the suture is performing no function and is

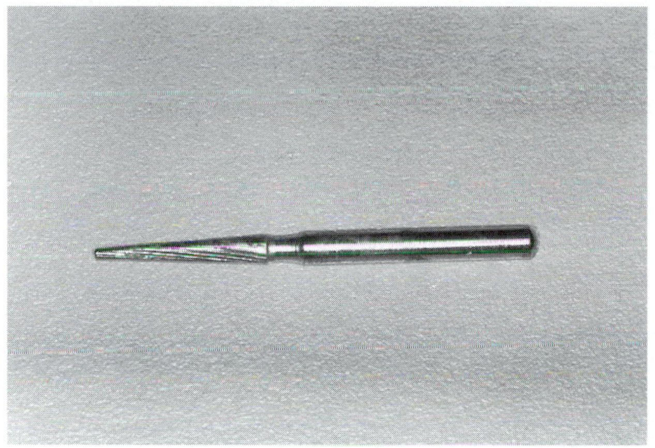

FIG. 19-54 Number 30 fluted composite finishing bur.

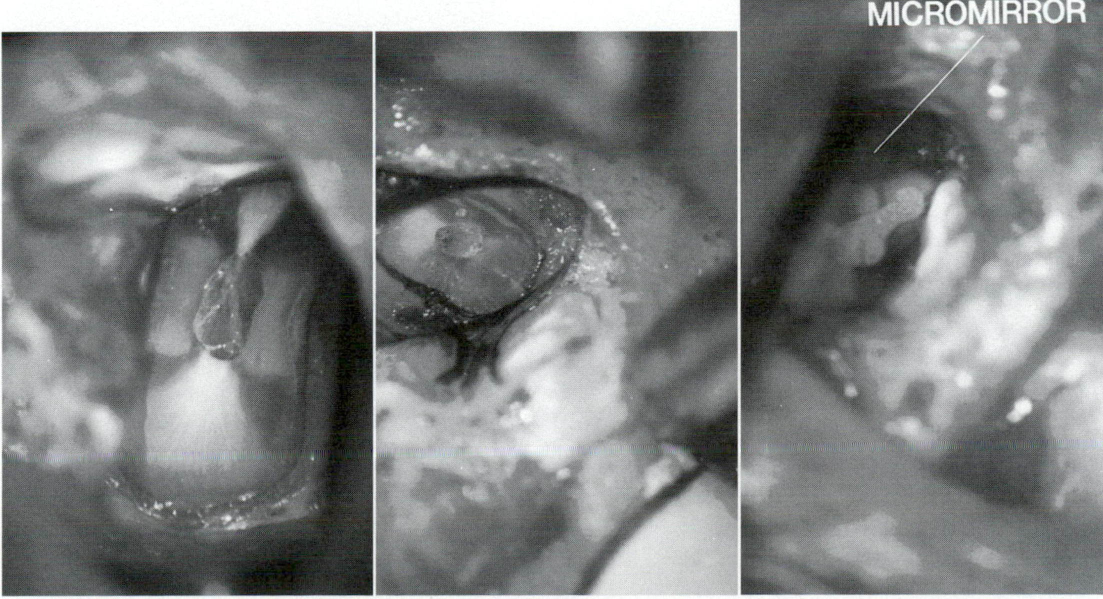

FIG. 19-55 Final inspection of retrofilling after finishing with a composite finishing bur. Smoothness and marginal integrity are checked.

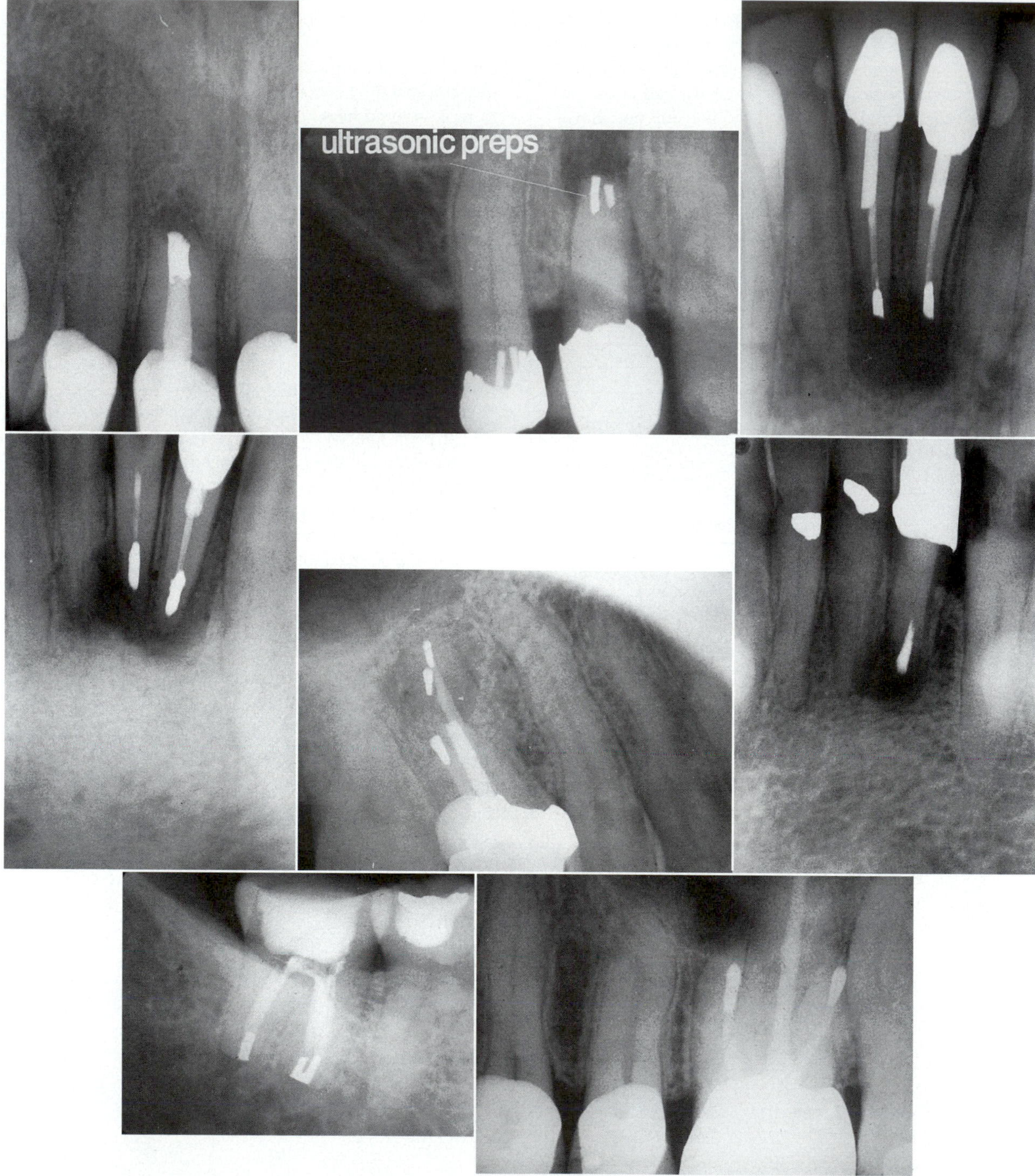

FIG. 19-56 Ultrasonic retropreparations show the conservative mesiodistal dimensions of the retropreparations and their placement up the longitudinal axis.

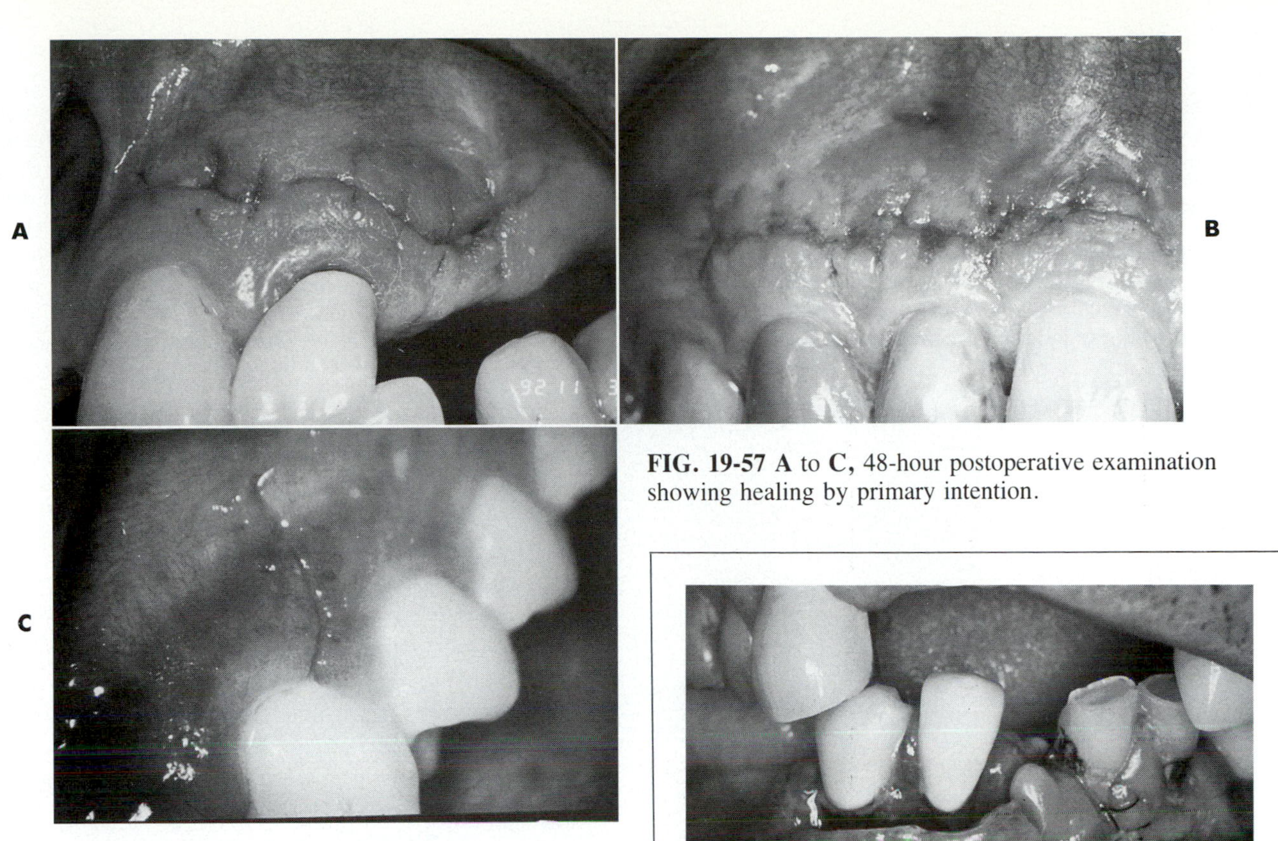

FIG. 19-57 A to **C,** 48-hour postoperative examination showing healing by primary intention.

FIG. 19-58 One-week postoperative checkup showing delayed healing by secondary intention.

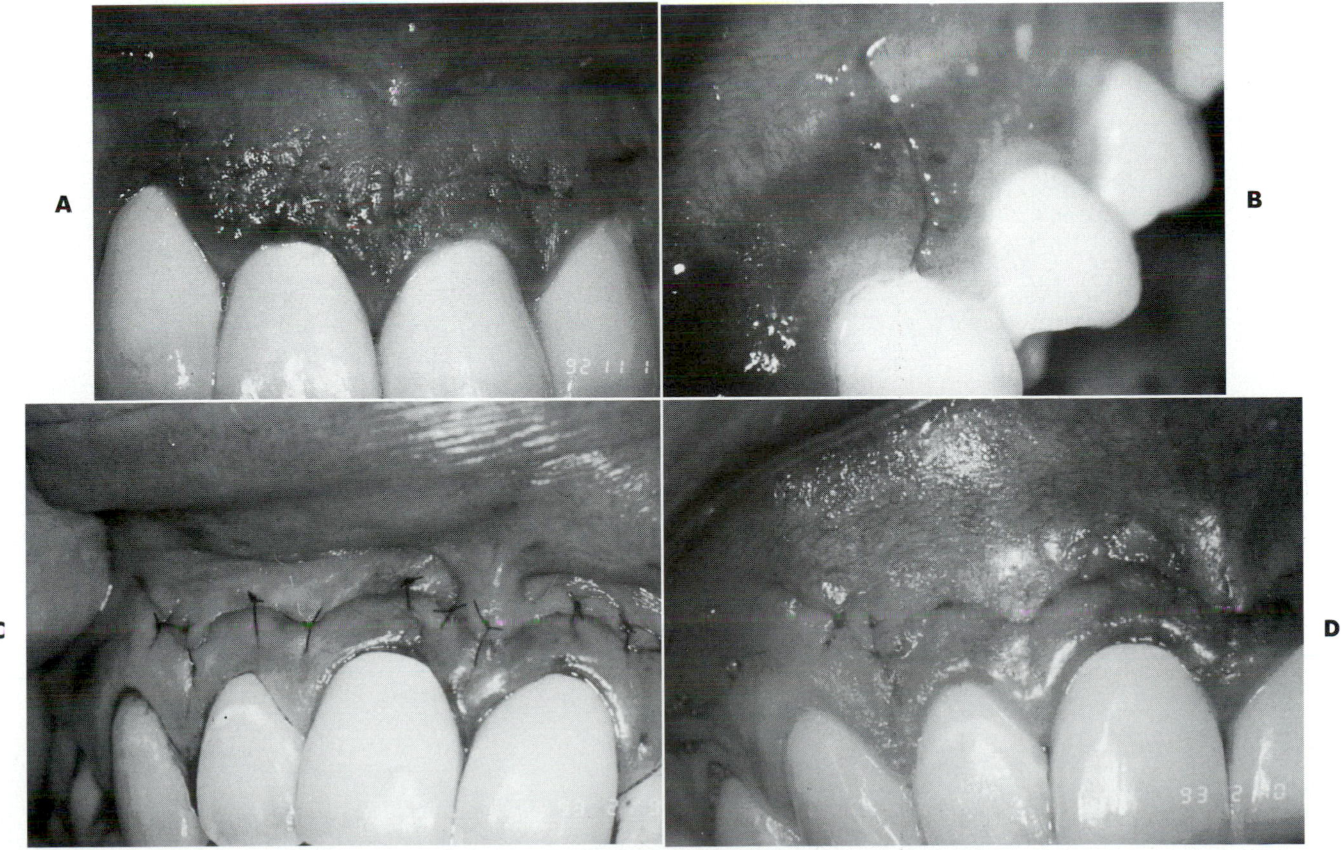

FIG. 19-59 A to **D,** 24-hour postoperative check demonstrating primary intention healing.

simply an irritant.[90] At 72 hours the entire length of suture is typically covered with a bacterial mat that is highly inflammatory to the wound site (Fig. 19-64).[127]

POSTOPERATIVE CARE

After suturing is complete, the surgeon should gently compress the surgical site for 10 to 15 minutes with moist gauze soaked in either chlorhexidene or saline. This procedure reduces clot thickness and achieves hemostasis. Postoperative instructions are given to the patient orally and in writing, and an ice pack is placed over the surgical site with instructions to apply it extraorally for 24 to 48 hours. The ice pack should be applied with light pressure and intermittently, not continuously. Continuous application of ice activates the body's protective mechanisms against frostbite by increasing blood flow to the area, thus increasing swelling.[52] Intermittent postoperative application of ice reduces the vascular rebound phenomenon, reduces postoperative swelling and edema,[51] and acts as

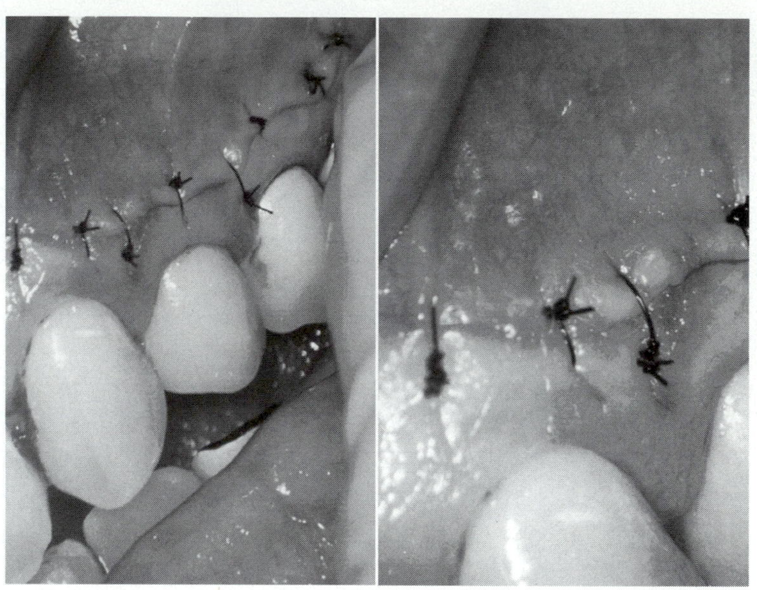

FIG. 19-60 Close apposition of wound edges facilitates primary closure. Careful placement of sutures reduces unnecessary trauma.

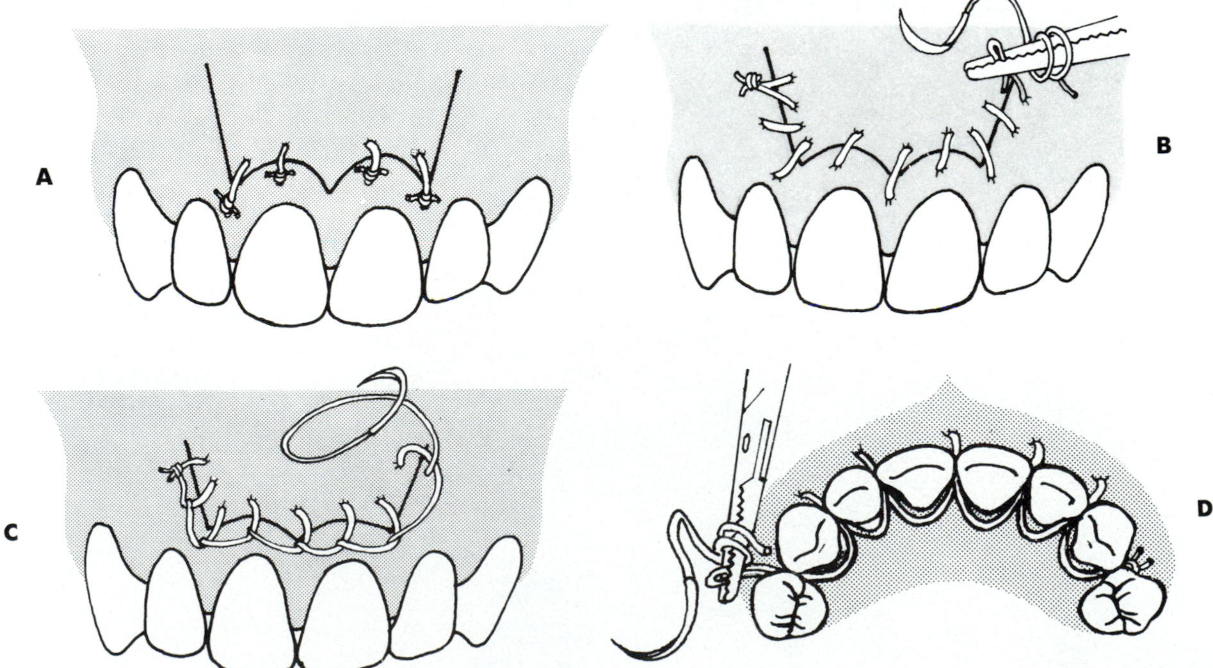

FIG. 19-61 Four suture techniques. **A,** Interrupted. **B,** Continuous mattress. **C,** Continuous blanket. **D,** Continuous sling.

an analgesic by interfering with pain fiber transmission. Patients should receive a postsurgical toothbrush with instructions on how to use it. The brush reduces plaque buildup without tearing or traumatizing the flap.

All patients should be contacted, preferably by the surgeon, that evening or if the surgery was performed late in the day the following morning. If this is not possible, patients should have a way of contacting their doctor by phone, should the need arise. Unlike most surgeons, dental surgeons release their patients immediately after surgery and there is very little recovery time or even adequate observation time. If a postsurgical problem occurs, the surgeon needs to be informed of it immediately so that corrective action can be taken.

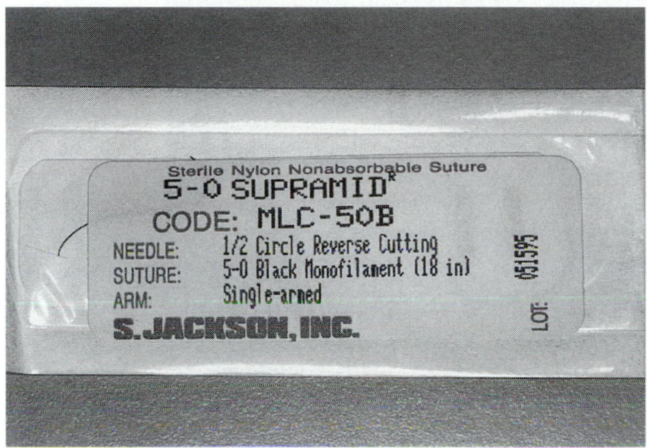

FIG. 19-62 Supramid nylon nonabsorbable suture.

POSTOPERATIVE COMPLICATIONS AND PATIENT MANAGEMENT

Possible postoperative sequelae include bleeding, infection, swelling, discoloration, pain, and delayed healing. Postsurgical bleeding and swelling can be managed by application of pressure with wet gauze or a wet chilled teabag (which contains tannic acid) for 20 to 30 minutes. If bleeding cannot be controlled by these measures, the patient should be seen by the doctor. If the doctor cannot control the bleeding with pressure techniques, a clotting deficiency should be suspected and the patient accompanied to the hospital for a hematologic workup. Postoperative pain after surgery is usually minimal and is managed appropriately with nonnarcotic analgesics.[31,76,142] Research has consistently shown that nonsteroidal antiinflammatory drugs administered preoperatively are more efficacious than opiate narcotics given after the pain develops.[30,31]

Presurgical administration of antibiotics is not indicated, and research shows that it may actually increase the probability of infection.[116,117] Surprisingly, postoperative infection is rare even though the procedure is performed in a sea of microorganisms. Most postoperative infections develop from either faulty aseptic technique or poor flap reapproximation and closure.[27,71,115]

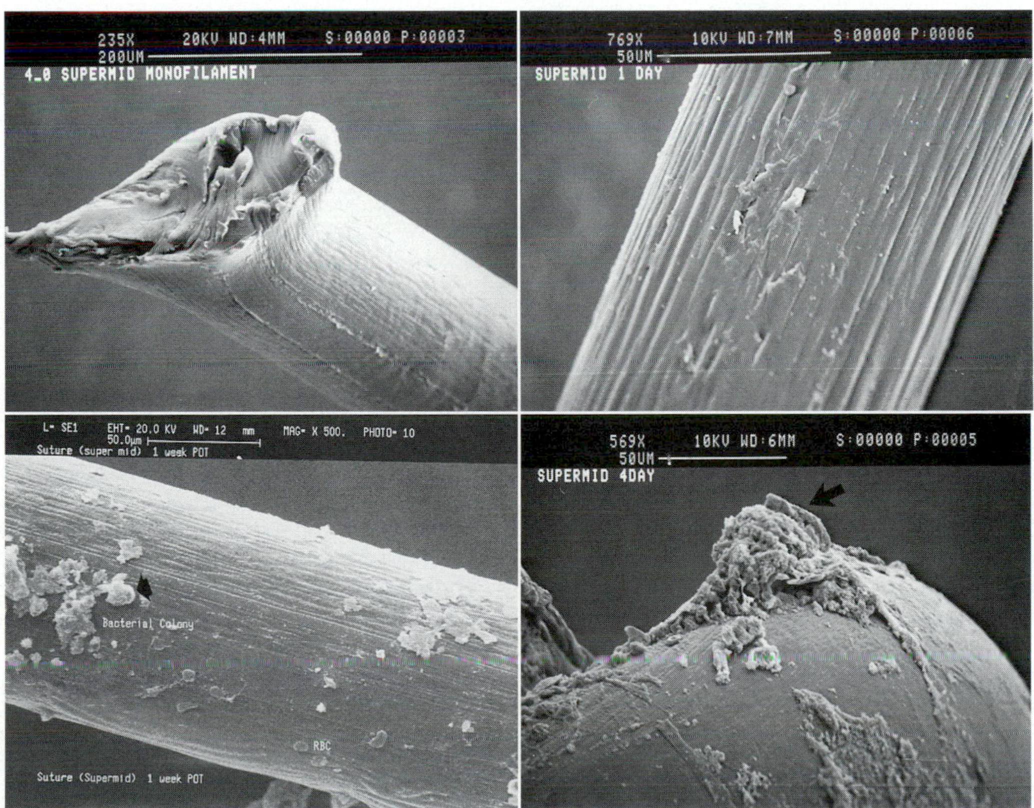

FIG. 19-63 Scanning electron micrographs of Supramid suture show minimal bacterial colonization. Bacterial colonization proceeds rapidly after 48 hours.

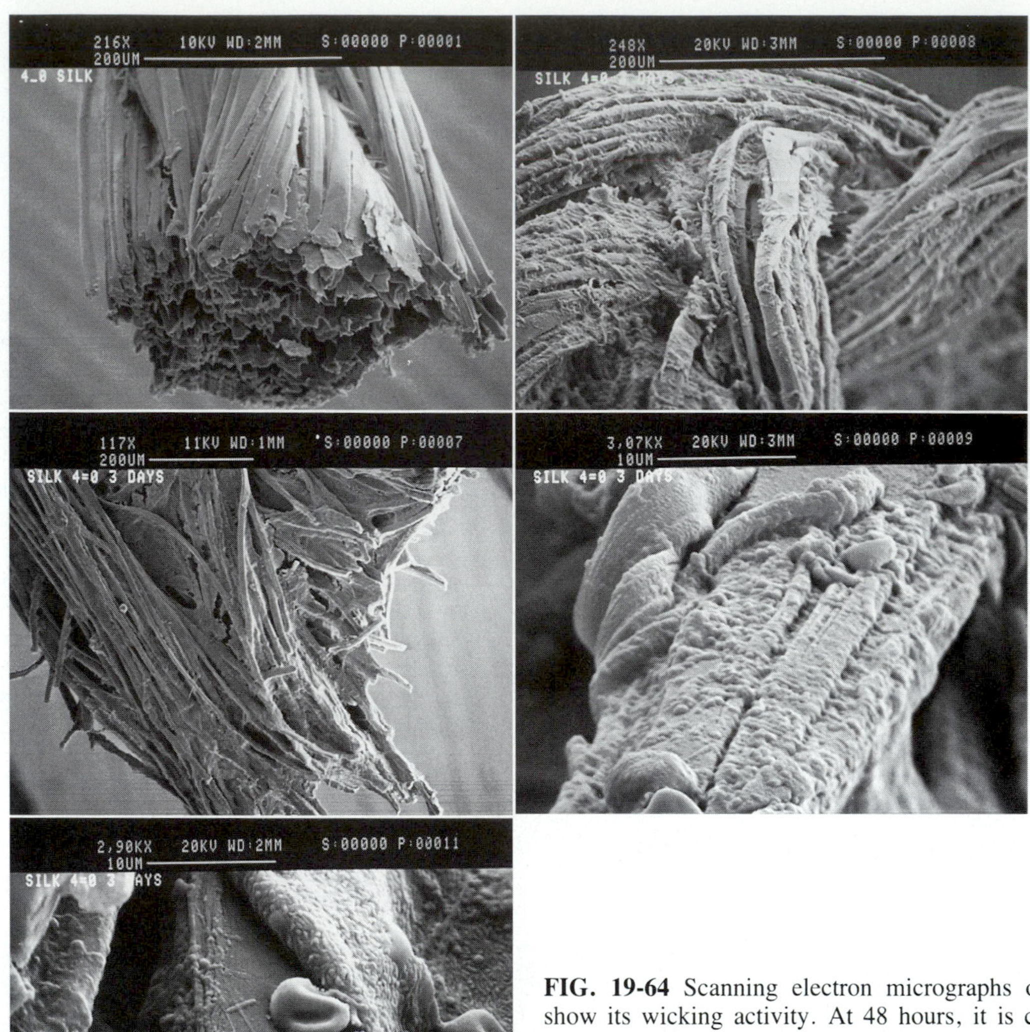

FIG. 19-64 Scanning electron micrographs of silk sutures show its wicking activity. At 48 hours, it is completely impregnated with bacterial colonies.

If infection is present, the antibiotic of choice is penicillin V potassium. If the patient is allergic to penicillin, erythromycin or clindamycin can be prescribed.[51] The patient should be monitored daily and the regimen changed if no improvement occurs. The only time antibiotics are routinely prescribed postoperatively, other than for medical reasons, is when during the surgical procedure the maxillary sinus or the floor of the nose has been perforated. These patients should begin taking antibiotics immediately postoperatively and continue for five days. These patients should also be covered with decongestants while the sinus membrane heals.

Postoperative care involves proper oral hygiene, chlorhexidene mouth rinses for four days, liquid food supplements (if needed), and rest. After the suture removal appointment, the patient should be checked again at 10 to 14 days, at which time all swelling and soreness should be gone. At six weeks, the soft tissue is evaluated again using a periodontal probe to check for a functional attachment.

Yearly recall for at least 2 years is suggested for follow-up care. It is not unusual to observe initial osseous healing after 2 years that is followed by periapical breakdown.[37]

Successful healing involves the cementogenic repair of the root apex, reestablishment of a functional periodontal ligament, and regeneration of apical alveolar bone (Fig. 19-65). Frequently, we must be satisfied with less than ideal healing, and many surgeries heal with a nonfunctional apical repair (i.e., a scar). Apical scars can be radiographically indistinguishable from recurrent disease, and such radiographic lesions should be monitored for changes in size and shape to determine if reentry is required. Postsurgical loss of function or symptomatic teeth with persistent periapical lesions indicate that the etiologic factors have not been eliminated by the surgery.

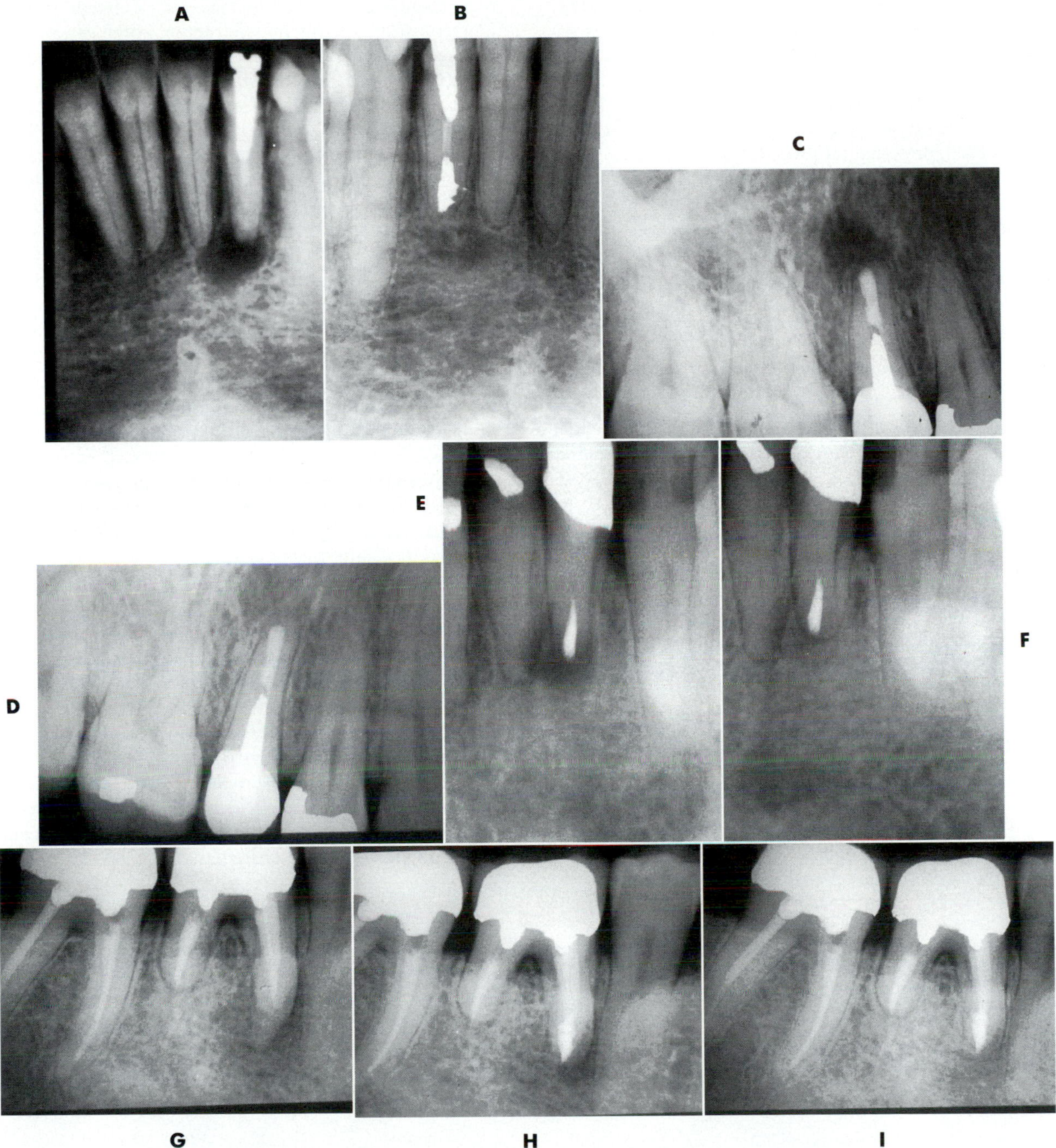

FIG. 19-65 A, Preoperative view shows large periapical lesion. **B,** Two-year recall shows regeneration of alveolar bone. **C,** Immediate postoperative radiograph shows Super EBA as a retrofilling material. **D,** Two-year recall examination shows resolution of the lesion and apical bone regeneration. **E,** Immediate postoperative radiograph shows Super EBA as a retrofilling material. **F,** One-year recall. **G,** Preoperative radiograph. **H,** Immediate postoperative radiograph with Super EBA retrofill. **I,** At 18-month recall there is good resolution of the lesion.

RECENT ADVANCES IN PERIRADICULAR SURGERY

The introduction of the operating microscope to endodontics has greatly enhanced the ability of the surgeon to inspect, prepare, and seal the apical ramifications. Before this technology was available, skillful manipulation of apical tissues required the use of high-powered loupes and surgical head lights (Fig. 19-66). Although these adjuncts afford the surgeon increased visibility, the surgical assistant frequently struggled with limited visibility and access. Because the range of magnification needed for periapical procedures varies from 3 to 30 times, the surgeon is forced to change loupes frequently during the procedure. The operating microscope (Fig. 19-67) provides commanding visual control over the surgical site for both the doctor and the first surgical assistant, in addition to providing five times the illumination of surgical head lights. This powerful tool enables the surgeon to change powers rapidly and with ease throughout the surgery. Having the first surgical assistant at the microscope permits the introduction of another pair of skilled hands into the surgical site and greatly facilitates the delicate procedures performed there. True surgical microscopes have the capability of adding documentation modules that allow simultaneous video and 35-mm photography with virtually no interruption in the surgical routine. This comprehensive documentation capability has applications in patient, doctor, and assistant education. It also provides a permanent record for insurance and legal purposes.[19]

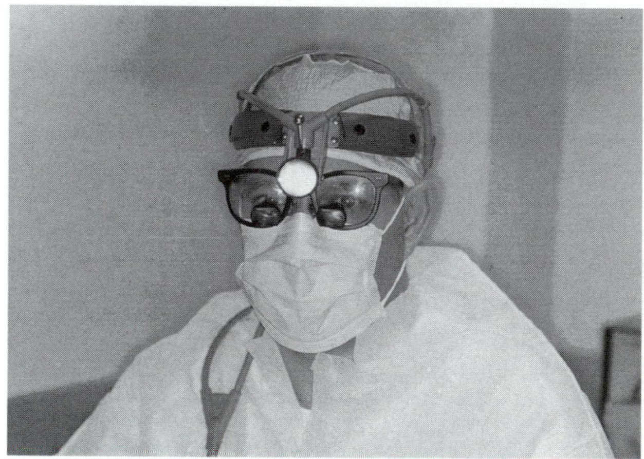

FIG. 19-66 Surgical head lamp and surgical telescopes provide the surgeon enhanced lighting and magnification.

The microsurgical approach to endodontic surgery has necessitated the development of a dedicated surgical armamentarium designed specifically for microsurgical procedures. The miniaturization of instruments to the appropriate scale allows the surgeon to take full advantage of the enhanced vision the microscope provides. Miniaturized optical-grade retromirrors (Excellence in Endodontics, Inc.) (Fig. 19-68) introduced into the surgical site allow examination in intimate detail of the apical anatomy of the beveled root system. These mirrors also permit close inspection of furcal defects and lateral root surfaces that previously were hidden from view. Particularly invaluable is the ability to inspect at high magnification and high illumination the lingual aspects of beveled roots, second canal systems, isthmuses, and aberrant portals of exit: all can be clearly seen (Fig. 19-69). Perhaps more important, the surgeon may decrease the bevel placed on these roots and can now section them more perpendicular to the long axis of the root. A highly skilled surgeon can section the root perpendicular to the long axis and inspect, prepare, and seal the root end indirectly, using a mirror (Fig. 19-70).

Working with upside-down images using a micromirror in tandem with an operating microscope demands a series of progressive skills that are mastered more easily by a dentist than by any other health professional. The development of microsurgical skills requires patience, practice, and an extraordinary amount of coordination among the surgical team. Achieving competence in this skill is well worth the effort and goes a long way toward reducing the level of stress that surgeons typically experience while performing difficult posterior surgery.

The application of the operating microscope not only to sur-

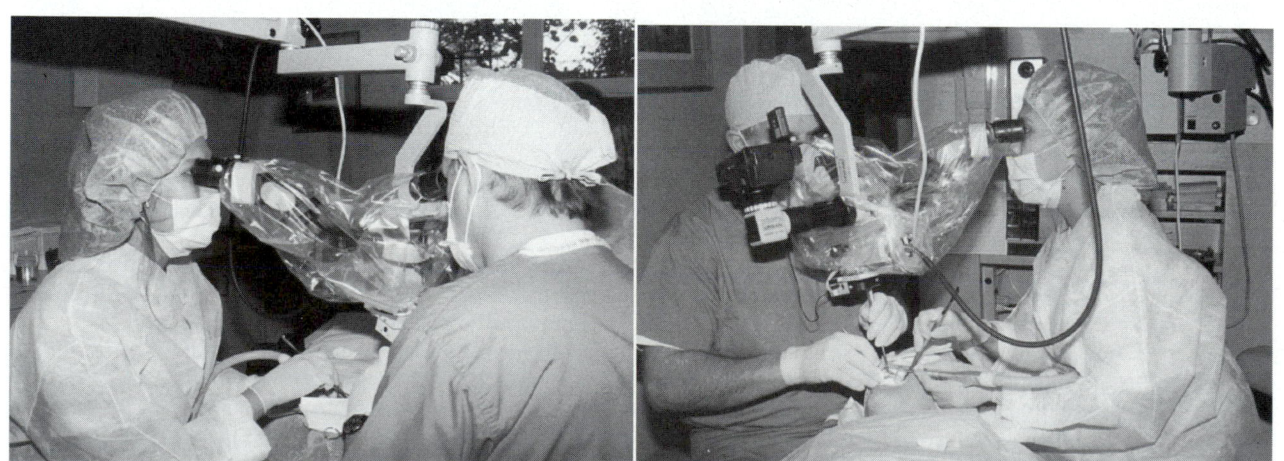

FIG. 19-67 A and **B,** True surgical operating microscope in use provides both doctor and first surgical assistant commanding visual control over the surgical site. The surgical operating microscope provides four to five times the light of surgical head lamps and varies the magnification from 3 to 30×.

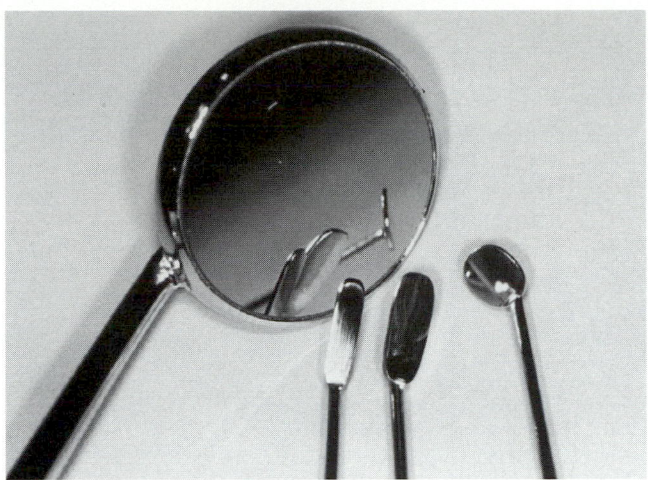

FIG. 19-68 Miniaturized optical-grade retromirrors.

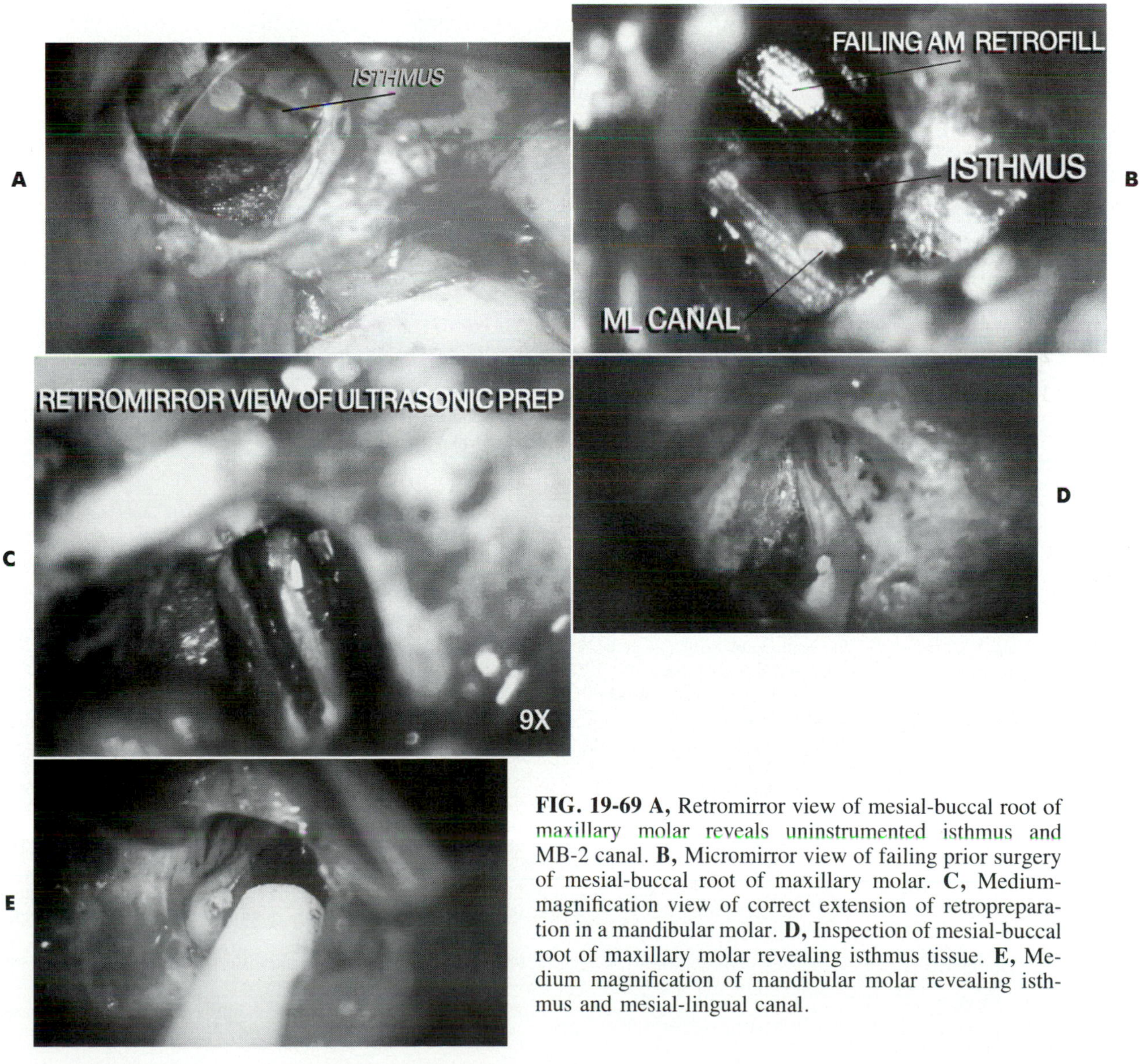

FIG. 19-69 A, Retromirror view of mesial-buccal root of maxillary molar reveals uninstrumented isthmus and MB-2 canal. **B,** Micromirror view of failing prior surgery of mesial-buccal root of maxillary molar. **C,** Medium-magnification view of correct extension of retropreparation in a mandibular molar. **D,** Inspection of mesial-buccal root of maxillary molar revealing isthmus tissue. **E,** Medium magnification of mandibular molar revealing isthmus and mesial-lingual canal.

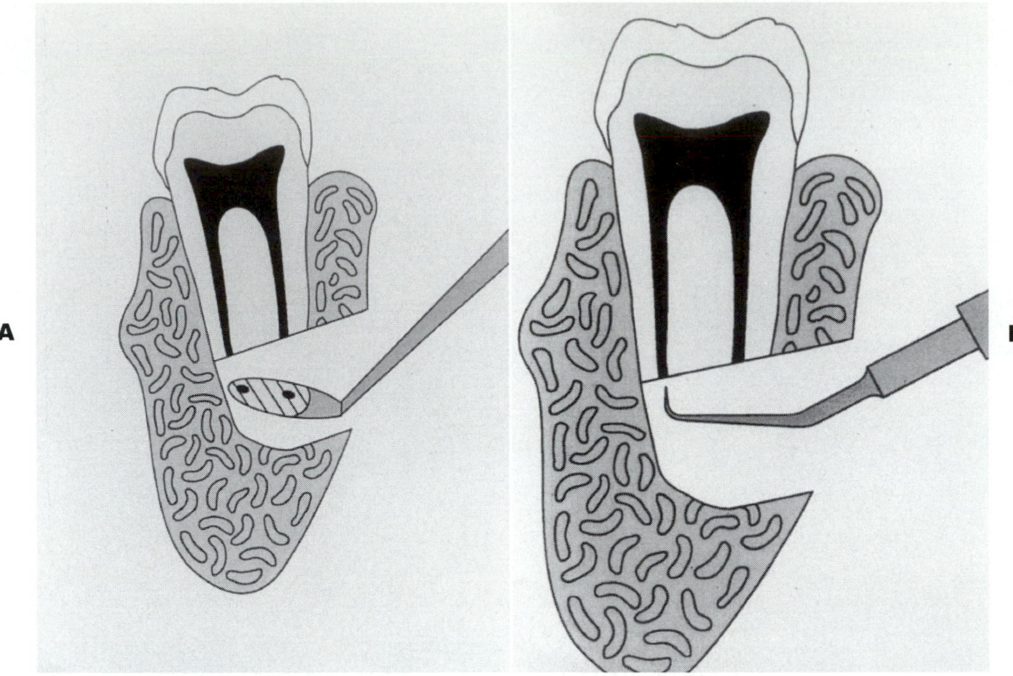

FIG. 19-70 A and **B,** Diagrammatic view of how a retromirror is used with a moderated bevel. The bevel is reduced, and all restorative procedures are done indirectly using the mirror.

gical endodontics but also to nonsurgical endodontics points to the next era in endodontics in which previously untreatable cases will be handled with great expertise by highly trained practitioners for the benefit of their patients. For the many benefits the operating microscope provides it represents the evolving state of the art and science in endodontics, but *it clearly does not represent the standard of care.*

REFERENCES

1. Arens DE, Adams WR, and DeCastro RA: Endodontic surgery, Philadelphia, 1981, Harper & Row.
2. Asboe-Jörgensen V, et al: Effect of chlorhexidene dressing on healing after periodontal surgery, J Periodontol 45:13, 1974.
3. Barber BCW, et al: Anatomy of root canals. II. Permanent maxillary molars, Aust Dent J 19:46, 1974.
4. Barber T, and Reisbick MH: Amalgam: past, present, future, J Am Dent Assoc 86:863, 1973.
5. Beltes P, et al: *In vitro* study of the sealing ability of four retrograde filling materials, Endod Dent Traumatol 4:82, 1988.
6. Bendra DL, et al: Leakage *in vitro* with IRM, high copper amalgam and EBA cement as retrofilling materials, J Endod 15:157, 1989.
7. Bennett CR: Monheim's local anesthesia and pain control in dental practice, ed 7, St. Louis, 1984, Mosby–Year Book.
8. Bergenholtz G, et al: Retreatment of endodontic fillings, Scand J Dent Res 87:217, 1979.
9. Beube FE: Study on reattachment of the supporting structures of the teeth, J Periodontol 18:55, 1947.
10. Beube FE: Factors in the repair of the alveolar bone and cementum, Oral Surg 2:379, 1949.
11. Block RM, and Bushell A: Retrograde amalgam procedures for mandibular posterior teeth, J Endod 8:107, 1982.
12. Block RM, and Lewis RD: Surgical treatment of iatrogenic canal blockages, Oral Surg 63:722, 1987.
13. Blomstedt B, and Osterberg B: Suture materials and wound infection, Acta Chir Scand 144:269, 1978.
14. Bloomquist DS: Pain control in endodontics, Dent Clin North Am 23:543, 1979.
15. Blum T: Life span of teeth whose roots have been resected, NY J Dent 15:60, 1945.
16. Burke IT: Retrofilling, Oral Surg 48:254, 1979.
17. Calderwood RG, et al: A comparison of the healing rate of bone after production of defects by various rotary instruments, J Dent Res 43:207, 1964.
18. Cambruzzi JV, and Marshall FJ: Molar endodontic surgery, J Can Dent Assoc 49:61, 1983.
19. Carr GB: Microscopes in endodontics, J Calif Dent Assoc 11:55, 1992.
20. Carr GB: Ultrasonic root-end preparation (Accepted for pub) J Endod, 1993.
21. Cobden RH, Thrasher EL, and Harris WH: Topical hemostatic agents to reduce bleeding from cancellous bone, J Bone Joint Surg 58:70, 1976.
22. Coolidge ED: Anatomy of the root apex in relation to the treatment problems, J Am Dent Assoc 1456, 1929.
23. Cooper SA, et al: Comparative analgesic potency of aspirin and ibuprofen, J Oral Surg 35:898, 1977.
24. Costick ER, Youngblood PJ, and Walden JM: A study of the effects of high-speed rotary instruments on bone repair in dogs, Oral Surg 17:563, 1964.
25. Cummings RR, et al: Endodontic surgery. In Ingle JI (ed): Endodontics, ed 3, Philadelphia, 1985, Lea & Febiger.
26. Cunningham J: The seal of root fillings at apicoectomy, Br Dental J 139:430, 1975.
27. Curren JB, Kennet S, and Young AR: An assessment of the use of prophylactic antibiotics in third molar surgery, Int J Oral Surg 3:1, 1974.
28. Curson I: Endodontics techniques—apical surgery, Br Dent J 121:470, 1966.
29. Dedolph TH, and Clark HB: A histological study of mucoperiosteal flap healing, J Oral Surg 16:367, 1958.

30. Dionne RA, and Cooper SA: Evaluation of preoperative ibuprofen for postoperative pain after removal of third molars, Oral Surg 45:851, 1978.
31. Dionne RA, et al: Suppression of postoperative administration of ibuprofen in comparison to placebo, acetaminophen and acetominorphin plus codeine, J Clin Pharmacol 23:37, 1983.
32. Dorn S, and Gartner A: Retrograde filling materials: a retrospective success-failure study of amalgam, EBA, and IRM, J Endod 16:1990.
33. Eames WB, et al: The effects of saliva contamination on dental amalgam, J Am Dent Assoc 86:652, 1973.
34. Ferguson MM, and Silverman S: Endocrine disease. In Jones JH, Mason DK (eds): Oral manifestations of systemic disease, London, 1980, WB Saunders.
35. Forrest L: Current concepts in soft connective tissue wound healing, Br J Surg 70:133, 1983.
36. Forssell H, et al: A follow-up study of apicoectomized teeth, Proc Finn Dent Soc 84:2:2, 1988.
37. Frank A, et al: Long-term evaluation of surgically placed amalgam filling, J Endod 18:391, 1992.
38. Frank A, et al: Clinical and surgical endodontics—concepts in practice, Philadelphia, 1983, JB Lippincott.
39. Friedman S, et al: Treatment results of apical surgery in premolar and molar teeth, J Endod 17:30, 1991.
40. Gabbiani G, et al: Granulation tissue as a contractile organ, J Exp Med 135:719, 1972.
41. Gage TW: Pharmacology of the autonomic nervous system. In Holyroyd SV, Wynn RL, and Requa-Clark B (eds): Clinical pharmacology in dental practice, ed 4, St Louis, 1988, Mosby–Year Book.
42. Gerstein H: Surgical endodontics. In Laskin DN (ed): Oral and maxillofacial surgery—II, St. Louis, 1985, Mosby–Year book.
43. Goldman HM, and Cohen DW: Periodontal therapy, ed 5, St Louis, 1973, Mosby–Year Book.
44. Gotthelf TS, and Rose LF: Diabetes mellitus. In Lynch MA (ed): Burket's oral medicine, ed 8, Philadelphia, 1984, JB Lippincott.
45. Green D: A stereo microscope study of 700 root apicies of maxillary and mandibular posterior teeth, OOO 22:375, 1960.
46. Grung B, et al: Periapical surgery in a Norwegian county hospital: follow-up findings of 477 teeth, J Endod 16:411, 1990.
47. Guldener PHA, and Langeland K: Endodontologie, Stuttgart, 1982, Georg Thieme Verlag.
48. Gutmann JL: Principles of endodontic surgery for the general practitioner, Dent Clin North Am 28:895, 1984.
49. Gutmann JL: Surgical procedures in endodontic practice. In Levine N (ed): Current treatment in dental practice, Philadelphia, 1986, WB Saunders.
50. Gutmann JL, and Harrison JW: Posterior endodontic surgery: anatomical considerations and clinical techniques, Int Endod J 18:8, 1985.
51. Gutmann JL, and Harrison JW: Surgical endodontics, Boston, 1991, Blackwell Scientific Publications.
52. Guyton AC: Textbook of medical physiology, ed 7, St. Louis, 1986, Mosby–Year Book.
53. Haasch GC, Gersteirn H, and Austin BP: Effects of two hemostatic agents on osseous *healing,* J Endod 15:310, 1989.
54. Hansen LS, and Silverman S: Localized tissue reaction to implanted amalgam: a review, J Calif Dent Assoc 10:33, 1982.
55. Harnish H: Apicoectomy, Berlin, 1975, Quintessenz Verlag-GmbH.
56. Harris M: Apicoectomy and retrograde amalgam in mandibular molar teeth, Oral Surg 48:405, 1979.
57. Harrison JW, and Jurosky KA: Wound healing in the tissues of the periodontium following periradicular surgery. II. The dissectional wound, J Endod 17:544, 1991.
58. Harrison JW, and Jurosky KA: Wound healing in the tissues of the periodontium following periradicular surgery. II. The incisional wound, J Endod 17:425, 1991.
59. Hartley F, et al: The success rate of apicoectomy—a retrospective study of 1,016 cases, Br Dent J 129:407, 1970.
60. Haupl K: Om rot-amputasjoner under saelig hensyntagen til rotfyllingsspormalet og operasjonsteknikken, Nor Tannlaegeforen Tid 42:37, 1932.
61. Hermann JB: Changes in tensile strength and knot security of surgical sutures *in vivo,* Arch Surg 106:707, 1973.
62. Hess W, and Zurcher E: The anatomy of the root canals of the permanent dentition, New York, 1925, William Wood & Co.
63. Hiatt WH, et al: Repair following mucoperiosteal flap surgery with full gingival retention, J Periodontol 39:11, 1968.
64. Hill TR: Surgical endodontics. In Harty FJ, and Roberts DH (eds): Restorative procedures for the practising dentist, Bristol, 1974, John Wright & Sons Ltd.
65. Hirsch J, et al: Periapical surgery, Int J Oral Surg 8:173, 1979.
66. Ighbaut J, et al: Progenitor cell kinetics during guided tissue regeneration in experimental periodontal wounds, J Periodont Res 23:107, 1988.
67. James GA: Simplified techniques in surgical periapical treatment, Dent Clin North Am 7:375, 1963.
68. Johnson LB, and Paffenbarger GC: The role of zinc in dental amalgams, J Dent Res 59:1412, 1980.
69. Jones NB: Dietary needs of the oral surgery patient with comparison of dietary supplements, J Oral Surg 28:892, 1970.
70. Kaplan SD, et al: A comparison of the marginal leakage of retrograde techniques, Oral Surg 54:583, 1982.
71. Karl RC, et al: Prophylactic antimicrobial drugs in surgery, N Engl J Med 275:305, 1966.
72. Kerekes K, and Tronstad L: Morphometric observations on the root canals of human molars, JOE 3:114, 1977.
73. Kirchoff DA: Localized argyria after a surgical endodontic procedure, Oral Surg 32:613, 1971.
74. Klinsberg J, and Butcher EO: Epithelial femetar in periodontal repair in the rat, J Periodontol 34:315, 1963.
75. Kohler CA, and Ramfjord SP: Healing of gingival mucoperiosteal flaps, Oral Surg 13:89, 1960.
76. Kusner G, et al: A study comparing the effectiveness of ibuprofen (Motrin), Empirin with codeine #3 and Synalgos-DC for relief of post-endodontic pain, J Endod 10:210, 1984.
77. Lavelle C, and Wedgewood D: Effect of internal irrigation on frictional heat generated from bone drilling, J Oral Surg 38:499, 1980.
78. Lemon RR, Steel PJ, and Jeansonne BG: Ferric sulfate hemostasis: effect on osseous wound healing. I. Left *in situ* for maximum exposure, J Endod, 1993 (in press).
79. Leubke RG, et al: Indications and contraindications for endodontic surgery, Oral Surg 7:97, 1964.
80. Leubke RG: Surgical endodontics, Dent Clin North Am 18:379, 1974.
81. Levine LH: Periodontal flap surgery with gingival fiber retention, J Periodontol 43:91, 1972.
82. Liggett WR, et al: Light microscopy, scanning electron microscopy and microprobe analysis of bone response to zinc and non-zinc amalgam implants, Oral Surg 49:263, 1980.
83. Lilly GE: Reaction of oral tissues to suture materials, Oral Surg 26:128, 1968.
84. Linghorne WJ, and O'Connell DC: Studies in the regeneration and reattachment of supporting structures of the teeth. I. Soft tissue reattachment, J Dent Res 29:419, 1950.
85. Linghorne WJ, and O'Connell DC: Studies in the regeneration and reattachment of supporting structures of the teeth. II. Regeneration of alveolar process, J Dent Res 30:604, 1951.
86. Little JW, and Falac DA: Dental management of the medically compromised patient, ed 3, St Louis, 1988, The CV Mosby Co.
87. Lucas CD: Root resection and apical canal filling after resection, Dent Summary 36:201, 1916.
88. Lucas CD: Technique of root resection, Dent Summary 6:793, 1919.
89. Lunskag J: Heat and bone tissue, Scand J Plast Reconstr Surg 9(suppl):1, 1972.
90. Mach SD, and Krizek TJ: Sutures and suturing—current concepts, J Oral Surg 36:710, 1978.
91. Majno G, et al: Contraction of granulation tissue *in vivo:* similarity to smooth muscle, Science 173:548, 1971.

92. Marcotte LR, Donson J, and Rowe NM: Apical healing with retrofilling materials amalgam gutta percha, J Endod 1:63, 1975.
93. Mason RM: Hemostatic mechanisms of microfibuillar collagen. In Proceedings of a symposium on avitene (MCH), Ft. Worth, Tex., 1975, Alcon Laboratories Inc.
94. Matsura ST: A simplified root-end filling technique, J Mich St Dent Assoc 44:40, 1962.
95. Melcher AH, et al: Synthesis of cementium-like tissue *in vitro* by cells cultured from bone: a light and electron microscope study, J Periodontal Res 21:592, 1986.
96. Messing JT, and Stock CJR: A colour atlas of endodontics, London, 1988, Wolfe Medical Pub Ltd.
97. Metcher AH, et al: Cells from bone synthesize cementum-like and bone-like tissue in vitro and may migrate into periodontal ligament in vivo, J Periodont Res 22:246, 1987.
98. Meyer VW: Die anatomic der wurzelkanäle, Dargestellt an mikroskopischen rekonstruktionsmodellen, Dtsch Zahnärztl Z 25:1064, 1970.
99. Michalls E: The role of surgery in endodontics, Br Dent J 118:59, 1965.
100. Mikkonen M, et al: Clinical and radiographic re-examination of apicoectomized teeth, Oral Surg 302:3, 1983.
101. Milam SB, and Grovannittii JA: Local anesthetics in dental practice, Dent Clin North Am 28:493, 1984.
102. Moberg LE: Electrochemical properties of corroded amalgams, Scand JJ Dent Res 441, 1987.
103. Moodnik R, et al: Retrograde amalgam filling: a scanning electron microscope study, J Endod 1:28, 1975.
104. Moorehead FB: Root-end resection, Dent Cosmos 69:463, 1927.
105. Morris ML: Healing of naturally occurring periodontal pockets about vital human teeth, J Periodontol 26:285, 1955.
106. Morris ML: Healing of naturally occurring periodontal pockets: preliminary report of the effects of external pressure, J Periodontol 32:202, 1961.
107. Nehammer CF: Surgical endondontics, Br Dent J 158:400, 1985.
108. Nespeca JA: Clinical trials with bupivacaine in oral surgery, Oral Surg 42:301, 1976.
109. Nicholls E: Retrograde filling of the root canal, Oral Surg 15:463, 1962.
110. Nicholls E: The role of surgery in endodontics, Br Dent J 118:59, 1965.
111. Okumura T: Anatomy of the root canal, In Trans 7, Int Dent Congress 1:170, 1926.
112. Omnell KA: Electrolytic precipitation of zinc carbonate in the jaw: an unusual complication after root resection, Oral Surg 12:848, 1959.
113. Osterberg B, and Blomstedt B: Effect of suture materials on bacterial survival in infected wounds, Acta Chir Scand 145:431, 1979.
114. Oynick J, and Oynick T: A study of a new material for retrograde fillings, J Endod 4:203, 1978.
115. Pack PD, and Haber J: The incidence of clinical infection after periodontal surgery: a retrospective study, J Periodontol 54:441, 1983.
116. Paterson JA, Cardo VA, and Stratigos GP: An examination of antibiotic prophylaxis in oral and maxillofacial surgery, J Oral Surg 28:753, 1970.
117. Pendrill K, and Riddy J: The use of prophylactic penicillin in peridontal surgery, J Periodontol 51:44, 1980.
118. Pricco DF: An evolution of bupivacaine in oral surgery, 35:126, 1977.
119. Proge MP, and Polson AM: Effect of root surfaces alterations on periodontal healing. I. Surgical denudation, J Clin Periodontol 9:428, 1982.
120. Quaranta M: Attuali orientamenti sulle possibilita e i limitidella chirugia periapicale, Riv Ital Stomatol 52:1015, 1983.
121. Register AA: Bone and cementum induction by dentin demineralized *in situ*, J Periodontol 44:49, 1973.
122. Register AA, and Burdick FA: Accelerated reattachment with cementogenesis to dentin demineralized in situ. I. Optimum range, J Periodontol 46:646, 1975.
123. Reit C, and Hirsch J: Surgical endodontic retreatment, Int Endod J 19:107, 1986.
124. Roberts DH, and Sowray JH: Local analgesia in dentistry, ed 2, Bristol, 1987, John Wright & Sons.
125. Rohrich RJ, and Spicer TE: Wound healing/hypertrophic scars and keloids. Selected readings in plastic surgery 4:1, 1986.
126. Ross JW: Retrograde root-filling in oral surgery, Trans Cong Int Assoc Oral Surg 4:98, 1973.
127. Rovee DT, and Miller CA: Epidermal role in the breaking strength of wounds, Arch Surg 96:43, 1968.
128. Ruben MP, et al: Healing of periodontal surgical wounds. In Goldman HM, and Cohen DW (eds): Periodontal therapy, ed 6, St. Louis, 1980, Mosby–Year Book.
129. Rud J, and Andreasen J: Operative procedures in periapical surgery with contemporaneous root fillings, Int J Oral Surg 1:297, 1972.
130. Ryan GB, et al: Myofiberblasts in human granulation tissue, Hum Pathol 5:55, 1974.
131. Schoonover IC, et al: Excessive expansion of dental amalgam, J Am Dent Assoc 29:1825, 1942.
132. Seifter E, et al: Impaired wound healing with streptozotain diabetes, Ann Surg 194:42, 1981.
133. Stock CJR, and Nehammer CF: Endodontics in practice, Br Dent Assoc 123, 1985.
134. Szeremeta-Brower TL, et al: A comparison of the sealing properties of different techniques: an autoradiographic study, Oral Surg 59:82, 1985.
135. Tanzilli JP, Raphael D, and Moodnik RM: A comparison of the marginal adaptation of retrograde techniques: a scanning electron microscope study, Oral Surg 50:74, 1980.
136. Tayler AC, and Campbell MM: Reattachment of gingival epithelium to the tooth, J Periodontol 43:281, 1972.
137. Telsch P: Development of raised temperatures after osteotomies, J Maxillofac Surg 2:141, 1974.
138. Thompson HC: Effect of drilling into bone, J Oral Surg 16:22, 1958.
139. Tronstad L, et al: Sealing ability of dental amalgams as retrograde fillings in endodontic therapy, J Endod 9:551, 1983.
140. Van Gunst ICA, and Hertog HJPM: On the relation between delayed expansion of amalgam and the composition of amalgam alloys, Br Dent J 103:428, 1957.
141. Van Winkle W, and Hastings JC: Considerations in the choice of suture material for various tissues, Surg Gynecol Obstet 135:113, 1972.
142. Vogel RI, and Gross JI: The effects of nonsteroidal anti-inflammatory analgesics on pain after periodontal surgery, J Am Dent Assoc 109:731, 1984.
143. Weine FS: Endodontic therapy, St. Louis, 1989, Mosby–Year Book.
144. Weine FS, and Gerstein H: Periapical surgery. In Weine FS (ed): Endodontic therapy, ed 4, St. Louis, 1989, Mosby–Year Book.
145. Weine F, et al: Canal configuration in the mesio-buccal root of maxillary first molar and its endodontic significance, Oral Surg 28:419, 1969.
146. Wirthlin MB: The current status of new attachment therapy, J Periodontol 52:529, 1981.
147. Zartner R, James G, and Burch B: Bone tissue response to zinc polycarboxylate cement and zinc-free amalgam, J Endod 2:203, 1976.

Self-assessment questions

1. Unless the benefit-risk ratio is high, surgery should be avoided by
   a. "brittle diabetics."
   b. dialysis patients.
   c. immunocompromised patients.
   d. all of the above.
2. Which of the following statements regarding the presurgical workup is false?
   a. It is performed by the surgical assistant.
   b. The patient is informed of the nature of the procedure.
   c. The patient's medical history is reviewed and blood pressure is checked.
   d. None of the above.
3. Maximum hemostasis is obtained by depositing anesthetic
   a. into the attached gingiva.
   b. into the papillae.
   c. into the alveolar mucosa.
   d. into all of the above.
4. 2% Lidocaine with 1:50,000 Epinephrine
   a. is contraindicated in the medically compromised patient.
   b. is administered after anesthesia is obtained.
   c. provides anesthesia and analgesia.
   d. is deposited in multiple injections into the vestibular tissues apical to the root apices.
5. The triangular/rectangular flap with sulcular incision
   a. provides the best access of all flaps.
   b. has no disadvantages.
   c. compromises the blood supply to the flap.
   d. elevation begins at the junction of the horizontal and vertical incision.
6. Which of the following statements concerning the triangular/rectangular flap with mucogingival incision is false?
   a. This flap is contraindicated with short roots.
   b. Survival of marginal gingiva depends on secondary blood supply.
   c. Because tissue reapproximation is simplified, scar formation is minimal.
   d. It is popular because marginal gingiva is undisturbed.
7. The most common cause of flap injury is
   a. insufficient extension of releasing incisions.
   b. excessive tension by sutures.
   c. using undermining elevation.
   d. improper retractor positioning.
8. Which of the following statements concerning apical curettage is true?
   a. Apical curettage is definitive treatment.
   b. Not all curetted soft tissue needs to be submitted for biopsy.
   c. Bony access should be enlarged to remove the lesion in toto.
   d. All of the above.
9. The angle of the beveled resected root
   a. should be sufficient to provide access to perform the retropreparation.
   b. is rarely greater than it appears to be.
   c. should be at 45 degrees to the facial surface.
   d. All of the above.
10. Ferric subsulfate
    a. is used to identify the complete outline of the root.
    b. is painted on the wall of the bony crypt to provide hemostasis.
    c. acts by causing intravascular coagulation.
    d. All of the above.
11. All beveled root canal fillings
    a. can be easily evaluated.
    b. leak.
    c. can be hermetically sealed by retrofilling without a magnification system.
    d. should be retrofilled only if there is an apparent incompletely sealed root canal system.
12. Which of the following is not a requirement for retropreparations?
    a. All isthmus tissue must be removed.
    b. In roots with one canal the shape is usually round.
    c. It must be parallel to the anatomic outline of the pulpal space.
    d. It must be at least 3 mm deep.
13. Ultrasonic root end preparations
    a. eliminate the bevel.
    b. facilitate ideal preparation.
    c. conserve root structure.
    d. All of the above.
14. Characteristics of an ideal retrofilling material include all of the following except
    a. long-term sealing ability.
    b. unaffected by moisture.
    c. slight expansion on setting.
    d. nonresorbable.
15. The retrofilling material that offers the most advantages to date is
    a. amalgam and cavity varnish.
    b. composite resin.
    c. IRM or EBA.
    d. polycarboxylate cement.
16. Sutures
    a. do not impede wound healing.
    b. ideally should be removed after 48 hours.
    c. are placed by proceeding from the attached tissue to the unattached tissue.
    d. All of the above.
17. Postoperative care does not include
    a. continuous application of an ice pack.
    b. chlorhexidene mouth rinses.
    c. written postoperative instructions.
    d. None of the above.
18. The operating microscope can
    a. enhance the ability of the surgeon to inspect, prepare, and seal the apex.
    b. be useful in patient education.
    c. provide a permanent record for insurance purposes.
    d. All of the above.

Chapter 20

The Management of Pain and Anxiety

Stanley F. Malamed

The problem of managing pain and anxiety in the practice of dentistry is a significant one. Studies have demonstrated that the major reason that over 50% of adult Americans do not seek routine dental care is fear of pain. Interviews with patients indicate that although they may not be in pain when they visit their dentist, the overwhelming majority truly believe that at some time during a dental appointment they will experience pain. The person most frequently cited as being responsible for this discomfort is the dentist.

Pain and anxiety are entirely different problems, yet at the same time they are closely related. Pain produced by dental treatment can usually be minimized or entirely prevented through thoughtful patient management and the judicious use of the techniques of pain control, especially local anesthesia. Anxiety, too, can usually be managed effectively; however, before anxiety can be managed, it must be recognized. Discovery of the cause of a patient's anxiety is the major factor in managing the problem. Once aware of a patient's fears, the dentist has many techniques available with which to care for the patient.

In most areas of dental treatment, the problem of anxiety control is greater than the management of pain. Pain control is usually readily obtained with a local anesthetic. Once effective pain control is established, anxiety control usually is more readily achievable. In endodontics more than in any other specialty of dentistry, pain control often proves to be more of a difficult problem than the management of anxiety. Because of this difficulty in achieving effective pain control, the patient undergoing endodontic treatment often anticipates the experience with a great deal of apprehension.

The following discussion covers the dual problems of pain control and anxiety control, with special emphasis on the pulpally involved tooth.

PAIN CONTROL

Although achieving adequate pain control for endodontic care is not usually difficult, there appear to be all too many instances when a satisfactory result eludes the doctor. The most likely explanation for the greater percentage of anesthetic failures in endodontics than in other areas of dental care lies in the tissue changes that commonly develop in and around pulpally involved teeth. To help better understand the problems associated with pain control in endodontics, a review of the mode of action of local anesthetics is presented.

Local Anesthetics—How They Work

The commonly employed injectable local anesthetics are weakly alkaline and poorly soluble in water. To make them clinically useful, they are combined with hydrochloric acid to form hydrochloride salts, which are soluble in water and acid in reaction.

In solution, the salts of local anesthetics exist in two forms: an uncharged molecule (RN) and a positively charged cation (RNH^+). The relative proportions of each ionic form depend on the pH of the solution in the cartridge and the tissue and on the pK_a of the specific anesthetic drug. The pK_a is the pH value at which a solution contains equal amounts of the un-ionized base and the cationic form of the drug.

The pK_a for a given anesthetic is a constant. The values for several local anesthetics are listed in Table 20-1. Because pK_a is a constant, the relative proportion of free base (RN) and charged cation (RNH^+) in the local anesthetic solution will depend on the pH of the solution.

$$RNH^+ \rightleftharpoons RN + H^+$$

As the pH of the anesthetic solution decreases (i.e., as it becomes more acid), hydrogen ion (H^+) concentrations increase and the equilibrium in the equation shifts toward the charged cationic form. Proportionally more cation will be present than free base. Conversely, if the pH of the solution is increased (more basic) the H^+ concentration decreases and a proportionally greater percentage of the local anesthetic exists in the free base form.

At normal tissue pH of 7.4, it can be seen (Table 20-1) that there is a greater proportion of anesthetic cation than of anesthetic base. Both forms of the anesthetic drug are essential for its anesthetic activity.[35,36]

For years it was thought that the un-ionized base form of the anesthetic solution was solely responsible for producing nerve block. Studies demonstrated that local anesthetics were more effective when prepared as alkaline solutions.[32,34] The cationic form was thought to be merely a convenient water-soluble vehicle, devoid of any anesthetic properties, for dispersion of the solution through tissues. It has been demonstrated, however, that several factors are involved in the ultimate anesthetic profile of a local anesthetic. These include (1) diffusion of the local anesthetic through the lipid-rich nerve sheath *(pK_a and lipid solubility)* and (2) binding of the local anesthetic at the receptor site *(protein binding, nonnervous tissue diffusibility,* and *intrinsic vasodilator activity)* (Table 20-2).[10] Researchers[35,36] evaluated the relationship between the pH of solutions, the presence or absence of a nerve sheath, and anesthetic activity. They concluded that both ionic forms of the anesthetic molecule are involved in the process of nerve sheath penetration and conduction block. The lipid-soluble uncharged (RN) base diffuses more easily through the nerve sheath than does the water-soluble cationic (RNH^+) form. Clinically, local anesthetics with a lower pK_a (more uncharged RN molecules) possess a more rapid onset of action than do those with a higher pK_a (Table 20-1).

The degree of lipid solubility appears to be important in determining the intrinsic anesthetic potency of a local anesthetic. Table 20-3 lists approximate lipid solubility of various local anesthetics. Increasing lipid solubility permits the anesthetic to penetrate the nerve membrane (which is 90% lipid) more easily.[5] This is reflected biologically as increased potency. Local anesthetics with greater lipid solubility produce more effective conduction blockade at lower concentrations than do less soluble drugs.

After penetration of the nerve sheath, a reequilibrium occurs between the base and cationic forms. Now, at the cell membrane itself, the charged cation binds to the protein receptor site in the sodium channel. Protein binding of the anesthetic molecule is responsible for (1) suppression of the electrophysiologic events occurring in propagation of a nerve impulse and (2) the duration of anesthetic activity. Proteins comprise approximately 10% of the nerve membrane. Local anesthetics (e.g., etidocaine, bupivacaine) possessing a greater degree of protein binding (Table 20-4)) than others (e.g., procaine) appear to attach more securely to protein receptor sites and are longer acting.

Figure 20-1 illustrates the sequence of events involved in peripheral nerve block in normal tissues. At a pH of 7.4, an anesthetic with a pK_a of 7.9 will reach equilibrium in the tissues with approximately 75% of its molecules in the cationic form and 25% in the base form. The base form can pass through the barrier to diffusion represented by the nerve sheath (epineurium) more readily than can the cationic form. Once the nerve sheath is penetrated, the RN molecules encounter a pH of 7.4 in the intracellular tissues surrounding the nerve membrane. The pH of the tissues within the epineurium and surrounding the nerve itself remains quite uniform even in the presence of marked changes in pH of extracellular tissues. This is due to the fact that the H^+ ion, like the anesthetic cation, cannot easily penetrate lipoid tissues. The pH of extracellular

TABLE 20-1. Dissociation constants (pK_a) of local anesthetics

Agent	pK_a	% base (RN) at pH 7.4	Approximate onset of action (min)
Mepivacaine	7.6	40	2 to 4
Etidocaine	7.7	33	2 to 4
Articaine	7.8	29	2 to 4
Lidocaine	7.9	25	2 to 4
Prilocaine	7.9	25	2 to 4
Bupivacaine	8.1	18	5 to 8
Tetracaine	8.5	8	10 to 15
Chloroprocaine	8.7	6	10 to 15
Procaine	9.1	2	14 to 18

TABLE 20-2. Summary of factors that affect local anesthetic action

Factor	Action affected	Description
pK_a	Onset	Lower pK_a = More rapid onset of action; more RN molecules present to diffuse through nerve sheath; onset time decreased
Lipid solubility	Anesthetic potency	Increased lipid solubility = Increased potency (Example: procaine = 1; etidocaine = 140) Etidocaine produces conduction blockade at very low concentrations whereas procaine poorly suppresses nerve conduction, even at higher concentrations
Protein binding	Duration	Increased protein binding allows anesthetic cations (RNH^+) to be more firmly attached to proteins located at receptor sites; thus duration of action is increased
Nonnervous tissue diffusibility	Onset	Increased diffusibility = Decreased time of onset
Vasodilator activity	Anesthetic potency and duration	Greater vasodilator activity = Increased blood flow to region = Rapid removal of anesthetic from injection site; thus decreased potency and decreased duration of anesthetic

TABLE 20-3. Lipid solubility of local anesthetics

Agent	Approximate lipid solubility	Usual effective concentration (%)
Procaine	1	2 to 4
Mepivacaine	1	2 to 3
Prilocaine	1.5	4
Lidocaine	4	2
Bupivacaine	30	0.5 to 0.75
Tetracaine	80	0.15
Etidocaine	140	0.5 to 0.75
Articaine	—	—
Chloroprocaine	—	—

TABLE 20-4. Protein-binding characteristics and duration of action of local anesthetics

Agent	Approximate protein binding	Approximate duration of action (min)
Procaine	5	60 to 90
Prilocaine	55	100 to 240
Lidocaine	65	90 to 200
Mepivacaine	75	120 to 240
Tetracaine	85	180 to 600
Etidocaine	94	180 to 600
Bupivacaine	95	180 to 600
Articaine	95	—
Chloroprocaine	—	—

fluid may therefore differ from the pH at the nerve membrane, and similarly the ratio of anesthetic base to cation at these sites may differ. In this environment reequilibration occurs with approximately 75% of the base reverting to the cation form, attaching to the receptor sites and producing neural blockade.

The "Pulpally Involved" Tooth

The problem of inadequate pain control during endodontics can be explained, in part, through changes occurring in periapical tissues. Pulpal and apical pathology (inflammation and/or infection) lead to a decrease of tissue pH in the region surrounding the involved tooth below what is normally found. Pus has a pH of 5.5 to 5.6. Because of this decreased pH, dissociation of the anesthetic solution favors the formation of a much larger proportion of cation relative to free base (Fig. 20-2). About 99% of a given drug (with a pK_a of 7.9) will be in the cationic form. Unfortunately this multitude of electrically charged RNH^+ cations is unable to migrate through the neural sheath. In the relative absence of the uncharged anesthetic base fewer anesthetic molecules reach the nerve membrane, where the intracellular pH remains normal and reequilibration between base and cation can occur. Fewer cations are present intracellularly, and the likelihood of incomplete anesthesia increases.

Solutions

One method of obtaining more intense anesthesia in an area of infection would be to deposit a greater volume of anesthetic into the region. A greater number (though still in the same low

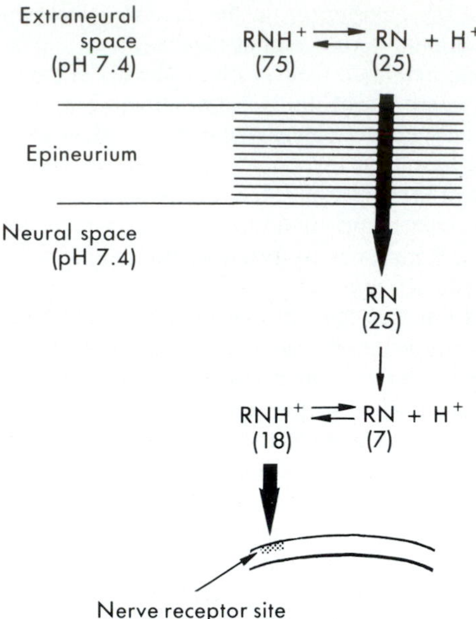

FIG. 20-1 Mode of action of a local anesthetic in normal tissue (pH 7.4). The anesthetic (pK_a = 7.9) is deposited in the extraneural tissues. Equilibrium occurs with approximately 75% of the molecules in the charged cationic form and 25% in base form. (Numbers in parentheses represent the proportion of anesthetic cation and base in extracellular and neural compartments.)

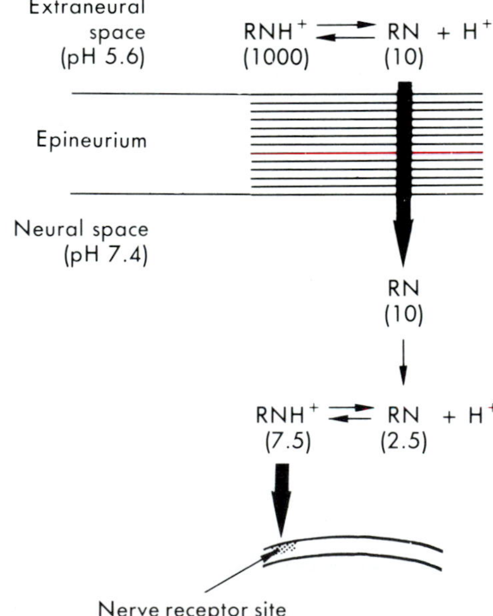

FIG. 20-2 Mode of action of a local anesthetic in an inflamed/infected area. The anesthetic (pK_a = 7.9) is deposited in the extraneural tissues (pH of 5.6). Equilibrium develops with approximately 99% of solution in the cationic form. Fewer anesthetic molecules pass through the epineurium to the neural space. The pH in the neural space is 7.4, and molecules reequilibrate. However, an insufficient number of molecules may be present, leading to a failure to produce profound clinical anesthesia.

percentage) of free base molecules would be liberated, with greater diffusion through the nerve sheath and a somewhat greater likelihood of achieving adequate pain control.

Although this procedure is somewhat effective, injection of anesthetic solutions into infected areas is undesirable because of the possibility of the spread of infection to a previously uncontaminated area. Deposition of the anesthetic into an area at a distance from the involved tooth is more likely to provide adequate pain control, because of the normal tissue conditions that exist there. Regional nerve block anesthesia is therefore a major factor in pain control for pulpally involved teeth.

There are also occasions, fortunately rare, when even regional block anesthesia at a distance from the infected tooth fails to produce adequate pain control. Omitting for a moment the most likely cause of this situation, faulty injection technique, Najjar[32] has proposed that inadequate pain control may be due to the fact that morphologic changes (e.g., neurodegenerative changes in the axon or the presence of inflammatory mediators) are developing. He states that morphologic changes in inflamed nerve, even at a distance from the actual inflammatory site, appear to be a significant barrier for normal electrolyte exchange at the membrane level. The net result is reinforcement of a nerve fiber's ability to generate action potentials. Studies[6,37] have demonstrated that inflammation potentiates peripheral nerve excitability.

Yet another unfortunate situation in endodontic pain control relates to the inflamed tooth that when anesthetized becomes asymptomatic but, on attempts to gain access to the pulp chamber and canals, becomes exquisitely sensitive to manipulation. Although no entirely satisfactory explanation exists for this circumstance, it may be explainable on the basis of an increase in the rate of stimulation to the nerve endings that occurs with use of the high- or low-speed handpiece. The degree of neural blockade may be adequate for a lower level of stimulation prior to preparation yet prove inadequate to block completely the rapid flood of impulses arising with use of the handpiece. This is equivalent to the so-called anesthetic window noted in obstetric anesthesia following epidural nerve block during delivery: The degree of pain control is quite adequate except during the most intense uterine contractions. The same intense increase in the rate of neural stimulation is thought to be responsible for this phenomenon in endodontics.

Local Anesthesia—Techniques

The tissue changes and their possible actions on the effectiveness of local anesthetics influence the choice of local anesthetic technique used in attempting to prevent discomfort during treatment. A variety of techniques are available in the maxilla and mandible.

Local infiltration (supraperiosteal injection)

Supraperiosteal anesthesia is described as a technique in which anesthetic is deposited *into* the area of treatment.[24] Small, terminal nerve fibers in the area are blocked and thus rendered incapable of transmitting impulses. Local infiltration anesthesia is commonly employed in maxillary teeth. Because of the ability of anesthetic solutions to diffuse through periosteum and the relatively thin cancellous bone of the maxilla this method of pain control will prove effective in endodontic procedures when infection (accompanied by local inflammation) is *not* present. Very often, however, when infection *is* present at the onset of an endodontic case and other anesthetic techniques must be relied on initially, infiltration anesthesia may prove effective at subsequent visits, provided effective cleaning and shaping of the root canals has been accomplished.

Supraperiosteal anesthesia is rarely effective in the adult mandible because of the inability of the anesthetic to penetrate the more dense cortical bone. In pediatric dentistry, infiltration anesthesia in the mandible is more successful. As a general rule, infiltration anesthesia in the mandible will be successful as long as the primary tooth remains. Once this tooth is replaced by a permanent tooth, regional block anesthesia should be considered initially.

In infiltration anesthesia the target area for deposition of the anesthetic is the apex of the tooth being treated. Only 0.6 to 0.9 ml of solution must be deposited for adequate pain control. Approximately 3 to 4 minutes is allowed to elapse before starting the procedure. On rare occasions, adequate pulpal anesthesia, even on pulpally uninvolved teeth, is not achieved following infiltration. From clinical experience it appears that the most common cause of this is the failure to deposit the anesthetic solution at or above the apical region of the tooth. The maxillary central incisor and canine, with relatively long roots, are most frequently involved in this situation. The first and second molars may, on rare occasion, have buccal root apices under the thick bone of the zygoma or medially flared palatal roots. A 27-gauge short needle is recommended.

Regional nerve block

It is quite possible that infiltration anesthesia will prove ineffective in blocking the transmission of painful stimuli in pulpally involved teeth. In these situations regional nerve block anesthesia is recommended. Nerve block is defined as a method of achieving regional anesthesia by depositing a suitable local anesthetic close to a main nerve trunk, preventing afferent impulses from traveling centrally beyond that point.[24] Nerve block anesthesia is likely to be successful when infiltration has failed since the anesthetic solution is being deposited some distance from the inflamed or infected tissue, where tissue pH and other factors are more nearly normal.

Several types of nerve block are useful in dentistry. Space does not allow for a detailed description of each, but a review of their effects does follow.

Maxillary anesthesia. Maxillary nerves that can be anesthetized include the posterior superior alveolar (PSA), the anterior superior alveolar, the greater palatine, the nasopalatine, and the second division or maxillary.

The *posterior superior alveolar* (PSA) nerve block, also called the zygomatic or tuberosity block, is indicated when pulpal anesthesia is required for the maxillary third, second, and first molars. In addition, the underlying buccal alveolar process, periosteum, connective tissue, and mucous membranes are anesthetized. During endodontic treatment, palatal infiltration is usually required for anesthesia of the palatal soft tissues. An additional infiltration of 0.6 ml into the buccal fold just anterior to the mesiobuccal root of the first molar is required in approximately 28% of patients to achieve complete anesthesia.

The *infraorbital* nerve block is an easy injection to administer, producing anesthesia of three nerves: the infraorbital, anterior superior alveolar, and middle superior alveolar. Dentally this block provides pulpal anesthesia for the central and lateral incisors, canine, and premolars, including their bony support and the soft tissues on the buccal surface. Palatal infiltration is usually necessary for anesthesia of the palatal soft tissues.

In both the posterior superior alveolar and the infraorbital nerve blocks, 0.9 ml of anesthetic is deposited at the target area. A 25- or 27-gauge long needle is employed in the infraorbital nerve block, and a 25- or 27-gauge short needle is recommended for the PSA nerve block.

Palatal anesthesia is often required during endodontic treatment and is also needed around the gingival margins of the tooth to be clamped. An adequate level of anesthesia can be obtained by infiltrating 0.3 ml of anesthetic into the palatal gingiva 3 to 5 mm below the gingival margin.

Larger areas of the palate seldom require anesthesia, but when necessary, two nerve blocks are available: the greater palatine and the nasopalatine.

The *greater* (or anterior) *palatine* nerve block provides anesthesia to both the hard and soft tissues ranging from the third molar as far anterior as the first premolar. In the region of the first premolar, partial anesthesia may be encountered as branches of the nasopalatine nerve overlap.

The *nasopalatine nerves* enter the palate through the incisive foramen, located in the midline just palatal to the central incisors and directly beneath the incisive papilla. They provide sensory innervation to the hard and soft tissues of the premaxilla as far distal as the first premolar, where fibers from the greater palatine nerve are encountered. A 27-gauge short needle is recommended for both palatal injections.

Because of the density of the palatal soft tissues and their firm attachment to bone, palatal injections are considered potentially traumatic. Palatal anesthesia can be achieved with a minimum of discomfort if care is taken throughout the procedure to ensure adequate topical anesthesia, adequate pressure anesthesia, slow penetration of tissues, continual slow deposition of solution, and injection of not more than 0.45 ml of solution.

A *maxillary* or *second division* nerve block, though rarely necessary, should be considered when other techniques of pain control prove inadequate because of infection accompanied by inflammation. This block provides anesthesia of the entire maxillary nerve peripheral to the site of injection: pulps of all maxillary teeth on the side of injection; buccal soft tissues and bone; hard palate on the injected side; and upper lip, cheek, side of the nose, and lower eyelid.

Two intraoral techniques are available for a maxillary nerve block.[26,34] The *first,* the high tuberosity injection, follows the same path as the posterior superior alveolar nerve block except that the depth of needle insertion is greater (1¼ inch vs. ¾ inch in the posterior superior alveolar). A 25-gauge long needle is used, and 1.8 ml of solution is deposited. The *second* intraoral approach[26] involves entering the greater palatine foramen, which is usually located palatally between the second and third maxillary molars at the junction of the alveolar process and the palatal bone. A 25-gauge long needle is carefully inserted into the foramen to a depth of 30 mm. Following aspiration, 1.8 ml of anesthetic solution is slowly deposited.

Mandibular anesthesia. Mandibular pulpal anesthesia is normally achieved through the inferior alveolar nerve block. Additionally, anesthesia of the buccal soft tissues and bone anterior to the mandibular molars is provided. The lingual nerve is usually anesthetized along with the inferior alveolar nerve. Anesthesia is achieved in the anterior two thirds of the tongue, the floor of the oral cavity, and the mucous membrane and mucoperiosteum on the lingual side of the mandible. A 25- or 27-gauge long needle is used and, following multiple negative aspirations, 1.5 ml of anesthetic solution is deposited.

Inferior alveolar nerve block. Successful inferior alveolar and lingual nerve block provides anesthesia to all mandibular tissues except the buccal mucous membrane and mucoperiosteum over the molars. If anesthesia of this region is required, the buccal nerve must be blocked. The buccal nerve is not anesthetized during inferior alveolar nerve block because it is a branch of the anterior division of the mandibular nerve; by contrast, the inferior alveolar and lingual nerves are branches of the posterior division. To block the buccal nerve, one uses a 25- or 27-gauge short or long needle and deposits 0.3 ml of anesthetic solution into the mucosa distal and buccal to the last molar in that quadrant.

In the absence of pulpal or periapical pathosis, inferior alveolar nerve block is successful (adequate pain control achieved) 80% to 85% of the time. Its rate of success diminishes significantly where disease exists. Because of the density of bone in the adult mandible, infiltration anesthesia is of little value; thus nerve block anesthesia becomes the primary avenue of pain control. When block anesthesia proves ineffective, fewer alternative techniques are available. There are, however, other nerve blocks that may succeed in the mandible.

Incisive nerve block. The incisive and mental nerves are terminal branches of the inferior alveolar nerve, arising at the mental foramen. The mental nerve, exiting from the mental foramen, provides sensory innervation to the skin of the lower lip and chin regions and the mucous membrane lining the lower lip; the incisive nerve, remaining within the mandibular canal, provides sensory innervation to the pulps of the premolars, canine, and incisors and the bone anterior to the mental foramen. Anesthesia of the region served by the *incisive nerve* should be considered when endodontic therapy is contemplated on premolars or other anterior teeth. A 25- or 27-gauge short needle is employed, and 0.6 to 0.9 ml of anesthetic is deposited outside the mental foramen. Finger pressure applied at the site of injection for 1 to 2 minutes following deposition ensures entry of solution into the mental foramen.

As mentioned previously, infiltration anesthesia is usually not effective in achieving pulpal anesthesia in the mandible. The sole exception is in the region of the lateral incisor, where up to 1 ml of anesthetic may be deposited into the mucobuccal fold at the level of the apex of the tooth. A 27-gauge short needle is recommended.

On occasion, adequate pain control is achieved in the mandible except in isolated areas. The area most often involved is the mesial root of the first molar. Successful pulpal anesthesia of third molars is frequently difficult to achieve because of the multiplicity of accessory innervations that are thought to exist. Indeed, adequate anesthesia is easier to obtain for third molar extraction than for restorative or endodontic procedures.

The mesial portion of the mandibular first molar not uncommonly is sensitive to painful stimuli when all other portions of the same tooth and adjacent structures are insensitive. Although many theories (involving the cervical accessory and transverse neck nerves) have been put forward to explain this situation, the mylohyoid nerve (a branch of the posterior division of the mandibular nerve) appears to be the culprit.[12] The mylohyoid nerve branches off the inferior alveolar nerve well above the inferior alveolar's entry into the mandibular foramen. It passes along the lingual border of the mandible in the mylohyoid groove, sending motor fibers to the anterior belly of the diagastric muscle. It has been demonstrated to contain sensory fibers, on occasion, that branch off and enter into the body of the mandible through small foramina on the lingual border of the mandible at about the second molar. These fibers presumably pass anteriorly through the body of the mandible to the mesial root of the first molar.

Whether or not the mylohyoid nerve is responsible, the problem of sensitivity in the inflamed first molar pulp can usually be alleviated with a 27-gauge short needle and 0.6 ml of anesthetic solution deposited against the lingual side of the mandible at the level of the apex of the mandibular *second* molar. Within 2 to 3 minutes, adequate anesthesia should be present. Although most often observed with the first molar, the problem of partial anesthesia can also occur with other teeth. Management consists of depositing 0.6 ml of solution at the apex of the tooth immediately *distal* to the involved tooth.

Mandibular block

A true mandibular (V3) block injection, one that provides adequate anesthesia of all sensory portions of the mandibular nerve (buccal, inferior alveolar, lingual, mylohyoid), can be obtained through the *Gow-Gates mandibular block*.[14,19] The target area is higher than in the traditional inferior alveolar nerve block technique: the lateral side of the neck of the mandibular condyle below the insertion of the lateral pterygoid muscle (Fig. 20-3).[14]

For this reason alone the success rate with the Gow-Gates mandibular block can be expected to be greater than that with the traditional approach, once the doctor learns the technique. Indeed, 97.25% of patients receiving the Gow-Gates block did not require supplemental anesthesia.[21] Other advantages of the Gow-Gates technique include a low positive aspiration rate (1.8%, compared with approximately 10% in the traditional technique) and no need for supplemental anesthesia (i.e., to the mylohyoid). A 25-gauge long needle is used in the Gow-Gates technique.

Two other techniques have been described that are effective in producing mandibular anesthesia, the periodontal ligament (PDL) injection (described below) and the Akinosi technique. The Akinosi (closed mouth) technique permits mandibular anesthesia to be obtained reliably in patients with extremely limited mandibular opening. It has proved effective in patients with trismus or severe infection.

Akinosi technique. A novel approach to mandibular anesthesia was described in 1977 by Akinosi.[2] This technique, a closed-mouth approach to mandibular anesthesia, is indicated especially when opening of the mandible is limited owing to infection, trauma, or trismus. Significant in endodontic therapy because of the possible presence of edema and/or infection, the Akinosi technique employs a 25-gauge or 27-gauge long dental needle held in the maxillary buccal fold on the same side of injection, at the height of the mucogingival junction of the last maxillary molar. Needle insertion occurs in the soft tissue on the lingual aspect of the mandibular ramus, immediately adjacent to the maxillary tuberosity. The needle is advanced almost parallel to the mandibular ramus for a distance of 25 mm (in the average-sized patient) at which point aspiration is attempted, and if negative, 1.8 ml of anesthetic solution deposited. The primary disadvantage to the Aki-

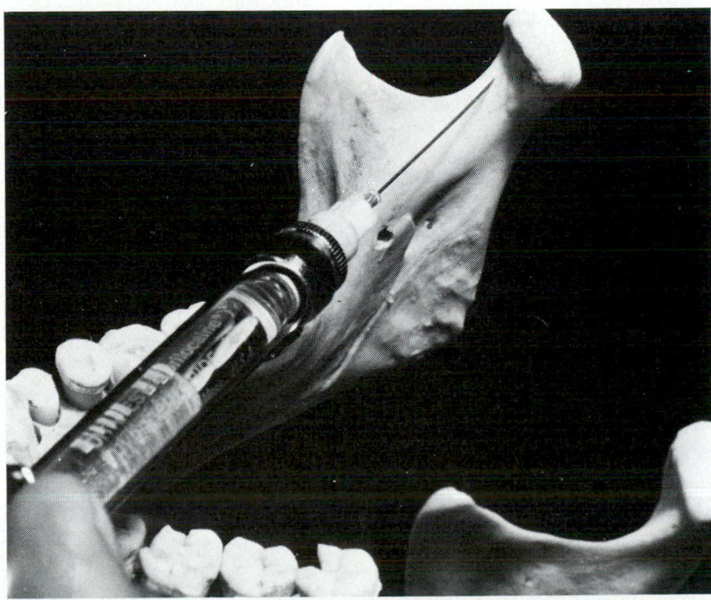

FIG. 20-3 Target area in the Gow-Gates technique is the lateral aspect of the neck of the condyle. (From Malamed SF: Handbook of local anesthesia, ed 3, St Louis, 1990, Mosby–Year Book.)

nosi technique is the absence of a bony contact to provide a landmark prior to injection of solution. However, the Akinosi mandibular block provides the clinician with a success rate approaching 80% to 85% (with practice!) in a situation (limited or no opening) in which in the past failure was almost guaranteed. Both motor and sensory anesthesia are obtained, permitting the patient to open wide, thus permitting treatment to commence.

Additional local anesthetic procedures

On occasion, the local anesthetic techniques just described fail to produce the required degree of pain control. There are other techniques that may then be employed to remedy the situation: the (1) PDL injection, (2) intraseptal injection, (3) intrapulpal injection, and (4) intraosseous injection.

Periodontal ligament injection. The PDL (or intraligamentary) injection is frequently used in restorative dentistry when isolated areas of inadequate anesthesia are present.[40] It may also be used alone to achieve pulpal anesthesia in a single mandibular tooth.[22] Advantages to its use in this manner include adequate pulpal anesthesia with a minimal volume of solution (0.2 to 0.4 ml) and the absence of lingual and lower lip anesthesia.

This technique may also prove effective in endodontically involved teeth. A 27-gauge short or a 30-gauge ultrashort needle is firmly placed between the periodontal ligament and the tooth to be anesthetized. With the needle bevel facing the root of the tooth, approximately 0.2 ml of anesthetic solution is deposited. Successful PDL anesthesia is usually indicated by resistance to the deposit of solution and by blanching (ischemia) of the tissues on injection. Multirooted teeth receive the injection (0.2 ml) on each root (Fig. 20-4).

Excessive volume of anesthetic can lead to complications, such as extrusion of the tooth.[33] Many devices (e.g., Ligmaject, Peripress) have been marketed to aid in this injection. Although they are effective, their success rate with this injection is equivalent to that with conventional syringes. The PDL injection is usually quite valuable as an adjunct to conventional nerve block techniques in endodontically involved teeth. Perhaps the only contraindication to its use would be insertion of the needle and deposition of anesthetic solution into an area of periodontal or periapical infection.

Intraseptal injection. The intraseptal injection, described by Saadoun and Malamed,[38] is a variation of the intraosseous injection. A 27-gauge 1-inch needle is inserted into the intraseptal tissue in the area to be anesthetized (Fig. 20-5). Although it is more frequently employed than the intraosseous injection, its success rate is not as high. Because of decreased bone density, it is more successful in younger patients. The needle must be firmly advanced into the cortical plate of bone. The soft tissues must be anesthetized prior to the needle insertion into bone. On injection, there must be considerable resistance to the advance of the plunger. Ease of administration usually means that the needle is located in the soft tissues, not bone. Resistance to injection as the solution is slowly forced under pressure into the cancellous bone is desirable. Enough solution must be administered to reach the periapical fibers (approximately 0.3 to 0.5 ml is recommended).

Intrapulpal injection. When the pulp chamber of a tooth has been exposed, either surgically or pathologically, the intrapulpal injection may be used to achieve adequate pain control.

A 25- or 27-gauge short or long needle is inserted into the pulp chamber or specific root canal as needed. Ideally the needle will be firmly wedged into the chamber or canal (Fig. 20-6). On injection, significant resistance is met and the solution must be inserted under pressure. Anesthesia is produced by the action of the anesthetic solution and by the applied pressure. There may be an initial brief period of sensitivity as the injection is started; but anesthesia usually occurs immediately thereafter, and instrumentation can proceed painlessly. When a snug fit of the needle in the canal is not possible, two procedures are used: (1) With the needle in the canal, warm white gutta-percha is inserted around it. After cooling, injection under pressure may proceed. (2) The anesthetic solution can be deposited in the chamber or canal, with anesthesia being produced by the chemical actions of the solution only. At least 30 seconds should elapse before an attempt is made to proceed with instrumentation. The former technique is preferred.

Intraosseous injection. Though rarely employed since the reintroduction of the PDL injection, the intraosseous injection can be effective in producing anesthesia adequate to permit opening of the pulp chamber, at which time intrapulpal anesthesia can be administered.

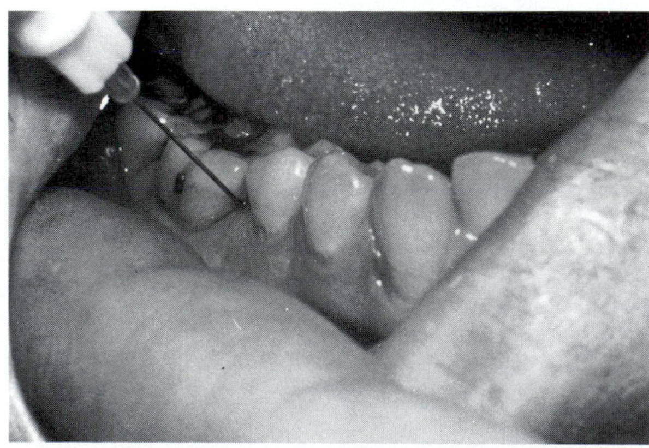

FIG. 20-4 To achieve anesthesia of the first molar, separate injections are required on the mesial and distal roots. (From Malamed SF: Oral Surg 53:118, 1982.)

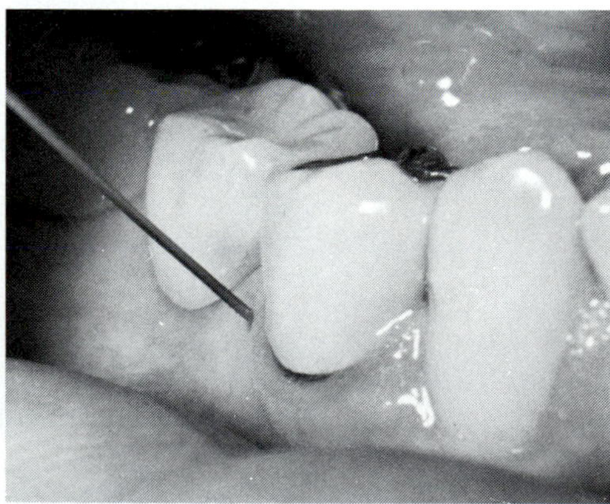

FIG. 20-5 In intraseptal injection a 27-gauge, 1-inch needle is inserted into the intraseptal bone distal to the tooth to be anesthetized. (From Malamed SF: Handbook of local anesthesia, ed 3, St Louis, 1990, Mosby–Year Book.)

To administer an intraosseous injection, the dentist must anesthetize the soft tissues and bone overlying the apical region of the tooth through local infiltration. A small incision (1 to 3 mm) is made down to the periosteum. By means of a small (No. ½ or 1) round bur, a hole is opened through the dense cortical plate of bone to the cancellous bone. Then with a 25-gauge short needle in the opening, approximately 1 ml of anesthetic solution is deposited (Fig. 20-7).

On occasion, a patient presents with a truly "hot" tooth. Then local infiltration, regional block anesthesia, and the other techniques described may prove ineffective. Intrapulpal anesthesia cannot be utilized until the pulp chamber is opened, which may not be immediately possible. The following sequence of treatment may be of value in this situation:

1. If a high-speed bur proves highly traumatic, a low-speed bur (though more time-consuming) may be less so.
2. Inhalation or intravenous sedation may help to allay anxiety and moderate the patient's responses to painful stimuli.
3. When the pulp chamber has been opened, direct intra-

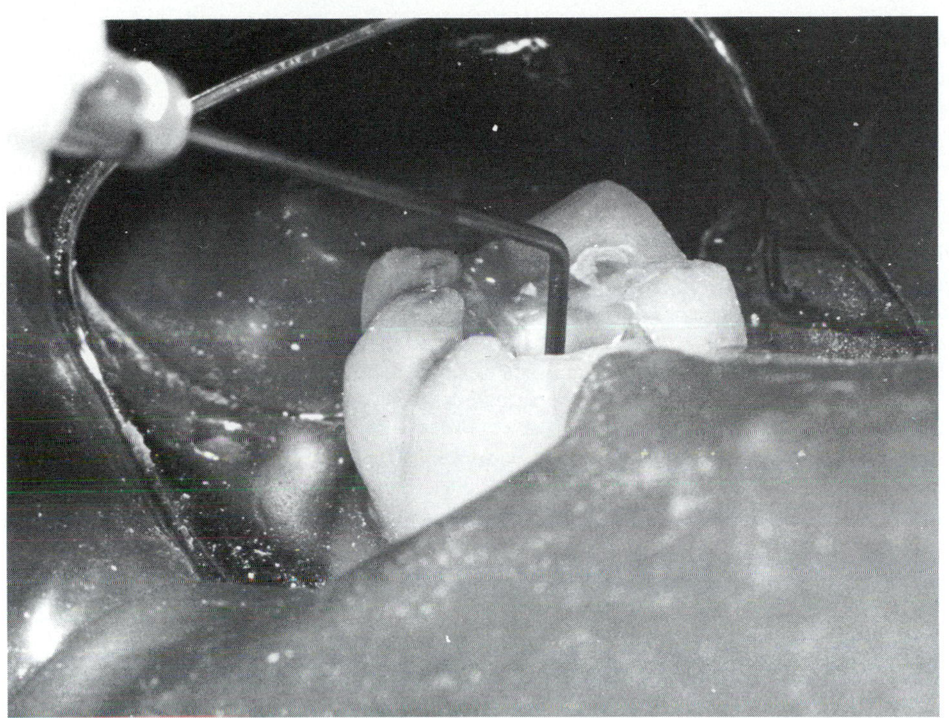

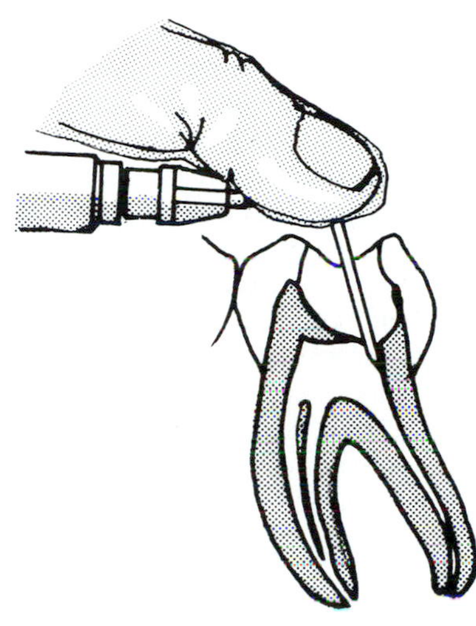

FIG. 20-6 In an intrapulpal injection the needle is inserted directly into the pulp chamber or a specific root canal. Ideally resistance is met and the solution is expressed under pressure. With the advent of intraligamentary anesthesia, this technique is seldom necessary to employ.

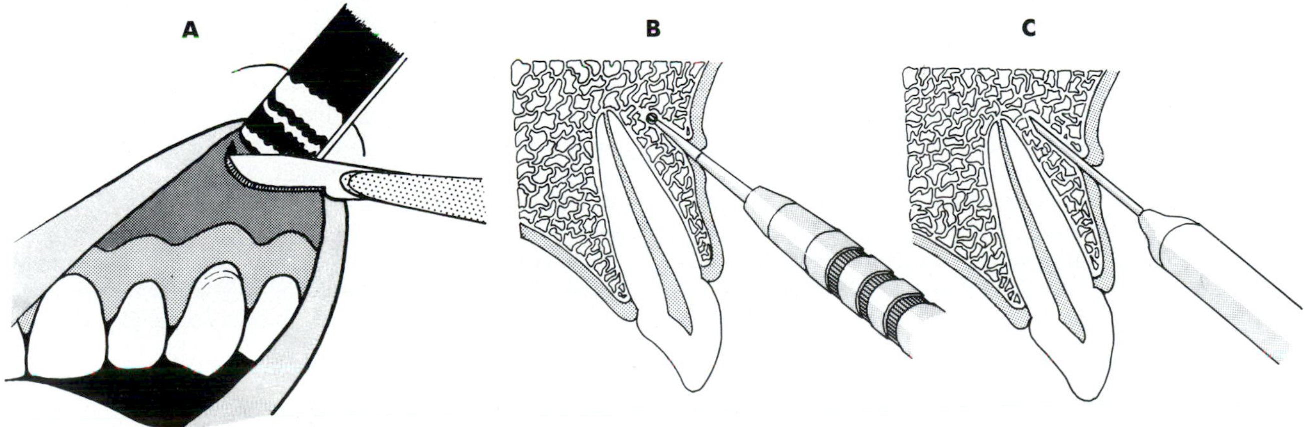

FIG. 20-7 An intraosseous anesthetic is used to obtain adequate pulpal obtundation only when other techniques have failed. The soft tissue over the site has previously been anesthetized through local infiltration. **A,** An incision is made down to the periosteum. **B,** By means of a small (½ or 1) round bur, a hole is opened in the cortical plate. **C,** A 25-gauge needle is placed in the opening, and anesthetic solution is deposited.

pulpal anesthesia usually can be administered and will prove effective.

4. If much pain persists, preventing further instrumentation, a small cotton pellet saturated with a vasoconstrictor-free local anesthetic solution (not topical anesthetic) is placed loosely in the tooth preparation. After a 30-second delay the pellet is pressed more snugly into the area of the pulpal exposure. Some sensitivity may exist, but within 2 or 3 minutes the area becomes less sensitive. The pellet is removed, and direct intrapulpal injection ensures adequate anesthesia.

Pain Control—Additional Considerations

In the overwhelming majority of endodontic procedures, if there is difficulty controlling pain at all, this happens only at the first appointment. Once the canals have been located and tissues extirpated, the requirement for pain control becomes minimal. Soft tissue anesthesia may be necessary for rubber dam application; however, if adequate tooth structure exists, even this is unnecessary. Instrumentation within a thoroughly debrided canal seldom requires anesthesia. Overextension of files beyond the apical foramen may produce a sensitivity that serves as an indicator to the doctor. If the patient overresponds to instrumentation, local infiltration or direct intrapulpal injection can be used.

In the filling of canals, considerable pressure may be exerted during condensation of the filling materials and may produce discomfort or pain. Local infiltration anesthesia should be considered before this procedure is started.

Electronic dental anesthesia

Electronic dental anesthesia (EDA) has received increasing attention in recent years. EDA devices provide clinical pain control via one or more methods, including the gate control theory of pain,[27] release of endorphins,[17] and/or release of serotonin.[7] Several studies[7,16,29] have demonstrated considerable clinical success with EDA in the areas of restorative, periodontal, and temporomandibular joint treatment. Clark and associates,[39] however, reported no success with EDA in the extirpation of vital pulp tissues.

The author has used EDA on nine patients who have had "hot" mandibular molars that could not be successfully anesthetized with local anesthetics alone or with local anesthesia plus inhalation sedation. The addition of EDA to these techniques provided adequate anesthesia to permit atraumatic entry into the pulp chambers, allowing extirpation of the tissues.

EDA alone in these situations may prove as effective (or ineffective) as local anesthesia alone, but in combination with local anesthetics (providing chemical anesthesia) and nitrous oxide and oxygen (producing an elevation of the pain threshold), EDA provides both a further elevation of pain threshold and an electrical block of pain impulses. These techniques are quite compatible and should be considered in difficult circumstances.

A number of EDA devices are currently marketed and have been approved by the U.S. Food and Drug Administration (FDA) for intraoral pain control. These include the Comfortron (M.D. Products, Ocala, Fla.), H-Wave Machine (Electronic Waveform Lab., Huntington Beach, Calif.), and the 3M Electronic Anesthesia Unit (3M, St. Paul, Minn.). The use of EDA as an adjunct for pain control is possible.

EDA recently received attention as a technique for postsurgical management. As yet unpublished studies demonstrate a significant decrease (or absence) of edema and pain in the postsurgical period when patients receive low-frequency electronic nerve stimulation immediately following apical (and other) surgery. (Local anesthesia was used for surgical pain control.) The requirement for postoperative analgesics was decreased in patients who received EDA.

Preoperative and postoperative pain control

The patient suffering from pulpitis most likely will have been taking oral analgesics for some time before the initial visit for endodontic treatment. The doctor should confirm, by asking the patient whether he or she is taking medication such as a nonsteroidal antiinflammatory drug (NSAID). A therapeutic blood level should be attained, if possible, prior to the initial endodontic visit. Ideally, two oral doses will have been taken by this time. The patient should continue to take the NSAID following treatment for a period of time determined by the treating doctor (1 or 2 days, depending on probable posttreatment discomfort). When prescribing analgesic drugs, the clinician should avoid writing "prn pain" in the instructions, for this suggests that the patient is not to take the drug unless he or she is feeling pain, when in fact the goal in managing surgical and posttreatment pain is to prevent it from recurring. Thus it is necessary for the patient to take oral doses on a regular basis (i.e., q4h or qid). When long-acting local anesthetics such as bupivacaine or etidocaine are administered in this manner, postendodontic discomfort is minimal.[18]

A telephone call from the doctor to the patient in the early evening on the day of treatment is valuable in minimizing posttreatment complications that may develop early the next morning. It is helpful to determine how the patient is doing, repeat posttreatment instructions, and reaffirm the importance of the patient's continuing to take prescribed medications (i.e., antibiotics and analgesics) as directed. Psychologically, such calls provide a tremendous boost to the patient in the immediate posttreatment period.

Pain control—suggested protocol for the emergency patient

Doctors contacted by a patient who is in acute pain have used the following protocol with considerable success in providing comfortable endodontic treatment in an "emergency."[39]

When initially contacted by telephone the doctor determines whether the patient has been taking oral analgesic medication. Most often, he or she has, but if not, therapy is started with an oral NSAID, preferably two doses prior to the appointment. Treatment should not be delayed, however, if this cannot be done. The initial goal will be to relieve the patient's acute problem, pain.

On arrival at the office, the patient should be seen as soon as possible after completion of the appropriate records (including a health history questionnaire). The dentist identifies which tooth is producing the problem (or, in some cases in which an immediate diagnosis is difficult, the area) and administers the appropriate injection technique to provide rapid onset of relief. Radiographs can be obtained following successful administration of the local anesthetic. The patient, no longer in pain, can return to the waiting area, if necessary, to await definitive treatment. Because the pain cycle has been interrupted the patient can relax, perhaps for the first time in several days.

Before the start of definitive endodontic treatment, it is suggested that the patient be reanesthetized, even if the original injection is still effective. All too often the use of the high-speed handpiece provokes even more intense pain than was present when the patient originally entered the office (the "anesthetic window"). Readministration of local anesthetic at this time serves to reinforce the anesthetic block, perhaps by providing additional RN molecules to diffuse into the neuronal tissue.

If the patient still experiences pain in spite of multiple local anesthetic administrations, the use of nitrous oxide–oxygen, carefully titrated to effect, is suggested. Nitrous oxide, at a 35% concentration, is equianalgesic to 10 mg of morphine or 50 mg of meperidine. It will not, in most cases, absolutely eliminate pain, but it will alter the patient's perception of pain, making it more tolerable.

In some few cases, however—most likely to develop in the mandibular molars—adequate pain control may still be unattainable even with the combined use of local anesthesia and inhalation sedation. It is in such situations that electronic dental anesthesia has been used with considerable success, thus far in a limited number of patients.

When the emergency treatment is completed and if the doctor thinks that there may be considerable posttreatment pain, the patient should be reanesthetized with a long-acting local anesthetic (etidocaine or bupivacaine), providing that the dosage of local anesthetic so far has been small enough to allow its administration. This can ensure up to 10 to 12 hours of posttreatment pain relief. The clinician should also reaffirm the importance of continued use of the oral analgesic medication, as directed, even though the patient might still be comfortable. It is easier to keep a patient free of pain than it is to eliminate pain once it recurs.

Again, it is helpful to telephone later the same day to determine how the patient is feeling. Minor problems can be managed more easily at this time, and postoperative instructions can be confirmed.

ANXIETY CONTROL

There are many causes of anxiety related to the dental situation; most frequently encountered is the fear of pain, and in no specialty of dentistry is the problem of pain control more acute than in endodontics. Because of this many patients are unusually apprehensive when faced with the need for endodontic treatment.

Yet most adult patients will not openly express their fears to the doctor. Rather, they sit in the dental chair, undergo dental care, and suffer in silence. Suppression of these anxieties is not always innocuous. Indeed, many potentially life-threatening situations may be precipitated by stress. Conditions ranging from hyperventilation and vasodepressor syncope to myocardial infarction have been encountered. Although usually of a relatively benign nature, syncope and hyperventilation can, if improperly managed, lead to significant morbidity, and possibly mortality.

Children, by contrast, do not have adults' inhibitions about the expression of apprehension. A child faced with an unpleasant situation will act "like a child": crying or screaming, perhaps even biting, kicking, or moving about in the dental chair. Significantly, healthy younger children rarely faint or hyperventilate.

Perhaps even more significant are the effects of unrecognized and unmanaged anxiety on the medically compromised patient. Patients with cardiovascular, respiratory, neurologic, and other metabolic disorders (thyroid disease, diabetes mellitus, adrenal disorders) cannot tolerate undue stress normally. They therefore represent an increased risk during dental care if they become apprehensive or feel pain.

Bennett[4] has stated, and others agree, that the greater the medical risk of the patient the more important it is to achieve adequate control of both pain and anxiety. The following discussion will present methods of recognizing anxiety in dental patients and will review the more common techniques of sedation, with special emphasis on their use during endodontic therapy.

Recognition of Anxiety

Most adult patients do not admit to being apprehensive about their pending dental treatment; therefore the task of exposing their anxiety becomes a form of detective work, the doctor and members of the office staff seeking clues.

A patient's previous dental history can aid in this regard. The patient with a history of many cancelled appointments for a variety of reasons may be hiding anxiety in this manner. In addition, the patient with a history of appointments for emergency treatment of painful situations should be suspect. Once the emergency treatment is completed (e.g., extraction, pulpal extirpation) and their pain relieved, the patient does not return until the next episode of dental pain.

Upon arrival in the dental office, the patient will often sit in the waiting room and discuss his or her fears of dentistry with other patients or with the office receptionist. The receptionist should therefore become conscious of statements made by patients concerning fears of dentistry. It is a rare patient indeed who will express these same fears to the doctor. The receptionist should be trained to advise the "chairside personnel" (i.e., the assistant, the doctor) that "Mrs. Smith mentioned to me she was terrified of injections" or that "she heard root canal work is very painful." Armed with this knowledge, the doctor and staff are better able to manage this patient's anxieties.

When an apprehensive patient is seated in the dental chair, other clues can be noted that relate to anxiety. The doctor should spend some time at each visit speaking with (not to) the patient. This permits the patient to speak up. Many patients complain that doctors do not allow (or do not seem to want) their patients to talk. Anxieties may be expressed at this time. Only a brief period need be devoted to this, but any time thus spent is well spent.

Touch your patient. The feel of the skin of apprehensive patients when you shake their hands can tell much. Cold, wet palms usually indicate anxiety.

Watch the patient. Apprehensive patients do not stop watching the doctor. They are afraid they will be "sneaked up on" and surprised (unpleasantly) with a syringe or some other instrument. The patient's posture in the chair is telling. Nonanxious patients appear comfortable in the chair, whereas apprehensive persons appear stiff, unrelaxed, on the verge of leaving the chair. The hands of nervous patients may firmly grip the arm rest of the chair in what has come to be known as the "white knuckle syndrome." They may clutch a handkerchief or shred a tissue without even being aware of it.

The forehead and arms of nervous patients may be bathed in perspiration despite effective air conditioning. Patients may even complain about the warmth of the room.

When these methods of recognizing anxiety in a dental office are employed, the situation takes on the aspect of a game: Can the doctor detect the patient's anxiety? Will the patient successfully keep his fears hidden from the doctor so as not to appear foolish? Unfortunately, on many occasions the patient wins. Then the doctor, unaware of the patient's anxieties, proceeds with the planned dental treatment only to discover that the patient was indeed apprehensive and faints at the sight of a local anesthetic syringe or pushes the doctor's hand away at a critical time in a procedure. Anxiety is obvious at this point, but the ideal time to detect it is *before* dental treatment begins.

The medical history questionnaire is a device that may be used to assist in the recognition of anxiety at an early stage. Corah[9] and Gale[13] determined which factors involved in dental treatment are most anxiety inducing in patients. They created an anxiety questionnaire to help determine a patient's degree of anxiety. The School of Dentistry of the University of Southern California has included several questions from this anxiety questionnaire in its medical history form[30]:

Do you feel very nervous about having dental treatment?

Have you ever had an upsetting experience in the dental office?

Has a dentist ever behaved badly toward you?

Is there anything else about having dental treatment that bothers you? If so, please explain.

These questions permit the patient to express his or her feelings about dentistry, perhaps for the first time. Many patients who would never verbally admit to anxiety answer these questions honestly. The addition of one or more questions concerning dental attitudes to the patient's completed medical history questionnaire is highly recommended.

Anxiety about dental care can usually be recognized through the use of the techniques just described. By so doing, the doctor is able to intervene and prevent the patient's anxiety from causing unwanted problems and complications during treatment.

Management of Anxiety

A variety of techniques for the management of anxiety in dentistry are available. Together these techniques are termed a spectrum of pain and anxiety control (Fig. 20-8). They represent a wide range, from nondrug techniques through general anesthesia. Although general anesthesia does have a useful place in this spectrum, its utilization today is quite limited outside the specialty of oral and maxillofacial surgery (and even within that specialty). Two reasons for decreased reliance on general anesthesia as a means of anxiety control have been the introduction and acceptance of the concept of conscious sedation in dentistry and the development within the past two decades of more highly effective drugs for the management of anxiety.

From a practical viewpoint, conscious sedation techniques present relatively safe, reliable, and effective methods of controlling anxiety with little or no additional risk to the patient. *Sedation* is defined as the decrease or elimination of anxiety in a conscious patient.[3] *Consciousness* is defined as the ability to respond appropriately to command with all protective reflexes intact including the ability to clear and maintain a patent airway.[3] In viewing the spectrum of pain control the reader can see that there are essentially two major types of sedation: those techniques involving the administration of drugs and techniques in which drug administration is not required. Techniques requiring drug administration are termed *pharmacosedation* and include the oral, intramuscular, inhalation and intravenous routes of drug administration. The term *iatrosedation* is applied to nondrug techniques—hypnosis, biofeedback, acupuncture, electroanesthesia, and the critically important "chairside manner."

Iatrosedation*

Before discussing the techniques of pharmacosedation, we must consider the *nondrug* techniques. The techniques of iatrosedation form the building blocks from which all pharmacosedative techniques grow. A relaxed and pleasant doctor-patient relationship will favorably influence the action of sedative drugs. Patients who are comfortable with a doctor either require a smaller dose of a given drug to achieve a desired

*This term, introduced by Dr. Nathan Friedman of the University of Southern California School of Dentistry, is defined as relaxing the patient through the doctor's behavior.

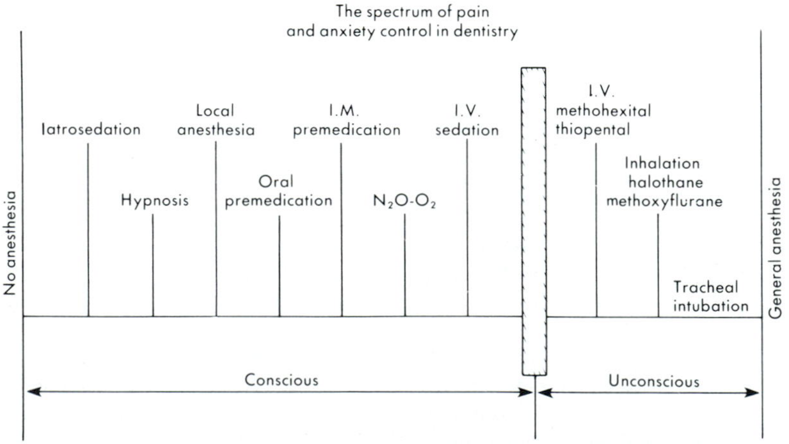

FIG. 20-8 Spectrum of pain and anxiety control in dentistry. Illustration of many of the techniques available in medicine and dentistry for patient management. Vertical bar represents the loss of consciousness. (From Malamed SF: Sedation: a guide to patient management, ed 2, St Louis, 1989, Mosby–Year Book.)

effect or respond more intensely to the usual dose. This is in contrast to patients who feel uncomfortable with a doctor. Their greater anxieties or fears cause them, either knowingly or unknowingly, to fight the effect of the drug, the result being poor sedation and an unpleasant experience for both the patient and the doctor.

A determined effort must be made by all members of a dental office staff to help allay the anxieties of the patient.

Pharmacosedation

Although iatrosedation is the starting point for all sedative procedures in a dental office, the level of anxiety present in many patients will prove too great to permit dental care to continue without the use of pharmacosedation. Fortunately, several effective techniques are available to aid in relaxing the apprehensive patient.

What goals are being pursued when pharmacosedative techniques are used? Bennett[4] has listed the following ones:

The patient's mood must be altered.
The patient must remain conscious.
The patient must be cooperative.
All protective reflexes must remain intact and active.
Vital signs must be stable and within normal limits.
The patient's pain threshold should be elevated.
Amnesia may be present.

These objectives comprise what might be considered ideal sedation for the dental patient.

There is a second important component to ideal sedation that must always be considered: The level of sedation must never reach beyond the level at which the doctor remains relaxed and capable of completing the dental procedure with uncompromised quality. Indeed, the quality of the dentistry on a sedated patient should be at least as high as, if not higher than, the quality of the same treatment on that patient without the use of pharmacosedation. Drug utilization in dentistry must never become an excuse for inferior quality dentistry. With adherence to these important criteria, the techniques discussed next may be employed safely and effectively.

Oral sedation. The most frequently employed technique of pharmacosedation, the oral route, offers some definite advantages over other techniques.

The oral route of drug administration is practically universally accepted by adult patients; in addition, it is one of the safest. Adverse drug reactions can and do arise following oral administration, but as a rule the intensity of the reaction is less than that seen following parenteral administration of the same drug.

The disadvantages of oral sedation tend to overshadow its advantages. Because of these disadvantages, the goals of oral sedation should be kept within well-defined limits of safety: slow onset of action (approximately 15 to 30 minutes), maximum clinical effect in about 60 minutes, long duration of action (3 to 4 hours), inability to titrate patient to the ideal sedation level, inability to rapidly increase or decrease the sedation level if need be, and the still impaired status of the patient at the termination of the procedure (requiring an adult to accompany the patient home). As can be seen from these, the administrator has little control over the ultimate effect of an orally administered drug on a patient.

Because of this lack of control, it is recommended that the oral route of sedation not be employed to achieve deep levels of sedation. Other, more controllable, techniques should be employed to achieve these levels. The uses to which oral sedation may safely be put include seeking conscious sedation (a) 1 hour before going to sleep the night before a dental appointment, if anxiety is severe and (b) 1 hour before scheduled dental treatment to help lessen preoperative anxiety.

Many drugs are available for use orally. It is strongly recommended that the reader consult a textbook[23] before prescribing any oral sedative drug to a patient—to determine correct dosage, contraindications, precautions, and other important information. In clinical experience the following drugs have proved to be the most effective in reaching the goals just enumerated: diazepam (Valium), oxazepam (Serax), hydroxyzine (Atarax, Vistaril), and hexobarbital (Sombulex, Pre-Sed) for preoperative anxiety control; flurazepam (Dalmane) or triazolam (Halcion) for hypnosis the night before dental treatment. Table 20-5 lists commonly employed oral antianxiety and sedative-hypnotic drugs. Additional information regarding drugs for oral sedation can be found in Chapter 12.

It must be remembered that the dental patient receiving oral sedatives must not be permitted to drive a motor vehicle either to or from the dental office.

Oral sedation may be required, especially at the first appointment, because of the preconceived ideas patients maintain about endodontic care. Proper use of iatrosedation and pain control usually obviate oral sedation at subsequent visits.

Intramuscular sedation. Intramuscular sedation is infrequently employed in dental practice.

Advantages of the intramuscular over the oral route include a more rapid onset of action for most drugs (approximately 10 to 15 minutes), maximum clinical effect within 30 minutes, and a more reliable drug effect for a given dose. Disadvantages include the inability to titrate to the ideal level of sedation, the inability to readily deepen the sedative effect if so desired, the inability to lighten the level of sedation, its long duration of action (3 to 4 hours for most drugs), and the need for an injection. The intramuscular route, like the oral route,

TABLE 20-5. Commonly used oral antianxiety and sedative-hypnotic drugs in dentistry

Drug group*	Proprietary name	Dose† (mg)
Barbiturates		
Hexobarbital	Pre-Sed Sombulex	250 to 500
Secobarbital	Seconal	100
Pentobarbital	Nembutal	50 to 100
Benzodiazepines		
Diazepam	Valium	5 to 10
Flurazepam	Dalmane	15 to 30
Oxazepam	Serax	15 to 30
Triazolam	Halcion	0.125 to 0.25
Others		
Chloral hydrate	Noctec Kessodrate Felsules	500 to 1500
Hydroxyzine	Atarax Vistaril	50 to 100

*Please see Chapter 12 for additional information.
†For a normal healthy 70-kg male. Patient response to these doses may vary; therefore the reader is advised to consult the drug insert for specific prescribing information before prescribing any drug.

lacks a degree of control that would be desirable. Therefore the level of sedation sought by intramuscular sedation should remain light to moderate. Only doctors trained in this technique of drug administration and in airway management should consider sedation via the intramuscular route.

When a drug is to be injected into a patient, it should be administered, if possible, intravenously where its clinical action will be more controllable, rather than by the less reliable intramuscular route.

Opioid analgesics such as meperidine (Demerol) are frequently employed via the intramuscular route for sedation. The benzodiazepine midazolam (Versed) is an effective agent, having received wide use as an intramuscular sedative since its introduction in 1986.[1,11,25]

In endodontics IM sedation is not contraindicated; however, if an x-ray unit is not readily available chairside, the patient will have to walk to the x-ray unit, possibly several times. Following IM injection he or she may require assistance in so doing. If the x-ray unit is present chairside, no such problem exists. Patients receiving any intramuscular CNS depressant must have an adult available to escort them home following treatment

Inhalation sedation. Nitrous oxide (N_2O) and oxygen (O_2) inhalation sedation is a remarkably controllable technique of pharmacosedation and is employed by 35% of practicing dentists in the United States.[20]

Because of its advantages over other sedation techniques, inhalation sedation is usually the method of choice when sedation is required. Recognized advantages include its rapid action (approximately 20 seconds, although 3 to 5 minutes may be required), the ability to titrate to the ideal level of sedation (N_2O is administered in 10% increments every 60 to 90 seconds until ideal sedation is achieved), the ability to rapidly lessen or deepen the level of sedation, total clinical recovery within approximately 3 to 5 minutes, and the ability to discharge most patients without any postoperative restrictions if the doctor so desires.

Disadvantages of inhalation sedation are few: the cost and size of the equipment, plus the need for intensive education of both doctor and staff in using the technique and attendant emergency measures.

Because of the degree of control maintained over inhalation sedation by the doctor, any level of conscious sedation compatible with the doctor's degree of experience can be achieved.

Although N_2O and O_2 inhalation sedation seems to be a nearly perfect technique, as with all drugs there will be times when the desired actions do not develop. Approximately 70% of all patients receiving N_2O-O_2 will be ideally sedated at a level between 30% and 40% N_2O, 15% will require less than 30% N_2O, and 15% will require more than 40%. Of this last 15% of patients, it may be said that some 5% to 10% will not be adequately sedated at any level of N_2O less than 70% to 75%. New inhalation sedation devices have a number of safety features incorporated into them whose basic goal is to prevent the patient from ever receiving less than 20% oxygen. Therefore it is probable that approximately 5% of patients receiving inhalation sedation will never become adequately sedated. If we add to this patients who are unable to breathe through the nose and those who have a very high level of anxiety, it is entirely possible that a failure rate of 10% to 15% could occur with inhalation sedation.

These comments are not meant to denigrate inhalation sedation. The purpose in stressing the possibility of failures is to illustrate that no technique, even inhalation sedation, is universally successful. Failures can and will occur whenever drugs are administered to patients. The drug administrator must know when to stop the administration. N_2O does not possess significant analgesic properties, although a degree of soft tissue analgesia develops in most patients at about 30% to 35% N_2O; therefore local anesthesia should be administered as it would be if inhalation sedation were not being used.

Inhalation sedation is entirely compatible with endodontic treatment. Indeed, the use of rubber dam converts most patients into nose breathers, facilitating the administration of N_2O-O_2. Inhalation sedation with N_2O-O_2 is a highly effective, easy to use, and safe technique of pharmacosedation. It is most effective for patients with mild to moderate anxiety. Failures may be noted in unusually apprehensive patients, but for these, other techniques are available.

In recent years several concerns have arisen relative to the use of N_2O and O_2 in dentistry. The first involves the effects on dental personnel of long-term exposure to low levels of N_2O. The use of scavenger-type devices to remove exhaled N_2O from the environment is recommended, despite the absence of definitive evidence of danger to dental personnel.[8] Another concern that must be noted is the abuse of N_2O by dental personnel. This has led to devastating effects, including peripheral sensory nerve deprivation.[28] N_2O is a potent anesthetic drug, not an innocuous vapor, and must not be abused. A third concern involves the use of any CNS depressant drug, including N_2O, on a patient of the opposite sex. Cases have been reported[19] in which the doctor was accused of sexual improprieties while the patient received N_2O-O_2. Two common threads appear: the patient received high concentrations of N_2O (in excess of 60%); and the doctor treated the patient without the benefit of a second person (auxiliary) present in the treatment room. Accusations such as these may easily be prevented by titrating nitrous oxide to the ideal sedation level and having an auxiliary, preferably of the same sex as the patient, present in the treatment area at all times.

Intravenous sedation. The goal in the administration of any drug (except, obviously, local anesthetics) is to get a therapeutic level of the drug in the bloodstream. The delays in onset of action noted with the preceding techniques were due to the slow absorption of drugs from the gastrointestinal tract and from muscle into the blood. It is apparent, then, that the direct administration of a drug into the venous circulation will result in a much more rapid onset of action and a greater degree of control than are found with other pharmacosedative techniques.

Only inhalation sedation, in which the inhaled gases rapidly reach the alveoli and capillaries, has an onset of action approaching that of intravenous sedation. A drop of blood requires approximately 9 to 20 seconds to travel from the hand to the heart and then to the brain. Patients can thus be readily titrated to an ideal level of sedation. The time required varies with the drug: intravenous diazepam or midazolam may require up to 4 minutes, whereas the Jorgensen technique may take 8 to 10 minutes. The level of sedation can easily be deepened if necessary; however, unlike inhalation sedation, it is impossible to lighten the level of intravenous sedation easily. Additional disadvantages of intravenous sedation include the possibility that potentially more dangerous situations will arise rapidly, especially if the technique is carried out improperly, the requirement of additional training for both doctor and office staff if the technique is to be safely employed,[3] the need for a responsible person to escort the patient from the dental office, and a considerable increase in liability insurance costs.

Venipuncture, a learned skill, requires practice and continued repetition if it is to be performed atraumatically. Once accomplished, the actual technique of intravenous sedation is quite simple. Because of the degree of control maintained by the doctor the level of sedation sought can vary from light to deep, depending on the experience of the doctor and the requirements of the patient.

Many techniques of intravenous sedation are available. Most involve sedative drugs and opioid analgesics or sedative-hypnotics and opioid analgesics. Although many drugs fit into these categories and may be used successfully for intravenous sedation, several techniques have become quite popular: intravenous benzodiazepine (midazolam or diazepam), benzodiazepine and opioid, and pentobarbital and opioid. Propofol, a rapid-acting, short-acting, nonbarbiturate sedative-hypnotic, has recently been added to the intravenous sedation armamentarium. Administered via a continuous infusion, the level of sedation can be carefully titrated, with return of the presedation state within 3 to 5 minutes of termination of the propofol infusion.

1. Until the introduction of midazolam in 1986, diazepam (Valium) was the most commonly used intravenous sedative in dentistry and medicine. Although they are similar agents, there are a number of important differences between them. Midazolam provides a significantly greater amnesic effect than diazepam, whereas diazepam appears to provide a greater degree of sedation. Water-soluble midazolam is much less likely to produce phlebitis than the lipid-soluble diazepam and may be administered via the intramuscular route with excellent effects expected. Midazolam appears to be approximately three to four times as potent as diazepam. Careful titration is recommended whenever midazolam is administered intravenously. Benzodiazepines do not possess analgesic properties, so local anesthesia must be administered for pain control.
2. Opioid agonists or opioid agonist/antagonists may be combined with antianxiety agents to produce more profound sedation and add a degree of analgesia. Because of their potential side effects (i.e., nausea, orthostatic hypotension, respiratory depression), opioids should be used only when needed and by doctors trained in their use. In endodontic treatment, in which establishing adequate pain control may be difficult, the use of opioids may, on occasion, be indicated. Opioids affect the way pain is interpreted by the central nervous system and produce a milder response than might otherwise be experienced. In combination with local anesthesia, opioids may help achieve adequate pain control in previously difficult situations.
3. Sedative-hypnotics (i.e., barbiturates) ought *not* to be employed as sole agents in intravenous sedation. While producing sedation these agents also *lower* the patient's pain reaction threshold, leading to an exaggerated response to painful stimuli. Instead of grimacing, a patient may jump in the chair, creating an unpleasant or potentially dangerous situation. To overcome this drawback, opioids are frequently administered along with sedative-hypnotics. Meperidine (combined with scopolamine) is injected following the sedative-hypnotic pentobarbital (Nembutal) in a technique termed the *Jorgensen technique*. For routine endodontic treatment this technique is too long acting, pentobarbital having a clinical duration of approximately 4 hours.

Intravenous sedation, particularly the shorter-acting techniques (i.e., midazolam, diazepam, diazepam or midazolam and opioid and propofol) are ideally suited for endodontic therapy. If the x-ray unit is located some distance from the patient, it may be both difficult and inconvenient to move the patient to the unit. During the early phase of the procedure, immediately after injection of the IV drug(s), the patient may also have difficulty maintaining an open mouth. Bite blocks should be available at this time.

Table 20-6 summarizes the recommended levels of sedation for the techniques discussed in this chapter.

Combined techniques. On occasion it may be necessary to consider combining several of the techniques just described. Some words of caution are in order.

Quite frequently the patient who requires either inhalation or intravenous sedation is apprehensive enough to need oral sedation, either the night before, or the day of, the dental appointment. There is no contraindication to this practice provided the level of oral sedation is not excessive *and* the inhalation or intravenous agents are carefully titrated. Because of

TABLE 20-6. Common routes of sedation in the dental office

Route of administration	Control: Titrate	Control: Rapid reversal	Recommended safe sedative levels
Oral	No	No	Light only
Rectal	No	No	Light only
Intramuscular	No	No	Adults: light, moderate Children: light, moderate, profound
Intravenous	Yes	No (most drugs) Yes (opiods)	Children*: light, moderate, profound Adults: light, moderate, profound
Inhalation	Yes	Yes	Any level of sedation

*There is little need for intravenous sedation in normal healthy children. Most children who permit a venipuncture will also permit a local anesthetic to be administered intraorally. Intravenous sedation is of great benefit, however, in management of handicapped children.
(From Malamed SF: Medical emergencies in the dental office, ed 4, St Louis, 1993, Mosby–Year Book.)

the level of oral sedative already in the blood, the requirement for other central nervous system depressants will usually be decreased. If "average" doses of inhalation or intravenous drugs are used without titration, an overdose may ensue. Titration is an important safety factor. When possible to titrate a drug, it is foolhardy not to.

The combination of intravenous and inhalation sedation should be avoided by all but the most experienced doctors. Too frequently reports are forthcoming of significant morbidity (and, on occasion, mortality) resulting from the ill-conceived conjoint use of these two potent techniques. Levels of sedation can vary rapidly, and unless constant effective monitoring is maintained, unconsciousness may develop with attendant airway problems before the doctor ever becomes aware of it. N_2O and O_2 may be employed successfully at the same appointment as intravenous sedation in the following manner: when a patient requiring intravenous sedation is apprehensive about venipuncture, N_2O and O_2 may be used to aid in establishing the intravenous infusion. Benefits of N_2O and O_2 during venipuncture include (1) a vasodilating effect, (2) anxiety-reducing actions, and (3) minor analgesic properties. After the establishment of an intravenous infusion, the patient must be given 100% oxygen and returned to their presedative state before any intravenous drug is administered.

Anxiety Control—Summary

Anxiety is common during dental treatment in general and endodontic treatment in particular. Although iatrosedative measures greatly aid in decreasing anxiety, pharmacosedative techniques may become necessary. A number of effective techniques are available in dental practice. The least potent, most controllable technique that allays anxiety should be used. Care must be observed, however, not to exceed the level of sedation at which the doctor feels capable of effectively and safely managing the patient. As a final note it should be remembered that no technique of sedation is always effective and that clinical failures are to be expected. When properly employed, the techniques of iatrosedation and pharmacosedation permit the doctor to manage successfully approximately 95% of patients seeking endodontic care without increasing the risk to the patient.

REFERENCES

1. Acute Pain Management Guideline Panel: Acute pain management: operative or medical procedures and trauma. Clinical practice guidelines. A HCPR Pub No. 92-0032, Rockville, Md., 1992, Agency for Health Care Policy and Research, Public Health Service, US Department of Health and Human Services.
2. Akinosi JO: A new approach to the mandibular nerve block, Br J Oral Surg 15:83, 1977.
3. American Dental Association, Council on Dental Education: Guidelines for teaching the comprehensive control of pain and anxiety in dentistry, J Dent Educ 36:62, 1972.
4. Bennett CR: Conscious sedation in dental practice, ed 2, St Louis, 1978, The CV Mosby Co.
5. Camejo G, et al: Characterization of two different membrane fractions isolated from the first stellar nerves of the squid *Dosidicus gigas,* Biochim Biophys Acta 193:247, 1969.
6. Chapman LF, Goodell H, and Wolff HG: Tissue vulnerability, inflammation, and the nervous system. Read at American Academy of Neurology, April, 1959.
7. Clark MS, et al: An evaluation of the clinical analgesia/anesthesia efficacy on acute pain using high frequency neural modulator in various dental settings, Oral Surg 63(4):501, April 1987.
8. Cohen F, et al.: Occupational disease in dentistry and chronic exposure to trace anesthetic gases, J Am Dent Assoc 101:21, 1980.
9. Corah N: Development of dental anxiety scale, J Dent Res 48:596, 1969.
10. Covino BJ: Physiology and pharmacology of local anesthetic agents, Anesth Prog 28:98, 1981.
11. Dormauer D, and Aston R: Update: midazolam maleate, a new water-soluble benzodiazepine, J Am Dent Assoc 106:650, 1983.
12. Frommer J, Mele FA, and Monroe CW: The possible role of the mylohyoid nerve in mandibular posterior tooth sensation, J Am Dent Assoc 85:113, 1972.
13. Gale E: Fears of the dental situation, J Dent Res 51:964, 1972.
14. Gow-Gates GAE: Mandibular conduction anesthesia: a new technique using extraoral landmarks, Oral Surg 36:321, 1973.
15. Gustainis JF, and Peterson LJ: An alternative method of mandibular nerve block, J Am Dent Assoc 103:33, 1981.
16. Hochman R: Neurotransmitter modulator (TENS) for control of dental operative pain, J Am Dent Assoc 116:208, 1988.
17. Hughes J: Identification of two related pentapeptides from the brain with potent opiate antagonist activity, Nature 258:577, 1975.
18. Jackson DL, Moore PA, and Hargreaves KM: Pre-operative nonsteroidal antiinflammatory medication for the prevention of postoperative dental pain, J Am Dent Assoc 119:641, 1989.
19. Jastak JT, and Malamed SF: Nitrous oxide sedation and sexual phenomena, J Am Dent Assoc 101:38, 1980.
20. Jones TW, and Greenfield W: Position paper of the ADA ad hoc Committee on trace anesthetics as a potential health hazard in dentistry, J Am Dent Assoc 95:751, 1977.
21. Malamed SF: The Gow-Gates mandibular block—evaluation after 4275 cases, Oral Surg 51:463, 1981.
22. Malamed SF: The periodontal ligament injection—an alternative to mandibular block, Oral Surg 53:118, 1982.
23. Malamed SF: Sedation: a guide to patient management, ed 2, St Louis, 1989, Times Mirror/Mosby College Publishing.
24. Malamed SF: Handbook of local anesthesia, ed 3, St Louis, 1990, Times Mirror/Mosby College Publishing Co.
25. Malamed SF, Quinn CL, and Hatch HG: Pediatric sedation with intramuscular and intravenous midazolam, Anesth Prog 36:155, 1989.
26. Malamed SF, and Trieger NT: Intraoral maxillary nerve block: an anatomical and clinical study, Anesth Prog 30:44, 1983.
27. Malamed SF, and Weine F: Profound pulpal anesthesia, Chicago, 1988, produced by the American Association of Endodontics (audiotape).
28. Malamed SF, et al: The recreational abuse of nitrous oxide by health professionals, J Calif Dent Assoc 8:38, 1980.
29. Malamed SF, et al: Electronic dental anesthesia for restorative dentistry, Anesth Prog 36:140, 1989.
30. McCarthy FM, Pallasch TJ, and Gates R: Documenting safe treatment of the medical-risk patient, J Am Dent Assoc 119:383, 1989.
31. Melzack R, and Wall PD: Pain mechanisms: a new theory, Science 150:971, 1965.
32. Najjar TA: Why can't you achieve adequate regional anesthesia in the presence of infection? Oral Surg 44:7, 1977.
33. Nelson PW: Injection system, J Am Dent Assoc 103:692, 1981 (letter).
34. Poore TE, and Carney FMT: Maxillary nerve block: a useful technique, J Oral Surg 31:749, 1973.
35. Ritchie JM, Ritchie B, and Greengard P: Active structure of local anesthetics, J Pharmacol Exp Ther 150:152, 1965.
36. Ritchie JM, Ritchie B, and Greengard P: The effect of the nerve sheath on the action of local anesthetics, J Pharmacol Exp Ther 150:160, 1965.
37. Rood JP, and Pateromichelakis S: Inflammation and peripheral nerve sensitization, Br J Oral Surg 19:67, 1981.
38. Saadoun AP, and Malamed SF: Intraseptal anesthesia in periodontal surgery, J Am Dent Assoc 111:249, 1985.
39. Shanes AM: Electrochemical aspect of physiological and pharmacological action in excitable cells. II. The action potential and excitation, Pharmacol Rev 10:165, 1958.
40. Walton RE, and Abbott BJ: Periodontal ligament injection: a clinical evaluation, J Am Dent Assoc 103:571, 1981.

Self-assessment questions

1. The duration of action of a local anesthetic can be increased by
   a. increasing its lipid solubility.
   b. increasing its protein-binding potential.
   c. decreasing its extra–neural tissue diffusibility.
   d. increasing its vasodilator activity.
2. Inadequate anesthesia in some cases of inflamed or infected pulps is due to
   a. a decrease in the tissue pH around the involved tooth.
   b. availability of more cations for binding at the receptor site.
   c. a larger proportion of the free base.
   d. a smaller proportion of the cation.
3. Supraperiosteal anesthesia is
   a. most effective in areas of infection.
   b. generally used for pulpal anesthesia of maxillary teeth.
   c. not effective for primary teeth in the mandibular arch.
   d. effective in areas of dense cortical bone.
4. The infraorbital nerve block does not anesthetize
   a. the maxillary premolar.
   b. the maxillary incisors.
   c. the palatal mucosa.
   d. the maxillary cuspid.
5. Partial anesthesia to the mesial of the mandibular first molar can be alleviated by
   a. anesthetizing the motor fibers of the mylohyoid nerve.
   b. depositing anesthetic on the buccal side at the level of the mesial apex.
   c. depositing anesthetic on the lingual side at the level of the apex of the second molar.
   d. all of the above.
6. Electronic dental anesthesia (EDA)
   a. has not been approved by the FDA for intraoral pain control.
   b. can be used without local anesthesia for pulp extirpation.
   c. has been successful as a technique for post–endodontic surgery patient management.
   d. has not been successful as an adjunct in treating "hot" mandibular molars.
7. Conscious sedation is a technique designed to
   a. control pain.
   b. control anxiety.
   c. control pain and anxiety.
   d. affect the patient's protective reflexes.
8. Oral sedation
   a. is the most frequently employed technique of pharmacosedation.
   b. is quick acting.
   c. is short acting.
   d. is least accepted by patients compared with other routes of drug administration.
9. Disadvantages of intramuscular sedation include
   a. inability to titrate to the ideal level of sedation.
   b. inability to deepen the level of sedation.
   c. inability to lighten the level of sedation.
   d. all of the above.
10. When sedation is required the most advantageous route of administration is
    a. oral.
    b. inhalation.
    c. intramuscular.
    d. intravenous.
11. Compared to diazepam (Valium), midazolam (Versed)
    a. provides an amnesic effect.
    b. is not as potent.
    c. requires no local anesthetic for pain control.
    d. provides a greater degree of sedation.
12. Which route of administration of conscious sedation requires no one to escort the patient from the office?
    a. Oral.
    b. Intravenous.
    c. Inhalation.
    d. None of the above.

Chapter 21

Bleaching of Vital and Pulpless Teeth

Ronald E. Goldstein
Van B. Haywood
Harald O. Heymann
David R. Steiner
John D. West

The last decade has been a time of widespread public acceptance and immense change for esthetic dentistry in general. During these years, bleaching continued to hold its century-old place as the simplest, most common, least invasive, and least expensive means available to dentists to lighten discolored teeth and eliminate or diminish many stains in both vital and pulpless teeth. Bleaching also underwent some important changes.

First of all, the numbers rose sharply. It is estimated that more than a million people had teeth bleached by dentists. Second, new methods continued to be introduced, providing a full circle to bleaching's long history. The earliest efforts at bleaching involved only a bleaching solution applied to the teeth. The first was oxalic acid, reported by Chappel in 1877, followed soon after by various forms of chlorine, until Harlan described what is believed to be the first use of hydrogen peroxide in 1884. (He referred to it as *hydrogen dioxide*.[60]) Once hydrogen peroxide was established as the most effective solution, the major advances focused on ways to facilitate the absorption of the bleaching agent. After initial efforts to speed the process using electric current and ultraviolet waves, Abbot in 1918 introduced an instrument to speed the chemical reaction by causing the temperature of the solution to rise.[60] Many improvements took place in this basic procedure in the next decades. In the 1980s we saw the introduction of another way to facilitate absorption of the bleaching agent, this by applying a weaker bleaching solution to the teeth for longer periods, usually by placing it in a retainer-like matrix that the patient wore for several hours daily over a period of weeks. As of 1994, more dentists are believed to be using night guard vital bleaching or matrix bleaching than any other methods. Combining matrix bleaching at home with in-office bleaching can lower costs while retaining the maximum control of results.

Third, the development of high-tech computer imaging has been another recent contribution to enhancing patient understanding, expectation, and, ultimately, satisfaction.

Fourth, bleaching increasingly took its place within broader dental treatment plans. For many patients, bleaching alone is sufficient to create dramatic changes in tooth appearance, sometimes in a single office visit. For others, however, it is used primarily in combination with other esthetic procedures, such as microabrasion or lightening a striated tooth before veneering or improving color of teeth adjacent to a new crown. In the 1980s and 1990s, new partnerships and referral patterns gave bleaching new roles as an adjunct to orthodontics, orthognathic surgery, endodontics, and restorative dental treatments as well as to treatments in dermatology and plastic and reconstructive surgery. In fact, an increasing number of dentists and other health professionals concerned with esthetics began asking all patients if they were satisfied with the color of their teeth.

The fifth and final measure of acceptance and change in bleaching in the past 10 years involves the availability and mass marketing of bleaching products to be used without dental evaluation and supervision. At least as many persons are believed to have purchased such products as received bleaching under a dentist's care. The commercial success of these do-it-yourself kits reflects the public's increased expectations for brighter teeth. But, as the concerned surveillance of the Food and Drug Administration (FDA) beginning in 1991 indicates,[1] the availability of over-the-counter home bleaching kits also reinforces the need for dentists to be informed and to educate their patients about the limits and dangers of bleaching before proper diagnosis of discoloration and radiographic examination of tooth soundness and possible defective restorations. These dangers include: possible hypersensitivity of teeth, perhaps because of cracks or caries or thinned enamel; irritation of gingiva, perhaps because the solution was left in too long by an overeager patient; ill-fitting matrices; and side effects such as allergic reactions.[16] Dental supervision is especially important because bleaching has been found to cause chemical softening of microfilled and hybrid composite resins, when the surface texture of composite resins was evaluated with scanning electron microscopy.[3] Dentists also need to educate patients about the advantages of dental supervision.

The interest in home bleaching for vital teeth also doubtless speeded the development and improvement of dentist-monitored combination office and home treatments, an outgrowth of matrix treatments in which patients were given a considerably greater hand in their own treatments. Sometimes called *power/home bleaching,* this approach offers initial in-office bleaching sessions, followed by a sequence of home treatments using a matrix fitted to the individual patient by the dentist.[16]

DETERMINING PATIENT APPROPRIATENESS FOR BLEACHING

The ideal teeth in our society have thick, even enamel with a bright, milky white appearance. Unfortunately, that bright, white look is usually seen only in healthy, fairly young people who have so far been spared all of the numerous genetic, environmental, medical, and dental insults that produce dingy or discolored teeth. Even this fortunate minority may experience wear and thinning of the enamel from overaggressive brushing and cleaning materials, acidic food and drink, and aging itself, all of which can diminish the covering power of the white enamel, letting more of the darker-hued dentin show through.[12]

Bleaching appears to work by oxidation, in which the bleaching agent enters the enamel/dentin of the discolored tooth and releases the molecules containing the discoloration. How *well* it works depends upon the cause of the stain and where, how deeply, how long the stain has permeated the structure of the tooth, and how well the bleaching agent can permeate to the source of the discoloration and remain there long enough to release deep stains.

For pulpless teeth, as described later in this chapter, stains can be attacked from the inside of the pulp chamber itself (if that is where the stain is), or high concentration bleaching agents can be applied to the surface and moderate heat used to activate the oxidation process, without concern for damage to the dead or nonexistent pulp. For vital teeth, however, stains can be attacked only from the surface, and there are stringent limits on temperature. Furthermore, the appropriateness of bleaching for vital teeth depends not only on the type and severity of stain but also on the unbroken surface, thickness, and other measures of health of the enamel.

For these reasons, diagnosis is the first, and perhaps the single most important, determinant of the success of bleaching for any discoloration. A good visual examination usually suggests the cause and extent of the discoloration and also the condition of the teeth and mouth in general. This examination should be combined with a medical history that focuses on any systemic problems or medications that might have affected or be affecting tooth coloration. You also should ask the patient about his or her use of tobacco and highly colored beverages or foods as well as any allergic reactions to hydrogen peroxide, plastic, or rubber. If your first view of the teeth and the answer to these questions suggest bleaching is an appropriate treatment, further testing will be necessary to determine any problems with the tooth structure that could affect tooth color, supply more helpful information for a diagnosis of causative factors, or make bleaching inappropriate.

Before proceeding further, however, take photographs of the staining, using an instant or 35-mm camera. Be sure to include a "constant" such as a shade tab in the photograph. This baseline data provide an excellent record of pretreatment for you to determine needed follow-up—and help the patient later to better recognize the cumulative effect of what may be an incremental, gradual improvement in tooth color.

The last dental workup should have been recent enough and thorough enough to completely reveal any periapical or other disease, caries, or defective restorations, and any enlargement of the pulp that would make the tooth unusually sensitive to heat. At this diagnostic examination, with bleaching in mind, the dentist verifies the vitality of teeth. If sensitivity was recorded at an earlier examination, those findings are compared with current ones. Radiographs and thermal and electric pulp tests may be necessary to answer questions of pulp size and vitality that will help determine what procedures to use in bleaching. Transillumination techniques permit the dentist to look at the teeth from different angles and observe the opacity, depth, and layers of any stains. Transillumination also can reveal caries, cracks, decalcified or hypocalcified areas, and areas of excess calcification. An intraoral video camera can be an especially effective means not only of seeing these defects on the television monitor but also of documenting your finding through a printout or video recording.

The next step in the diagnostic process is thorough prophylaxis. Ordinary cleaning of the teeth, even with the excellent pastes available to dentists today, does not remove deep stains, but a thorough prophylaxis using a Prophy-Jet may remove enough stain and plaque to satisfy the patient without bleaching. Its primary purposes, however, are to enable the dentist to see more clearly the extent of deep stain and to better prepare the teeth for treatment.

CAUSES OF DISCOLORATION

Extrinsic Discoloration

The most common discolorations are caused by dark-colored foods, beverages, or tobacco. Tobacco produces a yellowish brown to black discoloration, usually in the cervical portion of the teeth and primarily on the lingual surfaces. Marijuana may produce sharply delineated, slightly greenish rings around the cervical portion of the teeth next to the gingival margins. Chewing tobacco, on the other hand, frequently penetrates the enamel to produce even darker stains. Bleaching can be effective against all these stains if the enamel is even. Stains become more resistant to bleaching if the teeth have many pits, fissures, grooves or enamel defects. Bleaching can be effective in all these conditions, sometimes after a small number of treatments. If microcracks have allowed the stain to permeate the tooth, bleaching may not be effective and restorative treatment such as veneering or bonding may be indicated. Whatever esthetic treatment is chosen, the patient must be made to understand that its success will not stand up to continued use of the discoloring agent.

Dental Conditions That Cause Discoloration

The diagnostic examination may reveal dental problems that contribute to discoloration. Caries is a primary cause of pigmentation, appearing as opaque, white halo, or gray discoloration. Bacterial degradation of food debris in areas of tooth decay or decomposing filling can cause even deeper brown to black discolorations. Obviously all such problems must be corrected before bleaching begins. In some cases, repair may make bleaching unnecessary.

Dental restorations can also cause problems. Degraded tooth-colored restorations such as acrylics, glass ionomers, or composites can cause teeth to look gray and discolored. After the degraded restorations are replaced, bleaching can be an extremely effective way to remove the remaining discoloration. Restorations with metal amalgams, even silver and gold ones, may reflect shadows through the enamel, even when there has been no breakdown in the material. Replacing these restorations with less visible materials such as composite resin often changes the appearance of the tooth enough to satisfy the patient without bleaching; more often, it improves the results of bleaching. If the metal amalgams cannot be replaced because of the position of the restoration, bonding or laminating may be a better treatment.

The most troublesome staining from dental treatments are those from oils, iodines, nitrates, root canal sealers, pins, and other materials that have penetrated the dentinal tubules. The length of time the stain has been present determines the residual discoloration and can affect the eventual success of bleaching efforts.

Systemic Medications That Cause Permanent Discoloration

Tetracycline

The history of bleaching is inextricably tied to the widespread use of tetracycline antibiotics in midcentury. A virtual epidemic of distinctive yellow, brown, or gray stains occurred among people whose mothers had taken tetracycline while pregnant or who had themselves received it for as few as 3 days as a child. Much of what we know about the discoloration from systemic medication as well as the first widespread use of bleaching and subsequent development of modern bleaching techniques applicable to a wide variety of stains and discolorations occurred in response to this situation. Thanks to the dental profession's recognition of tetracycline's devastating effect on tooth formation, the FDA warned about the use of these antibiotics for pregnant women and children more than 30 years ago. Its use among the general public dropped precipitously, followed by a decline, the expected number of years later, in patients with tetracycline staining. Unfortunately, cases continue to be seen, especially among older patients. And tetracycline remains the only viable outpatient treatment for Rocky Mountain spotted fever and one of the most effective treatments for controlling secondary infection of the respiratory system often seen in children with cystic fibrosis.

Tetracycline provided dentists much insight into the mechanism by which medications could stain. Teeth are most susceptible to tetracycline discoloration during formation, beginning the second trimester in utero and continuing to roughly 8 years of age. It is believed that the tetracycline particles are incorporated into the dentin during calcification of the teeth, probably through chelation with calcium, which forms tetracycline orthophosphate.[44] The discoloration itself results from exposure of the teeth to sunlight, which is why the labial surfaces of the incisors tend to darken more quickly and intensely while the protected molars remain yellow longer.

A method for bleaching the discolored dentin of young adults who had undergone tetracycline treatment for cystic fibrosis was first published in 1970 by Cohen and Parkins[8] and remains the basis for much contemporary treatment. Its success spurred dentists concerned with esthetics to apply similar bleaching procedures to other stains and discolorations as well.

While not as common, tetracycline staining continues to be seen, and a medical history should include questions about use of it and of other medications. Tetracycline staining is extremely variable in its extent, color, intensity, and location, since the severity of stains depends on the time and duration of drug administration, and on which of more than 2000 patented formulations was administered. Fluorescence is necessary for precise diagnosis and description. Most cases fall into one of three major categories first proposed by Jordan and Boksman.[38]

First-degree tetracycline staining, a light yellow or light gray stain, uniformly distributed or concentrated in local areas, is highly amenable to bleaching. Good results frequently are achieved with power bleaching in four or fewer sessions. Second-degree tetracycline staining, similar but with darker or more extensive yellow or gray stains, requires more bleaching sessions for satisfactory results. Many dentists find a combination in-office/home matrix bleaching more effective.

Third-degree tetracycline staining, as described by Jordan and Boksman, is most intense, often dark gray or blue in color. Its most distinctive aspect is banding. The bands often remain evident even after extensive bleaching, so that satisfactory esthetic results may require veneering techniques with opaquers once the teeth have been lightened as much as possible by bleaching. It should be noted however, that up to 6 months of extended bleaching treatment for tetracycline shows promise of acceptable and enduring results.

Tetracycline stains that are simply too dark to attempt vital bleaching and for which bonding or laminating is a more appropriate place to begin may be classified as fourth degree.

Minocycline

The recent sudden appearance of ringlike stains on the teeth of adolescents and adults who have taken a semisynthetic derivative of tetracycline is a reminder of the power of medications given systemically to affect teeth coloration.[5] In addition to routine prescription for acne, minocycline is used for a variety of infections. Consequently, dentists can expect to see the number of cases rise and should include questions about its use in the medical history.

Since tetracycline is incorporated in the dentin during calcification of the teeth, adults whose teeth have already formed appear to be able to use it without risk of discoloration. Minocycline, in contrast, is absorbed from the gastrointestinal tract and combines poorly with calcium. Researchers at the National Institute of Dental Research believe the tooth pigmentation occurs because of minocycline's ability to chelate with iron and form insoluble complexes. Chung and Bowles[6] did a series of absorbance spectrum studies in vitro that provided evidence for the oxidative dissemination in minocycline that led to intrinsic dental staining. Another fascinating study by Dodson and Bowles[11] suggests the minocycline pigment produced in tissues is the same or very similar to that produced by ultraviolet radiation.

Like tetracycline, minocycline staining appears to be quite variable in degree and distribution, with less severe cases highly amenable to bleaching. More severe cases with heavy banding often require masking, ideally with porcelain lamination.

Fluoride

In areas where drinking water has a fluoride content in excess of four parts per million, a majority of children exposed for extensive periods between the third month of gestation through 8 years of age develop moderate to severe discoloration of the tooth surface, sometimes accompanied by loss of enamel. This condition was first described by Black and McKay in 1916,[4] but it took another 15 years before the cause was recognized. Today most cases are seen in the Southwestern United States, with fewer cases from the Eastern states, in areas where drinking water contains natural fluoride concentrations in excess of one part per million.[45] Use of fluoridated products, such as dentifrice, mouthwash, and vitamins, may increase this problem in areas where the fluoride concentration is close to this level.[18]

The type and degree of fluorosis problems depend on the intensity and duration of exposure, genetic vulnerability, and the point of the development of the enamel at which excessive fluoride intake occurs. The high concentration of fluoride is believed to cause a metabolic alteration in the ameloblasts, which results in a defective matrix and improper calcification. Histologic examination of the affected teeth shows a hypomineralized, porous subsurface enamel below a well-mineralized surface layer. This enamel hypoplasia is called *endemic enamel fluorosis* or *mottled enamel*. The premolar teeth are affected most often, followed by second molars, maxillary incisors, cuspids and first molars. Mandibular incisors are affected least. Where fluoride concentration is very high, primary teeth may also be affected.

Bleaching can work very well for most staining and discoloration problems of fluorosis, especially for simple fluorosis staining: brown pigmentation on a smooth enamel surface. It works less well with opaque fluorosis, in which flat gray or white flecks are visible on the enamel surface, or where there are white or opaque spots or multicolored stains. It lightens the teeth, but the whiter spots or banding may remain visible relative to the initial color. In such cases, and when staining is accompanied by pitting and other surface defects, treating with microabrasion, which is hydrochloric acid combined with pumice (Prema, Premier) may be best with which to begin. Bleaching is best viewed as a useful adjunctive treatment to lighten the teeth following removal of the offending brown or white spots. Eventually bonding or laminating may be necessary. Bleaching is rarely appropriate for teeth in which fluorosis has caused severe loss of enamel.

Systemic Conditions

Although relatively rare, some illnesses cause highly distinctive discoloration of the teeth by infusion of the dentin during critical stages of development. Children who suffer severe jaundice as infants may develop bluish gray or brown primary teeth as a result of postnatal staining of the dentin by bilirubin and biliverdin. Erythroblastosis fetalis, a result of Rh factor incompatibility between mother and fetus, frequently results in a pigmentation of the dentin of the infant's developing teeth. This occurs because of degradation of the excessive number of erythrocytes destroyed in Rh factor incompatibility. Porphyria causes excessive production of pigment that infuses the dentin, leaving primary and permanent teeth a dark purplish brown. Fortunately, this is an extremely rare condition.

Bleaching can be a useful treatment for most of these problems, depending on how light patients want their teeth to be. Other illnesses, however, cause discoloration of teeth by interfering with normal matrix formation or calcification of enamel. For these teeth, bleaching frequently cannot eradicate the white spots that disfigure the surface or is inappropriate because of weakness in the enamel. Such illnesses may be genetic, acquired, or environmental. Genetic conditions that sometimes cause enamel hypocalcification or hypoplasia include amelogenesis imperfecta and clefting of the lip and palate. Cerebral palsy, serious renal damage, severe allergies, and other acquired illnesses also interfere with the normal development of enamel, as do brain, neurologic, and other traumatic injuries. Children who do not have adequate vitamins A, C, and D, calcium, and phosphorus during the formative period sometimes develop enamel hypoplasia. The best treatment for most of these conditions is bonding or laminating.

Age-Related Discoloration

Part of the discoloration that almost inevitably accompanies aging is an extension of the genetic differences in natural tooth color and part is an accumulation of the insults and wear and tear experienced by the teeth. Years of coffee drinking and smoking have a cumulative effect, and these and other stains become even more visible because of inevitable cracking on the surface of the tooth, within its crystalline structure, and in the underlying dentin and pulp. In addition to wear and trauma on the teeth, amalgams and other restorations made years ago may begin to degrade. The best solution to this problem is first to replace the offending defective restoration, ideally with a tooth-colored restoration, then to evaluate whether bleaching on the labial surfaces will help to lighten the entire arch or the single tooth.

Another part of the discoloration, however, results from aging itself. Gradual thinning of the enamel may cause the facial surface of the tooth to appear flat, with a progressive shift in color owing to loss of the translucent enamel layer. Simultaneously, in response to the thinning of the enamel, a natural tooth protective mechanism begins to form secondary dentin, which is not only darker but less translucent. Thinned enamel and darkened dentin tend to create a darker, older-looking tooth.

Unless the enamel becomes too thin or worn, or cracking is too severe, bleaching works well against this age-related discoloration. In fact, bleaching often works *especially* well in older patients with yellow teeth because the pulp tends to shrink back in older teeth, making them less sensitive and affording the optional use of higher bleaching temperatures. The short time in the dental chair, the relatively low cost, and the relative lack of trauma also add to the appeal of bleaching for many older persons.

CONTRAINDICATIONS TO BLEACHING

- Too much sensitivity, because of severe erosion of the enamel, extremely large pulps, exposed root surfaces, the transient hyperemia associated with orthodontic tooth movement, or the patient's report of sensitivity. This may not be the same problem with matrix bleaching as with power bleach. In some cases, especially when the sensitivity is focused in the cervical areas, bleaching can still be used if the areas that are sensitive can be covered with a rubber dam and rubber dam substitute made by Den-Mat or Ultradent. In other cases, the cervical areas can be bonded with a slightly lighter composite, in the hopes that the remainder of the tooth will "more closely match" in color.
- Teeth with white or opaque spots. Bleaching usually does not remove such spots. Furthermore, many patients report the difference between the spots and the rest of the tooth varies during the course of the day, depending on a host of factors ranging from how dry the mouth is to the use of alcohol. A preferable treatment would be attempting to remove the white spot with microabrasion (Prema, Premier), bonding, or laminating. Haywood[33] says that the only truly effective means of removing, as opposed to covering, white spots is microabrasion, as described below. However, he adds, a combination of procedures, including bleaching of the adjacent teeth, can be used if the patient wants all of the teeth lighter.
- Extremely dark stains, especially those with banding or with uneven distribution. For example, with darker tetracycline stains, the majority of the bleaching takes place on the incisal half of the tooth, and it can be only partially overcome by selective bleaching and heat application. Consequently, veneering provides a better cover.

  White spots, banding, and dark stains may be partially bleached as a preliminary to bonding or veneering. Since this lightens the teeth somewhat, the contrast between the white spots and the teeth is diminished and this can improve the final result. But a recent study[55] suggests that special care needs to be taken when combining the two processes. They found that bleaching bovine teeth with peroxide reduced the adhesion of light-cured composite resin, regardless of whether the bleach was applied before or after etching. The residual peroxide in the dentinal tubules appeared to interfere with bonding, and even one full minute of washing with water did not eliminate the residual peroxide. A later study[49] led the editors of *Reality* to suggest that if bleaching is done on teeth that require only small restorations, then it is prudent to wait several weeks for remineralization before bonding, to improve bond strength. Haywood[33] says that 2 weeks wait between bleaching and bonding should prevent lowered shear strength.
- Teeth that have been bonded, laminated, or have extensive restorations. Teeth with extensive composite restorations may not have enough enamel to respond properly. In addition to the difficulty of bleaching a tooth to exactly match a restoration, bleaching chemicals can actually harm restorative materials. Koa and colleagues[39] believe bleaching materials should never come in contact with restorative materials. Their research found roughening on contact with all esthetic restorative materials, especially glass ionomers, although less to porcelain.
- Patients who are perfectionists or who do not have a good understanding of what bleaching can and cannot do for them. Bleaching is not perfect, since it merely changes color relative to highly variable depths and distributions of different stains on frequently imperfect teeth. You have only to thumb through today's popular magazines, replete with advertisements for inexpensive home bleaching kits touted by beautiful models with perfectly formed and colored teeth, to understand why your patients might not understand bleaching's ability and limits to provide white, even teeth. Computer imaging can help determine if the patient will be satisfied with the final result.

MICROABRASION: AN OPTION WHEN BLEACHING IS NOT EFFECTIVE

One of the more recent approaches to the challenge of intrinsically stained teeth and especially white spots is microabrasion. The first substance was 18% hydrochloric acid. Microabrasion actually removes 22 to 27 μm of the enamel per application by softening the enamel with hydrochloric acid and abrading it with a controlled abrasive technique. Prema (Premier Dental Products) compound, introduced in 1990, contains abrasive particles suspended with a low concentration of hydrochloric acid in a water-soluble gel and is applied to enamel with a hard rubber mandrill in a low-speed handpiece. A 1991 study by Scherer and colleagues [50] found that placing the Prema compound on facial enamel resulted in a more diffuse and milder etch patterns than straight 18 percent hydrochloric acid when compared by scanning electron microscopy. This was true for both 5- and 20-second treatments.

As described by Haywood[33] microabrasion is a possible second choice for certain discolorations that are not completely susceptible to bleaching. It also is an excellent way of permanently removing surface stains, and Haywood suggests a sequence of treatments in which dentist-prescribed, home-applied bleaching is followed by microabrasion if needed. If used for white spots, however, it may precede bleaching.

IN-OFFICE BLEACHING OF VITAL TEETH: FIRST DECISION

Incorporation into the Treatment Plan

Once the decision has been made to utilize bleaching, it is important to consider its sequence in the overall treatment plan for the patient. Generally, bleaching is the first treatment to be used after tissue management. Prophylaxis is always done initially and then any further periodontal treatment is undertaken.

Patients with soft tissue problems must be treated periodontically to control the inflammation before any bleaching is undertaken. The exception is when advanced bone loss is present and surgery will mean raising the tissue well into the root surface. In this case, it may be advisable first to bleach the tooth with adequate rubber dam protection. This would make it easier for the tissue to hold the dam in place at the C-E junction, rather than having the bleaching solution be exposed to the cervical root areas after periodontal therapy.

As discussed earlier, if using office power bleaching, damaged restorations should be repaired before bleaching, although consideration must be given to the color changes bleaching will produce. As for further restorations under consideration, many patients would like to obtain the maximum effect with bleaching before making a decision to proceed with restorative therapy. These patients should be reassured that *any* lightening produced by bleaching can be useful since it diminishes the amount of opacifier that will have to be incorporated into bonding or laminate veneer procedures.

If crowns or laminates are anticipated, it is important to wait at least 2 or 3 weeks after bleaching before taking the final shade, so as to match the shade with the bleached adjacent teeth. It is also important to warn the patient that additional bleaching may be necessary after several years in order to keep the adjacent or opposing teeth matched to the new crowns.

Preferably, bleaching takes place before orthodontics, especially if ceramic or metal brackets will be bonded to the teeth. The bonding impregnates the enamel and makes it more difficult to bleach the teeth. If this is not possible or if the patient previously had orthodontics, it is important to make certain all bonding material is removed from the tooth structure. This can be done with Prophy-Jet prophylaxis followed by mild acid etching before the first application of bleaching solution to better ensure that all the bonding material is removed.

Endodontists increasingly play an important role in esthetic dentistry. As the section on pulpless teeth in this chapter indicates, tooth color can vary widely, depending on the cause of pulp death, consequent treatment, and time. The endodontist is in a key position to query patients about their feelings about their tooth color. In fact, such questions should be included as part of a standard diagnostic input. And the endodontist's expertise is necessary in consultation with the general dentist concerned about the overall appearance of the patient's smile. Whether a single tooth or multiple teeth or the entire arch, the likely appearance of the nonvital tooth over the next few years must be conveyed to the referring dentist, who needs to know, for example, what will happen to an endodontically treated tooth that eventually receives a porcelain laminate. Will the tooth grow darker as the years go by, affecting the color of the laminated tooth and making it stand out? If so, will more opaquer have to be applied to that particular tooth restoration? In terms of bleaching, you may need to bleach that tooth somewhat more aggressively and plan for more frequent rebleaching.

And finally, of course, you need to consider if bleaching is going to be an adjunct for some other esthetic treatment. In these cases, bleaching should be done first. Some instances are obvious. For example, bleaching may help to improve the appearance of porcelain laminate veneers. When a great deal of opaquer has to be incorporated into the laminate or on the tooth itself, the resulting restoration often is artificial looking. Bleaching allows the shade of the base tooth to be lightened, providing a lighter and more natural-looking restoration. Bleaching also can be used on opposing or adjacent teeth, so that other more discolored or deformed teeth can be restored to a lighter shade than would otherwise be possible.

Choosing a Bleaching Solution

Oddly enough, of everything to do with bleaching, the agents themselves have changed least in the last hundred years or so. Abbot's discovery of the effectiveness of hydrogen peroxide has not been surpassed. Regardless of the innovations and improvements in equipment and delivery, some form of hydrogen peroxide remains the bleaching agent of choice. In most cases of in-office bleaching, a 30% to 35% concentration of hydrogen peroxide is the ideal mixture. Most matrix bleaching involves 3% hydrogen peroxide in the form of 10% to 15% carbamide peroxide.

One change which appears likely at present concerns the pH of hydrogen peroxide. A study[15] compared the effectiveness of regular dental bleaching agents, with a pH of 4.4, with that same agent at pH 9.0. After exposing two groups of 10 teeth each to the different pH mixtures for 15 minutes, Frysch et al concluded that bleaching teeth with hydrogen peroxide at pH 9.0 is more effective than using the usual acid pH of current peroxide-based bleaching agents.

Choosing a Bleaching Light

The choice of heating devices from the growing number available is in many ways a matter of personal preference and comfort. Some dentists prefer a photoflood lamp that focuses its rays on the labial surface of the tooth, providing light as well as heat (Fig. 21-1). Some manufacturers suggest using a polymerization light to accelerate the bleaching (see Fig. 21-5, *C*). Although this can work, it does require someone to hold it on each single tooth to be bleached. A dedicated bleaching light can simplify this procedure by allowing an assistant to monitor the result.

Hodosh and colleagues[36] prefer a rheostat-controlled solid state heating device with specially designed tips that allow the dentist to provide pin-point bleaching and heating in grooves, depressions, and smaller areas. If this individual metal-tip device is your choice, it is helpful to choose one with predictable temperatures (Fig. 21-2). These devices also require less time, with 10 minutes or less ordinarily being adequate to improve color noticeably.

Many dentists use the Illuminator (Union Broach), a state-of-the-art bleaching instrument that combines an activation light and activation wand for bleaching procedures on both vital and pulpless teeth (Fig. 21-3). A built-in sensor allows precise temperature of the bleaching light, elevating or lowering it as needed to maintain predetermined temperatures. The convenience of having both modalities within easy reach means the color of any darker tooth or teeth can be blended with extra heat by the bleaching wand following the overall in-office bleaching procedure.

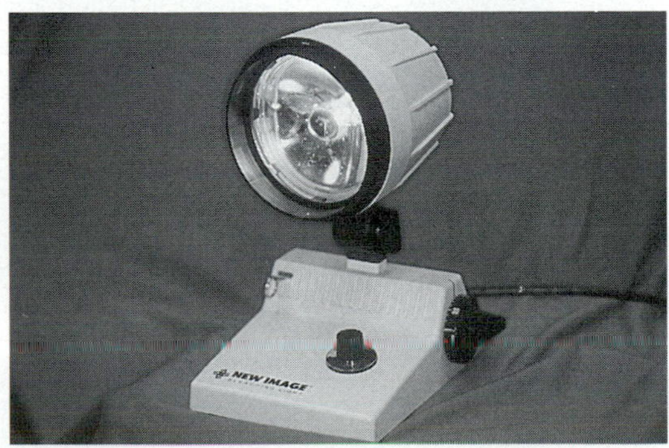

FIG. 21-1 This form of a bleaching light offers an easy way to adjust the beam of light since there is no metal frame encasing the bulb. It is placed approximately 13 inches from the teeth for 20 to 30 minutes and temperature adjusted for patient comfort throughout the treatment.

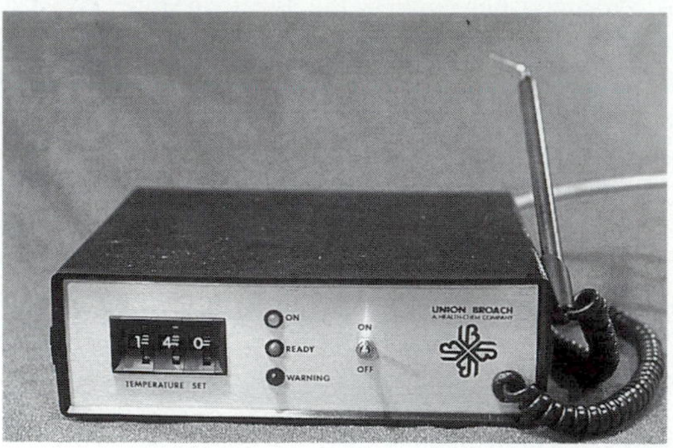

FIG. 21-2 The individual bleaching instrument was developed by the Indiana University School of Dentistry and consists of a heated tip which can be used for either external or internal bleaching of individual teeth.

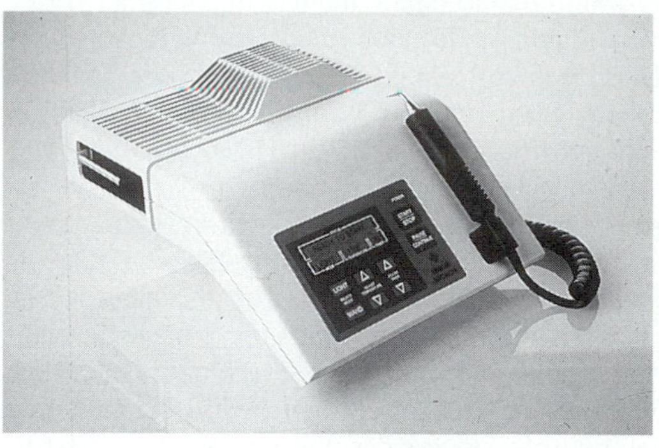

FIG. 21-3 The bleaching Illuminator is a combined bleaching light and heat wand that furnishes an LED readout for the most optimal combined bleaching instrument available today. (Courtesy Union Broach.)

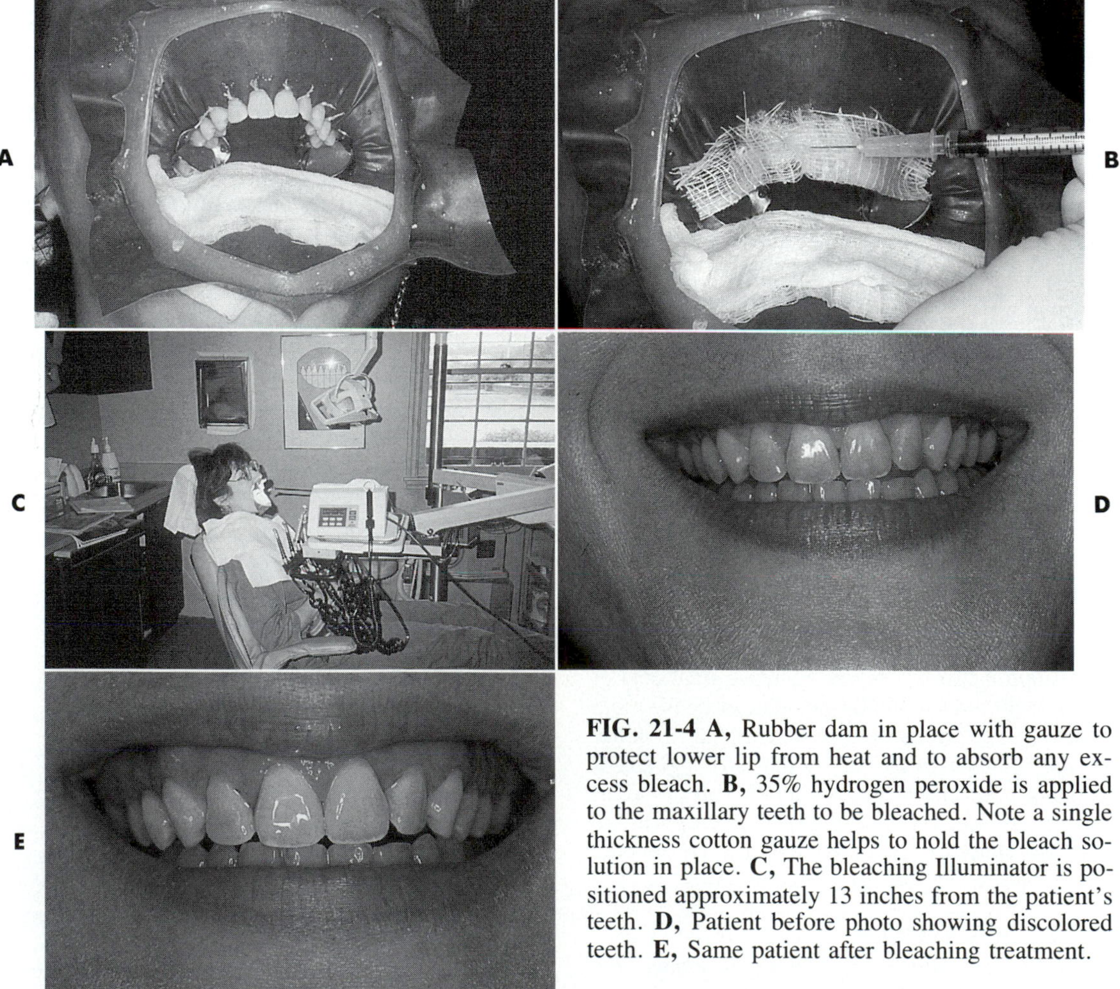

FIG. 21-4 A, Rubber dam in place with gauze to protect lower lip from heat and to absorb any excess bleach. **B,** 35% hydrogen peroxide is applied to the maxillary teeth to be bleached. Note a single thickness cotton gauze helps to hold the bleach solution in place. **C,** The bleaching Illuminator is positioned approximately 13 inches from the patient's teeth. **D,** Patient before photo showing discolored teeth. **E,** Same patient after bleaching treatment.

IN-OFFICE BLEACHING OF VITAL TEETH: STEP BY STEP GUIDELINES (FIG. 21-4)

Protecting the Patient and Dental Team

Before turning attention to the mouth, the patient's hands and clothes should be well protected with heavy plastic wrap. The importance of the patient's wearing safety glasses throughout the entire procedure, until he or she is told they can be removed, must be explained in detail to the patient; it can hardly be over emphasized since some of the most common injuries in a dental office involve the eyes.[9] All members of the dental team also must wear surgical rubber gloves and safety glasses as in all procedures.

Do not use any local anesthesia during bleaching! The patient's normal responses should be fully intact so that he or she can provide feedback about possible leakage through the rubber dam or if the heat becomes too intense. In those unusual cases in which otherwise appropriate patients absolutely refuse to go through bleaching without anesthesia, you will need to change the treatment plan. You may consider using matrix bleaching alone, or a bleaching compound that will not injure tissue if the dam should leak, or you may choose to proceed with in-office bleaching but using a lower level of heat and an increased number of bleaching visits. You also might consider using nonmetallic clamps to secure the rubber dam, thus reducing possible heat buildup in the clamps. Another alternative is to use an in-office technique of concentrated hydrogen peroxide with no heat or light.

The soft tissues of the mouth are protected by Oraseal (Ultradent) and a rubber dam (Fig. 21-5). Apply plain Oraseal to the gingiva—labially, buccally, lingually, and interproximally. The teeth to be bleached should be isolated with a rubber dam, and all teeth ligated with *waxed* dental floss. Form a protective pocket by turning the corners of the rubber dam and putting Oraseal on the proximal surfaces, only at the gingival areas, to act as an additional seal to prevent leakage. Also put Oraseal on any amalgams present to seal and help block out some of the heat that will be generated by the bleaching light. Arens suggests the dam be of dark color and heavy texture and that the holes be punched father apart than normal, to prevent the dam from sliding into the interproximal sulcus, exposing the papilla to the bleaching agent.[2]

Protecting the Soft Tissues in Preparation for Bleaching

To protect the patient's upper lip and adjacent tissue, place a piece of gauze saturated with cold water under the rubber dam. Also place gauze saturated with cold water over any metal clamps and the lower lip on top of the dam when bleach-

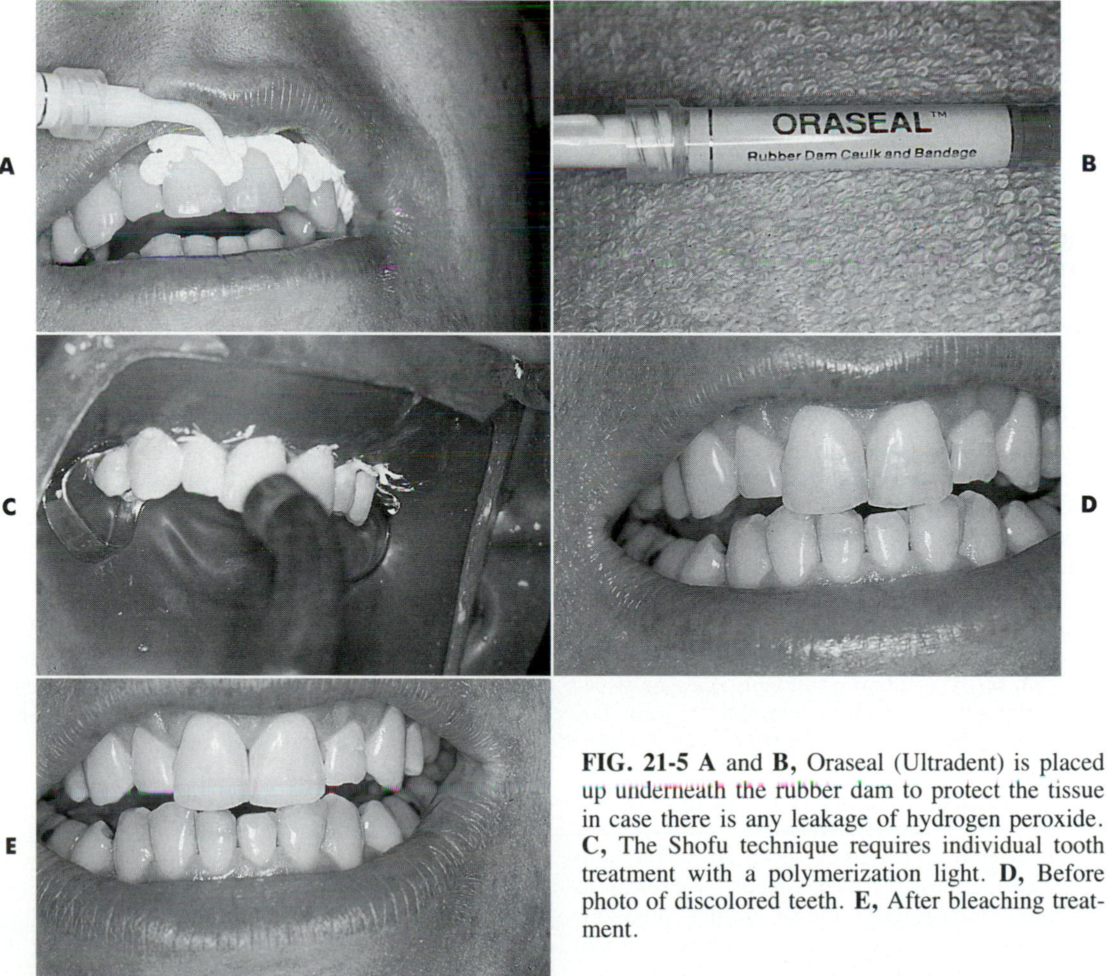

FIG. 21-5 A and **B,** Oraseal (Ultradent) is placed up underneath the rubber dam to protect the tissue in case there is any leakage of hydrogen peroxide. **C,** The Shofu technique requires individual tooth treatment with a polymerization light. **D,** Before photo of discolored teeth. **E,** After bleaching treatment.

ing maxillary teeth (Fig. 21-4, *A*). It is important to keep these gauze squares wet throughout the bleaching procedure, in order to protect the lips from the increased temperatures generated by the bleaching light.

Preparing the Teeth for Bleaching

The teeth will have been freed of all surface stains and plaque with Prophy-Jet during the earlier diagnostic period. Now, after the dam is in place, prepare the teeth for bleaching by first removing any excess varnish and jelly from the enamel surface and pumicing each tooth to remove any excess dam sealant or stain. Rinse thoroughly.

Bleaching can be accomplished without etching the enamel, and dentists like Hall[20] argue there is no advantage to etching the teeth before bleaching. Ten microns of enamel are lost during acid etching in addition to the 25 microns of enamel that are etched.[51] Furthermore, if the tooth is etched for bleaching, it generally must be polished after each appointment, removing an additional 5 to 50 microns of enamel. As Haywood points out, to not etch preserves the enamel, retaining the fluoride-rich surface layer of enamel, as well as shortening the appointment time.[33]

However, if your case suggests you need to enhance the penetrability of the bleaching solution, you can etch the enamel slightly first. Use a 35-37 percent buffered phosphoric acid to etch each tooth facially and lingually for five seconds. The increased ability of etching followed by bleaching to increase stain reduction has been noted by numerous clinicians, beginning with Boksman. In laboratory studies, Falkenstein[13] reported that the combination increased penetration on the calcium phosphate tetracycline molecule to reach up to 5-7 microns into the surface which is high.

Today, the desirability of etching is debated. If you *do* etch, rinse throughout for 20 seconds, then dry the teeth. They will appear chalky.

General Considerations for Applying the Bleaching Agent

The way in which bleaching solution is applied to the teeth will differ depending on the distribution of the discoloration. For discoloration which has affected some teeth or parts of teeth more striking than others, you literally paint the bleach on the tooth directly, concentrating on the pattern of staining. For more even distribution (such as most extrinsic stains and some systemically-caused discolorations), you can cover several teeth at once with gauze which you then infuse with the bleaching solution.

No matter what the approach, however, you want to leave some teeth untreated as controls in order to determine the effect of the treatment, both now and in follow-up. In working with pulpless teeth this is seldom a problem, since most patients only want the affected tooth to resemble the rest. For fluorosis-stained teeth, there may be unaffected teeth appropriate for controls. For more homogeneous discoloration such as that caused by medicines during the formation of the tooth, the mandibular teeth are acceptable controls.

And no matter what the condition or approach, you want to begin treatment on the most discolored teeth, proceeding to the less discolored. Good rules of thumb are that yellow or yellow-brown stains are easier to remove than gray and that incisal halves of teeth respond to bleach more quickly than cervical halves, due to the thinner dentin.

Homogeneous Discoloration

The application of the bleaching solution is identical for extrinsic staining, tetracycline, minocycline or other systemic causes of a consistent, homogeneous discoloration.

- After rinsing and drying the teeth as above, place on the dried teeth a piece of cotton gauze saturated with the hydrogen peroxide bleaching solution.
- Position a bleaching light (or the bleaching "Illuminator") approximately 13 inches from the teeth to be bleached, with the light shining directly on the teeth (Fig. 21-4, *C*). Begin with a rheostat setting of 5 (approximately 105 °F) and increase the temperature as long as the patient feels no sensitivity. The best results are achieved at the highest light and heat intensities, but temperatures slightly less than 115 degrees will bleach teeth, although at a slower rate. The usual range of temperatures for bleaching vital teeth is 115-140 degrees. Overheating can cause tissue damage.

  As the rheostat is being raised, ask the patient at each stage about his or her comfort, remembering that some patients will minimize initial discomfort in their eagerness to have brighter teeth. If the patient reports discomfort, check the sensitive spot or spots. Some tissue may need further covering with cold water-saturated gauze or the dam may have developed a small leak. If no area seems exposed, you will need to immediately lower the temperature to the highest degree with which the patient is comfortable, being certain to document the temperature used for the next bleaching session. Moving the light further back is another option to reduce the temperature, and this change too should be recorded exactly. These lower temperatures do not necessarily reduce your chance of success, although they probably do indicate you will have to provide additional number of treatments.
- Keep the gauze over the teeth being bleached continually wet with the bleaching agent by dispensing fresh bleaching solution from an eyedropper, syringe, or cotton swab (Fig. 21-4, *B*). The teeth to be bleached should be in continuous contact with a bleaching agent and light/heat for approximately 30 minutes.
- Remove the gauze and flush the teeth with copious amounts of *warm* water. Remove the floss by slipping an explorer under each knot to loosen it, or clip with a scalpel and pull the opened floss out with cotton pliers. As you remove the rubber dam, use a warm damp gauze to remove the excess Oraseal.

Heterogeneous Discoloration

The application of bleaching solution is similar for fluorosis-stained teeth and other conditions in which only selected teeth are affected or in which discoloration is uneven on the teeth. The main difference in treatment is the extra effort in dealing with the more concentrated stained areas.

- After rinsing and drying the teeth exposed through the rubber dam, cover the teeth to be bleached with gauze and apply a fresh solution of hydrogen peroxide to the stained area of the enamel of the teeth, beginning with the most heavily stained. Place the individual tooth instrument (bleaching wand) against the gauze covering the teeth for two to five minutes. Examine and repeat this sequence, of fresh hydrogen peroxide and application of the bleaching wand, until the desired shade is obtained.

- Flush with copious amounts of warm water. Remove the dam carefully, using a damp gauze to remove any excess Oraseal.

Finishing the Teeth

If you have etched the teeth, polish them with yellow-banded Shofu finishing wheels (Shofu contouring kit or Shofu quasite polishing cups).

If treatments extend over weeks, a protective interim seal will prevent or minimize new extrinsic stains during the follow-up period. Berman suggests 30 percent NaF (removable by flushing with water), or a varnish (removable with an organic solvent). He also suggests veneering the tooth with a thin coat of transparent sealant at the end of the bleaching sequence.

After the last treatment, polish with an impregnated rotary polishing wheel to achieve a high enamel luster (Shofu Composite Fine Mounted Disc).

BLEACHING PULPLESS TEETH

Bleaching Agents

Agents and techniques for bleaching discolored pulpless teeth have changed little in the last 30 years.[46,46a,53] The two bleaching agents most commonly used are Superoxol (30 to 35 percent hydrogen peroxide) and sodium perborate. Both are oxidizing agents. Superoxol has about twice the available oxygen as sodium perborate. This property makes it more reactive during bleaching and more likely to burn soft tissue.

Superoxol is heated directly within the pulp chamber in the thermocatalytic bleach or mixed with sodium perborate and sealed in the pulp chamber to form the walking bleach. Sodium perborate may be mixed with water as a less reactive type of walking bleach. Since their use causes few chairside problems what concern is there in using these agents to bleach teeth?

Resorption

Harrington and Natkin were the first to report a possible relationship between intracoronal bleaching of pulpless teeth and external cervical root resorption (Fig. 21-6).[21] Other studies found the incidence of cervical root resorption after bleaching ranged from 0 to 6.9 percent.[14,37] It could occur in as many as one of every 12 teeth bleached.

Originally, as noted in Walton's classic study,[56] it appeared that the combination of Superoxol and heat was initiating the resorption. However, in case reports subsequently published, two different characteristics were found in every instance of resorption.* One, the teeth became pulpless before the patient reached age 25. Two, no barrier had been placed between the endodontic filling material and the pulp chamber. Therefore, it appears that the age of the patient *at the time the tooth became pulpless* and the presence of a barrier may be as important as the type of bleaching agent and the use of heat during bleaching.

Etiology

In ten percent of all teeth, dentinal tubules communicate between the root canal system and the periodontal membrane space through defects at the cementoenamel junction (CEJ).[54] If the patient is young when the tooth becomes pulpless, the tubules will remain patent since formation of sclerotic dentin halts. These open tubules represent a conduit for the bleach solution to reach the periodontal ligament from the root canal system.

Since the dentinal tubules are oriented incisally, clinicians have advocated bleaching agents be placed apical to the labial CEJ to bleach the cervical third of the crown.[2,10,35] Three fac-

*References 10a, 14, 17, 19, 21, 37, 40a, 41, 41a, 44a.

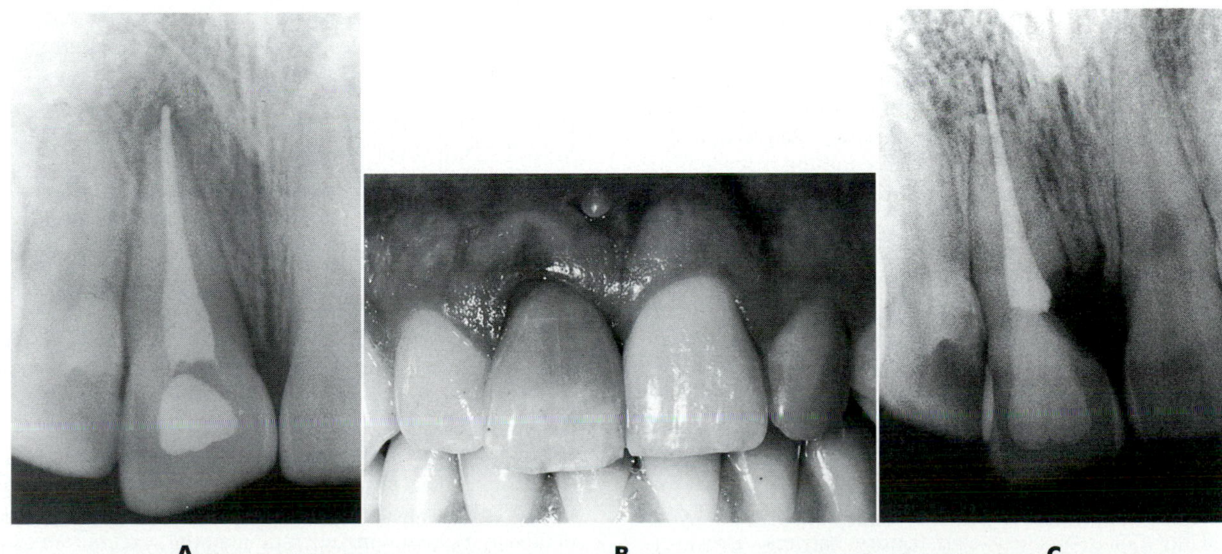

FIG. 21-6 Example of external cervical root resorption. **A,** Pre-bleach radiograph of a maxillary central. **B,** Color relapse after three years. **C,** Recall radiograph reveals resorption.

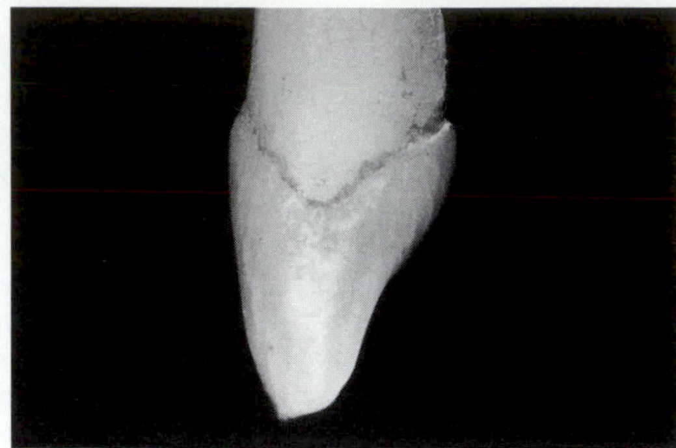

FIG. 21-7 Proximal view of the CEJ. A flat barrier, level with the labial CEJ, leaves a large area of uncovered proximal tubules.

tors, bleach placed apical to the CEJ, patent dentinal tubules in young pulpless teeth, and a defect in the cementoenamel junction may combine to allow the bleaching agent to diffuse into the periodontal ligament. An inflammatory reaction can be initiated, resulting in external cervical root resorption.[21]

Barrier

Clinicians have no control over the patient's age when a tooth becomes pulpless. They do have control over the location, shape and material of a bleach barrier between the filling material and the pulp chamber. The labial CEJ has been suggested as a guide to determine the barrier location.[48,57] The CEJ is not level but rather curves in an incisal direction on the proximal sides of the tooth (Fig. 21-7). If a flat barrier is placed, the proximal tubules are unprotected by the barrier material. This critical proximal area is where cervical root resorption begins.

Barrier Transfer

A barrier transfer is a simple, but important, step to help prevent external cervical root resorption. The intention is to cover the dentinal tubules apical to the epithelial attachment so that the bleaching agents are contained within the pulp chamber.

The barrier transfer technique refers to three periodontal probings made with a custom "transfer periodontal probe." This is a standard periodontal probe carefully curved to match the labial contour of the tooth. A labial recording is made from the epithelial attachment to the incisal edge of the tooth, followed by mesial and distal recordings. The internal level of the barrier is placed one millimeter incisal to the corresponding external probings of the epithelial attachment (Fig. 21-8). Now, the dentinal tubules can be blocked with a properly positioned barrier which covers the proximal area. The shape of the barrier from a facial view is a tunnel outline which should be verified radiographically (Fig. 21-9). The outline form from the proximal resembles a slope (Fig. 21-10). A radiograph of the intracoronal bleach barrier shows the distinct tunnel appearance (Fig. 21-11).[53a]

In preliminary studies, IRM, zinc oxyphosphate, and dentin sealants failed to create satisfactory barriers. However, Cavit and light-cured glass ionomer cements may offer promise as future barrier materials. More research is being done to identify the best barrier material.[10,43,48,52]

Resorption Repair

What can be done if no barrier is placed or the barrier fails and resorption occurs? There are five treatment options:

1. Calcium hydroxide therapy.
2. Forced orthodontic extrusion.
3. Surgery.
4. Extraction.
5. Submersion of the root.

Calcium hydroxide therapy. Two case reports indicate the resorption can be arrested using calcium hydroxide.[17,44a] In both instances, the defect was relatively small and the epithelial attachment was intact. If it is possible to probe through the sulcus to the level of the defect, calcium hydroxide therapy will not be successful.

Forced orthodontic extrusion. By extruding the root, the resorptive defect can be elevated coronal to crestal bone. Here it is accessible and can be included in a crown preparation or repaired.[34] Specific orthodontic criteria must be met for success.[40] The crown/root ratio must be 1:1 and the root should be non-tapering. Esthetic considerations due to the narrowness of the extruded root play a limiting role in choosing this approach. An orthodontic consultation is recommended.

Surgery. The most common approach to repair cervical defects is surgery. The resorption usually starts proximally and often wraps around toward the palatal. Both a labial and palatal flap are necessary for access. The lesion is cleaned, bony contouring accomplished, and the defect repaired. Esthetic concerns may arise due to bone loss and tissue changes. The tooth is more susceptible to fracturing.

Extraction. Extraction is the most common outcome when large resorptive defects are found. Patients are often very disappointed by the unexpected consequence. What was presented as a minor bleaching procedure has become extensive restorative treatment. A single tooth implant or a three-unit bridge is the prosthetic replacement. Esthetic difficulties arise if the labial cortical bone resorbs and the patient has a high smile line.

Submersion of the root. The coronal tooth structure and resorptive defect can be removed one to two millimeters below the cortical plates of bone, and tissue sutured over the surgical site.[58] Retaining the root may prevent the characteristic loss of labial bone so a more esthetic restoration can be achieved.

BLEACHING PROCEDURE

Step 1: Diagnose

Pulpal necrosis must be confirmed with pulp tests. Where previous endodontics treatment exists, verify healing and confirm that the root canal is obturated three dimensionally.

Step 2: Record Shade

A photograph and a shade guide provide legal and treatment references to measure the progress of color enhancement.

Step 3: Prepare Access Cavity

Access cavity design should follow normal straight line endodontics access guidelines. If root canal treatment is already completed and successful, then the access cavity is cleaned meticulously by removing necrotic material, excess root canal filling and endodontics sealer. Uncleansed pulp horns are most often a source for discoloration. Be sure to eliminate all debris from pulp horns.

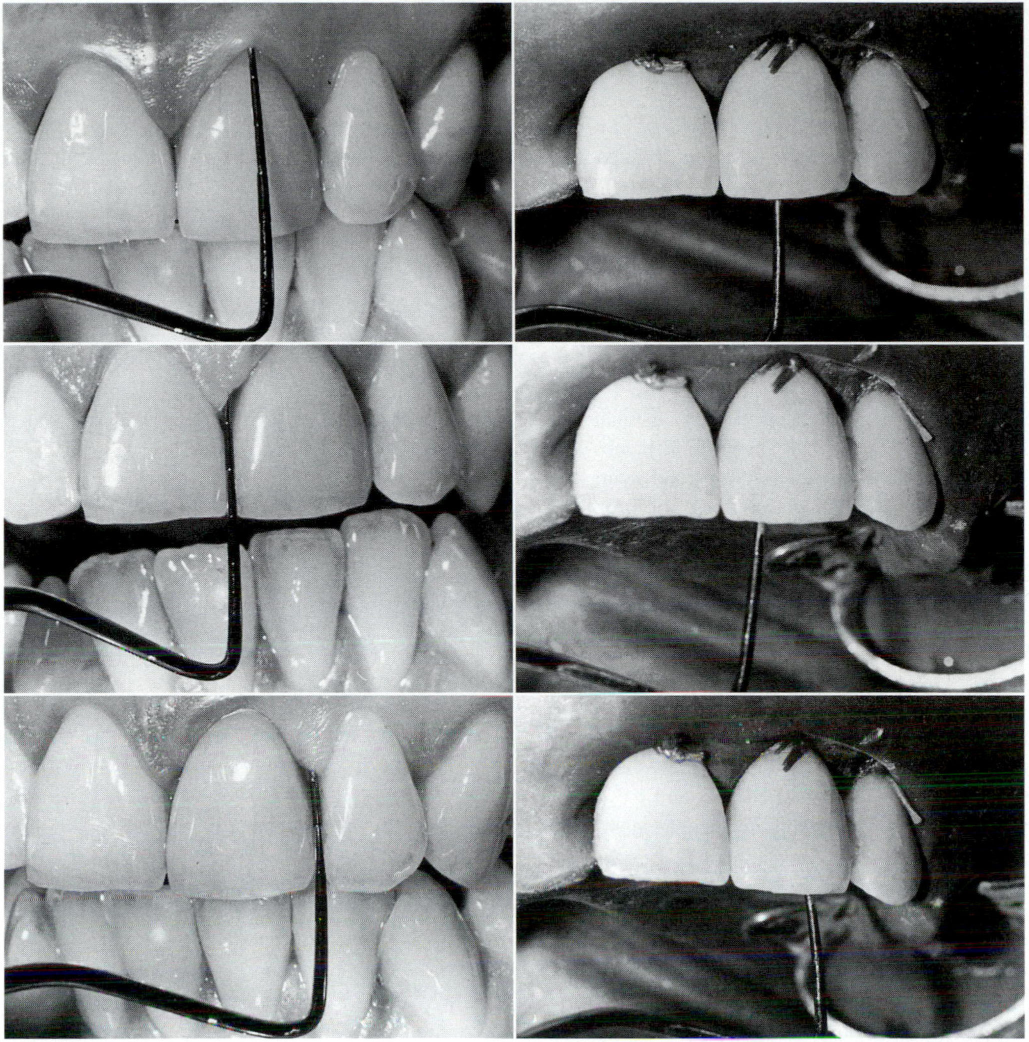

FIG. 21-8 Barrier transfer. The external level of the epithelial attachment is recorded at the labial, mesial, and distal. The intracoronal level of the barrier is placed 1 mm incisal to the corresponding external probing.

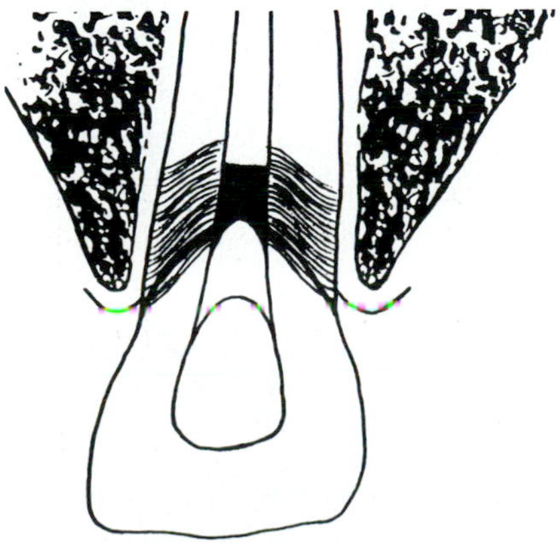

FIG. 21-9 Facial outline of the barrier resembles a tunnel.

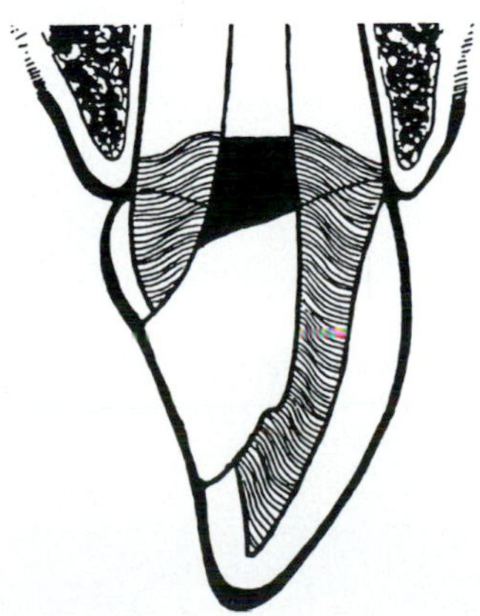

FIG. 21-10 Proximal outline appears as a slope.

Step 4: Record Barrier Probings

This step determines the location and shape of the barrier between the root canal obturation and the pulp chamber.

Step 5: Isolate the Tooth

After dental prophylaxis, isolate the tooth to be bleached with a well fitted rubber dam.

Step 6: Transfer Barrier Probing

Transfer the three external periodontal probings into the access cavity in order to create an outline for the internal barrier.

Step 7: Place Barrier Material

A glass ionomer barrier can be inserted into the chamber with a straight lentulo spiral and a slow speed hand piece. The correct incisal extension of the barrier is confirmed using the custom barrier probe. Drag the glass ionomer up the proximal walls, creating mesial and distal barrier wings. Light-cure the entire barrier.

If Durelon is used for barrier material, place a small cone on the end of an endodontics plugger and pack against the gutta-percha. The back of a spoon excavator is used to press Durelon against the proximal walls to the proper protective level. Use a wet cotton pellet to accelerate the setting time. The barrier should be at least 2 mm thick.

Step 8: Introduce Bleaching Solution

A cotton pellet placed against the labial access wall may then be saturated with Superoxol, or Superoxol may be deposited directly into the access cavity with a glass syringe fitted with a stainless steel needle.

Step 9: Thermocatalytically Activate Bleach

The analytic technology 5004 Touch 'n Heat (Analytic Technology, Redmond, Wash.) bleaching wand is introduced into the Superoxol. Use a no. 2 or 3 heat setting. Heat the solution for 2 minutes, then change the Superoxol and repeat one more time (Fig. 21-12). External brushes on the facial surfaces can enhance the bleaching effect. Heating should be no hotter than what a vital tooth could stand.

Step 10: Rinse and Close

After thermocatalytically bleaching the tooth, its true color should be evaluated after several days of rehydration. Rinse the chamber thoroughly and place a cotton pellet and Cavit. After the heat bleaching, if the shade is still too dark, place a walking bleach.

Step 11: Place Walking Bleach

Prepare a thick mix of sodium perborate and Superoxol, or sodium perborate and water. Fill the appropriate end of an amalgam carrier with the paste and pack it against the barrier and the labial surface (Fig. 21-13).

Step 12: Insert Temporary Seal

This step seems simple, but if the seal is not secure, leakage of the bleaching agent can occur. A 2 mm layer of Cavit produces an effective, efficient, and easy temporary. The first layer is wiped around the inner rim of the access cavity and the second layer is spread gently into the remaining concavity.

Step 13: Determine Duration of Walking Bleach

Leave the walking bleach in place for two to seven days or until the patient notices that the tooth is as light or slightly lighter than the adjacent teeth. Several applications may be necessary.

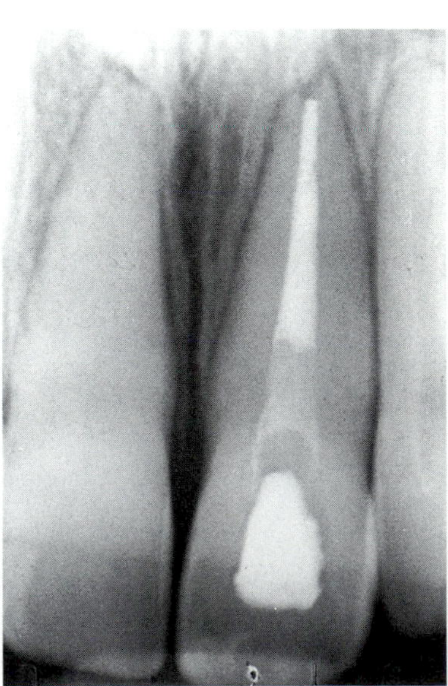

FIG. 21-11 Radiographic appearance of a bleach barrier.

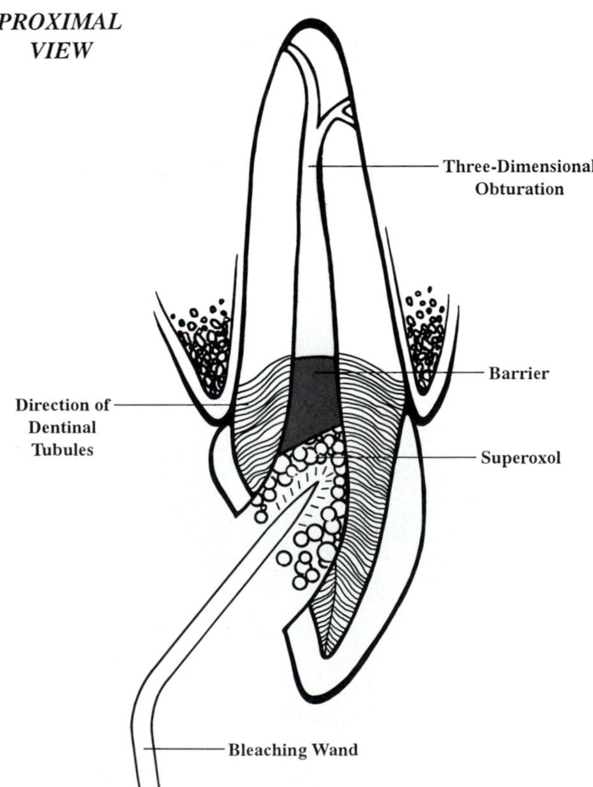

FIG. 21-12 Diagram of thermocatalytic bleach.

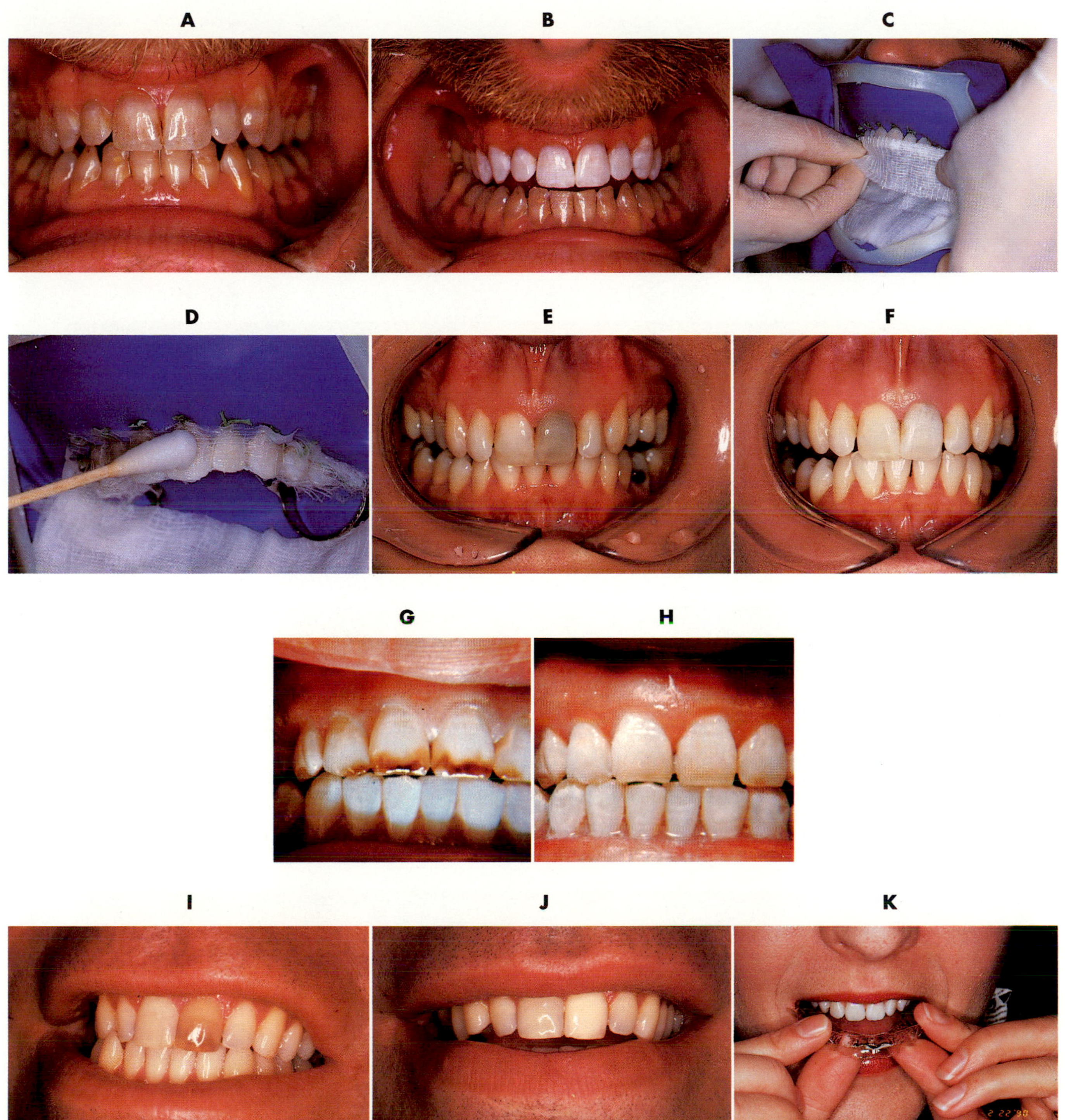

COLOR PLATE 2 A, Tetracycline stain. **B,** Same patient after three vital bleaching procedures. **C,** Application of gauze to anterior teeth that will be bleached. Dental floss is used to ligate each tooth that will be bleached. **D,** The gauze covering the surfaces of the teeth is continuously saturated throughout the procedure. **E,** Postendodontic discoloration, before treatment. **F,** Same patient after one in-office bleaching treatment. **G,** Endemic fluorosis stain. **H,** After the bleaching procedure. **I,** Vital discolored central incisor. **J,** Improved shade after one bleaching appointment. **K,** Matrix applied by patient for home bleaching technique. (**G** and **H** courtesy Dr. P. Colon.)

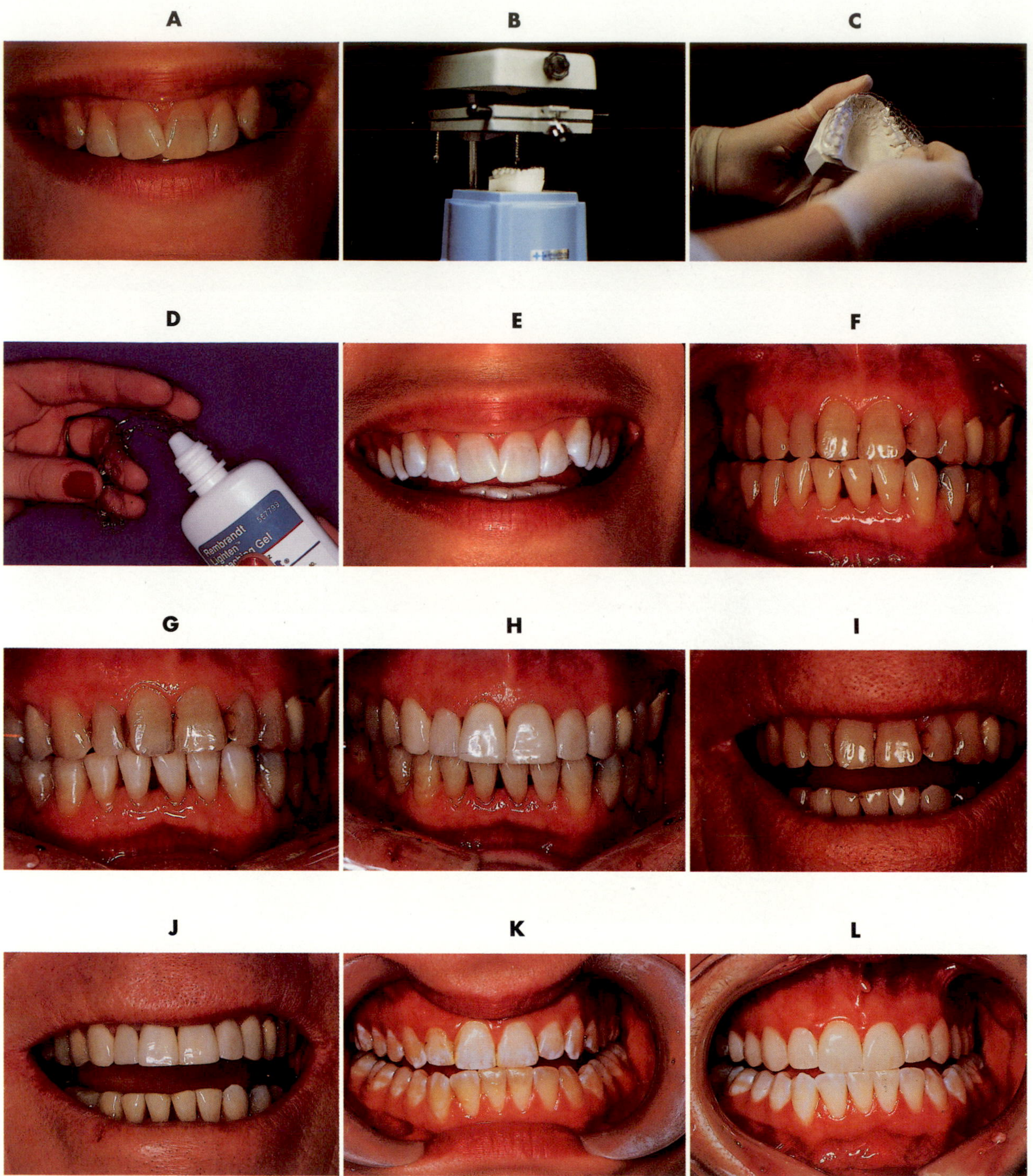

COLOR PLATE 3 A, This 30-year-old physician wanted lighter teeth within a short time. **B,** Patient's stone model on vacu-form press having matrix made. **C,** Matrix being pulled off the working cast to allow patient to have a controlled matrix bleach following in-office bleach. **D,** Bleaching solution being poured into matrix. **E,** Two in-office treatments, plus two weeks matrix bleaching, produced the above result. **F,** Sixty-five-year-old corporation president with darkly stained teeth. **G,** Lower teeth after one in-office "power" bleaching, consisting of 35% hydrogen peroxide and 30 minutes with the bleaching light. **H,** Patient after six maxillary porcelain laminates plus combination in-office and matrix bleach. **I,** Smile *before*. **J,** Smile *after* bleaching and laminates. **K,** Combination therapy with hypocalcification on maxillary incisors, dark lower and upper teeth. **L,** Patient after in-office bleaching and 10 porcelain laminates on maxillary incisors and bicuspids.

Step 14: Combination Bleaching

Thermocatalytic or a walking bleach may be used as separate methods or in combination to bleach a tooth. Which bleaching method is best? The effectiveness and rate of the bleaching change appears inversely proportional to the safety of the method. A walking bleach of sodium perborate and water bleaches teeth between 50 to 60% of the time, but no case reports of resorption have been associated with its use.[35,37,47]

The combination of Superoxol and heat followed by a walking bleach using a mixture of Superoxol and sodium perborate is effective in bleaching teeth about 90% of the time.[35] The impression is that an increased chance of resorption is possible with this combination (Fig. 21-14). However, if used with an adequate barrier and in a tooth which became pulpless in a patient older than 25 years, the chance of problems appears minimal.

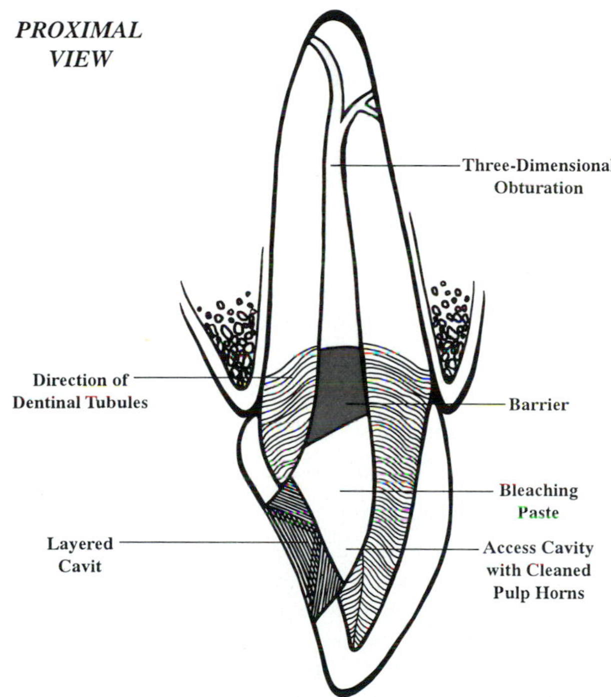

FIG. 21-13 Diagram of walking bleach.

Step 15: Restore Access

When the color of the tooth is satisfactory, seal the lingual access using an acid-etch light-cured composite. Light-cure from the labial surface, then the lingual surface. This may cause the composite to shrink toward the axial walls and reduce the rate of microleakage.[42]

Although acid-etching the cavosurface and the dentin and filling the chamber with a light-cured composite appears to reduce the rate of re-discoloration, microleakage remains a problem.[59] The extent to which it can be eliminated will determine the permanence of the bleaching effect.

RECOMMENDATIONS

Excellent Endodontic Treatment

Three-dimensional obturation of the root canal system is mandatory to prevent escape of the bleaching agent through underfilled foramina into the attachment apparatus.

Patient History

All published case reports of external cervical root resorption have manifested in patients whose teeth have become pulpless before age 25. Patient dentinal tubules appear to be a factor in permitting bleach to diffuse into the periodontal membrane space. It may be judicious to use sodium perborate and water when bleaching pulpless teeth in young patients or in teeth which became pulpless before age 25.

Barrier

The location, shape and material for a protective barrier are essential to the safe bleach.

No Etch

No significant difference exists between the color change in bleaching with or without prior internal chamber etching.[7] Etching opens the dentinal tubules and may increase the potential for external cervical root resorption if the barrier fails.

New Superoxol and Sodium Perborate

Bleaching agents lose their effectiveness over time. Superoxol may lose about 50% of its oxidizing strength in a six month period.[35]

Recalls

Resorption has been detected as early as six months after intracoronal bleaching.[10a] Most cervical root resorption has

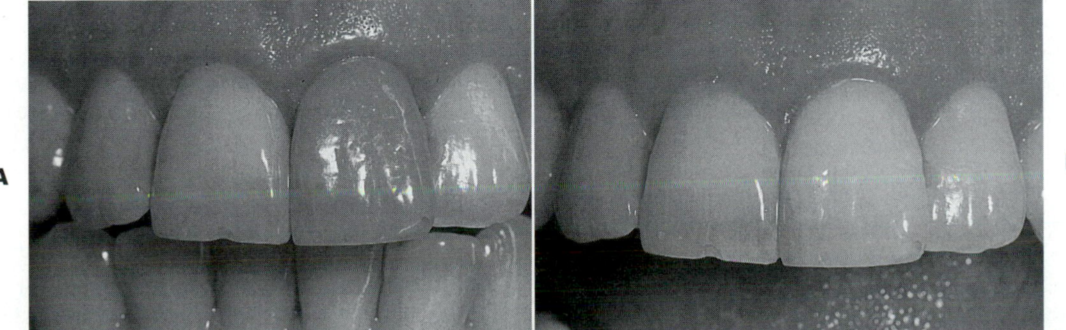

FIG. 21-14 A, Before intracoronal bleaching of pulpless tooth. **B,** After one treatment of thermocatalytic and walking bleach.

been detected after two years and was often too advanced to salvage the tooth. Early detection enhances the possibility of arresting or repairing the resorption.

Understanding the relationship of bleaching agents, cervical root resorption, and an intracoronal bleach barrier appears to be important in developing guidelines for a predictable and safe bleach.

NIGHTGUARD (MATRIX) VITAL BLEACHING

Nightguard vital bleaching or matrix bleaching uses an athletic-style vacuum-formed soft mouthguard and currently-available 10% carbamide peroxide-containing materials to bleach the teeth.[27] The nightguard vital bleaching technique (more appropriately called the "dentist-prescribed, home-applied" technique) is much less labor intensive, and requires less in-office time than other vital bleaching techniques. There are two basic regimens for the application of the whitening solutions: (1) sleeping with the nightguard filled with the bleaching material each night; and (2) wearing the loaded nightguard during the day (except the nightguard is removed for meals and oral hygiene) while changing the solution every 1.5-2 hours.[22] Treatment time usually consists of 4-6 weeks for night-time bleaching and 1-3 weeks for the daytime regimen of multiple applications. Either course of treatment or a combination of both may be used. There is no set regimen for treatment time that must be followed. Treatment results are basically time and dose related. The more the nightguard is worn, the faster the bleaching occurs. However, excessive extended wear beyond the prescribed treatment time should be avoided. There is no reason, nor is it desirable, to continue treatment with "touch-up" or periodic applications unless there is an obvious relapse of the initial results. Moreover, nightguard vital bleaching should be administered while under the supervision of a dentist. Faster results can be obtained by more frequent changing of the bleaching gel but limiting daily wearing of the matrix. For instance, the patient can change the solution every 20 minutes but wear the matrix one to three hours per day. The key is patient comfort, lifestyle, and material characteristics.

Prior to its introduction in the dental literature in 1989, this technique had been used since 1968, but no controlled clinical studies had been undertaken.[23] Laboratory studies published or in progress have shown no detrimental effects on teeth or restorations,[29,30] and animal/tissue studies have shown no untoward effects systemically or on oral tissues.[28] Human clinical studies have shown a 91% success rate, with most persons experiencing some lightening of their teeth.[26] However, not all teeth are responsive to the treatment, and not all patients respond at the same rate. As with all vital bleaching techniques, the only way to know definitely whether a patient's teeth will respond to the treatment is to attempt the treatment, with no guarantee of success. Some patient's teeth become very naturally white, other patient's teeth (especially those stained by tetracycline) achieve limited lightening (retaining the gray cast), while still others do not respond at all to bleaching. Tetracycline-stained teeth are the least responsive, brown fluorosed teeth respond moderately well, and teeth intrinsically discolored or discolored from aging, chromogenic foods (like coffee), or habits such as smoking bleach most effectively. Teeth in the two "less-responsive" categories often require extended treatment time to achieve the maximum benefit. It should be noted that other than experiencing a slight cleansing effect, existing composite or ceramic restorations do not lighten as a result of bleaching. Patients must be informed of this fact prior to treatment, since a mismatch of existing teeth-colored restorations with surrounding tooth structure may result if bleaching is successful.

No deleterious effects on any restorations have been reported, except for minor effects on composites. However, two common side effects have been noted in 66% of cases studied at the University of North Carolina using this bleaching treatment.[31]

First, for some persons, the peroxide solution may initially cause tissue irritation on the gingival papilla or gingival crest, much like a small burn or ulcer. This side effect often occurs during the first week of treatment, and resolves with no residual problems. Should any such pain or discomfort develop, the nightguard is removed, treatment suspended, and the dentist informed of this occurrence. Usually suspension of treatment for 1-2 days will resolve the problem unless the irritation is due to an ill-fitting nightguard. An office visit or a nightguard made from a new impression may be needed if the irritation persists.

The second side effect noted is that some teeth may become more sensitive to temperature changes during treatment. A complete return to normal sensation has been noted in all cases when treatment is terminated. Again, should the teeth be hypersensitive, the nightguard should be removed, treatment suspended, and the dentist contacted. Often, reducing exposure time will alleviate the problem and the bleaching treatment can be continued. The major limitations to wearing time are personal preference and the incidence or severity of tissue irritation and/or tooth sensitivity. None of the side effects have been shown to persist post-treatment in studies conducted at U.N.C.[32]

The bleaching result may be permanent, but is generally considered to be 1-3 years in duration. Re-treatment typically involves significantly less time than the original bleaching treatment.

First Appointment

Completion of the nightguard vital bleaching treatment usually will require three appointments. The initial appointment consists of an examination, including a medical and dental history, and determination of the probable cause of the discoloration (aging, drug-induced, intrinsic, smoking, chromogenic foods, fluorosis, etc.), as well as the prognosis of this treatment. This examination requires radiographs of the anterior teeth to determine the absence of any periapical pathology (along with electric pulp testing of questionable teeth), as well as to establish the baseline for treatment. Patient expectations and habits should be discussed and any consent forms and informative literature reviewed.[24] Advisement as to the need for replacement of other esthetic restorations should be determined at this time. *There are certain unknowns about this procedure at this time, especially regarding its longevity and efficacy.* However, longevity, as noted earlier, is considered to be 1 to 3 years, and efficacy is 91%. An impression of the arch to be treated is made, as well as photographs documenting the preoperative shade and condition of the teeth.

Only one arch should be treated at a time in order to maintain the other opposing arch as a standard for comparison to determine the ongoing effectiveness of treatment. If a removable partial denture (RPD) is present and the patient wishes to wear the nightguard both day and night, two impressions, with and without the RPD in place, will be made to fabricate two nightguards. One nightguard will be made for daytime with the RPD in place, and one for nighttime use with the RPD removed.

Laboratory Technique

An alginate impression of the arch to be treated is made and poured in cast stone. The impression should be made free of voids on or around the teeth by wiping alginate onto the teeth and gingival tissues prior to inserting the impression. After appropriate infection control procedures, the impression should be rinsed vigorously, then poured with dental stone. Incomplete rinsing of the infection-control chemicals from the impression may cause a softened surface on the stone, which may result in a nightguard which is slightly small and irritates tissue or teeth.

The resultant cast is trimmed around the periphery to eliminate the vestibule, and the base is thinned in the center portion of the cast. The cast generally must be lifted from the table of the cast-trimming machine in order to successfully remove the vestibule without damaging the teeth. The cast is allowed to dry, and any significant undercuts blocked out using a block-out material such as putty or clay.

The nightguard is formed on the cast using a heat/vacuum-forming machine (Fig. 21-15, *A*). After the machine has heated for 10 minutes, a sheet of soft, clear 0.020 to 0.035 inch nightguard material is inserted, and allowed to soften by heat until it sags approximately 1 inch. The top portion of the machine is then closed slowly and gently, and the vacuum allowed to form the heat-softened material around the cast. After sufficient time for adaptation of the material, the vacuum and heat are removed and the material allowed to cool while remaining on the stone cast.

Using a no. 12 surgical blade in a Bard-Parker handle, the nightguard is trimmed in a smooth straight cut about 3 mm from the most apical portion of the gingival crest of the teeth facially and lingually. The distance from the teeth is determined by tissue undercuts and frenum attachments. The excess material is removed first, then the horseshoe-shaped nightguard is removed from the cast. The edges of the guard are trimmed to a smooth texture with sharp, curved or serrated scissors until only about 2 mm of tissue are covered, and the tray does not engage tissue undercuts (Fig. 21-15, *B*). Some dentists elect to scallop the nightguard by cutting it to con-

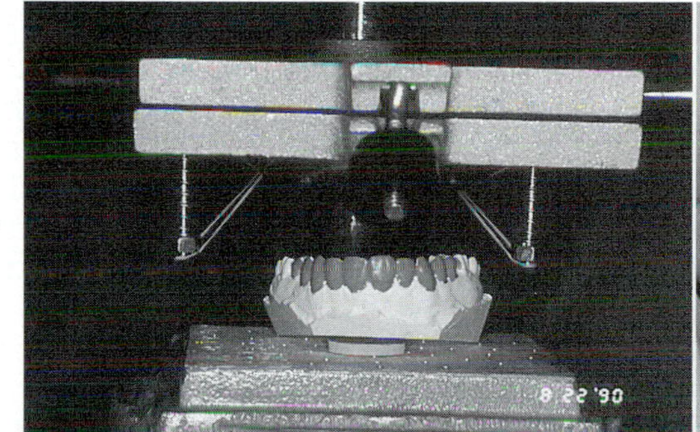

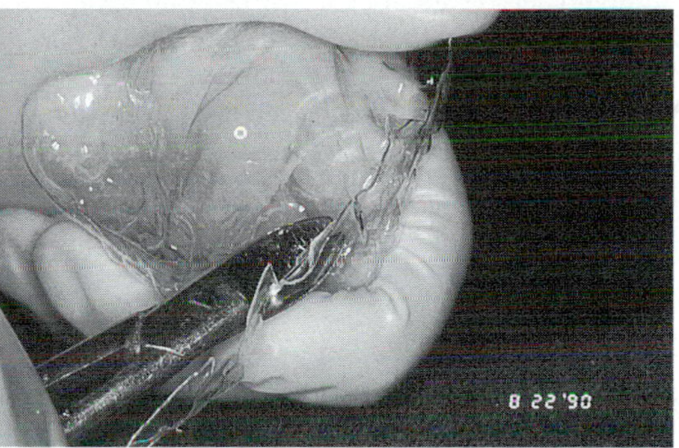

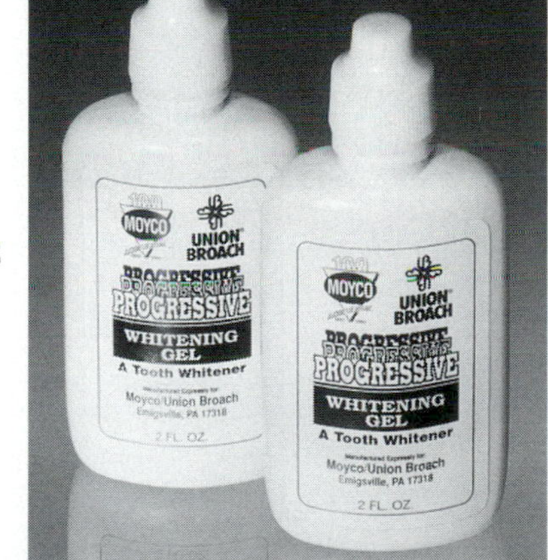

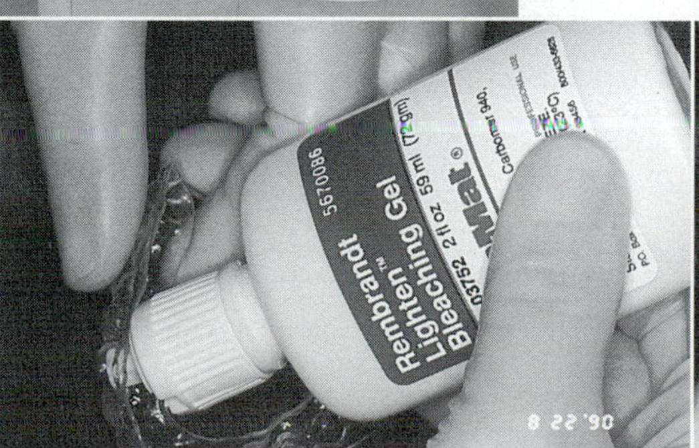

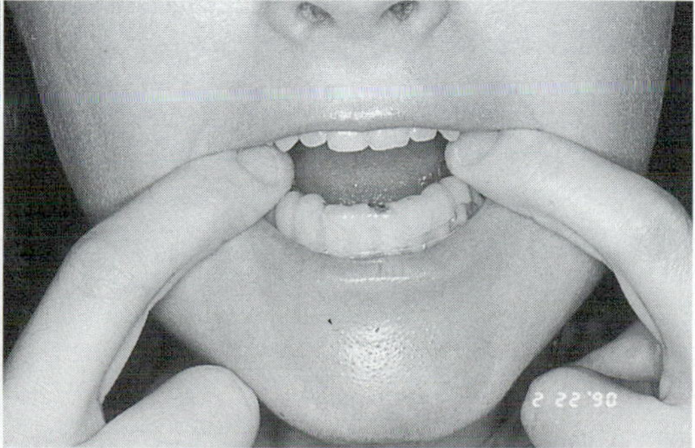

FIG. 21-15 A, The patient study cast has been painted with thickness material to serve as a spacer so that bleaching matrix will have room for reservoir of bleaching material. **B,** Trimming of the matrix material should be done to keep the bleaching solution away from the gingival tissue. **C,** Although most matrix bleaching materials are 10% carbamide peroxide, there are several, including the one pictured here, that contain 15% carbamide peroxide. **D,** Bleaching material being applied into the matrix. **E,** A patient applies the lower matrix containing bleaching material into the mouth.

form to the outline of the teeth, thus avoiding soft tissue contact. Other dentists form reservoirs on the facials of the teeth by placing spacers prior to nightguard fabrication. Reservoirs are important when using highly viscous bleaching materials.

Second Appointment

The second appointment involves inserting and fitting the nightguard and evaluating the occlusion. The nightguard is inserted into the mouth, and evaluated for rough edges or blanching of tissue. Problem areas are shortened or smoothed. The occlusion on the nightguard is evaluated with the patient in maximum intercuspation. If the patient is unable to obtain a comfortable intercuspation due to premature posterior tooth contacts, the occlusion may be improved by trimming the nightguard to exclude coverage of the most posterior teeth as needed to allow optimal anterior contact in maximum intercuspation. The edges of the nightguard on the palate should terminate in grooves or valleys where possible, rather than on the heights of soft tissue contours such as in the area of the incisive papillae. The patient should be instructed to avoid scratching the gingiva with fingernails during removal of the nightguard.

The patient is instructed in the application of the bleaching solution into the nightguard. Patients are instructed to apply 2 to 3 drops per tooth into each tooth area in the guard. The nightguard is inserted, and the excess expectorated (Fig. 21-15, *E*). There is generally a slight "medicine" taste to the material, and patients should be informed of this prior to the initial insertion. If the taste of the solution is deemed unpleasant, a cotton swab dipped in a mouthwash and dabbed on the tongue will minimize the bad taste. Patients should not rinse during treatment, but the nightguard should be removed for meals and oral hygiene.

A 10% carbamide peroxide material is recommended for this bleaching technique.[25] The bleaching solution will be provided to the patient, along with instructions for proper use. An orthodontic retainer case is given to the patient for storing the nightguard. The bleaching solution is usually replaced every 1½ to 2 hours during the day. If the nightguard is worn only at night, a single application of bleaching material at bedtime is indicated. If either of the two primary side effects occur, sensitive teeth or irritated tissue, the patient should reduce or discontinue treatment, and contact the dentist for determination of cause as earlier noted.

Third Appointment

The treatment will continue without further office visits until the desired shade is achieved, six weeks has passed, or a side effect needs attention, whichever comes first. A follow-up third appointment will determine whether the bleaching is successful or if it is desirable to continue treatment. This appointment may include postoperative photographs, a decision as to whether to treat the opposing arch, and instructions for future bleaching or restorative treatment needs. Retreatment at a later date using the same appliance is an option if there have not been significant changes in the teeth. However, it is the re-

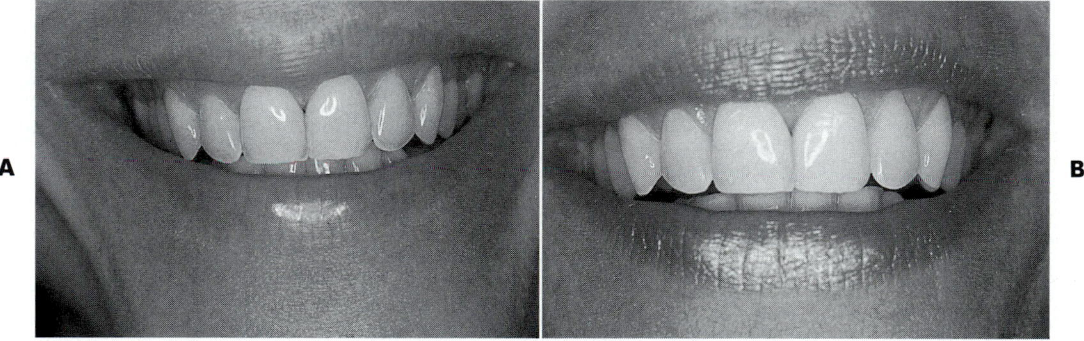

FIG. 21-16 A, Discolored teeth before bleaching. **B,** Approximately 3 weeks of home treatment obtained this result.

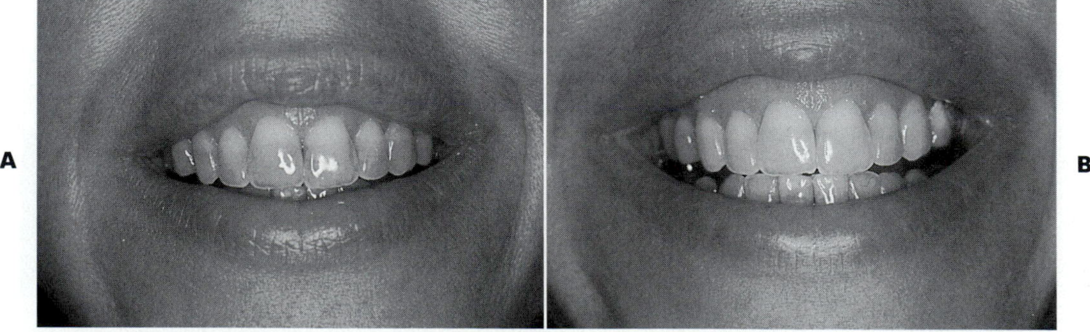

FIG. 21-17 A, Before bleaching shows tetracycline stain. **B,** After combined bleaching of 1 in-office and 3 weeks at-home matrix bleaching.

sponsibility of the patient to maintain possession of the nightguard. It should be stressed to the patient that any retreatment should only be performed under the supervision of a dentist.

A detailed consent form and letter explaining the bleaching treatment as outlined above is helpful, and can be mailed prior to the appointment if possible. Pre-mailing of information allows the dentist to focus more time on the examination and answering of questions. The patient should receive a copy of the consent form, which explains what is known or not known about the procedure as well as what other options they have for the treatment of their teeth.

Figures 21-16 and 21-17 show before and after bleaching comparisons.

REFERENCES

1. American Dental Association Position Statement on Tooth Whiteners, Chicago: ADA Council on Dental Therapeutics: September 13, 1991.
2. Arens D: The role of bleaching in esthetics, Dent Clin North Am 33:319, 1989.
3. Bailey SJ, and Swift EJ Jr: Effects of home bleaching products on composite resins, Quintessence Int 23:489, 1992.
4. Black GV, and McKay FS: Mottled teeth, an endemic developmental imperfection of the enamel of the teeth here-to-fore unknown in the literature of dentistry, Dent Cosmos 58:129, 1916.
5. Bowles WH: Personal communication, March 1991.
6. Bowles WH: Teeth discolored by minocycline, Dentistry Today, 5:4, 1986.
7. Casey LJ, et al: The use of dentinal etching with endodontic bleaching procedures, J Endod 15:535, 1989.
8. Cohen S, and Parkins FM: Bleaching tetracycline-stained vital teeth, Oral Surg 29:465, 1970.
9. Cooley R: Dilemma of discolored teeth due to tetracycline staining, Curr Dentistry 5:287, 1974.
10. Costas FL, and Wong M: Intracoronal isolating barriers: effect of location on root leakage and effectiveness of bleaching agents, J Endod 17:365, 1991.

10a. Cvek M, and Lindvall AM: External root resorption following bleaching of pulpless teeth with oxygen peroxide, Endod Dent Traumatol 1:56, 1985.

11. Dodson DL, and Bowles WH; Production of minocycline pigment by tissue extracts, Abstract No. 1267, J Dent Res 70:424, 1991.
12. Dzierzak J: Factors which cause tooth color changes: protocol for in-office "power bleaching," Pract Periodont Aesth Dent 2:15, 1991.
13. Falkensten RG: Tetracycline stain—treatable scourge, J Missouri Dent Assoc 56:17, 1976.
14. Friedman S, et al: Incidence of external root resorption and esthetic results in 58 bleached pulpless teeth, Endodont Dent Traumatol 4:23, 1988.
15. Frysch H, et al: Effect of pH adjustment on bleaching efficiency, Abstract No. 2248, J Dent Res 72(JADR Abstracts):384, 1993.
16. Garber DA, et al: Dentist-monitored bleaching: a combined approach, Pract Periodont Aesth Dent 3:22, 1991.
17. Gimlin DR, and Schindler WG: The management of postbleaching cervical resorption, J Endod 16:292, 1990.
18. Goldstein R: Bleaching teeth: new materials, new roles, J Am Dent Assoc 1987.
19. Goon W, Cohen S, and Borer R: External cervical root resorption following bleaching, J Endod 12:414, 1986
20. Hall DA: Should etching be performed as a part of a vital bleaching technique? Quintessence Int 22:679, 1991.
21. Harrington GW, and Natkin E: External resorption associated with bleaching of pulpless teeth, J Endod 5:344, 1979.
22. Haywood VB: History, safety, and effectiveness of current bleaching techniques and applications of the nightguard vital bleaching technique, Quintessence Int 23:471, 1992.
23. Haywood VB: Nightguard vital bleaching: a history and products update: Part 1, Esth Dent Update 2:63, 1991.
24. Haywood VB: Nightguard vital bleaching: a history and products update: Part 2, Esth Dent Update 2(5):82-85, 1991.
25. Haywood VB: Nightguard vital bleaching: current information and research, Esth Dent Update 1:7, 1990.
26. Haywood VB: Overview and status of mouthguard bleaching, J Esth Dent 3:157, 1991.
27. Haywood VB, and Heymann HO: Nightguard vital bleaching, Quintessence Int 20:173, 1989.
28. Haywood VB, and Heymann HO: Nightguard vital bleaching: how safe is it? Quintessence Int 22:515, 1991.
29. Haywood VB, Houck V, and Heymann HO: Nightguard vital bleaching: effects of varying pH solutions on enamel surface texture and color change, Quintessence Int 22:775, 1991.
30. Haywood VB, et al: Nightguard vital bleaching: effects on enamel surface texture and diffusion, Quintessence Int 21:801-6, 1990.
31. Haywood VB, Leonard RH, and Nelson CF: Effectiveness of nightguard vital bleaching (abstract 591), J Dent Res 71:179, 1992.
32. Haywood VB, Leonard RH, and Nelson CF: Nightguard vital bleaching longevity and side effects: 13 to 25 months data (abstract 835), J Dent Res 72:208, 1993.
33. Haywood VB: Bleaching of vital and nonvital teeth, Curr Opin Dent 142(March 2):142-149, 1992.
34. Heithersay GS: Combined endotontic orthodontic treatment of transverse root fractures in the region of the alveolar crest, Oral Surg 36:404, 1973.
35. Ho S, and Goerig AC: An in vitro comparison of different bleaching agents in the discolored tooth, J Endod 15:106, 1989.
36. Hodosh M: A new method of bleaching discolored teeth by the use of a solid state direct heating device, Dental Dig 76:344, 1970.
37. Holmstrup G, Palm AM, and Lambjerg-Hansen II: Bleaching of discolored root-filled teeth, Endod Dent Traumatol 4:197, 1988.
38. Jordan RE, and Boksman L: Conservative vital bleaching treatment of discolored dentition, Compend Contin Educ 5:803, 1984.
39. Koa EC, Peng P, and Johnston WM: Color changes of teeth and restorative materials exposed to bleaching (abstract 2436), J Dent Res 70:570, 1991.
40. Kokich VG: Enhancing restorative, esthetic, and periodontal results with orthodontic treatment. In S. Schluger et al (eds): Periodontal Disease, Philadelphia, 1990, Lea & Febiger.

40a. Lado EA, Stanley HR, and Weisman WI: Cervical resorption in bleached teeth, Oral Surg 55:78, 1983.

41. Latcham NL: Management of a patient with postbleaching cervical resorption. A clinical report, J Prosthet Dent Traumatol 65:603, 1991.

41a. Latcham NL: Postbleaching cervical resorption, J Endod 12:262, 1986.

42. Lemon R: Bleaching and restoring endodontically treated teeth, Curr Opin Dent 1:754, 1991.
43. McInerney ST, and Zillich R: Evaluation of internal sealing ability of three materials, J Endod 18:376, 1992.
44. Mello HS: The mechanism of tetracycline staining in primary and permanent teeth, J Dent Child 478, 1967.

44a. Montgomery S: External cervical resorption after bleaching a pulpless tooth, Oral Surg 57:203, 1984.

45. Murrin JR, and Barkmeier WM: Chemical treatment of vital teeth with intrinsic stain, Quintessence Int 13:6, 1982.
46. Nutting EB, and Poe GS: A new combination for bleaching teeth, J South Calif State Dental Assoc 31:289, 1963.

46a. Pearson HH: Bleaching of the discolored pulpless tooth, J Am Dent Assoc 56:64, 1958.

47. Rotstein I, et al: In vitro efficacy of sodium perborate preparation used for intracoronal bleaching of discolored nonvital teeth, Endod Dent Traumatol 7:177, 1991.
48. Rotstein I, et al: Effect of different protective base materials on hydrogen peroxide leakage during intracoronal bleaching in vitro, J Endod 18:114, 1992.

49. Ruse ND, et al: Preliminary surface analysis of etched, bleached, and normal bovine enamel, J Dent Res 69:1610, 1990.
50. Scherer W: Removal of intrinsic enamel stains with vital bleaching and modified microabrasion, Am J Dent 4:99, 1991.
51. Silverstone LM: The acid etch technique: in vitro studies with special reference to the enamel surface and the enamel-resin interface. In Proceedings of the International Symposium on Acid-Etch Techniques (1974: St. Moritz, Switzerland), Dogon IL and Silverstone LM, eds., St. Paul, Minn., North Central Publishers, 1975.
52. Smith JJ, Cunningham CJ, and Montgomery S: Cervical canal leakage after internal bleaching procedures, J Endod 18:476, 1992.
53. Spasser HF: A simple bleaching technique using sodium perborate, NY State Dent J 27:332, 1961.
53a. Steinor DR, and West JD: A method to determine the location and shape of an intracoronal bleach barrier, J Endodon (in press).
54. Ten Cate AR: Oral histology: development, structure, and function, ed 2, St Louis, 1985, The CV Mosby Co.
55. Torneck DC, et al: The influence of time of hydrogen peroxide exposure on the adhesion of composite resin to bleached bovine enamel, J Endod 16:123, 1990.
56. Walton RE, et al: External bleaching of tetracycline-stained teeth in dogs, J Endod 8:536, 1982.
57. Warren W, Wong M, and Ingram T: An in vitro comparison of bleaching agents on the crowns and roots of discolored teeth, J Endod 16:463, 1990.
58. Whitaker D, and Shankle R: A study of the histologic reaction of submerged root segments, Oral Surg 37:919, 1974.
59. Wilcox LR, and Diaz-Arnold A: Coronal microleakage of permanent lingual access restorations in endodontically treated anterior teeth, J Endod 15:584, 1989.
60. Zaragoza VMT: Bleaching of vital teeth: technique, EstoModeo 9:7, 1984.

Self-assessment questions

1. Which of the following is not helpful in determining if a patient is appropriate for bleaching?
   a. Recent periapical radiographs.
   b. Vitality tests.
   c. Transillumination.
   d. An intraoral camera.
2. The most difficult stains from dental treatment to bleach successfully are from
   a. amalgam restoration.
   b. root canal sealers.
   c. composite restorations.
   d. gold restorations.
3. Teeth are most susceptible to tetracycline staining from
   a. four months in utero to eight years of age.
   b. birth to seven years of age.
   c. seven months in utero until the third molars are formed.
   d. anytime during life.
4. As described by Jordan and Boksman, third degree tetracycline staining is
   a. dark gray or blue in color, with banding.
   b. dark yellow or gray in color.
   c. too dark to bleach.
   d. light yellow or gray in color.
5. Minocycline, in contrast to other tetracyclines,
   a. causes staining of enamel.
   b. causes discoloration in teeth after calcification.
   c. chelates with calcium to form tooth pigmentation.
   d. all of the above.
6. Fluorosis
   a. affects ameloblasts resulting in defective enamel development.
   b. most commonly affects premolars.
   c. is caused by drinking water containing fluoride concentrations in excess of one part per million.
   d. all of the above.
7. Which of the following is not a contraindication to bleaching?
   a. Dentin hypersensitivity.
   b. Teeth with white spots.
   c. Patients over 70 years of age.
   d. Patients who are perfectionists.
8. Which of the following statements concerning microabrasion is false?
   a. It is effective in treating white spots.
   b. The active ingredient is hydrochloric acid.
   c. It permanently removes surface stains.
   d. It can successfully treat some tetracycline stains.
9. Etching the enamel prior to bleaching
   a. enhances the penetrability of the bleaching solutions.
   b. shortens the appointment time.
   c. retains the fluoride-rich surface layer of enamel.
   d. all of the above.
10. The usual range of temperatures for bleaching vital teeth with a heat or light source is
    a. 100 to 115 degrees.
    b. 115 to 140 degrees.
    c. 140 to 160 degrees.
    d. 160 to as high as the patient can tolerate.
11. With vital bleaching
    a. both arches should be treated simultaneously.
    b. treatment should proceed from the less discolored teeth to the most discolored.
    c. incisal halves of teeth respond quicker than cervical halves.
    d. yellow-brown and gray stains are equally difficult to remove.
12. Which of the following is not necessary for vital bleaching?
    a. Patient wears safety glasses.
    b. Local anesthesia.
    c. Pumice prophylaxis.
    d. Polish teeth after last treatment.
13. The barrier material for bleaching pulpless teeth should be
    a. IRM.
    b. dental sealant.
    c. glass ionomer cement.
    d. zinc oxyphosphate.
14. Cervical resorption in bleached pulpless teeth may result from
    a. bleach placed apical to the CEJ.
    b. tooth becoming pulpless before patient reaches age 25.
    c. a defect in the CEJ.
    d. all of the above.
15. The most common treatment for cervical resorption following intracoronal bleaching is
    a. surgical repair.
    b. orthodontic extrusion.
    c. extraction.
    d. calcium hydroxide therapy.
16. Which of the following is not part of the bleaching procedure for endodontically treated teeth?
    a. Rubber dam isolation.
    b. Acid etching.
    c. Superoxol or sodium perborate.
    d. A heat source.

17. With nightguard vital bleaching
    a. the reported success rate is 75%.
    b. fluorosed teeth are the least responsive.
    c. the bleaching agent is 10% carbamide peroxide.
    d. patients with removable partial dentures can wear the nightguard only at night.
18. Unknowns about nightguard bleaching include all of the following except
    a. longevity
    b. effects on restorations.
    c. efficacy.
    d. none of the above.
19. Patient instructions during nightguard bleaching include
    a. replace bleaching solution every 3 to 4 hours.
    b. wear nightguard as long as possible.
    c. discontinue treatment and contact the dentist if teeth become hypersensitive.
    d. all of the above.
20. Following the second appointment, the nightguard bleaching patient should return to the office when
    a. the desired shade is achieved.
    b. six weeks have passed.
    c. if side effects need attention.
    d. all of the above, whichever comes first.

Chapter 22

Restoration of the Endodontically Treated Tooth

Galen W. Wagnild
Kathy I. Mueller

The goal of dental treatment is to provide optimal oral health, esthetics, and function. Therapeutic efforts should produce predictable treatment results that are easily maintainable and reliable over the long term. This objective applies to each tooth in the dentition, and more importantly to the dentition itself.

Endodontic therapy, restorative dentistry, and periodontal health are intimately related. Dental disease and restorative procedures affect the healthy pulp. Similarly, pulpal disease and endodontic therapy alter the attachment apparatus and the design of restorations.

The purpose of this chapter is to discuss this complex relationship and to describe treatment planning and procedures for restoring endodontically treated teeth with predictable clinical results.

RESTORATIVE DENTISTRY AND THE VITAL TOOTH

Effect of Restorative Procedures and Materials on the Pulp

The effect of dental restorative techniques and materials on the living pulp is reported in detail in Chapter 14. Teeth that require extensive restorations suffer pulpal injury from both the dental disease itself and from the treatment procedures used to restore the resultant damage. A number of precautions are listed in this excellent account that can help to reduce the harmful consequences of dental procedures on the pulp.

Postrestorative endodontic involvement

Damage to the pulp cannot be entirely eliminated from restorative dentistry.[4,34] As increasing amounts of tooth structure are removed for restorative preparations, the number of exposed dentin tubules increases dramatically. At the surface of the dentin, or the dentinenamel junction, dentin tubule density ranges between 15,000 and 20,000/mm^2. At the pulpal surface, the number of dentin tubules increases to 45,000 to 60,000/mm^2 and the diameter of each tubule increases. Therefore, deep preparations expose a large number of wide dentin tubules to trauma, dental materials, and bacterial products. Dentin permeability is greatest on thin axial surfaces, particularly mesial surfaces. These surfaces are often extensively reduced during preparation for full veneer crowns, and especially for fixed partial dentures involving mesially tipped abutments. Pulpal irritation becomes significant when the dentin thickness is reduced to 0.3 mm.[54]

Despite all safeguards, the process of tooth preparation and restoration is irritating to the pulp and the injury, at times, can be irreversible. Dental procedures are considered to be responsible for those endodontic complications in restored teeth that develop for no known reason. Abutment teeth have a higher risk of developing subsequent pulpal necrosis than vital teeth restored with single crowns, undoubtedly owing to the increased preparation required for parallelism. In a study of endodontic complications in restored teeth, approximately 0.3% of crowned teeth and 4.0% of abutment teeth became endodontically involved, when no caries, fracture, or other causative factor was present. When a cause was known, pulpal necrosis significantly increased. The combined effect of dental procedures and recurrent dental disease nearly quadrupled the rate of endodontic involvement for abutment teeth and increased the rate of teeth with single crowns more than 10-fold.[5]

Endodontic involvement increases in proportion to the degree of dental destruction and the complexity of the restoration. Teeth treated with a buildup and full veneer crown became necrotic roughly three times more frequently than those treated with a partial-coverage crown and 30 times more often than unrestored teeth.[17] In complex cases requiring periodontal-prosthetic reconstruction, 37% of teeth with advanced periodontal disease developed endodontic complications, compared with 19% of teeth with moderate periodontal disease.[19] This reflects a complicated interplay between multiple disease processes, more extensive tooth preparation, and the cumulative effects of previous dental breakdown and restoration.

Pulpal degeneration also increases with time following the insertion of the restorations. The pulpal insult initiated by the preparation and restoration procedures can continue undetected for many years. Among restored teeth that became endodontically involved for no known reason, only 12% deteriorated in the first three years after the restorative treatment. The necrosis rate increased to 38% in years 3 to 7 and 50% by years 7 to 12.[5]

This clear risk of increased endodontic involvement for teeth in need of restorations mandates careful prerestoration evaluation, particularly as the case's size and complexity increase. Endodontic intervention should be planned and integrated into a logical treatment sequence before any therapy is started. Both the patient and the clinician must be aware of the interdisciplinary nature of this approach.

Indications for prerestorative endodontic therapy

The evaluation of teeth to be restored should include these endodontic considerations: (1) the health of the root canal system, (2) the impact of planned restorative procedures on the pulp, and (3) the magnitude of the restorative effort. Instances in which restorative requirements significantly decrease the predictability of pulpal health or increase the chance for clinical failure should be managed with preventive endodontics.

Restorative procedures and the pulp

Teeth with healthy pulp systems are candidates for prophylactic endodontic therapy when restorative procedures requiring significant dentin removal are likely to endanger pulpal integrity. For example, vital teeth with minimal remaining tooth structure often require auxiliary retention for restorations. Retentive grooves, boxes, pins, and amalgam extensions are all placed at the expense of the dentin, and this can ultimately compromise vitality. Judicious endodontic therapy can be crucial to the success of the restoration when substantial tooth structure is missing. A tooth that has lost pivotal coronal dentin to caries, fracture, or old restorations may remain vital but exhibit insufficient supragingival tooth structure for retention of a new restoration. In this case the root canal system may be considered an extension of the restorative zone and the tooth is devitalized before placement of a dowel/core/crown restoration.

Substantial tooth preparation is common in cases with missing or malposed teeth, and this can jeopardize pulpal health. Preparation of nonparallel abutment teeth for fixed restorations entails extensive dentin removal from axial walls, which can encroach upon the pulp. Intracoronal attachments are also used to solve problems of missing or malposed teeth. However, the additional preparation needed for placement of the attachment within the confines of the crown can result in irreversible pulpal injury.

Periodontally involved teeth are at risk for pulpal involvement when crown margins are placed considerably apical to the cementoenamel junction (Fig. 22-1). The narrow circumference of the root dictates increased dentin removal in order to prepare tapered axial walls. The remaining layer of tooth structure overlying the pulp may be too thin to protect against irreversible degeneration from the combined effects of the tooth preparation process and potentially irritating restorative materials.

Preventive endodontics is also prescribed before restoration of periodontally involved vital teeth when root amputation or hemisection is planned in order to salvage portions of guarded teeth.[62] Similarly, teeth with significant periodontal bone loss can be endodontically treated and the roots retained to provide needed support for an overdenture.

Major occlusal corrections involving vital teeth may also dictate endodontic treatment before crown placement. Decreasing the occlusal height of a hypererupted tooth to restore a proper occlusal plane may necessitate devitalizing the tooth. Similarly, an unfavorable crown-root ratio is corrected by decreasing the clinical crown height through substantial occlusal reduction. Preventive endodontics should be considered in order to avoid access preparation through the crown at a later date.

Endodontic therapy should be planned in advance for teeth with fragile pulpal systems that require a cast restoration.[2] Treatment of chronic pulpitis is more efficient and effective when the tooth is devitalized before placement of a crown or bridge retainer. Vital teeth should be treated endodontically first if they have a guarded pulpal prognosis and would be dif-

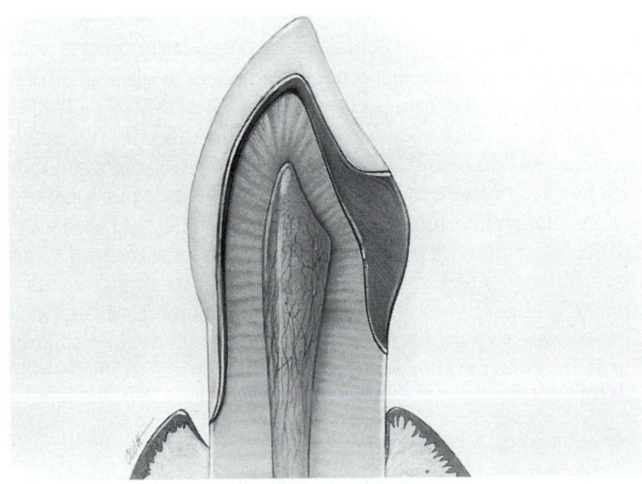

FIG. 22-1 Attachment loss often results in elongated clinical crowns. Restorative procedures require additional dentin removal from the axial walls and may be detrimental to pulpal vitality.

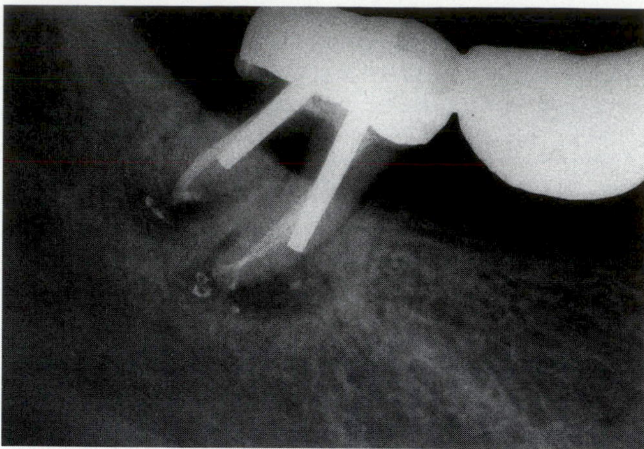

FIG. 22-2 Root anatomy dictates dowel location and dimension. The occlusal surface anatomy of this molar was used to project root location. Long axis dislocation of the restored crown and the root can result in dramatic clinical errors.

ficult to treat endodontically after completion of the planned restoration.

Magnitude of the restorative treatment

As the size and complexity of the restorative effort increase, the need for prerestoration endodontics simultaneously increases. Although it is possible to perform endodontic procedures after restorations are complete, the hazards associated with retroactive treatment are serious and should be prevented whenever possible. An access opening through an existing restoration structurally weakens the porcelain, disrupts the cement integrity, and removes dentin supporting the crown. Simply perforating the glazed surface of a porcelain fused to metal restoration may reduce porcelain strength by 50%.[41] Perforation of the occlusal porcelain and the metal coping can weaken the porcelain bond strength enough to cause separation of the porcelain veneer from the metal substructure. Endodontic access preparations can also remove a significant portion of the dentin core and vertical walls of the underlying preparation, compromising retention and resistance of the restoration.

In more compromised dentitions, occlusal requirements may alter the normal relationship of root anatomy to clinical crown in the restored dentition. The disorientation of crown morphology and underlying root form can lead to difficulty in endodontic access and result in excessive removal of coronal tooth structure. In the severe case, this disorientation can contribute to a mechanical perforation of the root (Fig. 22-2). These clinical realities may not much impact a treatment plan for a tooth that requires a single crown, but they may cause rapid destruction of a larger, more fragile and more complex restoration. These cases require prerestorative endodontic evaluation and the definitive treatment of strategic teeth with questionable pulpal prognosis.

Pretreatment evaluation

Before restorative therapy is instituted the tooth must be thoroughly evaluated to ensure success of the ultimate treatment goals. The tooth should be examined individually and in the context of its contribution to the overall treatment plan. Adjacent teeth, opposing teeth, and patient desires for treatment all should be considered. This survey includes endodontic, periodontal, restorative, and esthetic evaluations.

Endodontic evaluation

In addition to identification of nonvital teeth and the endodontic evaluation of vital teeth described above, the prerestorative examination should include an inspection of the quality of existing endodontic treatment. New restorations, particularly complex ones, should not be placed on abutment teeth with questionable endodontic prognosis.[3] Endodontic retreatment may be indicated for teeth that exhibit radiographic periapical disease or clinical symptoms of inflammation (see Chapter 24). Restorations that require a dowel need a dowel space, which is prepared by removing gutta-percha from the canal. Canals obturated with a silver cone or other inappropriate filling materials should be identified and endodontically retreated before the start of restorative therapy.

Periodontal evaluation

Maintenance of periodontal health is critical to the long-term success of endodontically treated and restored teeth. The periodontal condition of the tooth must be determined before initiation of endodontic therapy. In addition to a conventional periodontal examination, the effect of the planned restoration on the attachment apparatus must be considered. Many teeth suffer from significant structural defects that jeopardize coronal reconstruction. Extensive caries, tooth fracture, previous restorations, perforations, and external resorption can destroy tooth structure at the level of the periodontal attachment. Attempts to place restorative margins on solid tooth structure beyond these defects further invades the biologic attachment zone. Violation of the biologic width is invitation to failure of the clinical results (Fig. 22-3). A mutilated tooth in which restorative treatment would compromise the junctional epithelium or connective tissue attachment levels should be scheduled for periodontal crown lengthening surgery or orthodontic extrusion, in addition to endodontic and restorative procedures.[39,51]

Restorative evaluation

A restorative examination of the tooth should be performed before any definitive therapy is instituted. It is essential to determine if the tooth is restorable before endodontic treatment is performed. The strategic importance of a tooth should be determined before a final plan is formulated. Mutilated teeth may not warrant extensive treatment if adjacent healthy teeth are available as abutments. Conversely, the most distal tooth in a quadrant can be critical in avoiding a distal extension removable partial denture and merits extensive reconstructive efforts. Similarly, the success of a large restoration may depend on the availability of an intermediate abutment or a strategic tooth within a sextant.

In addition to the strategic position, the reliability of the tooth after restoration should be considered before it is included in a final treatment plan. The tooth to be retained must be able to withstand the functional forces placed upon it after reconstruction. Large amounts of missing tooth structure can be replaced with a cast restoration, a core, and possibly a dowel. However, a critical amount of solid coronal dentin is required, which must be encased in a metal coping for structural integrity of the restored tooth. This ferrule has been shown to significantly reduce the incidence of fracture in the

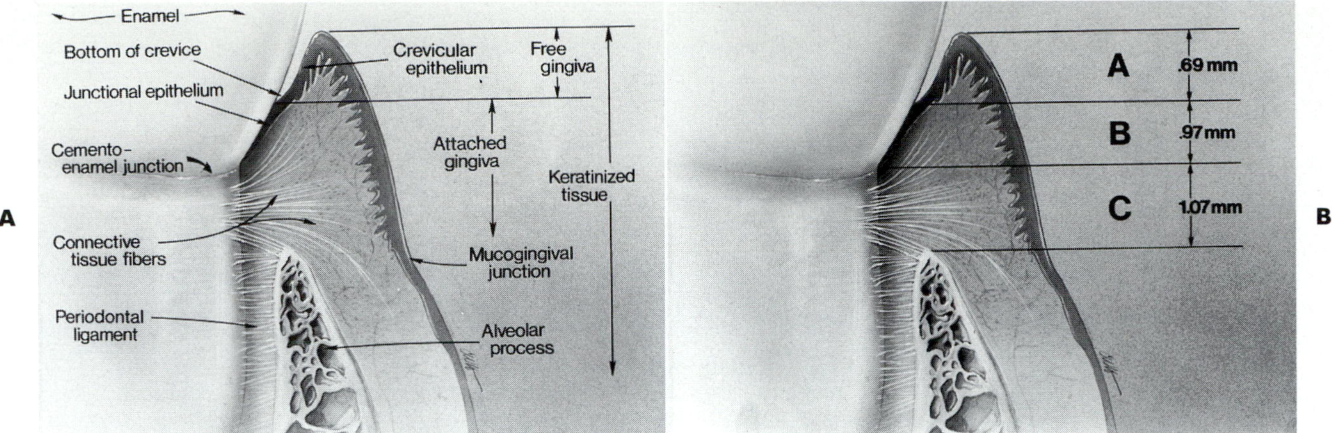

FIG. 22-3 A, Anatomy of the healthy attachment apparatus. **B,** Defective tooth structure necessitating margin placement into zones B and C are indications for crown-lengthening surgery or orthodontic extrusion. These zones contain the junctional epithelium and the connective tissue attachments.

root canal–treated tooth.[66] If sufficient solid tooth structure to accommodate a restoration with a ferrule is not available, the tooth should first be treated periodontally or orthodontically or extracted.

Esthetic evaluation

Potential esthetic complications should be investigated before initiation of endodontic therapy. Thin gingiva may transmit a shadow of dark root through the tissue. Metal dowels or amalgam placed in the canal results in unacceptable gingival discoloration from the underlying root. An aesthetically pleasing tooth that will not need a crown after endodontic treatment requires critical control of endodontic filling materials in the coronal third of the canal and the pulp chamber (Fig. 22-4). The color and translucency of most uncrowned teeth is adversely affected by opaque substances. Similarly, discoloration from gutta-percha can be visible in the coronal aspect of an endodontically treated tooth and should be limited to an apical level in the root. Endodontic and restorative materials in these aesthetically critical cases must be selected to provide the best health service with the least esthetic compromise.

The total evaluation of clinical problems should be completed before any definitive therapy is started. Treatment initiated because of an acute endodontic episode should be restricted to emergency care. After the tooth is stabilized, the clinician should return to the complete evaluation before continuing treatment. Accurate assimilation of endodontic, periodontal, restorative, and esthetic variables contributes to a rational, successful treatment outcome. There will be instances in which endodontic therapy could succeed, but failure would arise from other dental problems. These conditions should be detected and treated with an interdisciplinary approach, to maximize success. In the extreme case extraction may be indicated for teeth where endodontics could succeed but total completion of the treatment plan is impossible owing to periodontal or restorative deficiencies that cannot be corrected. These cases must be identified in the planning stage, and replacement of the condemned teeth must then be included in the overall treatment plan.

RESTORATIVE DENTISTRY AND THE NONVITAL TOOTH

Effects of Endodontics on the Tooth

Changes in endodontically treated teeth

The disease processes and restorative procedures that create the need for endodontic therapy affect much more than pulp vitality. The tooth structure that remains after endodontic treatment has been undermined and weakened by all of the previous episodes of caries, fracture, tooth preparation, and restoration. Endodontic manipulation further removes important intracoronal and intraradicular dentin. Finally, the endodontic treatment changes the actual composition of the remaining tooth structure. The combined result of these changes is the common clinical finding of increased fracture susceptibility and decreased translucency in nonvital teeth. As restorations for endodontically treated teeth are designed to compensate for these changes, it is important to understand the effects of endodontics on the tooth and the significance of each factor.

The major changes in the endodontically treated tooth include loss of tooth structure, altered physical characteristics, and altered esthetic characteristics of the residual tooth. The decreased strength seen in endodontically treated teeth is primarily due to the loss of coronal tooth structure and is not a direct result of the endodontic treatment. Endodontic procedures have been shown to reduce tooth stiffness by only 5%, whereas an MOD preparation reduces stiffness by 60%.[56] Endodontic access into the pulp chamber destroys the structural integrity provided by the coronal dentin of the pulpal roof and allows greater flexing of the tooth under function.[24] In cases with significantly reduced remaining tooth structure, normal functional forces may fracture undermined cusps or fracture the tooth in the area of the smallest circumference, frequently at the cementoenamel junction. The decreased volume of tooth structure from the combined effects of prior dental procedures creates a significant potential for fracture of the endodontically treated tooth.

The tooth structure remaining after endodontic therapy also exhibits irreversibly altered physical characteristics. Changes in collagen cross-linking and dehydration of the dentin result

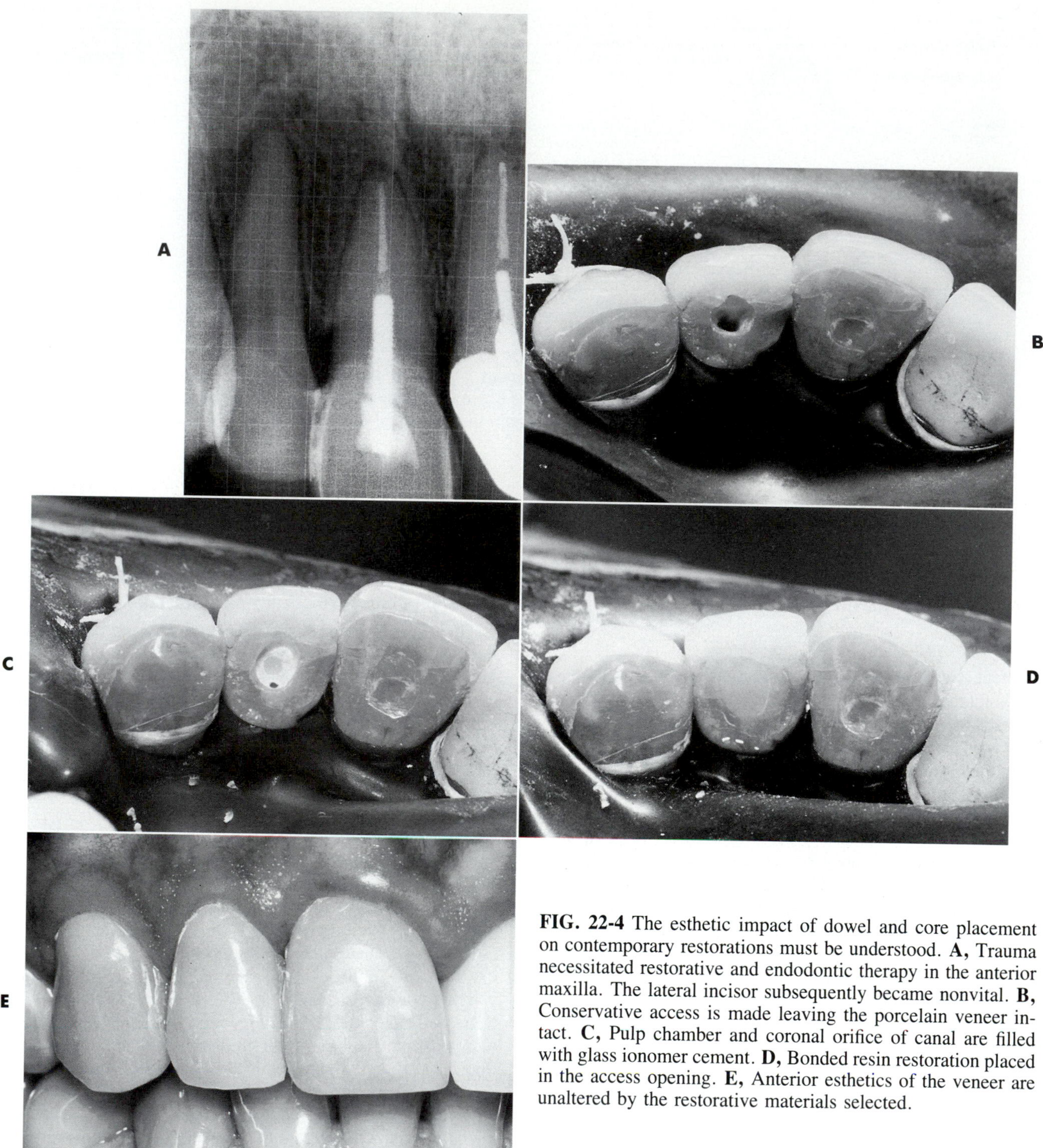

FIG. 22-4 The esthetic impact of dowel and core placement on contemporary restorations must be understood. **A,** Trauma necessitated restorative and endodontic therapy in the anterior maxilla. The lateral incisor subsequently became nonvital. **B,** Conservative access is made leaving the porcelain veneer intact. **C,** Pulp chamber and coronal orifice of canal are filled with glass ionomer cement. **D,** Bonded resin restoration placed in the access opening. **E,** Anterior esthetics of the veneer are unaltered by the restorative materials selected.

in a 14% reduction in strength and toughness of endodontically treated molars. Maxillary teeth are stronger than mandibular teeth, and mandibular incisors are the weakest.[24] The internal moisture loss has been shown to average approximately 9%, and it is greater in anterior teeth than in posterior ones.[1,27] This combined loss of structural integrity, loss of moisture, and loss of dentin toughness compromises endodontically treated teeth and necessitates special care in the restoration of pulpless teeth.

Esthetic changes also occur in endodontically treated teeth. Biochemically altered dentin modifies light refraction through the tooth and modifies its appearance. The darkening of nonvital anterior teeth is a well-known phenomenon. Inadequate endodontic cleaning and shaping of the coronal area also contributes to this discoloration by staining the dentin from degradation of vital tissue left in the pulp horns. Medicaments used in dental treatment and remnants of root canal filling material can affect the appearance of endodontically treated teeth.

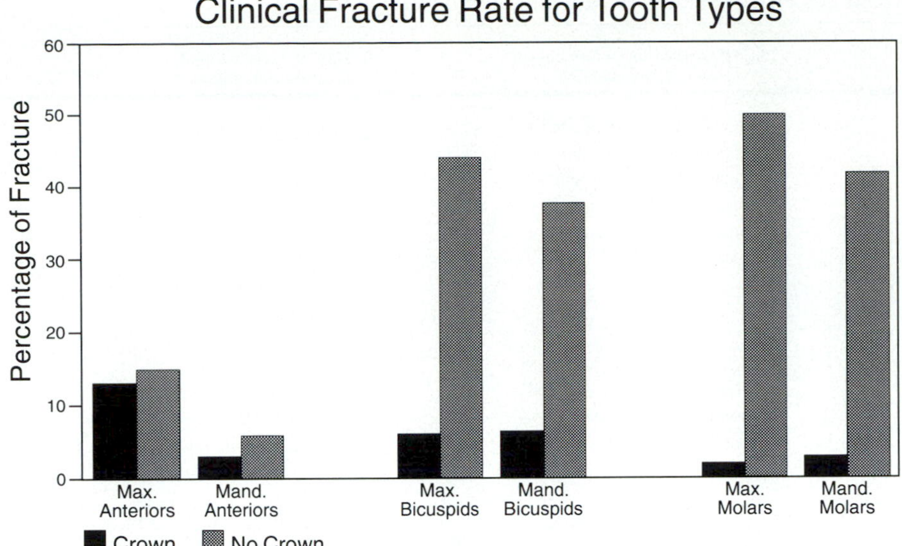

FIG. 22-5 Fracture of nonvital teeth increases in the posterior dentition when a coronal coverage restoration is not used.[70]

Treatment planning for restoration of nonvital teeth

All of the changes that accompany root canal therapy influence the selection of restorative procedures for endodontically treated teeth. Tooth structure loss can range from very minimal access preparations in intact teeth to very extensive damage that endangers the longevity of the tooth itself. A wide array of restorative materials and techniques are available to address problems presented by nonvital teeth at every point along this damage scale.

Restorative treatment decisions depend on the amount of remaining tooth structure, the functional demands that will be placed on the tooth, and the need for the tooth as an abutment in a larger restoration.[25,64] Posterior teeth carry greater occlusal forces than anterior ones, and restorations must be planned to protect posterior teeth against fracture (Fig. 22-5). The horizontal and torquing forces endured by abutments for fixed or removable partial dentures dictate more extensive protective and retentive features in the restoration.[70] Teeth with minimal remaining tooth structure are at increased risk for fracture, provide decreased retention for the restoration, and are in jeopardy for invasion of the periodontal attachment.

As the remaining tooth structure decreases and functional forces increase, greater restorative control is needed. Extensive damaged or missing tooth structure fundamentally alters the use of restorative procedures and the need for adjunctive treatment from the other specialties. Misunderstanding or misuse of integrated therapy can lead to an ever shortening cycle of treatment, breakdown, and retreatment.

Basic components used in restoration of nonvital teeth

Restorations for endodontically treated teeth are designed to replace the missing tooth structure and to protect the remaining tooth structure from fracture. The final restoration will include some combination of dowel, core, and coronal restoration. The selection of the individual components for the restoration depends on whether the nonvital tooth is an anterior or posterior tooth and whether significant coronal tooth structure is missing (Table 22-1). Not every endodontically treated tooth needs a crown or a dowel; some need all three components, and some need only an access seal for the coronal restoration. It is critically important to understand the clinical indications for each component, for overuse as well as underuse of dowels and crowns can increase the risk of unrestorable fracture. The purpose of each component, restoration design guidelines, and clinical procedures are described in the following sections.

Intact anterior teeth

Nonvital anterior teeth that have not lost tooth structure beyond the endodontic access preparation are at minimal risk for fracture and do not require a crown, core, or dowel.[69] Restorative treatment is limited to sealing of the access cavity.

Extensively damaged teeth

When a nonvital anterior or posterior tooth has lost significant tooth structure, a cast coronal restoration is required. An intermediary restoration, the dowel and core, is used to support and retain the crown. The final configuration of the restored tooth includes four parts (Fig. 22-6): (1) the residual tooth structure and its periodontal attachment apparatus; (2) the dowel material, located within the root; (3) the core material, located in the coronal area of the tooth; and (4) the definitive coronal restoration.

The dowel and core function together. The core replaces lost coronal tooth structure and provides retention for the crown. The dowel provides retention for the restorative material of the core and must be designed to minimize the potential for root fracture from functional forces. The crown restores function and esthetics and protects the remaining root and coronal structure from fracture. The specific design of each dowel and core is determined by the relative clinical need for each of these functions. The major design classifications are discussed in relation to their ability to satisfy these requirements.

TABLE 22-1. Material and design guidelines for prefabricated dowels and cores

	A. All coronal tooth remaining except access opening	B. Half or more coronal structure remaining	C. Less than half coronal structure remaining
Post	None. Bonded composite or glass ionomer in pulp chamber and canal entry of anterior tooth; bonded amalgam for posterior tooth.	Single-rooted teeth may require post as in **C;** multirooted teeth usually do not require prefabricated dowel. Bonded amalgam or composite in pulp chamber and coronal half of root canal.	Titanium or titanium alloy post
Bonding material in pulp chamber and canal	Bonded amalgam or bonded composite. GI bonds itself.	Same as **A.** GI questionable for core because of low strength, except in cases where significant tooth remains.	Same as **A**
Cement or other material in pulp chamber and canals	Cement not used. Bonded resin material or GI used in pulp chamber and canal entrance of anterior teeth. Bonded amalgam if posterior.	Cement not used. Bonded amalgam or composite placed as core. GI questionable for core because of low strength.	Resin cement for post (Imperva, Panavia, Resinment) *Or* Glass ionomer for post (Fuji I, Ketac-Cem, Shofu I) *Plus* Amalgam or composite core
Buildup material	Bonded resin restorative material or glass ionomer if anterior tooth.	Bonded spherical amalgam (Tytin, Valiant) *Or* Bonded composite (Core Paste, Fluoro-Core, Prosthodent, Ti-Core)	Same as **B**
Final restoration	None, unless needed for esthetic purposes.	Crown eventually	Crown eventually

Adapted from Guidelines for the restoration of endodontically treated teeth. Res Assoc Newslett 16:(11), 1992.

Dowel (post)

The dowel (Fig. 22-6) is a metal post or rigid restorative material placed in the radicular portion of a nonvital tooth. It functions primarily to aid retention of the restoration and secondarily to distribute forces along the length of the root. The dowel thus has a retentive role but does not strengthen a tooth.[25,37] Instead, the tooth is weakened if dentin is sacrificed to facilitate larger dowel placement. This is an important distinction, as significant damage can result from misplaced efforts to fortify roots with large dowels (Fig. 22-7). The foremost function of the dowel is to provide retention for the core and coronal restoration, and to do so without increasing the risk of root fracture.

Retentive role of the dowel

When a tooth has suffered significant coronal damage, insufficient sound tooth structure is left above the periodontal attachment to secure a restoration. The dowel within the residual root extends apically to anchor the materials used to support the crown. The root and dowel collectively can be considered an extension of the restorative zone.

In order to function, the retention must be clinically adequate between both the dowel and the root and between the dowel and the restorative core material. Dowel design, cementing media, and core material all affect the ability of dowels to be retained within the root and simultaneously to anchor the core during function. It is important, however, to distinguish between clinically adequate and excessive retention. Retention between the dowel and the root that is greater than necessary is not desirable and can lead to failure from untreatable root fracture rather than from loss of the restoration.[48,75]

Nonthreatening role of the dowel

Occlusal forces are transferred through the core to the dowel and ultimately along the length of the root. The dowel must be designed in such a way that it serves its retentive function without endangering the root or coronal integrity. The remaining dentin and dowel together must have adequate rigidity to withstand the functional load sustained by the tooth without deformation. Distortion of the dowel under function will result ultimately in the failure of the dowel, the remaining tooth structure, and the restoration.

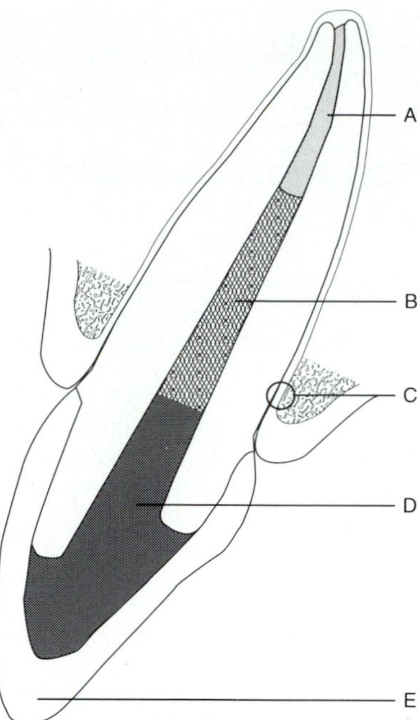

FIG. 22-6 The final configuration of the restored, endodontically treated tooth. The apical endodontic seal is preserved with 3 to 5 mm of gutta-percha **(A)**. The dowel **(B)** is the restorative material within the root. The core **(D)** replaces missing coronal tooth structure and retains the final coronal restoration **(E)**. Restorative and endodontic therapy must preserve the residual root and its attachment mechanism **(C)**.

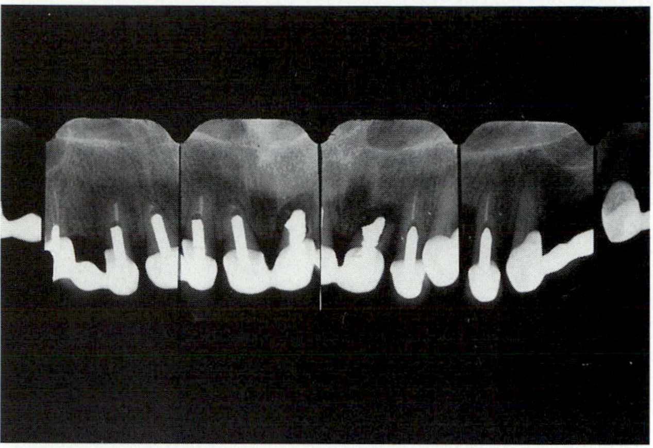

FIG. 22-7 Excessive dentin removal for the placement of large dowels weakens tooth structure.

The dowel must remain in the root for a successful restoration but must not damage the root in attempts to achieve maximum retention. Dowels should be retained by cementation to the dentin walls of the root; active engagement of the dowel space by screw threads is contraindicated. Maximum retention but maximum incidence of fracture are found with screw-type dowels.[9,18] In a clinical study, 40% of self-threaded dowels failed by angular and vertical root fracture, whereas almost 98% of cemented, parallel-sided dowels were successful.[68]

Dowel design

The nonthreatening and retentive capacity of the dowel depend on the appropriate combination of mechanical design features. The relevant variables are dowel length, taper, diameter, and surface configuration. Dowels are designed to take best advantage of each of these qualities; thus, no single approach or single system for the intermediary dowel and core restoration is sufficient for all cases.

Dowel classifications

The two major categories of dowels are preformed dowel systems (Fig. 22-8) and custom-cast dowels (Fig. 22-9). The proprietary preformed dowel systems include various sizes of ready made metallic dowels. Matching instrumentation is used to form a dowel space within the root (Fig. 22-10). The corresponding preformed metal dowel is secured to the root by a cementing medium, and a core is later formed from one of a variety of restorative materials.

A custom-cast dowel system utilizes a casting procedure to fabricate a one-piece metal dowel and core that has no interface between the dowel and the core. By using instrumentation that is paired with castable plastic patterns (Fig. 22-11), the dowel space is shaped to standard dimensions and may incorporate some customizing of the final dowel shape to that of the canal. A custom plastic or plastic and wax dowel and core pattern is produced, invested, and cast in a crown and bridge alloy. The final cast dowel and core is cemented to the residual tooth structure at a subsequent appointment.

Alternative custom dowel techniques are sometimes used, but generally they require increased fabrication time and are often technique sensitive. These include two-part dowel and core restorations for nonparallel roots, totally custom-tapered dowels, and other very individualized approaches to clinical problems.

Dowel length

Dowel retention is proportional to dowel length[60]; increasing the dowel length from 5.0 to 8.0 mm increases the retention by 47%.[33] The dowel length selected for a given root depends on a number of factors. Generally stated, the dowel should be long enough to satisfy clinical requirements without jeopardizing the root integrity. The standard parameters for dowel length in a tooth with normal periodontal support range between (1) two thirds of the length of the canal,[63] (2) the coronal length of the tooth,[63] and (3) half the bone-supported length of the root.[55] These guidelines are reasonable and clinically useful. The final length of the dowel in a periodontally healthy tooth is limited by two major variables, the root morphology and the need for sufficient apical seal in the root canal system.

Root morphology plays a great role in determining dowel length. The total root length is the most obvious factor in dowel length design. Equally important are root taper, root curvature, and cross-sectional root form. Clear and undistorted radiographs reveal root length, taper, and curvature. The root should have at least 1 mm of tooth structure remaining around the dowel in all directions in order to resist fracture or perforation (Fig. 22-12).[10] This concept dictates a shorter dowel in a tapered root, so that the apical extent of the dowel does not impinge on converging root walls. A longer dowel can safely be placed in a parallel-sided root of equal length. Root curvature

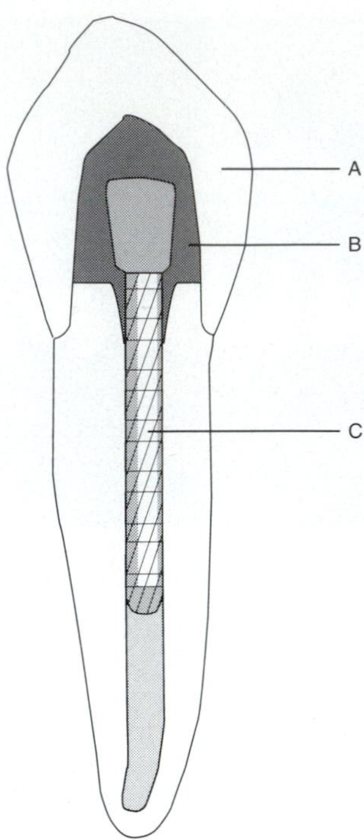

FIG. 22-8 The preformed dowel and core restoration. The preformed metal dowel **(C)** is cemented into the prepared dowel space. The core material **(B)** is retained by the dowel, by bonding to the tooth structure, by undercuts in the pulp chamber, and occasionally by auxiliary retentive pins, grooves, or boxes. The coronal restoration **(A)** provides the ferrule and restores esthetics and function.

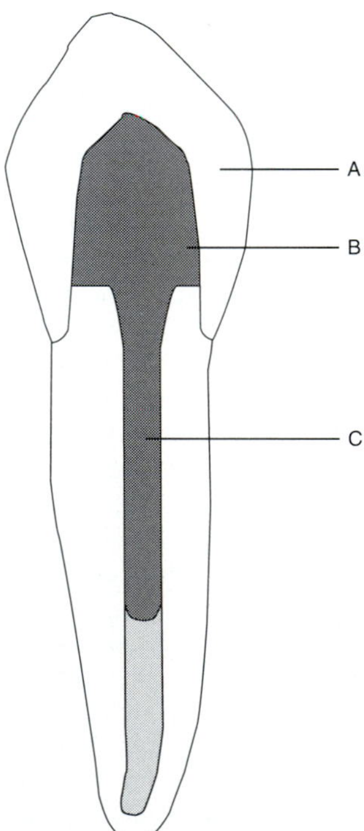

FIG. 22-9 The cast dowel and core restoration. The dowel **(C)** and the core **(B)** are cast of the same material and cemented to the tooth as a single unit. The coronal restoration **(A)** provides the ferrule and restores esthetics and function.

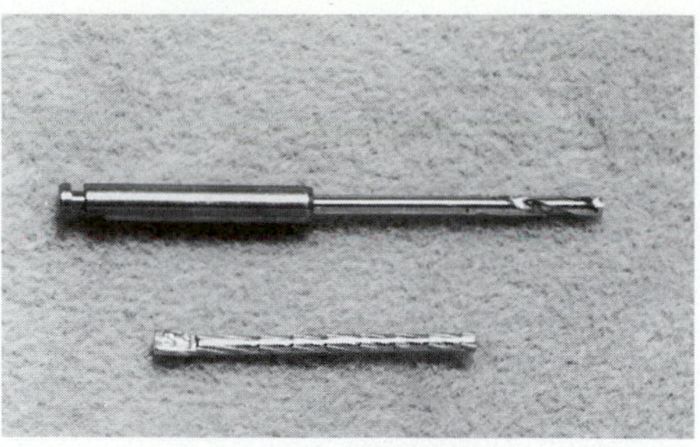

FIG. 22-10 Instrumentation used for fabrication of a preformed dowel. The drill refines the dowel space after initial gutta-percha removal. The corresponding preformed metal dowel should seat easily without active engagement of the dentin walls. (Para Post System, Whaledent International.)

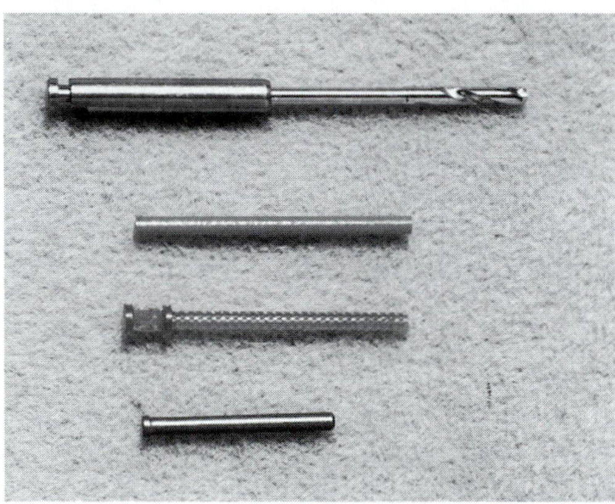

FIG. 22-11 Instrumentation used for fabrication of a cast dowel. *(From top)* The drill refines the dowel space after initial gutta-percha removal. The color-coded plastic impression dowel and plastic burnout dowel are used for the indirect technique; the plastic burnout dowel only is used for the direct cast dowel. The corresponding aluminum dowel is used to retain a provisional restoration. (Para Post System, Whaledent International.)

reduces dowel length in a similar manner; the greater the curve of the root and the more coronally located the curve, the shorter is the dowel. Cross-sectional root form cannot be evaluated by conventional radiographs alone. Thorough knowledge of root morphology for each tooth is mandatory for dowel placement. Furcations, both faciolingual and mesiodistal, along with developmental depressions, are present in predictable locations in the dentition (Fig. 22-13). Maxillary first molars have deep concavities on the furcal surface of 94% of the mesial buccal roots, 31% of distal buccal roots, and 17% of palatal roots. Mandibular first molars have root concavities on the furcal surface of all mesial roots and of 99% of distal roots.[6]

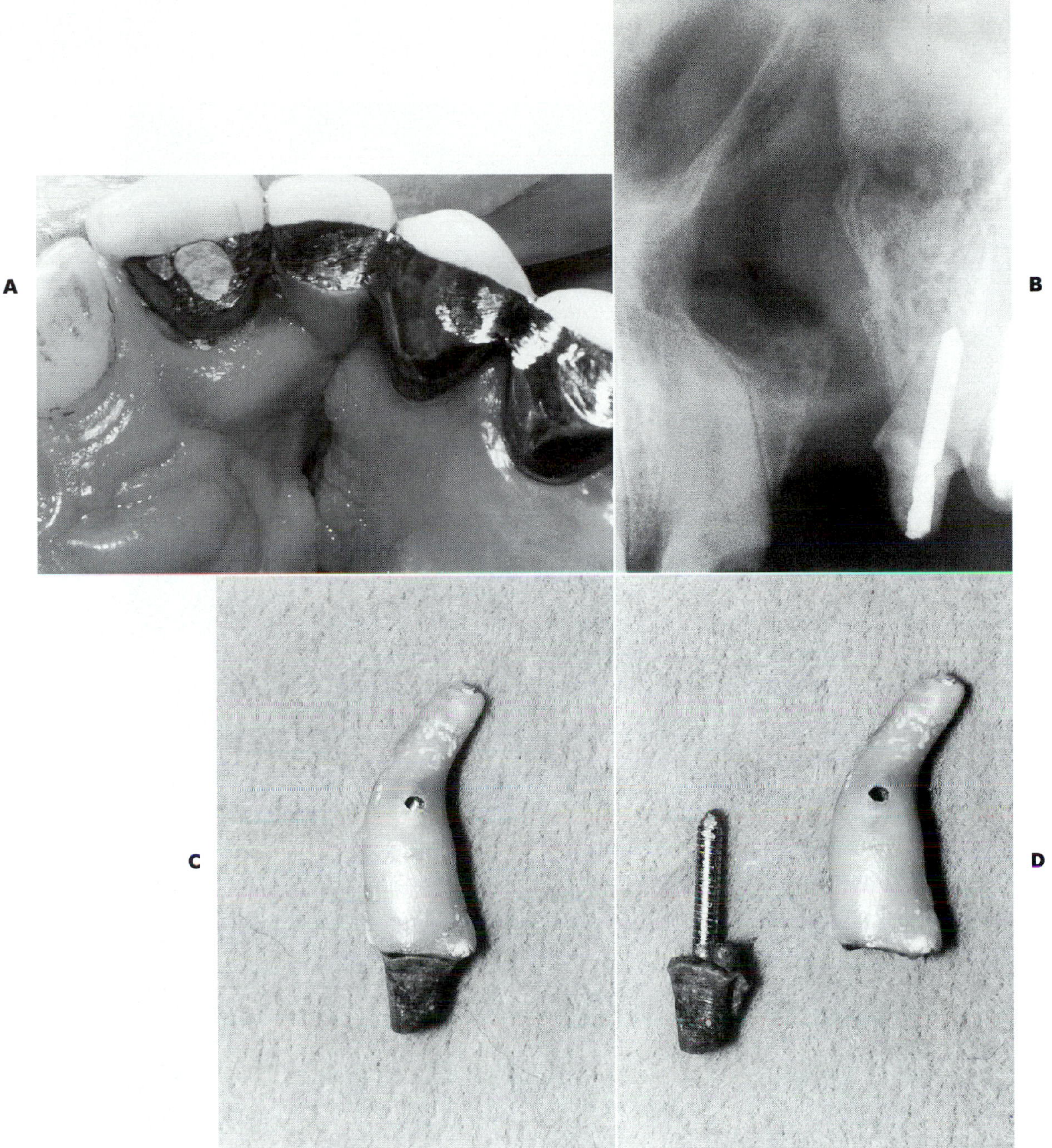

FIG. 22-12 Substantial tooth structure (at least 1 mm) must surround the dowel for strength. **A,** Persistent symptoms in the treated cuspid adjacent to the cleft were diagnosed as a root perforation. **B,** The radiograph appears to demonstrate an intact root surface. **C,** The extracted tooth reveals the dowel visible through the perforation. **D,** Dowel and core separation from the root verify that the perforation occurred at the apex of the dowel.

Maxillary first premolars have deep mesial concavities and slender roots with thin dentin.[24] Endodontically treated teeth with these root concavities require alteration of the length and placement of dowel materials, in order to eliminate thin dentinal walls or outright root perforations.[6,22,24]

The need to maintain adequate obturation is the second major limiting factor in dowel length. Retaining the last 3 to 5 mm of filling material at the apex is sufficient for the endodontic seal. A dowel placed closer to the apex than this distance, even when surrounded by adequate tooth structure, risks failure of the seal, and thus of the restoration effort (Fig. 22-14). Occlusal forces generate the least risk to the remaining tooth structure and surrounding bone when a dowel extends apical to the alveolar crest. Short dowels transfer forces to the unsupported root extending above the alveolus and can cause root fracture.[63]

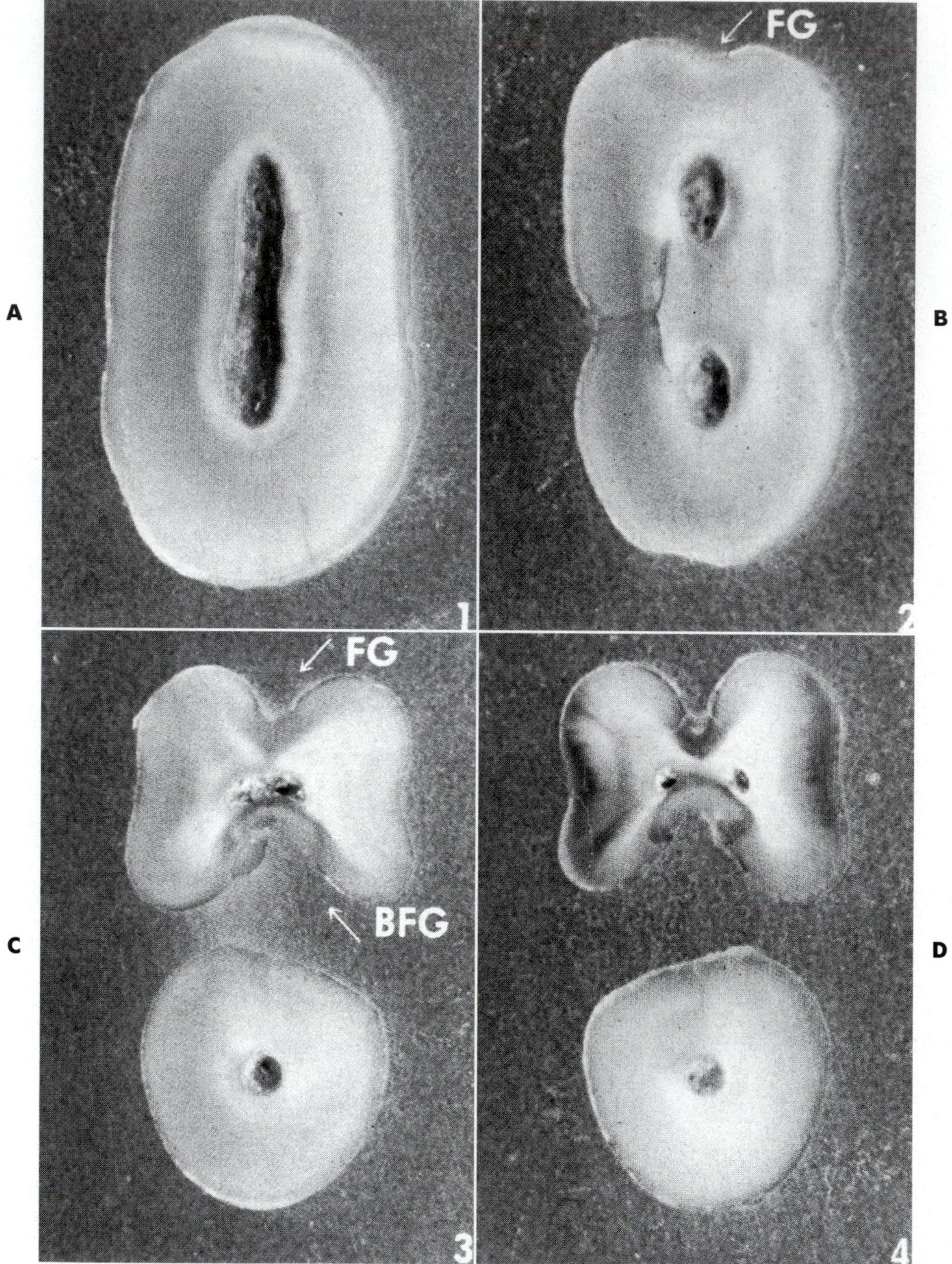

FIG. 22-13 Root anatomy has significant influence over dowel placement. **A,** The cross section of a maxillary first premolar at the cementoenamel junction; the buccal surface faces the top of the section. **B,** 2 mm apical to the CEJ; root irregularities and developmental depressions become apparent. **C,** 4 mm apical to the CEJ; the root has separated into buccal *(top)* and palatal roots and developmental grooves have deepened. **D,** 6 mm apical to the CEJ; the buccal root continues to demonstrate more accentuated depressions. Placement of a dowel in the buccal root risks perforation into the furcation of this tooth. The palatal root is a better choice for dowel placement. (From Int J Periodont Restor Dent 1:(5), 1981.)

When dowels are indicated they should be placed in roots that are round, straight, and long. Root anatomy of multirooted teeth is most suitable in the palatal roots of maxillary molars, palatal roots of maxillary premolars, and distal roots of mandibular molars.[1]

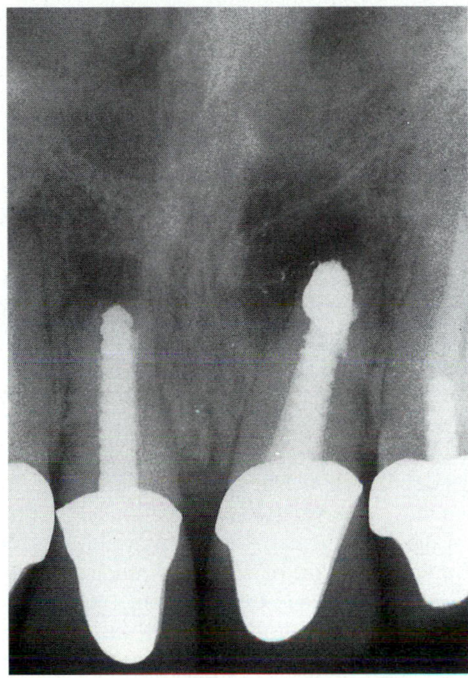

FIG. 22-14 Long, large-diameter dowels obliterate the apical seal and cause endodontic failure of two central incisors; 3 to 5 mm of intact endodontic seal must be retained at the apex.

Dowel shape

Placement of a parallel-sided dowel within the canal improves both the retention and the force distribution of the dowel. Parallel-sided dowels are two to four-and-one-half times as retentive as tapered ones.[30] Parallel-sided dowels also distribute functional loads to the root passively and are therefore indicated for the majority of cases.[13,74] Photoelastic studies have demonstrated that tapered dowels act like a wedge to exert significant lateral forces on the tooth structure.[32,66] These forces may ultimately result in a vertical root fracture. Tapered dowel form is generally reserved for the significantly tapered canal system, where use of a parallel-sided dowel would necessitate rigorous alteration of the radicular dentin walls. In these cases, the design of the crown is critical to protect against root fracture.

As root canal walls are not parallel, some preparation of the canal is required for a parallel-sided dowel. The taper of the canal system dictates how much tooth structure is to be removed for dowel placement. Instrumentation of the radicular dentin walls during dowel space preparation should be very conservative. Severely altering a tapered canal system to accept a parallel dowel defies the concept of preservation of tooth structure. This means that conservative parallel dowels in funnel-shaped canals will not contact the coronal aspect of the canal wall and will be surrounded by a layer of cement. It is no longer thought advisable to have intimate tooth-to-dowel contact in all areas of the restoration (Fig. 22-15).[65] To the contrary, tapered dowels that are closely adapted to the internal shape of the root canal are more likely to result in extensive root fracture than parallel-sided dowels.[66]

Dowel diameter

The dowel must be of sufficient diameter to resist functional forces.[63] Dowel-to-root dynamics are not improved by increasing the diameter beyond that point. A larger diameter gives little or no improvement in the dowel-to-root retention but significantly reduces the resistance of the tooth to fracture (Fig.

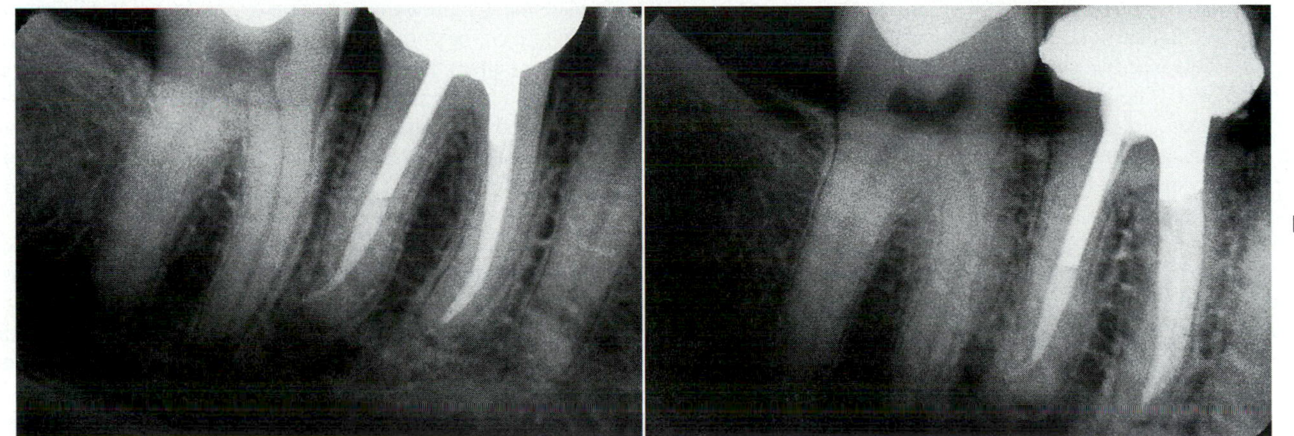

FIG. 22-15 Components of a successful restoration can be seen in these two radiographs of the same tooth. **A,** The gutta-percha seal is intact. Minimal dowel space instrumentation allows the dowel to be an extension of the canal system in the distal root. Cementing medium is evident in the larger, coronal opening of the distal canal. **B,** The mesial roots contain alloy condensed into the first 2 to 4 mm of the canal. The coronal restoration provides protection, function and, if needed, esthetics. (Courtesy Dr. Frank Casanova.)

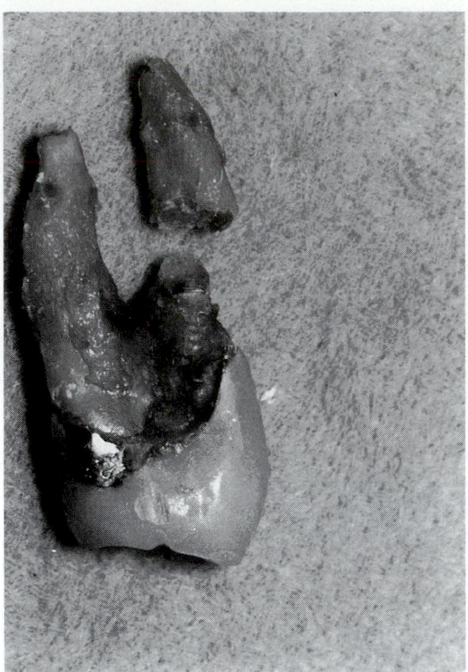

FIG. 22-16 Large dowel diameter in the buccal root resulted in a functional fracture of this premolar. Coronal to the fracture, the dowel can be seen through the thinned root surface. Excessive radicular dentin removal weakened the tooth.

22-16).[13] The preservation of dentin in the radicular areas takes precedence over the larger diameter dowel.

Surface configuration

The surface of a dowel can be smooth or serrated. Serrated surfaces provide mechanical undercuts for cement and significantly increase retention of parallel dowels over that of smooth surfaces.[11,75] Serrations can be horizontal with a single vertical vent channel, or fluted so that the serrations form a series of vents that reduce hydraulic forces generated during cementation.

The mechanical features that contribute the greatest retention are increased length, parallel sides, and a serrated surface of the dowel. The mechanical features that contribute most to the ability of the dowel to resist forces are increased length, parallel sides, and moderate diameter of the dowel. The most important aspect of fracture prevention, however, is not the dowel design but the final crown. The majority of early dowel and force studies were performed on unrestored teeth. The differences in fracture rate between various dowel designs disappeared when crowns were placed.[21] These findings were confirmed in a clinical study that showed that the presence of a dowel had little effect on the fracture rate of crowned teeth.[69]

Dowel materials

Materials used in dowel construction must be able to withstand functional stresses and resist corrosion and must not be harmful to the patient. Common dowel materials include alloys of gold, stainless steel, titanium, and dental amalgam.

The dentition in function is subject to intermittent forces loaded in multiple directions. The ramifications of this loading must be considered when selecting materials to reconstruct teeth after endodontic therapy. Important physical requirements for dowels include adequate stiffness, high yield strength, and favorable fatigue properties.[71] Stiffness is a combination of the modulus of elasticity of the component metal and the cross-sectional geometry of the dowel. Insufficient stiffness results in stress concentration, as the dowel repeatedly deforms and springs back under function. This stress concentration can ultimately cause fracture and failure of the tooth or restoration. The stiffness of the dowel also plays a role in the maintenance of marginal integrity of the coronal restoration. Dowel material that is not sufficiently rigid may force fragile restorative margins to accept high functional loads.[71] This can result in failure of the restorative material at the crown margin or degradation of the luting agent used to cement the restoration to the tooth. This marginal seal loss can result in caries at or under the margin.

Yield strength is the measure of resistance to permanent deformation.[15] Low–yield strength materials deform under lesser loads and transfer stresses to other portions of the restoration. Permanent deformation or bending of the dowel endangers the remaining tooth structure, the core material, the definitive restoration, and the cementing medium. Similarly, dowels possessing unfavorable fatigue properties are subject to premature failure when exposed to the repetitive stresses of oral function. This metal fatigue is manifested as a fracture of the dowel and it may lead to fracture of the tooth.

Dowel materials should be selected that are inert or highly resistant to the corrosive effects of oral fluids.[71] Corrosion resistance of the dowel material is important in a number of respects. An accumulation of corrosion products has been observed between dowels and fractured roots, fractured core material, and adjacent to discolored dentin and gingiva. Contact can occur between dowels and dentinal fluid or fluid microleakage at the tooth-restoration interface. A corrosive interaction between simulated oral fluid and certain pin and dowel alloys has been demonstrated in vitro.[67] Additional research is needed to determine the prevalence and clinical significance of dowel material corrosion. It is not clear whether corrosion is a cause or an effect of root fracture; nonetheless, procedures and materials that minimize the risk of corrosion should be selected.

The most significant corrosion occurs in stainless steel dowels that have been invested, heated, and allowed to cool. Heat treatment alters the microstructure of stainless steel and occurs with the now disputed technique in which a custom core is cast directly onto a preformed wrought metal dowel. In comparison, unheated stainless steel dowels do not exhibit similar deterioration. Custom cast dowels are fabricated from gold alloys and other conventional fixed prosthodontic metals. As these metals are generally nonreactive and the custom dowels are cast and not wrought, the issue of corrosion from heat treatment is eliminated. Preformed systems have traditionally relied on nickel–stainless steel alloys for dowel fabrication. These materials have met with much success in the renovation of endodontically treated teeth. They are economical, predictable clinical adjuncts to the restorative dentist. Recent concerns about the potential for sensitivity and allergy production by nickel alloys have been raised. Biocompatible titanium preformed dowels are less allergenic than nickel–stainless steel alloys. Titanium dowels, however, are significantly less radiopaque than the nickel-chrome alloys. The radiopacity of titanium dowels is similar to that of gutta-percha, and the image is further masked by zinc phosphate, polycarboxylate, and

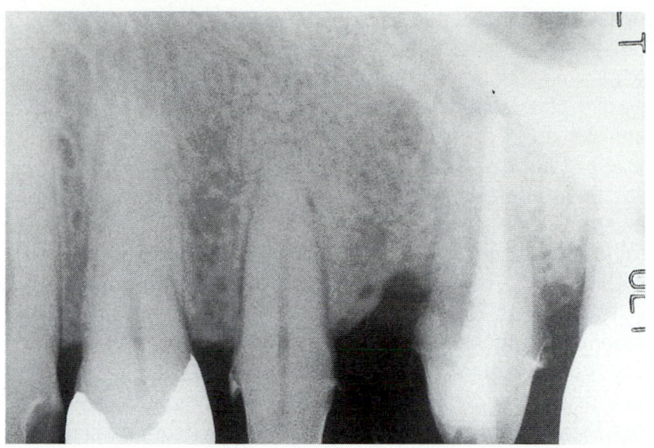

FIG. 22-17 Radiograph of a titanium dowel in the palatal root of the maxillary first molar. This material is more difficult to detect on radiographs than stainless steel or cast dowels.

other opaque cements.[23] Titanium dowels are difficult to distinguish in radiographs with densely condensed, gutta-percha–filled canals (Fig. 22-17). The titanium materials are also somewhat weaker than the nickel-chrome alloys. However, this difference is not clinically significant.[55]

In summary, conventional dowels should be passive and cemented into place. The residual dentin should undergo minimal alteration to accept the dowel. Length and diameter should be the least needed to withstand functional loading. Dowels should be cylindrical, with a serrated surface. They should be fabricated from materials that exhibit physical properties for long-term success and materials that do not corrode or otherwise break down and possibly endanger the patient. The dowel should be a rigid extension into the conservatively shaped root canal system, not an intrusion into the radiuclar dentin. The goal of dowel design is clinically sufficient retention of the dowel and maximum fracture resistance of the root, not the converse (Fig. 22-15).

Core

The core (Fig. 22-6) consists of restorative material placed in the coronal area of a tooth. This material replaces carious, fractured, or otherwise missing coronal structure and retains the final coronal restoration.

The core is anchored to the tooth by a direct connection of the core into the canal or through the endodontic dowel. The attachment between tooth, dowel, and core is mechanical, chemical, or both, as the core and dowel are usually fabricated of different materials.

The remaining tooth structure can also be altered to enhance retention of the core or to provide resistance to core rotation under function. Pins, grooves, and channels can be placed in the dentin in a position remote from the dowel space and keyways. However, these modifications all increase the core retention and resistance to rotation at the expense of tooth structure. In most cases, the irregular nature of the residual coronal tooth structure and the normal morphology of the pulp chamber and canal orifices eliminate the need for these tooth alterations. Using restorative materials that bond to tooth structure enhances retention and resistance without necessitating removal of valuable dentin. Therefore, if additional retentive or antirotation form for the core is deemed necessary, dentin removal should be kept to a minimum.

Desirable physical characteristics of a core include high compressive strength, dimensional stability, ease of manipulation, and short setting time. Contemporary cores include cast metal, amalgam, composite resin, and glass ionomer–silver materials.

Cast core

A cast core (Fig. 22-9) forming a one-piece dowel and core is a traditional and proven method of restoring endodontically treated teeth. This casting has superior physical characteristics at the core/dowel junction. Because the core is an integral extension of the dowel, the cast core does not depend on mechanical means for retention to the dowel. This construction avoids dislodgement of the core and crown from the dowel and root when minimal tooth structure remains. Selection of the dental alloy used in the casting allows control of core properties. Noble metals provide a noncorrosive final restoration. Increased stiffness and associated decreased dentin deformation can be obtained by casting ceramometal alloys or type IV gold.[79] When much tooth structure is missing, the core may be required to provide an antirotation function to the restoration. The cast dowel and core combination can utilize eccentric preparations in the dentin at the dowel-core interface or auxiliary retentive pins or cervical collar at the base of the core.[28] These antirotation features also increase core and crown retention.

The disadvantages of this cast dowel and core system, however, are considerable. The financial cost of providing this service is high, as two appointments are needed to complete the cast dowel and core. The laboratory expense, in time and materials, may be significant. The laboratory phase may also be somewhat technique sensitive in the core fabrication process. Casting a large core in contact with a small-diameter dowel pattern can result in porosity at the dowel-core interface. Fracture of the metal at this interface under function results in failure of the restoration. Attempts to circumvent this problem by casting a core to a proprietary stainless steel preformed dowel are contraindicated. The heating and casting procedures necessary in the laboratory degrade the physical characteristics of the stainless steel. Final qualities of this dowel-core restoration are not sufficiently strong or inert to withstand clinical forces over time. The cast dowel and core is indicated for small anterior and bicuspid teeth, as well as teeth with major coronal destruction. In addition, they may be used when functional forces on a tooth put the dowel-to-core retention at risk.

Amalgam core

Dental amalgam has many characteristics advantageous for core fabrication. Amalgam is very stable to thermal and functional stresses. As an intermediary material, this stability transmits minimal stress to the residual tooth structure and to the luting material of the final coronal restoration. Amalgam also presents a corrosion barrier that seals the tooth/alloy junction. The resultant low microleakage inhibits recurrent caries, coronal-apical endodontic contamination, and corrosion of the metals used in this dowel and core fabrication. High compressive strength, high tensile strength, and high modulus of elasticity are all hallmarks of dental amalgam that are ideal for a core material.[16,44]

Amalgam is easily manipulated and can set rapidly. Placement of a fast-setting, high-copper alloy core permits final crown preparation at the initial operative appointment. It is highly retentive when used in posterior teeth in conjunction with a preformed stainless steel dowel. Dowel retained amalgam cores in molars require more force to dislodge than cast dowel and cores.[37] The amalgam core demonstrates superior mechanical retention to tooth and dowel undercuts.[45] Additional retention and antirotation can be procured with auxiliary pins or dentin preparation. Bonded amalgam procedures enhance retention and further reduce microleakage by incorporating a layer of resin that chemically bonds to both dentin and metal.[12,47,61] A significant disadvantage of amalgam cores is the potential for corrosion and subsequent discoloration of the gingiva or remaining dentin. This core material can be used in almost all teeth where sufficient bulk of amalgam for strength is possible. Amalgam dowels should be avoided in teeth with high esthetic value.

Composite resin core

A third core material is composite resin, which is easy to manipulate and sets very rapidly. Preparation for the final restoration is readily accomplished during the core placement session. Additional retention and antirotation mechanisms are also easily achieved with auxiliary pins, dentin preparations, or dentin-bonding materials.[12]

Certain physical characteristics of the composite resins restrict routine use as core material to cases with significant remaining tooth structure. Polymerization shrinkage and contraction away from the tooth structure can result in core/tooth marginal opening and microcracks. These openings are potential avenues of extensive invasion for oral fluids following a break in marginal integrity of a final restoration or when a permanent restorative cement seal is lost. The microleakage phenomenon is greater with composite resins than with amalgam or glass ionomer materials. Composite resin is dimensionally unstable, and expansion in wet conditions can cause marginal openings or difficulty in seating final restorations. The thermal coefficient of expansion is two to ten times greater than that of tooth structure, which can affect the luting integrity and increase microleakage under the coronal restoration. A low modulus of elasticity allows deformation of composite resin under function, which can damage restorative margins, cause degradation of cement seals, or allow unacceptable load transfers to the dowel material. The composite resins should not be used as core materials in teeth with extensive structural damage. More than 2 mm of sound tooth structure should remain at the margin, and two dentin walls should be present for optimal composite resin core function.[2,16,53] Dentin-bonding agents and bonded composites all improve the physical characteristics and reduce microleakage of the composite resin core/tooth junction. No bonding agent, however, has been shown to entirely eliminate microleakage.[20,77,78]

Glass ionomer core

High-viscosity glass ionomer and glass ionomer–silver cements are core materials that employ adhesion to dentin. This chemical union improves retention of the restorations and reduces marginal leakage over that of unbounded amalgam or composite resin cores. The major benefit of glass ionomer materials is an anticariogenic quality derived from the presence of fluoride in the chemical composition.[16,42] Microleakage or other contact with oral fluids initiates fluoride ion release, which reduces the potential for recurrent caries.

The glass ionomer core materials are technique sensitive, and deviation from the manufacturer's recommendations can lead to failure of the core and of the final crown. Precise measurement and mixing procedures are important for obtaining maximum strength and adhesion of the restoration. Adhesive failure can result from contamination of the tooth surface with cutting debris, saliva, blood, or protein. Meticulous moisture control is vital. Excessive moisture results in solubility of glass ionomer components during the initial setting phase and reduces the marginal seal of the restoration. Conversely, excessive drying and desiccation of the tooth surface decreases the bond strength by reducing the dentin's "wettability" and interfering with intimate contact between the core and the tooth structure. Moisture must be excluded during the entire setting period, and the subsequent crown preparation procedures must be carefully executed to avoid heat production and cracking of the restorative material.

The physical characteristics of glass ionomer core materials limit their application to specific clinical conditions. The tensile strength and flexural strength of glass ionomer core material are lower than that of either amalgam or composite resin.[7] The fracture toughness is low, and the resulting brittleness contraindicates the use of glass ionomer buildups in thin anterior teeth or to replace unsupported cusps. Glass ionomer cores also exhibit low retention to preformed dowels.[45] Glass ionomer buildup materials can be used in posterior teeth in which (1) a bulk of core material is possible, (2) significant sound dentin remains, (3) additional retention is available with pins or dentin preparations, and (4) moisture control is assured.

Coronal-radicular core

An alternative to the traditional dowel and core for posterior teeth is the direct coronal-radicular restoration. This restoration consists of a core that replaces coronal tooth structure and extends 2 to 4 mm into the coronal portion of the canals.[50] The core is retained by a combination of the divergence of the canals in a multirooted tooth, the natural undercuts in the pulp chamber, adhesion with dentin-bonding agents, and retentive channels or preparations in the dentin.

The coronal-radicular core utilizes conventional restorative materials, including amalgam, composite resin, or glass ionomer–silver. The ease of manipulation and a rapid set of these core materials is an advantage. The buildup can be placed and prepared for a final coronal restoration in one visit. A single, homogenous material is used for the entire restoration, as opposed to the dual phases of a conventional preformed dowel and core. The coronal-radicular core is indicated for posterior teeth that have large pulp chambers and multiple canals for retention. The retention of coronal radicular alloy buildups in molars is equal to that of pin-retained amalgam cores.[31,43] The physical characteristics of alloy and composite resin allow this restoration to function well when as much as 50% of the coronal tooth structure has been lost. Greater amounts of tooth structure must be present if glass ionomer is used because of its low tensile strength. Because no dowel is present to distribute functional forces to the apical tooth structure, this restoration should be used cautiously in teeth that are abutments for large restorations generating high functional loads.

Dowel and core selection

Successful restoration of the endodontically treated tooth requires careful planning and meticulous instrumentation. Many of the dowel and core systems utilize common procedures, which will be presented together. Understanding the general technique of the major dowel and core subgroups allows the clinician to easily adapt to the specifics of a proprietary system in that group. It is not the object of this chapter to be an exhaustive compilation of available dowel systems.

Many factors affect the selection of a particular dowel and core system for tooth restoration. Two variables that have a major influence on this decision are the amount of remaining tooth structure and the functional stresses anticipated for the tooth. When a coronal restoration is indicated, the amount of tooth structure remaining after final preparation has the greatest importance in determining the design of the intermediary dowel and core. Tooth structure that appears adequate before the crown preparation may be grossly unsatisfactory after occlusal and axial reduction. Therefore, the initial crown preparation is first completed and the bulk and position of the prepared tooth structure are evaluated for dowel and core selection. Premature placement of an inappropriate dowel and core can create significant restoration problems.

The second major consideration in designing dowel and core restorations is the functional requirements of the tooth. Abutment teeth for removable partial dentures withstand greater stress and fracture more frequently than abutment teeth for fixed partial dentures or individual teeth within the dental arch. Consequently, endodontically treated abutment teeth for removable partial dentures require a dowel to distribute forces, as well as a core and a crown.[69] Fixed partial denture abutments and individual teeth can utilize pin-retained cores or coronal-radicular alloys without dowels, when volume of residual tooth structure permits.

Improper selection of the dowel and core system may result in clinical failure. Significant functional forces and minimal remaining tooth structure concentrate stresses at the core to dowel/tooth interface. Separation of the core material from the dowel and the tooth is common. The coronal restoration, with the core inside, separates from the dowel, which is retained in the root. A new core and crown may be fabricated if the existing dowel is satisfactory and increased retention is achieved with the added core material. If the existing dowel is unsatisfactory, removal is a delicate procedure. Persistent vibration with an ultrasonic cleaning device degrades the cement and allows withdrawal of the metal dowel (see Chapter 24). Extreme care must be used to protect the remaining tooth structure as additional dentin loss compounds the restorative problem. Forced removal of the dowel from the root may result in fracture of the root and loss of the tooth (see Chapter 24).

Coronal coverage

The final component of the endodontic reconstruction is the coronal restoration (Fig. 22-6). All coronal restorations reestablish function, restore esthetics, and isolate the dentin and endodontic fill materials from microleakage. Cast crowns are coronal restorations that fulfill all of these requirements and also distribute functional forces and protect the tooth against fracture.

As described earlier, the physical characteristics of the endodontically treated tooth differ from those of the vital tooth. Previous concern over the loss of dentinal resiliency assumed that all endodontically treated teeth became brittle and required a cast crown. Currently, the fundamental issue for fracture potential is the missing tooth structure and loss of architectural integrity of the remaining tooth. This view has altered the clinical criteria for placement of a coronal restoration. Depending on the tooth type and the degree of tooth structure decimated by previous disease, repair, and iatrogenic misadventures, the coronal restoration can range from a simple access seal to a crown that essentially replaces all of the coronal tooth structure (Table 22-1).

As a general rule, all endodontically treated posterior teeth and those anterior teeth that are structurally damaged should be restored with a crown. Crowns prevent a significant number of fractures in posterior teeth but do not similarly protect anterior ones (Fig. 22-5). In a large clinical study, the fracture rate for uncrowned bicuspids and molars was double that for those restored with crowns. The success rate for maxillary molars dropped from 97.8% for those with crowns to 50.0% for those without crowns. Anterior teeth are less at risk for fracture than posterior ones and showed no further improvement when restored with a crown. Maxillary anterior teeth exhibited a success rate of 87.5% for crowned teeth and 85.4% for uncrowned teeth. Therefore, endodontically treated anterior teeth do not require a crown or dowel unless extensive tooth structure is missing and integrity, function, and esthetics must be restored. The coronal restoration for endodontically treated intact anterior teeth consists of sealing the lin-

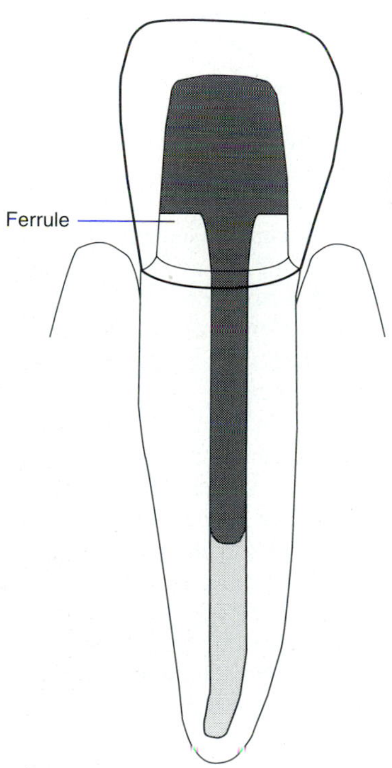

FIG. 22-18 The ferrule is an encircling band of metal usually provided by the coronal restoration. It greatly increases the resistance of a tooth to fracture. A ferrule should (1) be a minimum of 1 to 2 mm high, (2) have parallel axial walls, (3) totally encircle the tooth, (4) end on sound tooth structure, and (5) not invade the attachment apparatus of the tooth.

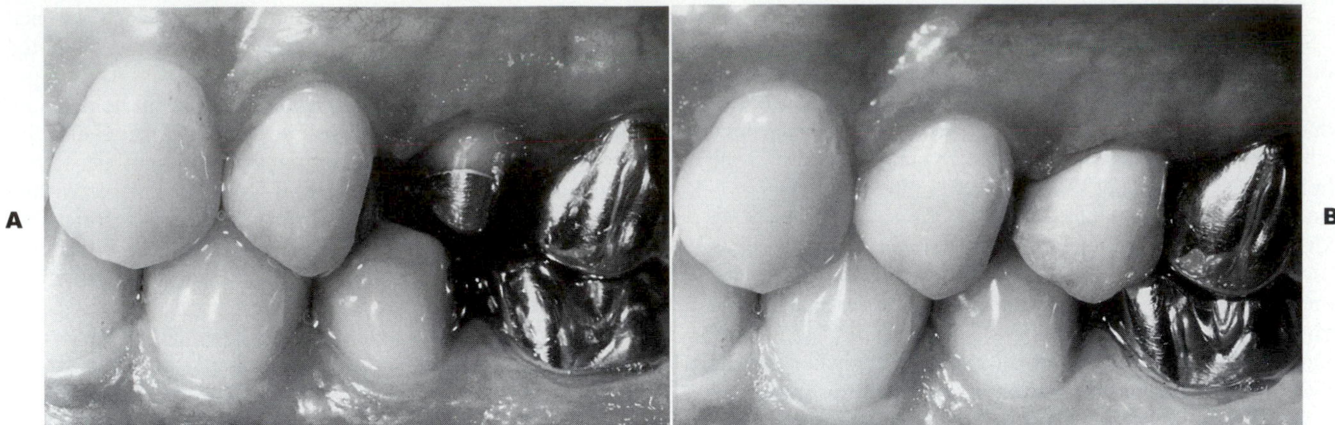

FIG. 22-19 The ferrule effect is provided by the coronal restoration. **A,** The second premolar with a preformed dowel and alloy core. **B,** The coping of the porcelain and metal crown supplies the ferrule. This encirclement significantly increases the fracture resistance of the tooth.

gual access cavity. Posterior teeth need coronal coverage to protect against fracture from occlusal forces, regardless of the amount of remaining tooth structure.[69]

Crown preparation for endodontically treated teeth is identical to that of vital teeth when substantial tooth structure remains. Once restored with a crown, the underlying sound tooth structure provides greater resistance to fracture than any dowel type or design. Natural tooth structure should be carefully preserved during all phases of dowel space and crown preparation.

For extensively damaged nonvital teeth the crown preparation design is critical. The minimal remaining tooth structure must be utilized effectively, so that the crown can restore function without harm to remaining root or to the periodontal attachment. The residual tooth between the core and the gingival sulcus must be structurally sound and a minimum of 2 mm high for the crown ferrule and margin. As caries, fracture, and other endodontic precedents can decimate the tooth to the tissue level, this amount of unaffected tooth structure often is not available, and adjunctive procedures are indicated first to obtain the necessary length.

The final coronal restoration provides added security to the tooth by consolidating the remaining cusps and prepared tooth structure and by creating a ferrule effect (Fig. 22-18). The ferrule is a metal band that encircles the external dimension of the residual tooth, similar to the metal bands around a barrel or a shovel handle. It is formed by the walls of the crown (Fig. 22-19) or cast telescopic coping (Fig. 22-20) encasing the gingival 1 to 2 mm of the axial walls of the preparation above the crown margin. A properly built ferrule significantly reduces the incidence of fracture in the nonvital tooth by reinforcing the tooth at its external surface and dissipating force that concentrates at the narrowest circumference of the tooth.[71] The ferrule also resists lateral forces from tapered dowels and leverage from the crown in function and increases the retention and resistance of the restoration. Crown preparations with a 1-mm coronal extension of dentin above the margin exhibit double the fracture resistance of preparations whose core terminates on a flat surface immediately above the margin.[46,66]

To be successful the ferrule must encircle a vertical wall of sound tooth structure above the margin and must not terminate on restorative material. The crown and crown preparation together must meet five requirements: (1) a minimum of 1 to 2 mm dentin axial wall height, (2) parallel axial walls, (3) the metal must totally encircle the tooth, (4) it must be on solid tooth structure, and (5) it must not invade the attachment apparatus.

A tooth whose remaining structure is insufficient to construct a ferrule, as described, should be evaluated for periodontal crown-lengthening surgery or orthodontic extrusion to gain access to additional root surface.[35] The lack of sufficient ferrule in the final restoration forces the core and the dowel to accept high functional stresses, often resulting in fracture due to material failure (Fig. 22-21).

The true extent of caries or other damage in a broken-down tooth can be difficult to determine before tooth preparation. Placement of a provisional restoration, or temporary crown, allows total evaluation of the tooth and supporting structures before committing the patient to definitive endodontics. As discussed in the section on Evaluation, structural, occlusal, and periodontal findings may condemn a tooth to extraction even though endodontic therapy can be successful. It is prudent to discover these facts before the canals are treated.

Provisional restorations

Once the decision is made to retain a tooth, crown preparation and provisional restoration in advance of endodontic treatment can assist the endodontic endeavor. Removal of this temporary crown at the endodontic appointment allows structural evaluation of the remaining coronal dentin and facilitates access entry to the chamber. When the procedure is completed, the provisional restoration is recemented and the function, esthetics, and protective qualities of the tooth are returned.

The provisional crown may also aid in rubber dam isolation. Left in place during root canal therapy, the provisional crown provides normal axial contours to the tooth and allows engagement of the rubber dam clamp. Access is then attained through the occlusal or lingual surface of the provisional restoration. A temporary material is used when the operative appointment for endodontics is complete.

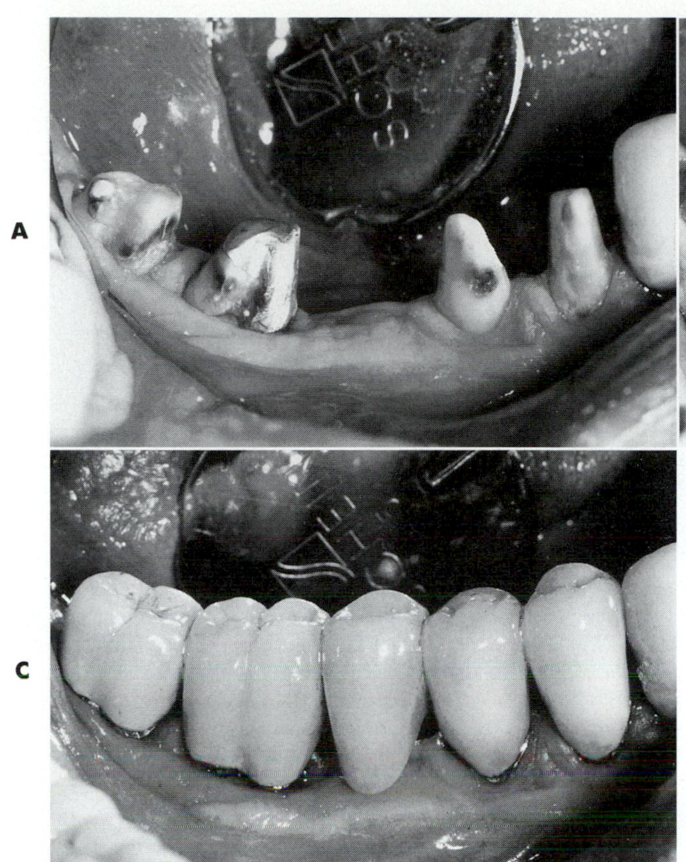

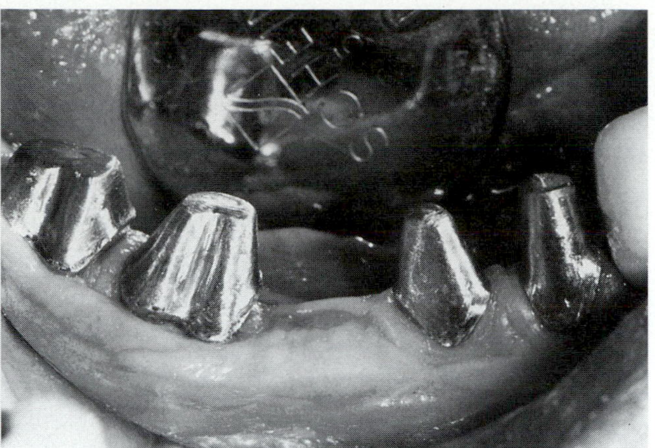

FIG. 22-20 The ferrule is produced by the primary coping. **A,** The second premolar and second molar both contain dowel and core restorations. **B,** The primary copings are seated. They encircle the tooth structure and provide the ferrule. **C,** The superstructure prosthesis is cemented. The superstructure does not add to the ferrule in this case.

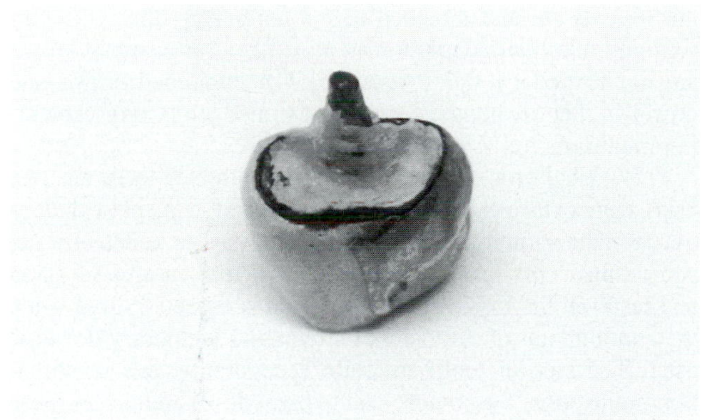

FIG. 22-21 A failed restoration with inadequate ferrule. The level of the core material is coincident with the restorative margin; functional forces were not resisted by adequate axial walls of sound tooth structure.

Finally, preendodontic preparation and provisionalization may assist in differential diagnosis. Proper diagnosis can be difficult when multiple clinical problems are present on the same tooth or on adjacent ones. Clarification of the true cause is aided by the removal of potential symptomatic variables, including caries, defective restorations, and cracked cusps. Decisions about the restorability of the tooth can be made and the tooth returned to temporary esthetics and function, before scheduling definitive endodontic treatment or extraction of the tooth.

Provisional crown fabrication techniques

Provisional crowns are fabricated using conventional fixed prosthodontic techniques and cementation procedures. Owing to its superior strength and color stability, methyl methacrylate acrylic resins should be used when crowns will be required to function over long periods of time. This is a stable material that allows various dental supportive therapies to be completed in an organized and controlled fashion without maintenance problems from breakdown of the acrylic resin. Temporary crowns formed from methyl methacrylate resins or cement-filled aluminum crown shells cannot be expected to provide the needed time and control to finish a prescribed treatment sequence.

After endodontic treatment, a provisional crown with attached temporary dowel can restore esthetics and function to the tooth with limited supragingival tooth structure until definitive restoration is possible (Fig. 22-22). Many proprietary dowel systems include aluminum temporary dowels for fabrication of dowel-retained provisional crowns. An appropriate temporary dowel is selected to fit the prepared dowel space. The dowel is seated and sized to fit within the confines of a crown shell or of the existing provisional crown. Slight internal relief in the crown allows resin material to attach to both the crown and the dowel. Undercuts within the tooth are blocked out or removed at the dowel-tooth interface. The tooth structure is lightly lubricated and a small amount of resin is placed in the relief area of the provisional crown. The crown is seated over the tooth and dowel and held in position until

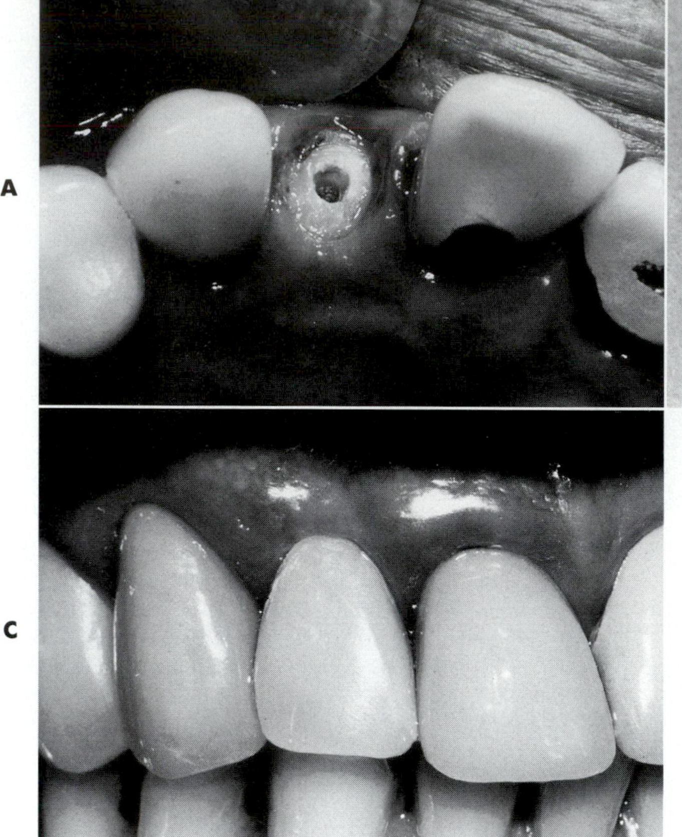

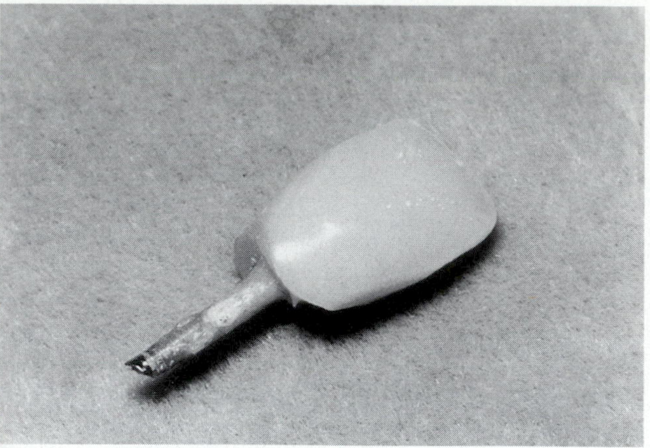

FIG. 22-22 Provisional crowns may be retained by temporary dowels until definitive therapy can be provided. **A,** A lateral incisor fractured below the level of the free gingival margin. **B,** Endodontic therapy was completed and a provisional crown fabricated with an aluminum dowel. **C,** The provisional restoration is in place. This procedure allowed time for orthodontic extrusion of the root. A final dowel, core, and coronal restoration was placed after sufficient tooth structure was present above the periodontal attachment.

the resin is set and attached to the temporary dowel. Occlusion and marginal adaptation of an existing provisional crown are not altered by this procedure. The combined crown and dowel is then cemented into place with a temporary cementing medium.

Provisional crowns for endodontically treated teeth must be used with extreme caution. Partial loss of cement seal does not provoke symptoms in the tooth and may go undetected for some time. This leakage can lead to severe carious invasion and result in the loss of the tooth. This is especially true when the combination of provisional crown and temporary dowel is used. The lack of tooth structure necessitating this combination predisposes the cement seal to breakdown and places these teeth at risk.

Dowel and core fabrication techniques

Numerous techniques are available for fabrication and placement of the dowel and core restoration. Most share the initial steps, including removal of gutta-percha and initial preparation of the dowel space. The procedures for each subgroup (preformed passive dowels and cast dowels) then diverge. The preformed systems then utilize common procedures for attachment of the core, a step that is unnecessary for cast dowel and core systems.

The first step for all types of dowel and core restorations is the removal of the gutta-percha from the dowel space. The amount of gutta percha to be removed is dictated by the desired dowel length, the bone height, and the root morphology, as discussed earlier. The procedure generally is best accomplished by the clinician providing the endodontic service, as that person has clear knowledge of the canal system's size and form. Removal of the filling material to form the dowel space should be completed in a passive manner, so as not to disturb the apical seal. A hot root canal plugger or electronic heating device can safely be used to remove gutta-percha.[26] It is important to heat the instrument hot enough to sear and remove the gutta-percha. An instrument that is too cool will melt the filling into a sticky mass that can dislodge the entire canal fill when the instrument is withdrawn. Extreme care must be taken so as not to injure the patient with the heated instruments.

Rotary instrumentation for gutta-percha removal is also available.[38] However, rotation instruments carry the risk of straying from the canal and cutting radicular dentin. This weakens the root structure and could result in lateral root perforation, particularly in the area of root flutings or concavities. If mechanical rotation is deemed necessary, instruments such as Peezo reamers or Gates-Glidden burs are indicated. They are designed to center themselves within the confines of the gutta-percha fill. However, occasional deviation into the dentin walls or dislodgement of the apical seal can occur.

The use of chemicals for gutta-percha removal should be discouraged. Containment of the chemical within the canal and total control to the desired depth are very difficult. The result of chemical removal may be leakage in the lateral canal complex or in the apical areas.

Some controversy exists about the timing of gutta-percha removal. Although some advocate a delay of 48 hours or more following final root canal filling before the dowel space is prepared, the current tendency is to complete both procedures at one sitting.[1] If the canal system is filled and the dowel space prepared at one appointment, vertical recondensation of the remaining apical fill material is indicated to ensure an intact seal.

The initial dowel space preparation procedure is similar for most dowel and core systems. The space cleared of gutta-percha has the form of the canal after cleaning and shaping and must be refined to the correct dimension and shape for the dowel. All of the proprietary systems are supplied with a series of drills to prepare the internal surface of the canal. The drills gradually increase the size of the canal, remove natural undercuts, and shape the canal to correspond with the provided dowel or dowel pattern. The drills are sized to match preformed metal dowels, preformed impression dowels, or preformed plastic dowel forms. The diameters of these drills and associated dowel forms are incremental from 0.7 to 1.7 mm. The goal at the refinement step is to establish a proper dowel space with a minimum of dentin wall alteration. Intimate contact of the dowel and dentin surface is not indicated for the passive dowel systems; adequate depth and cementation provide sufficient retention for these restorations. The drills provided for the internal refinement should be used with great caution. It is often possible to achieve necessary form in the dowel space by rotating the drills with finger force only. Correct depth can be measured with a periodontal probe or other small measuring device. The distance from a coronal landmark to the remaining gutta-percha is recorded. This measurement is transferred to the smallest drill for use in the canal; drills of progressively larger size are used until the apical 2 or 3 mm of dentin is engaged during rotation. Rotation with a dental handpiece is dangerous, as deviation from the cleared canal is easy and hazardous. In addition, power-driven instrumentation risks unnecessary enlargement of the canals and could damage the apical endodontic seal. The dowel space is now ready for the final clinical procedure, the actual dowel and core construction.

Cast dowel and core fabrication technique

Cast dowel and core restorations can be fabricated with either direct or indirect techniques. The procedures differ only in the means by which the dowel and core pattern is generated. Both utilize instrumentation and materials from the same proprietary systems (Fig. 22-11). In the direct technique, a castable dowel and core pattern is fabricated directly in the mouth, on the prepared tooth. The indirect technique utilizes an impression and stone die of the tooth for pattern fabrication. The pattern from either the direct or indirect technique is then invested and cast with gold or another crown and bridge alloy.

Using the direct technique, the final dowel and core pattern is fabricated during the first appointment. After the initial crown preparation and dowel space refinement, a preformed plastic dowel pattern is selected that corresponds to the last drill size used. This plastic rod is seated completely in the dowel space. The pattern should not bind on the internal walls of the root. If the passive fit is not achieved, a second pattern should be tried or the canal refined again. Passivity is important. After the dowel pattern is fitted, any necessary antirotation pins or dentin preparations are added, ensuring that they are parallel to the path of withdrawal. Undercuts should be eliminated by blocking out with glass ionomer cement or alloy rather than by removing valuable dentin. The tooth is lubricated lightly and the plastic dowel is seated. Self-curing acrylic resin or wax is added to the tooth to create a core attached to the dowel pattern. The final core shape is completed in the mouth by carving wax or preparing the hardened resin with a dental handpiece using copious water flow. The prepared pattern is removed from the tooth, the dowel orifice is protected with a cotton pledget and the provisional crown is cemented. If a dowel-retained provisional crown is used, no cement should be placed on the temporary dowel or in the canal (Fig. 22-23).

Using the indirect technique, a final impression of the prepared tooth and prepared dowel space is made during the first appointment. The final pattern is then fabricated on a die made from this impression. The crown margins need not be accurately reproduced at this stage unless a more complex telescopic dowel and core is planned. Again, proprietary systems provide matched drills, impression dowels, and laboratory casting patterns of various diameters. As a first clinical step, an impression dowel is selected and fitted to the refined dowel space. This impression dowel must seat easily in the prepared dowel space. Adhesive is applied to the coronal portion of the impression dowel and a final impression is made using conventional crown and bridge materials. The impression captures the form of the coronal tooth structure and picks up the impressional dowel. Total block out of undercuts need not be performed in the mouth at this time. The provisional crown is cemented in place and the patient is dismissed. A dental cast is fabricated with a die that precisely reproduces the prepared dowel space and the residual coronal tooth structure. In the laboratory, undercuts are corrected by block out on the cast. A preformed plastic dowel pattern is fitted into the die dowel space and wax is added to form the core. The final core shape is carved in the wax, and the dowel and core pattern is removed from the cast. Patterns generated from the both the direct and the indirect techniques are invested and cast in the same way. The final cast custom dowel and core is now ready for the patient's second appointment.

After removal of the provisional crown and temporary cement, the casting is carefully seated in the dowel space. It should slide easily into place without binding and without pressure. This is a passive dental restoration. Obstructions to easy seating should be detected by a silicone paste or paint-type disclosing medium and removed. This process is repeated until the casting seats completely and easily in the preparation. It is important to note that total marginal integrity between the casting and the tooth is not mandatory except as an indication of complete seating. This is an internal restoration; the entire cast dowel and core, along with the tooth structure of the ferrule, will be encapsulated by the coping of the final restoration. The final crown must have marginal integrity. The dowel and core restoration is now ready for cementation (see Cementation).

Preformed dowel and core fabrication technique

Preformed dowel and core combinations are an appropriate choice for most clinical situations, particularly for posterior teeth. They make up the vast majority of intermediary restorations placed in dental practice today. Though there are many variations, most systems contain preformed metallic dowels corresponding to the instrumentation used in refining the dowel space (Fig. 22-10). Once the dowel space preparation is complete, the matching metal dowel is easily selected by a numbering or color system. This dowel is placed in the finished

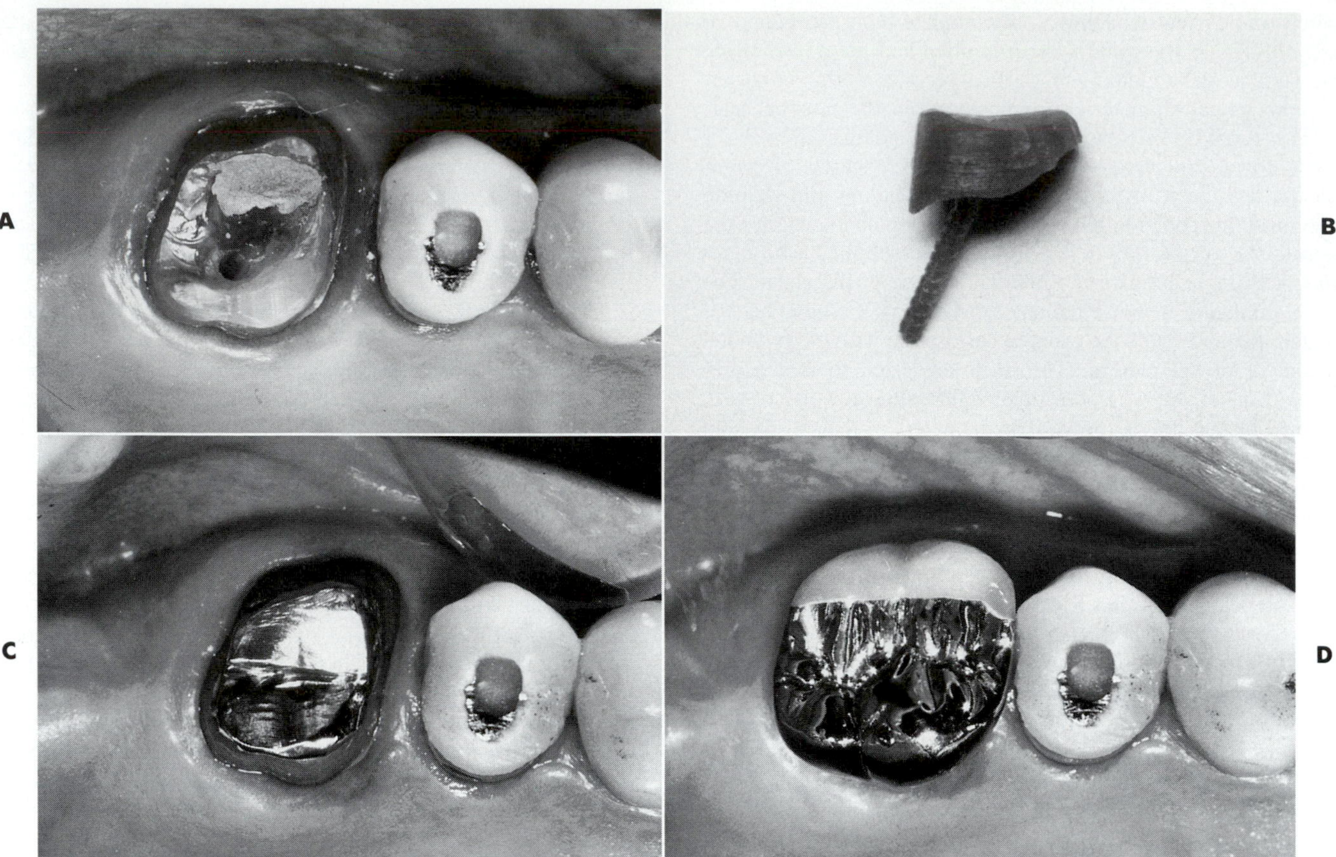

FIG. 22-23 The cast dowel and core restoration (direct technique). **A,** The tooth is prepared before final selection of a dowel and core system. The buccal canal undercuts are blocked out to form a path of withdrawal for the pattern without additional dentin removal. A plastic burnout dowel is fitted to the refined dowel space in the palatal root and resin is added to form the core portion of the pattern. **B,** The one-piece pattern is removed from the tooth and cast. **C,** Cast dowel and core is cemented in the preparation. **D,** The final coronal restoration is fabricated.

dowel space and should slide easily to the apical extension of the preparation. No binding and no force should be necessary to place this dowel. Resistance to seating should be removed by refining the dowel space; the preformed dowel should not be altered to fit the tooth, as any grinding on the apical area alters the dowel-root dynamics. Total seating is assessed by measuring the length of the dowel space from a fixed coronal landmark with a periodontal probe. This distance is transferred to the preformed dowel to confirm total embedding. Complete seating may also be confirmed by radiograph. After achieving a passive fit within the root, the excess coronal dowel metal must be shortened to an appropriate length. This must be completed before the dowel is cemented into the dowel space. Trimming the dowel after final cementation causes vibration and risks degradation of the cement, decreased retention, and possibly microleakage into the canal space. The dowel should be short of the internal occlusal surface of the final coronal restoration but must be long enough to retain the core. The dowel is now ready for cementation (Fig. 22-24) (see Cementation).

Core fabrication technique

After the dowel is luted to the root any necessary retentive and antirotation mechanisms are added. The minimal number of additional retentive devices should be used, as these pins, groves, and other dentin preparations remove tooth structure. Often the undercut nature of the remaining pulp chamber, the irregularity of the residual coronal tooth structure, and the angle at which the dowel exits the tooth are adequate to ensure core retention. These features, along with normal irregular cervical root anatomy, provide adequate antirotation to most restorations. The core material is then placed around the dowel, into the remaining pulp chamber, and built up to form the coronal restoration. A suitable matrix may be necessary. Manufacturer's instructions should be followed for mixing and placement of each of the core materials. Isolation from moisture contamination is vital during the core formation. Amalgam alloys, composite resins, and glass ionomer cements all require a dry field to obtain optimal physical characteristics. After the core material is set it can be prepared for the final coronal restoration. The dowel and any additional retentive de-

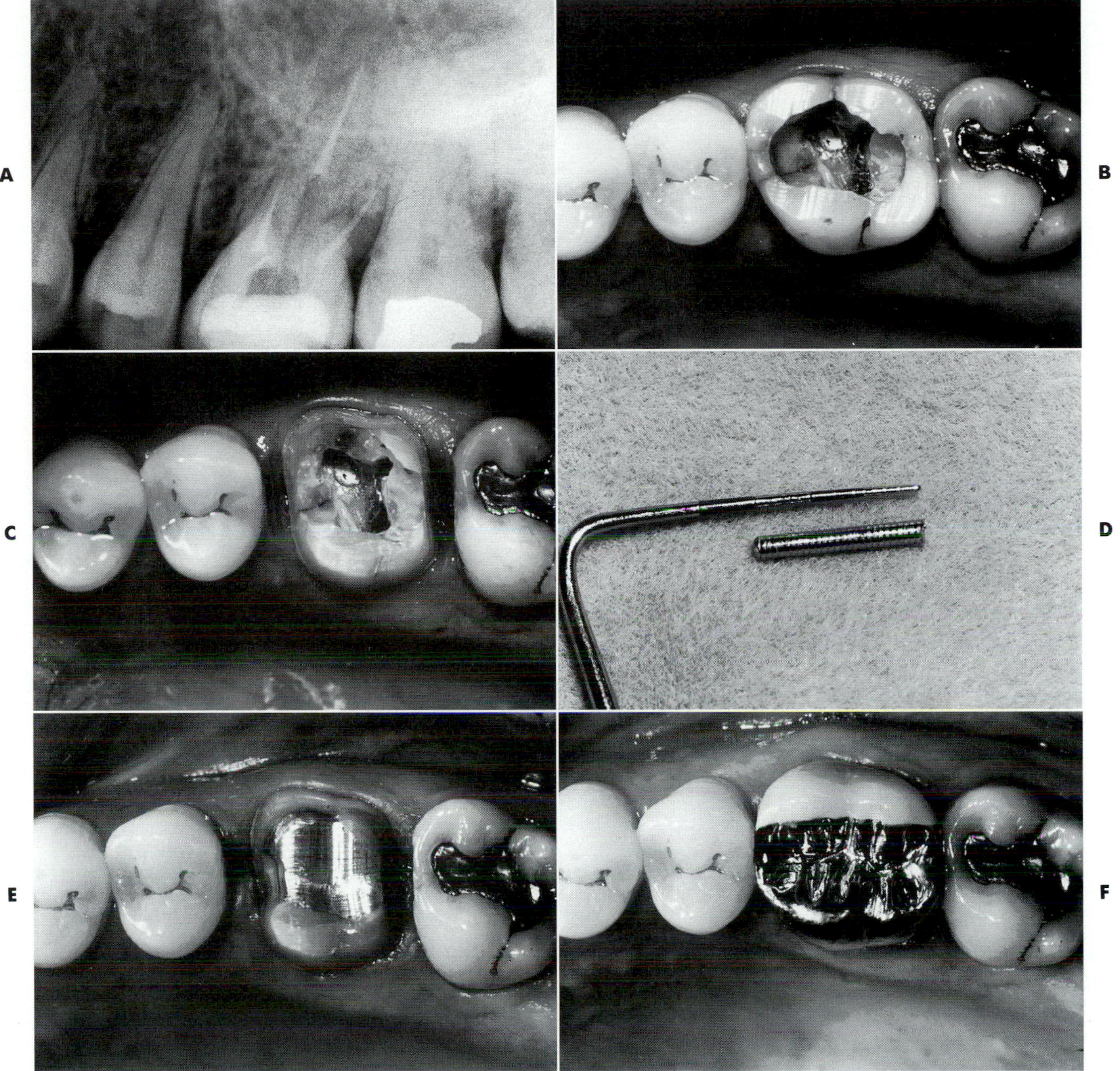

FIG. 22-24 The preformed dowel and alloy core. **A,** The postendodontic radiograph with a dowel space prepared in the palatal root. **B,** Occlusal view prior to preparation. The dowel and core system has not yet been selected. **C,** Final coronal preparation with sufficient tooth structure for a preformed dowel and alloy core. **D,** The dowel is cut to size prior to cementation using a periodontal probe to measure from a fixed coronal landmark to the base of the dowel space. **E,** Final preparation with the core in place. **F,** Final coronal restoration.

vices should not extend to the surface of the core when this preparation is completed. The tooth is now ready for the final coronal restoration.

Coronal-radicular restoration technique

The technique for coronal-radicular buildup (Fig. 22-25) of the nonvital tooth is straightforward. Because this restoration requires no dowel and because the restorative material is not rigid when placed, exact refinement of the coronal segment of the canals is not critical. Removal of 2 to 4 mm of gutta-percha from these canals is sufficient for preparation; no dentin need be altered. Undercuts and irregularities in the canal walls are actually advantages, as they increase retention of the restoration. Restorative materials can be bonded to the available tooth

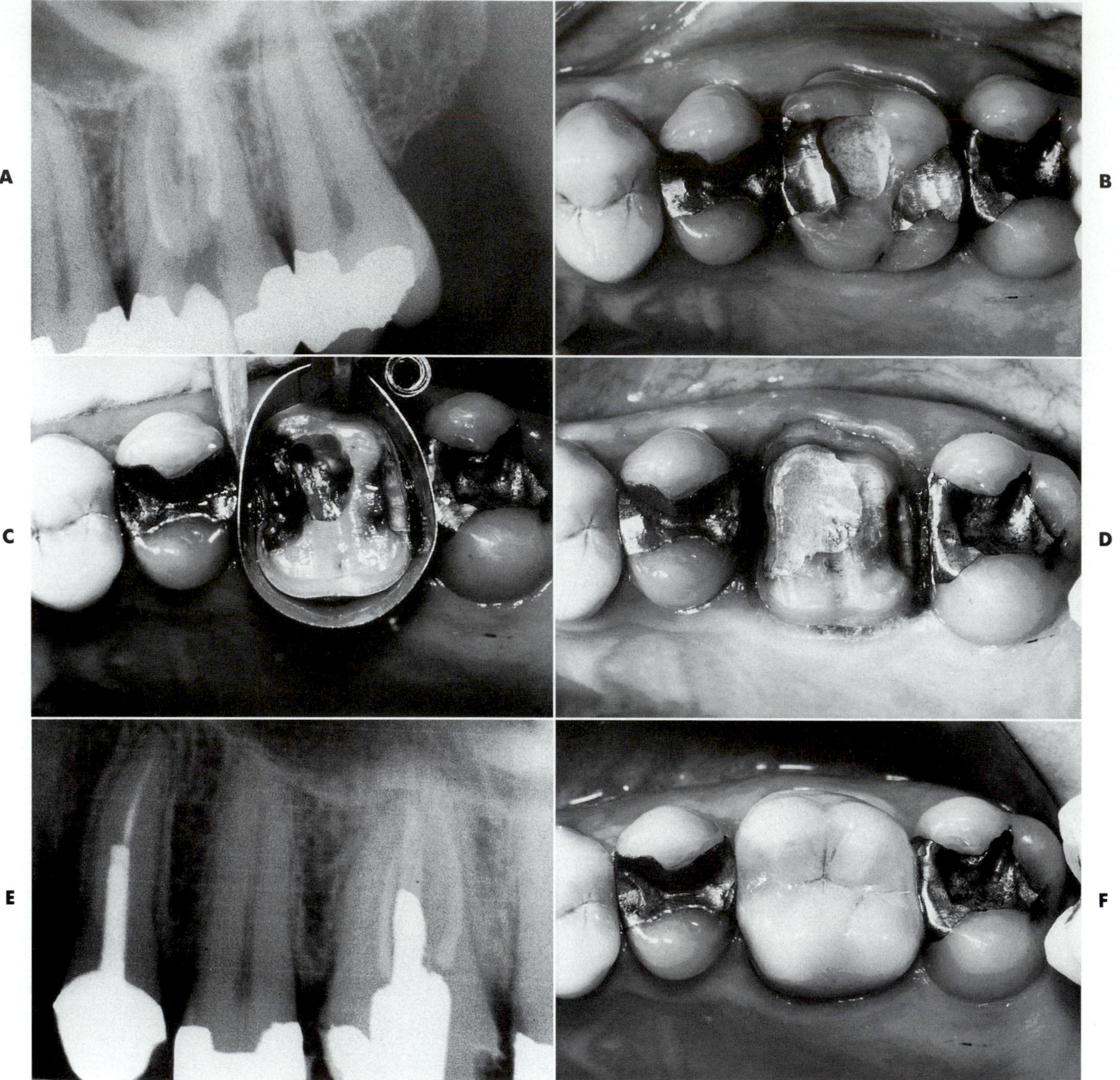

FIG. 22-25 The coronal radicular alloy. **A,** Postendodontic radiograph of maxillary first molar. **B,** Occlusal view prior to preparation. The dowel and core system has not yet been selected. **C,** Final coronal preparation with sufficient tooth structure for a bonded coronal radicular alloy. A matrix is used when condensing the alloy. **D,** Final preparation with core in place. **E,** Radiograph prior to final restoration. **F,** Final coronal restoration.

structure to increase retention, decrease microleakage, and potentially increase fracture resistance of the tooth. The tooth is now ready for the final coronal restoration.

Cementation

Dowel and core cementation materials have changed much in recent years. The ability to bond to dentin has significantly expanded the options available to the restorative dentist and has altered every phase of dowel and core restoration. Dowels can be cemented with zinc phosphate cement, glass ionomer cement, or resin cements. Use of a cement that bonds to the tooth structure, dowel, and core material offers obvious advantages.

Zinc phosphate cement is a traditional dental luting agent with a long and satisfactory clinical history. It provides retention through interlocking of small mechanical undercuts in the tooth structure and restorative materials. The retention is sufficient for well-designed dowels, cores, and coronal restorations but does not equal that of the chemically adhesive resin cements. This level of adequate but not excessive retention can be advantageous in the event of trauma or dowel removal, as loosening occurs by cement failure rather than by root fracture. The inability to chemically bond to residual tooth structure is also a disadvantage. Zinc phosphate cement retains the restoration but does not increase the resistance to fracture or inhibit marginal leakage by direct bond to the tooth.

Adhesive and resin cements differ from zinc phosphate in that they bond to tooth structure and to most dowel materials. This gives an added dimension to the luting agents used for dowel and core restorations. Glass ionomer cement bonds to dentin within the root and becomes incorporated into a glass ionomer core, forming a homogeneous unit. The anticariogenic effect of glass ionomer materials is a major advantage. The retention is similar to that of zinc phosphate cements, for a given dowel length and design.

Resin cements also bond to tooth structure and restorative materials. Current dentin bonding agents utilize various organic, hydrophilic, and hydrophobic components that react with both tooth structure and resin. These agents achieve chemical adhesion as well as micromechanical bonding to dentin collagen and tubules.[78]

Bond strengths achievable with resin cements can be very high. A study of resin cements found that parallel dowels cemented with a 4-META (4-methacryloxyethyl trimellitate anhydride) based cement are equal in retention to active or screw type dowels, without the inherent risk from screw threads in dentin. This cement-mediated maximum retention is not risk free, however, since 80% of the roots fractured when dowels were dislodged by force.[73] Conversely, adhesive cements may help the tooth resist fracture, as the dentin wall, cementing medium, and dowel become an integrated unit.[29] The retention of the core is also enhanced by dentin–bonded resin cements. Core materials of amalgam or composite resin can be bonded to the dentin, to the dowel, and to many cements used to lute the dowel.[36,48,49]

Fluid microleakage between tooth and restoration is inhibited by the cement bond, which is a major advantage over traditional, nonbonding cements. Control of this leakage is important to diminish recurrent caries around a restoration and to minimize coronal-apical contamination of the root canal system.

Manufacturer's instructions for the specific cement should be carefully observed in the precementation preparation of the canal, the dowel, and the tooth structure. Each class of dentin-bonding agents achieves adhesion through a different mechanism. Precise measuring and mixing operations are critical to the bonding capacity of these cements.

The general cementation procedures for insertion of dowel and core restorations are very similar, regardless of cement type. Once mixed, the cement is delivered to the dowel space with a lentulospiral, to ensure that all walls are coated. At the same time, the dowel or dowel and core are coated with a thin layer of cement; retention is greatest when both the dowel and the canal are coated, rather than either one alone.[57] The restoration should slide slowly and easily into place with light finger pressure. Most preformed dowels include a vent, generally a V-shaped groove, a flat surface, or spiral flutes in a round dowel. The vent allows dissipation of hydraulic backpressure during the cementation process. Excess cement must escape coronally, as the dowel nearly fills the dowel space. Significant pressure generation in nonvented cases may cause the root to crack during cementation.[52] Biting pressure to seat the restoration is not necessary. Tapping with a mallet or other instrument is absolutely contraindicated. Once the restoration is fully seated it should remain untouched until the cement has set passively. Manufacturers' instructions on total setting time should be followed precisely. When set, the excess cement is removed and the dowel/dowel and core portion of the restoration is complete.

Compromised tooth

Restoration of endodontically treated teeth becomes increasingly complex as the teeth or supporting structures become increasingly diseased. The compromises created by extensive loss of tooth structure alter the restorative procedures and affect the longevity of the tooth and the prosthesis. Mechanical requirements for structural integrity of the restoration and biologic requirements for the periodontal attachment apparatus often conflict. The narrow band of tooth structure that remains after severe breakdown is needed by both the restoration, for a ferrule, and the tissue, for periodontal health. Adjunctive procedures from other dental specialties may be needed before endodontic restoration of the severely damaged tooth.

Endodontic treatment can also become a form of adjunctive therapy to facilitate treatment of periodontally compromised teeth. Portions of teeth that otherwise may be candidates for extraction can sometimes be retained with hemisection or root amputation procedures. Periodontally guarded anterior teeth can be shortened and roots utilized as overdenture abutments. Adjunctive or supportive endodontic treatment is needed for these periodontal procedures. Dowel, core, and coronal restorations must also be designed for the new shape and function of the altered endodontic teeth.

Compromised tooth: posterior dentition

Teeth with diminished periodontal support may require integrated periodontal, endodontic, and restorative treatment. Moderate-to-severe attachment loss results in a significant alteration of crown-root ratio. The complexity due to diminished periodontal attachment is increased with multirooted teeth. The furcation involvement is common in the posterior dentition. Additionally, the loss of supporting tissues and periodontal therapy used to correct these problems often compromise restorative options.

Coronal preparation for both a path of withdrawal and reduction of the horizontal furcation invasion usually results in severe diminution of tooth structure. Establishment of a satisfactory taper for these teeth requires aggressive tooth preparation. The axial walls begin on the root surface, which has a smaller circumference than the cementoenamel junction. The axial walls must converge throughout the elongated clinical crown. This dentin removal brings the operative procedure, as well as the final restoration, close to the root canal system.

The problem is exacerbated in the multirooted tooth when restorative procedures attempt to diminish furcation invasions. Teeth that exhibit attachment loss apical to the root trunk have horizontal defects into the furcation area. Tooth preparation to minimize this dimension requires removal of significant tooth structure coronal to the furcation. The resultant "fluted" preparation is seen throughout the full length of the axial wall (Fig. 22-26). This procedure decreases the horizontal dimension of the furcation invasion but also increases pulpal morbidity. As

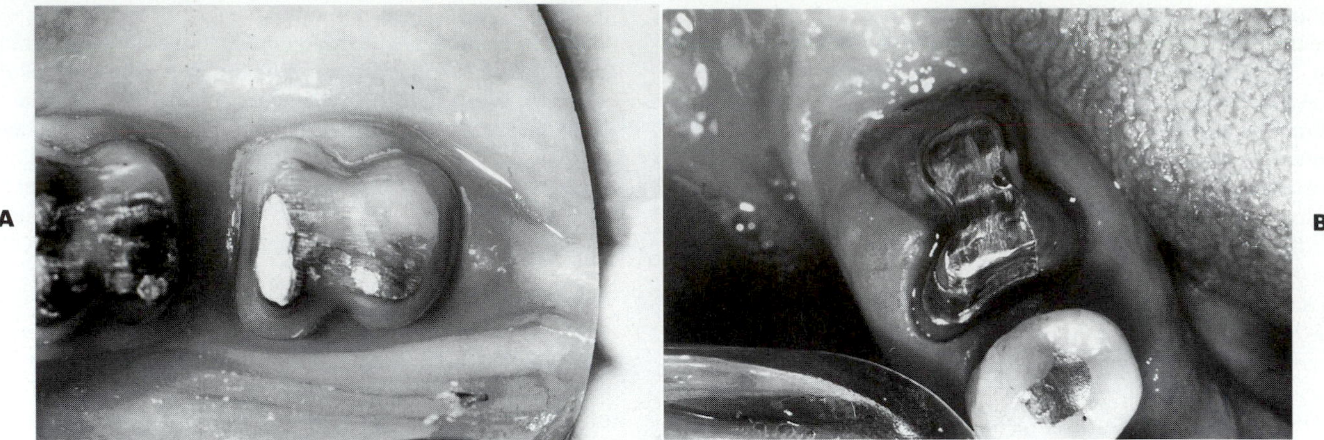

FIG. 22-26 Tooth preparation that is advantageous to the periodontium can prove deleterious to the pulp. **A,** Dentin reduction to decrease furcation invasions will bring the preparation and restoration in close proximity to the pulp chamber. **B,** Increased osseous destruction in the furcation results in exaggerated preparation designs.

discussed in the evaluation section of this chapter, preventive endodontics is indicated in cases with a strong suspicion of future pulpal involvement. The probability of pulpal degeneration in these teeth is statistically high.

When prerestorative root canal therapy is indicated for elongated, periodontally involved teeth, it is extremely important to retain as much radicular dentin as possible. These teeth are subject to fracture because of the increased leverage caused by greater crown length and the smaller diameter of root structure at the alveolar crest. Dowel placement may be needed for retention of the core; however conventional dowel guidelines do not apply in the restoration of the severely periodontally compromised tooth. The dowel is rarely as long as the clinical crown and often does not reach to the alveolar crest. Narrowing root morphology further limits the apical extension. The apical end of the dowel should not be at the level of the alveolar crest but should terminate above or below the alveolus. The bony crest and dowel terminus are both stress concentrators, and coincident placement increases fracture potential.[58]

Root amputation or tooth sectioning may be included in periodontal treatment of the multi-rooted tooth. The restorative strategy is significantly modified by this procedure. When the margin of the preparation is placed in the gingival crevice, all convexity on the axial wall must be removed. The root structure just coronal to the attachment level dictates the geometry of the restorative finish line. As the axial walls converge from the margin area, this outline form is retained. Thus, the morphology of the remaining root structure at the attachment level dictates the preparation design in the amputated or sectioned tooth (Figs. 22-27, 22-28). Concern for long-term structural integrity of the tooth is always heightened by this finding. Predictably, studies of these teeth reveal the major cause of failure over time to be root fracture, followed by recurrent periodontal disease, endodontic failure, caries, or loss of cement seal. As with periodontally sound teeth, the endodontic, periodontal and initial restorative preparation should be completed before selection of the dowel and core system. Again, maintenance of dentin is the primary goal. Anatomy of the remaining roots indicates the best location for dowel placement. Long, straight, and round roots of larger diameter should be selected for the dowel site. Determination of a cast dowel and core or a preformed system depends on the size of the core and the dentin removal required for a path of withdrawal. Adequate ferrule and exquisite control of occlusion are critical for the longevity of these teeth.

Anterior dentition

The cautions about restoration of periodontally compromised posterior dentition apply to the anterior sextants. Single root formation is an anatomic advantage in this area, as the furcation is eliminated; however, esthetic demands are a compounding issue. Margin placement above the free gingiva or minimal axial tooth reduction can lessen pulpal embarrassment in the posterior preparation. Heightened esthetic demands in the anterior dentition may not allow these compromises. Margin placement in the gingival crevice and full-depth facial reduction for veneering material may be esthetic requirements. The anterior sextant may also require connection to some or all of the posterior dentition. Paralleling these abutments usually mandates added dentin removal in the anterior segment. The cumulative effects of these insults on the anterior teeth may require preventive root canal therapy.

Anterior teeth with significant periodontal attachment loss may be retained as overdenture abutments. This option is available in the posterior areas, but is less frequently used. Guidelines for tooth selection and techniques for restoration of these teeth have been fully documented. Of importance here is the relationship between endodontics and restorative dentistry. The majority of these overdenture teeth function to support a removable prosthesis. Denture retention and lateral stability are minimal requisites. As such, functional forces to these abutments are directed mainly through the long axis of the tooth. Stress dissipation to the residual root through the use of a dowel is not required. These teeth may need only an obturating amalgam restoration in the canal system for a final restoration. A preparation depth of approximately 3 mm is sufficient to retain the alloy and seal the canal system. Coverage of the entire dome-shaped overdenture abutment is occasion-

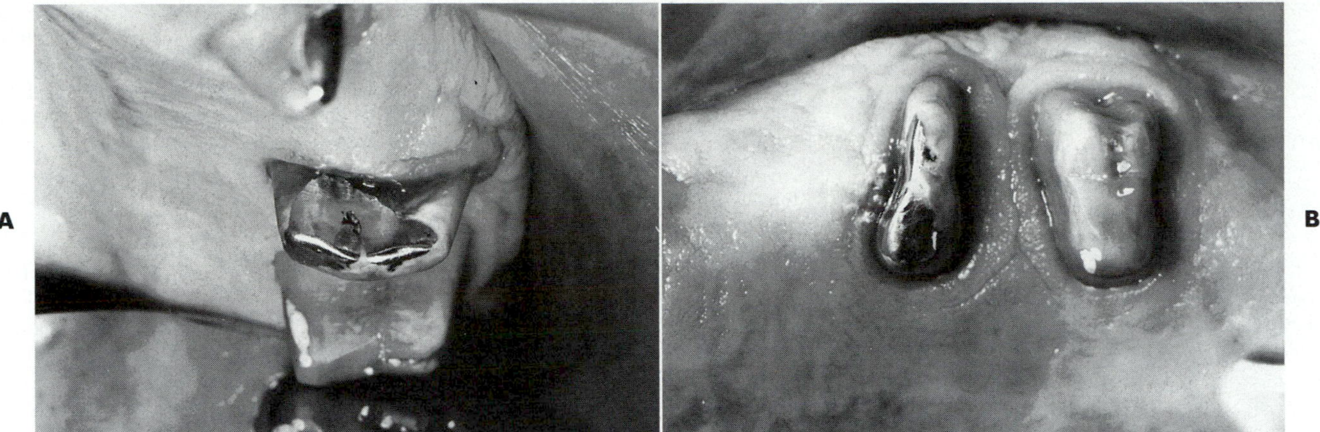

FIG. 22-27 A sectioned maxillary first molar with a preformed dowel and alloy core in place. **A,** The mesial view shows the core after removal of the mesiobuccal root. The alloy obliterates the pulp chamber and is separated from the attachment by the thin chamber floor. **B,** The root morphology and degree of periodontal attachment loss dictate margin geometry. Ultimate tooth reduction and preparation form converge from this level.

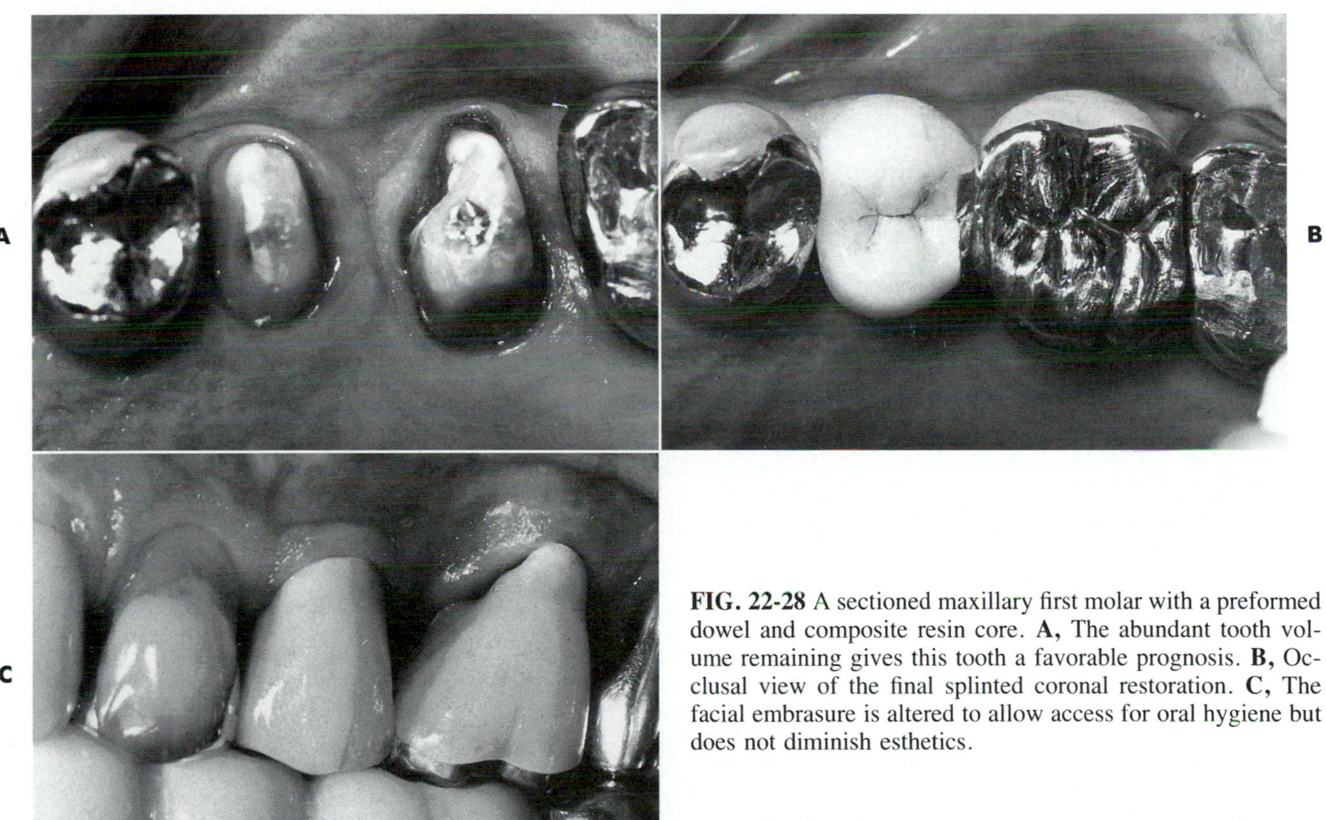

FIG. 22-28 A sectioned maxillary first molar with a preformed dowel and composite resin core. **A,** The abundant tooth volume remaining gives this tooth a favorable prognosis. **B,** Occlusal view of the final splinted coronal restoration. **C,** The facial embrasure is altered to allow access for oral hygiene but does not diminish esthetics.

ally indicated for caries control and restoration (Fig. 22-29). A dowel may be used in such a case to retain the coronal restoration; again force dissipation is minimal and the dowel length can be shortened. Only when the overdenture abutment is used for active retention of the prosthesis should guidelines for full-length dowels be followed. In addition to supplying support in a tissue-ward direction, these abutments also provide lateral stability and retain the prosthesis. Dowel placement distributes the functional load to the residual root and retains the precision attachment.[8]

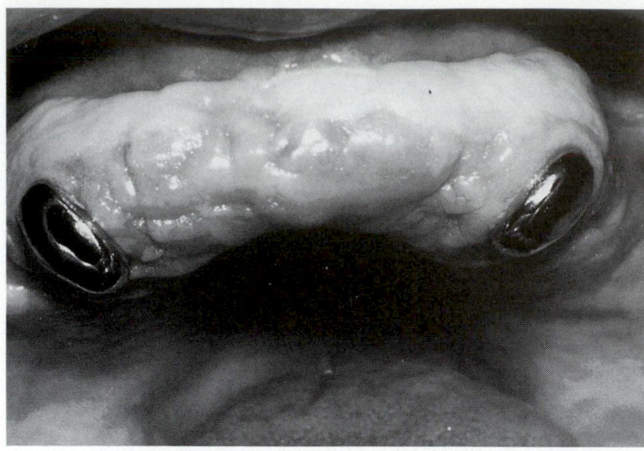

FIG. 22-29 Conventional overdenture teeth do not require dowels for stress distribution. Endodontic therapy is completed to allow reduction of the crown-root ratio. This case has cast gold copings for root coverage. In cases with sound tooth structure and low caries potential, bonded amalgam in the coronal segment of the canal is sufficient restoration.

Summary

The interrelationship between endodontics and restorative dentistry has been reviewed in this chapter. This connection is complex and requires a thorough understanding to produce consistent, successful clinical results. Treatment planning considerations presented for vital and nonvital teeth included endodontic, periodontal, restorative, and esthetic evaluations. Guidelines for restoration of the nonvital tooth and clinical techniques for this treatment were outlined. It is clear that recent advances in materials science have had a significant impact on the restoration of endodontically treated teeth. The ability to bond multiple restorative materials to each other and to tooth structure will continue to revolutionize this relationship in the future.

REFERENCES

1. Abou-Rass M: The restoration of endodontically treated teeth, new answers to an old problem, Alpha Omegan 75:68, 1982.
2. Abou-Rass M: The stressed pulp condition: an endodontic-restorative diagnostic concept, J Prosth Dent 48:264, 1982.
3. Abou-Rass M: Post and core restorations of endodontically treated teeth, Curr Opin Dent 2:99, 1992.
4. Barnett F: Pulpal response to restorative procedures and materials, Curr Opin Dent 2:93, 1992.
5. Bergenholtz G, and Nyman S: Endodontic complications following periodontal and prosthetic treatment of patients with advanced periodontal disease, J Periodontol 55:63, 1984.
6. Bower RC: Furcation morphology relative to periodontal treatment, J Periodontol 50:366, 1979.
7. Brandal JL, Nicholls JI, and Harrington GW: A comparison of three restorative techniques for endodontically treated anterior teeth, J Prosth Dent 58:161, 1987.
8. Brewer AA, and Morrow RM: Overdentures, St Louis, 1980, The CV Mosby Co.
9. Burns DA, et al: Stress distribution surrounding endodontic posts, J Prosth Dent 64:412, 1990.
10. Caputo AA, and Standlee JP: Pins and posts—why, when and how, Dent Clin North Am 20:299, 1976.
11. Colley IT, Hanmpson EL, and Lehman ML: Retention of post crowns, Br Dent J 124:63, 1968.
12. Cooley RL: Dentinal bond strength and microleakage of a 4-META adhesive to amalgam and composite resin, Quintessence Int 22:979, 1991.
13. Cooney JP, Caputo AA, and Trabert KT: Retention and stress distribution of tapered-end endodontic posts, J Prosth Dent 55:540, 1986.
14. Covey DA, and Moon PC: Shear bond strength of dental amalgam bonded to dentin, Am J Dent 4:19, 1991.
15. Craig, RG: Restorative dental materials, ed 9, St Louis, 1993, Mosby Co.
16. Engleman MJ: Core materials, CDA J 16:41, 1988.
17. Felton D: Long-term effects of crown preparation on pulp vitality (abstract 1139) J Dent Res 68 (spec issue):1009, 1989.
18. Felton DA, et al: Threaded endodontic dowels: effect of post design on incidence of root fracture, J Prosth Dent 65:179, 1991.
19. Ferrara A: Personal communication, January 1993.
20. Fitchie JG, et al: Microleakage of two dentinal bonding systems, Quintessence Int 21:749, 1990.
21. Gelfand M, Golman M, and Sunderman EJ: Effect of complete veneer crowns on the compressive strength of endodontically treated posterior teeth, J Prosth Dent 52:635, 1984.
22. Gher ME, and Vernino AR: Root anatomy: a local factor in inflammatory periodontal disease, Int J Periodont Restor Dent 5:53, 1981.
23. Goss JM, Wright WJ, and Bowles WF: Radiographic appearance of titanium alloy prefabricated posts cemented with different luting materials, J Prosth Dent 67:632, 1992.
24. Gutmann JL: The dentin-root complex: anatomic and biologic considerations in restoring endodontically treated teeth, SJ Prosth Dent 67:458, 1992.
25. Guzy GE, and Nicholls JI: In vitro comparison of intact endodontically treated teeth with and without endo-post reinforcement, J Prosth Dent 42:39, 1979.
26. Haddix JE, et al: Post preparation techniques and their effect on the apical seal, J Prosth Dent 64:515, 1990.
27. Helfer AR, Melnick S, and Schilder H: Determination of the moisture content of vital and pulpless teeth, J Oral Surg 34:661, 1972.
28. Hemmings KW, King PA, and Setchell DJ: Resistance to torsional forces of various post and core designs, J Prosth Dent 66:325, 1991.
29. Hussey DL: Resin retained posts, possible strengthening effects on dentine (Spec Abstr No. S54), J Dent Res 68: 1989.
30. Johnson JK, and Sakumura JAS: Dowel form and tensile force, J Prosth Dent 40:645, 1978.
31. Kane JJ, Burgess JO, and Summitt J: Fracture resistance of amalgam coronal-radicular restorations, J Prosth Dent 63:607, 1990.
32. Kantor ME, and Pines MS: A comparative study of restorative techniques in pulpless teeth, J Prosth Dent 38:405, 1977.
33. Krupp JD, et al: Dowel retention with glass ionomer cement, J Prosth Dent 41:163, 1979.
34. Langeland K, and Langeland LK: Pulp reactions to crown preparation, impression, temporary crown fixation and permanent cementation, J Prosth Dent 15:129, 1965.
35. Lenchner NH: Restoring endodontically treated teeth: ferrule effect and biologic width, Pract Periodont Aesth Dent 1:19, 1989.
36. Lorey R: Dentin adhesives and endodontic post retention (Spec Abstr No S52), J Dent Res 68: 1980.
37. Lovdahl PE, and Nicholls JI: Pin-retained amalgam cores vs. cast-gold dowel cores, J Prosth Dent 38:507, 1977.
38. Mattison GD, et al: Effect of post preparation on the apical seal, J Prosth Dent 51:785, 1984.
39. Maynard JG, and Wilson RD: Physiologic dimensions of the periodontium significant to the restorative dentist, J Periodontol 50:170, 1979.
40. McDonald AV, King PA, and Setchell DJ: An in vitro study to compare impact fracture resistance of intact root-treated teeth, Int Endod J 23:304, 1990.
41. McLean JW: The science and art of dental ceramics, vol 1, The nature of dental ceramics and their clinical use, Chicago, 1979, Quintessence Publishing Co.
42. McLean JW: Cermet cements, J Am Dent Assoc 120:43, 1990.
43. Mertz KA, Parker MW, and Pellew GB: Shear strength of two coro-

nal radicular amalgam and pin-retained amalgam, J Dent Res 66:289, 1987.
44. Michelich R, Nayyar A, and Leonard L: Mechanical properties of amalgam core buildups for endodontically treated premolars, J Dent Res 60:630, 1981.
45. Millstein PL, Ho J, and Nathanson D: Retention between a serrated steel dowel and different core materials, J Prosth Dent 65:480, 1991.
46. Milot P, and Stein RS: Root fracture in endodontically treated teeth related to post selection and crown design, J Prosth Dent 68:428, 1992.
47. Mojon P: Maximum bond strength of dental luting cement to amalgam alloy, J Dent Res 68:1545, 1989.
48. Nathanson D, and Ashayeri N: Effects of a new technique, CDA J 16:27, 1988.
49. Nathanson D, and Ashayeri N: New aspects of restoring the endodontically treated tooth, Alpha Omegan 83:76, 1990.
50. Nayyar A, Walton RE, and Leonard LA: An amalgam coronal-radicular dowel and core technique for endodontically treated posterior teeth, J Prosth Dent 43:511, 1980.
51. Nevins M, and Skurow HM: The intracrevicular restorative margin, the biologic width, and the maintenance of the gingival margin, Int J Periodont Restor Dent 2:31, 1984.
52. Obermayr G, et al: Vertical root fracture and relative deformation during obturation and post cementation, J Prosth Dent 66:181, 1991.
53. Oliva RA, and Low JA: Dimensional stability of composite used as a core material, J Prosth Dent 56:554, 1986.
54. Pashley DH: Clinical correlations of dentin structure and function, J Prosthet Dent 66:777, 1991.
55. Post and core—state of the art— '92, Clin Res Assoc Newslett 16:1, 1992.
56. Reeh ES, Messer HH, and Douglas WH, Reduction in tooth stiffness as a result of endodontic and restorative procedures, J Endodont 16:512, 1989.
57. Reel DC, et al: Effect of cementation method on the retention of anatomic cast post and cores, J Prosth Dent 62:162, 1989.
58. Reinhardt FA, et al: Dentin stresses in post-reconstructed teeth with diminishing bone support, J Dent Res 62:1002, 1983.
59. Rosenberg MM, et al: Periodontal and prosthetic management for advanced cases, Chicago, 1988, Quintessence Publishing Co.
60. Ruemping DR, Lung MR, and Schnell RJ: Retention of dowels subjected to tension and torsional forces: J Prosth Dent 41:159, 1979.
61. Scherer W, et al: Bonding amalgam to tooth structure: a scanning electron microscope study, J Esth Dent 4:199, 1992.
62. Schlugar S, Yuodelis RA, and Page RC: Periodontal disease, Philadelphia, 1977, Lea & Febiger.
63. Shillingburg HT, and Kessler JC: Restoration of the endodontically treated tooth, Chicago, 1982, Quintessence Publishing Co.
64. Sorensen JA: Preservation of tooth structure, CDA J 16:15, 1988.
65. Sorensen JA, and Engelman MJ: Effect of post adaptation on fracture resistance of endodontically treated teeth, J Prosth Dent 64:419, 1990.
66. Sorensen JA, and Engelman MJ: Ferrule design and fracture resistance of endodontically treated teeth, J Prosth Dent 63:529, 1990.
67. Sorensen JA, et al: Altered corrosion resistance from casting to stainless steel posts, J Prosth Dent 63:630, 1990.
68. Sorensen JA, and Martinoff JT: Clinically significant factors in dowel design, J Prosth Dent 52:28, 1984.
69. Sorensen JA, and Martinoff JT: Intracoronal reinforcement and coronal coverage: a study of endodontically treated teeth, J Prosth Dent 51:780, 1984.
70. Sorensen JA, and Martinoff JT: Endodontically treated teeth as abutments, J Prosth Dent 52:631, 1985.
71. Standlee JP, and Caputo AA: Biomechanics, CDA J 16:49, 1988.
72. Standlee JP, and Caputo AA: Endodontic dowel retention with resinous cements, J Prosth Dent 68:913, 1992.
73. Standlee JP, and Caputo AA: The retentive and stress distributing properties of split threaded endodontic dowels, J Prosth Dent 68:436, 1992.
74. Standlee JP, et al: Analysis of stress distribution by endodontic posts, Oral Surg 33:952, 1972.
75. Standlee FP, Caputo AA, and Hanson EC: Retention of endodontic dowels: effects of cement, dowel length, diameter and design, J Prosthet Dent 39:401, 1978.
76. Thorsteinsson TS, Yaman P, and Craig RG: Stress analyses of four prefabricated posts, J Prosth Dent 67:30, 1992.
77. Tjan AH, Grant BE, and Dunn FR: Microleakage of composite resin cores treated with various dentin bonding systems, J Prosth Dent 66:24, 1991.
78. Van Meerbeek B, et al: Dentin and enamel bonding agents, Curr Opin Dent 2:117, 1992.
79. Yaman P, and Thorsteinsson TS: Effect of core materials on stress distribution of posts, J Prosth Dent 68:416, 1992.

Self-assessment questions

1. Pulpal degeneration increases
   a. with the complexity of the restoration.
   b. with the degree of periodontal disease.
   c. with time, following insertion of the restoration.
   d. all of the above.
2. Endodontic access through existing crowns
   a. usually has no effect on porcelain strength.
   b. does not cause separation of the porcelain veneer from the metal substructure.
   c. often leads to excessive removal of coronal tooth structure.
   d. should not be performed.
3. During the restorative examination prior to endodontic therapy
   a. the strategic value of the tooth is of minor significance.
   b. a critical amount of solid coronal dentin is required.
   c. the ferrule has no effect on the incidence of root fracture.
   d. if insufficient tooth structure remains to withstand functional forces, the tooth should always be extracted.
4. In endodontically treated teeth
   a. decreased strength is due to the loss of coronal tooth structure.
   b. decreased strength is a direct result of the endodontic treatment.
   c. mandibular teeth are stronger than maxillary teeth.
   d. all of the above.
5. The dowel functions primarily
   a. to retain the core material.
   b. to strengthen the tooth.
   c. to distribute forces along the length of the root.
   d. to decrease the risk of root fracture.
6. Guidelines for dowel length in a tooth with normal periodontal support include
   a. two thirds of the length of the canal.
   b. the coronal length of the tooth.
   c. one half the bone-supported length of the tooth.
   d. all of the above.
7. Dowel features that contribute the greatest retention are
   a. increased length, parallel sides, and moderate diameter.
   b. increased length, taper, and serrated surface.
   c. increased length, parallel sides, and serrated surface.
   d. increased length, taper, and smooth surface.
8. Compared to nickel-chrome dowels, titanium dowels are
   a. stronger.
   b. less radiopaque.
   c. more allergenic.
   d. more economical.

9. The microleakage phenomenon is greatest with
   a. composite resin core.
   b. amalgam core.
   c. glass ionomer core.
   d. cast post and core.
10. Which material should be avoided in teeth with high esthetic value?
    a. Composite resin.
    b. Glass ionomers.
    c. Amalgam.
    d. Cast post and core.
11. Composite cores
    a. are anticariogenic.
    b. should be used only in teeth with significant remaining structure.
    c. are dimensionally stable.
    d. all of the above.
12. Which endodontically treated teeth always require a dowel, a core, and crown?
    a. Fixed partial denture abutments.
    b. Removable partial denture abutments.
    c. Individual teeth.
    d. None of the above.
13. The ferrule
    a. significantly reduces the incidence of fracture.
    b. must not terminate on restorative material.
    c. is a metal band encircling the external dimension of the residual tooth.
    d. all of the above.
14. For dowel space preparation
    a. gutta-percha is removed using heat, rotary instruments, or solvents.
    b. gutta-percha removal should be done 48 hours or more after root canal filling.
    c. intimate contact of the dowel and dentin is not necessary for passive dowel systems.
    d. to refine the dowel space dowel drills must be used in a dental handpiece.
15. Regarding cementation of the dowel
    a. zinc phosphate and glass ionomer cements increase resistance to fracture.
    b. zinc phosphate and resin cements inhibit marginal leakage.
    c. retention is greatest when both the dowel and canal are coated with cement.
    d. the dowel is seated with finger or biting pressure.
16. The major cause of failure of endodontically treated posterior teeth that are periodontally compromised is
    a. recurrent periodontal disease.
    b. root fracture.
    c. endodontic failure.
    d. caries.

Chapter 23

Pediatric Endodontic Treatment

Joe H. Camp*

Despite water fluoridation and emphasis on the prevention of caries, premature loss of primary and young permanent teeth continues to be common. The total prevention of caries is the ultimate goal of dentistry; but meanwhile, procedures must be utilized to preserve the primary and young permanent teeth ravaged by caries. This chapter deals with preservation of the primary and young permanent teeth that are pulpally involved. The objective of pulpal therapy is conservation of the tooth in a healthy state functioning as an integral component of the dentition.

Preservation of arch space is one of the primary objectives of pediatric dentistry. Premature loss of primary teeth may cause aberration of the arch length, resulting in mesial drift of the permanent teeth and consequent malocclusion. Whenever possible, the pulpally involved tooth should be maintained in the dental arch—provided, of course, that it can be restored to function, free of disease.

Other objectives of preserving primary teeth are to enhance aesthetics and mastication, prevent aberrant tongue habits, aid in speech, and prevent the psychologic effects associated with tooth loss. Premature loss of the maxillary incisors before age 3 has been shown to cause speech impairment that may persist in later years.[172]

Loss of pulpal vitality in the young permanent tooth creates special problems. Since the pulp is necessary for the formation of dentin, if the pulp is lost before root length is completed the tooth will have a poor crown-root ratio. Pulpal necrosis before the completion of dentin deposition within the root leaves a thin root more prone to fracture in the event of trauma. This situation also creates special problems in endodontic treatment, since endodontic techniques are usually not adequate to obturate the large blunderbuss canals. Additional procedures of apexification or apical surgery often become necessary to maintain the pulpless immature permanent tooth; the prognosis for permanent retention of the tooth is poorer than for the completely formed tooth.

In this chapter emphasis is on maintenance of pulpal vitality in the primary and young permanent teeth whenever possible to avoid many of the problems discussed elsewhere in this book.

Successful pulpal therapy in the primary dentition requires a thorough understanding of primary pulp morphology, root formation, and the special problems associated with resorption of primary tooth roots. Differences in the morphology of the primary and permanent pulps, in root formation, and in primary root resorption are covered later in this chapter. The reader is referred to Chapter 10 for a complete description of pulp and dentin formation.

DIFFERENCES IN PRIMARY AND PERMANENT TOOTH MORPHOLOGY (FIG. 23-1)

According to Finn[49] and Wheeler[233] the basic differences between the primary and the permanent teeth are these:

1. Primary teeth are smaller in all dimensions than the corresponding permanent teeth.
2. Primary crowns are wider from mesial to distal in comparison to their crown length than are permanent crowns.
3. Primary teeth have narrower and longer roots in comparison to crown length and width than do permanent teeth.

*The author wishes to thank Dr. Philip B. Edgerton for his contribution in revising this chapter.

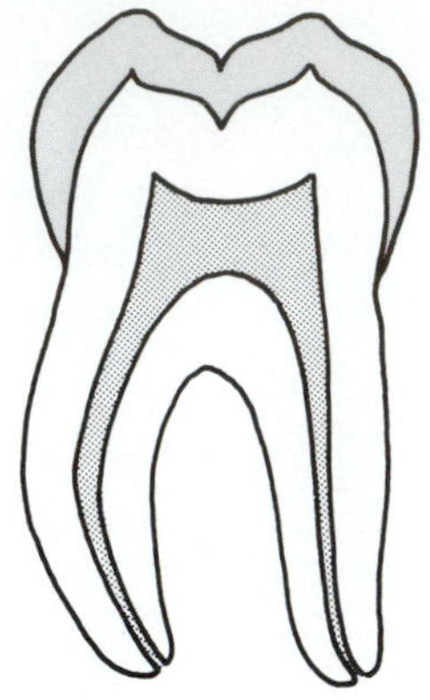
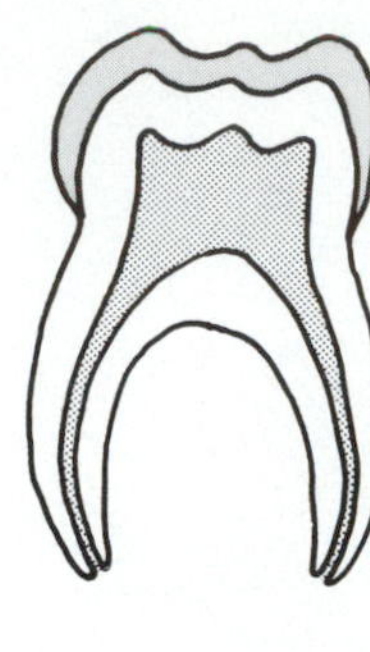

FIG. 23-1 Cross section of primary and permanent molars.

4. The facial and lingual cervical thirds of the crowns of anterior primary teeth are much more prominent than those of permanent teeth.
5. Primary teeth are markedly more constricted at the dentin-enamel junction than are permanent teeth.
6. The facial and lingual surfaces of primary molars converge occlusally so the occlusal surface is much narrower in the facial-lingual than the cervical width.
7. The roots of primary molars are comparatively more slender and longer than the roots of permanent molars.
8. The roots of primary molars flare out nearer the cervix, and they flare more at the apex, than do the roots of permanent molars.
9. The enamel is thinner, about 1 mm, on primary teeth than on permanent teeth and it has a more consistent depth.
10. The thickness of the dentin between the pulp chambers and the enamel in primary teeth is less than in permanent teeth.
11. The pulp chambers in primary teeth are comparatively larger than in permanent teeth.
12. The pulp horns, especially the mesial horns, are higher in primary molars than in permanent molars.

A detailed discussion of the anatomy of the individual primary root canals is presented later in this chapter.

Diagnosis

Before the initiation of restorative procedures on a tooth, a thorough clinical and radiographic examination must be concluded. The case history and any pertinent medical history must be thoroughly reviewed. Comprehensive coverage of diagnosis is to be found in Chapter 1, and the reader is referred to that chapter for a more in-depth discussion.

Good periapical and bitewing radiographs are essential to complete the diagnosis. Examination of the soft and hard tissues for any apparent pathosis is a routine part of the examination.

In the event that pulp therapy is required, the preoperative diagnosis is of utmost importance and should dictate the type of treatment to be carried out. If the pulpal status is not determined before operative procedures are begun and pulp therapy becomes necessary during the treatment, an adequate diagnosis may be impossible.

There are no reliable clinical diagnostic tools for accurately evaluating the status of the pulp that has become inflamed. An accurate determination of the extent of inflammation within the pulp cannot be made short of histologic examination.[202] Diagnosis of pulpal health in the exposed pulp of children is difficult, and the correlation between clinical symptoms and histopathologic conditions is poor.[126]

Although the diagnostic tests are admittedly poor for evaluating the degree of inflammation within the primary and young permanent pulp, they must always be performed to obtain as much information as possible to aid in the diagnosis before treatment is rendered. The recommended diagnostic tests for use in primary and young permanent teeth are discussed next.

Radiographs

Current radiographs are essential to examining for caries and periapical changes. Interpretation of radiographs is complicated in children by physiologic root resorption of primary teeth and by incompletely formed roots of permanent teeth. If one is not familiar with diagnosing radiographs of children or does not have radiographs of good quality, these normally occurring circumstances can easily lead to misinterpretation of normal anatomy for pathologic changes.

The radiograph does not always demonstrate periapical pathosis, nor can the proximity of caries to the pulp always be accurately determined. What may appear as an intact barrier of secondary dentin overlying the pulp may actually be a perforated mass of irregularly calcified and carious dentin overlying a pulp with extensive inflammation.[126]

The presence of calcified masses within the pulp is important to making a diagnosis of pulpal status (Fig. 23-2). Mild, chronic irritation to the pulp stimulates secondary dentin formation. When the irritation is acute and of rapid onset, the defense mechanism may not have a chance to lay down secondary dentin. When the disease process reaches the pulp, the pulp may form calcified masses away from the exposure site. These calcified masses are always associated with advanced pulpal degeneration in the pulp chamber and inflammation of the pulp tissue in the canals.[114,126]

Pathologic changes in the periapical tissues surrounding primary molars are most often apparent in the bifurcation or trifurcation areas rather than at the apices, as in permanent teeth (Figs. 23-2 and 23-3, *A*). Pathologic bone and root resorption is indicative of advanced pulpal degeneration that has spread into the periapical tissues. The pulpal tissue may remain vital even with such advanced degenerative changes.

Internal resorption occurs frequently in the primary dentition following pulpal involvement. It is always associated with extensive inflammation[70] and usually occurs in the molar root canals adjacent to the bifurcation or trifurcation area. Because of the thinness of primary molar roots, once the internal resorption has become advanced enough to be seen radiographically there is usually a perforation of the root by the resorption (Fig. 23-3, *B*). After the occurrence of perforation of the primary tooth root by internal resorption, all forms of pulpal therapy are contraindicated. The treatment of choice is extraction.

Pulp tests

The electric pulp tester is of little value in the primary dentition or in young permanent teeth with incompletely developed apices. Although it may indicate vitality, it will not give reli-

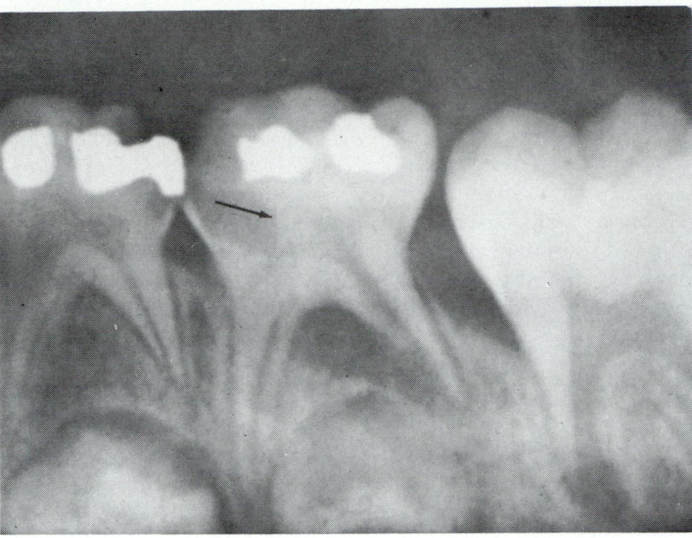

FIG. 23-2 Calcified mass in the pulp chamber. There is internal and external root resorption. The calcified mass *(arrow)* is an attempt to block a massive carious lesion. Because of resorption, this tooth should be extracted. Note the bone loss in the bifurcation area.

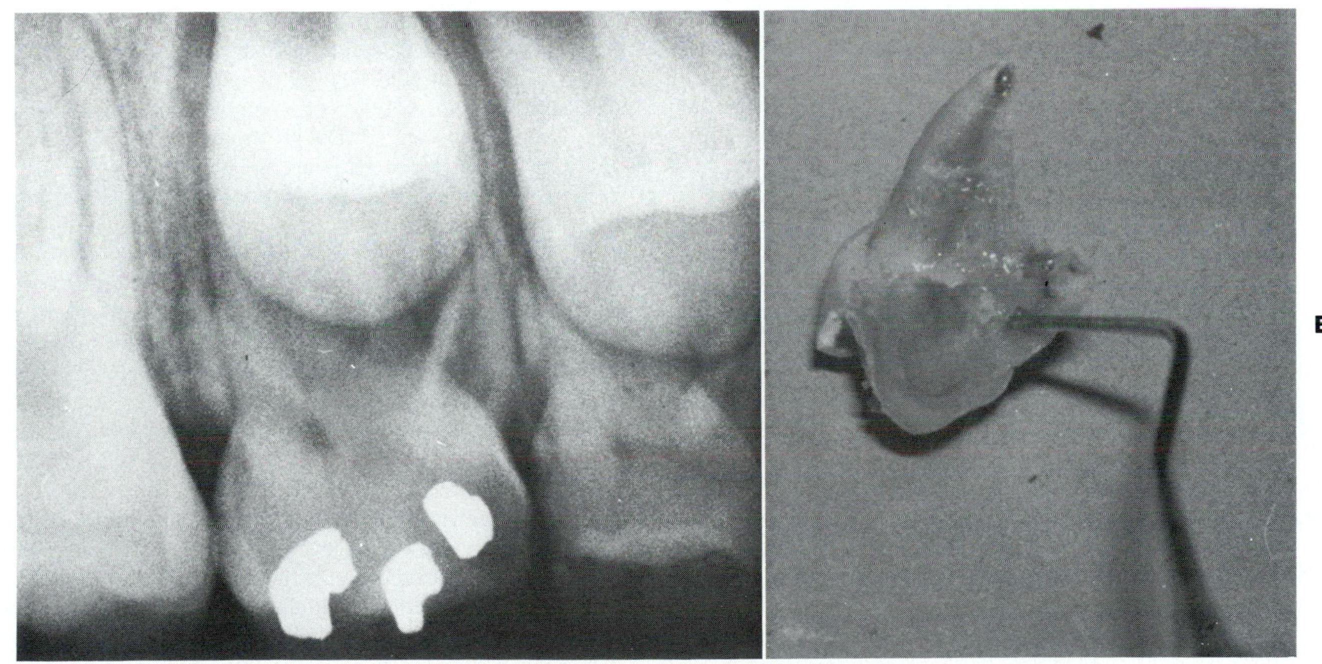

FIG. 23-3 Internal resorption due to inflammation from carious pulp exposure. **A,** Note the bone loss in the trifurcation and the internal resorption in the mesial root. **B,** Extracted tooth. Note the perforation of internal resorption. The probe is extended through the resorption defect.

able data as to the extent of inflammation within the pulp. Many children with perfectly normal teeth do not respond to the electric pulp tester even at the higher settings. Added to these factors is the unreliability of the response in the young child because of apprehension, fear, or management problems.

Thermal tests are also generally unreliable in the primary dentition for determining pulpal status.

Percussion and mobility

Teeth with extensive pulpal inflammation usually exhibit tenderness to percussion; however, this test is not very reliable in primary teeth of young children because of the psychologic aspects involved.

Tooth mobility is also not a reliable test of pulpal pathosis in primary teeth. During phases of active physiologic root resorption, primary teeth with normal pulps may have varying degrees of mobility. Furthermore, teeth with varying degrees of pulpal inflammation may have very little mobility.

Pulpal exposures and hemorrhage

It has been reported that the size of the exposure, the appearance of the pulp, and the amount of hemorrhage are important factors in diagnosing the extent of inflammation in a cariously exposed pulp. A true carious exposure is always accompanied by pulpal inflammation (see Chapter 14).[126,202] The pinpoint carious exposure may have pulpal inflammation varying from minimal to extensive to complete necrosis. However, the massive exposure will always have widespread inflammation or necrosis and will not be a candidate for any form of vital pulp therapy. Excessive hemorrhage at an exposure site or during pulp amputation is evidence of extensive inflammation. These teeth should be considered candidates for pulpectomy or extraction.

History of pain

A history of spontaneous toothache is usually associated with extensive degenerative changes in the pulp of a primary tooth[70]; nevertheless, absence of pain cannot be used to judge pulpal status, since varying degrees of degeneration or even complete necrosis of the pulp are seen without any history of pain.

Guthrie and associates[70] attempted to use the first drop of hemorrhage from an exposed pulp site as a diagnostic aid for determining the extent of degeneration within the pulp. A white blood cell differential count (hemogram) was made for each of 53 teeth included in the study. A detailed history, including percussion, electric pulp test, thermal tests, mobility, and history of pain, was obtained. The teeth were extracted and histologically examined. Upon correlation of the histologic findings with the hemogram and a detailed history, it was determined that percussion, electric and thermal pulp tests, and mobility were *unreliable* in establishing the degree of pulpal inflammation. The hemogram did not give reliable evidence of pulpal degeneration, even though teeth with advanced degeneration of the pulp involving the root canals did have an elevated neutrophil count. A consistent finding of the study, however, was advanced degeneration of pulpal tissue in teeth with a history of spontaneous toothache.

Primary teeth with a history of spontaneous, unprovoked toothache should not be considered for any form of pulp therapy short of pulpectomy or extraction.

INDIRECT PULP THERAPY

Indirect pulp therapy is a technique for avoiding pulpal exposure in the treatment of teeth with deep carious lesions in which there exists no clinical evidence of pulpal degeneration or periapical disease. The procedure allows the tooth to utilize the natural protective mechanisms of the pulp against caries. It is based on the theory that a zone of affected demineralized dentin exists between the outer infected layer of dentin and the pulp. When the infected dentin is removed, *the affected dentin can remineralize and the odontoblasts form reparative dentin,* thus avoiding a pulp exposure.[33]

Disagreement exists as to whether the deep layers of the carious dentin are infected. Several studies[104,111] showed deep carious lesions to be infected, whereas another[61] reported an area of softened and discolored dentin far in advance of bacterial contamination in acute caries. Still others[190,234] found that most organisms had been removed after the removal of the softened dentin although the incidence of bacterial contamination was higher in primary teeth than in permanent teeth; however, some dentinal tubules still contained small numbers of bacteria.

Kopel[108] summarized the results of various studies of the carious process and identified three distinct layers in active caries: necrotic soft dentin not painful to stimulation and grossly infected with bacteria, firm but softened dentin painful to stimulation but containing fewer bacteria, and slightly discolored hard sound dentin containing few bacteria and painful to stimulation.

In indirect pulp therapy the outer layers of carious dentin are removed. Thus most of the bacteria are eliminated from the lesion. When the lesion is sealed, the substrate upon which the bacteria act to produce acid is also removed. Exposure of the pulp occurs when the carious process advances faster than the reparative mechanism of the pulp. With the arrest of the carious process, the reparative mechanism is able to lay down additional dentin and avoid a pulp exposure.

Although carious dentin left in the tooth probably contains some bacteria, the number of organisms can be greatly diminished when this layer is covered with zinc oxide–eugenol or calcium hydroxide.[46,104]

The reparative and recuperative powers of the dental pulp have long been recognized in dentistry. In the mid-eighteenth century Pierre Fauchard advised that all caries in deeply carious sensitive teeth should not be removed because of the danger of pulpal exposure.[108] The principles of indirect pulp therapy were recognized as early as 1850.[72,89,235] These early investigators proposed leaving a layer of partially softened dentin to avoid exposure of the pulp and suggested that recalcification of areas of soft decalcified dentin could occur when the softened dentin was sealed under a filling. All these early investigators attributed their success to proper selection of cases. The techniques suggested were only for teeth without a history of pain or teeth in which slight inflammation was suspected. Although the techniques were empirical, the treatment was judged successful.

Dimaggio and Hawes[37,38] selected primary and permanent teeth that were free of clinical signs of pulpal degeneration and periapical pathosis and that appeared radiographically to have a pulp exposure if all the decay were removed. Upon removal of all decay, pulp exposure occurred in 75% of the teeth. In another group of teeth judged clinically to be the same as the first group, the authors achieved 99% success in avoiding pulp exposures with indirect pulp therapy. Reporting on an expanded number of teeth observed from 2 weeks to 4 years, their success rate remained at 97% for the indirect pulp therapy technique.[74]

Indirect pulp therapy has proved to be a very successful technique when cases are properly selected. Reports[103,147,216] show successes ranging from 74% to 99%. Differences in case selection, length of study, and type of investigation are responsible for the variations in success. Frankl's report[52] of pulp therapy in pediatric dentistry provides a complete review of the literature on indirect pulp therapy.

Indirect Pulp Therapy Technique

Indirect pulp therapy is utilized when pulpal inflammation has been judged to be minimal and complete removal of car-

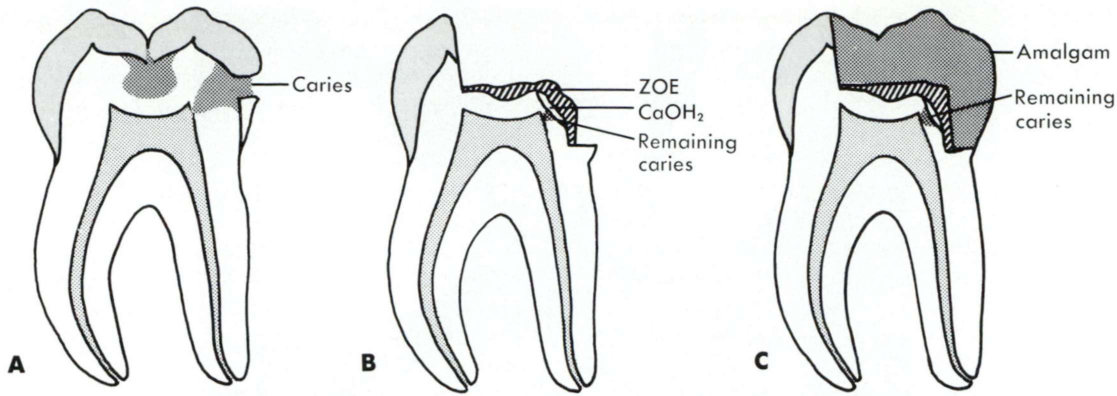

FIG. 23-4 Indirect pulp therapy. **A,** The pulp would probably be exposed if all caries were removed. **B,** All decay is eliminated except that just overlying the pulp. Calcium hydroxide—ZOE is placed over the remaining caries and deep carious excavation. ($Ca[OH]_2$ may be deleted and only ZOE placed.) **C,** The tooth is sealed with amalgam.

ies would probably cause a pulp exposure (Fig. 23-4, *A*). Careful diagnosis of the pulpal status is completed before the treatment is initiated. Any tooth judged to have widespread inflammation or evidence of periapical pathosis should receive endodontic therapy or be extracted.

The tooth is anesthetized and isolated with a rubber dam. All the caries except that immediately overlying the pulp is removed. Care must be taken to eliminate all the caries at the dentin-enamel junction. Because of its closeness to the surface, caries left in this area will likely cause failure. If there is communication of the caries with the oral cavity, the carious process will continue, resulting in failure.

Care must also be taken in removing the caries to avoid exposure of the pulp. A large round bur is best to remove the caries. The use of spoon excavators when approaching the pulp may cause an exposure by removal of a large segment of decay. Nevertheless, if used judiciously a spoon excavator is not contraindicated for removing caries near the dentin-enamel junction. All undermined enamel is not removed, for it will help retain the temporary filling.

After all caries except that just overlying the pulp has been removed, a sedative filling of either zinc oxide–eugenol (ZOE) or calcium hydroxide is placed over the remaining carious dentin and areas of deep excavation. The tooth may then be sealed with ZOE or amalgam (Fig. 23-4, *B, C*).

If the remaining tooth structure is insufficient to retain the temporary filling, a stainless steel band or temporary crown must be adapted to the tooth to maintain the dressing within the tooth (Fig. 23-5). If the dressing is lost and the remaining caries reexposed to the oral fluids, the desired effects cannot be achieved and a failure will occur.

If this preliminary caries removal is successful, the inflammation will be resolved and deposition of reparative dentin beneath the caries will allow subsequent eradication of the remaining caries without pulpal exposure.

The sedative dressing to be used in indirect pulp therapy may be either calcium hydroxide or ZOE. Studies have shown both materials to be effective and no compelling evidence has been presented that calcium hydroxide is superior to ZOE.[42,103,206]

The treated tooth is reentered in 6 to 8 weeks, and the remaining caries is extirpated. The rate of reparative dentin deposition has been shown to average 1.4 μm per day following cavity preparations in dentin of human teeth. The rate of reparative dentin formation decreases markedly after 48 days.[199] Dentin is laid down fastest during the first month following indirect pulp therapy and the rate then diminishes steadily with time. Pulpal floor depth reportedly has little effect on the amount of reparative dentin formed.[216] By contrast, another report[179] has stated that dentin formation is accelerated by thin dentin, that more dentin formation occurs with longer treatment times, and that greater dentin formation is observed in primary than in permanent teeth.

If the initial treatment was successful, when the tooth is reentered the caries will appear to be arrested. The color will have changed from a deep red rose to light gray or light brown. The texture will have changed from spongy and wet to hard, and the caries will appear dehydrated. *Practically all bacteria are destroyed under ZOE and calcium hydroxide dressing sealed in deep carious lesions.*[4,104]

Following removal of the remaining caries, the tooth may be permanently restored. The usual procedure of pulpal protection with adequate bases is, of course, mandatory before placement of permanent restorations.

DIRECT PULP CAPPING AND PULPOTOMY

Direct pulp capping and pulpotomy involve the application of a medicament or dressing to the exposed pulp in an attempt to preserve its vitality. Pulpotomy differs from pulp capping only in that a portion of the remaining pulp is removed before application of the medicament. These procedures have been employed for carious, mechanical, and traumatic exposures of the pulp—with reported high incidence of success as judged radiographically and by the absence of clinical signs and symptoms. Histologic examinations, however, have shown chronic inflammation under many carious pulp caps and diminished success rates.

Orban[150] described the histopathology of the pulp and concluded that the cells of the pulp were the same as those of loose connective tissue. He believed these cells could differentiate

A

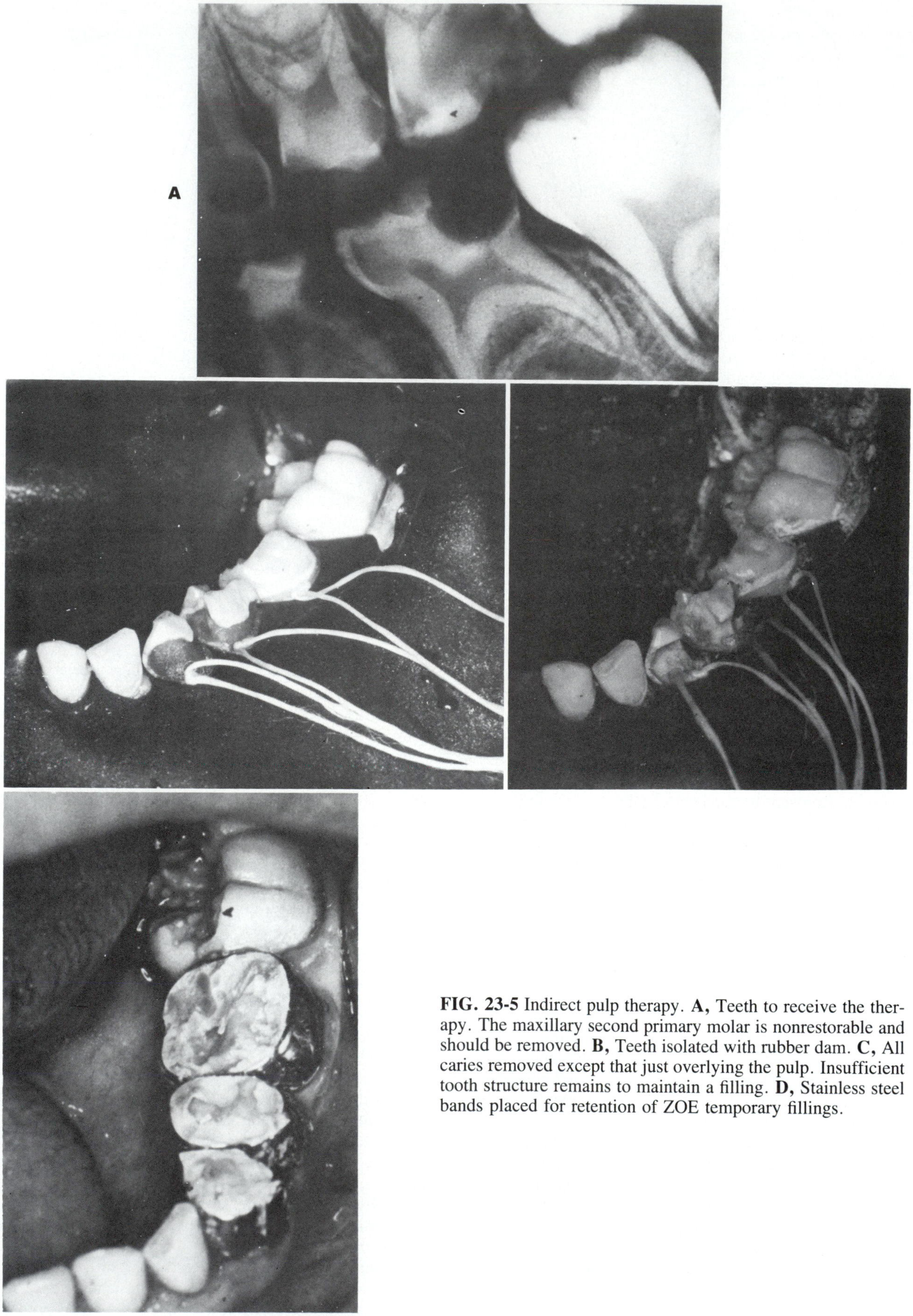

B

C

D

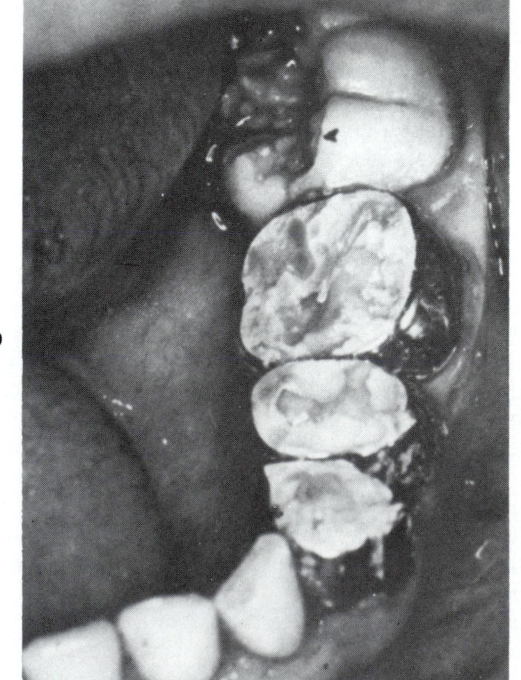

FIG. 23-5 Indirect pulp therapy. **A,** Teeth to receive the therapy. The maxillary second primary molar is nonrestorable and should be removed. **B,** Teeth isolated with rubber dam. **C,** All caries removed except that just overlying the pulp. Insufficient tooth structure remains to maintain a filling. **D,** Stainless steel bands placed for retention of ZOE temporary fillings.

and healing could occur in the dental pulp. In subsequent years much experimentation has taken place, with advocates both for and against pulp-capping and pulpotomy procedures.

Although disagreement exists concerning pulp capping and pulpotomy as permanent procedures in mature secondary teeth, it is universally accepted that vital technique must be employed in teeth with incompletely formed roots with exposed pulps. Once root formation has been completed, routine endodontic treatment may be performed.

Cvek[28,30,31] has reported that pulp capping and partial pulpotomy with calcium hydroxide on *traumatically exposed pulps* are successful 96% of the time. He found that the time between the accident and treatment was not critical as long as the superficially inflamed pulp tissue was removed prior to capping. The size of the exposure had no bearing on success or failure. The study included both mature teeth and teeth with incompletely formed roots. Continued calcification of the pulp following pulp capping was not a consistent finding; and when it occurred, it was usually within the first year. These findings have been substantiated by subsequent studies.[58,77,106]

Because of the normal aging of the dental pulp, chances of successful pulp capping diminish with age. Increases in fibrous and calcific deposits and a reduction in pulpal volume may be observed in older pulps. With age the fibroblast proliferation observed in the teeth of young animals is significantly reduced.[186]

Teeth with calcifications of the pulp chamber and root canals are not candidates for pulp-capping procedures. These calcifications are indicative of previous inflammatory responses or trauma and render the pulp less responsive to vital therapy.[11,29]

Agreement generally exists concerning pulp caps in young permanent teeth with blunderbuss apices, but there is disagreement as to whether mature permanent teeth should be pulp capped after a carious pulp exposure. Pulp capping after carious pulp exposure is widely accepted as the treatment of choice. Many clinicians believe that to obtain good results teeth must be carefully selected; pulp capping should be done only in the absence of a history of pain and when there is little or no bleeding at the exposure site.[126] However, other clinicians recommend extirpation of all cariously exposed pulps except those with incompletely formed apices, believing that although there may be no pain enough toxic products remain in the pulp to maintain the inflammation.[112]

These long-standing inflammations with circulatory disturbances are frequently accompanied by apposition and resorption of the canal walls and calcification in the pulp. The inflammation, calcification, apposition, and resorption may thrive under pulp caps, regardless of which material is used as the pulp-capping agent. In teeth with blunderbuss apices, some clinicians recommend pulp extirpation and filling of the canals after a pulp cap as soon as the apical foramen has closed because continued calcification may eventually render the canals unnegotiable.[112]

Few disagree that the ideal treatment for all carious pulp exposures on mature permanent teeth should be pulpal extirpation and endodontic treatment. It is unrealistic, however, to believe that this can be achieved in all cases. Extirpating the pulp is economically unfeasible in many cases and is time-consuming and difficult to accomplish in certain teeth. If vital pulp therapy fails, one usually still has the option of endodontic treatment.

Agreement exists that exposed caries on primary teeth should *not* be pulp capped. *Pulp-capping procedures in primary teeth should be reserved for teeth with mechanical exposures.* The pulpotomy procedure for primary teeth (see below) has been shown to be much more successful than pulp capping, and the time requirements for performing the procedures are similar. Therefore *it is recommended that carious pulp exposures on primary teeth not be pulp capped.*[114,201,202]

According to Seltzer and Bender[186] pulp capping should be discouraged for carious pulp exposures since microorganisms and inflammation are invariably associated. Macroscopic examination of such exposures is difficult, and areas of liquefaction necrosis may be overlooked. Because of accelerated aging processes in carious teeth and teeth having undergone operative procedures, they are poorer candidates for pulp caps than noncarious teeth; because of diminished blood supply, periodontally involved teeth are poor risks for pulp capping.

There is general agreement[33,126,186] that the larger the area of carious exposure the poorer the prognosis for pulp capping. With a larger exposure more pulpal tissue is inflamed and there is greater chance for contamination by microorganisms. With larger exposures there is also greater damage from crushing of tissues and hemorrhage, causing a more severe inflammation. However, when exposure occurs as a result of traumatic or mechanical injury to a healthy pulp, the size of the exposure does not influence healing.[28,154]

Location of the pulp exposures is an important consideration in the prognosis. If the exposure occurs on the axial wall of the pulp, with pulp tissue coronal to the exposure site, this tissue may be deprived of its blood supply and undergo necrosis, causing a failure. Then a pulpotomy or pulpectomy should be performed rather than a pulp cap.[197]

If pulp capping or pulpotomy is to be done, care must be exercised in removal of caries and/or dentin over the exposure site to keep to a minimum the pushing of dentin chips into the remaining pulp tissue. Studies have shown decreased success when dentin fragments are forced into the underlying pulp tissue.[11,99] Inflammatory reaction and formation of dentin matrix are stimulated around these dentin chips.[129] In addition, microorganisms may be forced into the tissue. The resulting inflammatory reaction can be so severe as to cause failure.

Experiments on germ-free animals have shown the importance of microorganisms in the healing of exposed pulp tissues; injured pulpal tissue contaminated by microorganisms did not heal whereas tissue in germ-free animals did heal regardless of the severity of the exposure.[98,153] Pulp procedures should always be carried out with rubber dam isolation and aseptic conditions to prevent introduction of microorganisms into the pulp tissue.

Marginal seal over the pulp-capping or pulpotomy procedure is of prime importance. The suggestion has been made[122] that major considerations for healing are respect for living tissue and the establishment of a tight marginal seal to prevent ingress of bacteria and reinfection. Healing and the formation of secondary dentin are inherent properties of the pulp. If allowed to do so, the pulp, like any connective tissue, will heal itself. Healing following pulp amputation has been shown to be essentially the same as initial calcification events that occur in other normal and diseased calcified tissues.[75] Factors promoting healing are conditions of the pulp at the time of amputation, removal of irritants, and proper postoperative care such as proper sealing of the margins.

After mechanical exposure of the pulp, an acute inflammation occurs at the exposure site. Blood vessels dilate, edema occurs, and polymorphonuclear leukocytes accumulate at the injury site. If the initial tissue damage is too severe, the pulp will become chronically inflamed, with eventual necrosis of the pulp. It has been shown, however, that repair can occur after pulp exposure. Mechanical exposures have a much better prognosis than do carious exposures because of the lack of previous inflammation and infection associated with the carious exposures. Repair depends on the amount of tissue destruction, the presence of hemorrhage, the patient's age, the resistance of the host, and other factors involved in connective tissue repair.[186]

After pulpal injury, reparative dentin is formed as part of the repair process. Although formation of a dentin bridge has been used as one of the criteria for judging successful pulp capping or pulpotomy procedures, bridge formation can occur in teeth with irreversible inflammation.[218] Moreover, successful pulp capping has been reported without the presence of a reparative dentin bridge over the exposure site.[180,229]

Pulp-Capping Agents

Many materials and drugs have been employed as pulp-capping agents. Materials, medicaments, antiseptics, antiinflammatory agents, antibiotics, and enzymes have been utilized as pulp-capping agents; but *calcium hydroxide is generally accepted as the material of choice for pulp capping.*[29,126,186]

Prior to 1930, when Hermann[80] introduced calcium hydroxide as a successful pulp-capping agent, pulp therapy had consisted of devitalization with arsenic and other fixative agents. Hermann demonstrated the formation of secondary dentin over the amputation sites of vital pulps capped with calcium hydroxide.

In 1938 Teuscher and Zander[213] introduced calcium hydroxide in the United States; they histologically confirmed complete dentinal bridging with healthy radicular pulp under calcium hydroxide dressings. Further reports[67,237] firmly established calcium hydroxide as the pulp-capping agent of choice. After these early works many studies have reported various forms of calcium hydroxide used, with success rates ranging from 30% to 98%.[52] The dissimilar success rates are attributed to many factors, including selection of teeth, criteria for success and failure, differences in responses among different animals, length of study, area of pulp to which the medicament was applied (coronally or cervically), and the type of calcium hydroxide employed.

When calcium hydroxide is applied directly to pulp tissue, there is necrosis of the adjacent pulp tissue and an inflammation of the contiguous tissue. Dentin bridge formation occurs at the junction of the necrotic tissue and the vital inflamed tissue. Although calcium hydroxide works effectively, the exact mechanism is not understood. Compounds of similar alkalinity (pH of 11) cause liquefaction necrosis when applied to pulp tissue. Calcium hydroxide maintains a local state of alkalinity that is necessary for bone or dentin formation. Beneath the region of coagulation necrosis, cells of the underlying pulp tissue differentiate into odontoblasts and elaborate dentin matrix.[186]

Occasionally, in spite of successful bridge formation, the pulp remains chronically inflamed or becomes necrotic. Internal resorption is a sometime occurrence following pulp exposure and capping with calcium hydroxide. In other cases complete dentin mineralization of the remaining pulp tissue occludes the canals to the extent that they cannot be penetrated for endodontic therapy if necessary. For these reasons pulpal extirpation and canal filling have been recommended as soon as root formation is completed after the use of calcium hydroxide[112,186] (Fig. 23-6). However, in view of the low incidence of this occurrence, it does not seem to be routinely justified unless necessary for restorative purposes.

It was postulated[237] that calcium would diffuse from a calcium hydroxide dressing into the pulp and participate in the formation of reparative dentin. Experiments with radioactive ions, however, have shown that calcium ions from the calcium hydroxide do *not* enter into the formation of new dentin. Radioactive calcium ions injected intravenously were identified in the dentin bridge. Thus it was established that *the calcium for the dentin bridge comes from the bloodstream.*[6,157,182] The action of calcium hydroxide to form a dentinal bridge appears to be a result of the low-grade irritation in the underlying pulpal tissue following application. This theory was supported by the demonstration of successful dentinal bridging after application of calcium hydroxide for short periods of time, followed by removal of the material.[32]

Different forms of calcium hydroxide have produced marked differences when applied to a pulp exposure.[156,211,220]

Commercially available compounds of calcium hydroxide in modified forms are known to be less alkaline and thus less caustic on the pulp. The reactions to Dycal, Prisma VLC Dycal, Life, and Nu-Cap have been shown to be similar.[197,198,211] The chemically altered tissue created by application of these compounds is resorbed first, and the bridge is then formed in contact with the capping material.[81,217,220] With calcium hydroxide powder (or Pulpdent) the bridge forms at the junction of the chemically altered tissue and the remaining subjacent vital pulp tissue. The altered tissue degenerates and disappears, leaving a void between the capping material and the dentinal bridge. This is the reason a bridge can be seen better radiographically with calcium hydroxide powder or Pulpdent than with the other commercial compounds. The quality of the dentin bridging was equally good with either material.

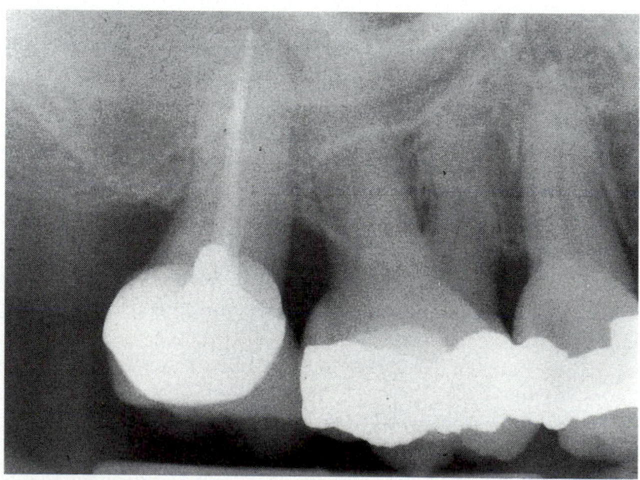

FIG. 23-6 Calcification of pulp chambers and root canals after calcium hydroxide pulp capping. The pulp chamber is completely obliterated, and the root canals partially obliterated. Because of calcification after the pulp capping, the root canals are extremely difficult to locate and negotiate.

Conflicting evidence has been reported on the success of Hydrex.[84,181,197] The resin catalyst in Hydrex caused pulpal necrosis when used as a direct pulp-capping agent.[185] MPC, a variation of Hydrex, has been shown to be a poor pulp-capping agent,[81,158] as was Prisma-Bond (a visible light–cured bis-GMA resin by the L.D. Caulk Co.).[159] Reolit, another hard-setting calcium hydroxide base, has proved unsuccessful in pulp capping, probably because of its neutral pH.[211]

The combination of calcium hydroxide in a methyl-cellulose base and metacresylacetate was shown to consistently produce bridging of regular reparative dentin with normal, uninflamed pulp tissue below the calcific barrier.[52,229]

The incorporation of antibiotics into pulp-capping agents to reduce or eliminate pulp infections has led to varying responses. Generally the antibiotic was ineffective in reducing inflammation or stimulating reparative dentin deposition.[21,64,127] There are dangers in using antibiotics as pulp-capping agents. Immunologic sensitization through pulp canals has been demonstrated. Induction of a hypersensitivity reaction may be a dangerous sequel to topically applied antibiotics.[186]

Corticosteroids have been incorporated into pulp-capping agents in attempts to reduce pain and inflammation.[16,21,50] Reparative dentin formation is inhibited by corticosteroids unless they are incorporated with calcium hydroxide. Reports have pointed out that although pain usually disappeared when the corticosteroids were used, these agents might have merely disguised and conserved a chronic inflammation and thus were not beneficial but just postponed the degeneration.[112,186] Combinations of corticosteroids and antibiotics have likewise proved of no value as pulp-capping agents.[88]

Isobutyl cyanoacrylate has been reported to be an excellent pulp-capping agent because of its hemostatic and bacteriostatic properties; at the same time it causes less inflammation than does calcium hydroxide.[13,15,32] However, it cannot be regarded as an adequate therapeutic alternative to calcium hydroxide since it does not produce a continuous barrier of reparative dentin following application to exposed pulpal tissue.[32] *N*-Butyl cyanoacrylate causes severe inflammation when used as a pulp-capping agent.[148]

Polycarboxylate cements have been reported to be well tolerated by pulp tissue, but they are initially irritating and do not stimulate formation of a dentin bridge.[43,127,176]

Other materials used as pulp-capping agents have included dentin,[142,225] albumin,[130] acid and alkaline phosphatase,[186] chondroitin sulfate,[186] chondroitin sulfate and collagen,[95] calcium-eugenol cement,[87] calcitonin (a calcium-regulating hormone),[194] barium and strontium hydroxide,[86] native enriched collagen solution,[17,57] and hydroxyapatite.[91]

An absorbable form of tricalcium phosphate ceramic has been reported to produce dentinal bridging when used as a pulp-capping agent in monkeys. The formation of a dentin bridge was enhanced when compared with that in a control using calcium hydroxide, and pulpal inflammation was minimal.[23,78] Tricalcium phosphate with magnesium and octocalcium phosphate induced formation of dystrophic dentin, whereas the addition of hydroxyapatite to tricalcium phosphate stimulated dentinal bridging superior to that produced with the use of calcium hydroxide.[93]

The use of ZOE applied directly to pulp tissue is a controversial tissue. As compared with calcium hydroxide, ZOE produced favorable results according to some researchers[110,183,229] but allowed chronic inflammation and eventual necrosis of pulp tissue to persist according to others.[70,124,184] Dentin bridge formation does not normally occur under ZOE pulp caps although it has been reported.[170,226]

Although capping inflamed pulps is not recommended, ZOE has been shown to be a more beneficial agent than calcium hydroxide under these circumstances.[218] Calcium hydroxide placed on acutely inflamed pulps leads to necrosis.

The ideal treatment for all carious exposures, except those in teeth with incompletely formed roots, might be pulp extirpation and root canal filling; nevertheless there are still indications for direct pulp capping. Economics, time, and difficulty of achieving root canal filling in certain teeth are a few of the reasons one may choose pulp capping over another form of pulp therapy. *The pulp capping material of choice at the present time remains calcium hydroxide*. If pulp capping is considered, one must consider all the factors discussed in this section to determine the prognosis of each case. In the event of failure of direct pulp capping, there is usually the option of endodontic therapy.

Pulp capping should *not* be considered for primary carious pulp exposures or for permanent teeth with a history of spontaneous toothache, radiographic evidence of pulpal or periapical pathosis, calcifications of the pulp chamber or root canals, excessive hemorrhage at the exposure site, or exposures with purulent or serous exudates.

PULPOTOMY

The pulpotomy procedure involves removing pulp tissue that has inflammatory or degenerative changes, leaving intact the remaining vital tissue, which is then covered with a pulp-capping agent to promote healing at the amputation site or an agent to cause fixation of the underlying tissue. The only difference between pulpotomy and pulp capping is that in pulpotomy additional tissue is removed from the exposed pulp. Traditionally, the term "pulpotomy" has implied removal of pulp tissue to the cervical line. However, the depth to which tissue is removed is determined by clinical judgment. All tissue judged to be inflamed should be removed in order to place the dressing on healthy, uninflamed pulp tissue. Better results are obtained if the amputation level is shallow because of better visualization of the working area. In multi-rooted teeth, the procedure may be simplified by removing tissue to the orifices of the root canals.

The difficulties of assessing the extent of inflammation in cariously exposed pulps have been previously discussed. However, several studies[31,76,77] have shown that inflammation is confined to the surface 2 to 3 mm of the pulp when traumatically exposed and left untreated for up to 168 hours. In experimental animals the results were the same whether the crowns were fractured or ground off. Direct invasion of vital pulp tissue by bacteria did not occur, even though the pulps were left exposed to the saliva. Under the same circumstances with cavity preparations into the teeth that left areas to impact food, debris, and bacteria in contact with the pulp, the inflammation ranged from 1 to 9 mm with abscess and pus formation.[31,76] The same results have been obtained in permanent teeth with incompletely formed roots as well as those with mature ones. Pulpotomy procedures for primary teeth are discussed later in this chapter.

Pulpotomy procedures using carbon dioxide laser[189] and electrosurgery[175,187,188,191] have been reported. Electrosurgical pulpotomies on primary teeth have produced results comparable to those found with the use of formocresol. The advantages of these techniques are the lack of hemorrhage and less mechanical damage to the underlying pulp. Although these procedures may hold promise, there has not yet been sufficient research to assess their validity.

Calcium Hydroxide Pulpotomy on Young Permanent Teeth

Despite the fact that vital pulp-capping and pulpotomy procedures for cariously exposed pulps in teeth with developed apices remain controversial, it is universally accepted that vital techniques be employed in those teeth with incompletely developed apices. Although many materials and drugs have been used as pulp-capping agents (described earlier), the application of calcium hydroxide to stimulate dentinal bridge formation in accidentally or cariously exposed pulps of young permanent teeth continues to be the treatment of choice.

The indirect pulp therapy technique should be used whenever possible with deep carious lesions in order to avoid exposure of the pulp (see p. 636). Every attempt should be made to maintain the vitality of these immature teeth until their full root development has been completed. Loss of vitality before root completion leaves a weak root more prone to fracture. Loss of vitality before completion of root length may leave a poor crown/root ratio and a tooth more susceptible to periodontal breakdown because of excessive mobility. If necessary, the remaining pulp tissue can be extirpated and conventional endodontic therapy completed when root formation has been accomplished.

Endodontic treatment is greatly complicated in teeth with necrotic pulps and open apices. Although apexification procedures have been perfected for these teeth, the treatment is extensive and costly for the patient and the resulting root structure is weaker than in teeth with fully developed roots. If the calcium hydroxide pulpotomy is not successful, the apexification procedure or surgical endodontics may still be performed.

Technique

After the diagnosis is completed, the tooth is anesthetized. If possible, pulpal procedures should always be performed under rubber dam isolation and aseptic conditions to prevent further introduction of microorganisms into the pulpal tissues. Care must be taken when placing the rubber dam on a traumatized tooth. If any loosening of the tooth has occurred, the rubber dam clamps must be applied to adjacent uninjured teeth. If this is impossible because of lack of adjacent teeth or partially erupted ones that cannot be clamped, careful isolation

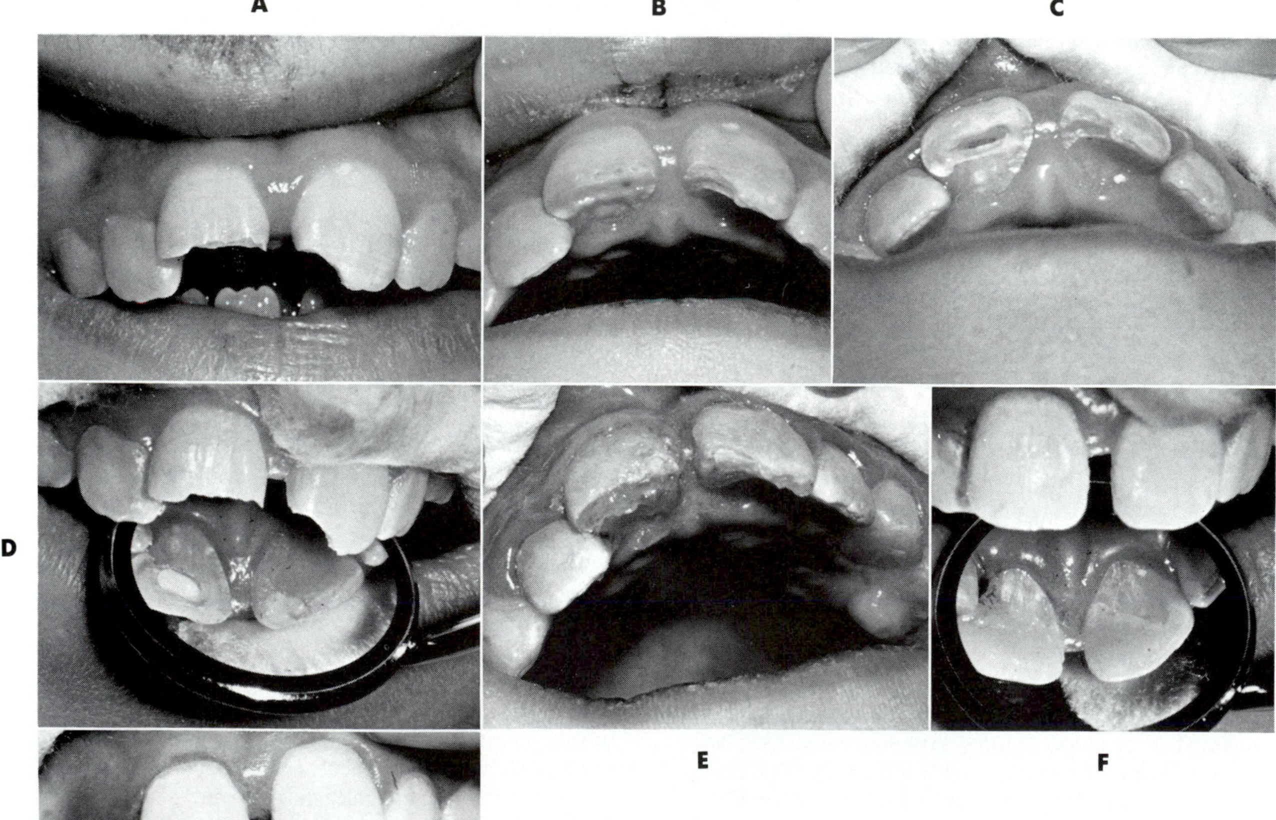

FIG. 23-7 Emergency treatment of fractured maxillary incisors. **A,** Initial examination 4 days after the trauma. **B,** Right central incisor with pulp exposure, left central with dentin exposure. **C,** Pulpotomy preparation after hemorrhage has been controlled with a moistened cotton pellet. **D,** Application of Dycal to the pulpal stump and exposed dentin. **E,** Acid etching of enamel. **F** and **G,** Completed acid etch resin restoration.

with cotton rolls and constant aspiration by the dental assistant may be utilized to maintain a dry field (Fig. 23-7).

In traumatically exposed pulps, only tissue judged to be inflamed is removed. Cvek[28] has shown that with pulp exposures resulting from traumatic injuries, regardless of the size of the exposure or the amount of lapsed time, pulpal changes are characterized by a proliferative response with inflammation extending only a few millimeters into the pulp. When this hyperplastic inflamed tissue is removed, healthy pulp tissue is encountered.[28] In teeth with carious exposure of the pulp, it may be necessary to remove pulpal tissue to a greater depth to reach uninflamed tissue.

The instrument of choice for tissue removal in the pulpotomy procedure is an abrasive diamond bur utilizing high speed and adequate water cooling. This technique has been shown to create the least damage to the underlying tissue.[68] Care must be exercised to ensure removal of all filaments of the pulp tissue coronal to the amputation site; otherwise, hemorrhage will be impossible to control. Following pulpal amputation, the preparation is thoroughly washed with physiologic saline or sterile water to remove all debris. The water is removed by vacuum and cotton pellets. Air should not be blown on the exposed pulp since it will cause desiccation and tissue damage.

Hemorrhage is controlled by slightly moistened cotton pellets (wetted and blotted almost dry) placed against the stumps of the pulp. Completely dry cotton pellets should not be used since fibers of the dry cotton will be incorporated into the clot and, when removed, will cause hemorrhage. Dry cotton pellets are placed over the moist pellets and slight pressure is exerted on the mass to control the hemorrhage. Hemorrhage should be controlled in this manner within several minutes (Fig. 23-7, *C*). It may be necessary to change the pellets to control all hemorrhage. If hemorrhage continues, one must carefully check to be sure that all filaments of the pulp coronal to the amputation site were removed and that the site is clean.

If hemorrhage cannot be controlled, amputation should be performed at a more apical level. Should it become necessary to extend into the root canals, a small endodontic spoon or round abrasive diamond bur may be used to remove the tissue on anterior teeth with single canals (Fig. 23-8). On posterior teeth, the use of endodontic files or reamers may be necessary if tissue is being amputated within the canals. *Obviously, extension of the amputation site is carried into the root canals only in teeth with blunderbuss apices.*

On teeth with blunderbuss apices, if tissue removal has been extended several millimeters into the root canals and hemorrhage continues, a compromise treatment should be considered. The hemorrhage is controlled with chemicals such as aluminum chloride or other hemostatic agents. Once hemorrhage is controlled, calcium hydroxide is placed in the canal against

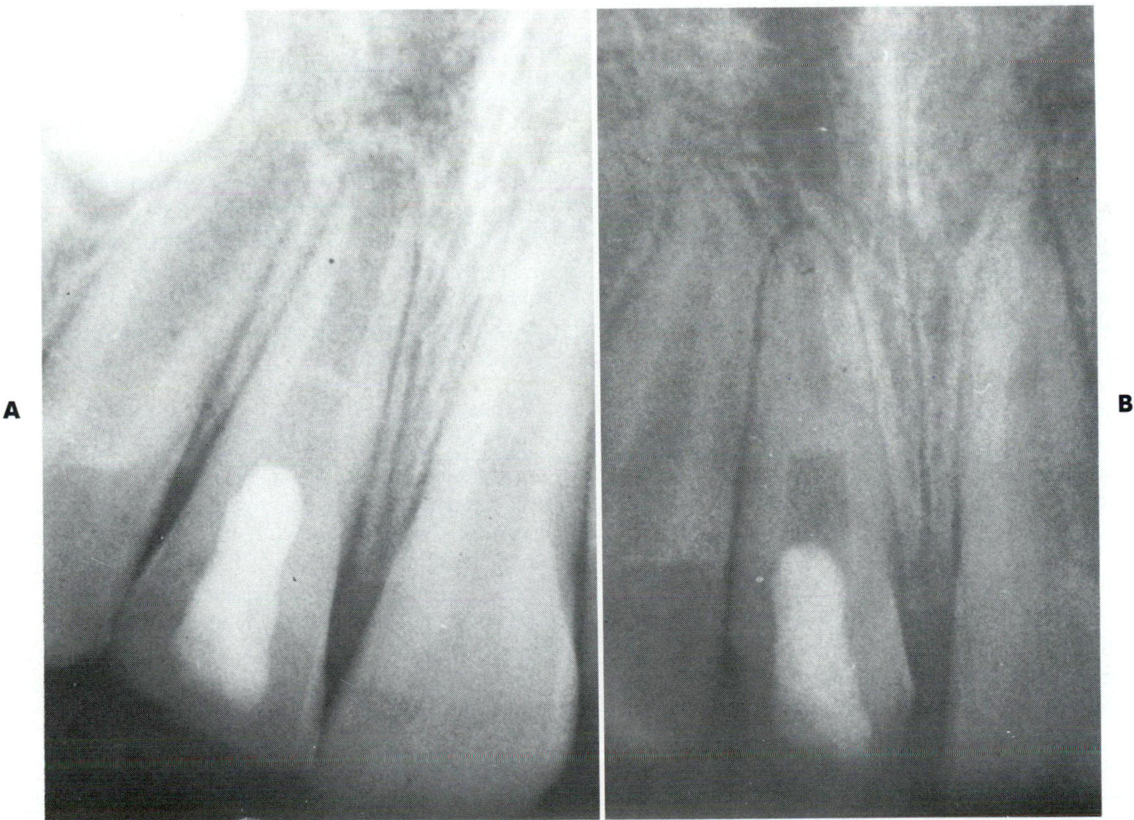

FIG. 23-8 Deep calcium hydroxide pulpotomy. **A,** Central incisor with an immature apex 10 weeks after a traumatic exposure of the pulp and a calcium hydroxide pulpotomy. Note the dentin bridge. **B,** Three years after pulpotomy. Note the thickening of the dentin bridge and the completion of root development. The tooth remained asymptomatic. No further endodontic treatment is indicated at this time.

the pulp stump and the tooth is sealed. These compromised teeth must be closely monitored for development of pathologic conditions. If necrosis of the remaining pulp tissue occurs, apexification procedures are instituted. If vitality is maintained, further root development with dystrophic calcification usually occurs. In these compromised cases, once the apex has formed, the tooth is reentered and conventional endodontic therapy is completed with gutta-percha obliteration.

In the normal pulpotomy procedure, once the hemorrhage has been controlled, a dressing of calcium hydroxide is placed over the amputation site (Fig. 23-7, *D*). If the pulpal amputation extends into the tooth only a few millimeters, the use of a hard setting material (e.g., Dycal or Life) is usually easiest. However, for deeper amputation, calcium hydroxide powder carried to the tooth in an amalgam carrier is the easiest method of application. The amalgam carrier is tightly packed with powder; then all but one fourth to one third of the pellet is expressed from the carrier and discarded. The remaining calcium hydroxide in the carrier is then expressed into the preparation site. The pellet of calcium hydroxide powder is carefully teased against the pulp stump with a rounded end plastic instrument. The entire pulp stump must be covered with a thin layer of calcium hydroxide. Care must be taken not to pack the calcium hydroxide into the pulp tissue, as this will cause greater inflammation and increase the chances of failure, or if pulpotomy is successful, there will be increased calcification of the remaining pulp tissues around the particles of calcium hydroxide.[221]

Pulpdent (calcium hydroxide in a methylcellulose base) may also be utilized for the pulpotomy procedure. If commercial preparations of calcium hydroxide are used, care must be taken to avoid trapping air bubbles when applying the material.

After the calcium hydroxide has been applied to the pulp stumps, a creamy mix of ZOE or other cement base must be flowed over the calcium hydroxide and allowed to set completely. When a composite resin restoration is to be utilized, eugenol compounds must be avoided since these interfere with a setting reaction of the composite. In these cases, a second layer of Dycal or Life is placed. After setting, the cement base layer should be thick enough to allow for condensation of a permanent restoration to effectively seal the tooth.

A permanent type of restoration should always be placed in the tooth to ensure the retention of the calcium hydroxide–cement base dressing. Unless a crown is necessary, amalgam is the material of choice for posterior teeth, and an etched composite restoration (Fig. 23-7, *E–G*) is preferred for anterior teeth.

Follow-up after pulp capping and pulpotomy

After pulp capping and pulpotomy, the patient should be recalled periodically for 2 to 4 years to determine success. Although the normal vitality tests such as electric and thermal sensitivity are reliable after pulp capping, they are usually not helpful in the pulpotomized tooth. Although histologic success cannot be determined, clinical success is judged by the absence of any clinical or radiographic signs of pathosis, the verification of a dentin bridge both radiographically and clinically, and the presence of continued root development in teeth with incompletely formed roots.

Controversy exists as to whether the pulp should be reentered after the completion of root development in the pulpotomized tooth. Some researchers[112,186] believe that pulp capping and pulpotomy procedures invariably lead to progressive calcification of the root canals. After successful root development, they advocate extirpation of the remaining pulp tissue and endodontic treatment. They recommend endodontic therapy because of the high incidence of continued calcification, which would render the canals nonnegotiable at some future time when endodontic therapy might be required because of disease. However, it has been my experience and others[30,58,77] that with good case selection, if a gentle technique is used in removing pulp tissue, care is taken to avoid contamination of the pulp with bacteria and dentin chips, and the dressing of calcium hydroxide is not packed into the underlying pulp tissue, progressive calcification of the pulp is an infrequent sequela of pulpotomy (Fig. 23-9).

In a follow-up study of clinically successful pulpotomies previously reported,[28] researchers[30] removed the pulps 1 to 5 years later for restorative reasons and found histologically normal pulps. They concluded that changes seen in the pulps do not represent sufficient histologic evidence to support routine pulpectomy after pulpotomy in accidentally fractured teeth with pulp exposures. Thus the routine reentry to remove the pulp and place a root canal filling after completion of root development is contraindicated unless dictated by restorative considerations such as the necessity for retentive post placement. Nevertheless, canal calcification, internal resorption, and/or pulp necrosis are potential sequelae of pulp-capping and pulpotomy procedures. Although unlikely, they are possible and the patient should be clearly informed.

In posterior teeth, where surgical endodontics is difficult, if continued calcification of the canal is observed following root closure, reentry of the tooth for endodontic therapy is recommended. In anterior teeth, if calcification of the canal has made conventional endodontics impossible, surgical endodontics may be performed with relative ease. Therefore, in anterior teeth, routine endodontic therapy following completion of root development is contraindicated unless clinical signs and symptoms of pathosis are present or unless such therapy is necessary for restorative procedures (placement of a post for retention of a crown because of missing tooth structure; Fig. 23-10).

Formocresol Pulpotomy on Young Permanent Teeth

Because of the reported clinical and histologic success with the formocresol pulpotomy on primary teeth, there has been much interest in this technique on young permanent teeth. Evidence of continued apical development following formocresol pulpotomy procedures on young permanent teeth with incompletely developed apices has been reported.[48,135,177,212] Several authors have reported better results with diluted formocresol. However, they reported a high incidence of internal resorption which increased in severity with longer periods of time.[56,155]

The formocresol procedure has appeal because there is a lack of calcification of the remaining pulp tissue as is sometimes seen with calcium hydroxide pulpotomy. After root completion, the tooth can easily be reentered, the pulp extirpated, and routine endodontic therapy performed. Contrary to these findings, one group of researchers[5] has shown calcification of the canals by continuous apposition of dentin on the lateral walls with equal frequency whether using calcium hydroxide

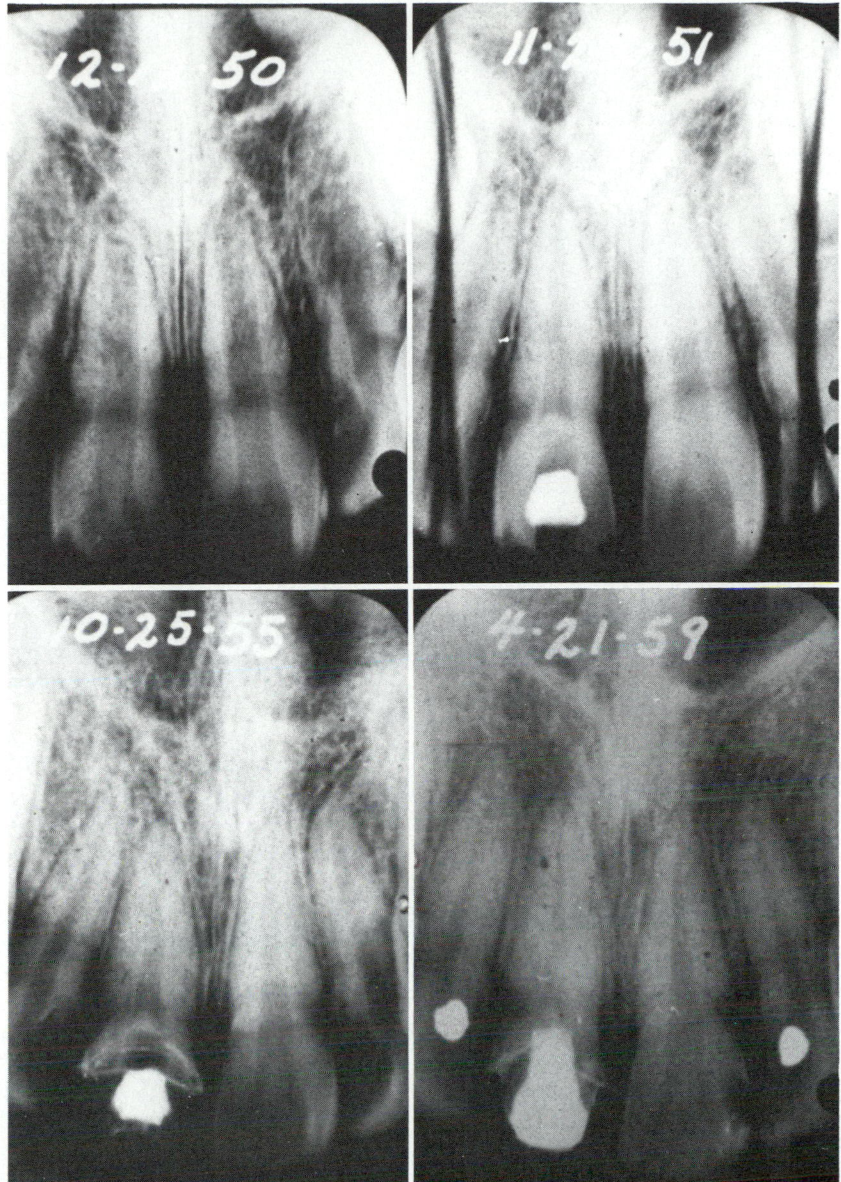

FIG. 23-9 Calcium hydroxide pulpotomy on a permanent incisor with an immature (or blunderbuss) apex. Traumatic exposure of the pulp of the central incisor was treated with a calcium hydroxide pulpotomy. The tooth at 1 year, 5 years, and 8½ years after pulpotomy remained asymptomatic. Root formation was completed, and the root canal appears to be of similar size to that of the adjacent incisor. (Courtesy Dr. Ralph McDonald.)

or formocresol. The only common demoninator to this reaction was the presence of dentin chips that had accidentally been pushed into the radicular pulp tissue.

A retrospective study using clinical and radiographic criteria reported successful results; however, there was a high degree of root canal obliteration by calcification which might preclude future root canal treatment.[212]

Other studies[101,134] have shown complete replacement of the pulp tissue with granulation tissue and the formation of osteodentin along the walls of the canals in permanent teeth following formocresol pulpotomies. The reaction was described as a healing rather than a destructive process, but persistent chronic inflammation was noted.

Although this treatment has been reported to be partly successful, it cannot be routinely recommended until further research showing the technique to be successful has been completed.

Formocresol pulpotomy procedures have been reported as temporary treatments on permanent teeth with necrotic pulps. Clinical success after 3 years has been reported.[215] The formocresol pulpotomy was performed rather than extraction when routine endodontic therapy could not be completed because of financial considerations. Complete endodontic treatment was advocated at a later date, with the formocresol pulpotomy used only as a *temporary* treatment.

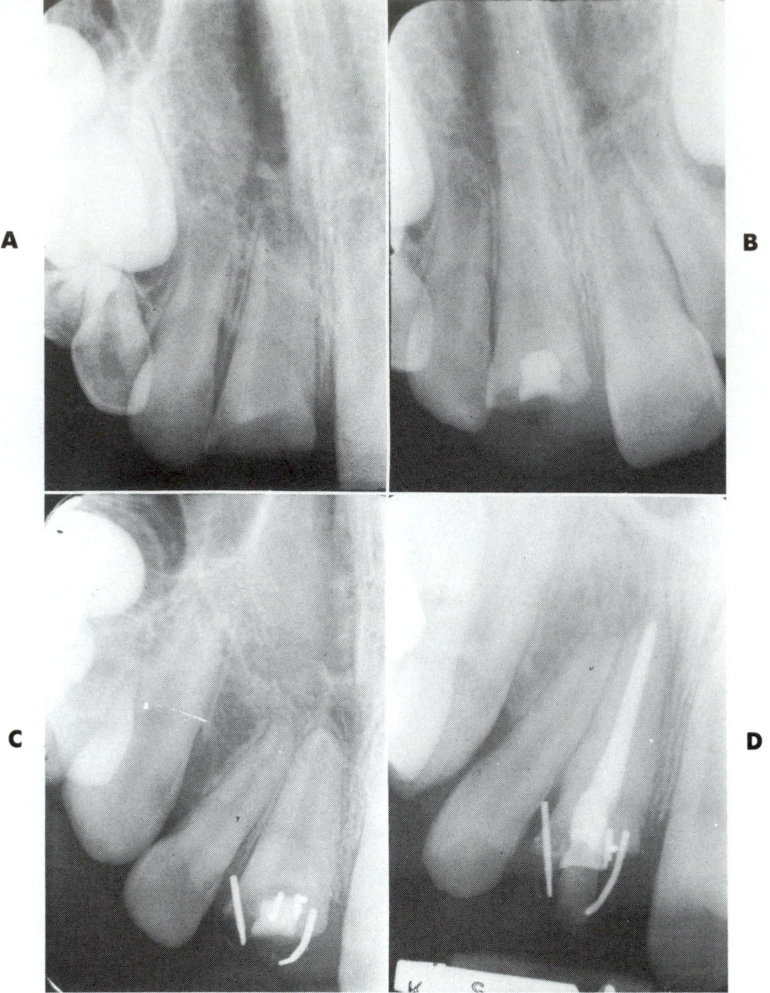

FIG. 23-10 Apexogenesis following calcium hydroxide pulpotomy. **A,** Traumatic injury has exposed the pulp in the maxillary central incisor before formation of the root was completed. **B,** Two months after calcium hydroxide pulpotomy, a dentin bridge has formed. **C,** Two and a half years after the pulpotomy, the root has completed its development. Note the lack of further pulpal calcification and a misplaced pin for retention of a temporary composite restoration. **D,** Root canal treatment has been completed so that the tooth may be permanently restored with a post and core and crown.

PULPOTOMY ON PRIMARY TEETH

Formocresol Pulpotomy on Primary Teeth

The use of formocresol in dentistry has become a controversial issue since reports of wide distribution of the medicament following systemic injection[137] and the demonstration of an immune response to formocresol-fixed autologous tissue implanted in connective tissues or injected into root canals.[18,214] However, the formocresol pulpotomy continues to be one treatment of choice for primary teeth with vital carious exposures of the pulp in which inflammation and/or degeneration are judged to be confined to the coronal pulp. The last reported world-wide survey of dental schools in 1987[7] showed a majority of pediatric dentistry departments and practicing pediatric dentists advocated the formocresol pulpotomy technique. Currently it is still widely taught and utilized in clinical practice. The current formocresol pulpotomy technique is a modification of that reported by Sweet in 1930.[209]

Histologic studies[121,123] have demonstrated the effects of formocresol on pulps of primary and permanent human teeth. Formocresol-saturated cotton pellets caused the surface of the pulp to become fibrous and acidophilic within a few minutes. After exposure to the formocresol for a period of 7 to 14 days, three distinct zones became evident: (1) a broad acidophilic zone of fixation, (2) a broad pale-staining zone with diminished cellular and fiber definition (atrophy), and (3) a broad zone of inflammatory cells concentrated at the pale-staining zone junction and diffusing apically into normal pulp tissue. There was no evidence of an attempt to wall off the inflammatory zone by fibrous tissue or calcific barrier. After 60 days to 1 year, the pulp was progressively fixed and the entire pulp ultimately became fibrous.

Subsequent investigations[44] showed that the effect of formocresol on the pulp varies depending on the length of time the drug is in contact with the tissue. After 5 minutes there was a surface fixation blending into normal pulp tissue apically. Formocresol sealed in contact with the pulp for 3 days caused calcific degeneration, and the technique was termed vital or nonvital, according o the length of time of the application. As a part of this report, the clinical data from Sweet's files were compiled and showed a 97% success rate.

The ingrowth of fibroblasts in tissue underlying formocresol-pulpotomized noncarious human primary canines has been reported.[35] At 16 weeks the entire pulp had degenerated and was being replaced with granulation tissue. Mild inflammation in addition to some calcific degeneration was noted.

Doyle and associates[39] compared calcium hydroxide and formocresol pulpotomies on mechanically exposed, healthy, primary dental pulps. A formocresol pellet was sealed in place 4 to 7 days, and the histologic study was conducted from 4 to 388 days. Of the 18 teeth in the calcium hydroxide group, only 50% were judged histologically to be successful; of the 14 teeth treated with formocresol, 92% were histologically successful. Radiographically the success rates were 64% and 93%, whereas the clinical success rates were 71% and 100% (calcium hydroxide versus formocresol pulpotomy). The authors were able to identify vital tissue in the apical third of the root canals after treatment with formocresol pulpotomies.

Studies of the effect of adding formocresol to the ZOE filling over the 5-minute formocresol-pulpotomized primary tooth[9,224] have shown no appreciable differences between cases in which formocresol was included in the cement and those in which it was not; and histologic investigations[171,196,224] have reported no significant differences between two-appointment and one-appointment (5-minute) formocresol pulpotomies.

Accumulation of formocresol has been demonstrated in the pulp, dentin, periodontal ligament, and bone surrounding the apices of pulpotomized teeth.[60,136] Formaldehyde was shown to be the component of formocresol that interacts with the protein portion of cells. The addition of cresol to formaldehyde appears to potentiate the effect of formaldehyde on protein.[143] In a study using human pulp fibroblast cultures, formaldehyde was shown to be the major component of formocresol causing cytotoxic effects and to be 40 times more toxic than cresol.[94]

Application of radioactive formocresol to amputated pulp sites has been shown to result in immediate absorption of the material. The systemic absorption was limited to about 1% of the applied dose, regardless of the amount of time the drug was applied. It was shown that formocresol compromised the microcirculation, causing vessel thrombosis, which limited further systemic accumulation.[136]

Animal experiments[18,214] have demonstrated that in vivo formocresol-fixed autologous tissue will produce an immune response when implanted into connective tissues or injected into root canals. The tissue became antigenically altered by formocresol and activated a specific cell-mediated lymphocyte response.

Other studies have demonstrated no evidence of this response in nonpresensitized animals,[192] and presensitized animals showed only a weak allergic potential.[223] This is in agreement with researchers[36] who have shown that formaldehyde demonstrated a low level of antigenicity in rabbits and as such would be an acceptable pulp medicament in regard to immunoreactive potential. Other investigators[117] studied lymphocyte transformation induced by formocresol-treated and untreated extracts of homologous pulp tissue in children with varying past experience with formocresol pulpotomies. Significant transformation responses were noted in over half the children, but they were unrelated to a clinical history of formocresol pulpotomy. Sensitization to pulp-related antigens was a common finding in the study. The authors concluded that formocresol pulpotomy does not induce significant immunologic sensitization to extracted antigens of homologous pulp or to pulp antigen altered by treatment with formocresol and therefore does not support other animal studies in which intense immunization schedules were used.[117] Clinical use of formocresol for many years without reports of allergic reaction has quite obviously substantiated this finding.

Concerns regarding the systemic effects of formocresol have also led to investigations concerning its possible embryotoxic and teratogenic effects.[53] In a study utilizing injections of 25% and 50% formocresol into chick embryos, significant increases were noted in mortality, structural defects, and retarded development.

After systemic administration of formocresol in experimental animals, it is distributed throughout the body. Metabolism and excretion of a portion of the absorbed formocresol occur in the kidneys and lungs. The remaining drug is bound to tissue predominantly in the kidneys, liver, and lungs. When administered systemically in large doses, acute toxic effects (including cardiovascular changes, plasma and urinary enzyme changes, and histologic evidence of cellular injury to the vital organs) were noted. The degree of tissue injury appeared to be dose related, with some of the changes being reversible in the early stages. The authors[137] were careful to point out that the administered doses were far in excess of those used clinically in humans and should not be extrapolated to clinical dental practice. In another study, the same authors emphasized that the quantities of formaldehyde absorbed systemically via the pulpotomy route were small and did not contraindicate the use of formocresol.[152]

A subsequent study[138] in which 16 pulpotomies (5-minute application of full-strength formocresol) were performed on a dog displayed early tissue injury to the kidneys and liver; however, cellular recovery could be expected since there was no evidence of the onset of an inflammatory reaction. In animals subjected to only one of four pulpotomies, there was no injury to the kidneys or liver. The heart and lungs of all the animals were normal. The authors pointed out that 16 pulpotomies expose a small dog to a much higher systemic level of formocresol than would several pulpotomies in a human. They further concluded that no clinical implications regarding the toxicity of absorbed formocresol should be drawn from this study. Other investigators[63] have shown that the effect of formocresol on pulp tissue is controlled by the quantity that diffuses into the tissue, and the quantity can be controlled by the length of time of application, the concentration used, the method of application, or a combination of all these factors.

With the use of isotope-labeled 19% formaldehyde, the presence of the drug was demonstrated in the lung, liver, kidney, muscle, serum, urine, and CO_2 following a 5-minute application to pulpotomy sites. The concentrations achieved in the tissues were equivalent to those found following an infusion of 30% of the amount placed in the pulp chamber.[163]

Another study utilizing ^{14}C-labeled formocresol showed that 12% of the material utilized in a 5-minute full-strength pulpotomy was recovered after 36 hours, chiefly from the teeth, plasma, urine, and also from the liver, kidneys, lungs, heart, and spleen.[73]

Implantation of undiluted formocresol-fixed tissue in animals causes necrosis of the surrounding connective tissues,[20] and dilution of the formocresol decreases the tissue irritation potential.[65] Investigations utilizing one-fifth concentration formocresol for pulpotomies have noted little difference as related to the initial effects on tissue fixation; however, earlier recovery of enzyme activity was apparent with the diluted formocresol than with the undiluted. Postoperative complications are reduced, and there is an improvement in the rate of recovery from the cytotoxic effects for formocresol when diluted.[118,119,207] It has been reported clinically that the same success is achieved with the diluted formocresol as with the undiluted.[55,131,132] *Therefore it is recommended that one-fifth concentration formocresol be utilized for pulpotomy procedures since it is as effective as and less damaging than the traditional preparation.*

One-fifth concentration formocresol is prepared in the following manner. The dilute solution is prepared by mixing three parts glycerin with one part distilled water. One part formocresol is then thoroughly mixed with four parts diluent.

A histologic study on teeth with induced pulpal and periapical pathosis[102] showed no resolution of inflammation or periapical pathosis after a 5-minute pulpotomy procedure. Canals with vital tissue exhibited more internal resorption than was reported by other researchers, and more apical resorption was seen in teeth with periapical and furcal involvement than was seen in teeth with vital pulps. Ingrowth of tissue was not observed in canals with necrotic tissue. Also noted was the lack of evidence of formocresol fixation of either apical or furcal lesions. Despite extensive inflammatory reactions around the apices of primary teeth close to the permanent tooth germs, no ill effects were observed on any tooth germs from the formocresol. Formocresol fixation was confined within the canals in all instances. Since the authors[102] concluded that the formocresol pulpotomy is an unacceptable procedure for teeth with pulpal and periapical pathosis, this study points out the importance of confining formocresol pulpotomies to primary teeth containing vital tissue in the root canals. Clinically, these results have also been substantiated.[212]

The fear of damage to the succedaneous tooth has been offered as an argument against formocresol pulpotomy on primary teeth. Studies have shown conflicting findings, ranging from the same incidence of enamel defects in treated and untreated contralateral teeth[133,174] to an increase in defects and positional alterations of the underlying permanent tooth.[128] It should be pointed out that studies of this nature are follow-up studies long after treatment, without knowledge of the existing status of the pulp prior to pulpotomy. Nor has anyone devised a study to ascertain the effects of the condition that necessitated the pulpotomy procedure. If the strict criteria outlined in this section are followed, the incidence of defects to the permanent teeth does not increase after formocresol pulpotomy.

Studies have shown that the exfoliation time of primary molars following formocresol pulpotomy is not affected.[133,222]

Indications and contraindications

The formocresol pulpotomy is indicated for pulp exposure on primary teeth in which the inflammation or infection is judged to be confined to the coronal pulp. If inflammation has spread into the tissues within the root canals, the tooth should be considered a candidate for pulpectomy and root canal filling or extraction. The contraindications for formocresol pulpotomy on a primary tooth are (1) a nonrestorable tooth, (2) a tooth nearing exfoliation or with no bone overlying the permanent tooth crown, (3) a history of spontaneous toothache, (4) evidence of periapical or furcal pathology, (5) a pulp that does not hemorrhage, (6) inability to control hemorrhage following a coronal pulp amputation, (7) a pulp with serous or purulent drainage, and (8) the presence of a fistula.

Technique (Fig. 23-11)

The formocresol pulpotomy is utilized on primary teeth whose roots are judged to be free of inflammation and/or infection. Compromise on this principle will lead to a diminished success rate and possible damage to the succedaneous tooth. Therefore the importance of a proper diagnosis cannot be overstressed.

After the diagnosis has been completed, the primary tooth is anesthetized and isolated with a rubber dam. All caries is removed. The entire roof of the pulp chamber is cut away with a high-speed bur and copious water spray. All the coronal pulp is removed with a bur or spoon excavator. Care must be exercised to extirpate all filaments of the coronal pulp. If any filaments remain in the pulp chamber, hemorrhage will be impossible to control. The pulp chamber is thoroughly washed with water to remove all debris. The water is removed by vacuum and cotton pellets.

Hemorrhage is controlled by slightly moistened cotton pellets (wetted and blotted almost dry) placed against the stumps of the pulp at the openings of the root canals. Completely dry cotton pellets should not be used since fibers of the cotton will be incorporated into the clot and, when removed, will cause hemorrhage. Dry cotton pellets are placed over the moist pellets, and pressure is exerted on the mass to control the hemorrhage. Hemorrhage should be controlled in this manner within several minutes. It may be necessary to change the pellets to control all hemorrhage. If hemorrhage occurs, carefully check to be sure that all filaments of the pulp were removed from the pulp chamber and that the amputation site is clean.

If hemorrhage cannot be controlled within 5 minutes, the pulp tissue within the canals is probably inflamed and the tooth is not a candidate for a formocresol pulpotomy. The clinician should then proceed with pulpectomy, or the tooth should be extracted.

When the hemorrhage has been controlled, one-fifth dilution formocresol on a cotton pellet is placed in direct contact with the pulp stumps. Fixation will not occur unless the formocresol is in contact with the stumps. The cotton pellet is blotted to remove excess formocresol after saturation and before the tooth is entered. Formocresol is caustic and will create a severe tissue burn if allowed to contact the gingiva.

The formocresol is left in contact with the pulp stumps for 5 minutes. When it is removed, the tissue will appear brown and no hemorrhage should be present. If an area of the pulp was not contacting the medication, the procedure must be repeated for that tissue. Small cotton pellets for applying the medication usually work best, since they allow closer approximation of the material to the pulp.

A cement base of ZOE is placed over the pulp stumps and allowed to set. The tooth may then be restored permanently. The restoration of choice is a stainless steel crown for primary

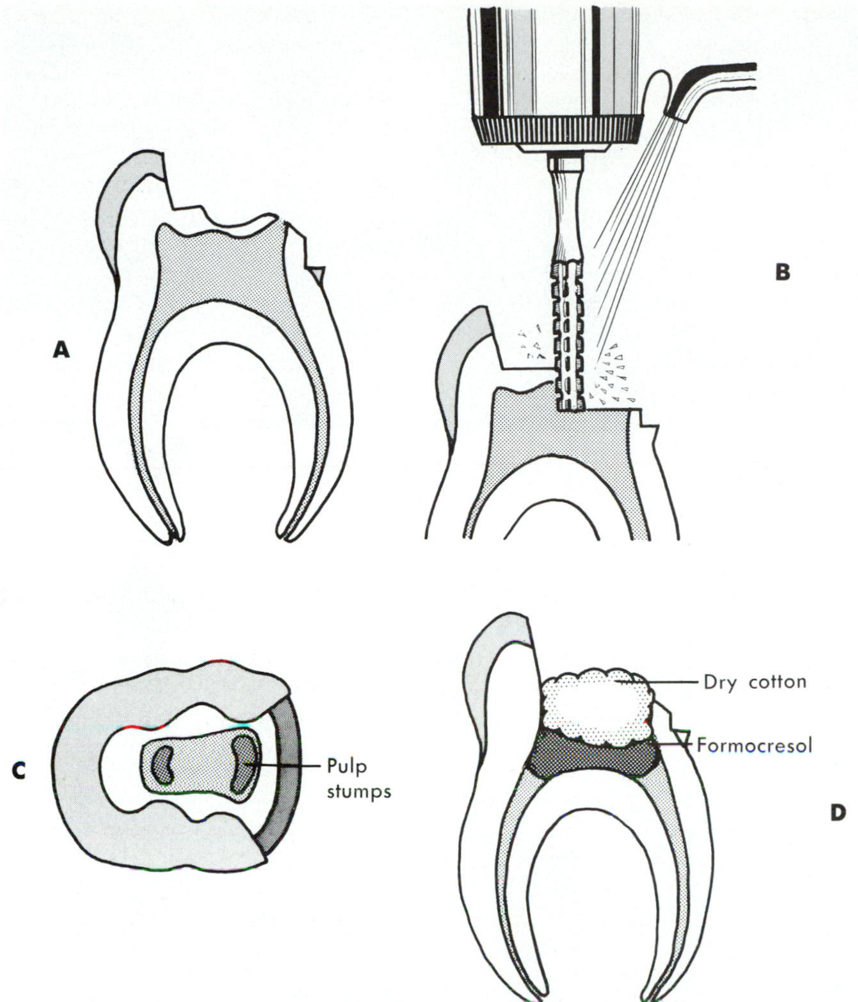

FIG. 23-11 Formocresol pulpotomy. **A,** Carious pulp exposure in the primary tooth. **B,** Removal of the roof of the pulp chamber. **C,** Pulp stumps after hemorrhage controlled. **D,** Formocresol application for 5 minutes. After fixation of the pulp stumps, a base ZOE is applied and the tooth is permanently restored.

molars. On anterior primary teeth a composite tooth-colored restoration is the treatment of choice unless the tooth is so badly broken down that it requires a crown.

With the formocresol, no dentin bridge formation occurs as with the calcium hydroxide pulpotomy (Fig. 23-12).

Failure of a formocresol pulpotomy is usually detected radiographically (Fig. 23-13). The first signs of failure are often internal resorption of the root adjacent to the area where the formocresol was applied. This may be accompanied by external resorption, especially as the failure progresses. In the primary molars a radiolucency develops in the bifurcation or trifurcation area. In the anterior teeth a radiolucency may develop at the apices or lateral to the roots. With more destruction the tooth will become excessively mobile. A fistula usually develops. It is rare for pain to occur with the failure of a formocresol pulpotomy. Consequently, unless patients receive follow-up checks after a formocresol pulpotomy, failure may be undetected. When the tooth loosens and is eventually exfoliated, the parents and child may consider the circumstances normal.

The development of cystic lesions following pulp therapy in primary molars has been reported.[178] An amorphous, eosinophilic material shown to contain phenolic groupings similar to those present in medicaments was found in the lesions. Other researchers[140] have observed furcal lesions in untreated pulpally involved primary molars containing granulomatous tissue with stratified squamous epithelium, suggesting the potential for cyst formation. In a subsequent study involving failed pulpotomized primary molars, most specimens were diagnosed as furcation cysts.[141] These findings point out the importance of follow-up to endodontic treatment on primary teeth.

Glutaraldehyde Pulpotomy

Evidence is rapidly accumulating that glutaraldehyde should replace formocresol as the medicament of choice for pulpotomy procedures on primary teeth. Numerous studies[36,210,230] have shown that the application of 2% to 4% aqueous glutaraldehyde produces rapid surface fixation of the underlying pulpal tissue, although its depth of penetration is limited. Unlike the varied response to formocresol, a large percentage of the

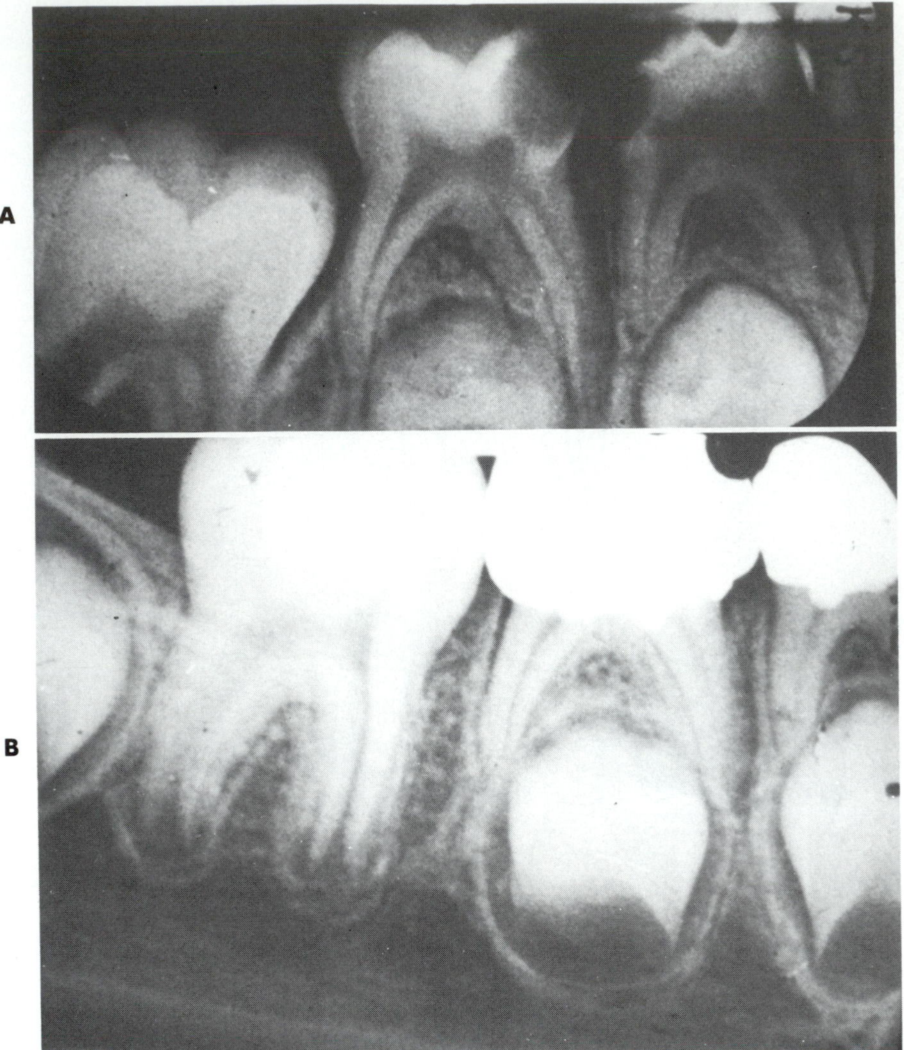

FIG. 23-12 Formocresol pulpotomy. **A,** Primary first and second molars with carious pulp exposures. **B,** Eighteen months after formocresol pulpotomy. Note the eruption of the permanent first molar.

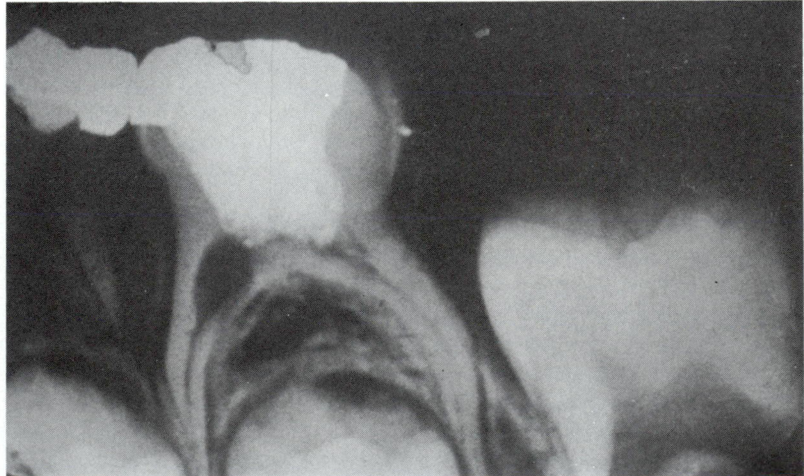

FIG. 23-13 Formocresol pulpotomy failure. Note the internal resorption in the mesial root and the radiolucency in the bifurcation.

underlying pulp tissue remained vital and was free of inflammation. A narrow zone of eosinophilic-stained and compressed fixed tissue was found directly beneath the area of application, which blended into vital normal-appearing tissue apically. With time, the glutaraldehyde-fixed zone is replaced through macrophagic action with dense collagenous tissue; thus the entire root canal tissue is vital.[109]

Glutaraldehyde is absorbed from vital pulpotomy sites but, unlike formocresol which is absorbed and distributed throughout the body within minutes of placement,[152] glutaraldehyde does not perfuse the pulpal tissue to the apex and will demonstrate less systemic distribution immediately after application.[34,115,231] Autoradiographs of isotope-labeled glutaraldehyde show that the drug is limited largely to the pulp space, with little evidence of escape outside the tooth following pulpotomy.[139] No differences have been reported in the incidence of enamel defects on succedaneous teeth with the use of formocresol- or glutaraldehyde-based pulpotomy techniques.[1]

Also unlike formaldehyde, which is mostly tissue bound with only a small fraction being metabolized, glutaraldehyde exhibits very low tissue binding and is readily metabolized. Glutaraldehyde is metabolized mostly in the kidney and lungs but is also found in liver, heart, and muscle tissues.[100,139] Glutaraldehyde is eliminated primarily in urine and expired in gases; 90% of the drug is gone within 3 days.[166]

Virtually no toxic effects have been shown following glutaraldehyde administration either via pulpotomy or systemic application. Large doses (up to 500 times the amount applied in a pulpotomy procedure) caused little toxic effect.[166] Cytotoxicity studies in human pulp fibroblasts showed 2.5% glutaraldehyde to be 15 to 20 times less toxic than formocresol or 19% formaldehyde.[94]

Isotope methods have shown that much of the glutaraldehyde distributed systemically is neutralized by oxidation to carbon dioxide, excretion by the kidney, and binding to plasma proteins.[169] It has also been shown that glutaraldehyde is not incorporated in the nuclear portion of fractionated liver cells, and it is felt to have little potential for chromosomal interference or mutagenicity.[168]

The concentrations of glutaraldehyde and formocresol that are necessary for adequate antimicrobial effect without excessive cytotoxic results have also been reported. A concentration of not less than 3.125% glutaraldehyde is recommended for adequate antimicrobial effect. At this concentration, less cytotoxic effect is exerted on surrounding tissues than by formocresol.[83] It has also been noted that the longer time required for tissue fixation by glutaraldehyde may make its cytotoxicity in clinical applications closer to that of formocresol than was previously reported.[208]

Although glutaraldehyde has been shown to produce antigenic products in much the same manner as formocresol,[164] it has a relatively low antigenicity[167] as compared with formocresol. Unfortunately, purified solutions of glutaraldehyde have been shown to be unstable.[162]

The indications, contraindications, and technique for the glutaraldehyde pulpotomy are the same as for the formocresol pulpotomy, except that glutaraldehyde is substituted for formocresol. Unfortunately, neither the optimal concentration of glutaraldehyde nor the amount of time of application has been conclusively established.

Investigators[62,116,165] have reported the effects of various concentrations and lengths of application of glutaraldehyde. Application of the glutaraldehyde through incorporation in ZOE led to a high failure rate, thus contraindicating this route of administration.[62] Buffering glutaraldehyde, increasing its concentration, and applying it for longer periods all enhance the degree of fixation. Only stronger solutions increase the depth of fixation.[116,165] Increased fixation gives greater resistance to removal and replacement of the fixed tissue. Weak concentrations and short application times lead to more severe inflammatory responses in the underlying pulpal tissue and to eventual failure.[116]

Their research has led Ranly and his associates[165] to recommend 4% buffered glutaraldehyde with a 4-minute application time, or 8% for 2 minutes.

In a 24-month follow-up of pulpotomies performed with 2% glutaraldehyde, the failure rate rose to 18% after 2 years, and the authors could not justify its use over formocresol.[59] Other authors have examined the evidence with regard to toxicity, mutagenicity, and systemic distribution, and do not recommend the substitution of glutaraldehyde for formocresol in pulpotomy technique.[47] The majority of training institutions continue to teach the formocresol technique, and a large majority of practicing pediatric dentists employ formocresol.[7]

Given comparable success rates and the undesirable effects of formocresol and glutaraldehyde, it would seem advisable to substitute the pulpectomy technique for the pulpotomy in primary teeth.[236]

PULPECTOMY IN PRIMARY TEETH

Primary Root Canal Anatomy

To complete endodontic treatment on primary teeth successfully, the clinician must have a thorough knowledge of the anatomy of the primary root canal systems and the variations that normally exist in these systems and to understand some of the variations in the primary root canal systems requires an understanding of root formation.

Root Formation

According to Orban[151] development of the roots begins after enamel and dentin formation has reached the future cementum-enamel junction. The epithelial dental organ forms Hertwig's epithelial root sheath, which initiates formation and molds the shape of the roots. Hertwig's sheath takes the form of one or more epithelial tubes (depending on the number of roots of the tooth, one tube for each root). During root formation the apical foramen of each root has a wide opening limited by the epithelial diaphragm. The dentinal walls taper apically, and the shape of the pulp canal is like a wide open tube. Each root contains one canal at this time, and the number of canals is the same as the number of roots. When root length is established, the sheath disappears but dentin deposition continues internally within the roots.

Differentiation of a root into separate canals, as in the mesial of the mandibular molars, occurs by continued deposition of dentin; this narrows the isthmus between the walls of the canals and continues until there is formation of dentin islands within the root canal and eventual division of the root into separate canals. During the process communications exist between the canals as an isthmus, then as fins connecting the canals. The reader is referred to Chapter 10 for a complete description of pulp and dentin formation.

As growth proceeds, the root canal is narrowed by continued deposition of dentin and the pulp tissue is compressed.

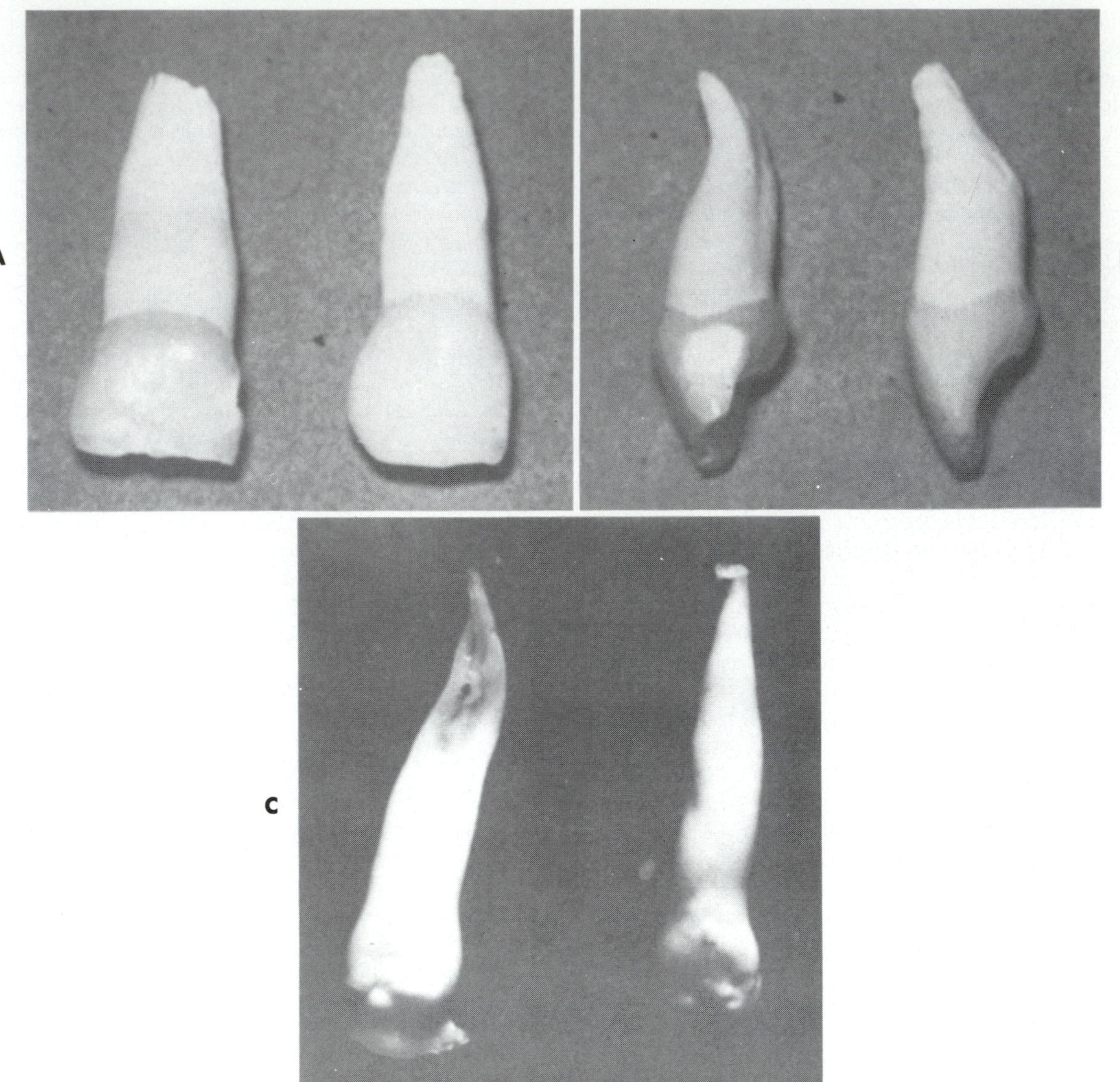

FIG. 23-14 Primary central incisors and silicone models of the pulp canals. **A,** Beginning resorption of the roots on the apical third of the lingual surfaces. **B,** Facial surfaces. **C,** Models. The pulp canals were injected with silicone and the tooth structure decalcified away, leaving a model of the root canal systems. Note the division of the canal on the right.

Additional deposition of dentin and cementum closes the apex of the tooth and creates the apical convergence of the root canals common to the completely formed tooth.

Root length is not completed until 1 to 4 years after a tooth erupts into the oral cavity. In the primary teeth the root length is completed in a shorter period of time than in the permanent tooth because of the shorter length of the primary roots.

The root-to-crown length of the primary teeth is greater than that of the permanent teeth. The primary roots are narrower than the permanent roots. The roots of the primary molars diverge more than those of the permanent teeth. This feature allows more room for the development of the crown of the succeeding premolar.[233]

The primary tooth is unique insofar as resorption of the roots begins soon after formation of the root length has been completed. At this time, the form and shape of the root canals roughly correspond to the form and shape of the external anatomy of the teeth. Root resorption and the deposition of additional dentin within the root canal system, however, significantly change the number, size, and shape of the root canals within the primary tooth.

It should be noted that most of the variations within the root canals of primary teeth are in the facial-lingual plane and that dental radiographs do not show this plane but show the mesial-distal plane. Therefore, when we view radiographs of primary teeth, many of the variations that are present are not visible.

Primary anteriors

The form and shape of the root canals of the primary anterior teeth (Figs. 23-14, 23-15) resemble the form and shape of

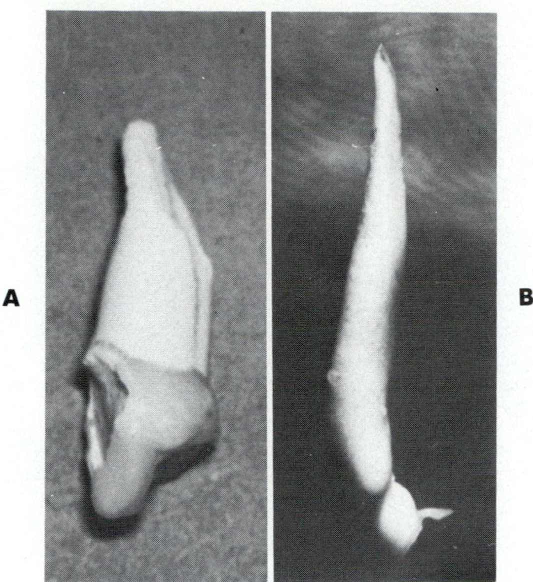

FIG. 23-15 Maxillary primary canine and silicone model of the root canal. **A,** Mesial surface. **B,** Model of the root canal.

the exteriors of the teeth. The permanent tooth bud lies lingual and apical to the primary anterior tooth. Owing to the position of the permanent tooth bud, resorption of the primary incisors and canines is initiated on the lingual surface in the apical third of the roots (Fig. 23-14, *A*).

Maxillary incisors. The root canals of the primary maxillary central and lateral incisors are almost round but somewhat compressed. Normally these teeth have one canal without bifurcations. Apical ramifications or accessory canals and lateral canals are rare but do occur[238] (Fig. 23-14).

Mandibular incisors. The root canals of the primary mandibular central and lateral incisors are flattened on the mesial and distal surfaces and sometimes grooved, pointing to an eventual division into two canals. The presence of two canals is seen less than 10% of the time. Occasionally lateral or accessory canals are observed.[238]

Maxillary and mandibular canines. The root canals of the maxillary and mandibular canines correspond to the exterior root shape, a rounded triangular shape with the base toward the facial surface. Sometimes the lumen of the root canal is compressed in the mesial-distal direction. The canines have the simplest root canal systems of all the primary teeth and offer few problems when being treated endodontically. Bifurcation of the canal does not normally occur. Lateral canals and accessory canals are rare[238] (Fig. 23-15).

Primary molars

The primary molars (Fig. 23-16) normally have the same number of roots and position of the roots as the corresponding permanent molars. The maxillary molars have three roots, two facial and one palatal; the mandibular have two roots, mesial and distal. The roots of the primary molars are long and slender compared with crown length and width, and they diverge to allow for permanent tooth bud formation.

The deposition of secondary dentin in primary teeth has been reported.[14,82,90] When formation of the roots of the primary molars has just been completed, only one root canal is present in each of the roots. After root formation the basic morphologic pattern of the root canals may change, producing variation and alterations in the number and size of the root canals due to the deposition of secondary dentin. This deposition begins at about the time root resorption begins. Variations in form are more pronounced in teeth that show evidence of root resorption.[82]

The most variation in the morphology of the root canals is found in the mesial roots of both maxillary and mandibular primary molars. This variation originates in the apical region as a thinning of the narrow isthmus between the facial and lingual extremities of the apical pulp canals. Subsequent deposition of secondary dentin may produce a complete separation of the root canal into two or more individual canals. Many fine connecting branches or lateral fibrils form a connecting network between the facial and lingual aspects of the root canals.

The variations found in the mesial roots of the primary molars are also found in the distal and lingual roots but to a lesser degree. Accessory canals, lateral canals, and apical ramifications of the pulp are common in primary molars—occurring in 10% to 20%.[82,238]

In the primary molars, resorption usually begins on the inner surfaces of the roots next to the interradicular septum. The effects of resorption on canal anatomy and root canal filling on the primary teeth will be discussed in detail later.

Maxillary first primary molar. The maxillary first primary molar has from two to four canals that roughly correspond to the exterior root form with much variation. The palatal root is often round; it is often longer than the two facial roots. Bifurcation of the mesial-facial root into two canals occurs in approximately 75% of maxillary first primary molars.[82,238]

Fusion of the palatal and distal-facial roots occurs in approximately one third of the maxillary primary first molars. In most of these teeth, two separate canals are present with a very narrow isthmus connecting. Islands of dentin may exist between the canals, with many connecting branches and fibrils (Fig. 23-16, *A*).

Maxillary second primary molar. The maxillary primary molar has two to five canals roughly corresponding to the exterior root shape. The mesial-facial root usually bifurcates or contains two distinct canals. This occurs in approximately 85% to 95% of maxillary second primary molars[82,238] (Fig. 23-16, *B*).

Fusion of the palatal and distal-facial roots sometimes occurs. These fused roots may have a common canal, two distinct canals, or two canals with a narrow connecting isthmus of dentin islands between them and many connecting branches or fibrils.

Mandibular first primary molar. The mandibular first primary molar usually has three canals roughly corresponding to the external root anatomy but may have two to four canals. It is reported that approximately 75% of the mesial roots contain two canals, whereas only 25% of the distal roots contain more than one canal[82,238] (Fig. 23-16, *C* and *D*).

Mandibular second primary molar. The mandibular second primary molar may have two to five canals but usually has three. The mesial root has two canals approximately 85% of the time, whereas the distal root contains more than one canal only 25% of the time[82,238] (Fig. 23-16, *E*).

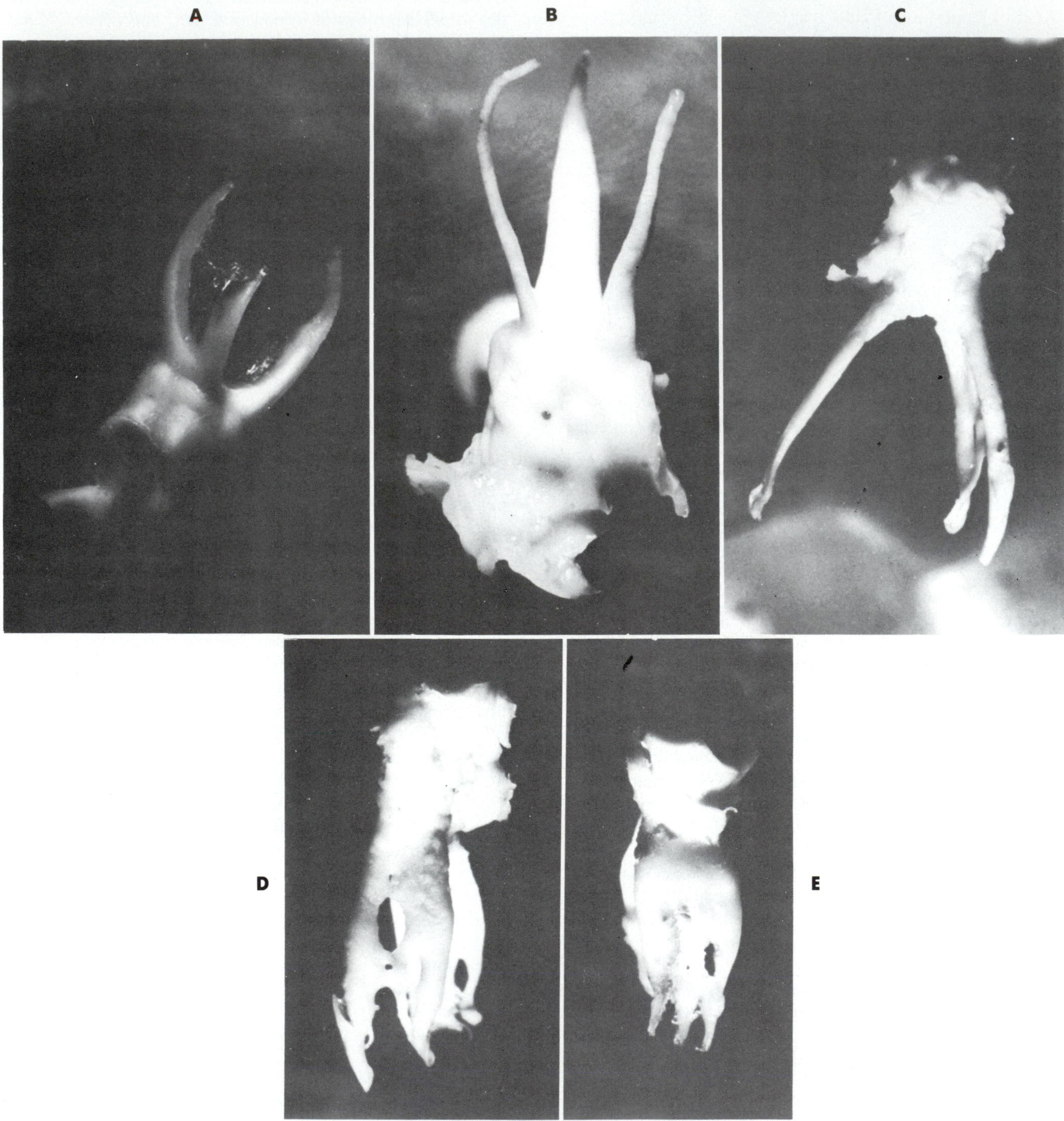

FIG. 23-16 Silicone models of the root canal systems of primary molars. **A,** Maxillary first molar. Note the fused distal and palatal roots. Note the thin fin connecting the roots. **B,** Maxillary second molar, facial surface. **C,** Mandibular first molar, facial view. **D,** Same tooth from the mesial surface. Note the connecting fibrils between the facial and lingual canals. **E,** Mandibular second molar, distal view. Three canals are present.

ROLE OF RESORPTION ON CANAL ANATOMY AND APICAL FORAMINA

In the newly completed roots of the primary teeth, the apical foramina are located near the anatomic apices of the roots. After the deposition of additional dentin and cementum, there are multiple apical ramifications of the pulp as it exits the root, just as in the mature permanent tooth.

Because of the position of the permanent tooth bud, physiologic resorption of the roots of the primary incisors and canines is initiated on the lingual surfaces in the apical third of the roots. In the primary molars, resorption usually begins on the inner surfaces of the roots near the interradicular septum.

As resorption progresses, the apical foramen may not correspond to the anatomic apex of the root but be coronal to it. Therefore radiographic establishment of the root canal length may be erroneous. Resorption may extend through the roots and into the root canals, creating additional communications with the periapical tissues other than through the apical foramina or lateral and accessory canals (Fig. 23-17).

Permanent Tooth Bud

The effects of primary endodontic therapy on the developing permanent tooth bud should be of paramount concern to the clinician.

Manipulation through the apex of the primary tooth is contraindicated since the permanent tooth bud lies immediately adjacent to the apex of the primary tooth. Overextension of root canal instruments and filling materials must be avoided. If signs of resorption are visible radiographically, it is advisable to establish the working length of endodontic instruments 2 or 3 mm short of the radiographic apex. The use of the radiographic paralleling technique with a long cone for maximum accuracy when measuring canal lengths is recommended.

Anesthesia is usually necessary for pulp extirpation and enlargement of the canals but is rarely needed when primary teeth are filled at a subsequent appointment. The response of the patient can sometimes be used as a guide to the approach to the apex and as a check to the length of the canal that was previously established radiographically. Hemorrhage after pulp removal indicates overextension into the periapical tissues.

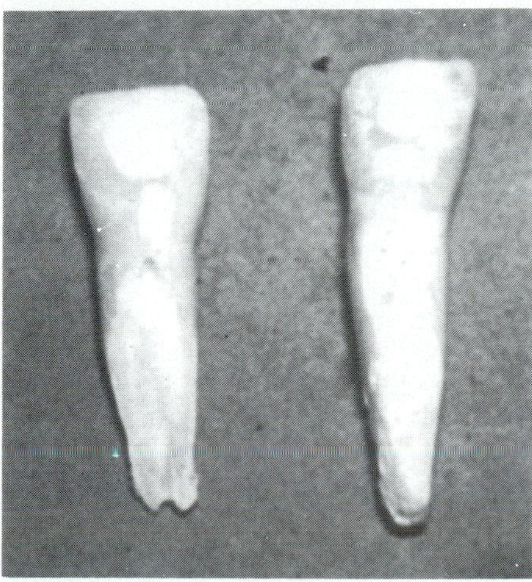

FIG. 23-17 These two primary mandibular incisors have lingual and apical resorption. Note that the left incisor has the apical foramen just beneath the cervical line whereas the right one has its apical foramen at the apex of the root.

The filling material utilized to obliterate the root canals on primary teeth must be absorbable so it can be absorbed as the tooth resorbs and so it offers no resistance or deflection to the eruption of the permanent tooth. *Materials such as gutta-percha or silver points are contraindicated as primary root canal fillers.*

Pulpectomy

Pulpectomy and root canal filling procedures on primary teeth have been the subject of much controversy. Fear of damage to developing permanent tooth buds and a belief that the tortuous root canals of primary teeth could not be adequately negotiated, cleaned, shaped, and filled have led to the needless sacrifice of many pulpally involved primary teeth.

Much has been written regarding potential damage to the developing permanent tooth bud from root canal fillings. While magnifying these dangers, many authors have advocated extraction of pulpally involved primary teeth and placement of space maintainers. However, there is no better space maintainer than the primary tooth. Also, nothing has been written concerning the damage of space maintainers on existing teeth in the mouth. For many space maintainers that are placed, adequate follow-up is not achieved because of the carelessness of either the patient or the clinician. Decalcification and rampant caries are frequent sequelae of loosened bands retained for extended periods of time. Poor oral hygiene around space maintainers contributes to increased decay and gingival problems. Deflection of erupting permanent teeth because of prolonged retention of space maintainers is sometimes encountered. Loss of space maintainers with resulting space loss can occur if the patient delays returning for treatment. These are a few of the problems that may be avoided by retention of the pulpally involved primary tooth when possible.

It has been reported[85] that while severe hypoplasia and disturbances in root development do not intensify, minor hypoplasia is increased in succedaneous teeth after root canal treatment of the primary precursors. However, all such studies are retrospective, involving erupted permanent teeth, and cannot ascertain damage as a result of injury or the infection that necessitated root canal therapy.

Economics has been advanced as an argument against endodontic treatment of primary teeth, but it is not a reasonable argument when compared with the cost of space maintainers, including the required follow-up treatment. In fact, endodontic treatment is probably the less expensive of the two alternatives when the entire treatment sequence is considered.

Success of endodontic treatment on primary teeth is judged by the same criteria that are used for permanent teeth. The treated primary tooth must remain firmly attached in function without pain or infection. Radiographic signs of furcal and periapical infection should be resolved, with a normal periodontal attachment. The primary tooth should resorb normally and in no way interfere with the formation or eruption of the permanent tooth.

Success rates ranging from 75% to 96% have been reported.[2,113,236] The usual means of studying root canal filling on primary teeth have been clinical and radiographic. There exists a great need for histologic study in this area.

Early reports of endodontic treatment on primary teeth usually involved devitalization with arsenic in vital teeth and the use of creosote, formocresol, or paraformaldehyde pastes in nonvital teeth. The canals were filled with a variety of materials, usually consisting of zinc oxide and numerous additives.[41,66,96,200]

The first well-documented scientific report of endodontic procedures on primary teeth was published by Rabinowitch in 1953.[161] A 13-year study of 1363 cases of partially or totally nonvital primary molars was reported. Only seven cases were failures. Most patients were followed for 1 or 2 years clinically and radiographically. Fillings of ZOE and silver nitrate were placed only after a negative culture was obtained for each tooth. Periapically involved teeth required an average of 7.7 visits to complete treatment; teeth with no periapical involvement required an average of 5.5 visits. Rabinowitch listed internal resorption and gross pathologic external resorption as contraindications to primary root canal fillings.

Another well-documented study reported a success rate of 95% in both vital and infected teeth using a filling material of thymol, cresol, iodoform, and zinc oxide.[2]

The reader is referred to Bennett[10] for a review of the techniques of partial and total pulpectomy.

In a well-controlled clinical study of primary root canals utilizing Oxpara paste as the filling material,[113] five preexisting factors were reported to render the prognosis less favorable: perforation of the furca, excessive external resorption of roots, internal resorption, extensive bone loss, and periodontal involvement of the furca. When teeth with these factors were eliminated, a clinical success rate of 96% was achieved. When all symptoms of residual infection were resolved before filling of the canals, the success rate improved. No radiographic evidence of damage to the permanent teeth was noted.

After reviewing the literature on root canal fillings on primary teeth, one is impressed with the lack of histologic material in this area. There exists a great need for further research on the subject.

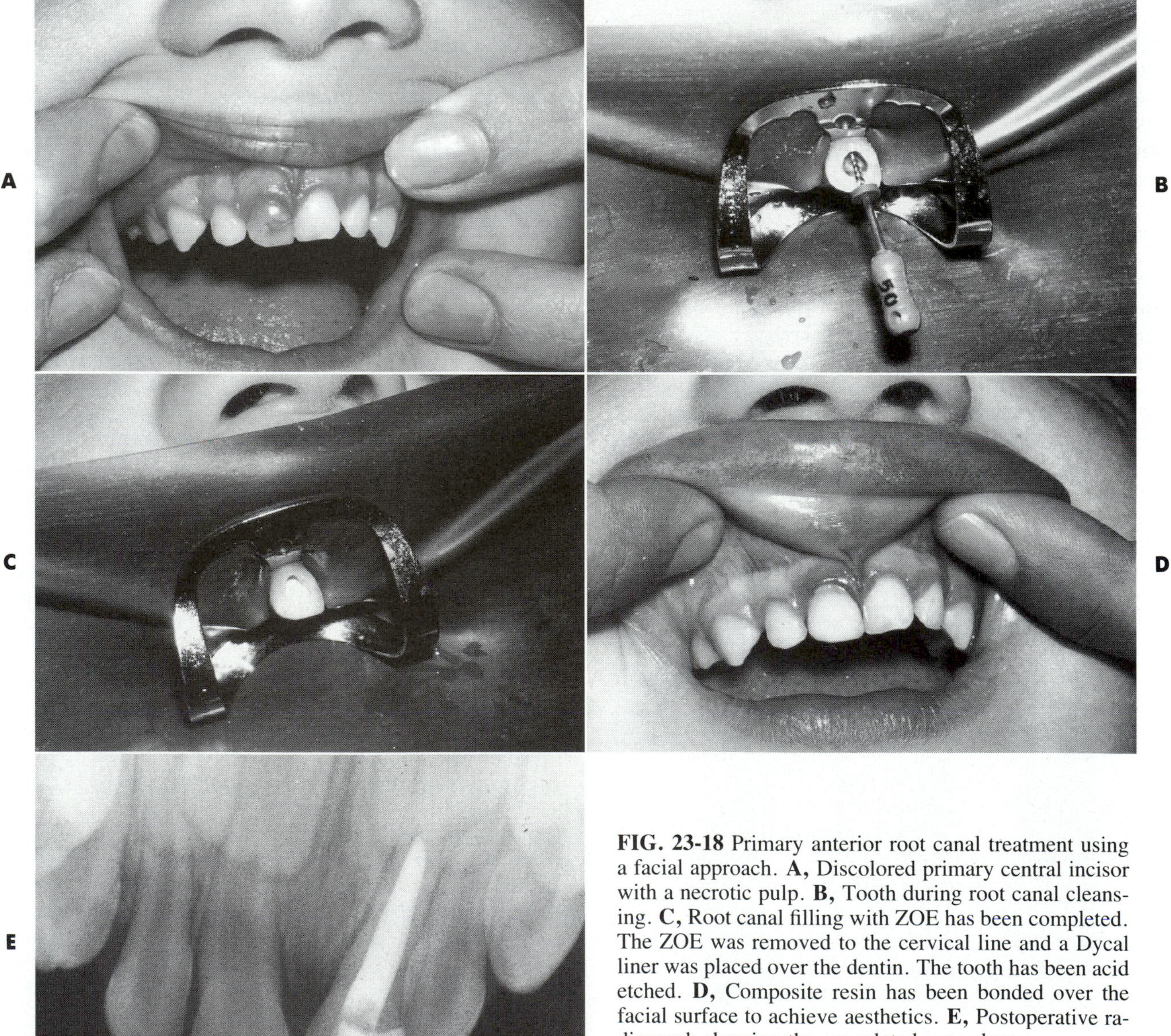

FIG. 23-18 Primary anterior root canal treatment using a facial approach. **A,** Discolored primary central incisor with a necrotic pulp. **B,** Tooth during root canal cleansing. **C,** Root canal filling with ZOE has been completed. The ZOE was removed to the cervical line and a Dycal liner was placed over the dentin. The tooth has been acid etched. **D,** Composite resin has been bonded over the facial surface to achieve aesthetics. **E,** Postoperative radiograph showing the completed procedures.

Contraindications for Primary Root Canal Fillings

Except for the following situations, all primary teeth with pulpal involvement that has spread beyond the coronal pulp are candidates for root canal fillings whether they are vital or nonvital:

1. A nonrestorable tooth
2. Radiographically visible internal resorption in the roots
3. Teeth with mechanical or carious perforations of the floor of the pulp chamber
4. Excessive pathologic root resorption involving more than one third of the root
5. Excessive pathologic loss of bone support with loss of the normal periodontal attachment
6. The presence of a dentigerous or follicular cyst

Internal resorption usually begins just inside the root canals near the furcation area. Because of the thinness of the roots of the primary teeth, once internal resorption has become visible radiographically, there is invariably a perforation of the root by the resorption (Fig. 23-3). The short furcal surface area of the primary teeth leads to rapid communication between the inflammatory process and the oral cavity through the periodontal attachment. The end result is loss of the periodontal attachment of the tooth, and ultimately further resorption and loss of the tooth.

Mechanical or carious perforations of the floor of the pulp chamber fail for the same reasons.

ACCESS OPENINGS FOR PULPECTOMY ON PRIMARY TEETH

Anterior Teeth

Access openings for endodontic treatment on primary or permanent anterior teeth have traditionally been through the lingual surface. This continues to be the surface of choice except for the maxillary primary incisors. Because of problems associated with the discoloration of endodontically treated primary incisors, it has been recommended to use a facial approach followed by an acid etch composite restoration to improve aesthetics (Fig. 23-18).[120] Bleaching techniques which are quite successful in permanent teeth are unsuccessful in primary teeth.

Many maxillary primary incisors requiring pulpectomy have discoloration caused by the escape of hemosiderin pigments into the dentinal tubules following a previous traumatic injury. Subsequent to pulpectomy and root canal filling, most primary incisors discolor.

The anatomy of the maxillary primary incisors is such that access may successfully be made from the facial surface. The only variation to the opening is more extension to the incisal edge than with the normal lingual access in order to give as straight an approach as possible into the root canal.

The root canal is filled with ZOE (see below), then the ZOE is carefully removed to near the cervical line. A liner of Dycal or Life is placed over the ZOE to serve as a barrier between the composite resin and the root canal filling. The liner is extended over the darkly stained lingual dentin to serve as an opaquer. The access opening and entire facial surface are acid-etched and restored with composite resin (Fig. 23-18).

Posterior Teeth

Access openings into the posterior primary root canals are essentially the same as those for the permanent teeth. (Chapter 7 contains a detailed description of access openings.) Important differences between the primary and permanent teeth are the length of the crowns, the bulbous shape of the crowns, and the very thin dentinal walls of the pulpal floors and roots. The depth necessary to penetrate into the pulpal chamber is quite less than that in the permanent teeth. Likewise, the distance from the occlusal surface to the pulpal floor of the pulp chamber is much less than in permanent teeth. In the primary molars, care must be taken not to grind on the pulpal floor since perforation is likely (Fig. 23-19).

When the roof of the pulp chamber is perforated and the pulp chamber identified, the entire roof should be removed with the bur. Since the crowns of the primary teeth are more bulbous, less extension toward the exterior of the tooth is necessary to uncover the openings of the root canals than in the permanent teeth.

Canal Cleaning and Shaping

Use of the rubber dam is essential in any endodontic procedure. As in permanent endodontic therapy, canal cleaning and shaping is one of the most important phases of primary endodontic therapy. The principles and techniques for permanent teeth described in detail in Chapter 8 are also advocated for primary teeth. The main objective of the chemical-mechanical preparation of the primary tooth is débridement of the canals. Although an apical taper to the canals is desirable, it is not necessary to have an exact shape to the canals as is necessary for gutta-percha fillings.

The importance of establishing a correct working length has been discussed (Chapter 8). To prevent overextension through the apical foramen, it is suggested that the working length be shortened 2 or 3 mm short of the radiographic root length, especially in teeth showing signs of apical root resorption.

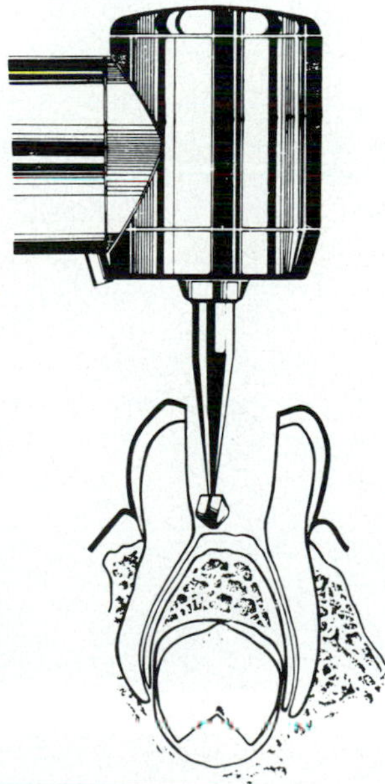

FIG. 23-19 Access opening in primary molar. A no. 4 round bur has been used to remove the roof of the pulp chamber and the dentin ledges over the canal orifices. Note the minimal length of the bur needed to penetrate to the pulpal floor. Caution must be exercised to avoid perforation of the pulpal floor. (From Goerig AC and Camp JH: Pediatr Dent 5:33, 1983.)

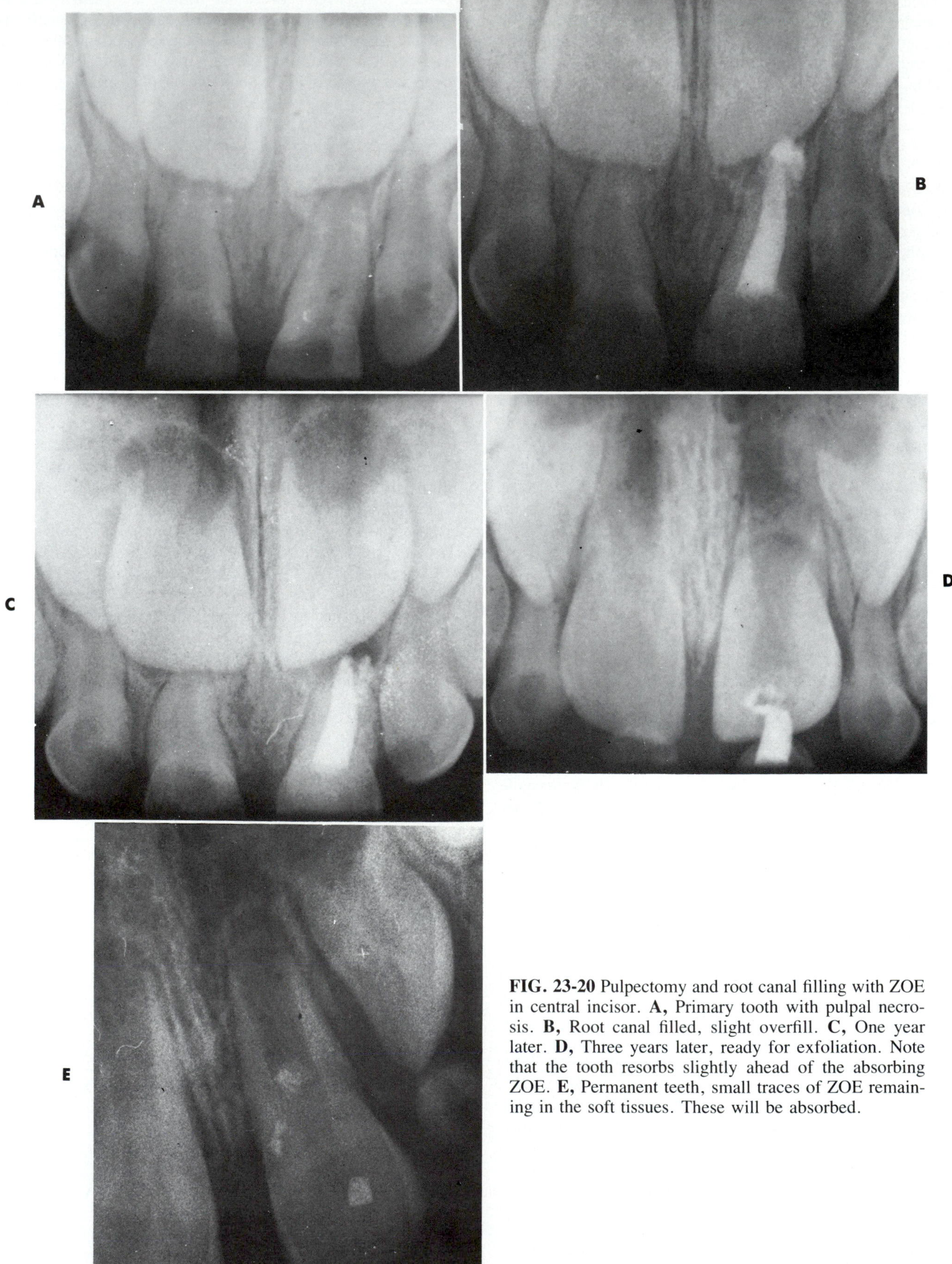

FIG. 23-20 Pulpectomy and root canal filling with ZOE in central incisor. **A,** Primary tooth with pulpal necrosis. **B,** Root canal filled, slight overfill. **C,** One year later. **D,** Three years later, ready for exfoliation. Note that the tooth resorbs slightly ahead of the absorbing ZOE. **E,** Permanent teeth, small traces of ZOE remaining in the soft tissues. These will be absorbed.

When working length is established (Fig. 23-22, *B*), the canal is cleaned and shaped as described in Chapter 8. The use of the Gates-Glidden drills is contraindicated; or if the drills are used, they must be confined simply to flaring the opening into the canals. Gates-Glidden drills should not be used in the canals because of the danger of perforation. Likewise, because of the thin walls of the roots, sonic and ultrasonic cleaning devices should not be utilized to prepare the canals of primary teeth.

Instruments should be gently curved to help negotiate canals, as described in Chapter 8. Shaping of the canals proceeds in much the same manner as is done to receive a gutta-percha filling. Care must be taken not to perforate the thin roots during cleaning and shaping procedures. The canals are enlarged several file sizes past the first file that fits snugly into the canal, with a minimum size of 30 to 35.

Since many of the pulpal ramifications cannot be reached mechanically, copious irrigation during cleaning and shaping must be maintained (Chapter 8). Débridement of the primary root canal is more often accomplished by chemical means than by mechanical means.[108] This statement should not be misinterpreted as a deemphasis of the importance of thorough débridement and disinfection of the canal. The use of sodium hypochlorite to digest organic debris and RC-Prep to produce effervescence must play an important part in removal of tissue from the inaccessible areas of the root canal system.

After canal débridement the canals are again copiously flushed with sodium hypochlorite and are then dried with sterile paper points; a pellet of cotton is barely moistened with camphorated parachlorophenol and sealed into the pulp chamber with a temporary cement.

At a subsequent appointment the rubber dam is placed and the canals reentered. As long as the patient is free of all signs and symptoms of inflammation, the canals are again irrigated with sodium hypochlorite and dried preparatory to filling. If signs or symptoms of inflammation are present, the canals are recleaned and remedicated and the filling procedure delayed until a later time.

Filling of the Primary Root Canals

The filling material for primary root canals must be absorbable so it will absorb as the roots resorb and will not interfere with the eruption of the permanent tooth. *The filling material of choice is ZOE without a catalyst.* The lack of a catalyst is necessary to allow adequate working time for filling the canals. The use of gutta-percha or silver points as primary root canal fillers is contraindicated.

The filling of the primary tooth is usually performed without a local anesthetic. This is preferable if possible so the patient's response can be utilized to indicate approach to the apical foramen. It is, however, sometimes necessary to anesthetize the gingiva with a drop of anesthetic solution to place the rubber dam clamp without pain.

The ZOE is mixed to a thick consistency and is carried into the pulp chamber with a plastic instrument or on a Lentulo. The material may be packed into the canals with pluggers or the Lentulo. A cotton pellet held in cotton pliers and acting as a piston within the pulp chambers is quite effective in forcing the ZOE into the canals. The endodontic pressure syringe[12,69] is also effective for placing the ZOE in the root canals.

Regardless of the method utilized to fill the canals, care should be used to prevent extrusion of the material into the periapical tissues. The adequacy of the obturation is checked by radiographs (Figs. 23-20 through 23-22).

In the event a small amount of the ZOE is inadvertently forced through the apical foramen, it is left alone since the material is absorbable.

When the canals are satisfactorily obturated, a fast-set temporary cement is placed in the pulp chamber to seal over the ZOE canal filling. The tooth may then be restored permanently.

In the primary molars it is advisable to place a stainless steel crown as the permanent restoration to prevent possible fracture of the tooth.

When the succedaneous permanent tooth is missing and the retained primary tooth becomes pulpally involved, the canals are filled with gutta-percha following pulpectomy. Since erup-

F

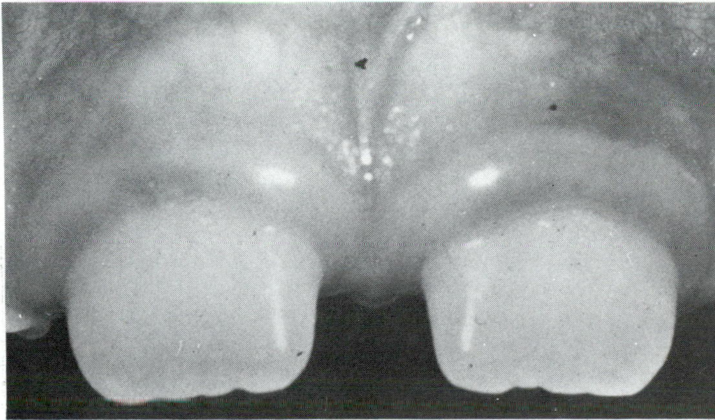

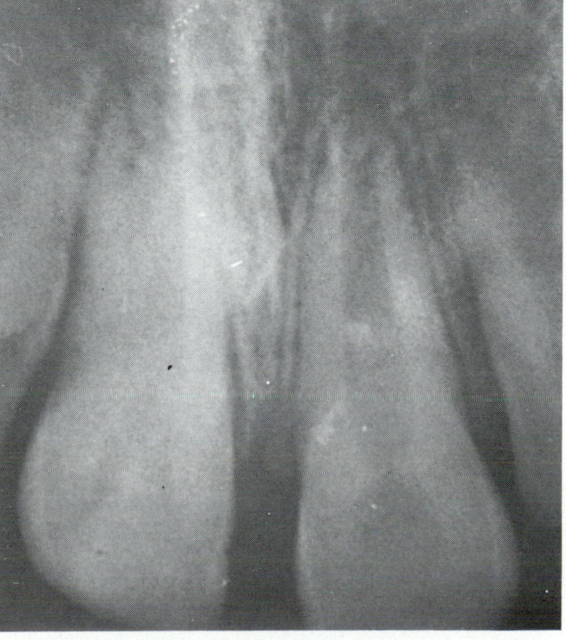

G

FIG. 23-20, cont'd F, The permanent central incisors newly erupted. Note that no defects are present on the crown even though there was a slight overfill of the primary root canal filling. **G,** Five years after pulpectomy and root canal filling. Note the normal apical closure and the almost total absorption of the ZOE remnants.

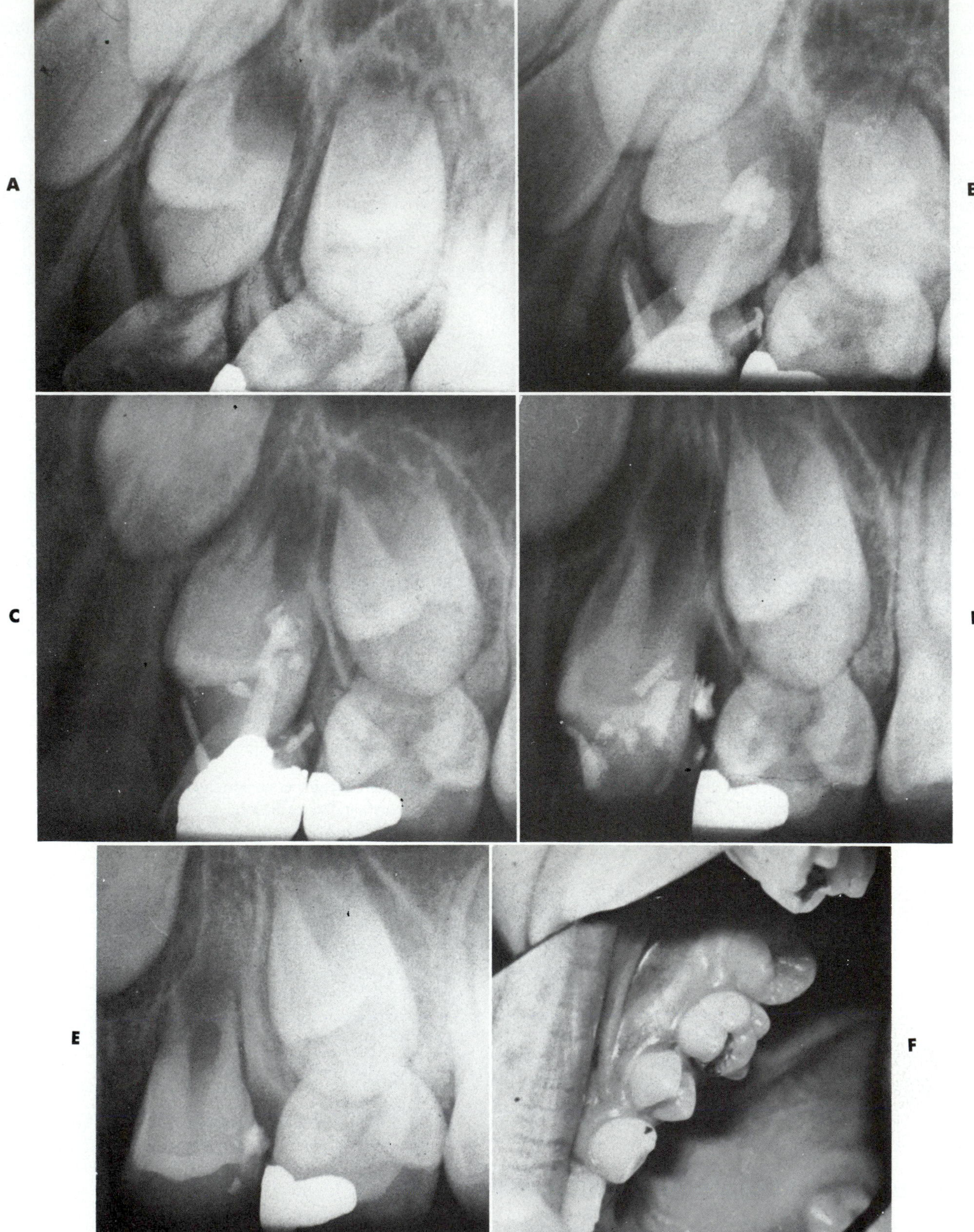

FIG. 23-21 Pulpectomy and root canal filling with ZOE in a maxillary posterior tooth. **A,** Carious exposure of a primary first molar. **B,** Root canals filled with ZOE. **C,** One year later. **D,** Two and one half years later. The tooth is ready to exfoliate. **E,** Erupted permanent premolar. Note the slight amount of ZOE retained in the soft tissue. The ZOE will undergo absorption. **F,** Note the permanent crown, free of defects.

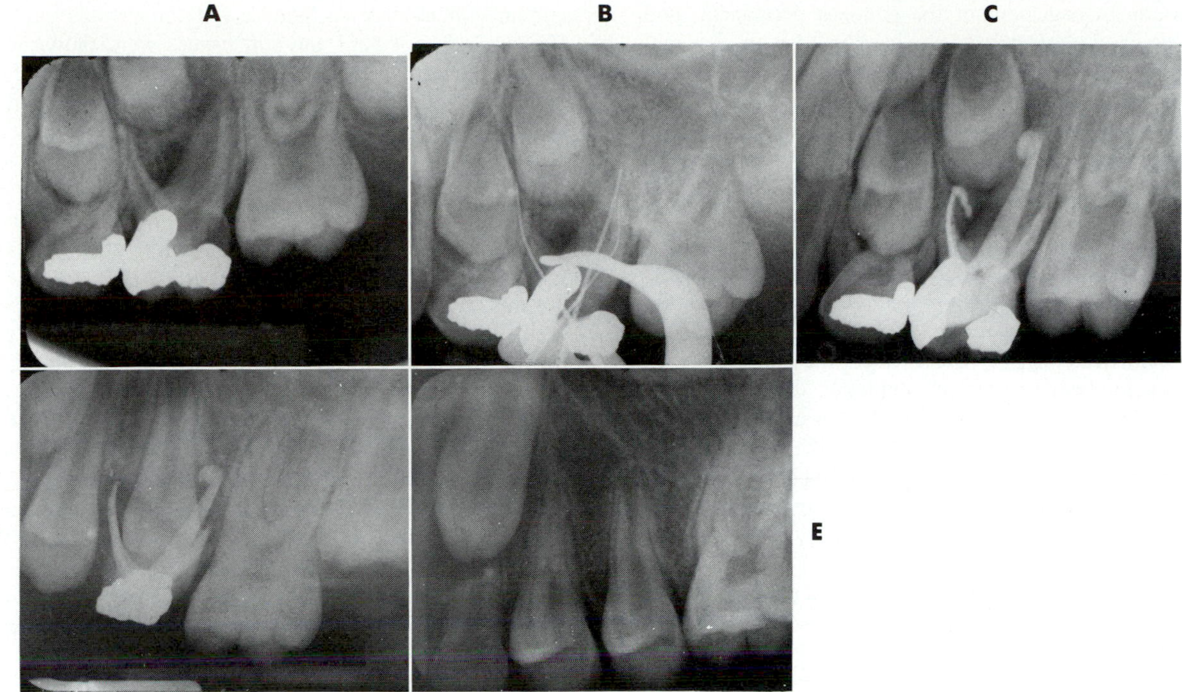

FIG. 23-22 Pulpectomy and root canal filling with ZOE in a maxillary primary second molar. **A,** Carious pulp exposure with a chronic abscess. Note the furcal and periapical radiolucencies. **B,** Instruments in place establishing the working length. **C,** Root canal filled with ZOE. **D,** Four and one half years following root canal treatment. The tooth is near exfoliation. **E,** One year later. The premolar is fully erupted and all traces of the ZOE have been resorbed.

tion of the permanent tooth is not a factor in these cases, gutta-percha is substituted for ZOE as the filling material of choice (Fig. 23-23).

Follow-up after Primary Pulpectomy

As previously stated, the rate of success following primary pulpectomy is high. However, these teeth should be periodically recalled to check for success of the treatment and to intercept any problem associated with a failure. While resorbing normally without interference with the eruption of the permanent tooth, the primary tooth should remain asymptomatic, firm in the alveolus, and free of pathosis. If evidence of pathosis is detected, extraction and conventional space maintenance are recommended.

It has been pointed out[203] that pulpally treated primary teeth may occasionally present a problem of overretention. After normal physiologic resorption of the roots reaches the pulp chamber, the large amount of ZOE present may impair the absorption and lead to prolonged retention of the crown. Treatment usually consists of simply removing the crown and allowing the permanent tooth to complete its eruption.

APEXIFICATION

A thorough knowledge of normal root formation is necessary to help one understand the processes involved in treating the pulpless permanent tooth with a wide-open immature apex.

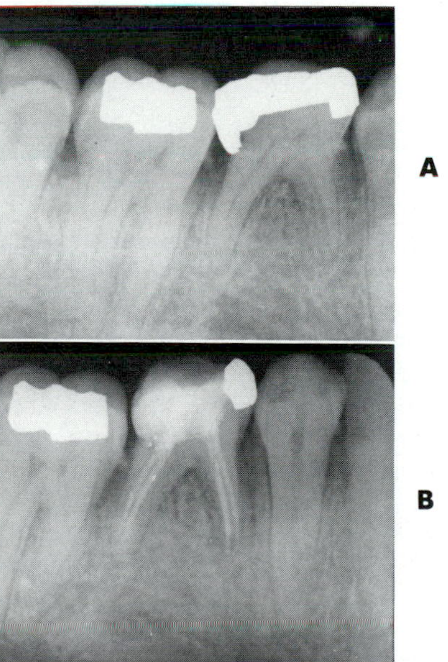

FIG. 23-23 Pulpectomy and root canal filling with gutta-percha in a retained mandibular primary second molar with no succedaneous permanent tooth. **A,** Carious exposure of pulp. **B,** Because the permanent premolar is absent, the root canals of the primary tooth were filled with gutta-percha rather than ZOE.

Endodontic management of the pulpless permanent tooth with a wide-open blunderbuss apex has long presented a challenge to dentistry. Prior to the introduction of apical closure techniques, the usual approach to this problem was surgical. Although the surgical approach was successful, the mechanical and psychologic aspects offered many contraindications. In the pulpless tooth with an incompletely formed apex, the thin fragile dentinal walls made it difficult to achieve an apical seal. When a portion of the root was removed to obtain a seal, the crown-root ratio was poor. Since this situation was usually present in the child patient, a less traumatic approach was desirable.

Many techniques have been advocated to manage the pulpless permanent tooth with an incompletely developed apex. The canals are cleaned and filled with a temporary paste to stimulate the formation of calcified tissue at the apex. The temporary paste is later removed after radiographic evidence of apical closure has been obtained and a permanent filling of gutta-percha is placed in the canal. The term *apexification* is used to describe this procedure.[205]

Many materials have been reported to successfully stimulate apexification. The use of calcium hydroxide for apexification in the pulpless tooth was first reported by Kaiser in 1964.[97] The technique was popularized by the work of Frank.[51] Since that time, $Ca(OH)_2$ alone or in combination with other drugs has become the most widely accepted material to promote apexification.

The calcium hydroxide powder has been mixed with camphorated parachlorophenol (CMCP), metacresyl acetate, Cresanol (a mixture of CMCP and metacresyl acetate), physiologic saline, Ringer's solution, distilled water, and anesthetic solution. Although some of these materials appear to enhance the action of the $Ca(OH)_2$ better than others, all have been reported to stimulate apexification. Most reports in the American literature[22,71,204] have advocated mixing the $Ca(OH)_2$ with CMCP or Cresanol, whereas reports from other parts of the world[27,125] show the same success using distilled water or physiologic saline as the vehicle with which the $Ca(OH)_2$ is mixed.

Materials like ZnO pastes,[25] antibiotic pastes,[8,79] Walkoff's paste,[19] and Diaket[54] have also been reported to promote apexification successfully. Similar results have been achieved after bleeding into the canal was stimulated by laceration of granulation tissue outside the canal.[149]

Attempts at apexification with calcium chloride[92] and barium hydroxide[195] have proved unsuccessful. However, the addition of barium sulfate to calcium hydroxide to enhance radiopacity has been shown to produce apexification. The recommended ratio of barium sulfate is one part added to eight parts calcium hydroxide.[227,228] Diatrizoate (organic iodine) has also been effectively utilized as a radiopaquer.[193] An endodontist's report[227] provides a better review of this literature.

In the teeth of humans and primates, tricalcium phosphate promotes apexification similar to that found with $Ca(OH)_2$.[107,173] The material has also been packed into the apical 2 mm of the canal to act as a barrier against which gutta-percha is condensed.[26] The treatment was achieved in one appointment. Using radiographic assessment, the authors reported successful apexification comparable to that achieved in multiple appointments with $Ca(OH)_2$.[26]

Collagen-calcium phosphate gel has been reported to produce apexification faster than $Ca(OH)_2$ in animals and humans. Various forms of hard and soft tissues were shown revitalizing pulpless root canals within 12 weeks. Formation of cementum, bone, and reparative dentin was noted within the connective tissue ingrowths; a normal periodontal ligament and the absence of ankylosis was also noted. The gel appears to function as an absorbable matrix, supporting hard tissue growth into the débrided root canals.[144-146] In contrast to this, however, another investigator[24] showed that collagen–calcium phosphate gel inhibits the reparative process, with extensive destruction of periapical tissues and no evidence of apexification. Despite the fact that this area of research shows promise for the future, at present it must be considered experimental.

Although apexification will occur with many materials, it has been reported even without the presence of canal filling material after removal of the necrotic pulp tissue.[45] The most important factors in achieving apexification seem to be thorough débridement of the root canal (to remove all necrotic pulp tissue) and sealing of the tooth (to prevent the ingress of bacteria and substrate). It has been noted that apexification will not occur when the apex of the tooth penetrates the cortical plate. To be successful, the apex must be completely within the confines of the cortical plates.[228]

Although highly successful, apexification should be the treatment of last resort in a tooth with an incompletely formed root. Attention should be focused on the maintenance of vitality in these teeth so that as much root length and dentin formation as possible can occur in the root. Indirect pulp therapy and vital pulp-capping and pulpotomy techniques have proved to be successful, aided by the tremendous blood supply present with the open apex. These procedures should be the treatment of choice if there is the possibility of success with any of them. When the tooth with an incompletely formed apex becomes pulpless or periapical disease has developed, apexification is the preferred treatment.

Apexification has been reported in an adult following failed conventional endodontic treatment and apicoectomy performed in childhood.[232] It has also been achieved during active orthodontic treatment.[3]

Determination of the extent of apical closure is many times difficult to ascertain. Radiographic interpretation of apical closure is often misleading. It must always be remembered that the dental radiograph is a two-dimensional picture of a three-dimensional object. Under normal conditions the dental radiograph shows the mesial-distal plane of the tooth rather than the facial-lingual plane. The facial-lingual aspect of the root canal, however, is usually the last to become convergent apically as the root develops. Therefore it is possible to have a dental radiograph showing an apically convergent root canal while in the facial-lingual plane the root canal is divergent (Fig. 23-24).

In teeth with vital tissue remaining in the root canal, techniques to maintain the vitality, rather than pulpectomy, should be utilized until complete root formation has occurred.

Technique

Diagnosis of pulpal necrosis in the tooth with an incompletely formed apex is sometimes difficult unless a frank exposure of the pulp chamber exists.

The usual cause of endodontic involvement in a tooth with an incompletely developed root is trauma. A detailed history

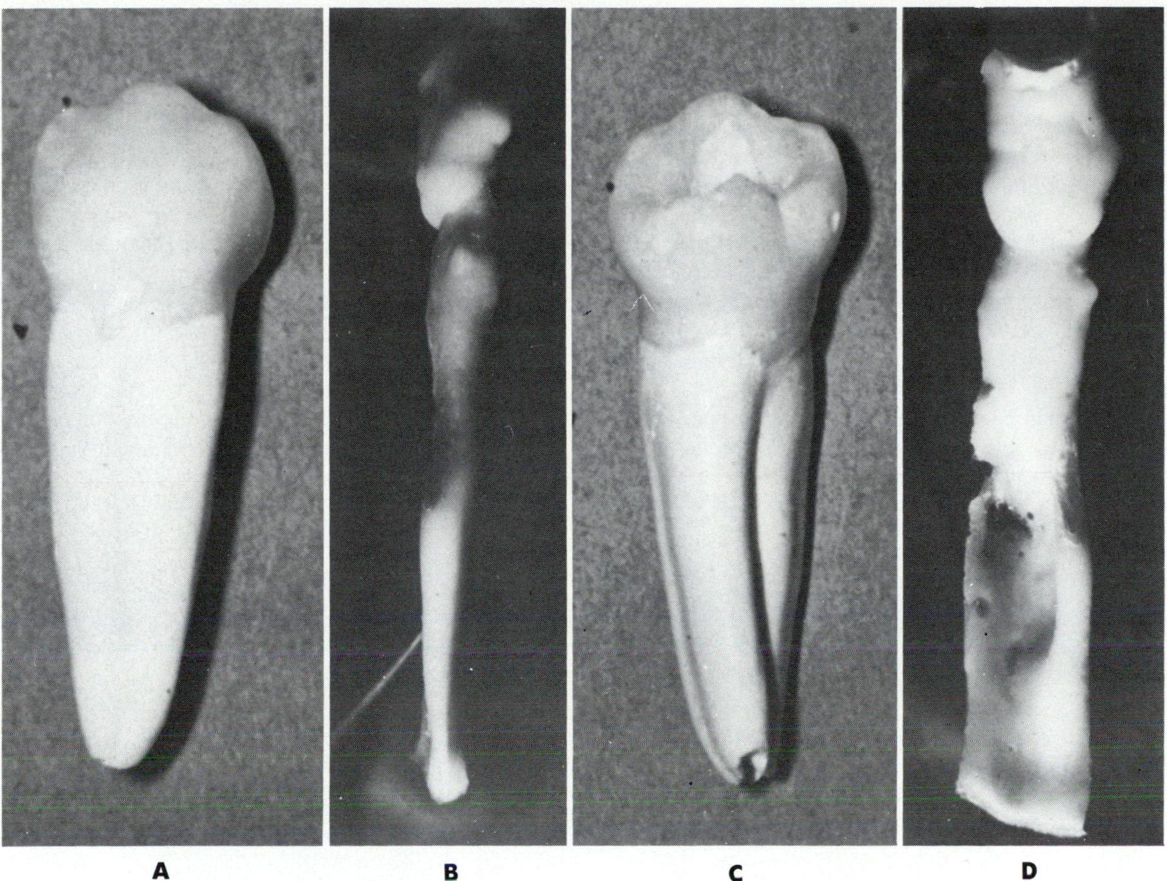

FIG. 23-24 Extracted mandibular premolar and silicone model of the root system. **A,** Facial view. **B,** Model from the facial surface. Note that the root canal diverges apically, which would correspond to the radiographic view of the tooth in the mouth. **C,** Lingual view. **D,** Model from the proximal view, apically divergent canal. With further development the root canal system will divide into two canals.

of any injury is of prime importance from both a diagnostic and a treatment point of view as well as documentation for insurance and dental-legal reasons.

Radiographic diagnosis of disease is complicated in these teeth because of the normal radiolucency occurring at the apex as the root matures. Comparison of root formation with that in contralateral teeth should always be considered.

The electric pulp tester usually will not provide meaningful data in teeth with incompletely formed roots. Thermal tests are more reliable for ascertaining vitality but may be complicated by the reliability of the response in the young child.

The presence of acute or chronic pain, percussion sensitivity, mobility, and any discoloration of the crown should be considered in the diagnosis.

In the tooth without a pulp exposure—if any doubt persists after all the foregoing tests have been completed—take a watch and wait approach before entering the tooth endodontically to be certain that conclusive evidence of pulpal necrosis exists. If dentin exposure is present, the tooth must be restored in such a manner as to prevent any further pulpal irritation.

In the apexification technique the canal is cleaned and sanitized in the routine endodontic manner. (See Chapter 8 for an in-depth discussion of this technique.) As in any endodontic procedure, the use of the rubber dam is mandatory.

The access opening is made as usual but may require some extension, especially in the anterior teeth, to accommodate the larger-sized instruments necessary to clean the root canals.

The length of the canal is established radiographically and the canal is cleaned as thoroughly as possible. Frequent irrigation with sodium hypochlorite helps remove debris from the canal. Since the coronal half of the root canal is of smaller diameter than the apical half, root canal instruments that are smaller than the canal space must be utilized. Thus, while mechanically cleaning and shaping the canal, lean the instruments toward each surface of the tooth to contact all surfaces of the root because the canal diverges apically. Sonic and ultrasonic devices are extremely helpful in debriding the canal.

After thorough débridement the canal is dried and just *barely* medicated with CMCP or some other suitable intracanal medicament. It is then sealed with a temporary cement.

If symptoms persist or any signs of infection are present at a subsequent appointment, or if the canal cannot be dried, the débridement phase is repeated and the canal is medicated with a slurry of $Ca(OH)_2$ paste and sealed.

When the tooth is free of signs and symptoms of infection, the canal is dried and filled with a stiff mix of $Ca(OH)_2$ and CMCP. The filling procedure is usually performed without the use of local anesthetic. This is preferable if possible so the patient's response can be utilized to indicate the approach to the apical foramen.

The material should be spatulated as little as possible since spatulation decreases the working time and may cause the material to set into a hard mass before the filling procedure is completed. If this happens, the canal may contain voids and should be recleaned and the filling procedure is then repeated.

The paste may be carried into the canal with an amalgam carrier, Lentulo spiral, disposable syringe, or endodontic pressure syringe. Pluggers are helpful for packing the material to the apex. The addition of some dry $Ca(OH)_2$ powder within the canal by means of an amalgam carrier will aid in condensing the paste of the apex. The canal should ideally be completely filled with the paste but should not be overfilled. The response of the patient is used as a guide in approaching the apex; however, because of differences in patient response, this method is not wholly reliable. Radiographic checks of the depth of the filling are essential to verify an adequate filling. The addition of small amounts of barium sulfate to the paste aids in radiographic interpretation without altering the response of the material.

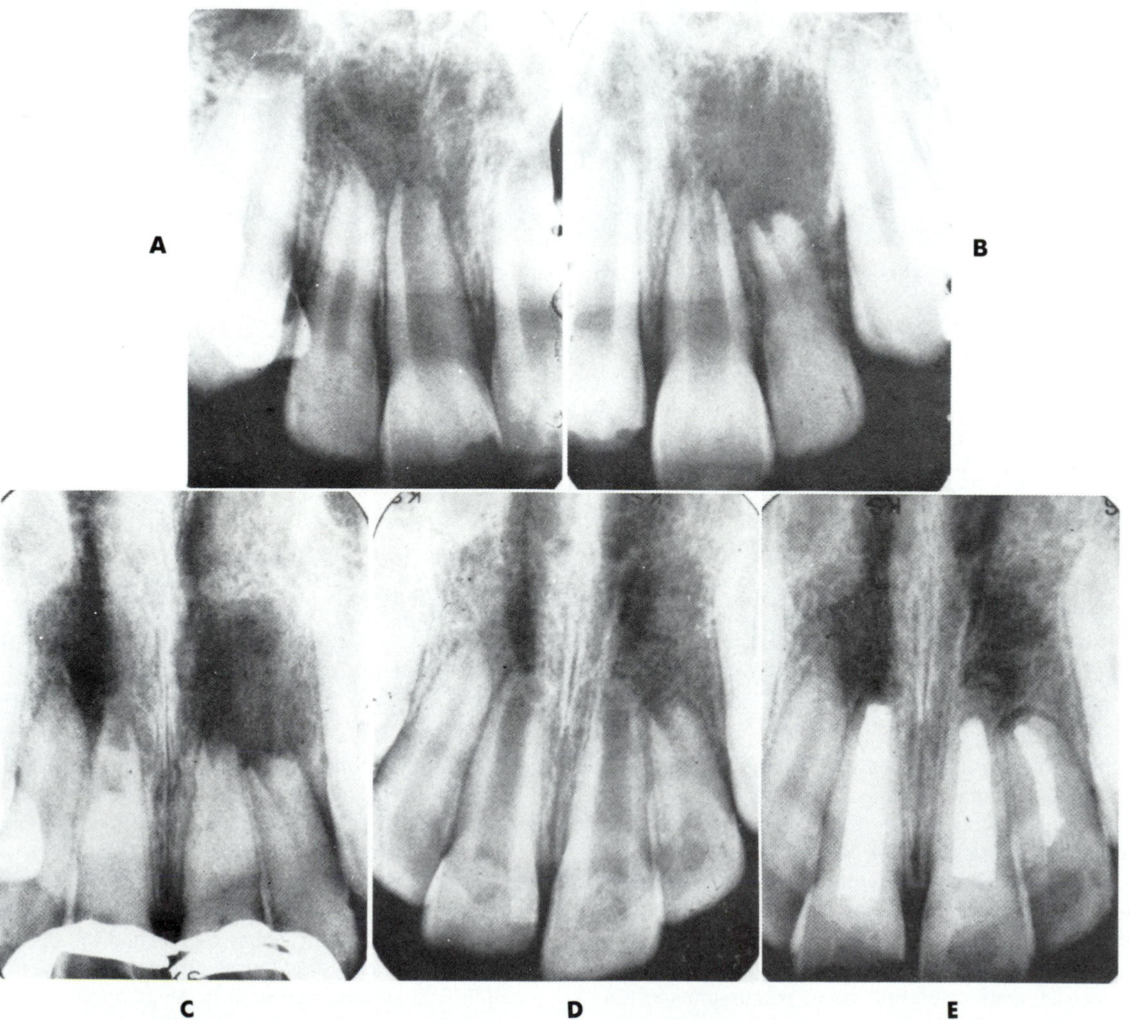

FIG. 23-25 Apexification in three permanent incisors, using calcium hydroxide—CMCP filling material. **A** and **B,** Open apices of the three incisors with periapical pathosis. Note the calcification that has occurred in the lateral incisor before pulpal necrosis. **C,** Calcium hydroxide—CMCP filling placed in two teeth. Note the void in the left incisor requiring further filling. **D,** Radiographic appearance of apexification a year later. **E,** Permanent root canal filling of gutta-percha after apexification.

Commercial pastes of $Ca(OH)_2$ may be used to fill the canals. In this technique, the paste is placed in the canal via the sterile needle supplied with the paste. The liquid portion of the paste is then absorbed with paper points placed into the canal. Injection and absorption of the liquid are repeated until filling of the canal is achieved. Condensation of the dried paste with pluggers is necessary to completely obliterate the canal space.

It has been reported that successful apexification can occur with an overfill of material; in fact, it has been reported that an overfill is preferable to an underfill.[22] In the event of an overfill, the material (being absorbable) is not removed from the apical tissues. The presence of an overfill rarely causes postoperative pain.

After the canal is filled, the access opening must be sealed with a permanent filling material. If the outer seal is defective, the calcium hydroxide paste is lost and recontamination of the canal will result. For this reason temporary-type cements should never be used to seal the tooth after the filling procedure. Composite resin or silicate cement is recommended for anterior teeth and amalgam for posterior teeth.

Periodic recall

The usual time required to achieve apexification is 6 to 24 months (average 1 year ± 7 months).[105] Factors that lead to increased time are the presence of a radiolucent lesion, interappointment symptoms, and loss of the external seal with reinfection of the canal. During this time the patient is recalled at 3-month intervals for monitoring of the tooth.

If any signs or symptoms of reinfection or pathology occur during this phase of treatment, the canal is recleaned and refilled with the $Ca(OH)_2$ paste. The patient is recalled until radiographic evidence of apexification has become apparent. Then the tooth is reentered and clinical verification of apexification is made by the failure of a small instrument to penetrate through the apex after removal of the $Ca(OH)_2$ paste. If apexification is incomplete, the canal is repacked with the $Ca(OH)_2$ paste, and the periodic recall continues (Fig. 23-25).

Histology of Apexification

The calcified material that forms over the apical foramen has been histologically identified as an osteoid (bonelike) or cementoid (cementum-like) material by investigators who have done apexification following periapical involvement of the treated teeth.[22,71,204] The formation of osteodentin after the placement of calcium hydroxide paste immediately on conclusion of a vital pulpectomy has also been reported.[40]

Histologic studies consistently report the absence of Hertwig's epithelial root sheath. Normal root formation usually does not occur following apexification. Instead, there appears to be a differentiation of adjacent connective tissue cells into specialized cells; there is also deposition of calcified tissue adjacent to the filling material. The calcified material is continuous with the lateral root surfaces. The closure of the

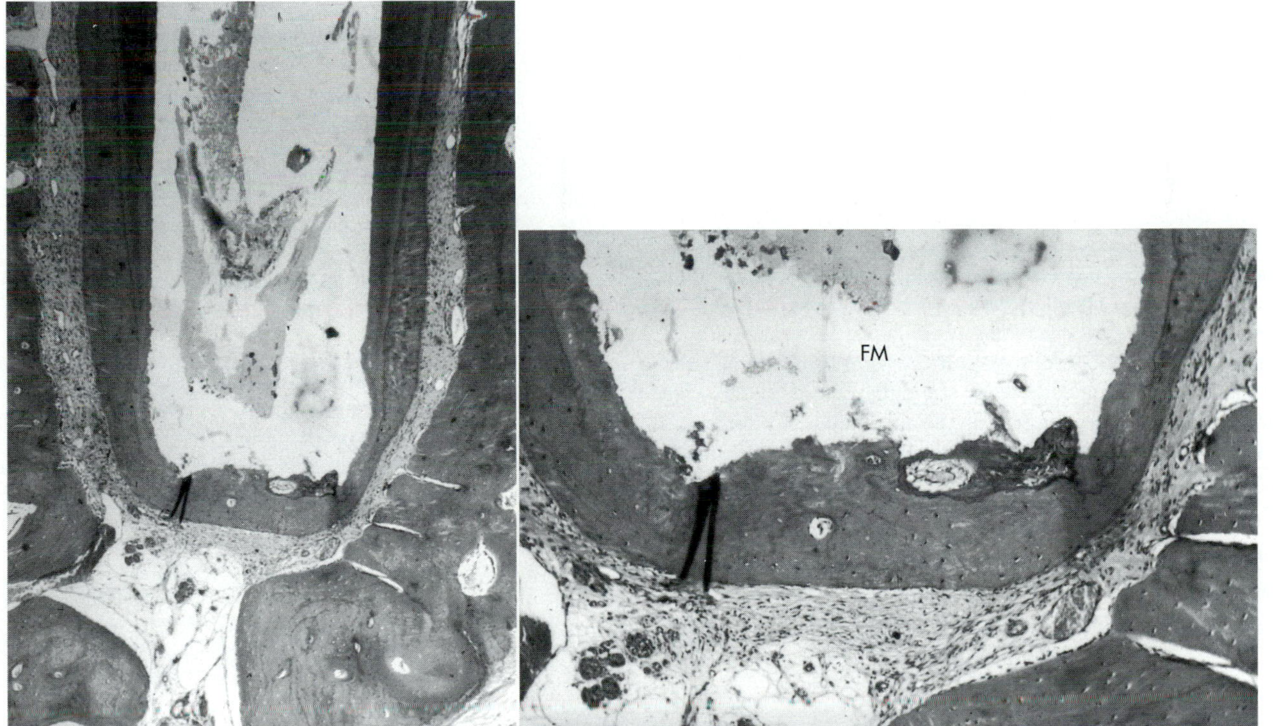

FIG. 23-26 Histologic sections of a dog's tooth after apexification. **A,** Cementum-like calcified tissue is closing the wide open apical foramen. Note the presence of debris within the canal due to inadequate cleaning of the canal before filling. **B,** Higher magnification showing cellular detail. The periodontal ligament *(P)* is free of inflammation. The filling material *(FM)*, calcium hydroxide—CMCP, was lost during processing. Note the presence of tissue communication through the calcified tissue. (H & E stain.)

apex may be partial or complete but consistently has minute communications with the periapical tissues (Fig. 23-26). For this reason apexification must always be followed by filling of the canal with a permanent root canal filling of gutta-percha.

Various types of apical closure have been reported in clinical studies of apexification. In view of the histologic evidence of subsequent studies, it would appear that these types of apical closure simply relate to the level to which the filling material was placed within or beyond the apical foramen.

Many of the failures of apexification have been shown histologically to arise from the difficulty of adequately cleaning and sanitizing the wide-open canals. The tooth with an apically divergent root canal is much more difficult to clean thoroughly than is the mature tooth, which becomes increasingly smaller as the apex is approached.

Although the formation of calcified tissue was noted in the presence of mild inflammation,[22] the results were consistently better in specimens that were free of inflammation. It is recommended therefore that the cleaning and filling procedure be done at separate appointments rather than in a single appointment. Likewise, ideally all signs and symptoms of infection and inflammation should be absent before the $Ca(OH)_2$ paste is placed.

Obturation with Gutta-Percha

After verification of successful apexification, the canal is thoroughly cleaned, care being taken not to damage the calcific barrier at the apex. The canal is then obturated with gutta-percha in the usual manner. Because of the large size of the canal, it may be necessary to prepare a customized gutta-percha point as described in Chapter 9. While the apexification procedure is highly successful, the root of such a tooth is weak and prone to fracture with subsequent injuries. Therefore apexification should be a treatment of last resort after all attempts at vital therapy have failed.

Restoration Following Apexification

Restoration of the immature tooth following obturation with gutta-percha should be designed to strengthen the tooth as much as possible. Placement of posts within the canal should be avoided unless no other means of restoration is obtainable. Preparation of a post space has been shown to weaken significantly the remaining tooth structure, whereas acid etching and placement of a composite resin strengthen the tooth, making it more resistant to fracture.[219] In the apexified tooth, the gutta-percha should be removed below the alveolar crest, the dentin acid etched, and bonded composite resin placed to strengthen the root.[160]

REFERENCES

1. Alacam A: Long-term effects of primary teeth pulpotomies with formocresol, glutaraldehyde–calcium hydroxide and glutaraldehyde–zinc oxide–eugenol on succedaneous teeth, J Pedodont 13:307, 1989.
2. Andrew P: The treatment of infected pulps in decisuous teeth, Br Dent J 98:122, 1955.
3. Anthony DR: Apexification during active orthodontic movement, J Endod 12:419, 1986.
4. Aponte AJ, Hartsook JT, and Crowley MC: Indirect pulp capping success verified, J Dent Child 33:164, 1966.
5. Armstrong RL, et al: Comparison of Dycal and formocresol pulpotomies in young permanent teeth in monkeys, Oral Surg 48:160, 1979.
6. Attala MN, and Noujaim AA: Role of calcium hydroxide in the formation of reparative dentin, J Can Dent Assoc 35:267, 1969.
7. Avram DC, and Pulver F: Pulpotomy medicaments for vital primary teeth: surveys to determine use and attitudes in pediatric dental practice and in dental schools throughout the world, J Dent Child 56:426, 1989.
8. Ball JS: Apical root formation in a non-vital immature permanent incisor, Br Dent J 116:166, 1964.
9. Beaver HA, Kopel HM, and Sabes WR: The effect of zinc oxide-eugenol cement on a formocresolized pulp. J Dent Child 33:381, 1966.
10. Bennett CG: Pulpal management of deciduous teeth, Pract Dent Monogr, p. 1, May-June, 1965.
11. Berk H, and Krakow AA: A comparison of the management of pulpal pathosis in deciduous and permanent teeth, Oral Surg 34:944, 1972.
12. Berk H, and Krakow AA: Endodontic treatment in primary teeth. In Goldman HM, et al, (eds): Current therapy in dentistry, vol 5, St. Louis, 1974, The CV Mosby Co.
13. Berkman M, et al: Pulpal response to isobutyl cyanoacrylate in human teeth, J Am Dent Assoc 83:140, 1971.
14. Bevelander G, and Benzer D: Morphology and incidence in secondary dentin in human teeth, J Am Dent Assoc 30:1079, 1943.
15. Bhasker SN, et al: Pulp capping with isobutyl cyanoacrylate, J Am Dent Assoc 79:640, 1969.
16. Bhasker S, Cutright DE, and Van Osdel V: Tissue response to cortisone-containing and cortisone-free calcium hydroxide, J Dent Child 36:1, 1969.
17. Bimstein E, and Shoshan S: Enhanced healing of tooth-pulp wounds in the dog by enriched collagen solution as a capping agent, Arch Oral Biol 26:97, 1981.
18. Block RM, et al: Cell-mediated immune response to dog pulp tissue altered by formocresol within the root canal, J Endod 3:424, 1977.
19. Bouchon F: Apex formation following treatment of necrotized immature permanent incisor, J Dent Child 33:378, 1966.
20. Brian JD, et al: Reaction of rat connective tissue to unfixed and formaldehyde-fixed autogenous implants enclosed in tubes, J Endod 6:628, 1980.
21. Brosch JW: Capping pulps with a compound of calcium phosphate, neomycin and hydrocortisone, J Dent Child 32:42, 1965.
22. Camp JH: Continued apical development of pulpless permanent teeth following endodontic therapy. Master's thesis, Bloomington, 1968, Indiana University School of Dentistry.
23. Chohayeb AA, Adrian JC, and Salamat K: Pulpal response to tricalcium phosphate as a capping agent, Oral Surg Oral Med Oral Pathol 71:343, 1991.
24. Citrome GP, Kaminski EJ, and Heuer MA: A comparative study of tooth apexification in the dog, J Endod 5:290, 1979.
25. Cooke C, and Rowbotham TC: Root canal therapy in nonvital teeth with open apices, Br Dent J 108:147, 1960.
26. Coviello J, and Brilliant JD: A preliminary clinical study of the use of tricalcium phosphate as an apical barrier, J Endod 5:6, 1979.
27. Cvek M: Treatment of non-vital permanent incisors with calcium hydroxide, Odontol Rev 23:27, 1972.
28. Cvek M: A clinical report on partial pulpotomy and capping with calcium hydroxide in permanent incisors with complicated crown fractures, J Endod 4:232, 1978.
29. Cvek M: Endodontic treatment of traumatized teeth. In Andreasen, JO: Traumatic injuries of the teeth, ed 2, Philadelphia, 1981, WB Saunders Co.
30. Cvek M, and Lundberg M: Histological appearance of pulps after exposure by a crown fracture, partial pulpotomy, and clinical diagnosis of healing, J Endod 9:8, 1983.
31. Cvek M, et al: Pulp reactions to exposure after experimental crown fracture or grinding in adult monkey, J Endod 8:391, 1982.
32. Cvek M, et al: Hard tissue barrier formation in pulpotomized monkey teeth capped with cyanoacrylate or calcium hydroxide for 10 and 60 minutes, J Dent Res 66:1166, 1987.

33. Dannenberg JL: Pedodontic-endodontics, Dent Clin North Am 18:367, 1974.
34. Davis MJ, Myers R, and Switkes MD: Glutaraldehyde: an alternative to formocresol for vital pulp therapy, J Dent Child 49:176, 1982.
35. Dietz D: A histological study of the effects of formocresol on normal primary pulpal tissue. Master's thesis, Seattle, 1961, School of Dentistry, University of Washington.
36. Dilley GJ, and Courts FJ: Immunological response to four pulpal medicaments, Pediatr Dent 3:179, 1981.
37. Dimaggio JJ, and Hawes RR: Evaluation of direct and indirect pulp capping, J Dent Res 40:24, 1962 (abstract).
38. Dimaggio JJ, and Hawes RR: Continued evaluation of direct and indirect pulp capping, J Dent Res 41:38, 1963 (abstract).
39. Doyle WA, McDonald RE, and Mitchell DF: Formocresol versus calcium hydroxide in pulpotomy, J Dent Child 29:86, 1962.
40. Dylewski JJ: Apical closure of non-vital teeth, Oral Surg 32:82, 1971.
41. Easlick KA: Operative procedures in management of deciduous molars, Int J Orthod 20:585, 1934.
42. Ehrenreich DW: A comparison of the effects of zinc oxide and eugenol and calcium hydroxide on carious dentin in human primary molars, J Dent Child 35:451, 1968.
43. El-Kafrawy AH, et al: Pulp reaction to a polycarboxylate cement in monkeys, J Dent Res 53:15, 1974.
44. Emmerson C, et al: Pulpal changes following formocresol applications on rat molars and human primary teeth, J South Calif Dent Assoc 27:309, 1959.
45. England MC, and Best E: Noninduced apical closure in immature roots of dogs' teeth, J Endod 3:411, 1977.
46. Fairbourn DR, Charbeneau GT, and Loesche WJ: Effect of improved Dycal and I.R.M. on bacteria in deep carious lesions, J Am Dent Assoc 100:547, 1980.
47. Feigal RJ, and Messer HH: A critical look at glutaraldehyde. Pediatr Dent 12:69, 1990.
48. Feltman EM: A comparison of the formocresol pulpotomy techniques and dycal pulpotomy technique in young permanent teeth. Master's thesis, Bloomington, 1972, School of Dentistry, Indiana University.
49. Finn SB: Morphology of the primary teeth. In Finn SB, et al (eds): Clinical pedodontics, ed 3, Philadelphia, 1967, WB Saunders Co.
50. Fiore-Donno G, and Baume LJ: Effects of capping compounds containing corticosteroids on the human dental pulp, Helv Odontol Acta 6:23, 1962.
51. Frank AL: Therapy for the divergent pulpless tooth by continued apical formation, J Am Dent Assoc 72:87, 1966.
52. Frankl SN: Pulp therapy in pedodontics, Oral Surg 34:293, 1972.
53. Friedberg BH, and Gartner LP: Embryotoxicity and teratogenicity of formocresol on developing chick embryos, J Endod 16:434, 1990.
54. Friend LA: The root treatment of teeth with open apices, Proc R Soc Med 59:1035, 1966.
55. Fuks AB, and Bimstein EC: Clinical evaluation of diluted formocresol pulpotomies in primary teeth of school children, Pediatr Dent 3:321, 1981.
56. Fuks AB, Bimstein E, and Bruchimn A: Radiographic and histologic evaluation of the effect of two concentrations of formocresol on pulpotomized primary and young permanent teeth in monkeys, Pediatr Dent 5:9, 1983.
57. Fuks AB, et al: Enriched collagen solution as a pulp dressing in pulpotomized teeth in monkeys, Pediatr Dent 6:243, 1984.
58. Fuks AB, et al: Partial pulpotomy as a treatment alternative for exposed pulps in crown-fractured permanent incisors, Endod Dent Traumatol 3:100, 1987.
59. Fuks AB, et al: Assessment of a 2 percent buffered glutaraldehyde solution in pulpotomized primary teeth of school children, J Dent Child 57:371, 1990.
60. Fulton R, and Ranly DM: An autoradiographic study of formocresol pulpotomies in rat molars using ^{3}H-formaldehyde, J Endod 5:71, 1979.
61. Fusayama T, Okuse K, and Hosoda H: Relationship between hardness, discoloration and microbial invasion in carious dentin, J Dent Res 45:1033, 1966.
62. Garcia-Godoy F, and Ranly D: Clinical evaluation of pulpotomies with ZOE as the vehicle for glutaraldehyde, Pediatr Dent 9:144, 1987.
63. Garcia-Godoy F, Novakovic DP, and Carvajal IN: Pulpal response to different application times of formocresol, J Pedodont 6:176, 1982.
64. Gardner DE, Mitchell DF, and McDonald RE: Treatment of pulps of monkeys with Vancomycin and calcium hydroxide, J Dent Res 50:1273, 1971.
65. Gazi HA, Nayak RG, and Bhat KS: Tissue-irritation potential of dilute formocresol, Oral Surg 51:74, 1981.
66. Gerlach E: Root canal therapeutics in deciduous teeth, Dent Surv 8:68, 1932.
67. Glass RL, and Zander HA: Pulp healing, J Dent Res 28:97, 1949.
68. Granath LE, and Hagman G: Experimental pulpotomy in human bicuspids with reference to cutting technique, Acta Odontol Scand 29:155, 1971.
69. Greenberg M: Filling root canals of deciduous teeth by an injection technique, Dent Dig 67:574, 1964.
70. Guthrie TJ, McDonald RE, and Mitchell DF: Dental hemogram, J Dent Res 44:678, 1965.
71. Ham JW, Patterson SS, and Mitchell DF: Induced apical closure of immature pulpless teeth in monkeys, Oral Surg 33:438, 1972.
72. Harris CA: The principles and practice of dental surgery, ed 4, Philadelphia, 1850, Lindsay & Blakiston.
73. Hata G, et al: Systemic distribution of ^{14}C-labeled formaldehyde applied in the root canal following pulpectomy, J Endod 15:539, 1989.
74. Hawes RR, Dimaggio JJ, and Sayegh F: Evaluation of direct and indirect pulp capping (abstract), J Dent Res 43:808, 1964.
75. Hayashi Y: Ultrastructure of initial calcification in wound healing following pulpotomy, J Oral Pathol 11:174, 1982.
76. Heide S: Pulp reactions to exposure for 4, 24 and 168 hours, J Dent Res 59:1910, 1980.
77. Heide S, and Kerekes K: Delayed partial pulpotomy in permanent incisors of monkeys, Int Endod J 19:78, 1986.
78. Heller AL, et al: Direct pulp capping of permanent teeth in primates using a resorbable form of tricalcium phosphate ceramic, J Endod 1:95, 1975.
79. Herbert WE: Three cases of disturbance of calcification of a tooth and infection of the dental pulp following trauma, Dent Pract 9:176, 1961.
80. Hermann BW: Dentinobliteran der Wurzelkanale nach der Behandlung mit Kalzium, Zahaertzl Rund 39:888, 1930.
81. Heys DR, et al: Histological considerations of direct pulp capping agents, J Dent Res 60:1371, 1981.
82. Hibbard ED, and Ireland RL: Morphology of the root canals of the primary molar teeth, J Dent Child 24:250, 1957.
83. Hill S, et al: Comparison of antimicrobial and cytotoxic effects of glutaraldehyde and formocresol, Oral Surg Oral Med Oral Pathol 71:89, 1991.
84. Hirschfeld Z, Sela J, and Ulmansky M: Hydrex and its effect on the pulp, Oral Surg 34:364, 1972.
85. Holan G, Topf J, and Fuks AB: Effect of root canal infection and treatment of traumatized primary incisors on their permanent successors, Endod Dent Traumatol 8:12, 1992.
86. Holland R, et al: Histochemical analysis of the dogs' dental pulp after pulp capping with calcium, barium and strontium hydroxides, J Endod 8:444, 1982.
87. Hørsted P, El Attar K, and Langeland K: Capping of monkey pulps with Dycal and a Ca-eugenol cement, Oral Surg 52:531, 1981.
88. Hume WR, and Testa Kenney AE: Release of ^{3}H-triamcinolone from Ledermix, J Endod 7:509, 1981.
89. Inglis OE: Can recalcification of dentin occur? A proposition, Pacific Dent Gaz 8:763, 1900.

90. Ireland RL: Secondary dentin formation in deciduous teeth, J Am Dent Assoc 28:1626, 1941.
91. Jaber L, Mascrès C, and Donohue WB: Electron microscope characteristics of dentin repair after hydroxylapatite direct pulp capping in rats, J Oral Pathol Med 20:502, 1991.
92. Javelet J, Torabinejad M, and Bakland LK: Comparison of two pH levels for the induction of apical barrier in immature teeth of monkeys, J Endod 11:375, 1985.
93. Jean A, et al: Effects of various calcium phosphate biomaterials on reparative dentin bridge formation, J Endod 14:83, 1988.
94. Jeng HW, Feigal RJ, and Messer HH: Comparison of the cytotoxicity of formocresol, formaldehyde, cresol, and glutaraldehyde using human pulp fibroblast cultures, Pediatr Dent 9:295, 1987.
95. Johansson BI, Persson I, and Manera P: Histologic effects of collagen and chondroitin sulfate as capping agents in amputated rat molar pulps, Arch Oral Biol 8:503, 1963.
96. Jordon ME: Operative dentistry for children, New York, 1925, Dental Items of Interest Publishing Co.
97. Kaiser JH: Management of wide-open canals with calcium hydroxide. Paper presented at the meeting of the American Association of Endodontics, Washington, DC, April 17, 1964. Cited by Steiner JC, Dow PR, and Cathey GM: Inducing root end closure of nonvital permanent teeth, J Dent Child 35:47, 1968.
98. Kakehashi S, Stanley HR, and Fitzgerald RT: The effects of surgical exposures of dental pulps in germ-free and conventional laboratory rats, Oral Surg 20:340, 1965.
99. Kalnins V, and Frisbie HE: Effect of dentin fragments on the healing of the exposed pulp, Arch Oral Biol 2:96, 1960.
100. Karp WB, Korb P, and Pashley D: The oxidation of glutaraldehyde by rat tissues, Pediatr Dent 9:301, 1987.
101. Kelley MA, Bugg JL, and Skjonsby HS: Histologic evaluation of formocresol and oxpara pulpotomies in rhesus monkeys, J Am Dent Assoc 86:123, 1973.
102. Kennedy DB, et al: Formocresol pulpotomy in teeth of dogs with induced pulpal and periapical pathosis, J Dent Child 40:44, 1973.
103. Kerkhove BC, et al: A clinical and television densitometric evaluation of the indirect pulp capping technique, J Dent Child 34:192, 1967.
104. King JB, Crawford JJ, and Lindahl RL: Indirect pulp capping: a bacteriologic study of deep carious dentine in human teeth, Oral Surg 20:663, 1965.
105. Kleier DJ, and Barr ES: A study of endodontically apexified teeth, Endod Dent Traumatol 7:112, 1991.
106. Klein H, et al: Partial pulpotomy following complicated crown fracture in permanent incisors: a clinical and radiographic study, J Pedodont 9:142, 1985.
107. Koenigs JF, et al: Induced apical closure of permanent teeth in adult primates using a resorbable form of tricalcium phosphate ceramic, J Endod 1:102, 1975.
108. Kopel HM: Pediatric endodontics, In Ingle JI and Beveridge EE, (eds): Endodontics, ed 2, Philadelphia, 1976, Lea & Febiger.
109. Kopel HM, et al: The effects of glutaraldehyde on primary pulp tissue following coronal amputation: an in vivo histologic study, J Dent Child 47:425, 1980.
110. Kozlov M, and Massler M: Histologic effects of various drugs on amputated pulps of rat molars, Oral Surg 13:455, 1960.
111. Langeland K: Management of the inflamed pulp associated with deep carious lesion, J Endod 7:169, 1981.
112. Langeland K, et al: Human pulp changes of iatrogenic origin, Oral Surg 32:943, 1971.
113. Laurence RP: A method of root canal therapy for primary teeth. Master's thesis, Atlanta, Ga. 1966, School of Dentistry, Emory University.
114. Law DB, Lewis TM, and Davis JM: Pulp therapy. In Law, DB et al, editors: An atlas of pedodontics, Philadelphia, 1969, WB Saunders Co.
115. Lekka M, Hume WR, and Wolinsky LE: Comparison between formaldehyde and glutaraldehyde diffusion through the root tissues of pulpotomy-treated teeth, J Pedod 8:185, 1984.
116. Lloyd JM, Seale NS, and Wilson CFG: The effects of various concentrations and lengths of application of glutaraldehyde on monkey pulp tissue, Pediatric Dent 10:115, 1988.
117. Longwill DG, Marshall FJ, and Creamer HR: Reactivity of human lymphocytes to pulp antigens, J Endod 8:27, 1982.
118. Loos PJ, and Han SS: An enzyme histochemical study of the effect of various concentrations of formocresol on connective tissues, Oral Surg 31:571, 1971.
119. Loos PJ, Straffon LH, and Han SS: Biological effects of formocresol, J Dent Child 40:193, 1973.
120. Mack RB, and Halterman CW: Labial pulpectomy access followed by esthetic composite resin restoration for nonvital maxillary deciduous incisors, J Am Dent Assoc 100:374, 1980.
121. Mansukhani N: Pulpal reactions to formocresol. Master's thesis, Urbana, 1959, College of Dentistry, University of Illinois.
122. Massler M: Pulp protection and preservation, Pract Dent Monogr 3, 1958.
123. Massler M, and Mansukhani H: Effects of formocresol on the dental pulp, J Dent Child 26:277, 1959.
124. Masterson JB: The healing of wounds of the dental pulp of man, Br Dent J 120:213, 1966.
125. Matsumiya S, Susuki A, and Takuma S: Atlas of clinical pathology, vol 1, Tokyo, 1962, The Tokyo Dental College Press.
126. McDonald RE, and Avery DR: Treatment of deep caries, vital pulp exposure, and pulpless teeth in children. In McDonald RE, and Avery DR (eds): Dentistry for the child and adolescent, ed 3, St Louis, 1978, The CV Mosby Co.
127. McWalter GM, El-Kafrawy AH, and Mitchell DF: Pulp capping in monkeys with a calcium hydroxide compound, an antibiotic and a polycarboxylate cement, Oral Surg 36:90, 1973.
128. Messer LB, Cline JT, and Korf NW: Long-term effects of primary molar pulpotomies on succedaneous bicuspids, J Dent Res 59:116, 1980.
129. Mjör IA, Dahl E, and Cox CF: Healing of pulp exposures: an ultrastructural study, J Oral Pathol Med 20:496, 1991.
130. Molven O: Dental pulp lesions covered with albumin, Oral Surg 30:413, 1970.
131. Morawa AP, et al: Clinical studies of human primary teeth following dilute formocresol pulpotomies (abstract), J Dent Res 53:269, 1974.
132. Morawa AP, et al: Clinical evaluation of pulpotomies using dilute formocresol, J Dent Child 42:360, 1975.
133. Mulder GR, van Amerongen WE, and Vingerling PA: Consequences of endodontic treatment of primary teeth. II. A clinical investigation into the influence of formocresol pulpotomy on the permanent successor, J Dent Child 54:35, 1987.
134. Mūniz MA, Keszler A, and Dominiguez FV: The formocresol technique in young permanent teeth, Oral Surg 55:611, 1983.
135. Myers DR: Effects of formocresol on pulps of cariously exposed permanent molars. Master's thesis, 1972, College of Dentistry, University of Tennessee.
136. Myers DR, et al: Distribution of ^{14}C-formaldehyde after pulpotomy with formocresol, J Am Dent Assoc 96:805, 1978.
137. Myers DR, et al: Acute toxicity of high doses of systemically administered formocresol in dogs, Pediatr Dent 3:37, 1981.
138. Myers DR, et al: Tissue changes induced by the absorption of formocresol from pulpotomy sites in dogs, Pediatr Dent 5:6, 1983.
139. Myers DR, et al: Systemic absorption of ^{14}C-glutaraldehyde from glutaraldehyde-treated pulpotomy sites, Pediatr Dent 8:134, 1986.
140. Myers DR, et al: Histopathology of furcation lesions associated with pulp degeneration in primary molars, Pediatr Dent 9:279, 1987.
141. Myers DR, et al: Histopathology of radiolucent furcation lesions associated with pulpotomy-treated primary molars, Pediatr Dent 10:291, 1988.
142. Nakashima M: Dentin induction by implants of autolyzed antigen-extracted allogeneic dentin on amputated pulps of dogs, Endod Dent Traumatol 5:279, 1989.
143. Nelson JR, et al: Biochemical effects of tissue fixatives on bovine pulp, J Endod 5:139, 1979.

144. Nevins AJ, et al: Revitalization of pulpless open apex teeth in rhesus monkeys, using collagen–calcium phosphate gel, J Endod 2:159, 1976.
145. Nevins A, et al: Hard tissue induction into pulpless open-apex teeth using collagen-calcium phosphate gel, J Endod 3:431, 1977.
146. Nevins A, et al: Induction of hard tissue into pulpless open-apex teeth using collagen-calcium phosphate gel, J Endod 4:76, 1978.
147. Nirschl RF, and Avery DR: Evaluation of new pulp capping agent in indirect pulp therapy, J Dent Child 50:25, 1983.
148. Nixon GS, and Hannah CM: N-butyl cyanoacrylate as a pulp capping agent, Br Dent J 133:14, 1972.
149. Nygaard-Østby B: The role of the blood clot in endodontic therapy: an experimental histologic study, Acta Odontol Scand 19:323, 1961.
150. Orban B: Contribution to the histology of the dental pulp and periodontal membrane with special reference to the cells of defense of these tissues, J Am Dent Assoc 16:965, 1929.
151. Orban BJ (ed): Oral histology and embryology, ed 4, St. Louis, 1957, The CV Mosby Co.
152. Pashley EL, et al: Systemic distribution of ^{14}C-formaldehyde from formocresol-treated pulpotomy sites, J Dent Res 59:603, 1980.
153. Paterson RC, and Watts A: Further studies on the exposed germ-free dental pulp, Int J Endod 20:112, 1987.
154. Pereira JC, and Stanley HR: Pulp capping: influence of the exposure site on pulp healing—histologic and radiographic study in dogs' pulp, J Endod 7:213, 1981.
155. Peron LC, Burkes EJ, and Gregory WB: Vital pulpotomy utilizing variable concentrations of paraformaldehyde in rhesus monkeys, J Dent Res 55:B129, 1976 (abstract no. 269).
156. Phaneuf RA, Frankl SN, and Ruben M: A comparative histological evaluation of three calcium hydroxide preparations on the human primary dental pulp, J Dent Child 35:61, 1968.
157. Pisanti S, and Sciaky I: Origin of calcium in the repair wall after pulp exposure in the dog, J Dent Res 43:641, 1964.
158. Pitt Ford TR: Pulpal response to MPC for capping exposures, Oral Surg 50:81, 1980.
159. Pitt Ford TR, and Roberts GJ: Immediate and delayed direct pulp capping with the use of a new visible light–cured calcium hydroxide preparation, Oral Surg Oral Med Oral Pathol 71:338, 1991.
160. Rabie G, et al: Strengthening and restoration of immature teeth with an acid-etch resin technique, Endod Dent Traumatol 1:246, 1985.
161. Rabinowitch BZ: Pulp management in primary teeth, Oral Surg 6:542, 1953.
162. Ranley DM: Glutaraldehyde purity and stability: implications for preparation, storage, and use as a pulpotomy agent, Pediatr Dent 6:83, 1984.
163. Ranley DM: Assessment of the systemic distribution and toxicity of formaldehyde following pulpotomy treatment. I, J Dent Child 52:431, 1985.
164. Ranley DM, and Lazzari EP: A biochemical study of two biofunctional reagents as alternatives to formocresol, J Dent Res 62:1054, 1983.
165. Ranley DM, Garcia-Godoy F, and Horn D: Time, concentration, and pH parameters for the use of glutaraldehyde as a pulpotomy agent: an in vivo study, Pediatr Dent 9:199, 1987.
166. Ranley DM, Horn D, and Hubbard GB: Assessment of the systemic distribution and toxicity of glutaraldehyde as a pulpotomy agent, Pediatr Dent 11:8, 1989.
167. Ranley DM, Horn D, and Zislis T: The effect of alternatives to formocresol on antigenicity of protein, J Dent Res 64:1225, 1985.
168. Ranley DM, Amstutz L, and Horn D: Subcellular localization of glutaraldehyde, Endod Dent Traumatol 6:251, 1990.
169. Ranley DM, and Horn D: Distribution, metabolism, and excretion of (^{14}C) glutaraldehyde, J Endod 16:135, 1990.
170. Ravn JJ: Follow-up study of permanent incisors with complicated crown fracture after acute trauma, Scand J Dent Res 90:353, 1982.
171. Redig DF: A comparison and evaluation of two formocresol pulpotomy techniques utilizing Buckley's formocresol, J Dent Child 35:22, 1968.
172. Riekman GA, and Elbadrawy HE: Effect of premature loss of primary incisors on speech, Pediatr Dent 7:119, 1985.
173. Roberts SC Jr, and Brilliant JD: Tricalcium phosphate as an adjunct to apical closure in pulpless permanent teeth, J Endod 1:263, 1975.
174. Rølling I, and Poulsen S: Formocresol pulpotomy of primary teeth and occurrence of enamel defects on the permanent successors, Acta Odontol Scand 36:243, 1978.
175. Ruemping DR, Morton TH Jr, and Anderson MW: Electrosurgical pulpotomy in primates—a comparison with formocresol pulpotomy, Pediatr Dent 5:14, 1983.
176. Safer DS, Avery JK, and Cox DF: Histopathologic evaluation of the effects of new polcarboxylate cements on monkey pulps, Oral Surg 33:966, 1972.
177. Sanchez ZMC: Effects of formocresol on pulp-capped and pulpotomized permanent teeth of rhesus monkeys. Master's thesis, Ann Arbor, 1971, University of Michigan.
178. Savage NW, et al: An histological study of cystic lesions following pulp therapy in deciduous molars, J Oral Pathol 15:209, 1986.
179. Sayegh FS: Qualitative and quantitative evaluation of new dentin in pulp capped teeth, J Dent Child 35:7, 1968.
180. Sayegh FS: The dentinal bridge in pulp-involved teeth. I, Oral Surg 28:579, 1969.
181. Sayegh FS, and Reed AJ: Correlated clinical and histological evaluation of Hydrex in pulp therapy, J Dent Child 34:471, 1967.
182. Sciaky I, and Pisanti S: Localization of calcium placed over amputated pulps in dogs' teeth, J Dent Res 39:1128, 1960.
183. Sekine N, Hasegawa M, and Saijo Y: Clinicopathological study of vital pulpotomy, Bull Tokyo Dent Coll 1:29, 1960.
184. Sela J, and Ulmansky M: Reaction of normal and inflamed dental pulp to Calxyl and zinc oxide-eugenol in rats, Oral Surg 30:425, 1970.
185. Sela J, Hirschfeld Z, and Ulmansky M: Reaction of the rat molar pulp to direct capping with the separate components of Hydrex, Oral Surg 35:118, 1973.
186. Seltzer S, and Bender IB: Pulp capping and pulpotomy. In Seltzer S and Bender IB (eds): The dental pulp, biologic considerations in dental procedures, ed 2, Philadelphia, 1975, JB Lippincott Co.
187. Shaw DW, et al: Electrosurgical pulpotomy—a 6-month study in primates, J Endod 13:500, 1987.
188. Sheller B, and Morton TH Jr: Electrosurgical pulpotomy: a pilot study in humans, J Endod 13:69, 1987.
189. Shoji S, Nakamura M, and Horiuchi H: Histopathological changes in dental pulps irradiated by CO_2 laser: a preliminary report on laser pulpotomy, J Endod 11:379, 1985.
190. Shovelton DS: A study of deep carious dentin, Int Dent J 18:392, 1968.
191. Shulman ER, Melver FT, and Burkes EJ Jr: Comparison of electrosurgery and formocresol as pulpotomy techniques in monkey primary teeth, Pediatr Dent 9:189, 1987.
192. Simon M, van Mullem PJ, and Lamers AC: Formocresol: no allergic effect after root canal disinfection in non-presensitized guinea pigs, J Endod 8:269, 1982.
193. Smith GN, and Woods S: Organic iodine: a substitute for $BaSO_4$ in apexification procedures, J Endod 9:153, 1983.
194. Smith HS, and Soni NN: Histologic study of pulp capping in rat molars using calcitonin, Oral Surg 53:311, 1982.
195. Smith JW, Leeb IJ, and Torney DL: A comparison of calcium hydroxide and barium hydroxide as agents for inducing apical closure, J Endod 10:64, 1984.
196. Spedding RH: The one-appointment formocresol pulpotomy for primary teeth, J Tenn Dent Assoc 48:263, 1968.
197. Stanley HR, and Lundy T: Dycal therapy for pulp exposure, Oral Surg 34:818, 1972.
198. Stanley HR, and Pameijer CH: Pulp capping with a new visible-light–curing calcium hydroxide composition (Prisma VLC Dycal), Oper Dent 10:156, 1985.
199. Stanley HR, White CL, and McCray L: The rate of tertiary (reparative) dentine formation in the human tooth, Oral Surg 21:180, 1966.

200. Stanton WG: The non-vital deciduous tooth, Int J Orthod 21:181, 1935.
201. Starkey PE: Methods of preserving primary teeth which have exposed pulps, J Dent Child 30:219, 1963.
202. Starkey PE: Management of deep caries of pulpally involved teeth in children. In Goldman HM, et al (eds): Current therapy in dentistry, vol 3, St Louis, 1968, The CV Mosby Co.
203. Starkey PE: Treatment of pulpally involved primary molars, In McDonald RE et al, editors: Current therapy in dentistry, vol 7, St Louis, 1980, The CV Mosby Co.
204. Steiner JC, and Van Hassel HJ: Experimental root apexification in primates, Oral Surg 31:409, 1971.
205. Steiner JC, Dow PR, and Cathey GM: Inducing root end closure of non-vital permanent teeth, J Dent Child 35:47, 1968.
206. Stewart DJ, and Kramer IRH: Effects of calcium hydroxide on the unexposed pulp, J Dent Res 37:758, 1958.
207. Straffon LH, and Han SS: Effects of varying concentrations of formocresol on RNA synthesis of connective tissue in sponge implants, Oral Surg 29:915, 1970.
208. Sun HW, Feigal RJ, and Messer HH: Cytotoxicity of glutaraldehyde and formaldehyde in relation to time of exposure and concentration, Pediatr Dent 12:303, 1990.
209. Sweet CA: Procedure for the treatment of exposed and pulpless deciduous teeth, J Am Dent Assoc 17:1150, 1930.
210. Tagger E, Tagger M, and Sarnat H: Pulpal reaction for glutaraldehyde and paraformaldehyde pulpotomy dressings in monkey primary teeth, Endod Dent Traumatol 2:237, 1986.
211. Tagger M, and Tagger E: Pulp capping in monkeys with Reolite and Life, two calcium hydroxide bases with different pH, J Endod 11:394, 1985.
212. Teplitsky PE: Formocresol pulpotomies on posterior permanent teeth, J Can Dent Assoc 50:623, 1984.
213. Teuscher GW, and Zander HA: A preliminary report on pulpotomy, Northwest Univ Dent Res Grad Q Bull 39:4, 1938.
214. Thoden Van Velzen SK, and Feltkamp-Vroom TM: Immunologic consequences of formaldehyde fixation of autologous tissue implants, J Endod 3:179, 1977.
215. Trask PA: Formocresol pulpotomy on (young) permanent teeth, J Am Dent Assoc 85:1316, 1972.
216. Traubman L: A critical clinical and television radiographic evaluation of indirect pulp capping, Master's thesis, Bloomington, 1967, Indiana University School of Dentistry.
217. Tronstad L: Reaction of the exposed pulp to Dycal treatment, Oral Surg 38:945, 1974.
218. Tronstad L, and Mjör IA: Capping of the inflamed pulp, Oral Surg 34:477, 1972.
219. Trope M, Maltz DO, and Tronstad L: Resistance to fracture of restored endodontically treated teeth, Endod Dent Traumatol 1:108, 1985.
220. Turner C, Courts FJ, and Stanley HR: A histological comparison of direct pulp capping agents in primary canines, J Dent Child 54:423, 1987.
221. Tziafas D, and Molyvdas I: The tissue reaction after capping of dog teeth with calcium hydroxide experimentally crammed into the pulp space, Oral Surg Oral Med Oral Pathol 65:604, 1988.
222. van Amerongen WE, Mulder GR, and Vingerling PA: Consequences of endodontic treatment in primary teeth. I. A clinical and radiographic investigation into the influence of the formocresol pulpotomy on the life-span of primary molars, J Dent Child 53:364, 1986.
223. van Mullen PJ, Simon M, and Lamers AC: Formocresol: a root canal disinfectant provoking allergic skin reactions in presensitized guinea pigs, J Endod 9:25, 1983.
224. Venham LL: Pulpal responses to variations in the formocresol pulpotomy technique: a histologic study. Master's thesis, Columbus, 1967, College of Dentistry, The Ohio State University.
225. Walsh M: Pulp reaction to anorganic bovine dentin. Master's thesis, Bloomington, 1967, Indiana University School of Dentistry.
226. Watts A, and Paterson RC: Pulp-capping studies with analar calcium hydroxide and zinc oxide-eugenol, Int Endod J 20:169, 1987.
227. Webber RT: Apexogenesis versus apexification, Dent Clin North Am 28:669, 1984.
228. Webber RT, Schwiebert KA, and Cathey GM: A technique for placement of calcium hydroxide in the root canal system, J Am Dent Assoc 103:417, 1981.
229. Weiss MB, and Bjorvatn K: Pulp capping in deciduous and newly erupted permanent teeth of monkeys, Oral Surg 29:769, 1970.
230. Wemes JC, et al: Histologic evaluation of the effect of formocresol and glutaraldehyde on the periapical tissues after endodontic treatment, Oral Surg 54:329, 1982.
231. Wemes JC, et al: Diffusion of carbon-14-labeled formocresol and glutaraldehyde in tooth structures, Oral Surg 54:341, 1982.
232. West NM, and Lieb RJ: Biologic root-end closure on a traumatized and surgically resected maxillary central incisor: an alternative method of treatment, Endod Dent Traumatol 1:146, 1985.
233. Wheeler RC: A textbook of dental anatomy and physiology, ed 4, Philadelphia, 1965, WB Saunders Co.
234. Whitehead FI, MacGregor AB, and Marsland EA: The relationship of bacterial invasions of softening of the dentin in permanent and deciduous teeth, Br Dent J 108:261, 1960.
235. Williams JL: The non-removal of softened dentine before filling, Int Dent J 20:210, 1899.
236. Yacobi R, et al: Evolving primary pulp therapy techniques, J Am Dent Assoc 122:83, 1991.
237. Zander HA: Reaction of the pulp to calcium hydroxide, J Dent Res 18:373, 1939.
238. Zurcher E: The anatomy of the root canals of the teeth of the deciduous dentition and of the first permanent molars, New York, 1925, William Wood & Co.

Self-assessment questions

1. The basic morphologic difference between primary and permanent teeth is that
   a. the thickness of dentin between the pulp and enamel is greater in primary teeth.
   b. the enamel is thicker on primary teeth.
   c. the pulp chamber is comparatively smaller in primary teeth than in permanent teeth.
   d. the pulp horns are higher in primary molars than in permanent molars.
2. Radiographically, in primary teeth
   a. pathologic changes in the periradicular tissues are most often apparent at the apices rather than the furcation in molars.
   b. the presence of calcified masses within the pulp is indicative of acute pulpal disease.
   c. the treatment of choice for internal resorption is extraction.
   d. pathologic bone and root resorption is always indicative of nonvital pulp.
3. Which of the following diagnostic tests are usually reliable for determining pulpal status in primary teeth?
   a. Thermal pulp tests.
   b. Electric pulp tests.
   c. Percussion testing.
   d. None of the above.
4. Indirect pulp therapy
   a. is indicated only in the treatment of teeth with deep carious lesions in which there is no clinical evidence of pulpal degeneration or periapical pathology.
   b. removes all the bacteria but not all the caries.
   c. includes placing calcium hydroxide or ZOE over the remaining caries and permanently restoring the tooth with amalgam.
   d. All of the above.

5. Direct pulp capping is recommended for primary teeth with
   a. carious exposures.
   b. mechanical exposures.
   c. calcification in the pulp chamber.
   d. All of the above.
6. Calcium hydroxide
   a. is the material of choice for direct pulp capping.
   b. may cause calcification of the remaining pulp tissue.
   c. does not enter into the formation of the dentin bridge.
   d. All of the above.
7. Formocresol pulpotomy on a primary tooth is indicated when
   a. there is a history of spontaneous toothache.
   b. the inflammation or infection is confined to the coronal pulp.
   c. the pulp does not hemorrhage.
   d. hemorrhage following coronal pulp amputation is uncontrollable.
8. Which of the following usually is *not* an indication of failure for a formocresol pulpotomy?
   a. Pain.
   b. Internal resorption of the root adjacent to the area where the formocresol was applied.
   c. Development of a periradicular radiolucency.
   d. Loosening of the tooth.
9. Formocresol pulpotomy as compared to glutaraldehyde pulpotomy
   a. is more successful.
   b. has more undesirable effects.
   c. is the technique taught at most dental schools.
   d. All of the above.
10. Which of the following statements concerning primary root canal anatomy is false?
    a. Root/crown ratio is smaller than that of permanent teeth.
    b. Roots are narrower than those of permanent teeth.
    c. Molar roots are more divergent than those of permanent molars.
    d. Roots are shorter than those of permanent teeth.
11. Considerations for endodontic treatment on primary teeth include
    a. profound anesthesia at the fill appointment.
    b. prevention of overinstrumentation and overfilling.
    c. three-dimensional obturation with gutta-percha.
    d. All of the above.
12. Which of the following is not a contraindication for root canal therapy of primary teeth?
    a. Radiographic evidence of internal resorption in the roots.
    b. Apical restoration involving the roots.
    c. Presence of a dentigerous or follicular cyst.
    d. Mechanical or carious perforation of the floor of the pulp chamber.
13. Access openings on primary incisors
    a. are from the facial surface.
    b. are from the lingual surface.
    c. are from the incisal surface.
    d. differ in location for maxillary and mandibular incisors.
14. Apexification is the treatment of choice for a permanent tooth with a wide-open apex when
    a. the pulp is necrotic.
    b. there is a history of spontaneous pain with a carious exposure.
    c. there is a large mechanical exposure with profuse pulpal bleeding.
    d. All of the above.

Chapter 24

Geriatric Endodontics

Carl W. Newton

Dental service requirements are determined by four demographic and epidemiologic factors: the population at risk, the incidence and prevalence of dental diseases, the accepted standards of care, and the perceived need and expectations toward dental health by the public.[10] As a result of the aging of the population, all of these factors are changing to one degree or another.

According to the U.S. Census Bureau, the number of persons aged 65 and over is expected to reach 35,000,000 by the year 2000, approximately 13% of the U.S. population.[50] The bureau also reported that 9% of those in the 65-and-over age group are 85 years or older. This figure will grow steadily to almost 17% by 2010. For census purposes, the geriatric population is generally divided into two groups, those 65 to 80 and those 80 and older.

The Social Security Administration (Fig. 24-1) shows the percentage distribution of the U.S. population by age from 1985 to 2020.[39] The oldest (85+) segment of the population will grow most rapidly before 2000.[26] The group aged 65 to 74 years will increase most rapidly between the year 2000 and 2020, as the post-World War II baby-boom generation enters the elderly category.

Until 1983, persons aged 65 and older made an average of 1.5 dental visits annually, a lower utilization rate than any other age group's.[48] Between 1983 and 1986, a 29% increase in visits by those 65 years and older was noted by the National Health Survey.[49] According to this survey, older adults currently make more visits per year, on average, than those in the "all ages combined" category. In the future, general dentists will routinely serve a growing number of older persons, who will account for ⅓ to ⅔ of their workload.[21]

Dental services, including root canal procedures, for the elderly population of the future are anticipated to be of two general types: (1) services for relatively healthy elderly who are functionally independent, and (2) services for elderly patients with complex conditions and problems who are functionally dependent.[26] The latter group will require care from practitioners who have advanced training in geriatric dentistry. This age group is being targeted in dental education programs and advanced training through improved curriculum, research, and publications on aging. The National Institute on Aging feels that all dental professionals should receive education concerning treatment of the elderly as part of basic professional education.

The purpose of this chapter is to discuss the effect of aging on the diagnosis of pulpal and periapical disease and successful root canal treatment. The quality of life for older patients can be significantly improved and reflected in their oral health and functions.

A simple pleasure in life is being able to eat what one wishes, and with age the simplest pleasures may become even more important, as does the need for proper diet and nourishment. Every tooth may be strategic, and old age is no time to be forced to replace sound teeth with removable appliances or dentures.

Consultation with elderly patients should help them overcome what may be a very limited knowledge of root canal treatment and lack of appreciation for regular dental care. Well-meaning friends and spouses who contend that their dentures are as good or better than their natural teeth may have had a lifetime of poor dental experiences or have forgotten what it is like to enjoy natural dentition.

The vast majority of elderly people engage in normal activity and can recognize and afford the value of good dentistry.

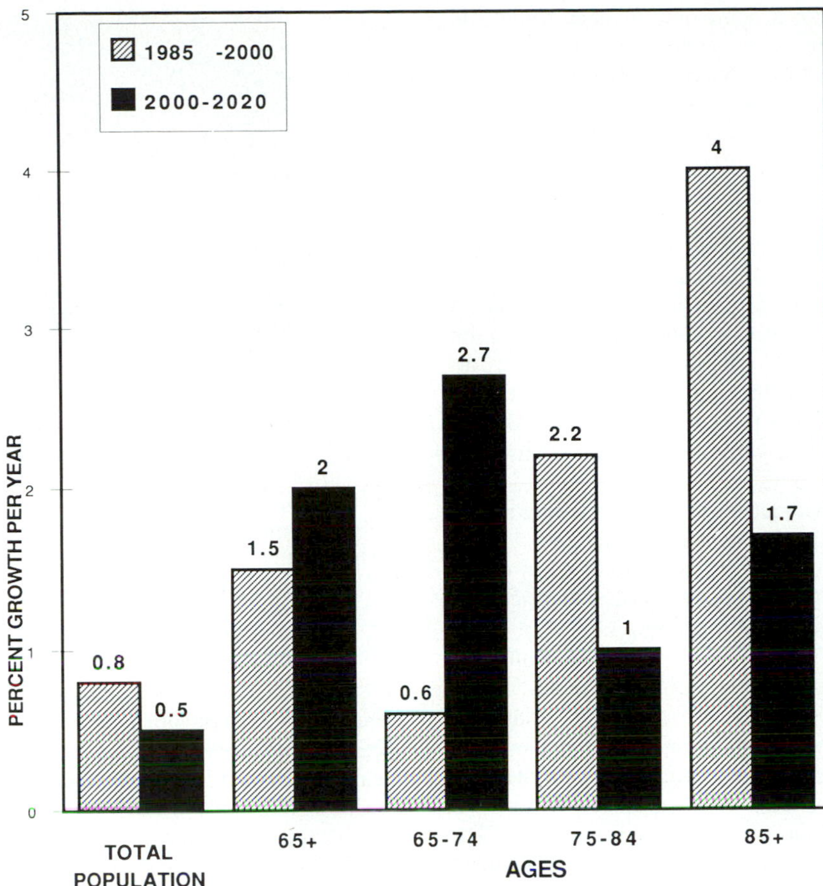

FIG. 24-1 Percentage growth rate and distribution of the U.S. population by age from 1985 to 2020.

Dentists should not presume that they know what is best for senior patients or what they can afford without the patient's full awareness. The needs, expectations, desires, and demands of older people may exceed those of any age group, and the gratitude shown by elderly patients is among the most satisfying of professional experiences.

The desire for root canal treatment among aging patients has increased considerably in recent years. Elderly patients are aware that treatment can be performed comfortably and that age is *not* a factor in predicting success.[2,44,46] Obtaining informed consent also requires that root canal treatment should be offered as a favorable alternative to the trauma of extraction and the cost of replacement. The distribution of specialists and the improved endodontic training of all dentists have broadened the availability of most endodontic procedures to everyone, regardless of age. Expanded dental insurance benefits for retirees and a heightened awareness of the benefits of saving teeth have encouraged many elderly patients to seek endodontia rather than extraction.

This chapter will compare the typical geriatric patient's endodontic needs with those of the general population. Pulp changes attributed to age are discussed in Chapter 11; their effects on clinical treatment will also be discussed.

MEDICAL HISTORY

A medical history should be taken before the patient is brought into the treatment room, and a standardized form should be used to identify any disease or therapy that would alter treatment or its outcome. Some older patients may need assistance in filling out the forms and may not be fully aware of their conditions or history. Vision deficits caused by outdated glasses or cataracts can adversely affect a patient's ability to read the typically small print on many history forms. Consultation with family, guardian, or physician may be necessary to complete the history, but the dentist is ultimately responsible for the treatment.

An updated history, including information on compliance with any prescribed treatment and sensitivity to medications, must be obtained at each visit and reviewed. Elders use more drugs than younger patients, and most of these medications are potentially important to the dentist.[22] The *Physicians' Desk Reference* should be consulted and any precaution or side effect of medication noted.

Although geriatric patients are usually knowledgeable about their medical history, some may not understand the implications of their medical conditions in relation to dentistry or may be reluctant to let the clinician into their confidence. Their perceptions of their illnesses may not be accurate, so any clue to a patient's conditions should be investigated.

Symptoms of undiagnosed illnesses may present the dentist with a screening opportunity that can disclose a condition that might otherwise go untreated or lead to an emergency. Management of medical emergencies in the dental office is best directed toward prevention rather than treatment.

Few families are without at least one member whose life has been extended as a result of medical progress. A great number have had diseases or disabilities controlled with therapies that may alter the clinician's case selection. Root canal treatment is certainly far less traumatic in the extremes of age or health than is extraction.

Chief Complaint

Most patients who are experiencing dental pain have a pulpal or periapical problem that will require root canal treatment or extraction. Dental needs are often manifested initially in the form of a complaint, which usually contains the information necessary to make a diagnosis. The diagnostic process is directed toward determining whether pulpal or periapical disease is present, whether palliative or root canal therapy is indicated, the vitality of the pulp, and which tooth is the source (see Chapter 1).

The clinician should, without leading, allow the patient to explain the problem in his or her own way. This gives the examiner an opportunity to observe the patient's level of dental knowledge and ability to communicate. Visual and auditory handicaps may become evident at this time.

Patiently encouraging the patient to talk about problems may lead into areas of only peripheral interest to the dentist, but it establishes a needed rapport and demonstrates sincere interest. A patient may exhibit some feelings of distrust if there is a history of failed treatments or if there are well-meaning denture-wearing friends or relatives who claim normal function and are now free of the need for dental treatment. The effect of the "focal infection" theory is still evident when other aches and pains cannot be adequately explained and loss of teeth is accepted as inevitable. The best patients are those who have already had successful endodontic treatment.

Most geriatric patients do not complain readily about signs or symptoms of pulp and periapical disease. A disease process usually arises as an acute problem in children, but assumes a more chronic or less dramatic form in the elderly. The *mere presence* of teeth indicates resistance to disease or proper maintenance. A lifetime of experiencing pains puts a different perspective on interpreting dental pain.

Pain associated with vital pulps (that which is caused by heat, cold, or sweets; or referred pain) seems to be reduced with age, and the severity of symptoms diminished. Heat sensitivity that occurs as the only symptom suggests a reduced pulp volume such as that occurring in the older pulps.[16] Pulpal healing capacity is also reduced, and necrosis may occur quickly following microbial invasion, again with reduced symptoms.

Although complaints are fewer, they are usually more conclusive evidence of disease. The complaint should isolate the problem sufficiently to allow the clinician to take a periapical radiograph before proceeding. Studying radiographs before an examination can prejudice rather than focus attention; accordingly they should be reviewed *after* the clinical examination has been completed.

Dental History

Search the patient's records and explore his or her memories to determine the history of the involved teeth or surrounding area. The history may be as obvious as a recent pulp exposure and restoration, or as subtle as a routine crown preparation 15 or 20 years ago. Any history of pain before or after treatments may establish the beginning of a degenerative process. Subclinical injuries caused by repeated episodes of decay and its treatment may accumulate and approach a clinically significant threshold that can be later exceeded following additional routine procedures. Multiple restorations on the same tooth are common (Fig. 24-2).

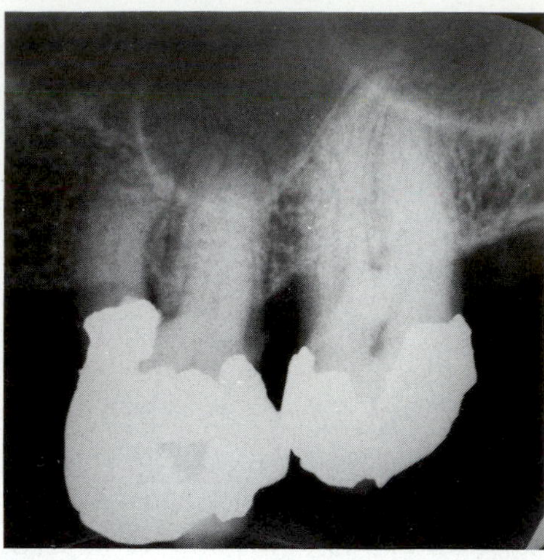

FIG. 24-2 Multiple restorations on this 74-year-old patient suggest repeated episodes of decay and restorative procedures whose pulpal effects can accumulate in the form of subclinical inflammation and calcification.

Recording information at the time of treatment may seem to be unnecessary busy work, but it could prove to be helpful in identifying the source of a complaint or disease many years later. Patients' recall of dental treatments is usually limited to a few years, but the presence of certain materials or appliances can sometimes date a procedure. Aging patients' dental histories are rarely complete and may indicate treatment by several dentists and at different locations.

Subjective Symptoms

The examiner can pursue responses to questions about the patient's complaint, the stimulus or irritant that causes pain, the nature of the pain, and its relationship to the stimulus or irritant. This information is most useful in determining whether or not the source is pulpal, whether it has extended to the apical tissues, and its reversibility, and can thus suggest what types of tests are necessary to confirm findings or suspicions. For further information the reader is referred to Chapter 1.

It is important to remember that pulpal symptoms are chronic in elderly patients, and other sources of orofacial pain should be ruled out when pain is not soon localized. Much of the information to be obtained from the complaint, history, and description of subjective symptoms can be gathered in a screening interview by the clinician's assistant or over the phone by the receptionist. The need for treatment can be established and can provide a focus for the examination.

Objective Signs

The intraoral and extraoral clinical examination provides valuable first-hand information about disease and previous treatment. The overall oral condition should not be overlooked while centering on the patient's complaint, and all abnormal

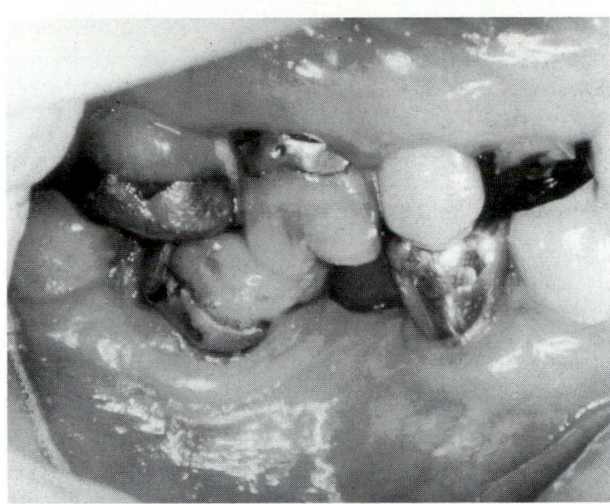

FIG. 24-3 Missing teeth and the subsequent tilt, rotation, and supereruption of adjacent and opposing teeth contribute to reduced functional ability and increased susceptibility to decay and periodontal disease.

conditions should be recorded and investigated. Exposures to etiologic factors that contribute to oral cancers accumulate with age, and many systemic diseases may initially manifest prodromal oral signs or symptoms.

Missing teeth contribute to reduced functional ability (Fig. 24-3). The resultant loss of chewing efficiency leads to a higher-carbohydrate diet of softer and more cariogenic foods. Increased sugar intake to compensate for loss of taste[13,24] and xerostomia[3] are also factors in the renewed susceptibility to decay.

Gingival recession, which creates sensitivity and is hard to control, exposes cementum and dentin that are less resistant to decay. A clinical study of 600 patients over age 60 showed that 70% had root caries and 100% had some degree of gingival recession.[51] The removal of root caries is irritating to the pulp and often results in pulp exposures or reparative dentin formation that affect the negotiation of the canal should root canal treatment later be needed (Fig. 24-4). Asymptomatic pulp exposures on one root surface of a multirooted tooth can result in the uncommon clinical situation of the presence of both vital and nonvital pulp tissue in the same tooth. Interproximal root caries is difficult to restore, and restoration failure as a result of continued decay is common (Fig. 24-5). Although the microbiology of diseases is not substantially different in different age groups, the altered host response during aging may modify the progression of these diseases.[47]

Attrition (Fig. 24-6), abrasion, and erosion (Fig. 24-7) also expose dentin through a slower process that allows the pulp to respond with dentinal sclerosis and reparative dentin.[41] Secondary dentin formation occurs throughout life and may eventually result in almost complete pulp obliteration. In maxillary anterior teeth, the secondary dentin is formed on the lingual wall of the pulp chamber[31]; in molar teeth the greatest deposition occurs on the floor of the chamber.[6] Although this pulp may appear to recede, small pulpal remnants can remain or leave a less calcific tract that may lead to a pulp exposure.

In general, canal and chamber volume are inversely proportional to age: as age increases canal size decreases (Fig. 24-8). Reparative dentin resulting from restorative procedures, trauma, attrition, and recurrent caries also contributes to diminution of canal and chamber size. In addition, the cementodentinal junction moves farther from the radiographic apex with continued cementum deposition (Fig. 24-9).[18] The thickness of young apical cementum[36] is 100 to 200 μm and increases with age to two or three times that thickness.[54]

The calcification process associated with aging appears clinically to be of a more linear type than that which occurs in a younger tooth in response to caries, pulpotomy, or trauma (Fig. 24-10). Dentinal tubules become more occluded with advancing age, decreasing tubular permeability.[23] Lateral and accessory canals can calcify, thus decreasing their clinical significance.

The compensating bite produced by missing and tilted teeth or attrition can cause temporomandibular joint dysfunction (less common in the elderly) or loss of vertical dimension. Any limitation in opening reduces available working time and the space needed for instrumentation.

The presence of multiple restorations indicates a history of repeated insults and an accumulation of irritants. Marginal leakage and microbial contamination of cavity walls is a ma-

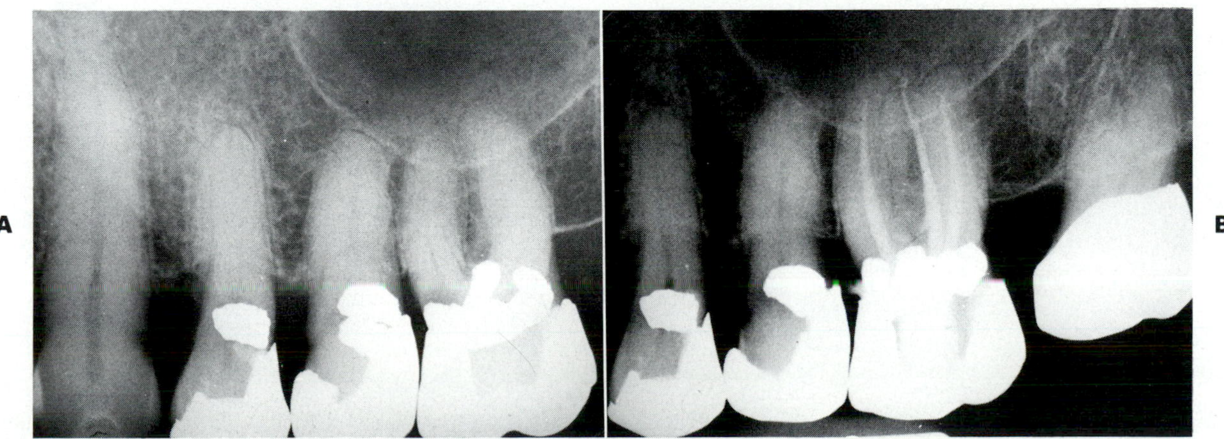

FIG. 24-4 Gingival recession exposes cementum and dentin, which is less resistant to decay. Root caries, **A,** often results in **B,** pulp exposures that require root canal treatment.

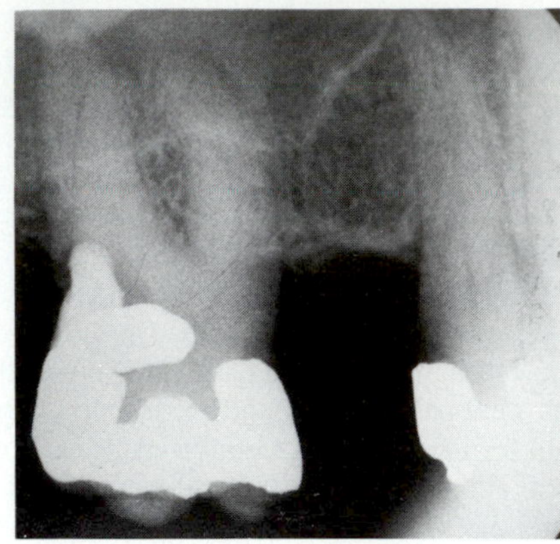

FIG. 24-5 Interproximal root decay is hard to restore and creates a very difficult isolation problem if root canal treatment is indicated.

jor cause of pulpal injury.[7] Violating principles of cavity design combines with the loss of resiliency that results from a reduced organic component to the dentin to increase susceptibility to cracks and cuspal fractures. In any further restorative procedures on such teeth, the clinician should consider the effect on the pulp as well as the effect on accessing and negotiating canals through such restorations if root canal therapy is indicated later.

Many cracks or craze lines (Fig. 24-7) may be evident as a result of staining, but they do not indicate dentin penetration or pulp exposure. Pulp exposures caused by cracks are less likely to present acute problems in older patients and often penetrate the sulcus to create a periodontal defect as well as a periapical one. If incomplete cracks are not detected early, the prognosis for cracked teeth in older patients will be questionable.

Periodontal disease may be the principal problem for dentate seniors.[9] The relationship between pulpal and periodontal disease (see Chapter 18) can be expected to be more signifi-

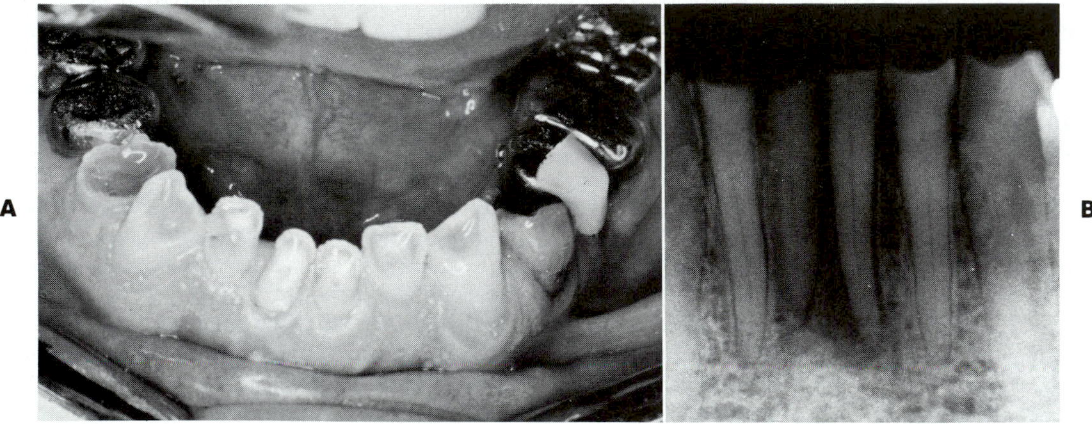

FIG. 24-6 A, Attrition exposes dentin through a slow process that allows the pulp to respond with reparative dentin, but pulp exposure eventually becomes clinically evident **(B).**

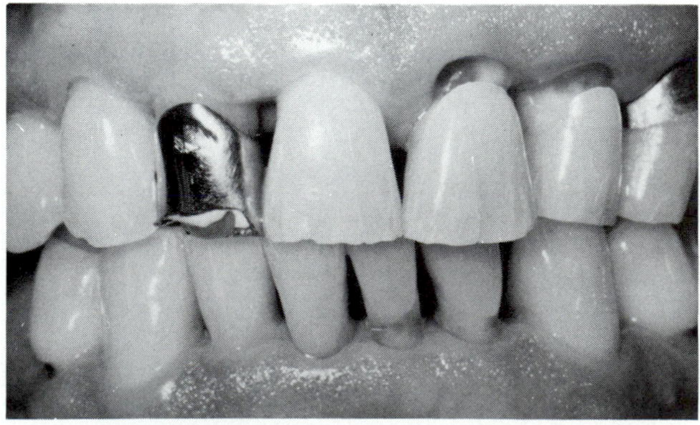

FIG. 24-7 Gingival recession also exposes cementum and dentin that is less resistant to abrasion and erosion, which can expose pulp or require restorative procedures that could result in pulp irritation.

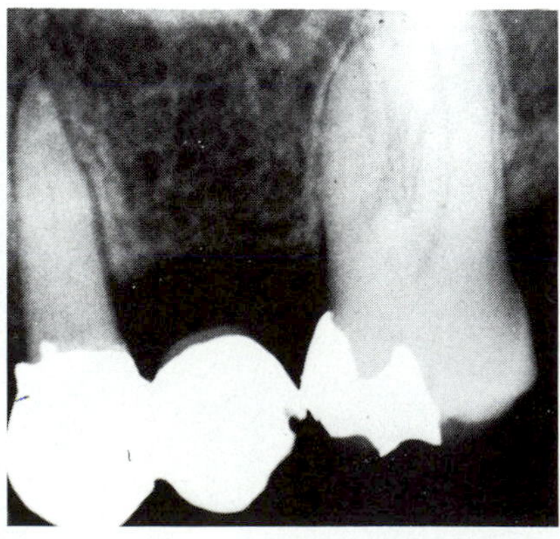

FIG. 24-8 In general, canal and chamber volume are inversely proportional to age: as age increases, canal size decreases. This maxillary molar illustrates reduced canal and chamber volume in an elderly patient.

cant with age. Retention of teeth alone demonstrates some resistance to periodontal disease. The increase in disease prevalence is largely attributable to an increase in the proportional size of the population who have retained their teeth.[20] The periodontal tissues must be considered a pathway for sinus tracts (Fig. 24-11). Narrow, bony-walled pockets associated with nonvital pulps are usually sinus tracts, but they can be resistant to root canal therapy alone when with time they become chronic periodontal pockets. Periodontal treatment itself can produce root sensitivity, disease, and pulp death.[19] In developing a successful treatment plan it is important to determine the effects on the pulp of periodontal disease and its treatment. The mere increase in incidence and severity of periodontal disease with age increase the need for combined therapy. The chronic nature of pulp disease demonstrated with sinus tracts can often be manifested in a periodontal pocket. Root canal treatment is commonly indicated before root amputations are performed. With age, the size and number of apical and accessory foramina are actually reduced as pathways of communication,[33] as is the permeability of dentinal tubules.

Examination of sinus tracts should include tracing with gutta-percha cones to establish their origin. Sinus tracts may have long clinical histories and usually indicate the presence of chronic periapical inflammation. They are excellent indicators of healing when they disappear following treatment. Presence of a sinus tract reduces risk of interappointment or postoperative pain, although drainage may follow canal débridement or filling.

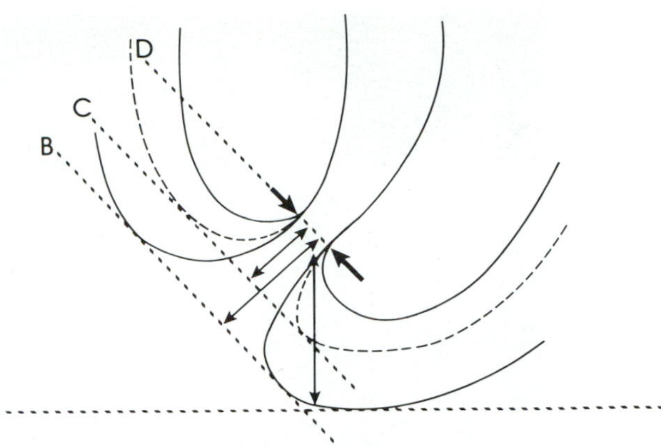

FIG. 24-9 The cementodentinal junction at *D* is the smallest diameter of the root canal system, and treatment at this point produces the smallest wound and greatest resistance to condensation during filling procedures. With continued cementum deposition throughout life, the distance from the anatomic apex increases (from *C* to *B*) as does the distance from the radiographic apex, *A*.

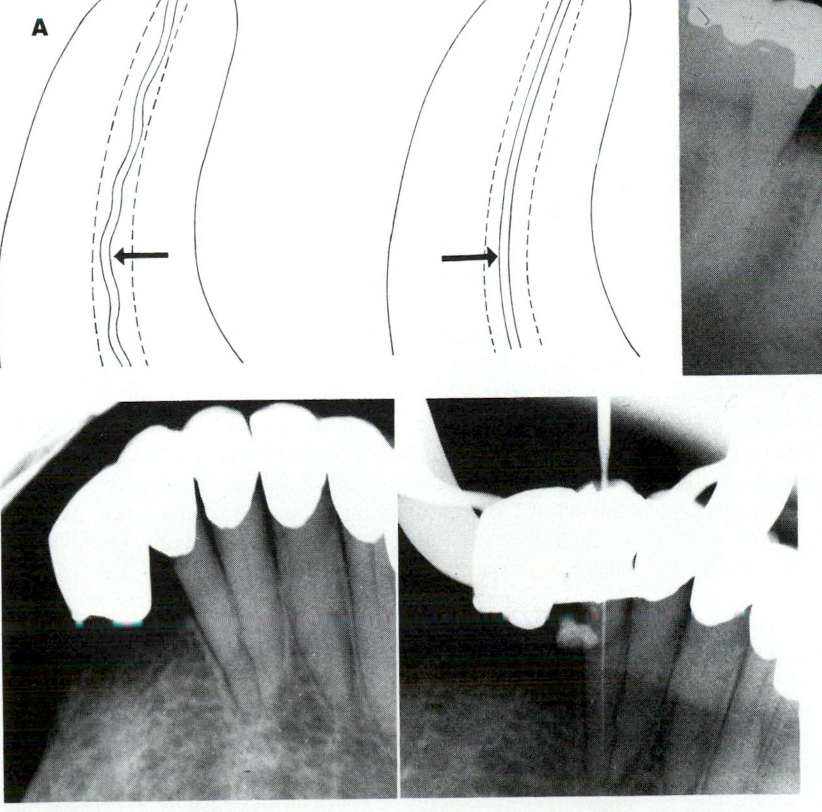

FIG. 24-10 A, The calcification process in aging appears clinically to be linear *(right)* and probably more easily negotiated than the irregular calcification diagrammatically illustrated *(left)* that occurs in a younger tooth. **B,** Treatment of this mandibular molar, with mesial canals calcified because of a pulp cap 15 years earlier, presents a much more difficult negotiation than **C** and **D,** the mandibular incisor in a 79-year-old patient.

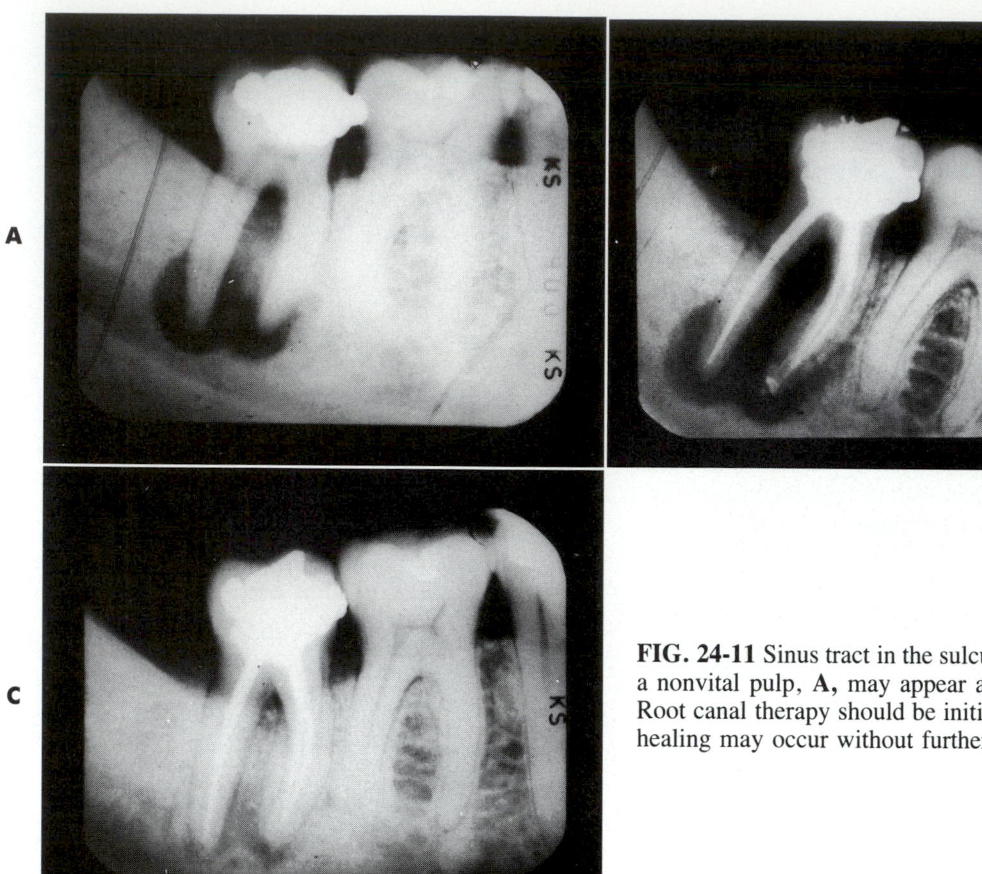

FIG. 24-11 Sinus tract in the sulcus of tooth no. 31 with a nonvital pulp, **A,** may appear as periodontal disease. Root canal therapy should be initiated, **B,** and complete healing may occur without further treatment, **C.**

Pulp testing

Information collected from the patient's complaint and history and from the examination may be adequate to establish pulp vitality and should direct the clinician toward the techniques that are most useful in determining which tooth or teeth are the object of the complaint.

Slow and gentle testing should be done to determine pulp and periapical status and whether palliative or definitive therapy is indicated. Vitality responses must correlate with clinical and radiographic findings and be interpreted as a supplement in developing clinical judgment. Techniques for clinical pulp-testing procedures are discussed in Chapter 1.

Transilluminating[32] and staining have been advocated as means to detect cracks, but their observation is of little significance in the absence of complaints because most older teeth, especially molars, will demonstrate some cracks. Vertically cracked teeth should always be considered when pulpal or periapical disease is observed and little or no cause for pulpal irritation can be observed clinically or radiographically. The chronic nature of periapical pathology caused by vertically cracked teeth indicates that it is longstanding, and the prognosis is questionable even when pocket depths appear normal. Periodontal pockets associated with cracks indicate a poor prognosis.

The reduced neural and vascular component of aged pulps,[5] the overall reduced pulp volume, and the change in character of the ground substance[40] create an environment that responds differently to both stimuli and irritants than that of younger pulps (Fig. 24-12).

There are fewer nerve branches in older pulps. This may be due to retrogressive changes resulting from mineralization of the nerve and nerve sheath (Fig. 24-13).[4] Consequently, the response to stimuli may be weaker than in the more highly innervated younger pulp.

There is no correlation between the degree of response to electric pulp testing and the degree of inflammation.[34] The presence or absence of response is of limited value and must be correlated with other tests, examination findings, and radiographs. Extensive restorations, pulp recession, and excessive calcifications are limitations in both performing and interpreting results of electric and thermal pulp testing. Attachments that reduce the amount of surface contact necessary to conduct the electrical stimulus are available from Analytic Technology,[27] and bridging the tip to small area of tooth sturucture with an explorer has been suggested.[29] Use of even this small electric stimulus in patients with pacemakers[52] is not recommended; any such risk would outweigh the benefit. The same caution holds true for electrosurgical units.

A test cavity is generally less useful as the test of last resort because of reduced dentin innervation. Vital pulps can sometimes be exposed with minimal pain; then the root canal treatment becomes part of the diagnostic procedure. Test cavities should be utilized only when other findings are suggestive but not conclusive.

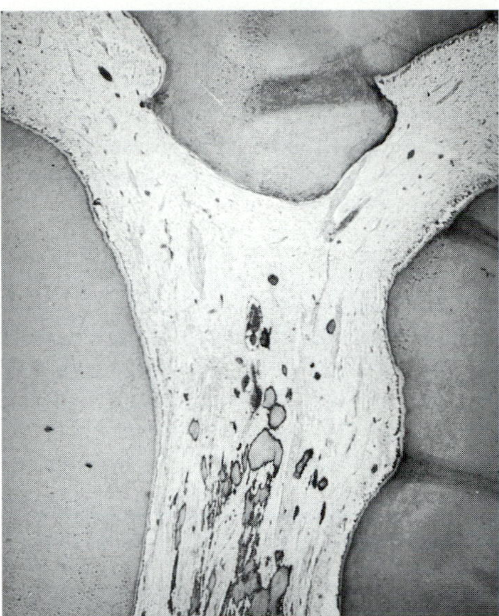

FIG. 24-12 There is a gradual decrease in the cellularity of older pulp tissue and the odontoblasts decrease in size and number and may disappear altogether in certain areas, particularly on the pulpal floor in multirooted teeth.

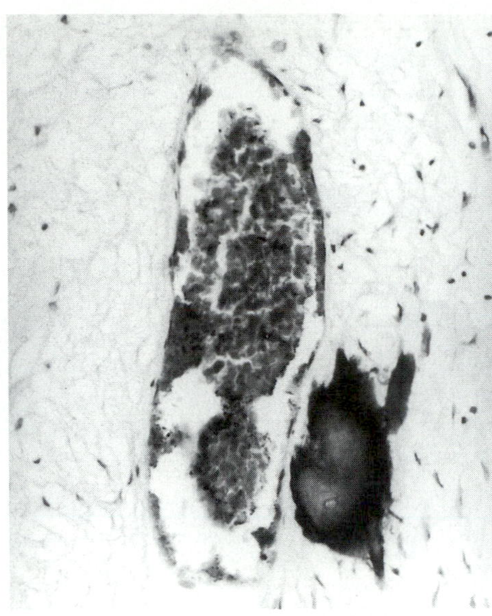

FIG. 24-13 Fibrosis appears to occur along the pathways of degenerated vessels and may serve as foci for pulpal calcification.

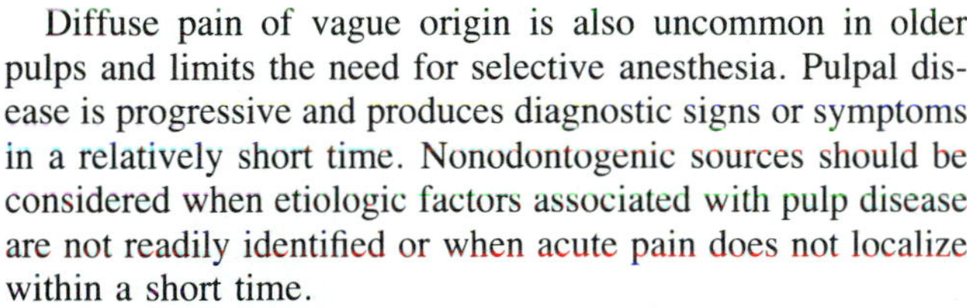

Diffuse pain of vague origin is also uncommon in older pulps and limits the need for selective anesthesia. Pulpal disease is progressive and produces diagnostic signs or symptoms in a relatively short time. Nonodontogenic sources should be considered when etiologic factors associated with pulp disease are not readily identified or when acute pain does not localize within a short time.

Discoloration of single teeth may indicate pulp death, but this is a less likely cause of discoloration with advanced age. Dentin thickness is greater and the tubules are less permeable to blood or breakdown products from the pulp. Dentin deposition produces a yellow, opaque color that would indicate progressive calcification in a younger pulp.

Radiographs

Indications for and techniques of taking radiographs do not differ much among adult age groups, although several physiologic, anatomic changes can significantly affect their interpretation. Film placement may be adversely affected by tori but can be assisted by the apical position of muscle attachments that increase the depth of the vestibule. Older patients may be less capable of assisting in film placement, and holders that secure the position should be considered. The presence of tori, exostoses, and denser bone (Fig. 24-14) may require increased exposure times for proper diagnostic contrast. The subjective nature of interpretation can be reduced with correct processing, proper illumination, and magnification.

The periapical area must be included in the diagnostic radiograph, which should be studied from the crown toward the apex. Angled radiographs should be ordered only after the original diagnostic radiograph suggests that more information is needed for diagnosis or to determine the degree of difficulty of treatment.

In older patients, pulp recession is accelerated by reparative dentin and complicated by pulp stones and dystrophic calcification. Deep proximal or root decay and restorations may cause calcification between the observable chamber and root canal.

The depth of the chamber should be measured from the occlusal and its mesiodistal position noted. Receding pulp horns apparent on a radiograph may remain microscopically much higher. Deep restorations or extensive occlusal crown reduction may produce pulp exposures that were not expected. The axial inclinations of crowns may not correlate with the clinical observation when tilted teeth have been crowned or become abutments for fixed or removable appliances. Access to the root canals is the most limiting condition in root canal treatment of older patients.

Canals should be examined for their number, size, shape, and curvature. Comparisons to adjacent teeth should be made. Small canals are the rule in older patients. A midroot disappearance of a detectable canal may indicate bifurcation rather than calcification. Canals will calcify evenly throughout their length unless an irritant (decay, restoration, cervical abrasion) has separated the chamber from the root canal. Retrograde fillings during apioectomies, more common during retreatment of older patients, indicate missed canals and roots as a common cause of failure.[1]

The lamina dura should be examined in its entirety and anatomic landmarks distinguished from periapical radiolucencies and radiopacities. The incidence of some odontogenic and nonodontogenic cysts and tumors characteristically increases with age and this should be considered when vitality tests do not correlate with radiographic findings. The incidence of osteosclerosis and condensing osteitis, however, decreases with age.[37]

Resorption associated with chronic apical periodontitis may significantly alter the shape of the apex and the anatomy of the foramen through inflammatory osteoclastic activity (Fig. 24-15).[8] The narrowest point in the canal may be difficult to

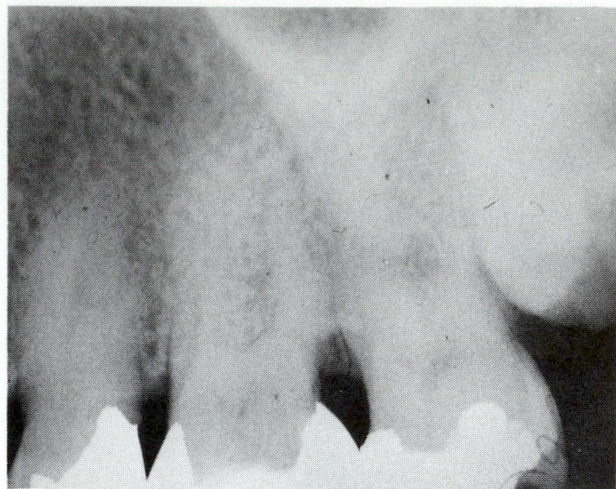

FIG. 24-14 Dense bone may indicate the need for increased exposure times to improve contrast needed to see canal and root anatomy.

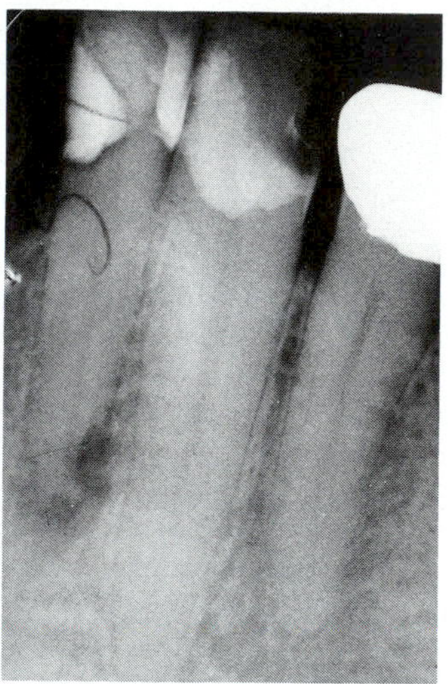

FIG. 24-15 Resorption associated with chronic apical periodontitis may alter the shape and the position of the foramen through osteoclastic activity. The narrowest point in the canal lies farther from the radiographic apex.

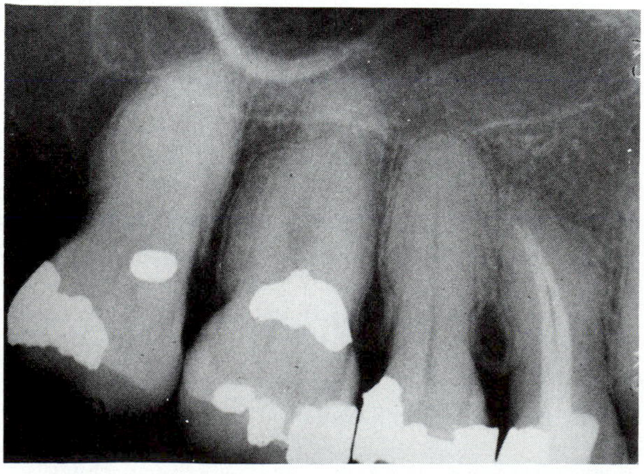

FIG. 24-16 Hypercementosis may completely obscure the apical anatomy and result in a constriction farther from the radiographic apex.

determine, and it will be positioned farther from the radiographic apex.

A continued normal rate of cementum formation may be demonstrated by a canal or foramen that appears to end or exit short of the radiographic apex, and hypercementosis (Fig. 24-16) may completely obscure the apical anatomy.[35]

DIAGNOSIS AND TREATMENT PLAN

A clinical classification that accurately reflects the histologic status of the pulp and periapical tissues is not possible—and not necessary beyond determining whether or not root canal treatment is indicated. A clinical judgment can be made, based on the patient's complaint, history, signs, symptoms, testing, and radiographs, as to the vitality of the pulp and the presence or absence of periapical pathology. This classification has not been shown to be a factor in predicting success,[12] interappointment or postoperative pain,[14] or the number of visits necessary to complete treatment[25] when the objectives of cleansing, shaping, and filling are clearly understood and consistently met. Of great clinical significance in treatment procedures is the assessment of pulp status in order to determine the depth of anesthesia necessary to perform the treatment comfortably.

One-appointment procedures offer obvious advantages to elderly patients (Fig. 24-17). The length of a dental appointment does not usually cause inconvenience, as may more numerous appointments, especially if a patient must rely on another person for transportation or needs physical assistance to get into the office or operatory.

Root canal treatment as a restorative expediency on teeth

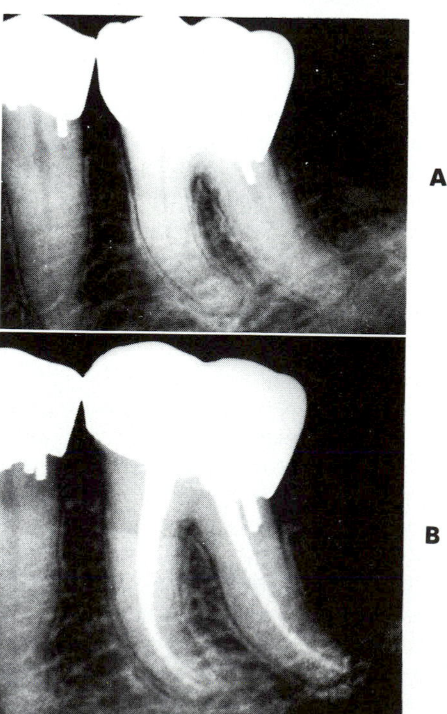

FIG. 24-17 A, Mandibular molar diagnosed with irreversible pulpitis in an 87-year-old patient who traveled 50 miles one way and was treated in one visit. **B,** Crown access restored at the same visit. Comfort of the patient was monitored and treatment was tolerated very well even though total chair time was 2 hours.

with normal pulps must be considered when cusps have fractured, or when supraerupted or malaligned teeth, intracoronal attachments, guideplanes for partial abutments, rest seats, or overdentures require significant tooth reduction. Predicting future need for root canal treatment and a practitioner's ability to perform treatment later is even more important, because the risk of losing the restoration during later access preparation increases with the thickness of the restoration and the reduction in canal size (Fig. 24-18). Because of a reduced blood supply, pulp cappings are not as successful in older teeth as in younger ones, and therefore are not recommended. The risk to the patient's future health and the effect it may have on his or her ability to withstand future procedures should also be considered. Endodontic surgery at a later time is not as viable an alternative as for a younger patient.

Consultation and Consent

Good communication should be established and maintained with all patients, regardless of whether or not they are visual or hearing impaired, or are fully responsible for making treatment decisions. Relatives or trusted friends should be included in consultations if their judgment is valued by the patient or needed for consent. Procedures should be explained so that they are completely comprehensible, and opportunities provided for questions and discussions. Obtaining signed consent to outlined treatment is encouraged and may be especially useful if the patient is forgetful.

Determining the patient's desires is as important as determining his or her needs and is required in obtaining informed consent. Priorities in treating pain and infection to properly and esthetically restore teeth to health and function should be unaffected by age (Fig. 24-19). A patient's limited life expectancy should not appreciably alter treatment plans and surely is no excuse for extractions or poor root canal treatment. It is important that each geriatric patient be well informed of risks and alternatives.

Acceptance of the eventual loss of teeth has been replaced by an understanding of the psychological and functional importance of maintaining dentition. Elderly patients whose lives have been changed for the worse by a previous surgical procedure may readily recognize the implications of the loss of teeth.

The capability of the clinician and the availability of endodontic specialists should also be considered. The obligation to offer root canal treatment as an alternative to extraction may exceed a clinician's ability to perform the procedure efficiently or successfully and referral may be indicated.

Obtaining informed consent prior to dental procedures usually is not a problem. However, medically compromised or cognitively impaired patients may make it difficult to acquire valid informed consent. Neuropsychiatric impairment may result in gross manifestations and indicate a reduced level of competency. Physicians or mental health experts should be consulted as needed, and no elective procedures performed until valid consent is established. Fortunately, acute pulpal and periapical episodes in which immediate treatment is indicated for pain or infection are less common than the low-grade signs and symptoms of chronic disease.

TREATMENT

The vast majority of geriatric patients who need and demand endodontic therapy are not institutionalized and are ambulatory. Institutionalized and nonambulatory patients require practitioners trained in those environments and facilities designed for access to dental health care. Such access is a benefit required in most institutions, but alternatives to root canal therapy may be the only services available. Extended health care facilities are now required to have dentists on staff before Medicare certification can be obtained. The dental office building, including both the interior design and the exterior approach, must be able to accommodate people with any handicapping condition.[28,55] Access for those who use ambulation aids such as canes, walkers, and wheelchairs should include comfort and safety in the parking lot, reception room, operatory, and rest room.

A physical and mental evaluation of the patient should determine the ideal time of day and length of time necessary to

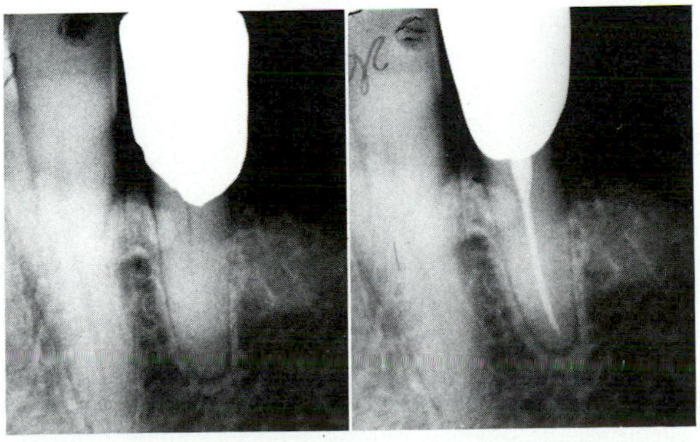

FIG. 24-18 A, Intracoronal attachments, guideplanes, and rest seats for partial abutments require significant tooth reduction and a bulk of metal that makes root canal treatment more likely and difficult. **B,** Successful treatment and preservation of the restoration when the canal is small is a challenge to the most skilled clinician.

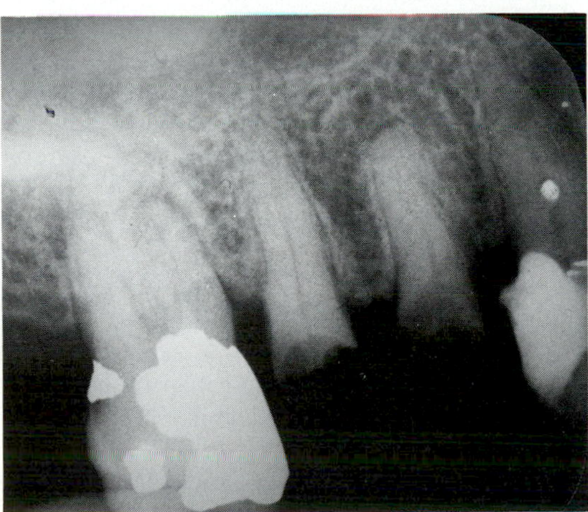

FIG. 24-19 This 84-year-old patient was pleased to find that all of these teeth could be saved with root canal procedures and crown and was eager to make the investment in time and money in spite of her limited life expectancy. Her concern focused on why these procedures had not been recommended by her previous dentist, whom she visited regularly.

schedule treatment. A patient's daily personal, eating, and resting habits should be considered, as well as any medication schedule. Morning appointments are preferable for some older patients, and their comfort, which will vary with the procedure indicated, dictates the length of the appointment. Some patients prefer late morning or early afternoon visits, to allow "morning stiffness" to dissipate.[11] They are more likely to tolerate long appointments better than most, although chair positioning and comfort may be more important for elders than for younger patients. Patients should be offered assistance into the operatory and into or out of the chair. Chair adjustments should be made slowly, and the ideal position established and used if possible. Pillows should be offered, as well as assistance in positioning them comfortably. Every effort should be made to accommodate the ideal position, even at some expense to the operator's comfort or access. The patient's eyes should be shielded from the intensity of the operator's light. If the temperature selected for the comfort of the office staff is too cool for the patient, a blanket should be available. As much work as possible should be performed at each visit, and a rest room break offered at intervals as the patient's needs indicate. Jaw fatigue is readily recognizable and may be the most limiting factor in a long procedure, requiring periods of rest; however, once such fatigue is evident, the procedure should be terminated as soon as possible. Bite blocks are useful in comfortably maintaining freeway space and reducing jaw fatigue.

Retired persons may rely on friends or relatives or public transportation and are very often early for appointments, but they are usually in no hurry once they arrive. Enough time should be scheduled to allow some social exchange, and a sincere personal interest should be demonstrated before proceeding. Allow patients to initiate handshakes, which may be very uncomfortable to arthritic joints. From a behavioral and management standpoint, geriatric patients are among the most cooperative, available, and appreciative.

Medically compromised patients among the elderly are at no more risk of complications than those in any other age group, and the chronicity of their diseases can alert the clinician to necessary precautions. It should again be recognized that for older people root canal therapy is far less traumatic than extraction.

The need for anesthesia is determined by the pulp vitality status and the cervical positioning of the rubber dam clamp. Aged patients more readily accept treatment without anesthesia and sometimes even need to be convinced that anesthesia is necessary for root canal treatment if their routine operative procedures have been performed without it. Teeth with necrotic pulps occasionally may be treated without anesthesia, if possible, to allow the patient's response to instrumentation through the apical foramen to determine file length or need for adjustment; this reduces the risk of overinstrumentation and inoculation of canal contents into the periapical tissue.

The cutting of dentin does not produce the same level of response in an older patient for the same reason that a test cavity is not as revealing during examination. The number of low threshold, high conduction velocity nerve endings in dentin are reduced or absent and do not extend as far into the dentin, and the dentinal tubules are more calcified.[5,40] A painful response may not be encountered until actual pulp exposure has occurred.

Anatomic landmarks that are used as guides to needle placement during block and infiltration injections are usually more distinguishable in older patients. Anesthetics should be deposited very slowly and skeletal muscle avoided if epinephrine is the vasoconstrictor. The effects of epinephrine should be considered when selecting anesthetics for routine endodontic procedures.

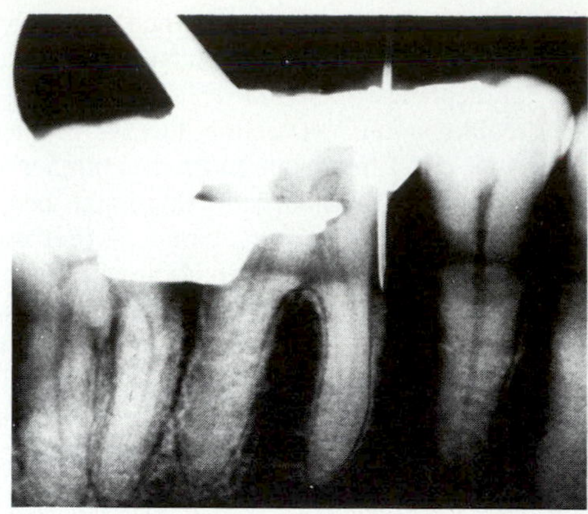

FIG. 24-20 Reduced width of the PDL makes needle placement for supplementary intraligamentary injections more difficult. Smaller needles may penetrate farther but bend more easily and may stick into root structure. Small amounts of anesthetic should be deposited slowly and under pressure with this technique.

The reduced width of the PDL[17] makes needle placement for supplementary intraligamentary injections more difficult (Fig. 24-20). Placing an anesthetic under pressure produces intraosseous anesthesia that extends to the apex as well as to adjacent teeth, but it also distributes small amounts of solution systemically.[38] Small amounts of anesthetic should be deposited during intraligamentary injections, and the depth of anesthesia checked before repeating. Like intrapulpal anesthesia, this type of anesthesia is not prolonged and the pulp tissue must be removed within 20 minutes.

The reduced volume of the pulp chamber makes intrapulpal anesthesia difficult. Initial pulp exposures are also hard to identify. Wedging a small needle into each canal to produce the necessary pressure for anesthesia is the method of last resort (Fig. 24-21). Every effort should be made to produce profound anesthesia. Patients should be encouraged to report any unpleasant sensation, and a prompt response should be made to any complaint. Patients should never be expected to tolerate pulpal pain.

Isolation

Single-tooth rubber dam isolation should be used whenever possible. Badly broken-down teeth may not provide an adequate purchase point for the rubber dam clamp and alternate rubber dam isolation methods should be considered (see Chapter 4). Multiple-tooth isolation may be used if adjacent teeth can be clamped and saliva output is low or a well-placed saliva ejector can be tolerated (Fig. 24-22). A petroleum-based lubricant for the lips and gingiva reduces chafing from saliva or perspiration beneath the rubber dam. Reduction in salivary flow and gag reflex reduces the need for a saliva ejector.

Canals should be identified and their access maintained if restorative procedures are indicated for isolation. The clinician should not attempt isolation and access in a tooth with questionable marginal integrity of its restorations. Fluid-tight isolation cannot be compromised when sodium hypochlorite is

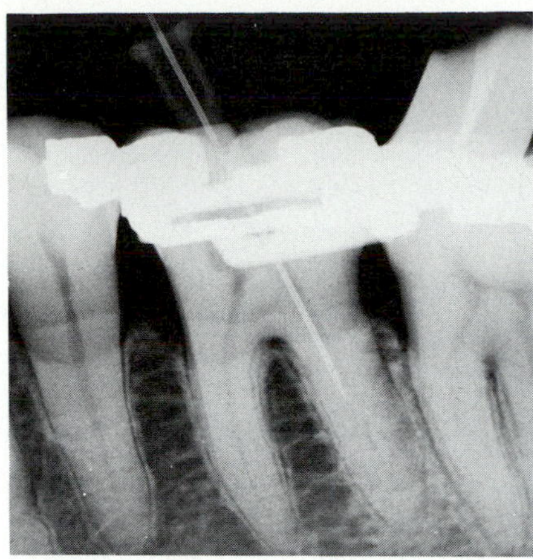

FIG. 24-21 Intraligamentary anesthesia is far superior to intrapulpal anesthesia, which is the method of last resort, and actual penetration into the canal may be necessary to generate sufficient pressure to produce profound anesthesia. Canal contents should be removed immediately because this is not a long-lasting anesthesia.

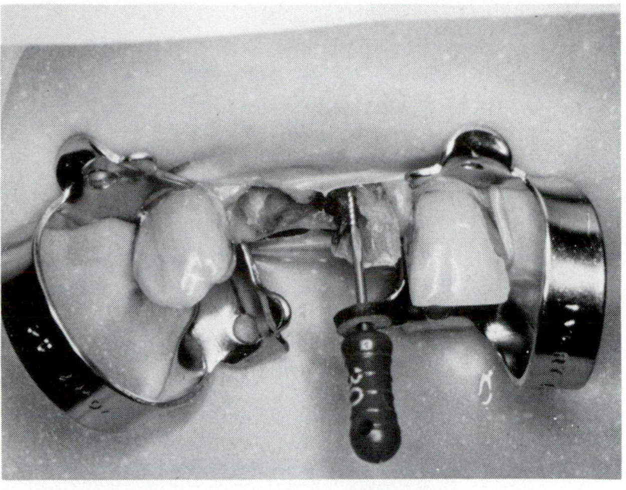

FIG. 24-22 Multiple tooth isolation techniques protect the patient from instruments but do not provide the fluid-tight environment preferred for the safe use of sodium hypochlorite.

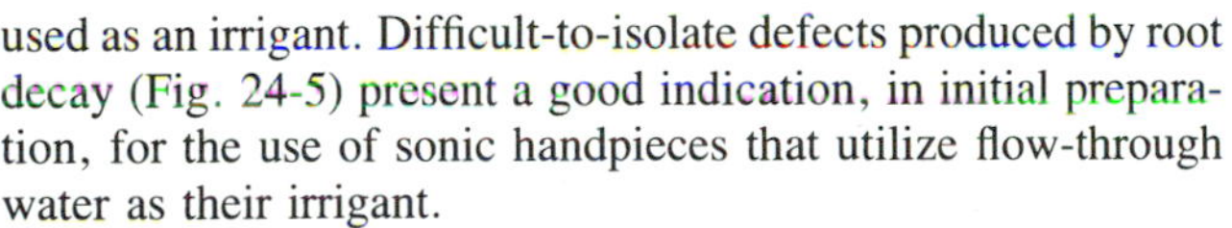

used as an irrigant. Difficult-to-isolate defects produced by root decay (Fig. 24-5) present a good indication, in initial preparation, for the use of sonic handpieces that utilize flow-through water as their irrigant.

The many merits of single-visit root canal procedures described in Chapter 4 should again be considered when isolation is compromised. The few benefits of multiple-visit treatment are further reduced if an interappointment seal is difficult to obtain.

Access

Adequate access and identification of canal orifices are probably the most difficult parts of root canal treatment on aged teeth. Although the effects of aging and multiple restorations may reduce the volume and coronal extent of the chamber or canal orifice, its buccolingual and mesiodistal position remain the same and can be predicted from radiographs and clinical examination. Canal position, root curvature, and axial inclinations of roots and crowns should be considered during the examination (Fig. 24-23). The effects of access on existing restorations and the possible need for actual removal of the restoration should be discussed with the patient before proceeding. Coronal tooth structure or restorations should be sacrificed when they compromise access for preparation or filling (Fig. 24-24). The reader is referred to Chapter 7 for more details on proper access openings.

Magnification in the range of 2.5 to 3.5× (e.g., Designs for Vision) has become a common tool and can be designed to fit the clinician's most comfortable working distance. The most recent introduction of endodontic microscopes offers clear magnification of 25× or greater.

Pain, bleeding, disorientation of the probing instruments, or an unfamiliar feel to the canal may indicate a perforation (Fig. 24-25). The size of the perforation and the extent of contamination determine the success of repair and do not necessarily indicate failure.

A lengthy, unproductive search for canals is fatiguing and frustrating to both the clinician and the patient. Scheduling a

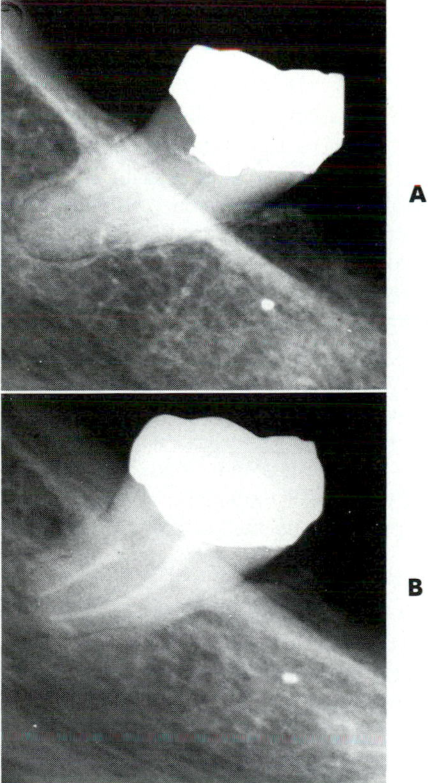

FIG. 24-23 A, This mandibular third molar in a 78-year-old patient has tilted mesially and has been restored with a full crown, upright to allow a path of insertion for a removable partial denture. **B,** Successful root canal treatment is the primary objective; retaining the crown, when possible, also represents significant savings to the patient. This crown will be replaced; a post space has been prepared.

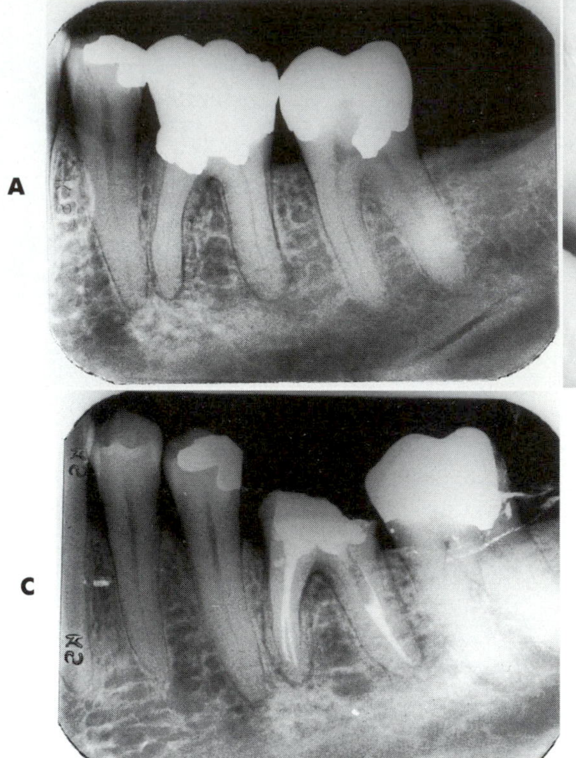

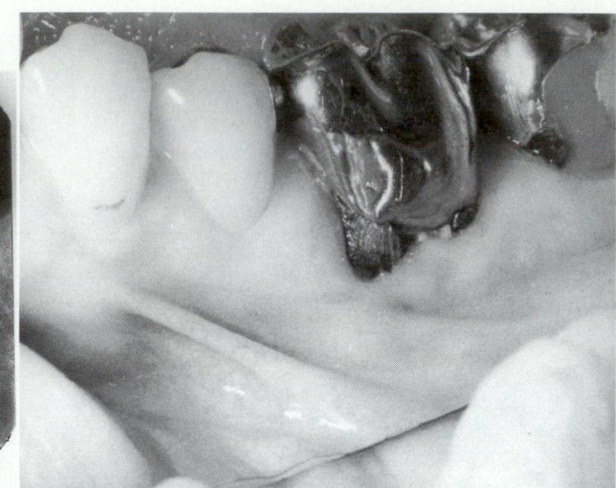

FIG. 24-24 Patient presents with calcified canals, **A,** and a full gold crown with margins on buccal root alloy restorations, **B.** Access to all canals required crown removal, **C.**

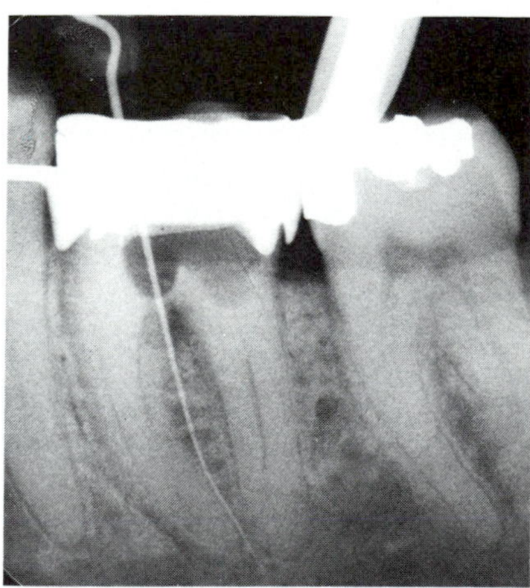

FIG. 24-25 Pain, bleeding, or disorientation of the probing instrument may indicate a perforation and should be immediately investigated radiographically. Repair is possible when the opening is pinpointed and the periodontal tissues are still normal.

second attempt at this procedure is often productive. Personal clinical experiences and judgment will determine when the search for the canals must be terminated and alternatives to nonsurgical root canal treatment considered.

Modifications to enhance access vary from widening the axial walls to increasing visibility or light, to complete removal of the crown.[43] Alterations may be indicated after canal penetration to the apex if tooth structure interferes with instrumentation or filling procedures.

Very few canals of older teeth, even maxillary anteriors, have adequate diameter to allow the safe and effective use of broaches. Older pulps may give a clinical appearance that reflects their calcified, atrophic state with the stiffened, fibrous consistency of a wet toothpick. Any broached canals should be thoroughly instrumented at the same appointment.

Preparation

The calcified appearance of the canals resulting from the aging process presents a much different clinical situation than that of a younger pulp in which trauma, pulpotomy, decay, or restorative procedures have induced premature canal obliteration. Unless further complicated by reparative dentin formation, this calcification appears to be much more concentric and linear. This allows easier penetration of canals, once they are found. An older tooth is more likely to have a history of earlier treatments, with a combination of calcifications present. For a description of cleaning and shaping root canals, the reader is referred to Chapter 8.

The length of the canal from the actual anatomic foramen to the dentinocemental junction (DCJ) increases with the deposition of cementum throughout life.[18] The advantage of this situation in the treatment of teeth with vital pulps is countered by the presence of necrotic, infected debris in this longer canal when periapical pathosis is already present. The actual cementodentinal junction width or most apical extent of the dentin, remains constant with age.[42]

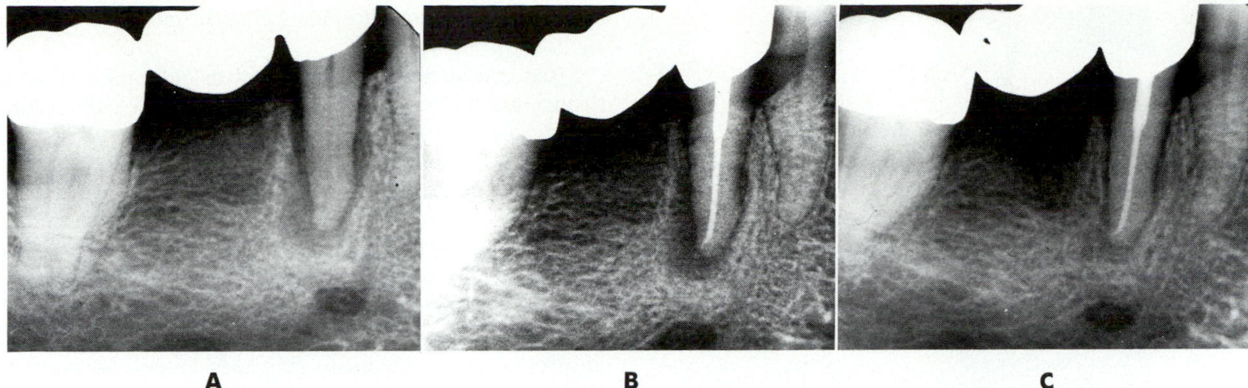

FIG. 24-26 A, A long-standing periapical radiolucency with a draining sinus tract indicated the need for root canal treatment on this fixed bridge abutment of an 80-year-old patient. **B,** Routine root canal treatment shows a foramen that exits to the distal. **C,** One-year recall examination shows bone remineralizing well and continued function of the fixed appliance.

Since this DCJ is the narrowest constriction of the canal, it is the ideal place to terminate the canal preparation. This point may vary from 0.5 to 2.5 mm from the radiographic apex and be difficult to determine clinically. Calcified canals reduce the operator's tactile sense in identifying the constriction clinically, and reduced periapical sensitivity in older patients reduces the patient's response that would indicate penetration of the foramen. Increased incidence of hypercementosis, in which the constriction is even farther from the apex, makes penetration into the cemental canal almost impossible. Apical root resorption associated with periapical pathosis further changes the shape, size, and position of the constriction.

The frequency and intensity of discomfort following instrumentation has not been shown to be related to the amount of preparation, the type of interappointment medication or temporary filling,[14] pulp or periapical status,[12] whether or not the root canal filling is completed at the same appointment,[25] tooth number, or age.[44] The more constricted dentinocemental junction permits a much smaller pulp wound and resists penetration with even the initial small files. Dentin debris creates a matrix early in the preparation[53] and further reduces the risk of overinstrumentation or the forcing of debris into the periapical tissues,[30] which could cause an acute apical periodontitis or abscess. Further access to periapical tissues through the canal is likewise limited.

Obturation

For the elderly patient, the prudent clinician selects gutta-percha filling techniques that do not require unusually large midroot tapers or generate pressure in this area, which could result in root fracture. The reader is referred to Chapter 9 for the most appropriate technique to use to seal the canal.

The role of the dentinal plug and its effect on the apical seal and success has been discussed. The likelihood of plug formation increases when the apex is constricted or when a file length is established at a distance from the radiographic apex and canals are calcified. These characteristics are all common in older teeth. The plug may create its own seal, contribute to a solid matrix for producing a condensed gutta-percha seal, and reduce the effects of overinstrumentation and filling.[30]

Coronal seal plays an important role in maintaining the apically sealed environment and has significant impact on long-term success.[45] Even a root-filled tooth should not have its canals exposed to the oral environment. Permanent restorative procedures should be scheduled as soon as possible and intermediate restorative materials selected and properly placed to maintain a seal until then. Glass ionomer cements are of value for this purpose when mechanical retention is not ensured with the preparation.

Success and Failure

Repair of periapical tissues following endodontic treatment in older patients is determined by most of the same local and systemic factors that govern the process in all patients. With vital pulps, periapical tissues are normal and can be maintained with an aseptic technique, confining preparation and filling procedures to the canal space. Infected, nonvital pulps with periapical pathology must have this process altered in favor of the host tissue, and repair will be determined by the ability of this tissue to respond. Factors that influence repair will have their greatest effect on the prognosis of endodontic therapy when periapical pathology is present (Fig. 24-26).

With aging, arteriosclerotic changes of blood vessels increase and the viscosity of connective tissue is altered, making repair more difficult.[34] The rate of bone formation and normal resorption decreases with age, and the aging of bone results in greater porosity and decreased mineralization of the formed bone. A 6-month recall period to evaluate repair radiographically may not be adequate; it may take as long as 2 years to produce the healing that would occur at 6 months in an adolescent.

Studies that suggest a difference in success between age groups must note the smaller numbers usually in this older treatment group and the local factors that make treatment difficult. Overlooked canals are a more common cause of failure in older patients (Fig. 24-27), which explains the increased clinical indications for retrograde fillings when surgical treatment is attempted.[1] Heat sensitivity as an isolated symptom may indicate a missed canal. For further information on assessing failures and possible retreatment, the reader is referred to Chapter 25.

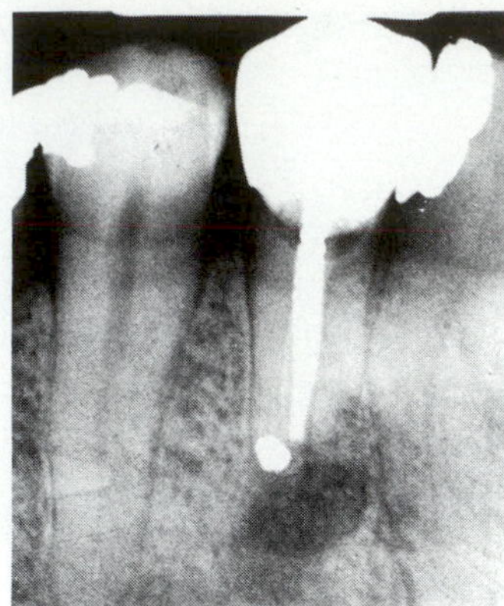

FIG. 24-27 Overlooked canals are a more common cause of failure in older patients, which explains increased clinical indications for retrograde fillings when surgical treatment is performed.

ENDODONTIC SURGERY

Considerations and indications for endodontic surgery are not much affected by age. The need for establishment of drainage and relief of pain are not common indications for surgery. Anatomic complications of the root canal system such as calcified canals, nonnegotiable root curvatures, extensive apical root resorption, and pulp stones occur with greater frequency in older patients. Perforation during access, losing length during instrumentation, ledging, and instrument separation are iatrogenic treatment complications associated with treatment of calcified canals.

Medical considerations may require consultation but do not contraindicate surgical treatment when extraction is the alternative. In most instances surgical treatment may be performed less traumatically than an extraction, which may also result in the need for surgical access to complete root removal. A thorough medical history and evaluation should reveal the need for any special considerations, such as prophylactic antibiotic premedication, sedation, hospitalization, or more detailed evaluation.

Local considerations in treatment of older patients include an increase in the incidence of fenestrated or dehisced roots and exostoses (Fig. 24-28). The thickness of overlying soft and bony tissue is usually reduced, and apically positioned muscle attachments extend the depth of the vestibule. Less anesthetic and vasoconstrictor are needed for profound anesthesia. Tissue is less resilient, and resistance to reflection appears to be diminished. The oral cavity is usually more accessible with the teeth closed together, because the lips can more easily be stretched. The apex can actually be more surgically accessible in older patients. Ability to gain such access varies with the skill of the surgeon; however, some areas are unreachable by even the most experienced.

The position of anatomic features such as the sinus, floor of the nose, and neurovascular bundles remains the same, but their relationship to surrounding structures may change when teeth have been lost. The need may arise to combine endodontic and periodontic flap procedures, and every effort should be made to complete these procedures in one sitting.

When apicoectomy is to be performed, the surgeon must consider whether the root that will be left is long enough and thick enough for the tooth to continue to remain functional and stable. This factor is especially important when the tooth will be used as an abutment. Detailed surgical procedures are presented in Chapter 19.

Ecchymosis is a more common postoperative finding in elderly patients and may appear to be extreme (Fig. 24-29). The patient should be reassured that this condition is normal and that normal color may take as long as 2 weeks to return. The blue discoloration will change to brown and yellow before it disappears. Immediate application of an ice pack following surgery reduces bleeding and initiates coagulation, to reduce the extent of ecchymosis, and later application of heat helps to dissipate the discoloration.

RESTORATION

Root canal treatment saves roots and restorative procedures save crowns. Combined, these procedures are returning more

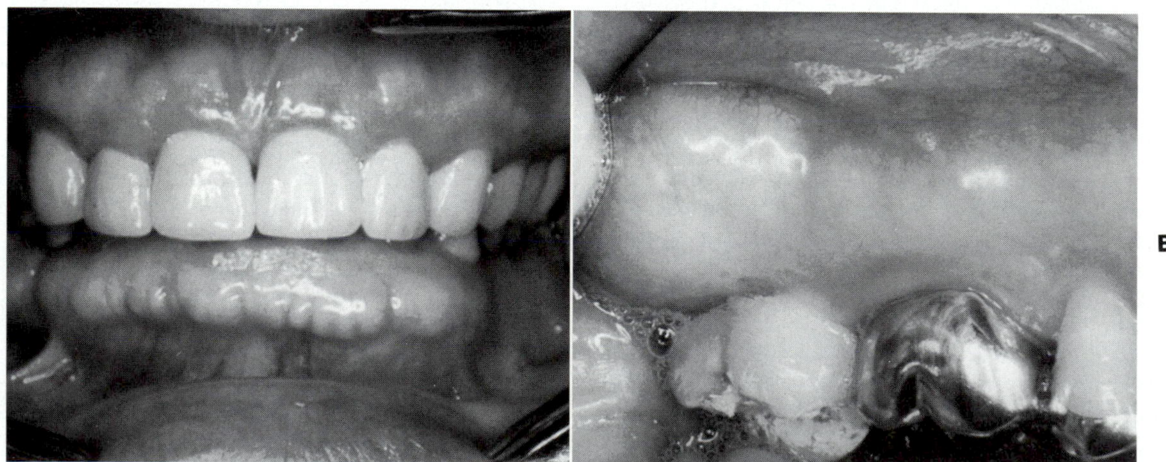

FIG. 24-28 Exostoses, as illustrated in this mandibular anterior, **A,** and maxillary molar, **B,** covered with thin tissue that can easily be torn during flap reflection, as well as the more obvious heavy bone and its effect on surgical access.

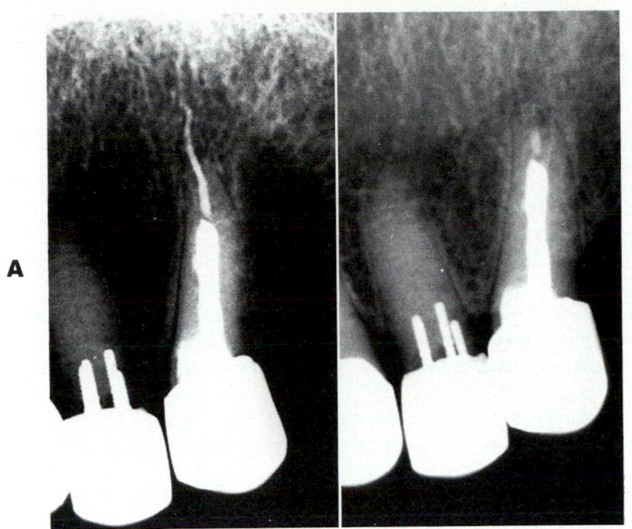

FIG. 24-29 A, Surgical treatment of this overextended filling in an 89-year-old woman will require a deep incision, because of the length of the tooth, with involvement of tissues that will likely cause ecchymosis. The amount of bone reduction necessary and total time the flap is elevated also affect the amount of bruising. **B,** This root apex was fenestrated and the overfill was in the soft tissue.

teeth to form and function than was thought possible just a few decades ago. General considerations and procedures for postendodontic restoration are detailed in Chapter 22.

The value of the tooth, its restorability, its periodontal health, and the patient's wishes should be part of the evaluation preceding endodontic therapy. The restorability of older teeth can be affected when root decay has limited access to sound margins or reduced the integrity of remaining tooth structure (Fig. 24-30). There can also be insufficient vertical and horizontal space when opposing or adjacent teeth are missing.

In conclusion, it can be seen that geriatric endodontics will gain a more significant role in complete dental care as our aging population recognizes that a complete dentition, and not complete dentures, is a part of their destiny.

REFERENCES

1. Allen RK, Newton CW, and Brown CE Jr: A statistical analysis of surgical and nonsurgical endodontic retreatment cases, J Endod 15:261, 1989.
2. Barbakow FH, Cleaton-Jones P, and Friedman D: An evaluation of 566 cases of root canal therapy in general dental practice: postoperative observations, J Endod 6:485, 1980.
3. Baum BJ: Evaluation of stimulated parotid saliva flow rate in different age groups, J Dent Res 60:1292, 1981.
4. Bernick S: Effect of aging on the nerve supply to human teeth, J Dent Res 46:694-699, 1967.
5. Bernick S, and Nedelman C: Effect of aging on the human pulp, J Endod 3:88, 1975.
6. Bhaskar H: Orban's oral histology and embryology, ed 5, St Louis, 1962, Mosby–Year Book.
7. Browne RM, and Tobias RS: Microbial microleakage and pulpal inflammation: a review, Endod Dent Traumatol 2:177, 1986.
8. Delzangles B: Scanning electron microscopic study of apical and intracanal resorption, J Endod 14:281, 1989.
9. Douglas CW, Gammon MD, and Orr RB: Oral health status in the U.S.: prevalence of inflammatory periodontal disease, J Dent Educ 49:365, 1985.
10. Douglas CW, and Furino A: Balancing dental service requirements and supplies: epidemiologic and demographic evidence, J Am Dent Assoc 121(5):587, 1990.
11. Ettinger R, Beck T, and Glenn R: Eliminating office architectural bar-

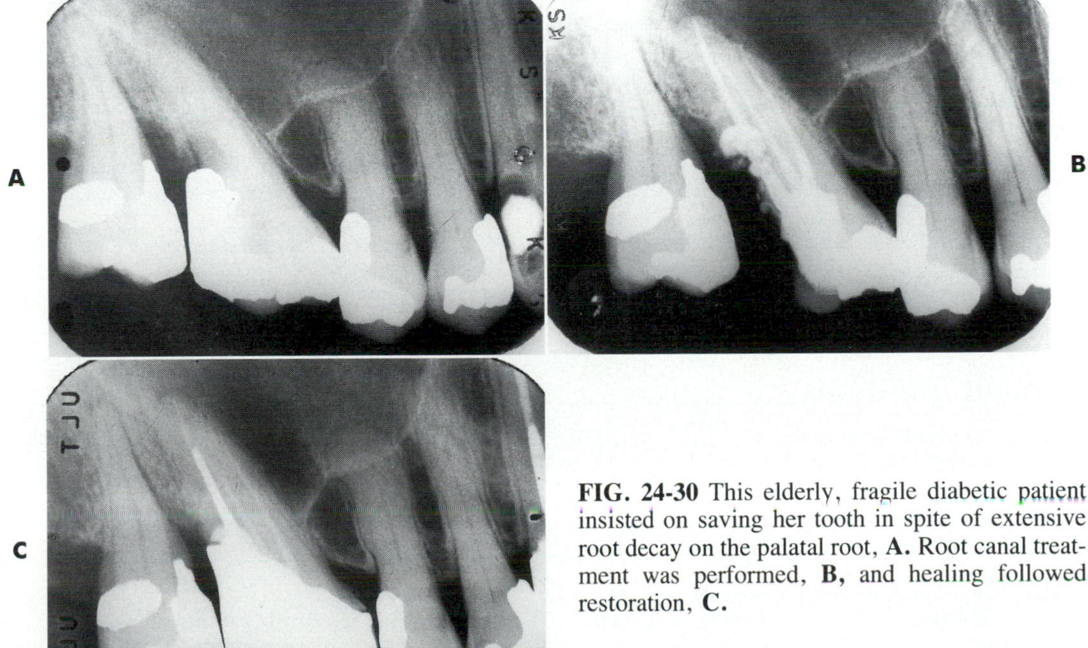

FIG. 24-30 This elderly, fragile diabetic patient insisted on saving her tooth in spite of extensive root decay on the palatal root, **A.** Root canal treatment was performed, **B,** and healing followed restoration, **C.**

riers to dental care of the elderly and handicapped, J Am Dent Assoc 98(3):398, 1979.
12. Ferguson SA: A statistical analysis of 2500 endodontic cases at Indiana University School of Dentistry and in private practice. Unpublished master's thesis, Indianapolis, 1981, Indiana University School of Dentistry.
13. Frank ME, Hettinger TP, and Mott AE: The sense of taste: neurobiology, aging, and medication effects, Crit Rev Oral Biol Med 3(4):371, 1992.
14. Harrison JW, Baumgartner JC, and Svec TA: Incidence of pain associated with clinical factors during and after root canal therapy. I—Interappointment pain, J Endod 9:385, 1983.
15. Ingle JI: Geriatric endodontics, AO 79:47, Fall 1986.
16. Kier DM, et al: Thermally induced pulpalgia in endodontically treated teeth, J Endod 17:38, 1991.
17. Klein A: Systematic investigations of the thickness of the periodontal ligament, Ztschr Stomatol 26:417, 1928.
18. Kuttler Y: Microscopic investigation of root apexes, J Am Dent Assoc 50:544, 1955.
19. Lowman JV, Burke RS, and Pelleu GB: Patent accessory canals: incidence in molar furcation region, Oral Surg 36:580, 1973.
20. MacNeil RC: The geriatric patient: a periodontal perspective, J Ind Dent Assoc 70:24, 1991.
21. Meskin LH: Economic impact of dental service utilization by older patients, J Am Dent Assoc 120:665, 1990.
22. Miller CS: Documenting medication use in adult dental patients: 1987-1991, J Am Dent Assoc 123:41, 1992.
23. Miller WA, and Massler M: Permeability and staining of active and arrested lesions in dentine, Br Dent J 112:187, 1962.
24. Moeller TM: Sensory changes in the elderly, Dent Clin North Am 33:29, 1989.
25. Mulhern JM, et al: Incidence of post-operative pain after one appointment endodontic treatment of asymptomatic pulpal necrosis in single-rooted teeth, J Endod 8:370, 1982.
26. National Institute on Aging: Personnel for health needs of the elderly through year 2020. Report to Congress. Washington, DC, US Government Printing Office, 1, 14, 1987.
27. Newton CW, and Zunt SL: Endodontic intervention in the traumatic bone cyst, J Endod 13:405, 1987.
28. Palmer C: New Federal law will ban discrimination, ADA News 21(11):1-2, 1990.
29. Pantera EA, Anderson RW, and Pantera CT: Use of dental instruments for bridging during electric pulp testing, J Endod 18:37, 1992.
30. Patterson SM, et al: The effect of an apical dentin plug in root canal preparation, J Endod 14:1, 1988.
31. Philippas GG, and Applebaum E: Age changes in the permanent upper canine teeth, J Dent Res 47:411, 1968.
32. Polson AM: Periodontal destruction associated with vertical root fracture, J Periodontol 48:27, 1977.
33. Rubach WC, and Mitchell DF: Periodontal disease, accessory canals and pulp pathosis, J Periodontol 36:34, 1965.
34. Seltzer S: Endodontology, ed 2, Philadelphia, 1988, Lea & Febiger.
35. Seltzer SS, and Bender IB: The dental pulp, ed 3, Philadelphia, 1984, JB Lippincott Co.
36. Selvig KF: The fine structure of human cementum, Acta Odontol Scand 23:423, 1965.
37. Shafer WG, Hine MK, and Levy BM: A textbook of oral pathology, ed 3, Philadelphia, 1974, WB Saunders Co.
38. Smith GN, and Walton RE: Periodontal ligament injections: distribution of injected solutions, Oral Surg 55:232, 1983.
39. Social Security Administration, 1985.
40. Stanley HR, and Ranney RR: Age changes in the human dental pulp. I—The quantity of collagen, Oral Surg 15:1396, 1962.
41. Stanley HR, et al: The detection and prevalence of reactive and physiologic sclerotic dentin, reparative dentin and dead tracts beneath various types of dental lesions according to tooth surface and age, J Oral Pathol 12:257, 1983.
42. Stein TJ, and Corcoran JF: Anatomy of the root apex and its histologic changes with age, Oral Surg, Oral Pathol, Oral Med 69:238, 1990.
43. Streiff JT, and Gerstein H: Access cavity preparation. In: Techniques in clinical endodontics, Philadelphia, 1983, WB Saunders Co.
44. Strindberg L: The dependence of the result of pulp therapy on certain factors: an analytic study based on radiographic and clinical follow-up examinations, Acta Odontol Scand 14(suppl 21): 1956.
45. Swanson K, and Madison S: An evaluation of coronal microleakage in endodontically treated teeth. I—Time periods, J Endod 13:56, 1987.
46. Swartz DB, Skidmore AE, and Griffin JA: Twenty years of endodontic success and failure, J Endod 9:198, 1983.
47. Tenovuo J: Oral defense factors in the elderly, Endod Dent Traumatol 8:93, 1992.
48. U.S. Department of Health and Human Services: Use of dental services and dental health, United States: 1986. Washington, DC, 1988, Government Printing Office. Publication No. 88-1593 (National Health Survey; series 10; no. 165.)
49. U.S. Department of Health and Human Services: Personnel for health needs of the elderly through year 2020. September 1987 report to Congress. Bethesda, Md, 1987, U.S. Public Health Service, NIH Publication No. 87-2950.
50. U.S. Census Bureau: US current population reports. US Census Bureau publication no 952. Washington, DC, 1984, US Government Printing Office.
51. Wallace MC, Retief DH, and Bradley EL: Prevalence of root caries in a population of older adults, Geriodontics 4:84, 1988.
52. Woodly L, Woodworth J, and Dobbs JL: A preliminary evaluation of the effect of electric pulp testers on dogs with artificial pacemakers, J Am Dent Assoc 89:1099, 1974.
53. Yee RDS, et al: The effect of canal preparation on the formation and leakage characteristics of the apical dentin plug, J Endod 10:308, 1984.
54. Zander H, and Hurzeler B: Continuous cementum apposition, J Dent Res 37:1035, 1958.
55. Zitterbart PA: The changing face of dental practice, J Ind Dent Assoc 71:8, 1991.

Self-assessment questions

1. Periapical radiographs should be reviewed
   a. before discussion of the chief complaint.
   b. after discussing the chief complaint with the patient.
   c. just before the clinical examination.
   d. after completing the clinical examination.
2. With aging,
   a. lateral canals become more clinically significant.
   b. gingival recession exposes cementum and dentin, which is less resistant to decay.
   c. the cementodentinal junction moves closer to the radiographic apex with continuous apical remodeling.
   d. All of the above.
3. Which pulp tests have limited diagnostic value in geriatric patients?
   a. Electric pulp tests.
   b. Test cavity.
   c. Selective anesthesia.
   d. All of the above.
4. Cracked teeth
   a. are rare in geriatric patients.
   b. will not have pulpal or periodontal disease unless the cause of pulpal irritation is evident
   c. with periapical disease and normal pocket depths have an excellent prognosis following root canal therapy.

   d. when associated with periodontal pockets have a poor prognosis.
5. In geriatric patients
   a. there is a direct correlation between the degree of response to electric pulp testing and the degree of inflammation.
   b. there is a reduced volume and increased neural component of the pulp.
   c. tooth discoloration usually is not indicative of pulpal death.
   d. diffuse pain of vague origin is common.
6. In the geriatric patient, with increasing age, radiographically
   a. the incidence of condensing osteitis increases.
   b. the incidence of odontogenic and nonodontogenic cysts increases.
   c. the apical constriction is closer to the radiographic apex.
   d. All of the above.
7. Regarding endodontic treatment in aged patients,
   a. one appointment procedures are advantageous.
   b. frequent appointments of short duration are preferable.
   c. root canal treatment is more traumatic than extraction.
   d. intraligamentary injection is the recommended technique for obtaining anesthesia.
8. The frequency and intensity of discomfort following instrumentation is *not* related to
   a. the amount of preparation.
   b. pulp or periapical status.
   c. whether or not the root canal is filled at the same appointment.
   d. All of the above.
9. In evaluating success and failure of endodontic therapy in aged patients, one must consider that
   a. the bone of the aged patient is more mineralized than that of a younger patient.
   b. overlooked canals are seldom a problem because they are usually calcified.
   c. as long as 2 years may be necessary to produce healing that would occur at 6 months in an adolescent.
   d. cold sensitivity is the only symptom that may indicate a missed canal.
10. Endodontic surgery in geriatric patients
   a. requires more anesthetic and vasoconstrictor than in younger patients.
   b. is usually indicated to establish drainage or for relief of pain.
   c. produces postoperative ecchymosis more commonly than in younger patients.
   d. seldom requires the placement of a retrograde filling.

Chapter 25

Endodontic Failures and Re-treatment

Adam Stabholz
Shimon Friedman
Aviad Tamse

THE EXTENT OF ENDODONTIC FAILURES

Reports on Endodontic Treatment Results

What are the success and failure rates for root canal treatment? Over the 30 years since Strindberg's comprehensive study,[125] much effort has been invested in attempts to answer this basic question. In different studies the success rate ranges from 53%[45] to 95%.[76,86] The higher figure suggests that almost every endodontic treatment succeeds, whereas the lower figure indicates that almost every second case fails. This discrepancy cannot be explained in the context of a modern, scientifically based form of therapy such as the endodontics we practice today.

Data from 20 different studies representing the work on endodontic success and failure of investigators from eight different countries are presented in Tables 25-1 and 25-2. The year of the study, author, number of teeth included, operator, follow-up period, and treatment results are presented in Table 25-1. All these studies investigated at least one factor that might have influenced treatment results. In several studies eight or more such factors were evaluated. The factors are coded and listed for each study. Remarks are introduced to highlight special points whenever they were considered contributory. Table 25-2 presents 22 factors whose potential influence on the endodontic success rate was evaluated in the reviewed studies. Strindberg[125] classified the various factors he examined as biologic and therapeutic. Since then, various researchers have related additional factors to endodontic success. In Table 25-2 each factor is related to the studies that evaluated it and their agreement or disagreement about the factor's influence on the treatment results. The factors are listed in accordance with the frequency of their mention in the literature.

A review of the factors that were evaluated by three or more different authors reveals disagreement rather than agreement about their influence on endodontic success. The influence on treatment results of several other factors (e.g., extension of filling material, obturation quality, and observation period) is largely agreed upon. The presence of periapical pathosis prior to treatment is a significant factor, too, according to most authors. However, all authorities agree that neither the location of a treated tooth in the maxilla or mandible nor the type of filling material is significant, and most believe that age and sex have no effect on treatment results.

Variability of Reported Treatment Results

Table 25-1 demonstrates that there is considerable variation in observation period from one study to another. Is this fact significant? Can we assume that the quality of obturation and the apical extension of the filling material are therapeutic factors that are directly related to the technique used by the operator? Are the treatment results achieved by qualified specialists superior to those of undergraduate students? Were teeth in the studies mainly ones involved with periapical pathosis, or not? Did the investigators assess their results clinically or radiographically? Did they use comparable criteria for their assessments? Were their radiographic evaluations objective? Should we compare results of different studies at all in our search for the extent of endodontic failures?

To understand the extent of endodontic failures an analysis of the major reasons responsible for the variability of the re-

TABLE 25-1. Characteristics of reports on endodontic success and failure

Year	Authors	Number of cases (teeth)	Operator	Follow-up period (yr)	Reported treatment results (%)			Factors studied that related to results	Remarks
					Success	Uncertain	Failure		
1956	Strindberg[125]	529	Author	4	87	2	11	a,b,c,d,f,g,i,k,q,s,t*	
1961	Grahnen & Hansson[31]	763	Students	4-5	81	—	19	a,b,c,e,h,i	
1963	Seltzer et al.[106]	2921	Authors	≥½	80	—	20	a,b,d,l,m	
1963	Zeldow and Ingle[147]	42	Faculty	2	83.3	—	16.7	l	Nonvital teeth only, with positive cultures prior to obturation
1964	Bender et al.[9]	706	Authors	2	82	—	18	a,b,g,l,m	
1964	Grossman et al.[36]	432	Students	1-5	90	1	9	a,d,f,j	Success rate represents the mean value between nonvital and vital teeth
1965	Ingle[43]	1229	Students and practitioners	2	91.5	—	8.5	c,d,e,v	
1969	Storms[124]	158	Students	1	81	14	5	a,b,d,f,h,i,l,p,q	
1970	Harty et al.[37]	1139	Faculty and students	≥½	90	—	10	b,d,f,n	Anterior teeth only; postgraduate student patients
1970	Heling & Tamse[39]	213	Students	1-5	70	—	30	a,b	
1974	Selden[103]	1571	Author	0.5	94	—	6	a,c,g	
1976	Adenubi & Rule[1]	870	Hospital staff	5-7	88.2	4.8	7	a,b,e,f,g,h,j,k,n	Anterior teeth only; all patients under 16 years
1978	Jokinen et al.[45]	1304	Students	2-7	53	13	34	a,b,c,d,e,g,h,j,p	
1979	Kerekes & Tronstad[50]	501	Students	3-5	91	4	5	a,c,d,f,g,i,o,u	"Number of cases" represents number of roots
1980	Barbakow et al.[4]	566	Practitioners	≥1 and up	87.4	5.7	6.9	a,b,c,d,i	
1983	Morse et al.[76]	220	Author	0.5-3	94.5	—	5.5	a,b,c,h	Results analyzed per 458 canals also
1983	Oliet[81]	338	Author	≥1.5	89	—	11	a,b,c,d,e,o	153 teeth treated in single visits
1983	Swartz et al.[127]	1007	Students	≥1	87.8	—	12.2	a,b,c,d,e,k,p	
1986	Pekruhn[86]	925	Author	1	94.8	—	5.2	a,c,r	Single visit only
1989	Petersson et al.[89]	3383	Practitioners	—	74	—	26	b,f	Results based on radiographic survey only

See Table 25-2 for explanation of codes.

TABLE 25-2. Biologic and therapeutic factors reported to potentially influence success or failure*

Code	Factor	Influence on success or failure	
		Yes	No
a	Apical pathosis	1, 9, 36, 39, 45, 50, 76, 86, 106, 124, 125, 127	31, 81, 89, 103
b	Extension of filling material	1, 4, 9, 31, 37, 39, 45, 76, 81, 89, 103, 124, 125, 127	
c	Tooth type (anteriors, premolars, and molars)	31, 39, 45, 125, 127	4, 43, 50, 76, 81, 86, 103
d	Age	36, 37, 103	4, 43, 45, 50, 81, 124, 125, 127
e	Sex	127	1, 31, 43, 45, 125
f	Obturation quality	1, 36, 37, 50, 89, 124, 125	
g	Observation period	1, 9, 45, 50, 125	103
h	Tooth type (maxillary or mandibular)		1, 31, 45, 76, 124
i	Pulp vitality	31, 124, 125	4, 50
j	Type of intracanal medication	36, 45	1
k	Type of filling material		1, 31, 125, 127
l	Bacterial status of root canal before obturation	147	9, 103, 124
m	Obturation technique		9, 103
n	Procedural periapical disturbances	1, 37	
o	Number of treatment sessions		50, 81
p	Postoperative restoration	45, 127	124
q	Patient's general health status		124, 125
r	Preoperative pain		86
s	Postoperative pain		125
t	Apical resorption	125	
u	Length of endodontic session		50
v	The operator		43

*The factors are presented in descending order of frequency at which they were investigated in the reviewed studies.

ported data is required. These reasons are related to the design of the studies, the endodontic techniques employed in them, the qualifications of the operators who perform the treatment, and the complexity of the included cases. They are also related to the observation period in each study, and to the criteria that were used for evaluating treatment results.

Design of Studies

As long as investigators use different criteria for evaluating success and failure, a wide variation in reported treatment results will exist.

Different evaluation methods of treatment results

Most investigators used radiographic and clinical findings to evaluate treatment results. Several used only radiographic findings,[49,53,89] whereas others used histologic examination.[78,108,109] There are problems associated with each of these evaluation methods, as well as with the correlation between them.[6,97,109] Clinical evaluation often relies on subjective findings, such as report of pain or discomfort upon percussion, that are subject to individual variation.[76] However, resorting to only a radiographic evaluation may allow pathosis that is clinically evident but produces no radiographic manifestation to be overlooked (Fig. 25-1).[8] Using a histologic examination for routine evaluation is impractical. Moreover, its value is limited because of the need for interpretation of the findings.[18,97,108] Unfortunately, there is only limited correlation between various evaluation methods for endodontic treatment results. In teeth with periapical radiolucencies considered in the studies, there was a definite correlation between clinical, radiographic, and histologic findings, whereas no such correlation existed in teeth without periapical radiolucencies.[8]

Recall rate

One researcher[86] observed that the recall rate in most studies of endodontic success varied from 11% to 74%, whereas some reports did not mention the recall rate at all. He suggested that the success-failure ratio in the unexamined portion of the population could not be assumed to be the same as that in the examined portion. Furthermore, he found that more than 80% of the endodontic failures were asymptomatic, thus dismissing the argument that endodontic failures are more likely to be presented for recall evaluation than endodontic successes because of persistent discomfort. He concluded by saying that, to be considered valid, studies of failure in any clinical discipline must contain adequate numbers of recalls, and that at the very least inclusion of the original sample should be mandatory.[86]

The recall rate in Strindberg's study[125] was the highest reported so far. He suggested that pain during treatment may have been the cause of the patients' refusal to return for follow-up examination, because the patient may have ascribed a painful experience to a lack of skill on the part of the dentist. Another investigator[103] analyzed the patient's response to recall appeal and concluded, "Those patients whose root canals had been left open prior to definitive treatment and those whose canals required re-treatment were much more likely to return for recall evaluation than other patients." In any case, various clinical situations should not be considered as influencing the analysis of treatment results unless it is proved that they directly affect the treatment success rate.

Inclusion of extracted teeth in the study material

When teeth are extracted because of persisting pain after endodontic therapy the cause is usually treatment failure, but oc-

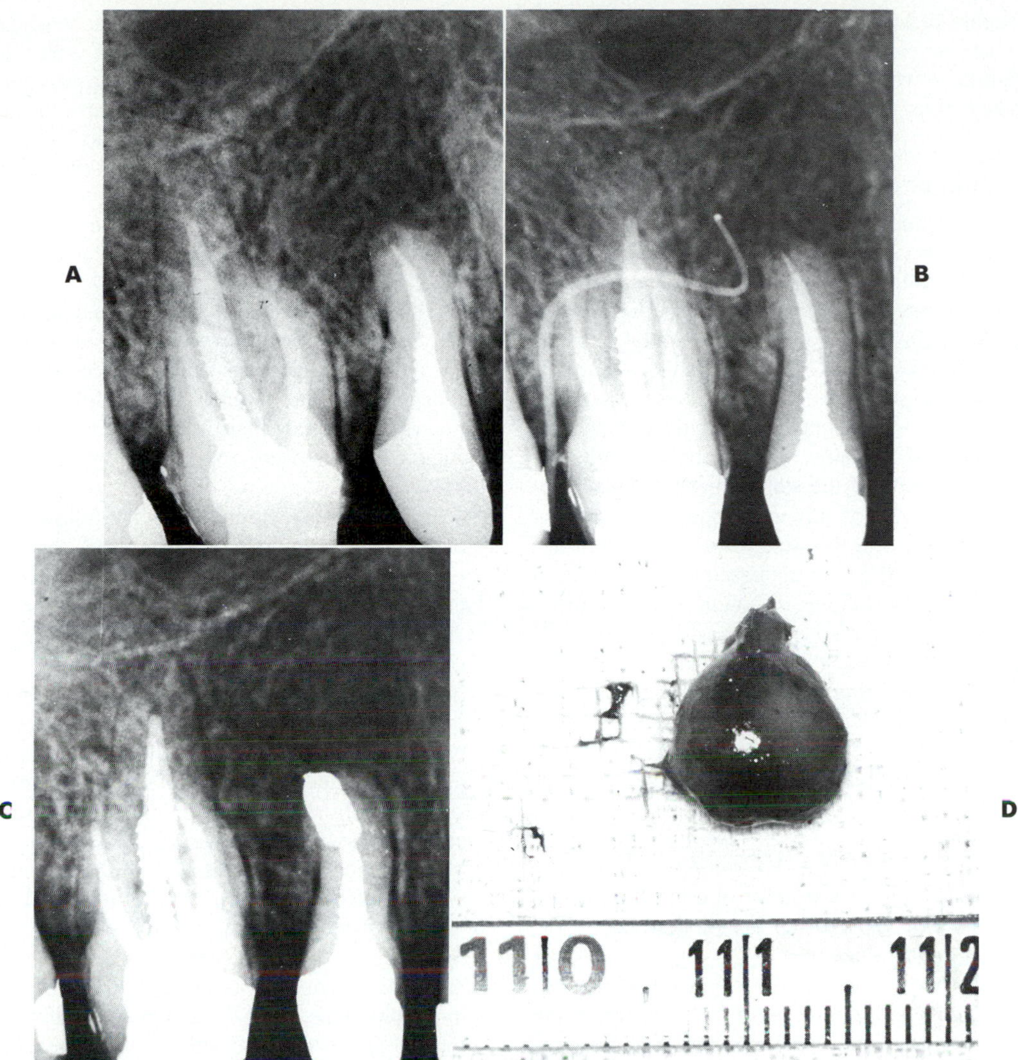

FIG. 25-1 Extensive pathology not clearly manifested radiographically. **A,** Preoperative radiograph of patient with sinus tract located in the alveolar mucosa between the maxillary first and second molars, referred for retreatment of the distobuccal root of the maxillary first molar. **B,** Contradictory to initial diagnosis, the sinus tract is traced with gutta-percha to the maxillary second premolar. **C** and **D,** The pathologic tissue was removed surgically, with subsequent apicoectomy and amalgam retrofilling. The lesion is larger than expected from the radiographs and was histologically confirmed to be a cyst.

casionally it may be the result of crown or root fractures.[8] Furthermore, teeth in which moderate to intense pain persists during treatment are often extracted too. This fact may be significant in the assessment of endodontic treatment results, since extracted teeth "are rarely included in the analysis of endodontic failures, and yet they probably constitute a significant number of failures."[8] Yet, when they are included in the study material, the indiscriminate identification of extracted teeth with endodontic failures may falsify the data as well.[76]

Periapical pathosis

Tables 25-1 and 25-2 demonstrate clearly the widespread agreement that the preoperative presence of periapical pathosis reduces the endodontic success rate. In their classical study Seltzer and associates[106] reported 92% success in teeth without periapical pathosis and 76% success in teeth with such pathosis. Other authors reported similar discrepancies, citing such figures as 78% to 65%[39] and 96% to 86%.[112]

It was pointed out in a more recent study[50] that in previous studies teeth with periapical radiolucencies constituted between 18% and 64% of the material. Such a significant difference in the inclusion of a potentially "failing" factor in the studies may explain why the results of those studies also differ significantly.

Multiplicity of Factors Affecting Treatment Results

The large number of influencing factors does not by itself cause variation in treatment results. However, their possible reciprocal influence may lead to conflicting results. Strindberg[125] remarked on these possibilities of reciprocal influence between the different factors thus: "It is clear that in the study of the influence of the various factors on the therapeutic results, the association between the various explanatory variables must be eliminated, thus giving the pure effect of each variable."

Treatment Techniques

The effect of endodontic treatment technique on the success rate has been clearly demonstrated.[50] After the introduction of Ingle's standardized technique[42] to a Norwegian dental school, a 10% higher success rate was reached than had been shown in the previous long-term studies at the same school. The investigators stated, "In this comparison all variables like teachers, biologic philosophy, materials, and medicaments were the same. Only a change in instruments and technique had taken place. It may be assumed, therefore, that the better results obtained after the introduction of the standardized technique really were due to superiority of this technique." The greatest increase in the success rate in this study was recorded in anterior teeth, from 78% to 91%. An increased success rate as a result of improvement of technique, although without statistical significance, was also reported in the Washington study.[43]

The most prominent therapeutic factors shown in Table 25-2 are apical extension of the filling material and obturation quality. These two factors were examined in several studies, producing unanimous agreement that they do influence treatment results. Both factors are directly related to treatment technique.[50]

Qualification of Operators and Difficulty of Cases

It may be agreed that the qualifications of an undergraduate student are different from those of an experienced specialist. Table 25-1 presents the qualifications of the operators in each study. It appears that any comparison of studies in which students performed root canal treatment with those in which the operators were specialists would be irrelevant. Such a comparison can be justified only when it is based on a study designed to examine just this variable. The effect of this variable on the results must have been taken for granted, however, since only one study attempted to evaluate it.[43] The Washington study[43] concluded that there was no statistically significant difference in success rates between cases treated by undergraduate students and those treated by dentists in private practice. The explanation to this finding was, "Most of the university clinic cases failed because of errors in treatment, whereas the majority of the private practice cases failed because of errors in case selection."

Naturally the easy cases, whenever possible, find their way to undergraduate clinics, whereas experienced dentists and endodontists treat more complex cases, which also have a more doubtful prognosis. In other words, the difficulty of the treated cases may also contribute to the wide variation in the reported treatment results.

Observation Period

Table 25-1 demonstrates that in almost half of the studies the treatment results were evaluated 1 year or less after the completion of treatment. The period of postoperative observation advocated by various investigators varies between 6 months to 4 years.[37] One researcher[80] reviewed the literature and recommended that a 2-year follow-up period may be considered adequate. The Washington study[43] was based on a 2-year recall analysis, claiming that it became apparent that the 6-month and 1-year radiographs were useless for analysis because in middle-aged and elderly patients periapical repair frequently was not complete. Comparable conclusions were suggested by other researchers[50] who presented a significantly higher success rate when evaluating results 3 years after treatment than after 6 months or 1 year.

Another study[45] showed that the endodontic success rate was low in the first 3 years and became higher and more stable at later observations.

The two last studies[45,50] categorized the treatment results not only as success or failure but also as doubtful or uncertain. As the number of successful cases increased with time, there was a decrease in the number of doubtful cases. This can be explained by the fact that the process of healing may be slow.[45] Similar results were reported in young patients in another study.[1]

Strindberg[125] recommended that follow-up examinations be performed at regular intervals and that the postoperative progress be followed until a fairly stabilized condition is established. In his opinion, a minimum of 4 years is the desirable follow-up period. However, it was suggested that healing may still occur in cases regarded as failures even after 4 years if the observation period is prolonged.[25] One group[9] added an interesting angle to the discussion of the optimal observation period. Comparing the 6-months and 2-year follow-up results, they found that in teeth without areas of rarefaction there was a statistically significant difference in the success rate. At the end of 6 months there was 92.7% success, which dropped to 88.8% 2 years after treatment. In teeth with preoperative areas of rarefaction they did not observe a difference in the incidence of repair after 6 months and 2 years. They postulated that it takes 6 to 24 months for a developing granuloma to break down enough periapical bone to become visible on radiographs. One study[103] disagreed with all the others, establishing that 6-month results were as reliable statistically as those of 18 months for the determination of overall healing. The first international conference on endodontics[35] dealt with this dilemma and recommended a 1- to 2-year period of observation. There appears to be a consensus that the results obtained after an observation period shorter than 1 year are unacceptable. Thus, the success rate of a given study may depend on the ratio between the cases evaluated after 6 to 12 months and those evaluated after a longer period. It was suggested also that the validity of results obtained 1 year after treatment of vital cases should be questioned.[9]

Criteria for Definition of Treatment Results

Use of different criteria in studies

"There is no agreement on the definition of success or failure of endodontic treatment inasmuch as there is no agreement on criteria."[109] The same principal authors who made that statement also reappraised the criteria in another publication.[8] They suggested the following criteria for successful endodontic therapy are more realistic than those previously in vogue, admitting that they are not inclusive or conclusive.

1. Absence of pain or swelling.
2. Disappearance of fistula.
3. No loss of function.
4. No evidence of tissue destruction.
5. Radiographic evidence of an eliminated or arrested area of rarefaction after 6 to 24 months.

In one study indicating 53% success, the lowest of all published rates, "cases in which the area of an initial rarefaction had definitely become smaller, but in which bone repair was incomplete, were classified as *doubtful*."[45] This group constituted 13% of the total material. Other investigators[36,50,124] also defined cases with a decrease in the size of a preexisting periapical pathosis as doubtful or uncertain. It must be pointed out that similar findings would have been interpreted by Bender and associates[8] and other researchers[76,103,127] as successful, entirely changing the reported results. Some investigators[31,86,125] believe that a complete restoration of the periapical bone should take place before a case is declared successful. In fact, Bender and associates[8] agreed that rating as successful only perfectly healed cases would result in a drop in the success rate to as low as 39% to 62%, depending on the study in question. In their view, it is erroneous to expect that a considerably reduced rarefaction will continue to shrink and fill in completely after a prolonged observation period.

Other researchers[76] also suggested that progressive repair after 1 year was acceptable evidence of success, considering the fact that it may frequently take several years for complete bone repair to be evident radiographically. They also pointed out that in vital cases periapical widening of the periodontal space was accepted as success in some studies,[50,103,125] was not acceptable in others,[37,39] and was considered doubtful in some.[36] They explained that the relatively high success rate in their study in teeth with a periapical rarefaction may be related to their definition of success, which allowed both complete periapical repair *and* a discernible decrease in the size of the lesion, whereas others considered the latter cases to be doubtful or failures. As long as investigators use different criteria for evaluating success and failure, this fact alone will contribute to the wide variation in reported treatment results.

Fallibilities of radiographic interpretation

The importance of radiographic evaluation in determining endodontic success or failure cannot be overemphasized. It is a universal tool in the assessment of treatment results without which no claim of success could be justified. Since the radiographic evaluation plays a basic role in the assessment of treatment results, any fallibility associated with the interpretation of radiographs directly distorts the reported rates of success and failure. The following factors that influence fallibility should be considered:

1. Change in angulation.
2. Quality of film.
3. Lack of radiographic changes.
4. Proximity to anatomic landmarks.
5. Radiolucency of periapical scar tissue.
6. Personal bias and disagreement between different interpreters.

Bender and associates[8] showed that a change in angulation can often reduce the size of the image of a lesion, or even make it disappear. This will lead to a false assessment of treatment results, and the mistaking of failure for success. Conversely, a lesion that does not show up on the preoperative radiograph can appear on a follow-up radiograph that is exposed in a different angulation. Faulty interpretation as a result of a change of angulation in the horizontal or vertical planes may increase or decrease the apparent number of failures or successes in a given sample. In addition, differences in exposure and developing conditions can produce differences in film density that can directly distort judgments of success or failure.

There may be swelling and pain, necessitating incision and drainage, without any radiographic evidence (Fig. 25-1).[8] "This condition prevails if the labial bone plate is extremely thin and the amount of bone destroyed is not great enough to produce a contrast that can be visualized on the roentgenogram."[8] Furthermore, in the apical portion of the root bone can be completely denuded without producing radiographic changes.[8] Lutwak[61] suggested that at least 50% of the bone must be decalcified in order for a lesion to be evident on the radiograph. Bender and associates[6] further demonstrated that the size of radiographic rarefaction does not correlate with the actual amount of bone destruction. Accordingly, the validity of basing the evaluation of endodontic treatment results solely on radiographic interpretation has been questioned.[127]

The interpretations of radiographic changes may be difficult because of the proximity of anatomic landmarks.[76] The maxillary sinus, mental foramen, and inferior alveolar canal may mimic periapical pathosis. The superimposition of the zygoma or other radiopaque landmarks may conceal the periapical area so that changes cannot be observed (Fig. 25-2).[130]

The occurrence of periapical healing without radiographically demonstrable bony restoration should not be overlooked,[37] because periapical repair might be by connective tissue rather than bone.[36,87] Bender and associates[8] claimed that such conditions exist but only in a small number of cases. They found healing through the formation of scar tissue in only 2 of 100 specimens.

As infrequent as this kind of healing may be, it would still affect the interpretation of endodontic treatment results because such cases may be considered failures, whereas in every respect other than the radiographic appearance they are a success.

Personal bias also influences the interpretation of the radiographs.[8] One examiner may not consider the widening of the periapical periodontal ligament space of a tooth he or she treated to be a manifestation of failure, whereas an indepen-

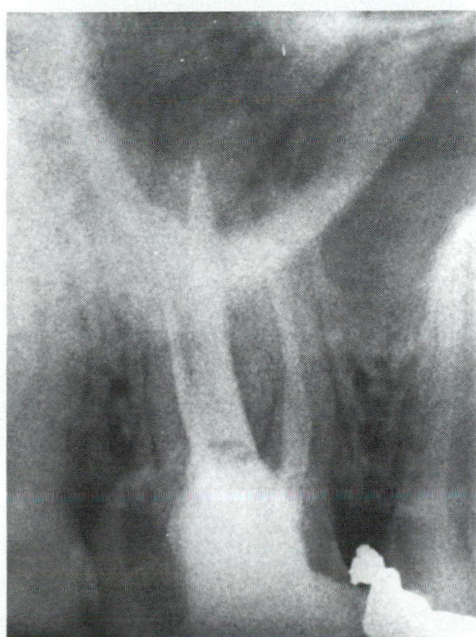

FIG. 25-2 Superimposition of the zygomatic bone on the periapical areas of the buccal roots of the mandibular first molar does not permit the determination of the treatment results.

dent evaluator may interpret the radiographic evidence more strictly.[8] This dilemma of radiographic interpretation was demonstrated by Goldman and associates,[30] who showed that when six examiners read posttreatment radiographs independently and without consulting one another, they agreed on fewer than half of the cases. This conclusion was also reached by other researchers.[27,146]

CAUSES OF ENDODONTIC FAILURES

The causes of endodontic failures have been classified differently by several authorities. Grossman[33] divided the causes into four categories: poor diagnosis, poor prognosis, technical difficulties, and careless treatment. Another researcher[16] listed several alternatives for the differential diagnosis of endodontic failures. His acronym, POOR PAST, stands for "*p*erforation, *o*bturation, *o*verfill, *r*oot canal missed, *p*eriodontal disease, *a*nother tooth, *s*plit, and *t*rauma," all of which may cause endodontic failure. In the Washington study,[43] the causes of failure were classified into three main groups. Apical percolation, as a result of incomplete obturation and unfilled canals, accounted for 63.5% of failures. Operative errors, such as root perforation, gross overfilling, and broken instruments, made up 14.5%. Errors in case selection, and treatment of cases with root resorption or coexisting periodontal pathology, constituted 22%.

Seltzer[104] attributed endodontic failure largely to local factors, the majority of which are associated with the operative procedures of root canal therapy. Thus, errors during instrumentation and obturation may inadvertently affect the periapical tissues and subsequently lead to failure. In his classification, local factors associated with operative procedures included infection, poor débridement, excessive hemorrhage, mechanical and chemical irritation, incomplete and overextended root canal fillings, mechanical perforations, and broken instruments. Other local factors included morphologic considerations, root fractures, preoperative periapical lesions, metal corrosion, and periodontal involvement.

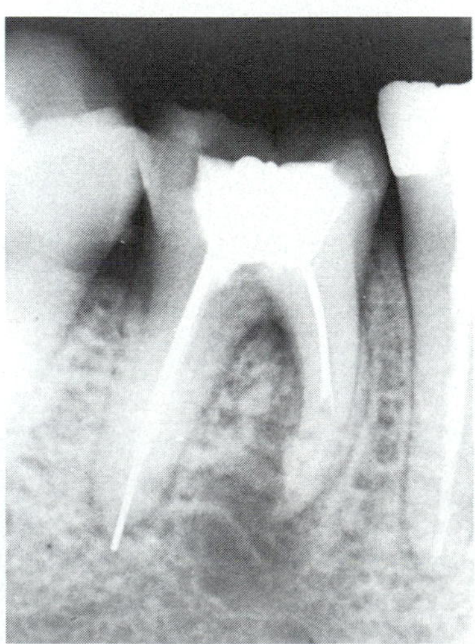

FIG. 25-3 Endodontic failure possibly associated with several factors. Poor canal preparation, insufficient obturation, corrosion products from silver points, or a leaky coronal restoration may have contributed to the failure of endodontic therapy.

Faced with an endodontic failure, the clinician must try to establish the possible cause of the problem, so that it may be treated successfully. Sometimes the cause of failure can be identified easily, but in many cases a cause is not evident. Often it is a combination of factors that cause failure. An example of such a situation is demonstrated in Figure 25-3, in which failure might have been caused by improper instrumentation, inadequate obturation of the canal with the silver cone, or the corrosive products from the cone.

The various procedures associated with root canal therapy can be divided into three treatment phases: preoperative, operative, and postoperative. Since endodontic failure can be related to each one, the causes for failure will be classified as preoperative causes, operative causes, and postoperative causes.

Preoperative Causes

Failure of endodontic therapy can be the result of misdiagnosis, poor case selection, or a poor prognosis, all of which are preoperative considerations. Mistaken diagnosis does not necessarily result in treatment failure of a treated tooth, but rather in the failure of treating the patient. "Misdiagnosis" in this context means that endodontic treatment was instituted without identification of the true origin of the pathology (Fig. 25-4). Consequently the pathology remains untreated and symptoms continue. Furthermore, in many instances such persistence of symptoms may again be misinterpreted as failure of the treatment that was performed.

Diagnosis

Incorrect diagnosis usually results from a misinterpretation or lack of information, either clinical or radiographic. Misinterpretation of pain or of the results of vitality tests, and misdiagnosis of oral lesions such as sinus tracts or of periodontal disease can all lead to endodontic therapy in the wrong tooth. The same may result from the misinterpretation of the radiographs of superimposed structures and bony lesions.[46]

Radiographs are also the principal tool for preoperatively assessing the anatomic configuration of the root canal system. Failure to recognize the radiographic manifestation of various canal system aberrations, such as multiple canals or dilacerations, often results in mistreatment, and, subsequently, in failure (Fig. 25-5). The importance of radiographic evaluation and the pitfalls of radiographic interpretation were emphasized and discussed previously. A condition that is often misdiagnosed, and one that results in treatment failure, is the vertical root fracture.

Awareness, knowledge, and experience are necessary to recognize the clinical and radiographic signs of this entity. What is perplexing about diagnosing vertical root fractures is that their manifestations often resemble disease of endodontic or periodontal origin.[59,71] In vital teeth certain prevailing symptoms are indicative of pulpal pathology.

When vertical root fractures are left untreated, the pulp becomes necrotic and earlier symptoms give way to periapical rarefaction, periodontal abscesses, sinus tracts, and mobility,[59,71] all of which may be mistaken for pathologies of pulpal or periodontal origin. A periodontal pocket may form as a result of chronic inflammation along the fracture line. Essentially, such pockets are sinus tracts extending to the end of the fracture; however, a periodontal pocket alongside the fracture generally appears in a late stage, and in such cases bone loss

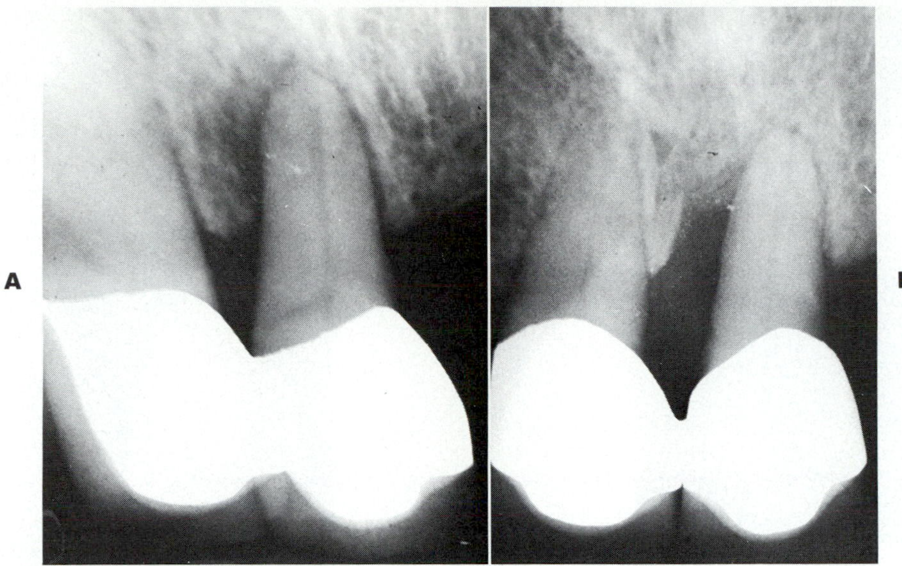

FIG. 25-4 Misdiagnosis of the origin of a lesion. **A,** The maxillary central incisor was referred for endodontic therapy, for what was radiographically diagnosed by the referring dentist as a chronic apical abscess. **B,** Positive vitality testing, periodontal probing, and a differently angulated radiograph proved the lesion to be of periodontal origin.

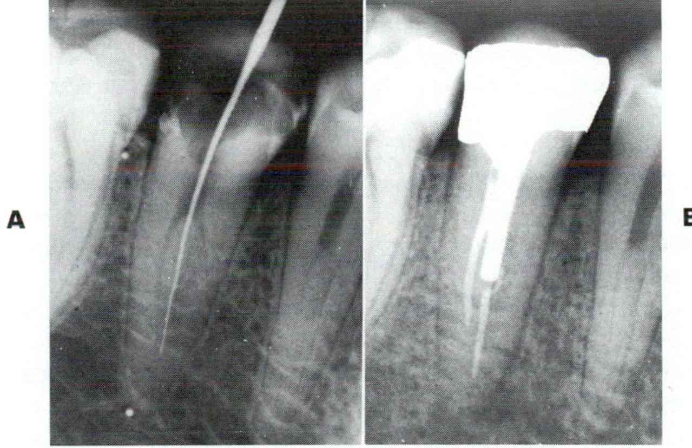

FIG. 25-5 Radiographic misinterpretation of canal system morphology. **A,** Operative radiograph of a mandibular second premolar with three canals. **B,** Unawareness of the anatomic aberration resulted in failure.

alongside the fracture may also be demonstrated radiographically (Fig. 25-6).[90] Radiographic evidence of periodontal disease-like bone loss was found in 75% of vertical fracture cases, apical radiolucency in 22%, and displacement of root segments in 3%.[71] In another study, radiographic evidence of fracture could be found in only 30% of the cases.[99] Another radiographic manifestation of a vertical root fracture may be a hairlike line that is evident if the angulation of the x-ray beam is right (Fig. 25-7).[15]

Case selection

The purpose of case selection is to determine the feasibility and practicality of treatment, so as to avoid treating cases that

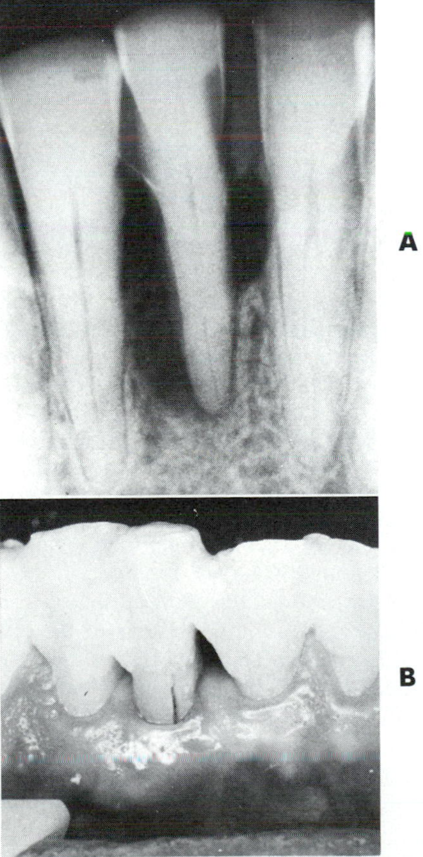

FIG. 25-6 Late-stage manifestation of vertical root fracture. **A,** Radiographic evidence of advanced bone loss on the distal aspect of the root, the result of vertical root fracture. **B,** Clinical view confirming the fracture.

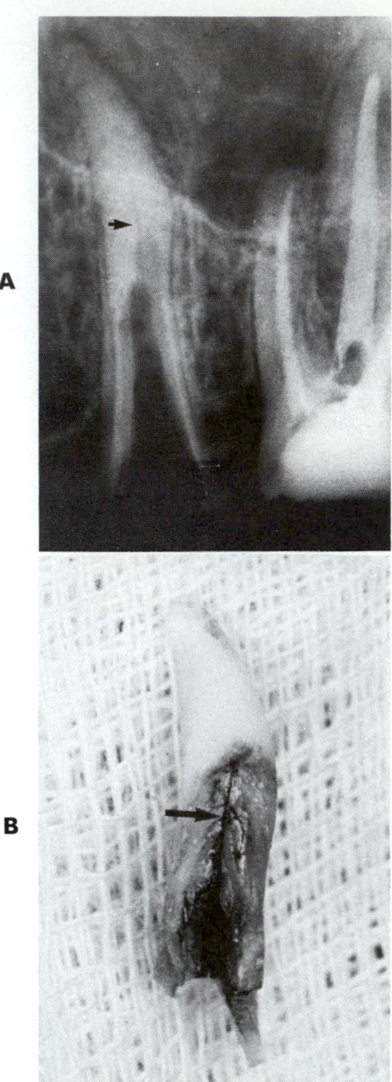

FIG. 25-7 Radiographic manifestation of vertical root fracture. **A,** Preoperative radiograph of a maxillary second premolar. A hairlike fracture line may be mistaken for the root canal *(arrow).* **B,** The fracture line demonstrated after tooth extraction *(arrow).*

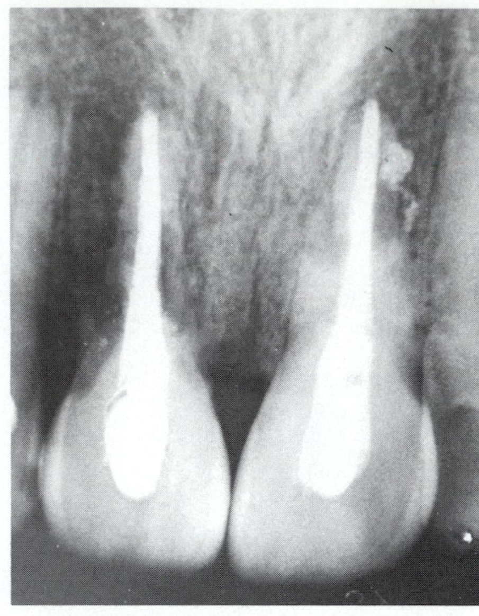

FIG. 25-8 Failure associated with replantation 3 years previously of both traumatically avulsed maxillary central incisors. Treatment was instituted in accordance with the rationale of this procedure, which recognizes its poor prognosis.

will fail regardless of the quality of treatment. Therefore, case selection (Chapter 3) is one of the most significant factors affecting endodontic treatment results.[43] In the Washington study,[43] 22% of the failures were attributed to mistaken case selection. The more rigid the criteria of the operator in case selection, the greater the chances for successful results,[128] whereas treatment of all cases without case selection criteria increases the chances of failure. Failures caused by poor case selection may be divided into those that are predictable and those that are not. Failures that could have been predicted result from misjudgment of the feasibility and practicality of the treatment.

They are related to the evaluation of the patient's cooperation and of the technical difficulties in the course of treatment, such as unnegotiable canals, root resorption, or the impossibility of restoring the tooth. Unpredictable failures related to case selection may be caused by conditions that are not considered to be contraindications to therapy, which yet deteriorate during or following therapy so as to cause failure. These may be secondary periodontal involvement, occlusal trauma, or transformation of the periapical lesion to an apical cyst.

Prognosis

Prognosis can be defined as the prediction of long-term treatment results. This consideration is based on the clinical condition of the tooth and on the quality of the treatment. At times, as in some cases of tooth avulsion, the prognosis is recognized as being poor, and yet treatment is justifiably attempted against all odds (Chapter 16). The loss of the tooth in such cases may be expected; although it constitutes a failure, it is not comparable to a routine endodontic failure (Fig. 25-8). In other cases the endodontic prognosis may depend on the outcome of additional therapy, as in cases of combined periodontal-endodontic lesions.[16] In such cases failure may occur if the periodontal treatment is unsuccessful (Fig. 25-9).[109]

Operative Causes

Operative errors in the course of therapy caused approximately 76% of failures in the Washington study material,[43] making them the major cause of endodontic treatment failure. Operative procedures in endodontic therapy are aimed at obtaining mechanical and biologic objectives, assuring thorough cleansing and shaping of the root canal system (Chapter 8). Neglecting to observe those objectives may result in treatment failure, and the operative causes may be divided accordingly.

Failure to obtain mechanical objectives

Mechanical objectives are related to endodontic cavity preparation (i.e., access cavity and canal shaping). Endodontic cavity preparation, in its broad sense, facilitates the cleansing of the canal system and its obturation in three dimensions. An improper access cavity may be either under- or overextended,

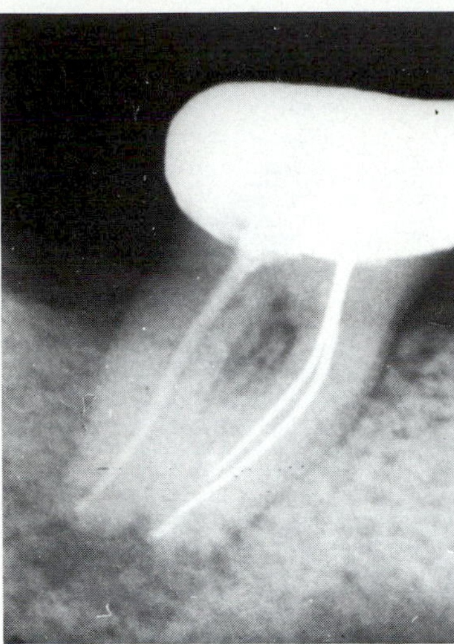

FIG. 25-9 Prognosis of coexisting periodontal and endodontic involvement. Endodontic failure in the mandibular second molar may have been facilitated by inadequate or unsuccessful periodontal therapy.

resulting from failure to derive its outline design from the internal anatomy of the pulp chamber (Chapter 7). Underextending the access cavity may lead to overlooking a root canal. In addition, it restrains the convenience during instrumentation and may result in insufficient shaping of the canal,[104] or even breakage of endodontic instruments.

Whether or not a broken instrument affects treatment results depends largely on the stage of canal preparation when it breaks and the status of the remaining pulp stump.[21] In vital pulp cases, as well as after thorough instrumentation, the chances for failure are less than in other cases (Fig. 25-10).[21,35] Another consequence of an underextended access preparation may be the retention of tissue in the pulp chamber.[104] Such pulp remnants may constitute a continuing irritation and produce a discoloration of the crown (Chapter 21). Both such sequelae are forms of failure. Overextended access cavities are prepared at the sacrifice of dentin, the excessive reduction of which weakens the teeth,[136] so that fractures may occur.[100] Another error in access preparation may be perforation of the pulp chamber walls or floor, with increased potential for failure (Fig. 25-11).

The other facet of endodontic cavity preparation is the shaping of the canal to a cylindroconical shape, with a continuous taper and a sound apical constriction. An error that occurs frequently in this stage is failure to maintain the canal's curvature. It may result in various alteration forms of the canal morphology (Chapter 7) and have a detrimental effect on the quality of the obturation and on the treatment results (Fig. 25-12). Extreme deviation from the original canal shape or overzealous flaring of curved canals may result in perforation of the root (Fig. 25-13).

In a recent study[75] the sealing ability of three different materials used to repair lateral perforations was evaluated by autoradiography. Although EBA cement provided a better seal than silver glass-ionomer and amalgam, microleakage could be demonstrated in all tested groups. In some cases a perforation may be sealed and corrected in a nonsurgical way,[48] but its

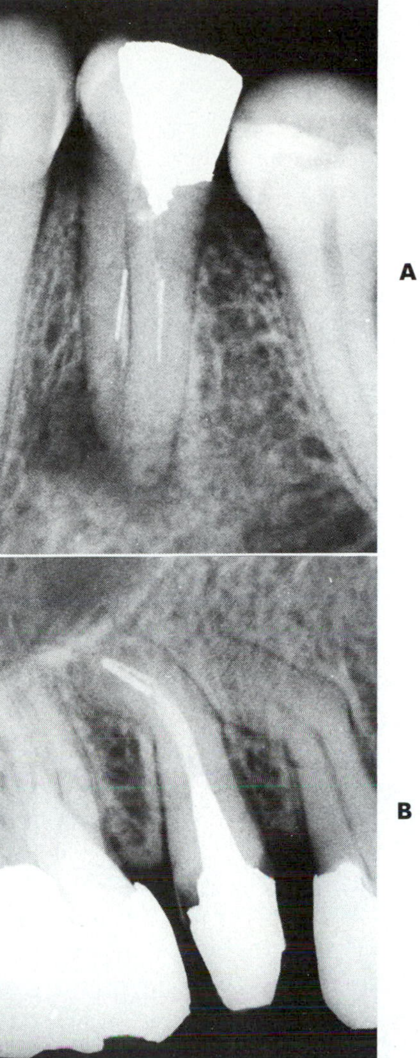

FIG. 25-10 Failures associated with intracanal breakage of instruments. **A,** Breakage before completion of instrumentation in a necrotic tooth usually results in failure. **B,** Failure may not necessarily occur after breakage in a vital tooth or a thoroughly instrumented one.

irritating effect on the supporting tissues may cause a lesion to develop[107] that can no longer be treated successfully.

Failure to attain biologic objectives

Biologic objectives include removal of all potential irritants from the root canal space and the control of infection and periapical inflammation. Together with the mechanical objectives they constitute the entire endodontic therapy; while the canal is being shaped it is also cleansed of organic debris.

This is considered a critical requirement for successful therapy,[33] because remaining pulpal debris may irritate the periapical tissues and jeopardize periapical repair. It has been established that the presence of bacteria in the root canal has a detrimental effect on endodontic treatment results.[25,56] Lin and associates[57] recently showed a correlation between bacterial infection in the root canal system and the presence of periradicular rarefaction in endodontic failures. Intracanal infection,

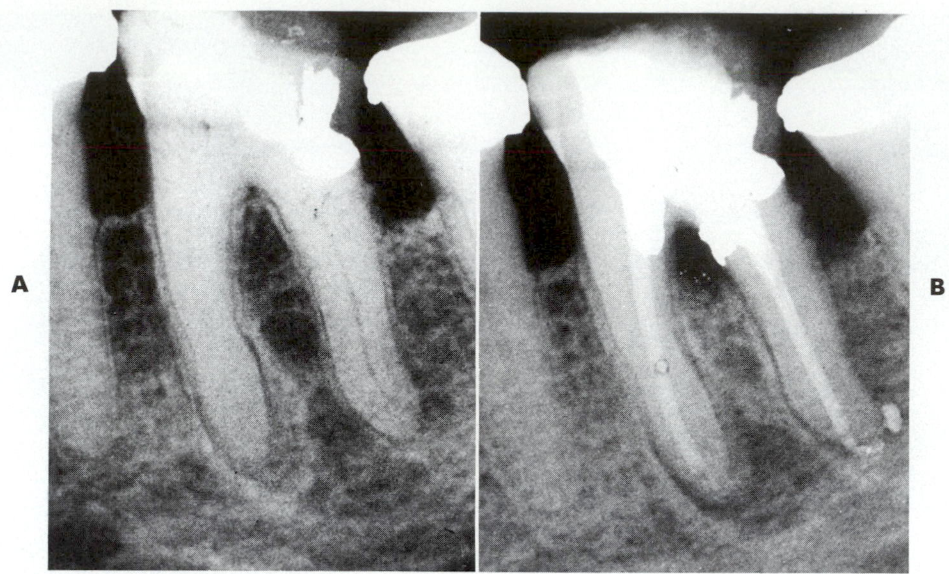

FIG. 25-11 Failure associated with erroneous access cavity preparation. **A,** Preoperative radiograph of a mandibular first molar indicated for endodontic therapy. **B,** Two perforations of the pulp chamber floor during access preparation resulted in failure.

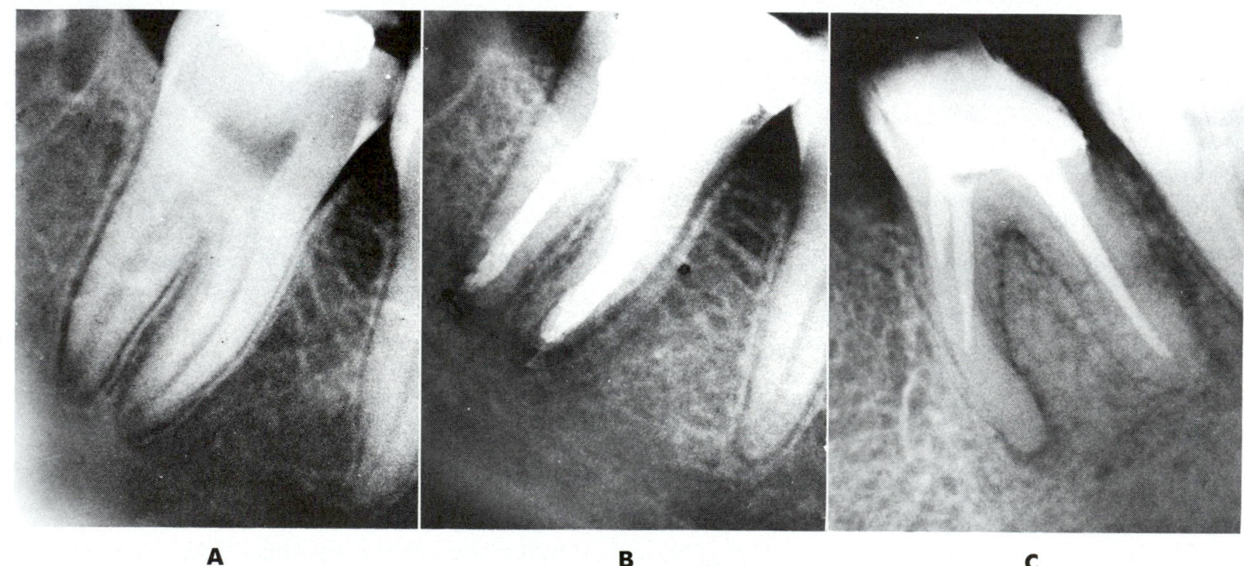

FIG. 25-12 Failure associated with erroneous canal shaping. **A,** Preoperative radiograph of a mandibular second molar with a moderately curved mesial root. **B,** Extreme "zipping" of the mesial canals resulted in compromised obturation and failure. **C,** Ledging of the canal resulted in failure because apical third of the canal being untreated.

more than any other factor, causes periapical inflammation and tissue destruction, the degree of which depends on host resistance and bacterial virulence and population.[104] However, studies on root canal instrumentation have concluded that complete removal of all debris from the canal is unfeasible.[65] It was demonstrated that healing of the periapical tissues could take place despite incomplete canal débridement and in the presence of microorganisms.[68,105,108] Nevertheless, the requirement of an aseptic technique and root canal disinfection remain the biologic basis of endodontic therapy. Failure to cleanse and disinfect the root canal, as well as failure to maintain an aseptic technique, is a dominant cause of endodontic failure.

The control of periapical inflammation also calls for confinement of the operative procedures to the canal space, which affords a better chance for periapical repair.[106,128] Occasional

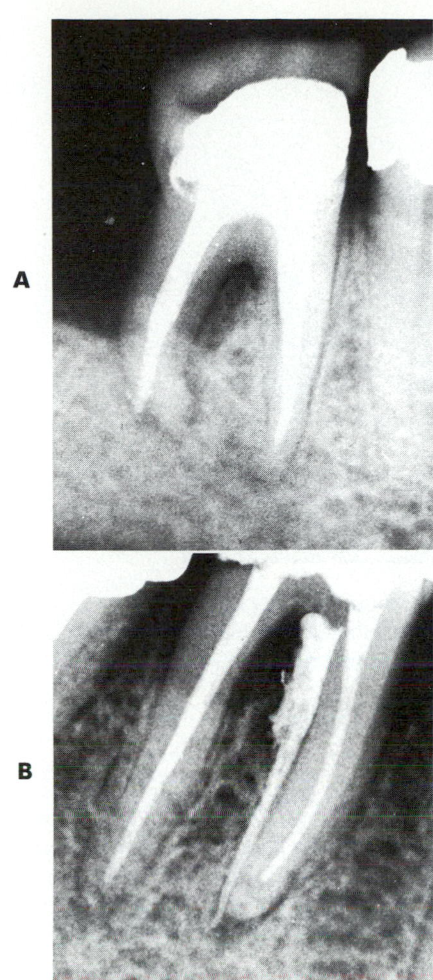

FIG. 25-13 Failures associated with perforations. **A,** Failure to maintain the curvature in the distal root of a mandibular first molar. **B,** Careless use of Gates-Glidden burs resulted in perforation of the mesial root in a mandibular first molar.

overinstrumentation causes periapical hemorrhage and usually only mild transitory inflammation, whereas continuous overinstrumentation provokes an inflammatory response capable of resorbing the hard tissues of tooth and bone.[110] Proliferation of epithelial rest cells of Malassez can occur, leading to formation of an apical cyst.[104] Overinstrumentation may also carry microorganisms from the root canal to the periapical tissues, which in turn may cause a severe inflammatory response and endanger the outcome of therapy.[104] Even with overinstrumentation periapical inflammation may occur as a response to the presence of debris pushed beyond the confinement of the canal space. Dentin and cementum chips were found in the periapical tissues of teeth in which endodontic treatment has failed.[143]

Periapical inflammation can also be provoked by overextended root canal filling (Fig. 25-14). The severity of the reaction depends on the type of material, its setting stage, and the amount.[82] Whereas gutta-percha is tolerated well by the tissue,[83] some sealer cements are irritating and even toxic.[77] Silver cones may also be irritating, especially when they become corroded.[111]

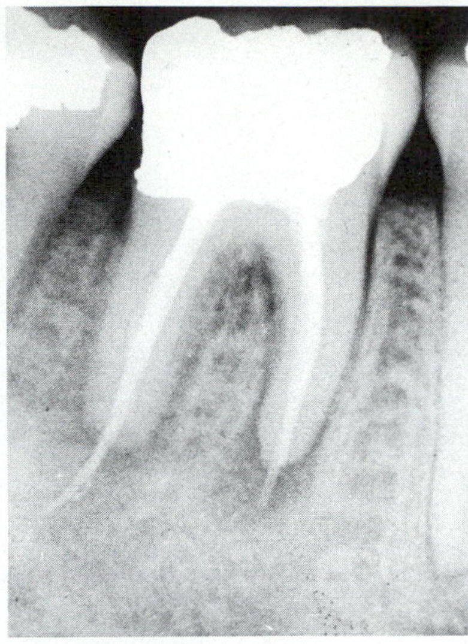

FIG. 25-14 Failure associated with an overextended and poorly obturated root filling, which may act as a foreign body, causing inflammation in the periapical tissues.

The basic requirement of canal obturation, as shown in Chapter 9, is to seal the canal space hermetically to the cementodentinal junction. Compromised obturation may cause treatment failure even if all the other clinical steps are performed satisfactorily.[33] Errors that occur during the obturation stage are the result of poor canal shaping or of improper selection and use of root filing techniques (Fig. 25-15). Poorly condensed obturation, either underfilled or underextended, has been related directly to apical percolation.[43] Furthermore, it is believed that a hermetic seal of the root canal system is intended primarily to prevent microbial leakage from the oral cavity and subsequent reinfection.[104] In periodontally involved teeth, reinfection may occur also via the exposed lateral canals.[104] These theories may explain the causative effect of poor obturation on endodontic failures.

Postoperative Causes

Postoperative sequelae can cause endodontic failure, or create lesions that are interpreted as endodontic failure. Such postoperative causes include trauma and fracture, superimposed nonendodontic involvement, and a poorly designed final restoration or lack of any restoration. The longevity of the endodontically treated tooth is at risk without a final restoration. Restoration of the crown is necessary for function and aesthetics, without which therapy does not achieve its goals. It also prevents leakage from the oral cavity into the canal system that can break the apical seal, causing failure of the treatment.[127] In recent years in vitro studies[63,126,134] showed correlation between poorly designed, or unrestored, crowns of endodontically treated teeth and leakage of dyes and bacteria through the root canals. A post-type restoration may also cause endodontic failure when aseptic technique is not maintained or if the root is perforated in the course of post preparation (Fig. 25-16). A particularly common error occurs when the remaining canal obturation after post preparation is not sufficient to provide an adequate apical seal.[93]

Another facet of postendodontic restoration is the preven-

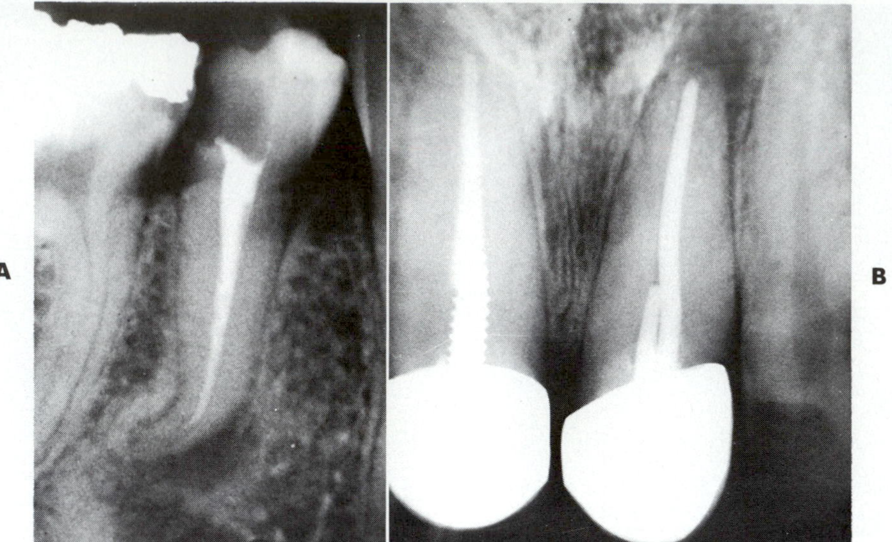

FIG. 25-15 Failures associated with inadequate root canal obturation. **A,** Poor shaping and short obturation caused by underextended access cavity in the mandibular second premolar resulted in failure. **B,** Poor execution of obturation techniques in a maxillary central incisor resulted in underfilled obturation and subsequent failure.

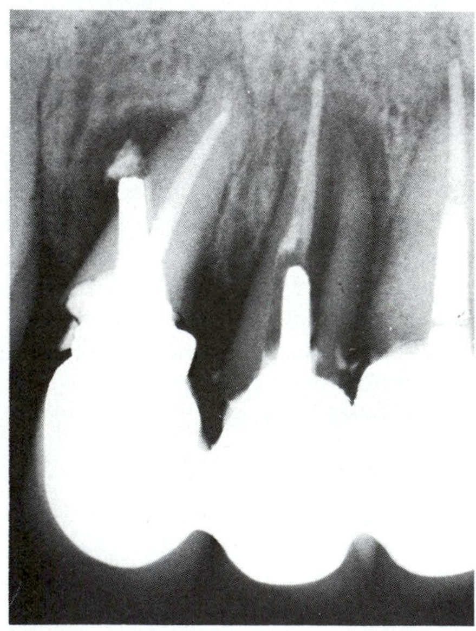

FIG. 25-16 Failures associated with post restorations. Perforation during post preparation in the maxillary lateral incisor and excessive pressure during post placement in the central incisor are causing irreparable damage.

tion of occlusal trauma. According to Seltzer,[104] there is an increased incidence of failure among cases that are treated endodontically and restored with either single crowns or bridge units. Periapical healing of an endodontically treated tooth may be impaired in the presence of constant trauma.[104]

One of the potential postoperative causes of failure that has not been given much emphasis is the vertical root fracture. Not only are endodontically treated teeth weakened by considerable loss of tooth substance, but the chance of fracture is increased as a result of the desiccation of the dentin.[5,38] Fractures and their consequences are usually manifested postoperatively. Nevertheless it has been stated, based only on anecdotal reports, that fractures can actually occur during root canal obturation.[58,72,129]

Fractures are known to result also from the prosthetic reconstruction of endodontically treated teeth. Excessive preparation of a root canal for a post weakens the tooth and has been shown to increase its susceptibility to fracture.[136] Lateral pressure during placement of posts may also cause fracture (Fig. 25-16).[71,84,92] The use of tapered, threaded screw posts is particularly harmful. These posts are designed to be slightly wider than the prepared canal; during placement they cut into and wedge the dentin.

Such posts create considerable lateral forces that, when coupled with the torque of mastication, precipitate root fracture (Fig. 25-17). Volumetric expansion of endodontic posts caused by corrosion and thermal change has also been postulated[3,98] as a cause of vertical root fractures. However, it is quite possible that the corrosion of posts associated with root fractures may have been the result, rather than the cause, of fracture.[88]

The difficulty in diagnosing vertical root fractures may be the reason for the limited attention they have received in past discussions of endodontic failure. Careful diagnostic analysis of failed cases may well lead to increased recognition of the significance of vertical root fracture as a cause of endodontic failure. Investigators[90] described three major types of bony lesions that may be associated with vertical root fracture. A halolike lesion around the root tip extending to midroot level resembles the appearance of a simple endodontic failure, especially when the obturation has not fulfilled the accepted criteria (Fig. 25-18).

Angular periodontal defects of variable width extending apically from the crestal bone (Fig. 25-17), or a widened peri-

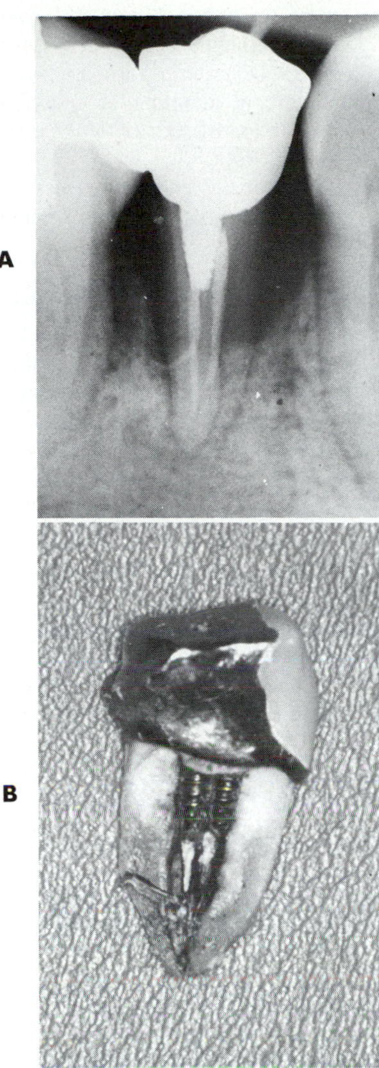

FIG. 25-17 Failure associated with screw posts. **A,** Fractured mandibular second premolar demonstrating bilateral angular periodontal defects, being traced with gutta-percha. **B,** Same tooth after extraction. The root fracture resulted from the use of two screw posts.

odontal ligament space (Fig. 25-19), may appear on one side of the root or on both. Such lesions may be mistaken for bony defects resulting from periodontal disease. In a clinical study on 36 cases of vertical root fracture, Testori and associates[132] found that the sign most often revealed by x-ray was a radiolucent periradicular band.

Endodontic failure may result from a nonendodontic origin, regardless of adequate endodontic therapy. Examples are deleterious effects from orthodontic treatment and periodontal disease.

Endodontic treatment results can be controlled and predicted only to a certain extent, and failures can and will occur even in the best-managed endodontic cases. Often, it may not be possible to identify with certainty the exact cause of failure. In other cases there may be a combination of causes. Although the identification of a particular causative factor in endodontic failure may be speculative, attempts to relate a failure to specific causes are of much academic and clinical importance. The academic value of this attitude is that further progress may be made in recognizing the causes of endodontic failure, which can lead to improving the predictability of endodontic therapy. Clinically, the feasibility of successfully treating a failed case depends on the elimination of the cause of failure, and only by doing so can we expect to correct endodontic failures predictably.

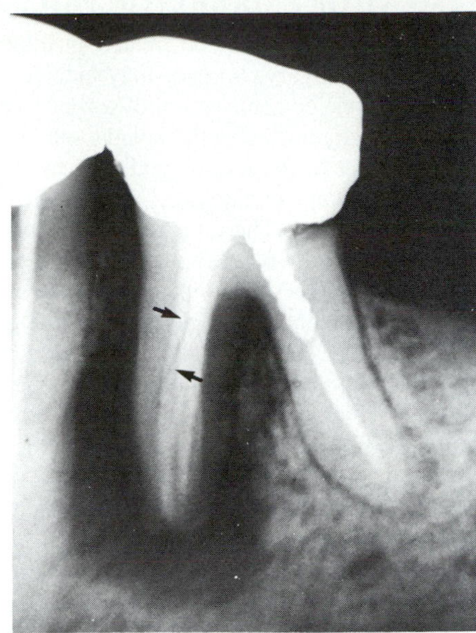

FIG. 25-18 Failure associated with vertical root fracture. The halolike bone loss is pathognomonic of root fracture but may be mistaken for a large periapical lesion caused by simple endodontic failure. Note the hairlike fracture line that is superimposed on the obturation *(arrows).*

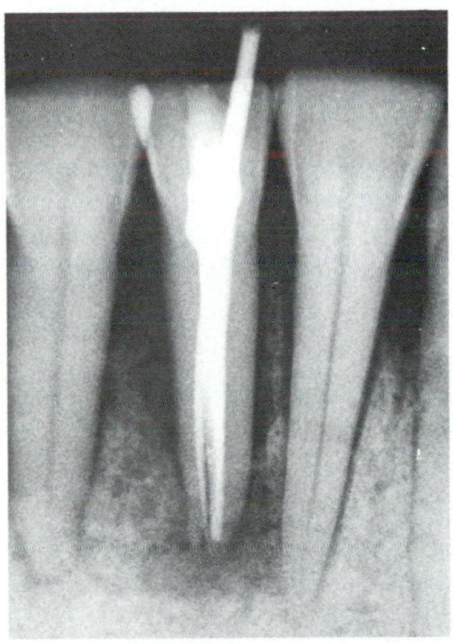

FIG. 25-19 Vertical root fracture manifested by bilateral widening of the periodontal ligament space, as well as by periapical radiolucency. A sinus tract is being traced with gutta-percha.

RETREATMENT OF ENDODONTIC FAILURES

Endodontic failure cases may be treated in either of two ways: retreatment or surgery. Surgery may include extraction of the tooth, resection, or hemisection of a root (see Chapter 18), all of which mean removal of the failed tooth or root without attempting to treat it. Surgery may also be used to correct endodontic failures by apical curettage, apicoectomy, and retrofilling of the root canals. These procedures are presented in detail in Chapter 19, and, so, are not discussed here.

Endodontic retreatment varies in many respects from primary endodontic treatment. The objectives of therapy remain the same, but the fact that the tooth was treated previously without success raises several unique considerations: First, the teeth that require retreatment usually have already been restored, and the restoration has to be damaged to regain access to the root canals. Second, in particular situations retreatment may be considered to technically improve a root filling that radiographically appears to be unsatisfactory, but a better result is not always obtainable[11] and the effort often results in frustration. Third, in retreatment also "iatrogenic factors have to be dealt with,"[55] and they present technical and therapeutic challenges beyond those encountered during primary treatment. Finally, the prognosis for retreatment is considerably poorer than that for primary treatment.[2,10] These considerations are accentuated by increased patient concern about the necessity of repeating a treatment. Consequently, the patient may develop higher awareness and expectations of success than in routine, primary endodontic treatment.

All these considerations complicate the subjective interpretation of information involved in the process of case selection,[94,133] resulting in considerable variation in the opinions of clinicians about the treatment of endodontic failures.[89,94,113] When general dental practitioners were asked in surveys to suggest the treatment for specific endodontic failures, their treatment plans varied from no treatment to extraction.[94,113] Such lack of consensus demonstrates the need for establishing firmer criteria for case selection in endodontic failures.

In recent years, retreatment has accounted for an increasing portion of endodontic treatment procedures, primarily because of (1) the development of criteria for case selection[22]; (2) guidelines for the treatment planning of endodontic retreatment[118]; and (3) introduction of specific techniques that facilitate retreatment.[24]

The following section of this chapter discusses the distinctive features of endodontic retreatment with reference to these three aspects.

Criteria for Case Selection in Retreatment

The first step in considering retreatment is to establish a diagnosis based on clinical and radiographic evaluation. Various criteria may be used for this purpose; however, each clinician should apply consistent criteria for routine definition of endodontic treatment results. Care must be taken at this stage not to neglect differential diagnosis, since several clinical entities may resemble endodontic failure.[7,16] The final diagnosis may be *failure*[109,121] or *success*.[8,121] However, among successful cases some have to be considered *potential failures* (Fig. 25-20).[2]

Established failure

All cases of endodontic failure are associated with pathosis, and occasionally symptoms, which necessitates treatment. There is leeway only in the choice of treatment,[121] either nonsurgical (retreatment) or surgical.[8,16,121] The selection of treatment depends on the feasibility of establishing coronal access to the canals, which would be required for retreatment (Fig. 25-21).

Cast restorations may obstruct conventional access to the canals (Fig. 25-21, *A*). Their removal may endanger the integrity of the tooth,[43] or they may be considered too costly to remake. Cases of endodontic failure in which establishing coronal access is considered unfeasible require *surgery*.[12]

Whenever coronal access to the canals is considered feasible, either *retreatment* or *surgery* may be selected (Fig. 25-

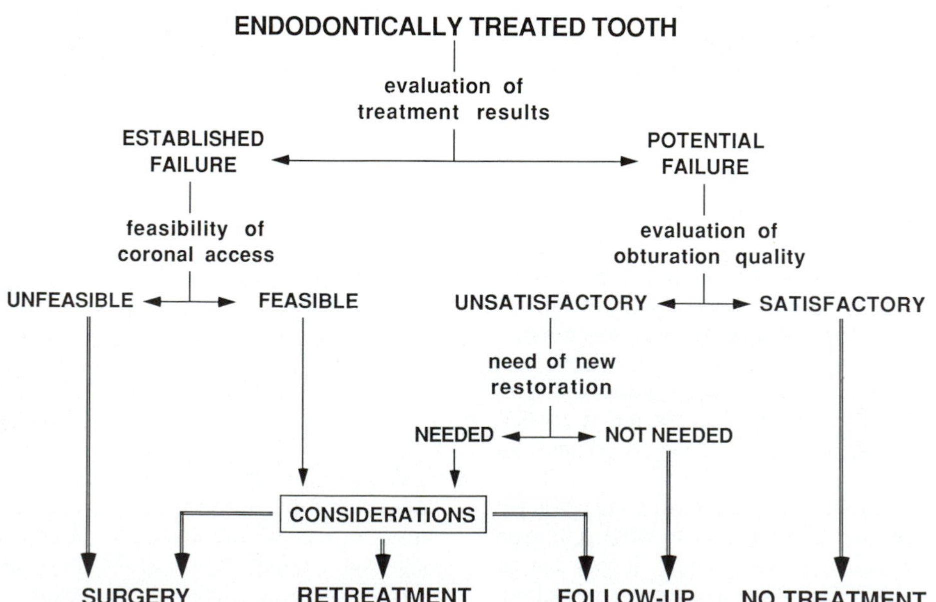

FIG. 25-20 A schematic outline of the considerations and criteria for case selection in endodontic retreatment. (From Friedman S, and Stabholz A: J Endod 12:28, 1986.)

21, *B*). The decision should be based on specific clinical and radiographic considerations, which will be discussed subsequently.

Success and potential failure

Successful endodontic cases should not usually require further treatment. Nevertheless, apparent success may result after unsatisfactory therapy.[105,128] In such cases failure may become manifest at a later stage (Fig. 25-22).[109] "Prediction of possible future failure must be considered as a reason for retreatment, although many of these cases were and could continue to be clinical and radiographic successes."[2] However, cautious consideration is advocated, since such cases may become complicated or fail as a result of retreatment attempts (Fig. 25-23).[11] The potential for failure in apparently successful cases relates to the quality of the endodontic therapy and the demand for prosthetic restoration. Retrospective assessment of the quality of endodontic therapy generally consists of only radiographic evaluation of the obturation.[55] Such factors are observed as the obturation of all root canals, the apical extension of the root filling, and its density. Thus, the obturation may be considered to be *satisfactory* or *unsatisfactory*.

Successful endodontic cases with satisfactory root canal obturation should be considered true successes, and as such they require *no treatment*.

It is when the obturation is unsatisfactory that a presently successful case should be considered a potential failure. Because future failure may be triggered by prosthetic intervention (Fig. 25-22),[45] these cases should be evaluated in the light of the prosthetic treatment plan. When a new prosthetic restoration is not indicated, there is no indication for endodontic

A

B

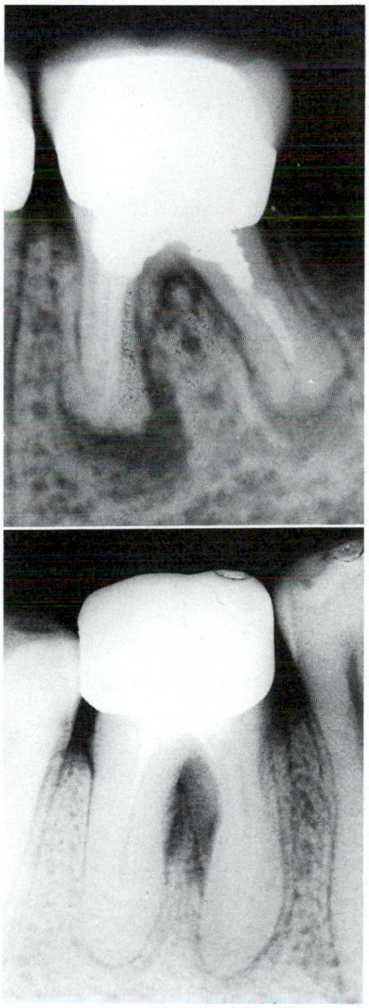

FIG. 25-21 Retreatment of established failure. **A,** Retreatment via coronal access may be considered unfeasible when a satisfactory restoration has to be sacrificed, or when there is risk of damaging the tooth during removal of the restoration. **B,** Coronal access for retreatment can be gained at the cost of a faulty restoration without endangering the tooth. (From Friedman S, and Stabholz A: J Endod 12:28, 1986.)

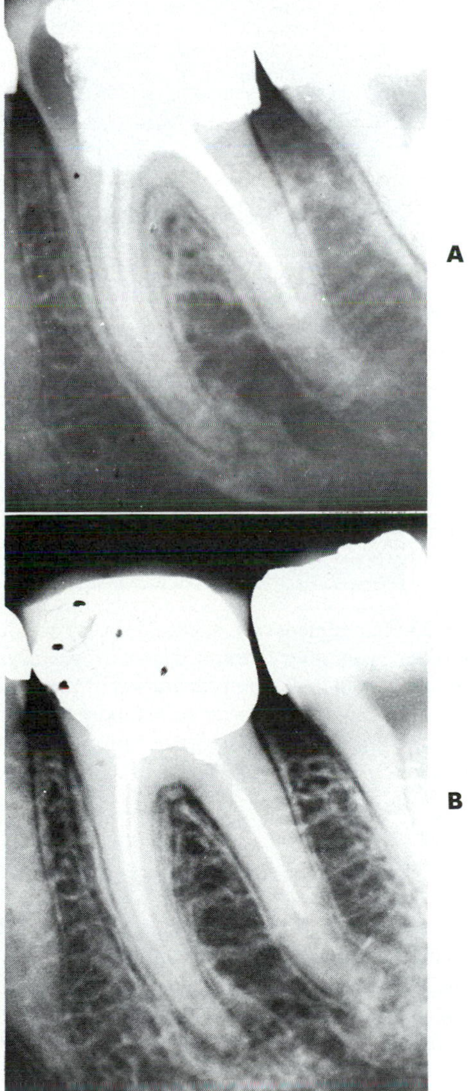

FIG. 25-22 Endodontic success after unsatisfactory therapy should be considered a potential failure, which may manifest itself later. **A,** The success of poor endodontic therapy in a mandibular first molar was confirmed radiographically and clinically 3 years after therapy. **B,** Periapical radiolucencies 8 months after the construction of a new prosthetic restoration indicate that the endodontic therapy has failed.

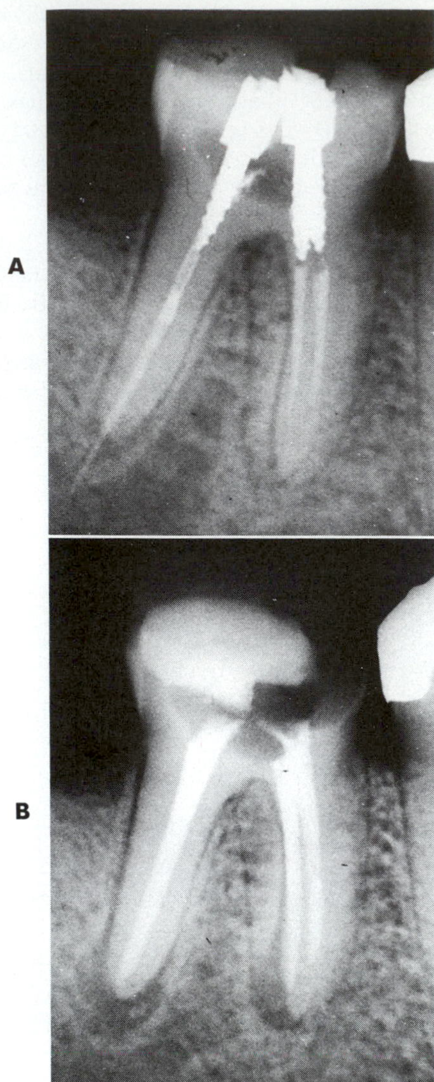

FIG. 25-23 Retreatment of a successful case resulting in failure. **A,** Four years after therapy the tooth was asymptomatic. Retreatment was indicated in preparation of the tooth for a cast restoration. **B,** Six months after retreatment the appearance of radiolucent periapical areas suggests failure. (From Friedman S, and Stabholz A: J Endod 12:28, 1986.)

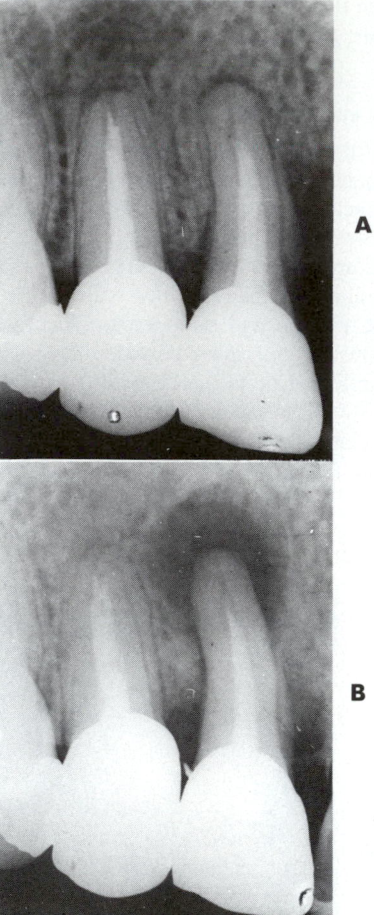

FIG. 25-24 Late manifestation of endodontic failure. **A,** Both maxillary premolars were endodontically treated and restored 10 years before this routine radiograph was taken. Despite poor therapy the teeth were comfortable with minute periapical widening of the periodontal ligament space. **B,** Two years later symptoms evolved, with a dramatic change in the periapical radiographic appearance of the first premolar (12 years after therapy).

retreatment, either,[16] but awareness is required of the possible delayed manifestation of failure (Fig. 25-24).[1,109] Therefore, although retreatment is not indicated at present, continued *follow-up* is recommended.

The cost and effort involved in prosthetic restorations dictate that the treated teeth should offer a sound endodontic prognosis (Fig. 25-22). Furthermore, a prosthetic restoration may prohibit or complicate the access should endodontic retreatment be indicated in the future (Fig. 25-21).[118] Therefore, before a prosthetic restoration is applied to a tooth with poor obturation, even though it may appear radiographically and clinically successful, either *retreatment* or *follow-up* is to be considered. The decision is based on the same considerations as those used in cases of failure.

Clinical and Radiographic Considerations

Case history

As with every other therapeutic approach, the case history is of utmost importance for selecting the treatment of choice. The case history is helpful in recognizing the nature of a case, healing potential, pathogenesis, and urgency of treatment. The record of previous endodontic treatment such as possible calcifications after pulpotomies (Fig. 25-25, *A*) or repeated failures of surgery or retreatment (Fig. 25-25, *B*) may suggest restrictions to further treatment attempts.[137] Early radiographs, time elapsed since previous treatment, and previous symptoms are all related to the case history and should be considered whenever available. Attempts should be made to differentiate between poor therapy and therapy compromised because of objective clinical limitations.

Clinical situation

The presence or absence of symptoms and their severity determine the urgency of treatment. Discomfort may occasion-

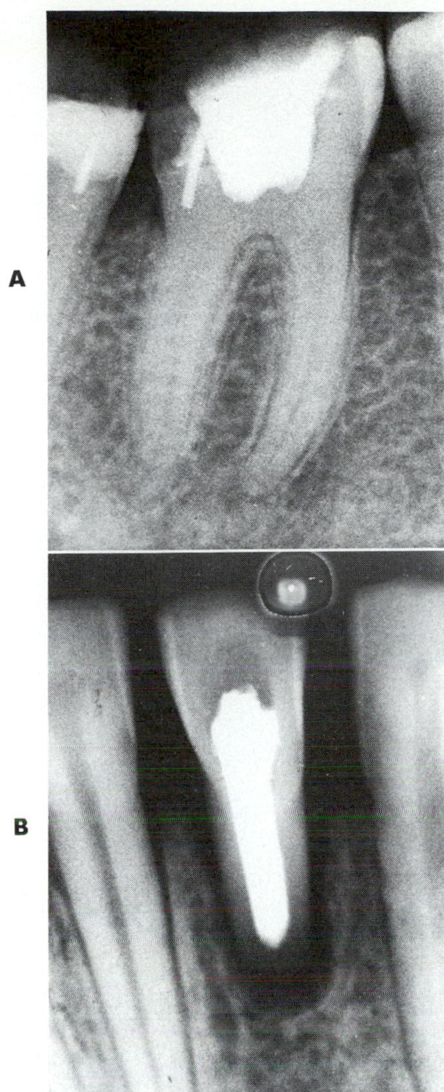

FIG. 25-25 Consideration of previous therapy. **A,** Pulpotomy in the mandibular first molar resulted in calcification of the root canals, which may prohibit successful endodontic therapy. **B,** Case history of this mandibular central incisor revealed that nonsurgical and surgical retreatments were both repeated twice, suggesting that further such attempts are likely to fail. (From Friedman S, and Stabholz A: J Endod 12:28, 1986.)

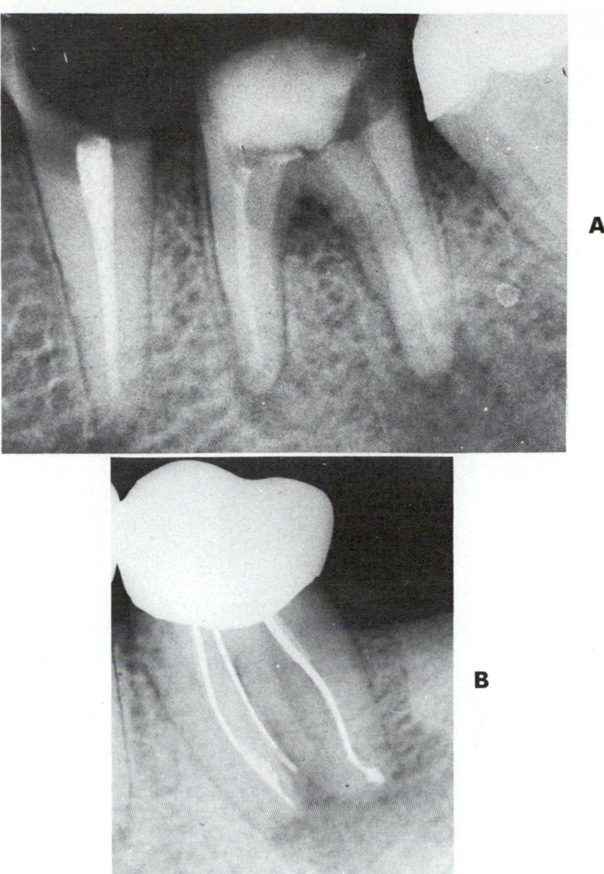

FIG. 25-26 Consideration of clinical situation. **A,** Massive breakdown of these teeth's crowns suggests that the feasibility of restoring them should be confirmed prior to retreatment. **B,** Combined endodontic-periodontal lesion involving the mandibular second molar. The periodontal prognosis should be questioned before retreatment is undertaken. (From Friedman S, and Stabholz A: J Endod 12:28, 1986.)

ally dictate the choice of surgical treatment over the lengthier retreatment. Both retreatment and surgery of teeth that cannot be satisfactorily restored must be avoided (Fig. 25-26, *A*).

In cases with periodontal involvement, endodontic surgery may be contraindicated because of an unfavorable crown-root ratio (Chapter 20), and retreatment may be the therapy of choice. However, the prognosis for combined endodontic-periodontal therapy should be assessed before retreatment is initiated (Fig. 25-26, *B*).[34]

Anatomy

Endodontic failure is frequently caused by untreated canals, which are more amenable to endodontic retreatment than to surgical retrofilling techniques. Therefore, the radicular anatomy of each case, especially those with aberrant configuration, must be carefully examined to disclose possible unfilled canals, for which retreatment may be preferable (Fig. 25-27, *A*). Pronounced canal curvature, calcifications, or divergences may be difficult to negotiate in retreatment (Fig. 25-27, *B*). Indiscriminate attempts at retreatment in such canals often fail,[109] whereas surgery may be successful.

Root canal filling

Several aspects of the root canal filling may be taken into consideration with regard to retreatment: *(a)* The *apical extension* is evaluated in relation to the root apex and the site of the pathologic lesion. Often a short filling appears to be readily retreatable farther apically, but this may be impossible to accomplish in many cases.[11] The chances of coronally retrieving an overextended filling are even slimmer (Fig. 25-28). *(b)* The *density* is directly related to the difficulty of removing the filling material from the root canal. Whenever possible, the density should be examined clinically, because it often does not correlate with the radiographic image. *(c)* The *type of fill-*

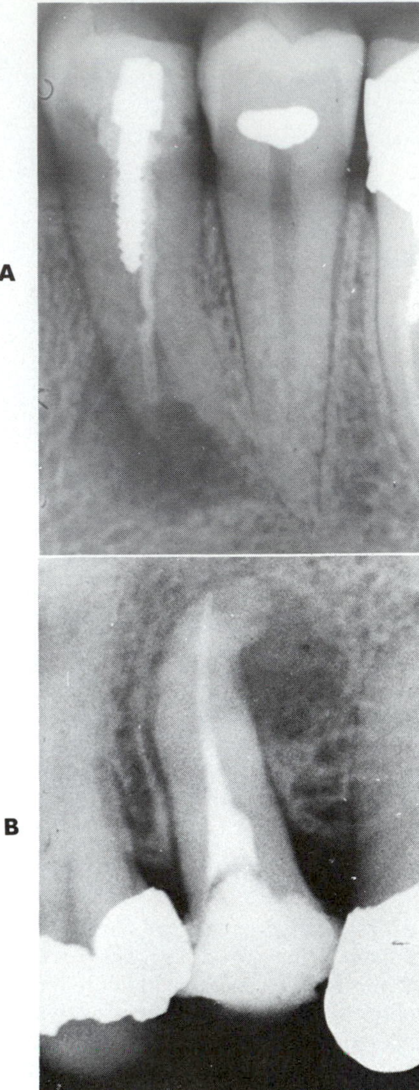

FIG. 25-27 Consideration of root anatomy. **A,** Failure associated with an untreated second root canal in a mandibular first premolar. Endodontic retreatment is the treatment of choice, with a better prognosis than apical surgery. **B,** The chances to improve the apical obturation in this maxillary second premolar are poor because of its anatomic configuration. Surgery may offer a better prognosis than retreatment in such cases.

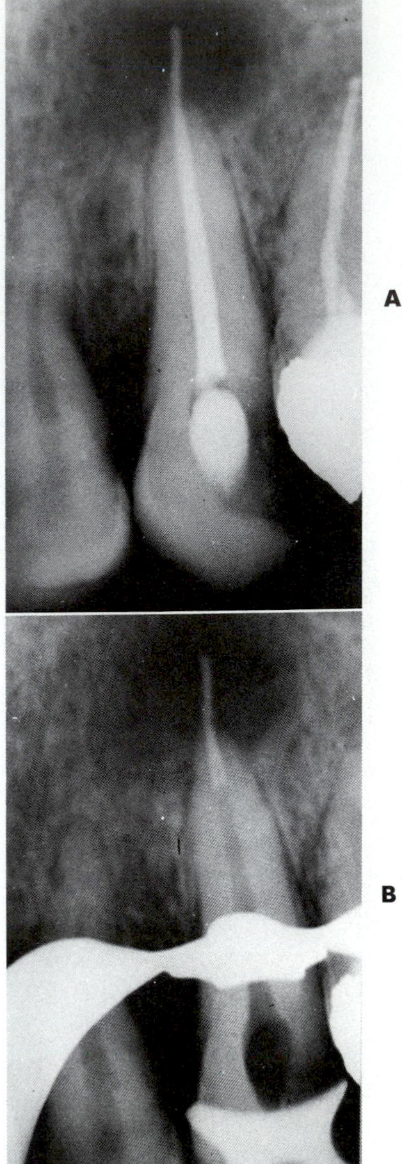

FIG. 25-28 Consideration of overextended obturation. **A,** Removal of gutta-percha was attempted in retreatment of this maxillary canine. **B,** The overextended portion of gutta-percha separated at the apical level and could no longer be removed via the root canal. (From Friedman S, and Stabholz A: J Endod 12:28, 1986.)

ing material is important because removal of each type of material poses specific difficulties. Some materials, such as zinc phosphate cement, may be impossible to remove, making retreatment unfeasible. The retreatment of teeth with various root filling materials is discussed further in this chapter.

Intraradicular and extraradicular interference

Endodontic failure may be associated with separated instrument fragments[32,109] that would have to be removed or bypassed if retreatment is performed. The chances of doing either successfully depend mainly on their location.[21] Occasionally it may be prudent to avoid retreatment so as to prevent complications from attempts to overcome inaccessible broken instruments (Fig. 25-29, *A*).[21] Perforations of the root or pulp chamber offer a poor prognosis (Fig. 25-29, *B*).[16] Although some perforations may be filled from within the tooth, others require external access and may dictate surgical treatment rather than retreatment. If the presence of a ledge is suspected it may be impossible to renegotiate the canal successfully (Fig. 25-29, *C*),[11] and additional damage may result. When the chances to renegotiate the canal are assessed to be poor, surgery may be preferred over retreatment. External root resorption, particularly of the replacement type (see Chapter 17), may not be predictably arrested[109]; therefore its presence may be considered a contraindication for retreatment (Fig. 25-29, *D*). In specific cases, endodontic failure may be caused by bac-

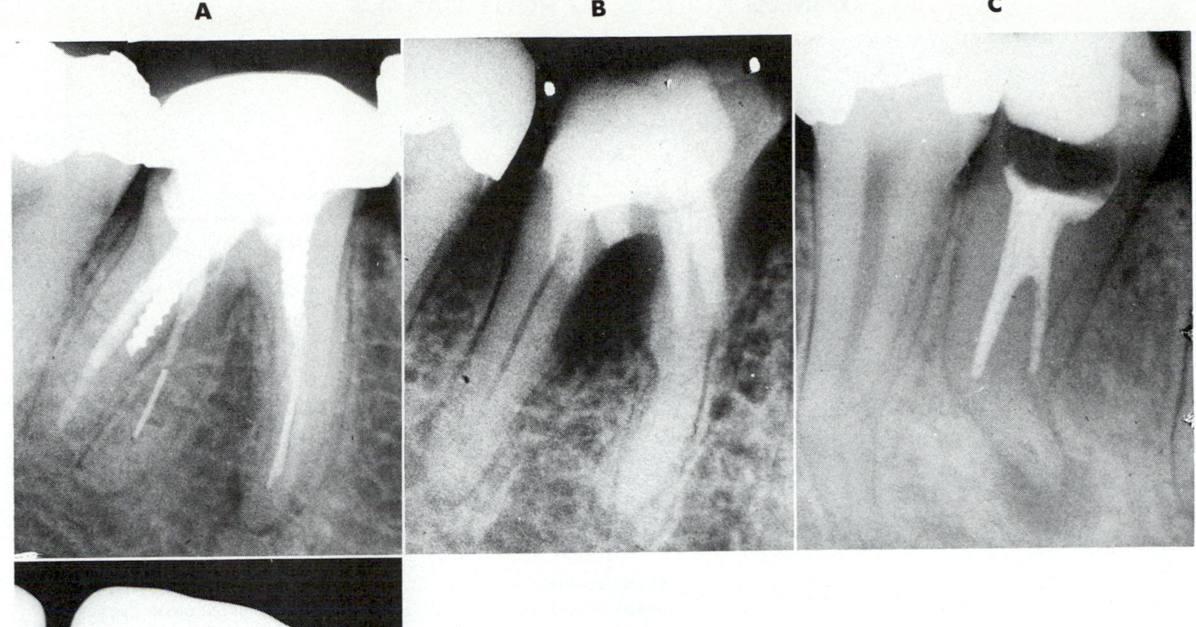

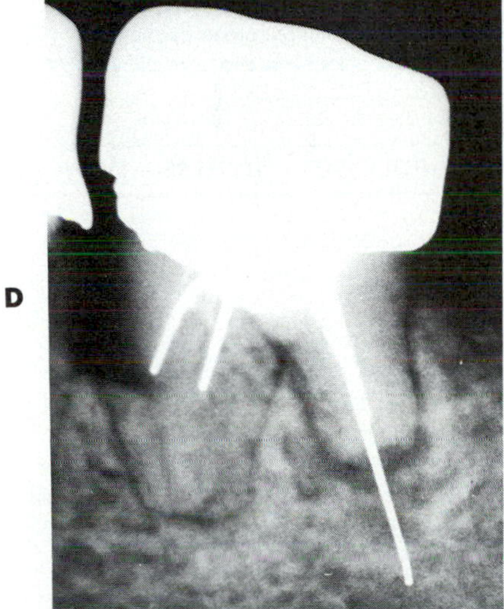

FIG. 25-29 Consideration of factors reducing the chances of retreatment success. **A,** Fragments of instruments separated inaccessibly in the canal. **B,** Perforations of the root canal system. **C,** Ledges in curved root canals. **D,** Progressive external root resorption. (From Friedman S, and Stabholz A: J Endod 12:28, 1986.)

teria harbored on the outer aspect of the root tip that do not respond to routine root canal treatment.[135] In such cases surgery should be preferred.

Possible complications

Many of the complications associated with regaining access to root canals in previously restored teeth and instrumenting obstructed root canals are discussed in detail further in this chapter. These, and the possible complications from endodontic surgery, have to be weighed against one another, so that each case is treated with the least probability of complication.

Cooperation of the patient

Because it is a lengthier procedure than surgery, endodontic retreatment requires the full cooperation of the patient.[102] Furthermore, the patient is required to cooperate in a repetition of a previously unsatisfactory treatment that may have undermined his or her trust, often without even realizing the necessity for retreatment. The patient should be informed about the available treatment alternatives and should participate in the choice of treatment.[22]

Capability of the clinician

In the further sections of this chapter are discussed specific retreatment techniques. Some require considerable experience.[2,102] The clinician, whether experienced or not, whether general practitioner or specialist, should evaluate each case from the perspective of his or her own capability.[55] In doubtful cases, clinicians should consult an endodontist, whom they may consider to be more experienced than themselves.

Conclusion of considerations

In endodontic retreatment both the patient and the clinician are exceptionally concerned about the chances of success.[133] For this reason the prognosis must be assessed carefully, considering all the factors discussed. This assessment must recognize all alternative treatments, including surgical modalities[121] and osseointegrated implants, and their possible advantages in specific cases.

Retreatment Planning

In addition to their root canals being obturated, the majority of teeth for which retreatment is indicated have been re-

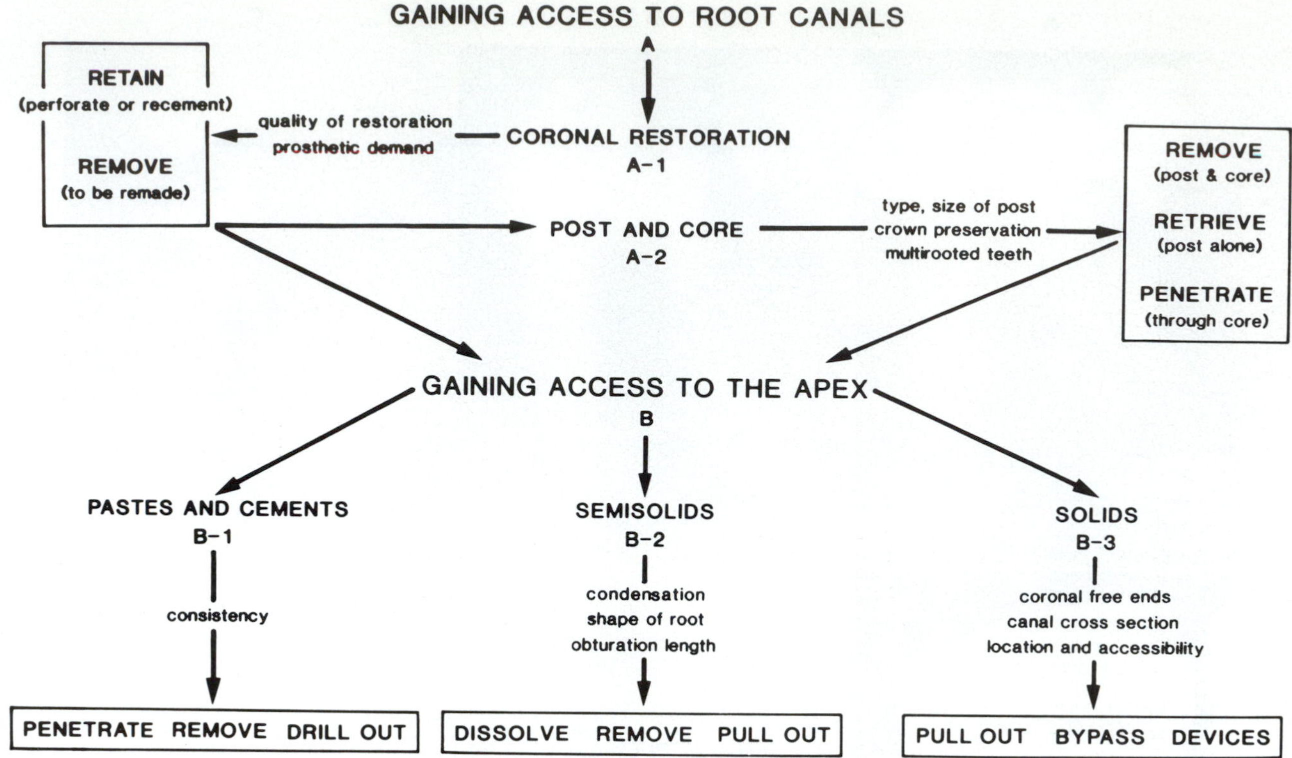

FIG. 25-30 A schematic outline of the considerations and guidelines for endodontic retreatment planning. (From Stabholz A, and Friedman S: J Endod 14:607, 1988.)

stored. Thus, endodontic retreatment first involves gaining access to the root canals, and later gaining access to the apical foramina.[118]

Any of various treatment modalities may be chosen for coping with the restoration as well as with the obturation, all of which have advantages and disadvantages related to endodontic therapy. The guidelines for retreatment planning are presented schematically in Figure 25-30.

Gaining access to root canals

As mentioned previously, a large percentage of endodontic failures result from operative errors, one of which is incorrect endodontic cavity preparation.[43] Often the access cavity found in association with endodontic failures is underextended and must be reevaluated and improved before reinstrumentation of the canals is begun.[64] For the purpose of retreatment, extensive convenience form has to be established to allow further shaping of the previously enlarged canals and to facilitate removal of the obturation materials.[64]

Two types of restorations have to be considered before access to root canals can be established in pulpless restored teeth. The tooth crown usually has a coronal restoration that may frequently be supported by a post and core.

Coronal restoration. The coronal restorations in endodontically treated teeth may consist of simple or complex fillings of any of several materials. Such restorations do not require particular consideration in regard to endodontic retreatment. More extensive restorations (e.g., fixed partial prostheses) cover the outer and inner tooth and increase the chances for error during access preparation. In addition, options to retain satisfactory prosthetic restorations that are costly to remake should be explored as a service to patients. Depending on the type of cementation, the cast restorations may be removed without damage so that they may be recemented after retreatment. However, during attempts to do so there is always some risk of breaking the tooth. If the restoration is to remain in place, endodontic access can be established by perforating the restoration and later repairing the access perforation *in situ*.[14] The pros and cons of retreatment through a prosthetic restoration, as opposed to removing it, relate to several factors:

Tooth morphology. Tooth morphology may be better realized if the prosthetic restoration is removed. Access cavity preparation through a prosthetic restoration is more complicated and time consuming and may result in irreparable procedural damage.[73]

Radiographs. More radiographic information about the coronal part of the tooth may be obtained if the prosthetic restoration is removed.[73] This includes the identification of perforations, coronal extension of silver cones, and possible calcifications in the canal orifices, as well as the dimensions of the pulp chamber (Fig. 25-26, *B*).

Vertical fractures. The relation of vertical root fractures to endodontic failures was discussed previously in this chapter. Inasmuch as a fracture is difficult to diagnose, its absence should be verified before retreatment is initiated. With the restoration removed a vertical fracture may be visualized, whereas with the crown in position a fracture may be overlooked.

Endodontic cavity. The principles of endodontic cavity preparation, particularly in regard to outline form, convenience form, and removal of remaining carious dentin, may be better

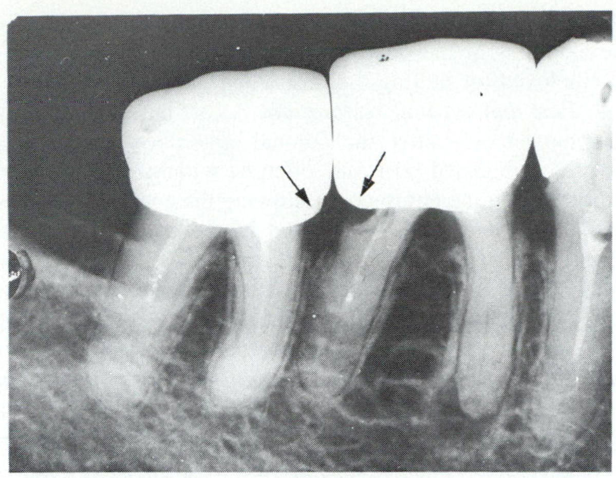

FIG. 25-31 Poor marginal adaptation and secondary caries *(arrows)* in mandibular first and second molars will allow leakage if crowns are retained during retreatment. (From Stabholz A, and Friedman S: J Endod 14:607, 1988.)

accomplished by establishing direct access than through a prosthetic restoration.[43]

Tooth isolation. A satisfactory restoration facilitates the placement of the rubber dam and temporary filling. Conversely, an ill-fitting restoration or secondary caries allows leakage beneath the rubber dam that is difficult to control (Fig. 25-31).[43]

Tooth function. With the restoration in place patient comfort, uncompromised function, and aesthetics are maintained.

These considerations suggest that the following guidelines should be used in planning retreatment of a restored tooth. *Remove* restorations of poor quality, particularly those with poor marginal adaptation or secondary caries and those that are intended in the prosthetic treatment plan to be replaced. *Retain* satisfactory restorations that should not be replaced, by either accessing through and later repairing them or removing them so that they can later be recemented. When function or aesthetics have to be maintained or when isolation is expected to be difficult and the present restoration is reasonably satisfactory, it may be retained temporarily to facilitate retreatment comfort even if it is designated for future replacement.

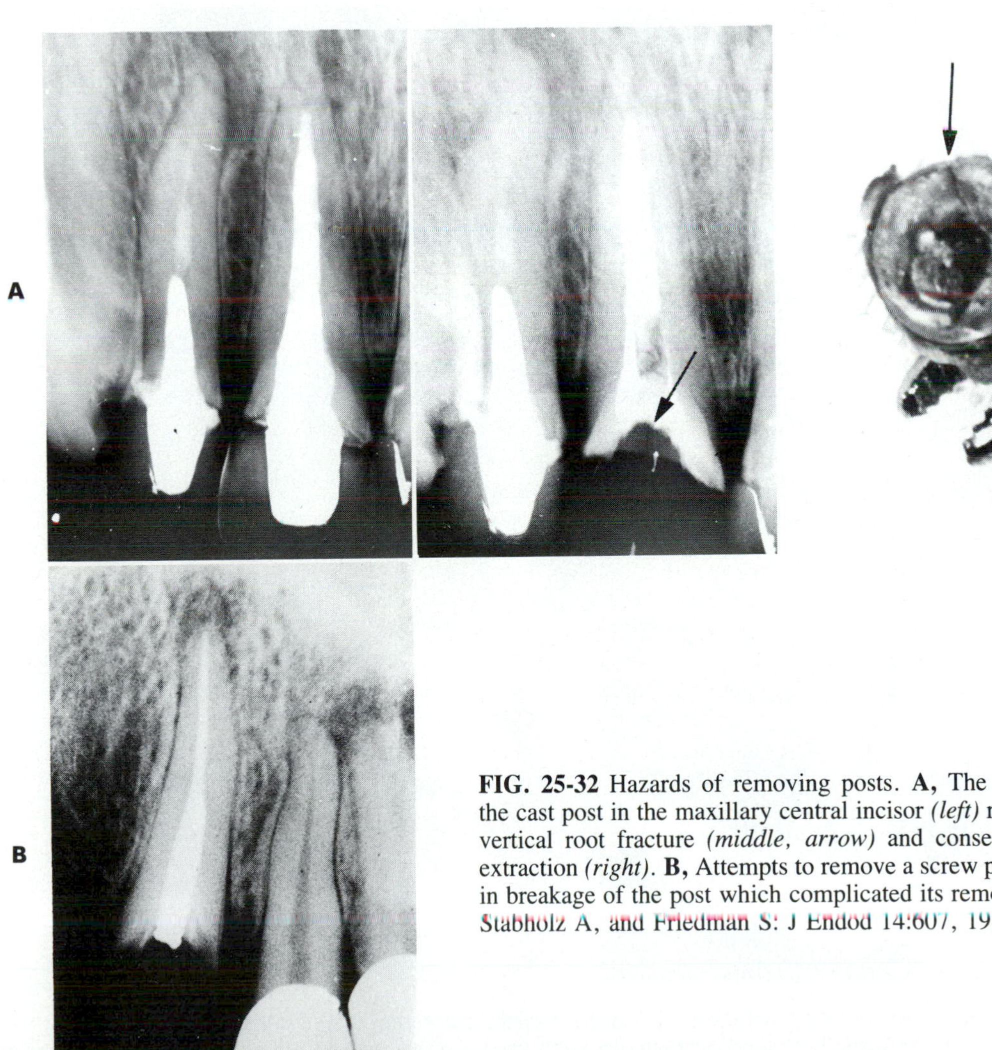

FIG. 25-32 Hazards of removing posts. **A,** The removal of the cast post in the maxillary central incisor *(left)* resulted in a vertical root fracture *(middle, arrow)* and consequent tooth extraction *(right)*. **B,** Attempts to remove a screw post resulted in breakage of the post which complicated its removal. (From Stabholz A, and Friedman S: J Endod 14:607, 1988.)

Post and core. Some literature suggests that a radicular post space weakens the tooth[100,136]; nevertheless, it is a common practice to restore pulpless teeth with posts and cores. A complete discussion of posts and cores will be found in Chapter 22. To gain access to the root canals in need of retreatment, the clinician must remove or perforate the post and the core, taking into consideration the following factors:

1. Hazards of removing the post. Having been weakened by a prepared radicular post space, the tooth may fracture when a cast post is removed (Fig. 25-32, *A*).[43] Removing a threaded post may be less dangerous, the risk being proportional to the amount of surface contact between the post and the dentin. A post may also break inside the root and become difficult to remove (Fig. 25-32, *B*).

2. Reducing post retention. The application of ultrasonic vibration to a post can weaken its retention and facilitate removal.[26] Whenever necessary, coronal dentin walls retaining the post may be reduced to eliminate post retention.

3. Forceful pulling of posts. Applying forces to cast posts in attempts to remove them increases the risk of root fracture. This risk is minimized if the forces are applied strictly along the long axis of the post,[62] and special devices may have to be employed for pulling the post along its long axis.[62,119,123]

4. Post and coronal restoration. A cast post and core may be removed only after the coronal restoration has been removed. A threaded post may often be withdrawn alone without sacrificing the entire core, allowing the coronal restoration to be retained in place, supported by the core and the tooth structure (Fig. 25-33). As governed by these considerations, the following guidelines are suggested for endodontic retreatment of teeth restored with posts and cores. Depending on the type, length, and width of the post, and the wall contact of the core, *the retention should be reduced before attempts are made to remove the post and core,* and special devices may be employed to facilitate removal. When it is indicated to preserve a coronal restoration supported by a threaded post, access through the core may be established in order *to retrieve the threaded post alone*. In multirooted teeth whose posted canal does not require retreatment and when removal of the post is contraindicated, it is suggested that the clinician *penetrate*

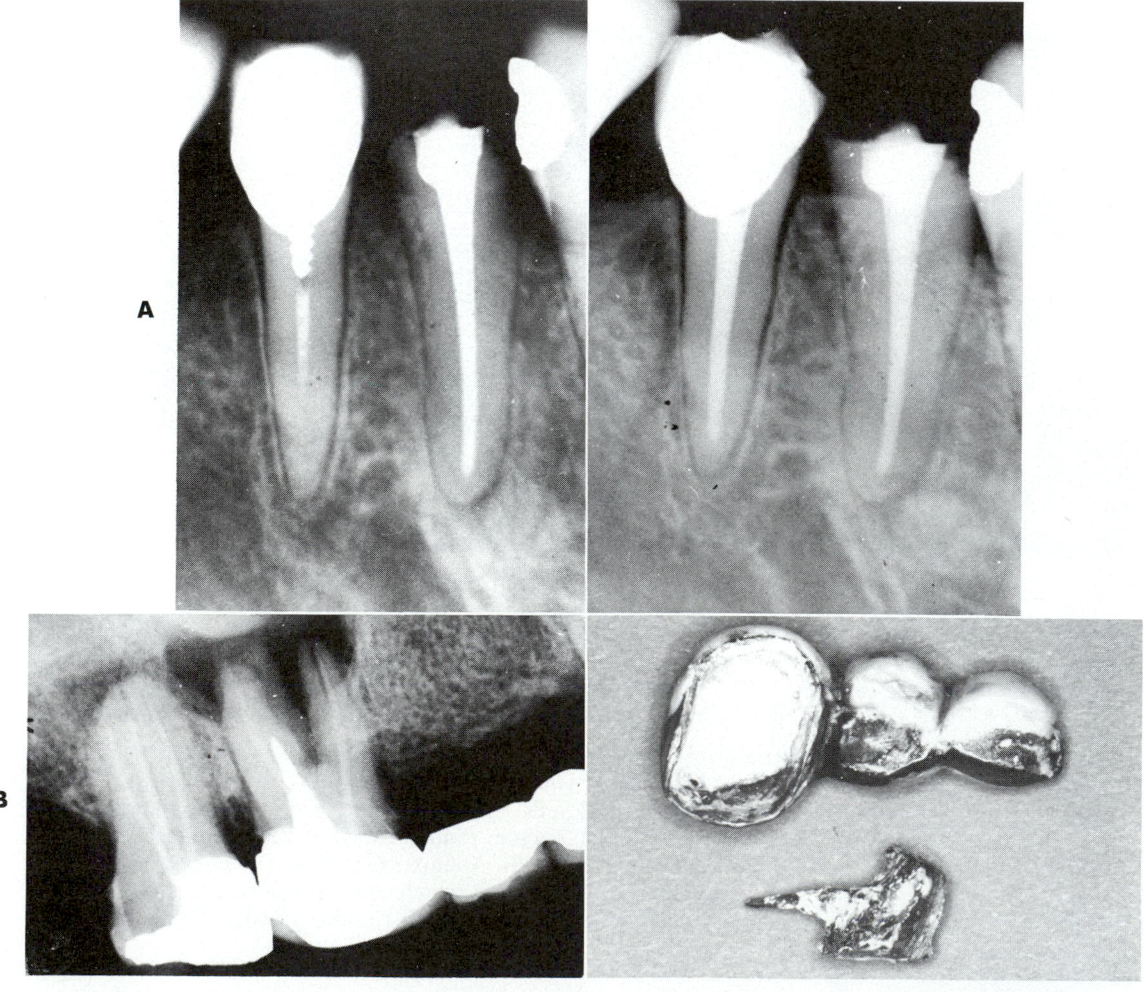

FIG. 25-33 Interrelationship of the post and the coronal restoration in retreatment. **A,** The screw post in the mandibular second premolar *(left)* has been removed to allow retreatment without removing the crown and the complete core *(right)*. **B,** To allow the removal of the cast post and core *(left)* for the purpose of retreatment in the maxillary first molar, the bridge had to be removed *(right)*. (From Stabholz A, and Friedman S: J Endod 14:607, 1988.)

through the core to gain access to the canals in need of retreatment without removing the post (Fig. 25-34).

Gaining access to the apical foramen

In nonsurgical retreatment access to the apex can be regained only after the filling materials are removed from the canal. During canal instrumentation, the usual resistance of the dentin walls to the instruments is coupled with additional resistance by the filling materials.[118] This increased resistance may result in an undesired alteration of the retreated canal morphology. The treatment plan for removing the filling materials must be tailored to prevent errors of this nature.

Various materials have been recommended and used for filling root canals, but they cannot all be discussed in this chapter. From a study of 1300 retreatment cases performed in the United States, in which 53.6% of the teeth were originally obturated with gutta-percha, 20.6% with pastes, and 9.5% with silver points,[2] it would appear that these are the most frequently encountered filling materials in retreatment. The materials may be broadly classified as pastes and cements, semisolid materials, and solid ones. The following guidelines are suggested for removing them for endodontic retreatment.

Pastes and cements. A retrospective analysis of retreatments suggests that the frequency of using pastes for root ca-

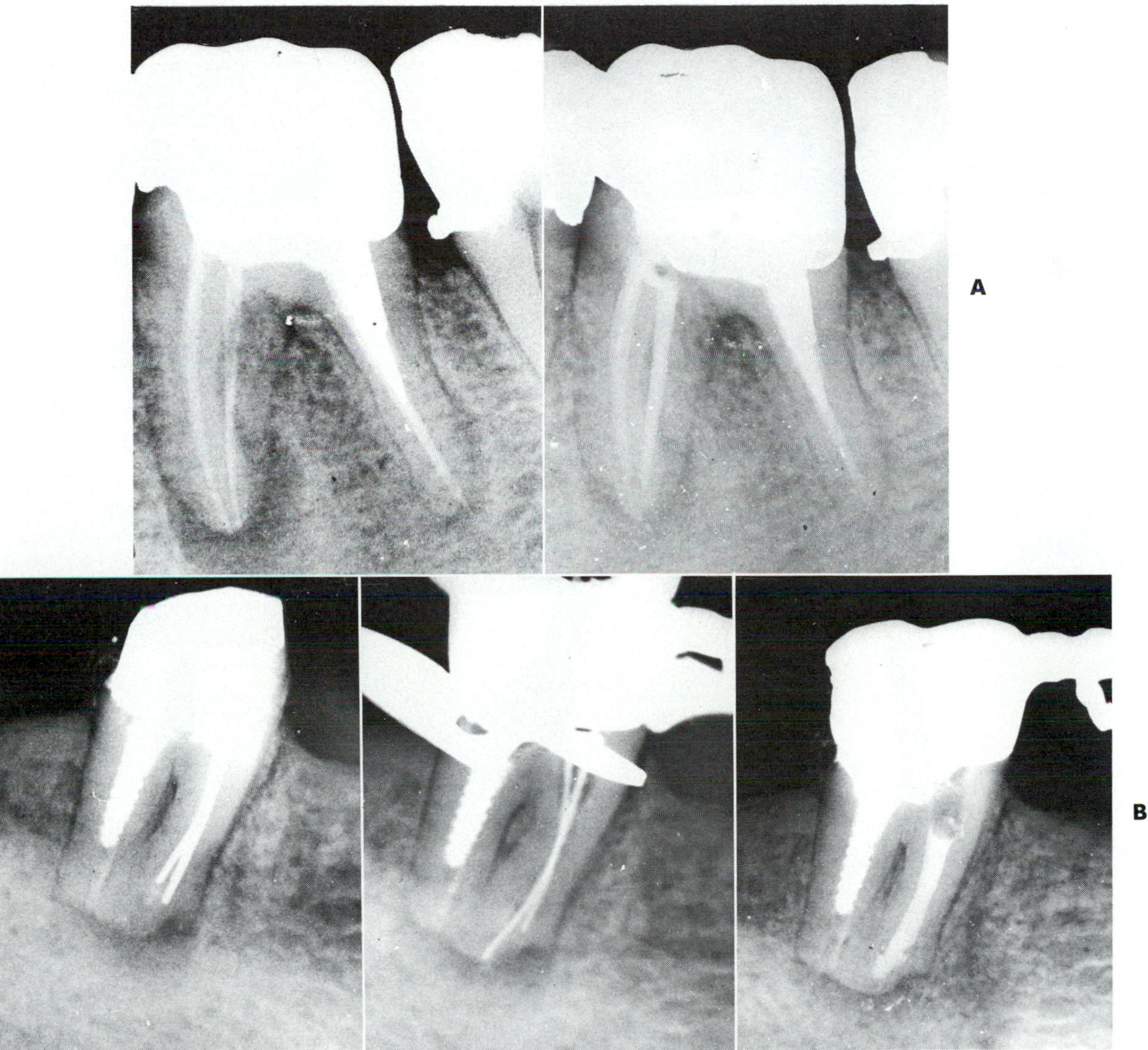

FIG. 25-34 Partial retreatment of multirooted teeth restored with post and core. **A,** Mesial canals in the mandibular first molar restored with a cast post and core and a crown *(left)* have been successfully retreated (*right,* follow-up 1 year) without removing the cast post and core. **B,** Preoperative radiograph *(left)* of the mandibular second molar abutment restored with a screw post and amalgam core. To facilitate proper isolation the bridge was recemented and the mesial canals were retreated through an access cavity perforating the crown and core *(middle)*. Concern about breaking the distal root dictated that the oversized post remain in place. Retreatment was completed successfully (*right,* follow-up 6 months). (From Stabholz A, and Friedman S: J Endod 14:607, 1988.)

nal obturation is not decreasing.[2] Although some pastes may be dissolved with common solvents, hard cements such as N-2, glass ionomer, and zinc phosphate do not yield themselves to solvents.[29,123] The feasibility of removing pastes and cements from the root canal depends on the consistency of the material, which, unfortunately, cannot be assessed by radiographs alone and has to be tested clinically.

Soft-setting pastes. The clinician should attempt initially to *penetrate* soft-setting pastes with routine endodontic instruments.[123]

Hard-setting cements. Ultrasonic endodontic devices can disperse hard cements[44,51,120] and should be used to *remove* them.

When this appears to be unfeasible or unsuccessful, attempts should be made to *drill out* the cement, but only to a depth that is considered safe, to avoid root perforation. Failure to penetrate the cement and to instrument the entire canal may necessitate surgery (Fig. 25-35).[55]

Semisolid materials, gutta-percha. Gutta-percha may be dissolved with various solvents to facilitate removal,[131] though since the majority of the available solvents are either toxic, harmful or inefficient,[140,143] their use should be avoided whenever possible. The treatment plan for retreating gutta-percha root fillings depends on the following considerations:

1. Quality of condensation. The fastest way to retreat a poorly condensed obturation is to *pull out* the gutta-percha through the access opening (Fig. 25-36). In a well-condensed obturation it is necessary to *dissolve* the gutta-percha. In ei-

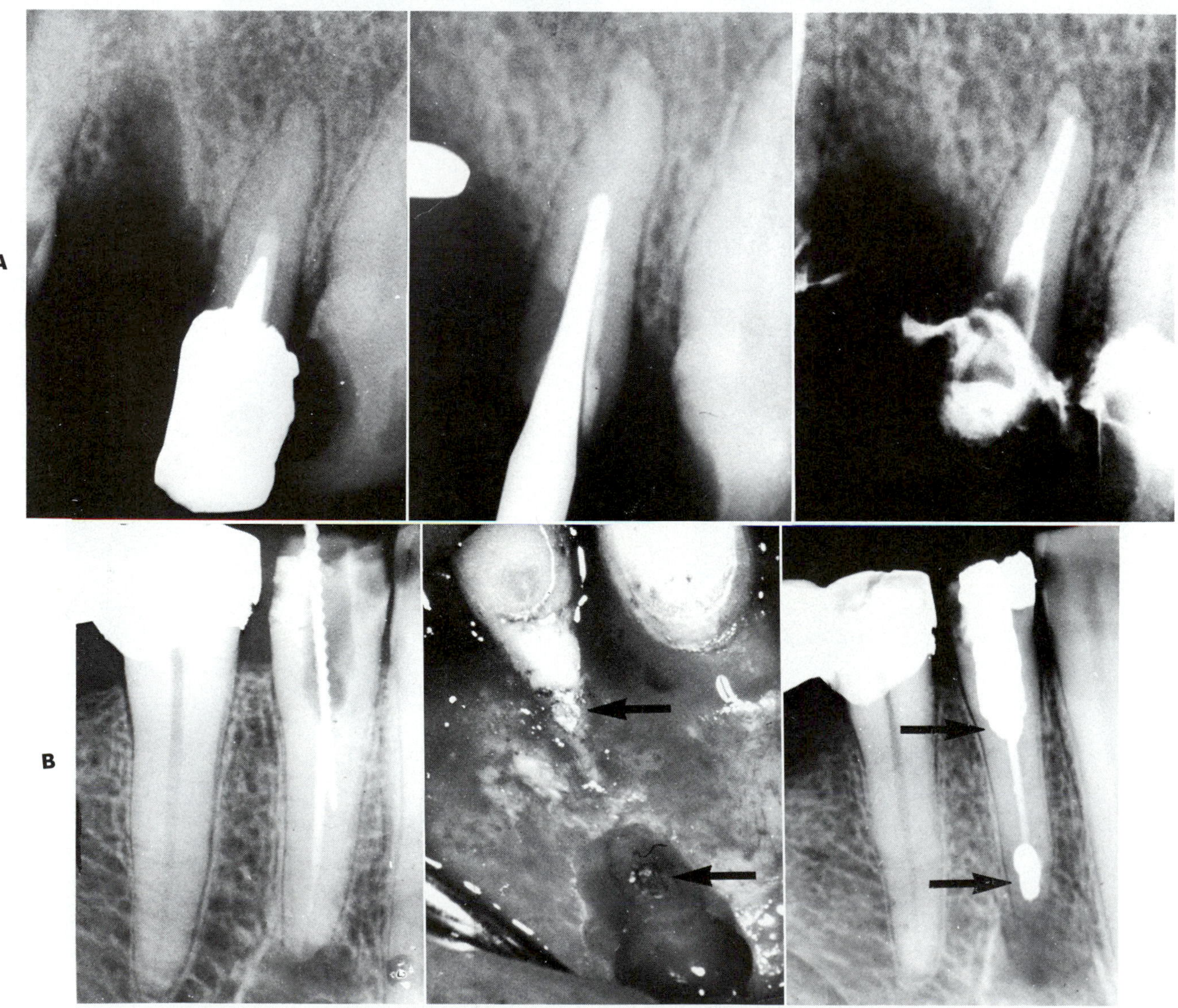

FIG. 25-35 Retreatment of hard cement root fillings by drilling. **A,** Preoperative radiograph of the maxillary lateral incisor indicated for retreatment in preparation for a new restoration *(left)*. The cement root filling was drilled out *(middle)*, and retreatment was completed satisfactorily *(right)*. **B,** Attempts to drill out the hard cement root filling in the mandibular first premolar resulted in a perforation *(left)* that necessitated surgical retrofilling of the canal and the perforation *(middle* and *right, arrows)*. (From Stabholz A, and Friedman S: J Endod 14:607, 1988.)

ther case the coronal portion of the obturation may be drilled out, with a Gates-Glidden or Peeso bur.

2. Shape of root canal. In curved canals it is advisable to *dissolve* the gutta-percha, so as to allow resistance-free negotiation of the canal curvature without ledging or perforation (Fig. 25-37). In readily accessible, straight canals it is expeditious to *remove* the gutta-percha with rotary endodontic instrumentation.

3. Length of obturation. In root canals that were prepared and filled considerably short of their apices, particularly curved ones, ledges may have formed at the apical end of the obturation.[118] To prevent further ledging of the canal in such cases it is necessary to *dissolve* the gutta-percha (Fig. 25-37). Overextended gutta-percha must not be dissolved but rather bypassed carefully with the hope of *pulling out* the overextending cones in one piece. A convenient coronal pathway should be established to allow removal (Fig. 25-38).[91]

Solid materials and obstructing objects. The treatment plan for removing obstructing solid objects depends on the feasibility of either grasping them with an extracting device[21] or bypassing them with endodontic instruments.[21] Both procedures may be expedited by application of ultrasonic vibration.[40,79,114] Retreating the accessible portion of the canal without removing the object is another possibility; the prognosis is related to the presence or absence of canal infection, and it may be poor in the presence of periapical breakdown.[21]

The following guidelines are suggested for planning retreatment of solid materials.

Coronal free ends. Coronal ends of silver points that extend into the pulp chamber are visible in radiographs of uncrowned teeth. They should be preserved and grasped to *pull out* the cones.[123] In the presence of amalgam cores the coronal ends of silver points cannot be isolated; therefore the entire core should be separated and removed with the points embedded in the amalgam (Fig. 25-39). Silver points without accessible coronal ends should be managed in the same manner as broken instruments.[52,123]

Canal cross section. When root canals are not expected to be quite round in cross section, attempts should be made to *bypass* the obstructing object (Fig. 25-40). Bypassed objects may then be loosened and retrieved, or remain integrated in the new canal obturation (Fig. 25-41).[21]

Location of object and accessibility. The removal of obstructing objects that are unlikely to be retrieved, as previously suggested, should be attempted with special grasping devices. The safe use of such devices is related to the location of the object.[21] Because of their rigid design the use of grasping devices is restricted to rather large, straight roots and to objects located coronally in the canal.[79,114] Their use in the middle and apical portions of the root canal may weaken the tooth or result in perforation (Fig. 25-42).[21,114]

Retreatment Techniques

Numerous techniques have been suggested in the literature for retreatment of root canals, and they cannot all be discussed in this chapter. This review focuses on discussion of those techniques that are considered the most practical. They are presented according to the root filling material they are proposed to retreat.

Retreatment of pastes and cements

Soft-setting pastes. Normally soft-setting pastes do not interfere with negotiation of the root canal throughout its entire length with regular endodontic instruments. Therefore, their removal does not require specific techniques. In such cases instrumentation of the root canal with the use of copious irriga-

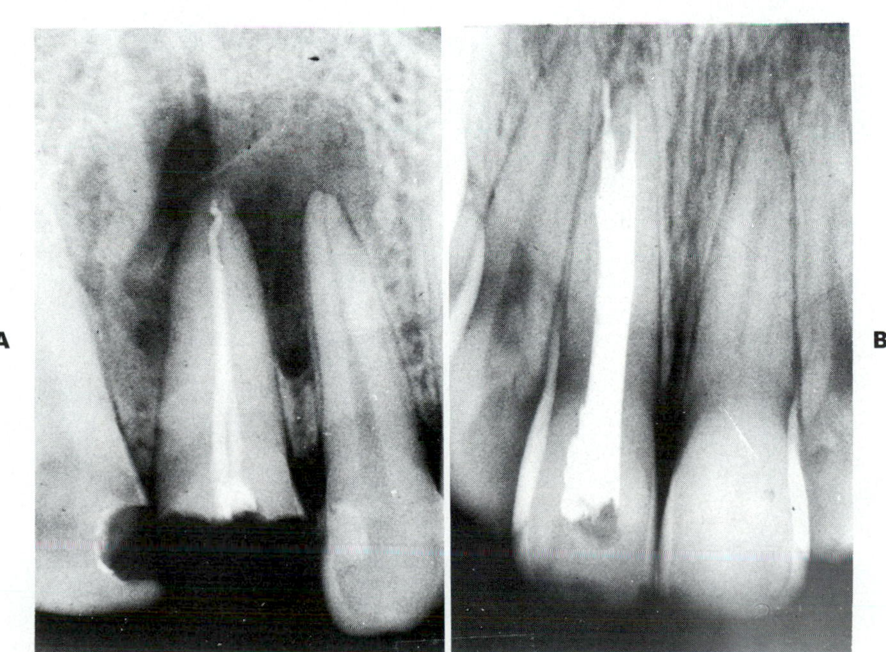

FIG. 25-36 Gutta-percha retreatment planning considering its density. **A,** Attempts should be made to pull out poorly condensed gutta-percha without dissolving it. **B,** Well-condensed gutta-percha mass requires dissolving to facilitate its removal up to the apical portion of the canal. (From Stabholz A, and Friedman S: J Endod 14:607, 1988.)

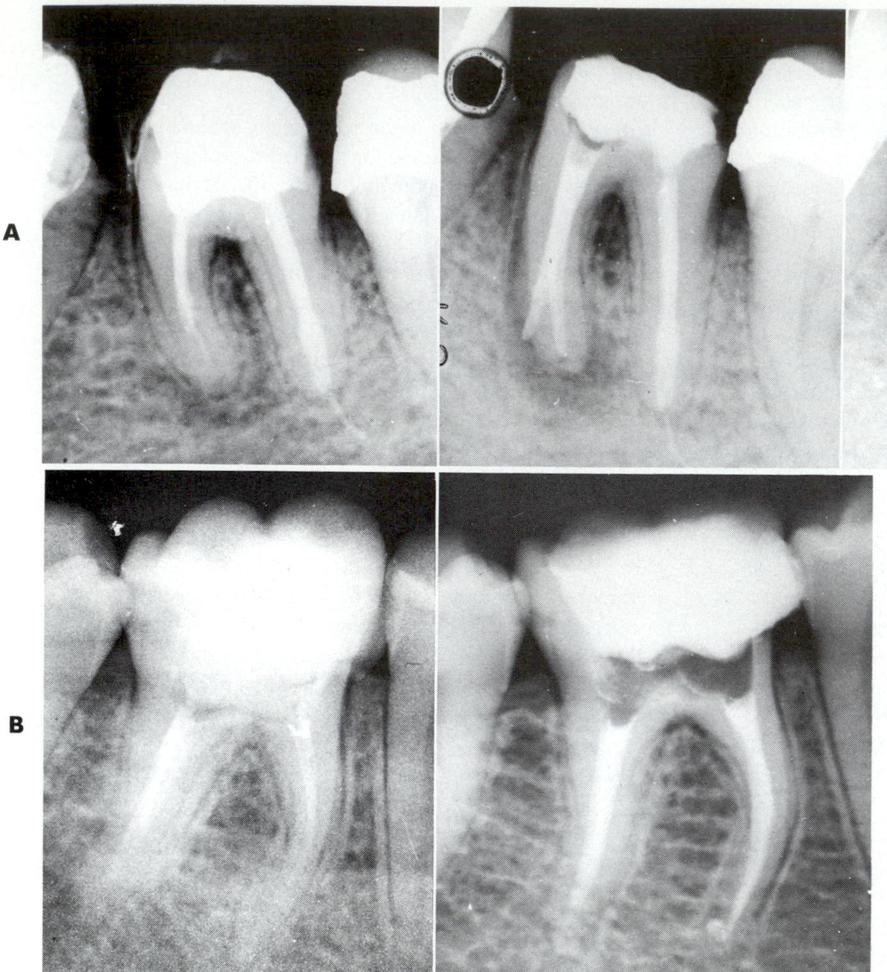

FIG. 25-37 Gutta-percha retreatment planning, including consideration of the root shape. **A,** Retreatment without dissolving the gutta-percha in the mesial canals of the mandibular first molar *(left)* resulted in perforation and treatment failure *(middle)*. Consequently, the untreated apical portion of the canal was retrofilled surgically, and the perforating excess gutta-percha was removed *(right)*. **B,** Satisfactory retreatment of the mandibular first molar with curved mesial canals facilitated by dissolving the gutta-percha. (From Stabholz A, and Friedman S: J Endod 14:607, 1988.)

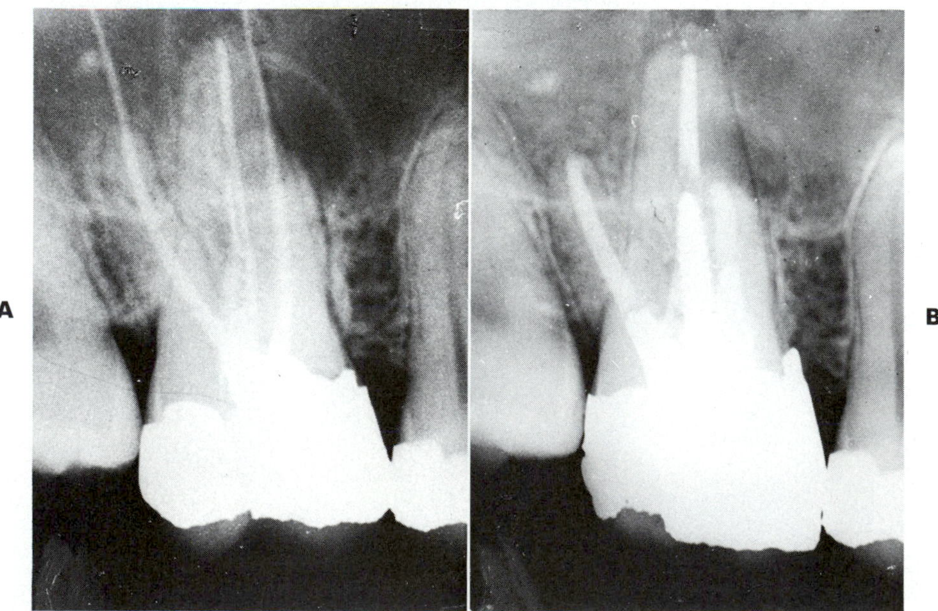

FIG. 25-38 Retreatment of overextended gutta-percha root filling. **A,** Preoperative radiograph of maxillary first molar with considerably overextended gutta-percha in both buccal roots. **B,** Retreatment was completed via the root canals, including removal of the overextended material (follow-up 4 months). The endodontic access cavity was widened to allow ample convenience. (From Stabholz A, and Friedman S: J Endod 14:607, 1988.)

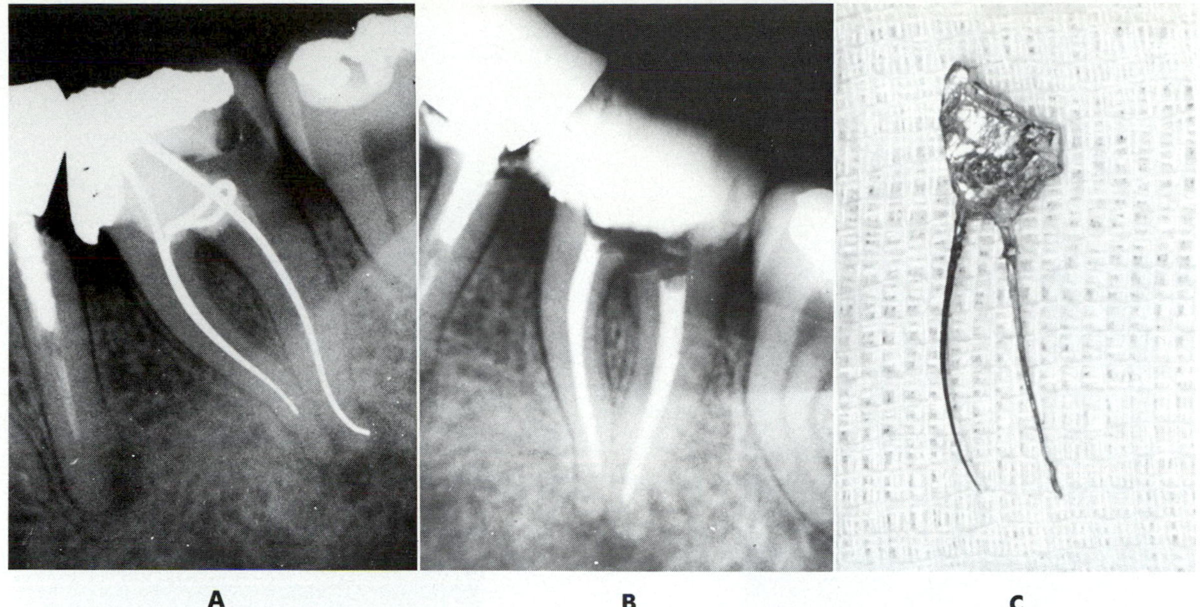

FIG. 25-39 Silver cones extending into the pulp chamber. **A,** Coronal ends of silver cones in the mandibular second molar can be identified in the pulp chamber. **B,** By grasping the coronal ends the operator can pull out the cones to allow retreatment. The coronal ends of silver cones blend with the amalgam core and cannot be isolated. The core may be separated and removed in one piece, **C,** with the possibility of removing the silver cones with it. (From Stabholz A, and Friedman S: J Endod 14:607, 1988.)

tion suffices to remove the paste.[123] However, to some extent, even soft-setting pastes may exert resistance during instrumentation, which may result in an undesired shaping of the canal.[118]

Hard-setting cements. If possible, hard-setting cements should be dissolved.[29,123] When this is not possible, their removal may be attempted by either of the following two techniques.

Dispersion by ultrasonic vibration. Endosonic files are placed in the orifice of the obturated canal and activated with light apical pressure.[44,51,120] The ultrasonic vibration pulverizes the cement, while the continuous irrigation flushes out the dispersed particles. This procedure is gradually continued apically, until the entire obturation is removed. It is time consuming,[44,51] and files may break.[51] In a curved canal the apex may be transported; therefore the pathway of retreatment must be frequently monitored radiographically.[44] Ultrasonic devices with a higher vibration frequency are better suited for this technique.[44]

Drilling with rotary instruments. Hard cements may be drilled out by rotary endodontic instruments, such as Beutelrock or engine reamers, or by burs.[29,123] Drilling in the canal carries a high risk of perforating the root, as drilling depth should be limited.[29] Intermittent radiographic monitoring is mandatory to control the direction of drilling (Fig. 25-43). To allow drilling in the desired direction the convenience form has to be extended. Probing should be attempted frequently to negotiate the canal further apically by regular endodontic instruments.[29] Occasionally this may become possible even before the most apical portion of the paste-filled canal is reached,[29] since voids are often present in paste obturations.[13]

Retreatment of gutta-percha

The coronal portion of gutta-percha obturations should always be drilled out, preferably by means of endodontic drills such as the Gates-Glidden or Peeso. This simple step has a triple advantage[64]: the usually most condensed coronal portion of the obturation is removed quickly, while a reservoir is provided for the solvents that may have to be used next, and an improved convenience form is obtained for negotiating the root canal.[54] To remove the coronal portion of the obturation the use of a hot spreader or heat carrier was also suggested.[29] Although some gutta-percha may be removed in this fashion, creating a limited space for further negotiation and for solvents, no more convenience is provided by this technique. Gutta-percha may be dissolved or removed in its solid form.

Techniques for dissolving gutta-percha. Dissolving avoids the use of excessive force in the negotiating of gutta-percha–obturated canals.[23] Extrusion of solvent into the periapical tissues should be prevented.[29]

Solvents of gutta-percha. Gutta-percha is soluble in chloroform, methylchloroform, carbon disulfide, carbon tetrachloride, benzene, xylene, eucalyptol oil, halothane, and rectified white turpentine.[47,143] The solubility of various brands of gutta-percha varies.[131] There is also a difference in the solvents' dissolving efficiency.[131,140,143]

Chloroform—The most effective and widely used of the solvents, chloroform evaporates rapidly and is therefore a useful chairside material.[74] It is, however, a potential carcinogen.[69,95,117] Although its carcinogenic effect in humans has been questioned[17] and its use in dentistry is not strictly prohibited in most countries,[69] it would appear advisable to refrain from using it. Furthermore, chloroform is toxic and may

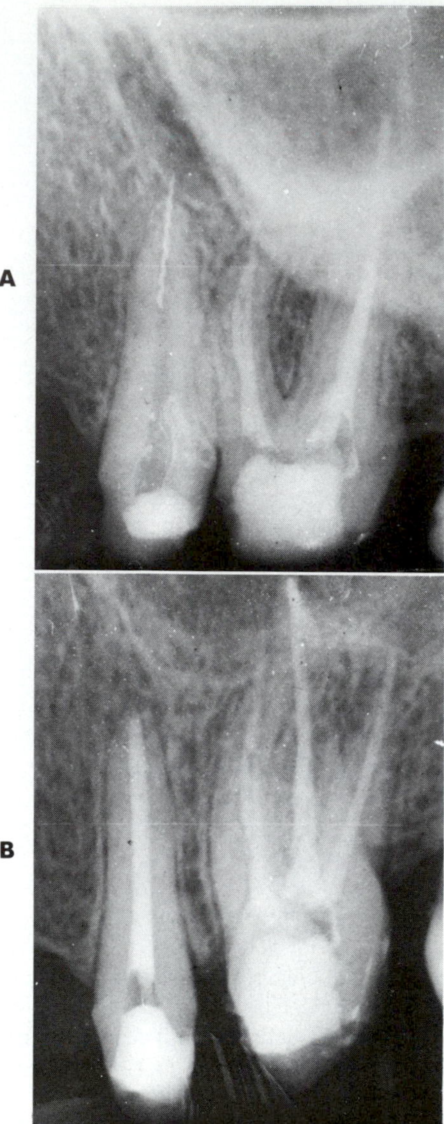

FIG. 25-40 Retreatment of a broken instrument in an oval-shaped canal. **A,** A broken instrument extending through the apical foramen of the maxillary second premolar, the canal of which is usually oval in cross section. **B,** The instrument was bypassed and removed, and retreatment completed. (From Stabholz A, and Friedman S: J Endod 14:607, 1988.)

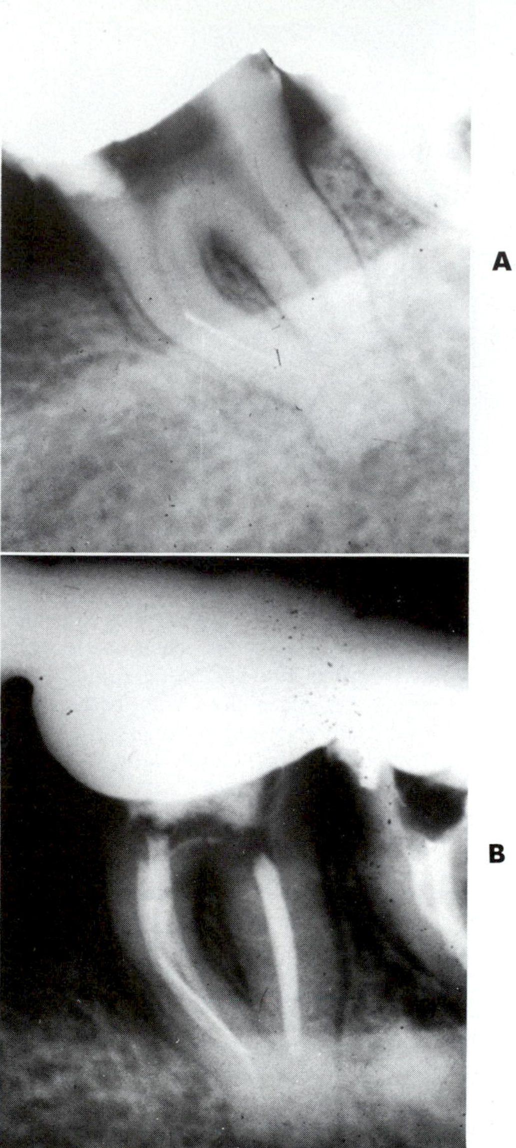

FIG. 25-41 Bypassing a broken file. **A,** No. 20 K-file separated in a mesiobuccal canal of a mandibular second molar. Attempts to grasp the file are unadvisable because of its location and the pronounced root curvature. **B,** The broken file was bypassed and both the mesial canals are obturated successfully while the file remains in the mesiobuccal canal. (From Friedman S, et al: J Endod 16:543, 1990.)

be harmful to the periapical tissues.[83,115,140] It has also been suggested that repeated exposure to chloroform vapors may have adverse health effects for clinicians and staff.[69]

Xylene—Xylene is highly toxic[143] and evaporates too slowly to be used at chairside. However, it has been advocated for dissolution of gutta-percha between treatment sessions, used as an intracanal medication.[131] Its dissolving effect on gutta-percha is considerably poorer than that of chloroform.[131]

Eucalyptol—Eucalyptol is somewhat less irritating than chloroform[77] and is antibacterial.[60,66] However, it is toxic when ingested[85] and is the least effective gutta-percha solvent.[131,140,144] Only when heated is its effectiveness comparable to that of chloroform.[140]

Methyl chloroform—Methyl chloroform was named the best alternative to chloroform for the retreatment of gutta-percha.[140] It is nonflammable, not carcinogenic, and less toxic than chloroform. Its dissolving efficiency is poorer than that of chloroform yet superior to that of xylene and eucalyptol.[140] An industrial solvent, it may have to be tested further before being used clinically.[143]

Halothane—A volatile anaesthetic agent of relatively low toxicity with a long history of medical application, halothane was recently suggested for dissolving gutta-percha.[41,143] It is less effective than chloroform.[41,143] The use of the solvents

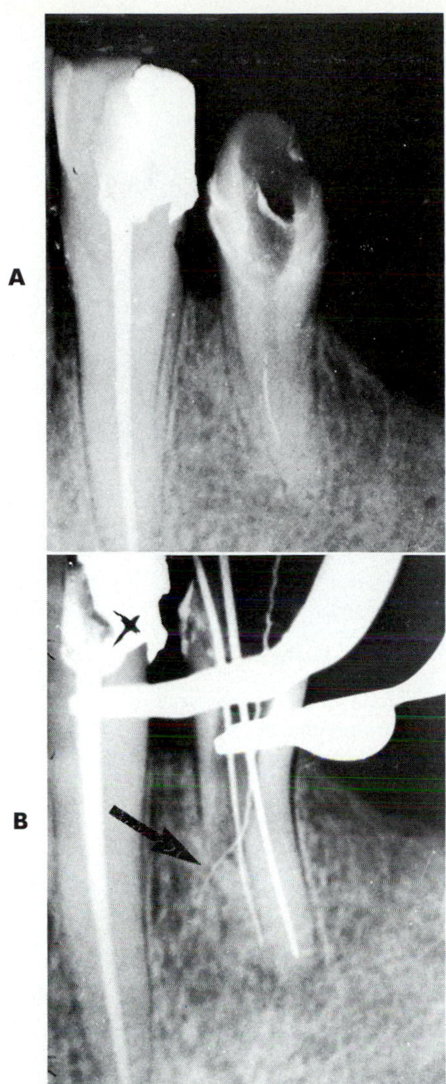

FIG. 25-42 Retreatment of an inaccessible broken instrument. **A,** A broken instrument in the apical half of a thin root in a two-rooted mandibular first premolar. **B,** The use of an extracting device (Masserann Kit) resulted in removal of the instrument, but also in a perforation of the root *(arrow)*. (From Stabholz A, and Friedman S: J Endod 14:607, 1988.)

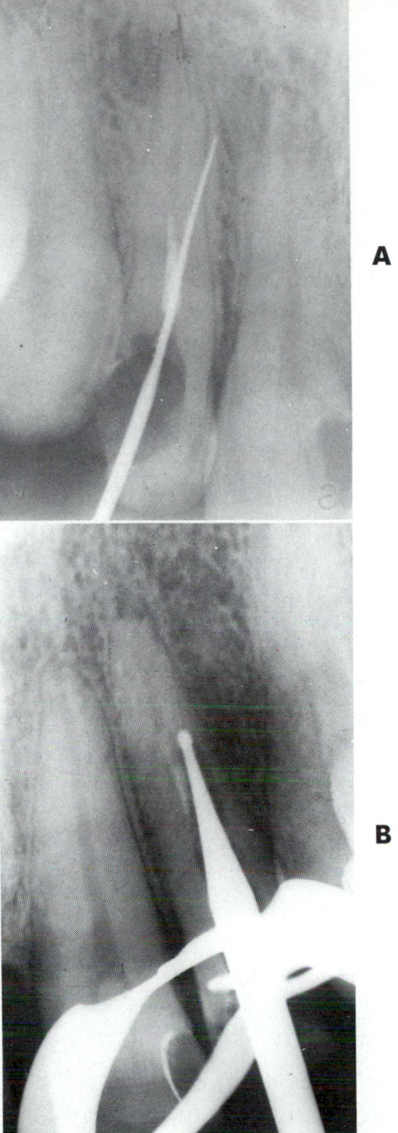

FIG. 25-43 Retreatment of hard cement obturation with rotary instruments. **A,** Use of engine reamer resulted in root perforation. **B,** Radiographic control of the use of a bur. (From Friedman S, et al: J Endod 16:543, 1990.)

has to be supplemented by further means of negotiating the canal and removing the softened material from it. Several techniques have been mentioned for this purpose.

Hand instrumentation. This is the most commonly practiced technique, although it is time consuming and occasionally yields limited results.[142]

Following the introduction of solvent, the canal is negotiated with files or reamers to the desired length. The working length is estimated from the preoperative radiograph and must be confirmed radiographically during instrumentation of the canal.[64] Occasionally this is difficult, since the files are not distinguished clearly enough from the gutta-percha to observe their ends (Fig. 25-44).[23] An aid in this stage may be the use of an electronic apex locator.

Automated instrumentation. The automated handpieces developed for endodontic use do not offer any advantage in the retreatment of gutta-percha. The only notable exception is the reported possibility of bypassing gutta-percha canal obturations with the Canal Finder and chloroform (Fig. 25-45).[23] This technique is fast and safe, and short-filled curved canals may be negotiated beyond the obturation.[23] Thus, a length radiograph may be obtained at an early stage, without the need to first instrument the canal extensively to remove the bulk of material from it (Fig. 25-46).[23] The Canal Finder system also has a built-in apex locator that may be used as an aid in preventing overinstrumentation with this technique.

Ultrasonic instrumentation. Ultrasonic instrumentation following softening with chloroform does not facilitate the removal of gutta-percha from the root canal,[142] even when continuous irrigation with a solvent is used.[141]

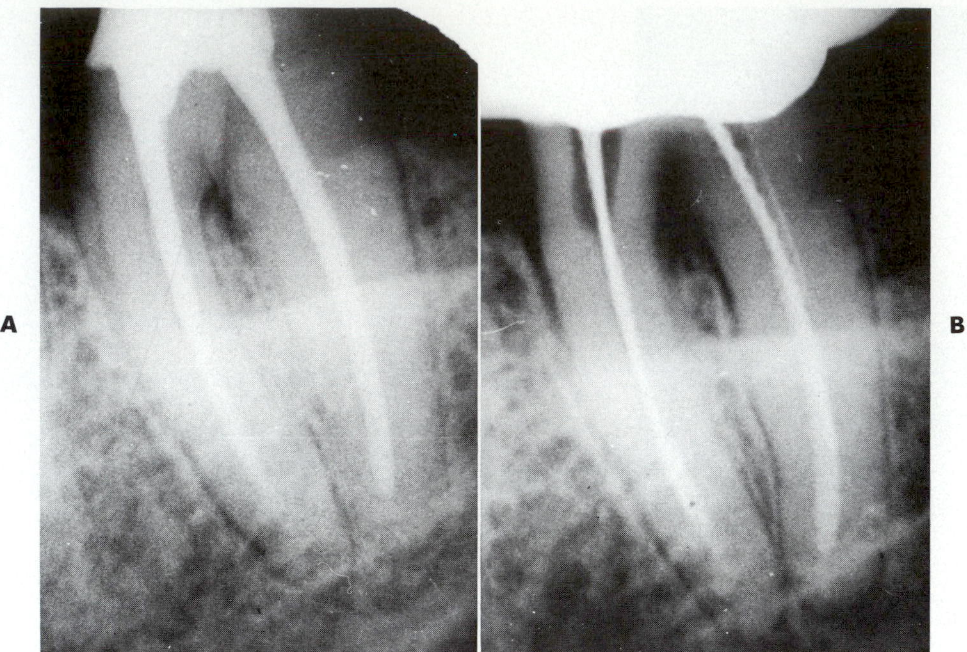

FIG. 25-44 Establishing working length in retreatment of gutta-percha–filled canals. **A,** Preoperative radiograph of mandibular second molar obturated with gutta-percha. **B,** No. 30 files cannot be visualized clearly enough to establish the working length. (From Friedman S, et al: J Endod 15:432, 1989.)

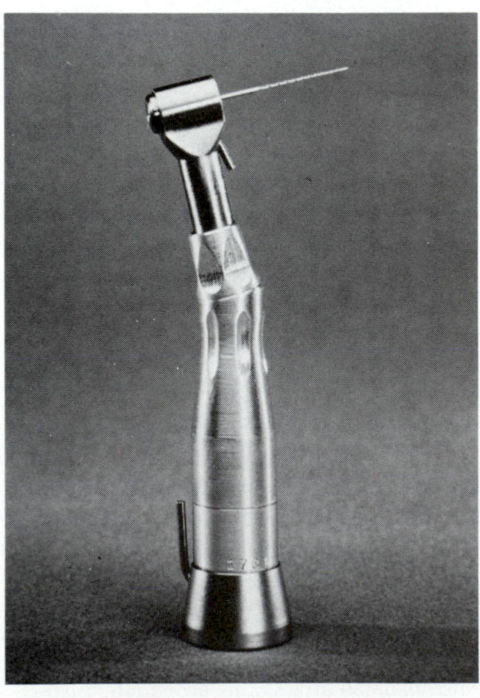

FIG. 25-45 The Canal Finder system offers an advantage in retreatment of gutta-percha, using its pathfinding K-files in combination with chloroform to bypass the root filling in curved, shortly obturated canals.

Solid gutta-percha techniques. Gutta-percha in solid form may be removed from the root canal by means of rotary instruments, or pulled out in one piece by hand instruments (Fig. 25-47).

Pulling out gutta-percha. This is the technique of choice whenever the gutta-percha is poorly condensed.[29] Reamers or K files are used to bypass the obturation,[29] and Hedström files are engaged into the loosely condensed gutta-percha cones, which are then retrieved in one piece by pulling back the instrument (Fig. 25-47). When successful, it is the easiest and fastest means of removing gutta-percha. The files have to be gently threaded into the gutta-percha,[123] so as to prevent pushing it periapically (Fig. 25-48). The same technique is useful in retrieving overextended gutta-percha through the root canal (Fig. 25-48). At times it may become necessary to bypass the gutta-percha with the file beyond the apical foramen to assure that the overextended gutta-percha does not separate at the apex.

Rotary removal of gutta-percha. Removal of gutta-percha with rotary instruments is safe only in straight canals.[118] It may be justified only when the gutta-percha appears to be well condensed and the use of solvents is contraindicated. The fine, flexible Beutelrock reamers should be preferred to engine reamers for this purpose (Fig. 25-47). Such rotary instruments may readily perforate the root; therefore they should be driven slowly into the gutta-percha and advanced freely without being forced in any direction by the operator. These instruments are also fragile, and their incorrect use may result in breakage inside the canal. Another rotary instrument, the GPX, was designed specifically for removing gutta-percha from root canals. Although it is supplied in sizes from No. 25 to larger, this in-

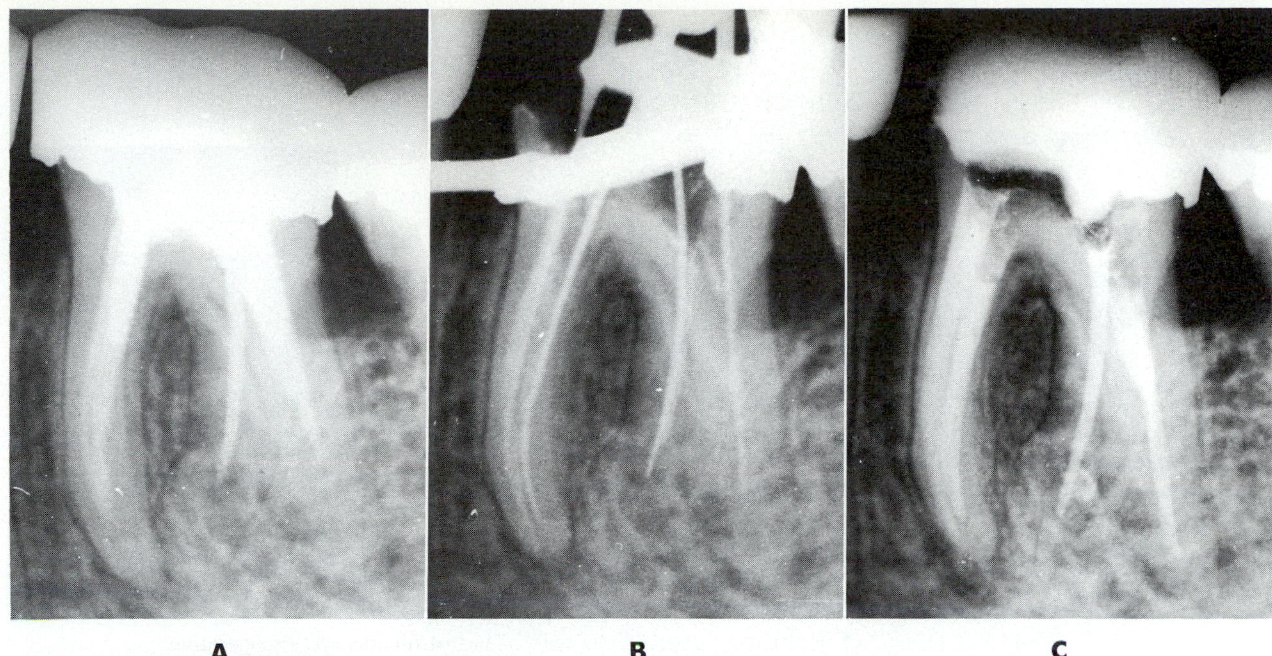

FIG. 25-46 Retreatment of gutta-percha with the Canal Finder. **A,** Preoperative radiograph of mandibular first molar with four curved canals that require retreatment. **B,** All canals were negotiated with Canal Finder K-files and chloroform beyond their obturation level, before most of the gutta-percha was removed and without transportation. The working length may now be established accurately. **C,** Completion of retreatment. (From Friedman S, et al: J Endod 15:432, 1989.)

strument is inflexible, and can not be recommended for use in curved canals.

Retreatment of solid objects

The techniques discussed below are necessary only when a solid object, either a silver point or a fragment of an instrument or post, cannot be easily grasped and pulled out. A readily accessible solid object may be withdrawn from the canal by a variety of instruments, including Stieglitz or Perry pliers,[123,139] a hemostat, a modified Castroviejos needle holder,[20,91] or a Caulfield silver point extractor.[91] Ultrasonic vibration facilitates this technique, particularly if the object is cemented in the canal.[29,52,70] According to one report[40] more than 50% of silver cones may be removed in this fashion.

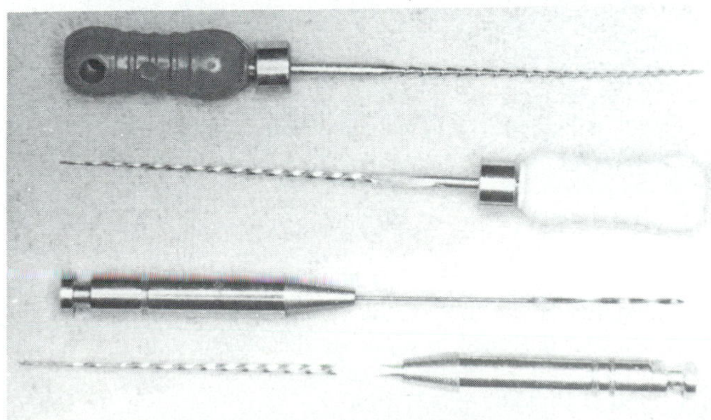

FIG. 25-47 Some of the instruments that may be used in retreatment of solid gutta-percha. *From bottom to top:* Engine reamer, Beutelrock, reamer, Hedström file.

Whenever the object cannot be grasped, attempts should be made to bypass it,[21] to possibly facilitate its removal or allow completion of canal therapy without its removal (Fig. 25-41).[40] Several techniques may be useful in this procedure.

Bypassing with hand instruments. Reamers and files may be used to bypass an obstructing object in the root canal[122] and solvents may be used to soften its cementation.[26,91] Occasionally, friction with the files results in retrieval of the object (Fig. 25-49).[29,52] Multiple Hedström files may be inserted alongside the bypassed instrument and twisted around it so as to provide sufficient grip for its retrieval.[43,91] Normally this is a lengthy procedure. Intermittent irrigation, alternating sodium hypochlorite with hydrogen peroxide or RC-Prep, may float the object coronally through the effervescence they create.[122]

Bypassing with automated and ultrasonic instruments. Silver cones that cannot be bypassed with hand files may be bypassed and subsequently retrieved by the Canal Finder.[40] In difficult cases silver cones and broken instruments may be successfully retrieved by means of ultrasonic instrumentation, combining vibration with copious irrigation.[40,79,114] The relative ease with which this technique is performed suggests that "the use of an ultrasonic scaler in silver cone retreatment cases should be considered a primary method rather than a secondary method."[52] However, as with any use of the endosonic device, file breakage and perforation are possible complications.[79] Furthermore, an object may be pushed apically (Fig. 25-50), occasionally even beyond the apex.[79]

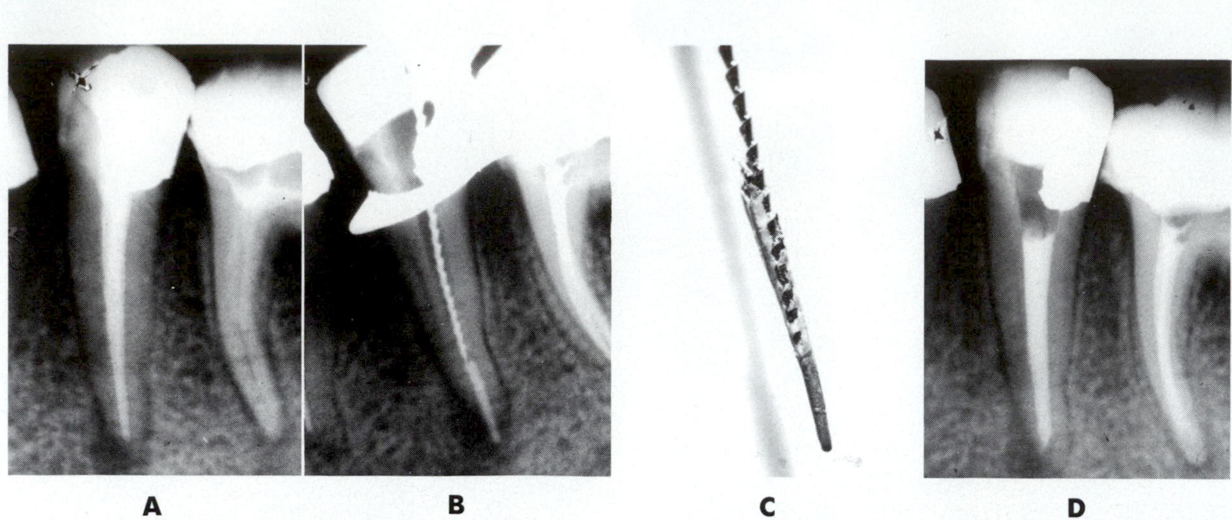

A B C D

FIG. 25-48 Retreatment of undissolved gutta-percha with hand instruments. **A,** Preoperative radiograph of mandibular second premolar in need of retreatment. **B,** Careless use of files resulted in periapical displacement of gutta-percha. **C,** Overextended gutta-percha was retrieved with a Hedström file. **D,** Retreatment completed successfully after removal of all gutta-percha. (From Friedman S, et al: J Endod 16:543, 1990.)

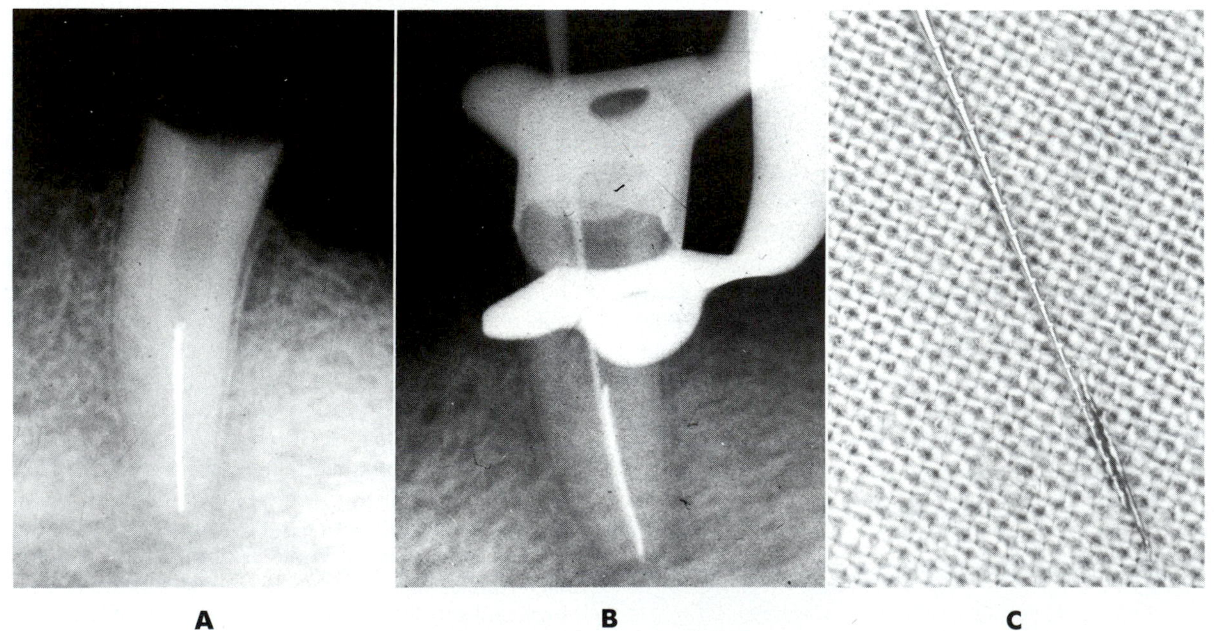

A B C

FIG. 25-49 Bypassing and retrieving a broken file with hand instruments. **A,** Radiograph of mandibular second premolar with broken file obstructing the apical half of the canal. Note the flared access preparation in the coronal aspect of the root designed to facilitate the convenience form. **B,** Bypassing the broken instrument with a K-file. **C,** Retrieval of the broken instrument with a Hedström file. (From Friedman S, et al: J Endod 16:543, 1990.)

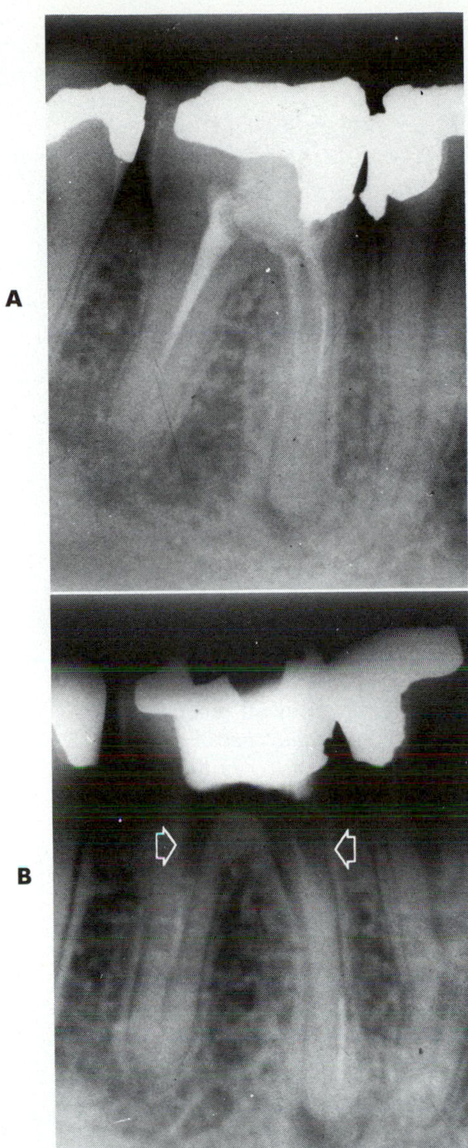

FIG. 25-50 Displacement of a broken file during retreatment. **A,** Preoperative radiograph of mandibular first molar with broken file in the mesiobuccal canal. **B,** Attempts to bypass the file with endosonic instruments resulted in its being pushed apically. Note the coronal flaring of the canals with Gates-Glidden burs *(arrows)* to facilitate a convenient access. (From Friedman S, et al: J Endod 16:543, 1990.)

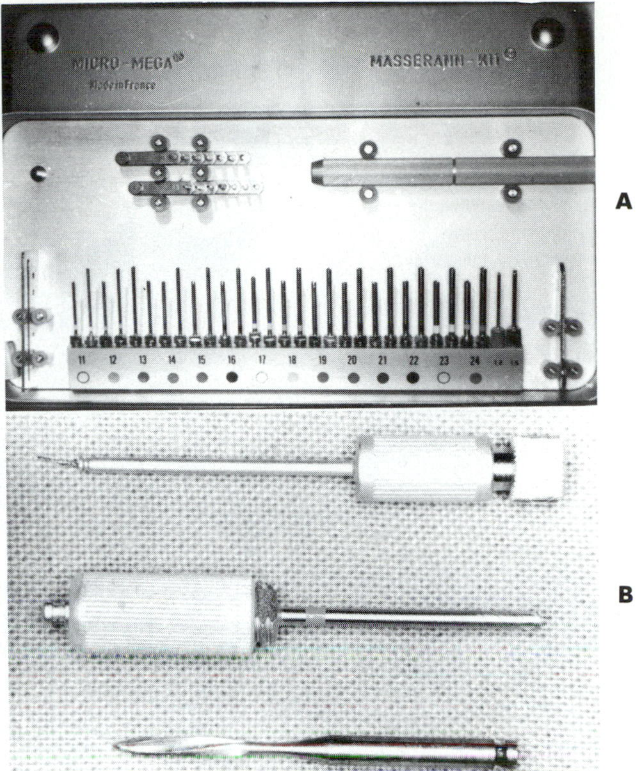

FIG. 25-51 The Masserann Kit is the most comprehensive device for the removal of obstructing objects from root canals, such as files, silver points, or broken posts. **A,** The complete set. **B,** Particular instruments.

Special grasping devices. Numerous devices, ideas, and tricks have been suggested for retrieving foreign objects from root canals. Among these, the Masserann technique[67] has received most attention.

Masserann and alternative extractors. The Masserann kit consists of an extractor into which the object to be retrieved is locked. An assortment of end-cutting trepan burs are used in anticlockwise rotation, to provide access for the extractor (Fig. 25-51).[19,67,101] The trepans are large and rigid and can be used safely only in the coronal portions of large, straight roots.[24,114,138] Frequent radiographic monitoring is mandatory, and ample convenience form must be established so that the desired direction can be maintained toward the target object (Fig. 25-52).[24] Neglect of these precautions, or use of the trepans in curved roots or apical locations, will result in root perforation.[21,26] This technique also requires considerable sacrifice of radicular dentin,[24,138] thus making the tooth more susceptible to fracture (Fig. 25-53).[21,136]

The Masserann technique is significantly more successful in anterior teeth than in posterior teeth,[101] it is time consuming,[101] and, all together, it is believed to be inferior to the ultrasonic technique.[79] The recently introduced Endo Extractor differs from the Masserann only by using a cyanoacrylate adhesive to lock the object into the extractor.[28,116] Therefore, the same precautions and limitations apply to this modality as to the Masserann technique.

Wire loop technique. A thin steel wire is inserted into a 25-gauge hypodermic needle. On the sharp side of the needle a loop is formed, and on its other side the free ends of the wires are pulled to tighten the loop. The needle is placed in the canal so that the loop contacts the broken instrument, then the loop is tightened and the instrument may be retrieved by pulling the needle back. To obtain positive results with this technique the object must be exposed enough to be grasped by the wire loop,[96] and at this stage it probably could be engaged by other extracting systems as well.

By closely adhering to the principles of diagnosis, case selection, access opening, cleaning, shaping, and sealing root canals, the clinician can avoid the anguish of attempting to snatch success from the jaws of endodontic failure.

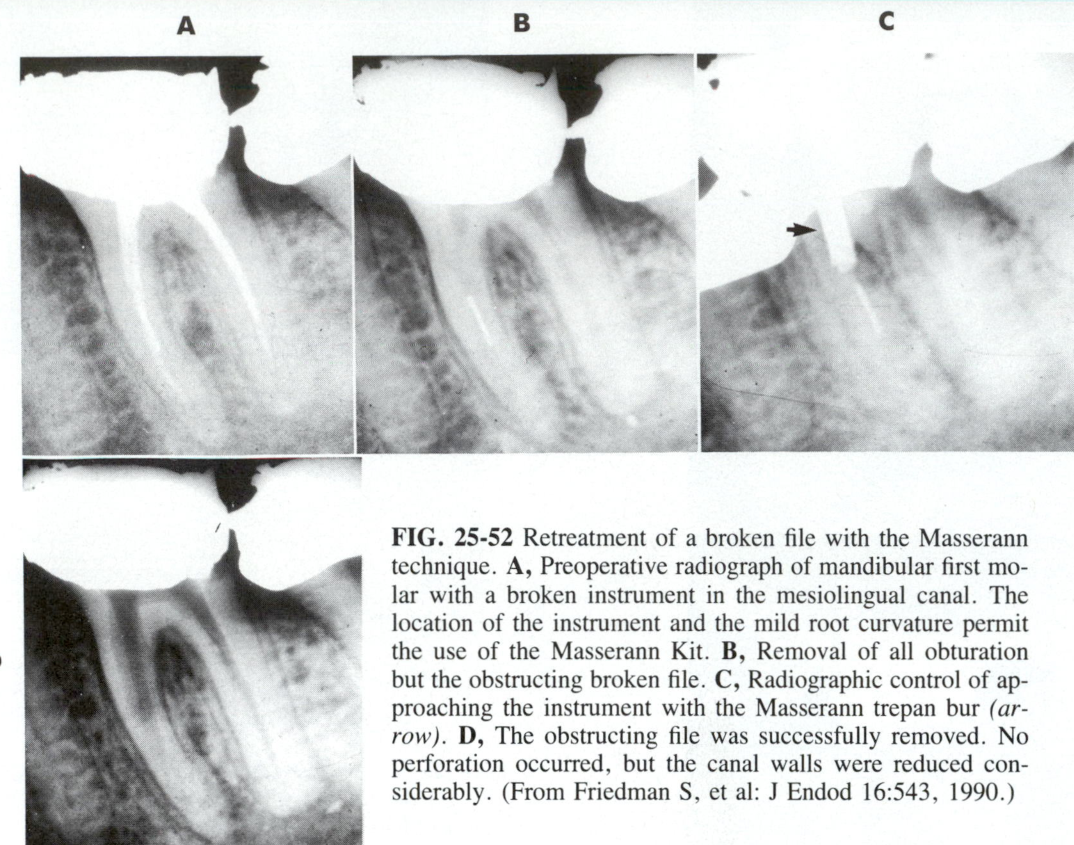

FIG. 25-52 Retreatment of a broken file with the Masserann technique. **A,** Preoperative radiograph of mandibular first molar with a broken instrument in the mesiolingual canal. The location of the instrument and the mild root curvature permit the use of the Masserann Kit. **B,** Removal of all obturation but the obstructing broken file. **C,** Radiographic control of approaching the instrument with the Masserann trepan bur *(arrow)*. **D,** The obstructing file was successfully removed. No perforation occurred, but the canal walls were reduced considerably. (From Friedman S, et al: J Endod 16:543, 1990.)

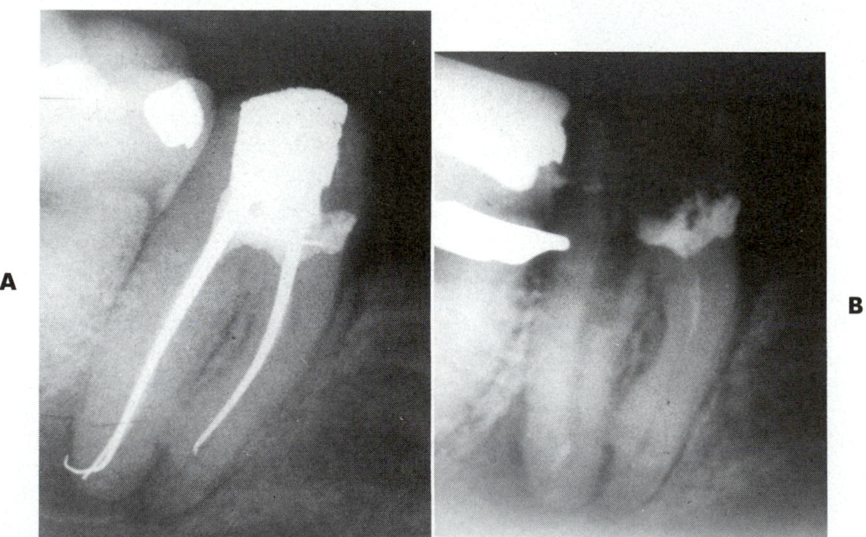

FIG. 25-53 Retreatment of a silver cone with the Masserann technique. **A,** Preoperative radiograph of mandibular second molar obturated with large-size silver cones. The distal root is obturated with two cones, one of which is overextended and twisted around the apex. **B,** The Masserann Kit was used successfully in the distal root to retrieve the silver cones, resulting in a significant sacrifice of dentin in the coronal portion of the root.

REFERENCES

1. Adenubi JO, and Rule DC: Success rate for root fillings in young patients: a retrospective analysis of treated cases, Br Dent J 141:237, 1976.
2. Allen RK, Newton CW, and Brown CE: A statistical analysis of surgical and nonsurgical endodontic retreatment cases, J Endod 15:261, 1989.
3. Angmar-Mansson B, Omnell KA, and Rud J: Root fractures due to corrosion, Odontol Rev 20:245, 1969.
4. Barbakow FH, Cleaton-Jones P, and Friedman D: An evaluation of 566 cases of root canal therapy in general dental practice. II. Postoperative observations, J Endod 6:485, 1980.
5. Bender IB, and Freedlend JB: Adult root fracture, J Am Dent Assoc 107:413, 1983.
6. Bender IB, and Seltzer S: Roentgenographic and direct observation of experimental lesions in bones. I, J Am Dent Assoc 62:152, 1961.
7. Bender IB, Seltzer S, and Freedland J: The relationship of systemic diseases to endodontic failures and treatment procedures, Oral Surg 16:1102, 1963.
8. Bender IB, Seltzer S, and Soltanoff W: Endodontic success: a reappraisal of criteria. I and II, Oral Surg 22:780, 1966.
9. Bender IB, Seltzer S, and Turkenkopf S: To culture or not to culture? Oral Surg 18:527, 1964.
10. Bergenholtz G, et al: Influence of apical overinstrumentation and overfilling on re-treated root canals, J Endod 5:310, 1979.
11. Bergenholtz G, et al: Retreatment of endodontic fillings, Scand J Dent Res 87:217, 1979.
12. Block RM, and Bushel A: Retrograde amalgam procedures for mandibular posterior teeth, J Endod 8:107, 1982.
13. Block RM, Pascon EA, and Langeland K: Paste technique retreatment study: a clinical, histopathologic, and radiographic evaluation of 50 cases, Oral Surg 60:76, 1985.
14. Burell WD, and Goldberg AT: Vented endodontic-access crowns, J Prosthet Dent 32:267, 1974.
15. Cameron CE: The cracked tooth syndrome, J Am Dent Assoc 93:971, 1976.
16. Crump MC: Differential diagnosis in endodontic failure, Dent Clin North Am 23:617, 1979.
17. Davidson IWF, Summer DD, and Parker JC: Chloroform: a review of its metabolism, teratogenic, mutagenic, and carcinogenic potential, Drug Chem Toxicol 5:1, 1982.
18. Davis MS, Joseph SW, and Bucher JF: Periapical and intracanal healing following incomplete root canal fillings in dogs, Oral Surg 31:662, 1971.
19. Feldman G, et al: Retrieving broken endodontic instruments, J Am Dent Assoc 88:588, 1974.
20. Fors UGH, and Berg JO: A method for the removal of broken endodontic instruments from root canals, J Endod 9:156, 1983.
21. Fors UGH, and Berg JO: Endodontic treatment of root canals obstructed by foreign objects, Int Endod J 19:2, 1986.
22. Friedman S, and Stabholz A: Endodontic retreatment: case selection and technique. I. Criteria for case selection, J Endod 12:28, 1986.
23. Friedman S, Rotstein I, and Shar-Lev S: Bypassing gutta-percha root fillings with an automated device, J Endod 15:432, 1989.
24. Friedman S, Stabholz A, and Tamse A: Endodontic retreatment and technique. III. Retreatment techniques, J Endod 16:543, 1990.
25. Frostell G: Clinical significance of the root canal culture. In Grossman LI (ed): Transactions, third international conference on endodontics, Philadelphia, 1963, University of Pennsylvania.
26. Gaffney JL, Lehman JW, and Miles MJ: Expanded use of the ultrasonic scaler, J Endod 7:228, 1981.
27. Gelfand M, Sunderman EJ, and Goldman M: Reliability of radiographical interpretations, J Endod 9:71, 1983.
28. Gettleman BH, et al: Removal of canal obstructions with the Endo Extractor, J Endod 17:608, 1991.
29. Gilbert BO, and Rice RT: Re-treatment in endodontics, Oral Surg 64:333, 1981.
30. Goldman M, Pearson AH, and Darzenta N: Endodontic success: who's reading the radiograph? Oral Surg 33:432, 1972.
31. Grahnen H, and Hansson L: The prognosis of pulp and root canal therapy: a clinical and radiographic follow-up examination, Odontol Revy 12:146, 1961.
32. Grossman LI: Fate of endodontically treated teeth with fractured root canal instruments, J B Endod Soc 2:35, 1968.
33. Grossman LI: Endodontic failures, Dent Clin North Am 16:59, 1972.
34. Grossman LI: Endodontic practice, ed 10, Philadelphia, 1981, Lea & Febiger.
35. Grossman LI (ed): Transactions, First international conference on endodontics, Philadelphia, 1953, University of Pennsylvania.
36. Grossman LI, Shepard LI, and Pearson LA: Roentgenologic and clinical evaluation of endodontically treated teeth, Oral Surg 17:368, 1964.
37. Harty FJ, Parkins BJ, and Wengraf AM: Success rate in root canal therapy: a retrospective study of conventional cases, Br Dent J 70:65, 1970.
38. Helfer AR, Melnick S, and Schilder H: Determination of the moisture content of vital and pulpless teeth, Oral Surg 34:661, 1970.
39. Heling B, and Tamse A: Evaluation of the success of endodontically treated teeth, Oral Surg 30:533, 1970.
40. Hullsman M: The retrieval of silver cones using different techniques, Int Endod J 23:298, 1990.
41. Hunter KR, Doblecki W, and Pelleu GB: Halothane and eucalyptol as alternatives to chloroform for softening gutta-percha, J Endod 17:310, 1991.
42. Ingle JI: A standardized endodontic technique utilizing newly designed instruments and filling materials, Oral Surg 14:83, 1961.
43. Ingle JI: Endodontics, ed 3, Philadelphia, 1985, Lea & Febiger.
44. Jeng HW, and El Deeb ME: Removal of the hard paste fillings from the root canal by ultrasonic instrumentation, J Endod 13:295, 1987.
45. Jokinen MA, et al: Clinical and radiographic study of pulpectomy and root canal therapy, Scand J Dent Res 86:366, 1978.
46. Kaffe I: In Goaz PW, and White SC (eds): Oral radiology, ed 2, Saint Louis, 1987, Times Mirror/Mosby College Publishing.
47. Kaplowitz GJ: Evaluation of gutta-percha solvents, J Endod 16:539, 1990.
48. Kaufman A: Conservative treatment of root perforations using apex locator and thermatic compactor: case study of a new method, J Endod 15:267, 1989.
49. Kerekes K: Radiographic assessment of an endodontic treatment method, J Endod 4:210, 1978.
50. Kerekes K, and Tronstad L: Long-term results of endodontic treatment performed with a standardized technique, J Endod 5:83, 1979.
51. Krell KB, and Neo J: The use of the ultrasonic endodontic instrumentation in the retreatment of a paste-filled endodontic tooth, Oral Surg 60:100, 1985.
52. Krell KV, Fuller MW, and Scott GL: The conservative retrieval of silver cones in difficult cases, J Endod 10:269, 1984.
53. Kuttler Y: Analysis and comparison of root canal–filling techniques, Oral Surg 48:153, 1979.
54. Leeb J: Canal orifice enlargement as related to biomechanical preparation, J Endod 9:463, 1983.
55. Lewis RD, and Block RM: Management of endodontic failures, Oral Surg 66:711, 1988.
56. Lin LM, et al: Clinical, radiographic, and histologic study of endodontic treatment failures, Oral Surg 11:603, 1991.
57. Lin LM, Skribner JE, and Gaengler P: Factors associated with endodontic treatment failures, J Endod 18:625, 1992.
58. Lindauer PA, et al: Vertical root fractures in curved roots under simulated clinical conditions, J Endod 15:345, 1989.
59. Lommel TJ, et al: Alveolar bone loss associated with vertical root fructure, Oral Surg 45:909, 1978.
60. Low D, Rowal BD, and Griffin WJ: Antibacterial activity of essential oils, Planta Med 26:184, 1974.
61. Lutwak L: Symposium on osteoporosis, Am Geriatr Soc 13:115, 1969.

62. Machtou P, Sarfati P, and Cohen AG: Post removal prior to retreatment, J Endod 15:552, 1989.
63. Magura ME, et al: Human saliva coronal microleakage in obturated root canals. An in vitro study, J Endod 17:324, 1991.
64. Mandel E, and Friedman S: Endodontic retreatment: a rational approach to root canal instrumentation, J Endod 18:565, 1992.
65. Mandel E, Machtou P, and Friedman S: Scanning electron microscope observation of canal cleanliness, J Endod 16:279, 1990.
66. Maruzella JC, and Sicurella NA: Antibacterial activity of essential oil vapors, J Am Pharm Assoc 49:692, 1960.
67. Masserann J: Entfernen metallisher Fragmente aus Wurtzelkanalen, J Br Endod Soc 5:55, 1971.
68. Matsumia S, and Kitamura M: Histopathological and histobacteriological studies of the relation between the condition of sterilization of the interior of the root canal and the healing process of periapical tissues in experimentally infected root canal treatment, Bull Tokyo Dent Coll: 1:1, 1960.
69. McDonald MN, and Vire DE: Chloroform in the endodontic operatory, J Endod 18:301, 1992.
70. Meidinger DL, and Kabes BJ: Foreign object removal utilizing the CaviEndo ultrasonic instrument, J Endod 11:301, 1985.
71. Meister F, Lommel TJ, and Gerstein H: Diagnosis and possible causes of vertical root fracture, Oral Surg 49:243, 1980.
72. Meister F, et al: An additional clinical observation in two cases of vertical root fracture, Oral Surg 52:91, 1981.
73. Metzger Z, and Shperling I: Iatrogenic perforation of the roots of restoration-covered teeth, J Endod 7:232, 1981.
74. Metzger Z, Assif O, and Tamse A: Residual chloroform and plasticity in customized gutta-percha master cones, J Endod 14:546, 1988.
75. Moloney LG, Feik SA, and Ellender G: Sealing ability of three materials used to repair lateral root perforations, J Endod 19:59, 1993.
76. Morse DR, et al: A radiographic evaluation of the periapical status of teeth treated by the gutta-percha–eucapercha endodontic method: a one year follow-up study of 458 root canals, Oral Surg 55:607, 1983.
77. Morse DR, et al: A comparative tissue toxicity evaluation of the liquid components of gutta-percha root canal sealers, J Endod 7:545, 1981.
78. Muruzabal M, and Erausquin J: The process of healing following endodontic treatment in the rat molar. In Grossman LI (ed): Transactions, fifth international conference on endodontics, Philadelphia, 1973, University of Pennsylvania.
79. Nagai O, et al: Ultrasonic removal of broken instruments in root canals, Int Endod J 19:298, 1986.
80. Nicholls E: Assessment of the periapical status of pulpless teeth, Br Dent J 114:453, 1963.
81. Oliet S: Single-visit endodontics: a clinical study, J Endod 9:147, 1983.
82. Olsson B, Sliwkowski A, and Langeland K: Intraosseous implantation for biological evaluation of endodontic materials, J Endod 7:253, 1981.
83. Olsson B, and Wennberg A: Early tissue reaction to endodontic filling materials, Endod Dent Traumatol 1:138, 1985.
84. O'Reilly PMR: Management of a vertically fractured endodontically treated tooth, Oral Surg 60:208, 1985.
85. Patel S, and Wiggins J: Eucalyptus poisoning, Arch Dis Child 55:4.05, 1980.
86. Pekruhn RB: The incidence of failure following single-visit endodontic therapy, J Endod 12:68, 1986.
87. Penick EC: Periapical repair by dense fibrous connective tissue following conservative endodontic therapy, Oral Surg 14:239, 1961.
88. Peterson KB: Longitudinal root fracture due to corrosion of an endodontic post, J Can Dent Assoc 37:66, 1971.
89. Petersson K, et al: Endodontic status and suggested treatment in a population requiring substantial dental care, Endod Dent Traumatol 5:153, 1989.
90. Pitts DL, and Natkin E: Diagnosis and treatment of vertical root fracture, J Endod 9:338, 1983.
91. Plack WF, and Vire DE: Retrieval of endodontic silver points, Gen Dent 32:124, 1984.
92. Plant JJ, and Uchin RA: Endodontic failures due to vertical root fractures: two case reports, J Endod 2:53, 1976.
93. Portell FR, et al: The effect of immediate versus delayed dowel space preparation on the integrity of the apical seal, J Endod 8:154, 1982.
94. Reit C, and Grondahl H-G: Endodontic retreatment decision making among a group of general practitioners, Scand J Dent Res 96:112, 1988.
95. Reuber MD: Carcinogenicity of chloroform, Environ Health Perspect 31:171, 1979.
96. Roig-Greene JL: The retrieval of foreign objects from root canals: a simple aid, J Endod 9:394, 1983.
97. Rowe AHR, and Binnie WH: Correlation between radiological and histological inflammatory changes following root canal treatment, J Br Endod Soc 7:57, 1974.
98. Rud J, and Andreasen JO: A study of failures after endodontic surgery by radiographic, histologic and stereomicroscopic methods, Int J Oral Surg 1:311, 1972.
99. Rud J, and Omnell KA: Root fractures due to corrosion, Scand J Dent Res 78:397, 1970.
100. Sails SG, et al: Patterns of indirect fracture in intact and restored human premolar teeth, Endod Dent Traumatol 3:10, 1987.
101. Sano S, Miyake K, and Osada T: A clinical study on the removal of the broken instrument in the root canal using Masserann Kit, Kanagawashigaku 9:50, 1974.
102. Scharwatt BR: The general practitioner and the endodontist, Dent Clin North Am 23:747, 1979.
103. Selden HS: Pulpoperiapical disease: diagnosis and healing: a clinical endodontic study, Oral Surg 37:271, 1974.
104. Seltzer S: Endodontology, ed 2, Philadelphia, 1988, Lea & Febiger.
105. Seltzer S, and Bender IB: Cognitive dissonance in endodontics, Oral Surg 20:505, 1965.
106. Seltzer S, Bender IB, and Turkenkopf S: Factors affecting successful repair after root canal therapy, J Am Dent Assoc 67:651, 1963.
107. Seltzer S, Sinai I, and August D: Periodontal effects of root perforations prior to and during endodontic procedures, J Dent Res 49:332, 1970.
108. Seltzer S, et al: A histological evalution of periapical repair following positive and negative root canal cultures, Oral Surg 17:507, 1964.
109. Seltzer S, et al: Endodontic failures: an analysis based on clinical, roentgenographic, and histologic findings—I and II, Oral Surg 23:500, 1967.
110. Seltzer S, et al: Biological aspects of endodontics. III. Periapical reactions to root canal instrumentation, Oral Surg 26:534, 1968.
111. Seltzer S, et al: A scanning electron examination of silver cones removed from endodontically treated teeth, Oral Surg 33:589, 1972.
112. Sjogren U, et al: Factors affecting the long-term results of endodontic treatment, J Endod 16:498, 1990.
113. Smith JW, Crisp JP, and Torney DL: A survey: controversies in endodontic treatment and re-treatment, J Endod 7:477, 1981.
114. Souyave LCJ, Inglis AT, and Alcalay M: Removal of fractured endodontic instruments using ultrasonics, Br Dent J 159:251, 1985.
115. Spangberg L, and Langeland K: Biologic effects of dental materials. I. Toxicity of root canal–filling materials on Hela cells in vitro, Oral Surg 35:402, 1973.
116. Spriggs K, Gettlemen B, and Messer HH: Evaluation of new method for silver point removal, J Endod 16:335, 1990.
117. Squire RA: Ranking animal carcinogens: a proposed regulatory approach, Science 214:877, 1981.
118. Stabholz A, and Friedman S: Endodontic retreatment: case selection and technique. II. Treatment planning for retreatment, J Endod 14:607, 1988.
119. Stamos DE, and Gutman JL: Revisiting the post puller, J Endod 17:466, 1991.

120. Stamos DE, Stamos DG, and Perkins SK: Retreatodontics and ultrasonics, J Endod 14:39, 1988.
121. Stewart GG: Evaluation of endodontic results, Dent Clin North Am 11:711, 1967.
122. Stewart GG: Chelation and flotation in endodontic practice: an update, J Am Dent Assoc 113:618, 1986.
123. Stock CJR, and Nehammer CF: Negotiation of obstructed canals: bleaching of teeth, Br Dent J 158:457, 1985.
124. Storms JL: Factors that influence the success of endodontic treatment, J Can Dent Assoc 35:83, 1969.
125. Strindberg LZ: The dependence of the results of pulp therapy on certain factors: an analytic study based on radiographic and clinical follow-up examination, Acta Odontol Scand 14(suppl 21), 1956.
126. Swanson K, and Madison S: An evaluation of coronal microleakage in endodontically treated teeth. Part I, Time periods, J Endod 13:56, 1987.
127. Swartz DB, Skidmore AE, and Griffin JA: Twenty years of endodontic success and failure, J Endod 9:198, 1983.
128. Szajkis S, and Tagger M: Periapical healing in spite of incomplete root canal debridement and filling, J Endod 9:203, 1983.
129. Tamse A: Iatrogenic vertical root fractures in endodontically treated teeth, Endod Dent Traumatol 4:190, 1988.
130. Tamse A, Kaffe I, and Fishel D: Zygomatic bone and process interference with correct radiographic diagnosis in maxillary molars, Oral Surg 50:563, 1980.
131. Tamse A, et al: Gutta-percha solvents: a comparative study, J Endod 12:337, 1986.
132. Testori T, Badino M, and Castagnola M: Vertical root fractures in endodontically treated teeth: a clinical survey of 36 cases, J Endod 19:87, 1993.
133. Thoden Van Velzen SK, Duivnvoorden HJ, and Schuurs AHB: Probabilities of success and failure in endodontic treatment: a Bayesian approach, Oral Surg 52:85, 1981.
134. Torabinejad M, Ung B, and Kettering JD: In vitro bacterial penetration of coronally unsealed endodontically treated teeth, J Endod 16:566, 1990.
135. Tronstad L, Barnett F, and Cervone F: Periapical bacterial plaque in teeth refractory to endodontic treatment, Endod Dent Traumatol 6:73, 1990.
136. Trope M, Maltz DO, and Tronstad L: Resistance to fracture of restored endodontically treated teeth, Endod Dent Traumatol 1:108, 1985.
137. Weine FS: Endodontic therapy, ed 3, St Louis, 1982, Mosby–Year Book.
138. Weine SW, and Rice RT: Handling previously treated silver point cases: removal, retreatment, and tooth retention, Compend Contin Educ Dent 7:652, 1986.
139. Weisman MI: The removal of difficult silver cones, J Endod 9:210, 1983.
140. Wennberg A, and Orstavik D: Evaluation of alternatives to chloroform in endodontic practice, Endod Dent Traumatol 5:234, 1989.
141. Wilcox LR: Endodontic retreatment: ultrasonics and chloroform as the final step in reinstrumentation, J Endod 15:125, 1989.
142. Wilcox LR, et al: Endodontic retreatment: evaluation of gutta-percha and sealer removal and canal reinstrumentation, J Endod 13:453, 1987.
143. Wourms DJ, et al: Alternative solvents to chloroform for gutta-percha removal, J Endod 16:539, 1990.
144. Yanchich PP, Hartwell GR, and Portell FR: A comparison of apical seal: chloroform versus eucalyptol-dipped gutta-percha obturation, J Endod 15:257, 1989.
145. Yusuf H: The significance of the presence of foreign material periapically as a cause of failure of root canal treatment, Oral Surg 54:566, 1982.
146. Zakariasen KL, Scott DA, and Jensen JR: Endodontic recall radiographs: how reliable is our interpretation of endodontic success or failure and what factors affect our reliability? Oral Surg 57:343, 1984.
147. Zeldow BJ, and Ingle JI: Correlation of the positive culture to the prognosis of endodontically treated teeth: a clinical study, J Am Dent Assoc 66:9, 1963.

Self-assessment questions

1. Which of the following is not significant in evaluating treatment results?
   a. The extension of filling material.
   b. The location of the treated tooth.
   c. The obturation quality.
   d. The presence of periapical pathosis before treatment.
2. In evaluating treatment results, the consensus on the minimum period of observation was
   a. at least 6 months.
   b. 6 months to a year.
   c. at least 1 year.
   d. at least 2 years.
3. Pitfalls associated with radiographic interpretation of success or failure include
   a. change in angulation.
   b. lack of radiographic changes.
   c. personal bias.
   d. All of the above.
4. Which of the following statements concerning radiographs is true?
   a. Swelling and pain, necessitating incision and drainage, may occur without any radiographic indication.
   b. At least 30% of the bone must be decalcified for a lesion to be evident radiographically.
   c. The size of the lesion on the radiograph is indicative of the actual amount of bone destruction.
   d. Complete denudation of bone over the root apex is always evident radiographically.
5. Underextending the access cavity preparation may lead to
   a. a missed canal.
   b. breakage of endodontic instruments.
   c. discoloration of the crown.
   d. All of the above.
6. Bony lesions that may be associated with vertical root fracture include
   a. a widened periodontal ligament space on one or both sides of the root.
   b. a halo-like lesion around the root apex extending to midroot.
   c. an angular periodontal defect extending apically from the crestal bone.
   d. All of the above.
7. Endodontic retreatment
   a. is as technically challenging as original treatment.
   b. has a poorer prognosis than original treatment.
   c. is performed only on endodontic failures.
   d. has different objectives than primary treatment.
8. Clinically successful cases with radiographically unsatisfactory obturation
   a. should always be retreated.
   b. should be retreated only if a new prosthetic restoration is planned.

c. should be considered for retreatment or follow-up if a new prosthetic restoration is planned.
d. should only be considered for follow-up if no new restoration is planned.

9. Which of the following aspects of the root canal filling is not a factor in determining whether an endodontic failure should be retreated or surgically treated?
a. time since obturation.
b. apical extension of filling material.
c. density of filling material.
d. type of filling material.

10. Removal of existing prosthetic restorations before retreatment
a. is always indicated.
b. permits more radiographic information to be obtained.
c. will not aid in revealing a vertical fracture.
d. All of the above.

11. To remove soft-setting pastes, they should initially be penetrated by
a. sonic instruments.
b. ultrasonic instruments.
c. routine endodontic instruments.
d. solvents.

12. Overextended gutta-percha should be removed
a. by pulling it out in one piece.
b. surgically.
c. with rotary instruments.
d. with solvents.

13. During retreatment the coronal portion of gutta-percha should be
a. dissolved with solvents.
b. drilled out.
c. removed by heat.
d. removed using ultrasonics.

14. Chloroform
a. is the most effective gutta-percha solvent.
b. is prohibited for use in dentistry in most countries.
c. has no adverse effects on clinicians.
d. All of the above.

15. Which solvent, when heated, is as effective as chloroform?
a. Xylene.
b. Methyl chloroform.
c. Halothane.
d. Eucalyptol.

16. The technique of choice for removing poorly condensed gutta-percha is
a. automated instrumentation.
b. hand instrumentation.
c. ultrasonic instrumentation.
d. rotary instrumentation.

17. The Masserann kit technique for removing solid objects
a. is not time consuming.
b. is more successful in posterior teeth than in anterior ones.
c. requires frequent radiograph monitoring.
d. is better than the ultrasonic technique.

PART FOUR

ISSUES IN ENDODONTICS

Chapter 26

Ethics in Endodontics

James T. Rule
Robert M. Veatch

INTRODUCTION

Stephen Cohen

Excellence in clinical endodontic practice involves making both good technical decisions about what treatment is needed and value-based decisions about what course of action serves the individual patient best. Most discussions about what is best for a patient are reduced to the dictum "Do the right thing."

The knowledge and information needed for making good technical decisions are the core of what *Pathways of the Pulp* offers its readers. Because the editors believe that the issues and considerations that inform each individual judgment of what serves the patient best are just as important as good technical decisions, we have invited Dr. James Rule and Dr. Robert Veatch, authors of the superb new text, *Ethical Questions in Dentistry* (Quintessence, 1993), to provide an initial exploration of the ethical content of daily endodontic practice.

Public trust of endodontics and endodontic practitioners is based on our providing the highest quality care for every patient. We conclude *Pathways of the Pulp* with this thought-provoking discussion of ethics as a critically important light that guides us on the pathway to excellence.

OPENING REMARKS

Every day of their professional lives, dentists face decisions that have ethical implications. Most often the issues involve the utilization of complicated diagnostic or technical skills in the delivery of patient care. The way these skills are used is based on the values of both the dentist and the patient. Every recommendation by a dentist and every agreement by a patient has ethical substance, in its potential for patients to be helped or harmed or their wishes and values to be respected or ignored. Sometimes a practitioner's recommendation may conflict with what the patient wants. Sometimes what the patient wants may sound foolish to the dentist. How the dentist responds to these problems and many others determines the character of a dentist's practice.

Some situations occur so often that they may not even be recognized as having ethical content. Other times, the circumstances are complex and the answers are not readily apparent. In both situations a background in philosophical ethics can be helpful in making sound decisions. Unfortunately, while technologic advances and changes in societal perspectives over the last 20 years have increased the ethical challenges inherent in dentistry, dental schools have been relatively slow to respond. Further, although at present 80% of all dental schools offer courses in ethics, the emphasis in many is on jurisprudence.

This does not mean that dentists are not interested in or disturbed about ethical issues. In recent years, published reports have shown concerns about poor quality of care, violations of public trust, flagrant advertising, self-regulation, informed consent, interactions with impaired or incompetent colleagues, financial interactions with patients and insurance companies, and other matters. Dental practitioners have developed a variety of approaches, including the reliance on values instilled during dental school, discussions with colleagues and consideration of the American Dental Association Code of Ethics, and their own personal standards, to resolve these problems. The purpose of this chapter is to provide a brief orientation to a more general approach to ethical reasoning and problem solving using illustrations related to endodontics.

THE NATURE OF ETHICAL PROBLEMS

What constitutes an ethical problem, as opposed to a clinical, scientific, or legal problem? It might appear that some problems are purely clinical or scientific; however, such a view is illusory if by that we mean that clinical or scientific decisions can ever be made without some value judgment. Every clinical, scientific, or legal problem involves an evaluative component. Evaluations can often be identified by the words that are used—*good, bad, right, wrong, should, ought,* or *must*. Sometimes words that are not as conspicuously evaluative nonetheless convey value judgments. Claiming that an effect is a *benefit* or that a treatment is *indicated* conveys such a judgment, as does identifying an effect as a *harm* or a *side effect*. Of course, not all evaluations are moral ones. Some value judgments are esthetic, cultural, or merely matters of personal taste. Certain evaluations, however, are indeed ethical. Most of us can rely on common sense to tell the difference between ethical and other kinds of evaluations. The formal criteria of ethical evaluations are beyond the scope of this presentation. What is critical to know at this point is that all clinical or scientific decisions require evaluations.[15] Decisions are easy when the difference between good and bad is clear cut. In other situations, decisions are more difficult and choices must be made between one good and another or between the lesser of two evils.

Evaluation may become an ethical issue when the dentist realizes that the evaluation involves a trade-off between conflicting values. For example, the dentist may highly value his or her ability to reduce pain using local anesthesia, whereas the patient may fear the side effects of the anesthetic, may object to its duration, or may simply tolerate dental pain. It is clear that there is no definitively correct value judgment here. The value judgment of the dentist and the patient may conflict. The dentist who does what he or she thinks is best for the patient could end up violating the autonomy of the patient.

VALUES IN CLINICAL DENTAL ETHICS

In 1988 Ozar and colleagues[12] published a report that presents seven value categories held by the dental profession and describes how values are important in clinical decision making. The authors also propose a ranking of the values to help clarify the decision-making process when values conflict. The values, in descending order, are as follows: (1) life and health, (2) appropriate and pain-free oral functioning, (3) patient autonomy, (4) preferred practice values, (5) esthetic values, (6) cost, and (7) other external factors.

The very existence of these values, as well as their ranking, is controversial, both within the dental profession and outside it. For example, a certain minute risk of life is taken whenever local anesthesia is used in the name of pain-free dentistry, yet most dentists believe that risk is justified. Others may place patient autonomy above dental health and appropriate functioning. Patients may elevate external (nondental) factors above all the other values listed. Furthermore, according to some ethical systems, any of these values should be subordinated to other ethical concerns that have nothing to do with values at all. For now, however, it will be helpful to summarize one version of a possible list of values.

Life and Health

The sustaining of life and the promotion of overall health is the central concern of all practitioners and patients. Under most circumstances dentists should not undertake treatment that will jeopardize the life or health of patients.

Appropriate and Pain-Free Oral Function

This complex and important value has two broad aspects to it. First, practitioners value actions that are appropriate for such factors as age, health, and home care compliance. These values include the basics of disease prevention and the maintenance of oral health. For a patient who, for reasons of physical limitations, cannot possibly meet normal standards of cooperation, the dentist might conclude it is unethical to begin any treatment whose success depends on patient cooperation.

The second aspect deals with comfort in oral function. Some dentists and patients rank the long-term expected benefits in function over other values. An example can be seen in a patient who is referred to an endodontist for an apicoectomy on a lower first molar that serves as the distal abutment of a bridge but that has extensive bone loss so that only 3 to 4 mm of bone remains. In such a situation the endodontist might consider it unethical to perform the apicoectomy, recommending instead an extraction and the construction of the bridge using the second molar as the abutment, even though the patient might demand that the tooth be saved.

Patient Autonomy

In the context of health care, autonomy refers to the ability of competent patients to make their own health care decisions that reflect their own values and goals. Ozar and co-workers[12] give the example of a patient who refuses further treatment on a tooth and requests that it be extracted. The tooth in question has received several other procedures and now requires endodontic treatment and a crown. The dentist believes the tooth can be saved and disagrees with the patient's choice. In this situation, the tooth is already compromised, and although the dentist disagrees with the extraction, the request is reasonable and can be complied with.

Preferred Practice Values

During their formal education, dentists receive powerful messages about treatment choices. Examples include the restoration of carious teeth rather than extraction (when possible) and the use of direct pulp caps in mechanical exposures rather than more extensive pulp therapy. Preferred practice values rank higher in many dentists' minds than those of cost or esthetics, but according to Ozar's group,[12] they are less important than patient autonomy. In addition, those who agree place high value on patients' being fully aware of alternatives where they exist. And in many situations where the patient chooses a treatment not favored by the dentist, the concept of preferred practice values suggests that the dentist should comply.

Esthetic Values

Dentists recognize that facial and intraoral appearance are important to patients, and they routinely consider esthetic factors in their treatment recommendations. On the other hand, dentists are not likely to place their concern for esthetics over considerations of pain-free oral functioning in the event of incompatibility between the two.

Cost

Ordinarily one thinks of cost as being mainly the patient's concern, but it can influence the recommendations of the dentist as well. Dentists may fail to recommend certain treatments because they know, or at least believe, that the patient will be unable to afford it. However, dentists usually consider cost as a lower-ranking value in their recommendations to patients. An example is an endodontist who is asked to retreat a maxillary first molar because an abscess of a second mesialbuccal canal was missed during the first treatment. On the basis of expected long-term success, the endodontist may recommend nonsurgical endodontic therapy rather than an apicoectomy, even though the retreatment would be more costly if it also involved replacing an existing porcelain-fused-to-metal crown.

External Factors

Considerations that are not purely dental ones often enter in to the dentist's decision-making process. This broad category includes social and cultural influences, public welfare, factors of social justice, and even the dentist's own personal responsibilities. Ozar's group[12] recognize that certain external factors may take precedence in the hierarchy and at times may be more important than, for example, cost or esthetic factors.

The role of values in ethical decisions in dentistry is a complicated and controversial issue. In order to be clear on their role and to understand more systematic alternatives to approaching ethical decision making, we need to examine some of the basics of ethical principles.

ETHICAL PRINCIPLES

Over the last two decades, principles such as autonomy, nonmaleficence, beneficence, and justice have been accepted as basic principles.[2,11,16] Briefly stated, these principles require that all actions (including those by health care providers) demonstrate

Regard for self-determination (respect for autonomy)
Avoidance of doing harm (nonmaleficence)
Promotion of well-being (beneficence)
Fairness in the distribution of goods and harms (justice).

Other principles are sometimes included with these, including veracity, fidelity, avoidance of killing, and perhaps privacy and confidentiality.[4] Some of these are combined, or one may be treated as derivative of another. Autonomy, veracity, and fidelity may be combined into the principle of respect for persons. Confidentiality may be derived from the general principle of fidelity.

Autonomy

The moral principle of autonomy provides the underpinning for broad concepts such as the right to privacy, freedom of choice, and the acceptance of responsibility for one's actions.[2,11,16] It is the moral principle that supports one's freedom to think, judge, and act independently, without undue influence. Although the notion of autonomy grew out of the Western idea of political self-rule, in medical ethics it gives rise to a duty to permit individuals to make informed decisions about factors affecting their health. Issues of autonomy, especially as they pertain to questions of informed consent, are at the heart of many ethical dilemmas that occur in dentistry. In dentistry, a patient who values the preservation of her teeth may be deprived of that opportunity if her dentist assumes she will want an abscessed tooth removed because he believes she cannot afford endodontic treatment.

The principle of autonomy sometimes conflicts with other principles, as in a situation where a dentist's conviction that the patient is better off saving teeth is in opposition to a patient's adamant wishes to have extractions and dentures. The management of such conflicts is a source of controversy. Some view autonomy as the highest-ranking principle, one that must remain inviolate. Many people, however, recognize that autonomy must be limited, at least in some cases in which autonomous action will do harm to others. More controversial are cases, such as the one mentioned above, in which acting autonomously upsets others or offends their moral standards. The patient's preference for dentures conflicts with the standards of the dentist.

The resolution of these conflicts depends on one's understanding of the priority of the principles. Some people hold that autonomy has equal priority with the principles of beneficence, nonmaleficence, justice, and the others.[3] In this view one can make a moral choice only after assessing the implications of all the relevant principles. Others give autonomy an absolute priority over beneficence when only the welfare of the autonomous actor is at stake while recognizing the need to balance autonomy when the rights or welfare of others is affected.[16]

Nonmaleficence

The principle of nonmaleficence holds that an action is wrong insofar as it inflicts harm on others. This principle is commonly thought to be a cornerstone of the Hippocratic Oath, appearing as the admonition, "Above all, do no harm."[7] However, the Hippocratic Oath itself, though it states that the physician should benefit the sick and protect them from harm, does not give supremacy to nonmaleficence. Issues of nonmaleficence abound in dentistry, as in all professions. A general dentist with limited endodontic skills considers doing a molar root canal himself rather than referring to an endodontist. An oral surgeon wonders about referring a small (probable) squamous cell carcinoma of the skin to a plastic surgeon or doing the biopsy himself.

Beneficence

Beneficence is the principle that actions are moral insofar as they enhance welfare.[11] It is interwoven with nonmaleficence in a continuum that extends from doing no harm to the prevention and removal of harm and the doing of good.[8] Despite the connection between these concepts, there is an important difference between them in the nature of the action required. In most instances nonmaleficence requires only restraint from harmful acts. An example is the restraint from recommending esthetic bonding when it is obvious that the patient does not believe there is an esthetic problem.[9] Beneficence, on the other hand, is more likely to require positive, definitive action, which places certain demands on the time or other resources of the individual.

Most ethical theories would consider beneficence an obligation that may be overridden by other, more compelling considerations. In fact, some approaches to the problem of conflict among ethical principles so radically subordinate beneficence that it would never be justified to violate someone's autonomy simply to do him good.

In medicine and dentistry beneficence has traditionally been considered the cornerstone on which the profession functions.[14] Its central role is generally affirmed by professional codes of ethics from the Hippocratic Oath to the Principles of Ethics of the American Dental Association.

As clinicians consider the expression of beneficence to their patients, it is obvious that the process involves the balancing of benefits against harms. This situation occurs when, in the process of providing benefit, it is necessary to inflict harms to a greater or lesser degree. An example is the consideration of an apicoectomy for the treatment of a mandibular premolar where there is a risk of permanent paresthesia. Sometimes the balancing process is very difficult, as when mandibular resection is being considered in the presence of the malignant ameloblastoma.

Justice

The principle of justice has to do with three closely related ideas: (1) treating people fairly, (2) giving people what they deserve, and (3) giving people that to which they are entitled.[2] Since these ideas are subject to broad interpretations, the concept of justice is extremely complex and controversial. With respect to the dispensing of scarce dental health care resources, should people get dental care because they need it, because they want it, because they are handicapped, because they are employed (or unemployed), because they can afford it, or for other reasons?

The preceding discussion shows the major role that justice has in discussions of public policy. The principles of beneficence, nonmaleficence, and respect for autonomy also figure in these discussions. How these principles relate to the principle of justice depends on one's strategy for resolving conflict among principles. One approach would be to balance the competing claims. Another would be to attempt to order the principles in some fashion. Still another one is to balance autonomy and justice but to rank them both over beneficence and nonmaleficence.[16]

Similarly, justice, though particularly relevant in public policy discussions, also plays an important role in decisions that must be made in the dental practitioner's office. Is a patient who is not in your practice entitled to emergency care (especially in the middle of the night)? Should second-rate treatment be instituted when full fees cannot be afforded? Should you accept a request to provide limited free endodontic services to a nursing home just when your practice is getting busy?

Other Ethical Principles

These four principles—autonomy, nonmaleficence, beneficence, and justice—together have received predominant attention in contemporary health care ethics. Other principles, however, are included in many medical ethical theories and often prove decisive in ethical issues faced by dentists. Particularly important for ethical considerations in dentistry are the principles of veracity and fidelity.

Veracity

One characteristic of actions, rules, and practices that are judged *right* is that they involve telling the truth and not telling lies. The Hippocratic tradition used to judge truth telling to patients based on considerations of whether the truth would help or hurt the patient, but since 1980 the American Medical Association has been committed to dealing honestly with patients, without regard to whether honesty also produces benefit and avoids harm.[1]

Fidelity

Another aspect sometimes subsumed under the rubric of respect for persons is fidelity. This is the belief that it is morally right to keep promises, both implicit and explicit. Fidelity may be the source of duties of health professionals to their patients. Additionally, fidelity is believed by some to be the foundation of the duty of confidentiality. According to them, health professionals make a promise to patients to keep certain information confidential. Breaking confidence is really breaking faith. Of course, much hinges on exactly what is promised, and that discussion is, unfortunately, beyond the scope of this presentation.

ETHICAL DECISION MAKING

In approaching the analysis of ethical issues, we suggest that better ethical decisions will occur if an established method of analysis is used. An orderly approach to decision making allows us to take into consideration variations and conflicting views that may exist among personal values, conscience, religious convictions, professional codes of ethics, legal constraints, and the viewpoints of patients. A four-step approach to ethical decision making in dentistry is presented below.

Protocol for Ethical Decision Making[10,13]

As you consider the dilemma that you face, you must first make sure that the resolution of the issues actually depends on ethical considerations. Sometimes what appears to be an ethical dispute really hinges on disagreements or misunderstandings of the facts of the case. You should determine that there is clarity and agreement on all of the relevant facts. Once that is accomplished, these four steps should be followed.

Step 1: Naming the alternatives

List the possible alternatives. Keep in mind the possible consequences—to the patient, yourself, and others. This will be dealt with further in step 4. Include all aspects of the circumstances in your considerations, including dental, medical, social, and psychological. At this stage include all options that are possibilities, even those that seem immoral, as long as they could be plausible to the patient or to some health professional. There will always be some options that are beyond reason for everyone considering the alternatives. Eliminating these from consideration already constitutes a moral judgment. In order to keep such judgments to a minimum at this point, include all options that any relevant decision maker considers plausible.

Step 2: Identifying the ethical considerations

Consider the ethical implications of each alternative. Identify the ethical principles involved and determine the role of beneficence, nonmaleficence, respect for autonomy, justice, and other principles. Once you have determined the role of beneficence and nonmaleficence, you may also want to determine the greatest balance of good over harm.

Step 3: Weighing the considered judgments of others

After you have begun applying the principles to the alternatives, as a guide to your deliberations and a check against your own judgment, consider what your professional group believes to be ethical in this situation. Its view may or may not be morally correct, but it at least tells you what your colleagues have concluded in similar situations. You may also wish to consider the statements of codes of dental ethics from other countries or the codes of other health professions on similar topics, as well as the views of other organizations—religious, civic, political, social—that might have ethical views relevant to the question at hand.

Moreover, if as part of becoming a professional or a member of these other groups you have made certain morally binding commitments, keep in mind that those commitments must be evaluated in the context of the principle of fidelity and its implication that it is right-making to keep such commitments. Thus, the promises you have made in the process of assuming certain roles may be relevant to deciding what ought ethically to be done.

Step 4: Ranking alternatives

Sometimes the process of working through steps 2 and 3 establishes that one of your alternatives satisfies the ethical requirements of the case better than all the others. Often, however, your analysis will show that various principles, rules, or values (and the courses of action that follow from them) are in conflict. In these situations additional analysis is sometimes required. One approach would be to determine your general position about conflict among principles and to apply it to the specific case. For example, some people attempt to rank certain principles as precedent over others. Other people simply consider all principles equally weighty and attempt to make an intuitive judgment on how to resolve conflict. Others prefer to reason by analogy from cases for which moral judgments are clear. On the basis of such analysis, select the course of action that best resolves the conflicts.

CASE STUDIES

Dentists who manage endodontic problems confront a variety of ethical dilemmas. Sometimes the issues involve questions about interactions with patients; often they involve problems with colleagues. The following two cases illustrate both situations.

A Marginal Need for Treatment[5]

Dr. Virginia Seyler was treating a 39-year-old woman who had been referred by her general dentist for endodontic treatment of a painful lower left third molar. Dr. Seyler felt the problem would be readily managed despite some problems in access. The patient did not like the idea of losing any of her teeth and had accepted her dentist's recommendations for endodontics without hesitation.

Dr. Seyler, on the other hand, thought the patient would be better off if the lower third molar were extracted rather than treated endodontically. Its mesial marginal ridge was in occlusal contact with only the distal marginal ridge of the upper second molar. Otherwise no other occlusal contact existed between those teeth. The lower third molar was virtually useless from a functional standpoint. All in all Dr. Seyler thought that the treatment was not worth the cost and discomfort to the patient.

Dr. Seyler wondered what she should tell her patient, who clearly seemed to want the endodontic treatment. Additionally, Dr. Seyler was reluctant to suggest that the tooth be extracted because she did not want to offend the general dentist who had been a steady source of referrals for a long time.

A Communication Problem[6]

Dr. John Knowles was an endodontist who was seeing a 35-year-old man referred by a general dentist for the treatment of a mandibular first molar. The tooth had a 3 by 4 mm radiolucency at the apex of its mesial root. However, there also was vertical periodontal bone loss along the mesiobuccal aspect of the mesial root deep enough to communicate with the periapical lesion and to complicate the treatment significantly. To make matters worse, there was generalized vertical bone loss throughout the mouth.

Dr. Knowles knew that the patient had been seeing the referring dentist for almost 20 years, yet the periodontal situation was in an inexcusable state. He felt the patient needed to know about his condition, but he did not want to ruin the patient's relationship with his dentist. Another problem was that the dentist was a regular source of referrals, and he did not want to jeopardize that relationship.

Discussion

Both Dr. Seyler and Dr. Knowles are faced with decisions about what to tell their patient and how to handle the problem with the referring dentist. Their situations are similar in that they both are in the awkward position of disagreeing with their patient's dentist. However, the cases differ greatly in the nature of the disagreement. Dr. Seyler thinks the referring dentist made only an error of judgment. In her opinion, the proposed treatment is functionally unnecessary and the patient would be better off having the tooth extracted. On the other hand, she recognizes that a case can be made for the endodontics (and the subsequent necessary crown) if the patient either fears extraction or values the retention of teeth, despite the inconvenience and increased cost of treatment.

In Dr. Knowles' case, he is concerned about incompetence. He sees problems on two counts, neither of which is known to the patient. One is the recommendation for endodontics on a tooth that also needs significant periodontal treatment; the other is the patient's long-standing generalized periodontal condition.

Taking into account the difference in the nature of the problems between the two cases, consider first what the endodontists ought to tell their patients. What would the patients want to know about their condition? If the patients would want a complete and frank appraisal, could this knowledge complicate the relationships either between the patient and his or her referring dentist or between the endodontists and their referral sources? If frank disclosure was judged to be helpful to the patient but potentially damaging to the relationships the endodontists have with their referral sources, what are the ethical considerations in deciding what to do? Another issue brought up in Dr. Knowles' case is the scope of responsibility that an endodontist has for the general well-being of the patient. Should Dr. Knowles inform his patient of the generalized periodontal condition, even though it has nothing to do with the reasons for which the patient was referred?

Besides the interactions with their patients, the endodontists also need to consider how they should handle their problems with the referring dentists. Should the endodontists communicate with their referral sources about their concerns? It seems plausible that the difference of opinion that Dr. Seyler has with her colleague could be handled without difficulty. But what about Dr. Knowles? Is it best for the general dentist to know about Dr. Knowles' concerns even if that disclosure were to jeopardize a source of patient referrals? Are there approaches that Dr. Knowles could take that would allow his concerns to be expressed without running the risk of losing his referral source?

REFERENCES

1. American Medical Association: Code of medical ethics: current opinions of the council on ethical and judicial affairs of the American Medical Association, Chicago, Ill, 1992, American Medical Association.
2. Beauchamp TL, and Childress JF: Principles of biomedical ethics, ed 3, New York, 1989, Oxford University Press.
3. Brody B: Life and death decision making, New York, 1988, Oxford University Press.
4. Childress JF: The normative principles of medical ethics. In Veatch RM (ed): Medical ethics, Boston, Mass, 1989, Jones & Harcourt.
5. Cohen S: Personal communication, 1993.
6. Cohen S, and Jones OJ: Personal communication, 1993.
7. Edelstein L, et al (eds): Ancient medicine: selected papers of Ludwig Edelstein, Baltimore, Md, 1967, Johns Hopkins University Press.
8. Frankena WK: Ethics, ed 2, Englewood Cliffs, NJ, 1963, Prentice-Hall.
9. Gilbert JA: Ethics and esthetics, J Am Dent Assoc 117:490, 1988.
10. McCullough L: Ethical issues in dentistry. In Hardin JF (ed): Clark's clinical dentistry, Philadelphia, 1988, JB Lippincott Co.
11. National Commission for the Protection of Human Subjects of Biomedical and Behavioral Research. The Belmont report: ethical principles and guidelines for the protection of human subjects of research, Washington, DC, 1978, US Government Printing Office.
12. Ozar DT, et al: Value categories in clinical dental ethics, J Am Dent Assoc 116:365, 1988.
13. Ozar DT: Model for ethical decision making. Informal distribution through PEDNET, 1989.
14. Pellegrino ED, and Thomasma DC: For the patient's good, New York, 1988, Oxford University Press.
15. Veatch RM: Case studies in medical ethics, Cambridge, Mass, 1977, Harvard University Press.
16. Veatch RM: A theory of medical ethics, New York, 1981, Basic Books.

Answers to Self-Assessment Questions

Daniel B. Green
H. Robert Steiman
Richard E. Walton

Chaper 1: Diagnostic Procedures

1a	6c	11a
2b	7b	12d
3b	8b	13b
4b	9b	14c
5d	10d	

Chapter 2: Orofacial Dental Pain Emergencies

1c	6b	11c
2b	7c	12c
3c	8a	13c
4b	9b	14c
5c	10c	

Chapter 3: Nonodontogenic Facial Pain and Endodontics

1d	6d
2c	7c
3d	8d
4c	9c
5b	10c

Chapter 4: Case Selection and Treatment Planning

1a	6b	11d
2b	7c	12c
3b	8a	13c
4c	9c	14d
5a	10c	15a

Chapter 5: Preparation for Treatment

1d	6c	11a
2b	7b	12c
3b	8c	13d
4c	9d	
5b	10c	

Chapter 6: Armamentarium and Sterilization

1b	6a
2b	7b
3a	8b
4d	9b
5c	10c

Chapter 7: Tooth Morphology and Access Openings

1b	6b	11a
2d	7b	12c
3c	8c	13d
4c	9c	14b
5a	10b	

Chapter 8: Cleaning and Shaping the Root Canal System

1c	6c	11b	16b
2c	7b	12c	17c
3d	8d	13d	18a
4a	9c	14b	
5b	10b	15c	

Chapter 9: Obturation of the Root Canal System

1a 6a
2c 7c
3d
4b
5c

Chapter 10: Records and Legal Responsibilities

1d 6a
2b 7a
3c 8b
4d 9d
5b

Chapter 11: Pulp Development, Structure, and Function

1c 6d 11a 16a 21c
2c 7c 12d 17a
3b 8d 13d 18d
4a 9b 14d 19d
5b 10d 15c 20d

Chapter 12: Periapical Pathology

1d 6c 11d 16d
2c 7a 12c
3d 8b 13a
4b 9a 14d
5c 10a 15b

Chapter 13: Microbiology and Immunology

1c 6c 11c 16d
2b 7b 12b 17d
3b 8c 13a
4b 9c 14a
5b 10a 15d

Chapter 14: Instruments, Materials, and Devices

1b 6d 11c 16d
2a 7a 12d
3c 8a 13a
4b 9a 14c
5d 10a 15c

Chapter 15: Pulpal Reaction to Caries and Dental Procedures

1d 6d 11a 16a
2c 7c 12a 17d
3d 8b 13b 18b
4c 9a 14d 19d
5a 10d 15c 20b

Chapter 16: Traumatic Injuries

1c 6b 11a 16d 21d
2a 7b 12d 17c 22a
3c 8b 13c 18d 23a
4c 9a 14c 19a
5c 10d 15d 20a

Chapter 17: Root Resorption

1a 6a 11a 16c
2a 7c 12b 17a
3c 8b 13c 18d
4b 9a 14d
5c 10c 15d

Chapter 18: Endodontic-Periodontal Relations

1b 5d
2a 6a
3d 7d
4b 8c

Chapter 19: Surgical Endodontics

1c 6c 11b 16b
2a 7d 12b 17a
3c 8c 13d 18d
4b 9a 14c
5a 10c 15c

Chapter 20: The Management of Pain and Anxiety

1b 6c 11a
2a 7b 12c
3b 8a
4c 9d
5c 10b

Chapter 21: Bleaching of Vital and Pulpless Teeth

1d 6d 11c 16b
2b 7c 12b 17c
3a 8d 13c 18b
4a 9a 14d 19c
5b 10b 15a 20d

Chapter 22: Restoration of the Endodontically Treated Tooth

1d 6d 11b 16b
2c 7c 12b
3b 8b 13d
4a 9a 14c
5a 10a,c 15c

Chapter 23: Pediatric Endodontic Treatment

1d 6d 11b
2c 7b 12b
3d 8a 13c
4a 9c 14a
5b 10a

Chapter 24: Geriatric Endodontics

1d 6b
2b 7a
3d 8d
4d 9c
5c 10c

Chapter 25: Endodontic Failures and Re-treatment

1b 6d 11c 16b
2c 7b 12a 17c
3d 8c 13b
4a 9a 14a
5d 10b 15d

Index

C

D

J

K

L

M

N